Amurotu

An Invitation to Health

TWELFTH EDITION

DIANNE HALES

THOMSON

WADSWORTH

Australia • Brazil • Canada • Mexico • Singapore • Spain • United Kingdom • United States

THOMSON

WADSWORTH ™

An Invitation to Health, 12th Edition
Dianne Hales

Executive Editor: NEDAH ROSE
Development Editor: PAT BREWER
Assistant Editor: KARI HOPPERSTEAD
Editorial Assistant: COLIN BLAKE
Technology Project Manager: DONNA KELLEY
Marketing Manager: JENNIFER SOMERVILLE
Marketing Assistant: MICHELE COLELLA
Marketing Communications Manager: BRYAN VANN
Project Manager, Editorial Production: ANDY MARINKOVICH
Creative Director: ROB HUGEL
Art Director: LEE FRIEDMAN
Print Buyer: JUDY INOUYE
Permissions Editor: JOOHEE LEE

Production Service: THE BOOK COMPANY
Text Designer: JOHN WALKER
Photo Researcher: MYRNA ENGLER PHOTO RESEARCH, INC.;
   NATALIE RICHMOND
Copy Editor: YONIE OVERTON
Illustrator: HESPENHEIDE DESIGN
Cover Designer: GIA GIASULLO
Cover Image: COPYRIGHT © VINCENT BESNAULT/ZEFA/
   CORBIS
Cover Printer: COURIER CORPORATION/KENDALLVILLE
Compositor: G & S TYPESETTERS, INC.
Printer: COURIER CORPORATION/KENDALLVILLE

Printed in the United States of America
1 2 3 4 5 6 7 10 09 08 07 06

Thomson Higher Education
10 Davis Drive
Belmont, CA 94002-3098
USA

For more information about our products, contact us at:
Thomson Learning Academic Resource Center
1-800-423-0563

For permission to use material from this text or product,
submit a request online at **http://www.thomsonrights.com**.
Any additional questions about permissions can be submitted
by e-mail to **thomsonrights@thomson.com**.

Library of Congress Control Number: 2005934428

ISBN 0-495-01147-9

To my husband Bob, and my daughter, Julia, who make every day an invitation to joy.

Myrna Engler, In Memoriam

Brief Contents

Contents

© Kelly Harriger/CORBIS

© Bob Schatz/Getty Images

SECTION II HEALTHY LIFESTYLES 103

SECTION III RESPONSIBLE SEXUALITY   207

© Michael Dwyer/Stock, Boston

SECTION IV AVOIDING HEALTH RISKS   301

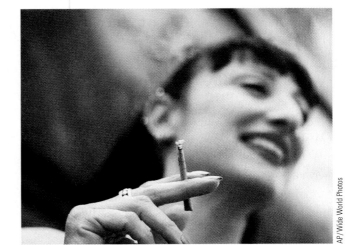

CHAPTER 13   TOBACCO USE, MISUSE, AND ABUSE   366

SECTION V PROTECTING YOUR HEALTH   389

CHAPTER 14   DEFENDING YOURSELF AGAINST INFECTIOUS DISEASES   390

CHAPTER 17   HEALTH-CARE CONSUMERISM AND COMPLEMENTARY/ ALTERNATIVE MEDICINE **488**

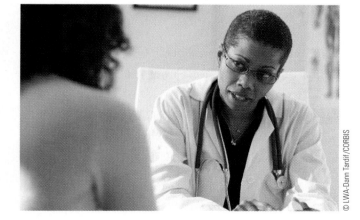

© LWA-Dann Tardif /CORBIS

Key Features

Preface

TO THE STUDENT

This textbook is an invitation to you—an invitation to a healthier, happier, fuller life. Every day you make choices that can affect both how long and how well you live. The knowledge you acquire in this course will help you make better choices, ones that will have a direct impact on how you look, feel, and function—now and for decades to come.

Perhaps you are in good health and think you know all you need to know about how to take care of yourself. If so, take a minute and ask yourself some questions:

- How well do you understand yourself? Are you able to cope with emotional upsets and crises? Do you often feel stressed out?

- How nutritiously do you eat? Are you always going on—and off—diets?

- Do you exercise regularly?

- How solid and supportive are your relationships with others? Are you conscientious about birth control and safe-sex practices?

- Do you occasionally get drunk or high? Do you smoke?

- What do you know about your risk for infectious diseases, heart problems, cancer, or other serious illnesses?

- Are you a savvy health-care consumer? Do you know how to evaluate medical products and health professionals?

- How much do you know about complementary and alternative medicine?

- If you needed health care, do you know where you'd turn or how you'd pay?

- Have you taken steps to ensure your personal safety at home, on campus, and on the streets?

- Can you improve your odds for living a long and healthy life?

- What are you doing today to prevent physical, psychological, social, and environmental problems in the future?

As you consider these questions, chances are there are some aspects of health you haven't considered before—and others you feel you don't have to worry about for years. Yet the choices you make and the actions you take now will have a dramatic impact on your future.

Your health is your personal responsibility. Over time, your priorities and needs will inevitably change, but the connections between various dimensions of your well-being will remain the same: The state of your mind will affect the state of your body, and vice versa. The values that guide you through today can keep you mentally, physically, and spiritually healthy throughout your lifetime. Your ability to cope with stress will influence your decisions about alcohol and drug use. Your commitment to honest, respectful relationships will affect the nature of your sexual involvements. Your eating and exercise habits will determine whether you develop a host of medical problems.

An Invitation to Health, 12th Edition, is packed with information, advice, recommendations, and research, and provides the first step in taking full charge of your own well-being. An important theme of this book is prevention. Ultimately, the power of prevention belongs to you—and it's a lot easier than you might think. You could simply add a walk or workout to your daily routine. You could snack on fruit instead of high-fat foods. You could cut back on alcohol. You could buckle your seat belt whenever you get in a car. These things may not seem like a big deal now, yet they could make a crucial difference in determining how active and fulfilling the rest of your life will be.

Knowledge alone can't assure you a lifetime of well-being. The rest depends on you. The skills you acquire, the habits you form, the choices you make, the ways you live day by day will all shape your health and your future. You cannot simply read this book and study health the way you study French or chemistry. You must decide to make it part of your daily life.

This is our invitation to you.

—*Dianne Hales*

TO THE INSTRUCTOR

The only constant in life is change. The same is true for *An Invitation to Health.* A great deal has changed over the lifetime of this book—in medical research, in the field of health, on college and university campuses, in the nation and the world. What has not changed is the commitment we share to prepare students to make informed, thoughtful choices that will help them live longer, healthier, happier, fuller lives.

For more than 25 years, it has been my privilege to work closely with health educators around the country toward this goal. *An Invitation to Health* contains the insights, perspectives, and wisdom of many people. Each edition has been enriched by what we've learned before. In this twelfth edition, much has changed—but the essentials remain the same.

As I point out to students, health—unlike physics or

history—is not a subject that they must memorize and master, but one to be both learned and lived. Often for the first time in their lives, students in a university health class become aware of the importance of personal responsibility for their health and acquire the skills they need to protect their well-being and prevent serious health problems.

By its very nature, health is an interactive course. Every topic of every lecture prompts questions. Every week brings health news that students are eager to discuss and debate. This edition of *An Invitation to Health* offers even more features designed to intrigue and involve your students. Every chapter begins with a campus-based vignette illustrating the relevance of the material to a student's life. Every chapter incorporates research on college students or college-age in-dividuals; these findings are highlighted by an icon. In addition, the redesigned "Student Snapshot" feature reports recent data on the health, habits, and concerns of today's college students. The American College Health Association's comprehensive *National College Health Assessment* is the source for many of the statistics.

Although your students may not be aware of it, this textbook works to promote change in indirect as well as direct ways. Simply reading the text and taking a health course can have a significant impact. One reason is what psychologists call the *exposure effect*. The more that individuals see, hear, or read about a topic, the more positively they view it. Because of the sheer quantity of information your students receive in the classroom and in their readings, they will want to heed at least some of the suggestions for change.

Once they do, another law of influence kicks in: the consistency principle. Students begin to see themselves as individuals who have control over their actions and who can change the way they think and behave. Without any conscious effort, their commitment to change grows, and the process of change takes on a momentum of its own.

The twelfth edition of *Invitation to Health* introduces two new chapters: one on behavioral change and one on weight management. "Changing for Life" (Chapter 2) provides a primer in behavioral change, including coverage of the transtheoretical model of change, the stages of change, and the keys to successful change. In addition, it discusses risky behaviors on campus and provides guidance on setting goals and changing bad health habits.

With excess weight emerging as the number-one public health threat of the twenty-first century, "Taking Control of Your Weight" (Chapter 7) presents current information on the worldwide obesity epidemic, explores its causes, reports the latest research on the dangers to health, explains popular approaches to losing weight, and offers advice on achieving and maintaining a healthy weight. This chapter also includes a comprehensive discussion of eating disorders.

As always, this edition defines health in the broadest sense of the word—not as an entity in itself but as a process of discovering, using, and protecting all possible resources within the individual, family, community, and environment. It presents the most recent, state-of-the-science information on medical research, along with the fundamental background students need to understand and apply these findings.

Many chapters have been extensively revised, updated, and reorganized. "Psychological Health" (Chapter 3) includes major new sections on spirituality, sleep, the mind-body connection, gender and depression, and attention disorders. "Personal Nutrition" (Chapter 6) has been completely rewritten, based on *Dietary Guidelines for Americans, 2005,* with new sections on using the MyPyramid System, glycemic index and glycemic load, vitamins, and the eating habits of college students. "Communicating and Relating" (Chapter 8) features new material on social health, hooking up, dysfunctional relationships, emotional abuse, infatuation, the transition into adulthood, cohabitation, same-sex relationships and marriage, and divorce.

"Alcohol Use, Misuse, and Abuse" (Chapter 12) includes new sections on alcohol poisoning, abstinence, moderate drinking, binge drinking, college drinking, and controlling your drinking. In "Defending Yourself Against Infectious Diseases" (Chapter 14), students will find updates on influenza, meningitis, SARS, the STI risk continuum, HIV, and AIDS.

As I tell students, *An Invitation to Health* can serve as an owner's manual to their bodies and minds. By using this book and taking your course, they can acquire a special type of power—the power to make good decisions, to assume responsibility, and to create and follow a healthy lifestyle. This textbook is our invitation to them to live what they learn and make the most of their health and of their lives.

This textbook also is an invitation to you as an instructor. I invite you to share your passion for education and to enter into a partnership with the editorial team at Wadsworth. We welcome your feedback and suggestions. Please let us hear from you at http://thomsonedu.com/health. I personally look forward to working with you toward our shared goal of preparing a new generation for a healthful future.

OVERVIEW OF THE TWELFTH EDITION: LIFE SKILLS FOR CHANGE

The keystone of this edition is behavioral change and life skills. This new emphasis reflects the growing recognition of the need for improving health behaviors and teaching students the best ways to make healthy changes both now and in the future.

While every edition of *An Invitation to Health* has included strategies and tools for change, the twelfth edition greatly expands this material. A new chapter, "Changing for Life," introduces students to the latest insights into behavioral change, including how people change, the stages of change, and change processes.

With its theme of behavioral change and life skills, the twelfth edition introduces a new student-focused feature: "Your Life Coach." In every chapter this feature presents practical information on how to make healthful changes. Examples include "Going for Your Goals" (Chapter 2), "Coping with Stress" (Chapter 4), "Get a Grip on Emotional Eating" (Chapter 7), "Building Healthy Relationships" (Chapter 8), "Taking Charge of Alcohol Use" (Chapter 12), and "Staying Healthy Longer" (Chapter 18).

In addition, each chapter includes "Your Action Plan," which follows the chapter health survey so students can recognize the behaviors they need to change and implement changes successfully. Examples include "Your Action Plan for Stress Management" (Chapter 4), "Your Action Plan for Responsible Drinking" (Chapter 12), "Your Action Plan for Protecting Yourself from Medical Mistakes and Misdeeds" (Chapter 17), and "Your Action Plan for Personal Safety on Campus" (Chapter 19).

Following the "Self Survey" and "Health Action Plan" is another new feature, "Case in Point," which illustrates a specific student's action plan for making a behavioral change, such as losing weight or resisting peer pressure.

This edition has another two new features in addition to "Your Life Coach" and "Case in Point." A new critical thinking feature, "You Decide," provokes analysis and discussion of a hot topic related to health, such as abortion or same-sex marriage. "Learn It/Live It" summarizes the chapter in a unique and practical advice format so that students can see not only the main points in a chapter but how to apply their new knowledge to their own lives.

In addition, we've retained, updated, and enhanced other popular features, including the chapter "FAQ," "Self Survey," "Strategies for Change/Strategies for Prevention," "Student Snapshot," and "Savvy Consumer" sections.

 This edition includes gender-specific information in every chapter, flagged with icons representing men and women. As in previous editions, icons also indicate material related to students and campus life and to cultural or racial diversity.

Because the health sciences advance so rapidly, all of the chapters have been updated with the most current research, including many citations published in 2005 and incorporating the latest available statistics. The majority come from primary sources, including professional books, medical, health, and mental health journals, health education periodicals, scientific meetings, federal agencies and consensus panels, publications from research laboratories and universities, and personal interviews with specialists in a number of fields. In addition, "Internet Connections" presents reliable Internet addresses where students can turn for additional information and a suggested exercise using InfoTrac® College Edition, an online library of hundreds of academic journals and popular periodicals.

Following is a chapter-by-chapter listing of some of the key topics that have been added, expanded, or revised for the twelfth edition:

Chapter 1: Your Invitation to Health

- New section: How Healthy Are Americans?
- New section: Healthy Campus 2010
- New section: How Healthy Are Today's Students?
- Your Life Coach: Staying Healthy on Campus
- New section: Health in the Twenty-First Century
- New FAQ section: What Can I Do to Improve my Health If My Racial Background Puts Me at Risk?

Chapter 2: Changing for Life— New chapter this edition

- Making Healthy Changes
- The Transtheoretical Model of Change
- The Keys to Successful Change
- Your Life Coach: Going for Your Goals
- Risky Behaviors on Campus
- Recovering From a Relapse
- Learn It/Live It: Changing for Good

Chapter 3: Psychological Health

- Your Life Coach: Achieving Your Maximum Potential
- How Can I Find Happiness?—Revised
- New section: Spirituality
  - With subsections: Can Prayer Keep Us Healthy?—Revised
  - Expressing Gratitude—New
  - Forgiveness—New
- Major changes in Sleep section, with new subsections: Why Sleep Matters, What Happens When We Sleep?, Sleep Disorders, Insomnia, Breathing Disorders, Movement Disorders, Circadian Rhythm Sleep Disorders.
- Revised section: How Much Sleep Do I Need?
- New section: Who Develops Mental Disorders?
- New section: The Mind-Body Connection
- New section: Is Exercise a Good Treatment for Psychological Problems?
- New section: Gender and Depression
- New section: Are Antidepressants Dangerous?
- Attention Disorders—Revised

Chapter 4: Personal Stress Management

- New section: Five Categories of Stressors
- Updated section: Stress Effects on Physical Health
- Your Life Coach: Coping With Stress
- Updated section: Stress Effects on Psychological Health

Chapter 5: The Joy of Fitness

- New sections distinguishing health-related fitness and performance-related fitness
- New section: Fitness and the Dimensions of Health
- New section: Working Out on Campus: Student Bodies in Motion

- Section on the benefits of physical activity completely updated, including new subsection on Sexuality
- New section: Exercise Guidelines for Americans
- New section: How Can I Separate Fitness Facts from Fiction?
- New Savvy Consumer: Watch Out for "Pump Fiction"
- New section: Stepping Out: Walk the Walk with subsections: Why Walk? and America on the Move
- Your Life Coach: Overcoming Exercise Excuses
- Performance-Enhancing Drugs revised and updated
- New section: Does Stretching Improve Athletic Performance?
- New section: Mind-Body Approaches, with three subsections: Yoga, Pilates, T'ai Chi

Chapter 6: Personal Nutrition

- Completely revised based on *Dietary Guidelines for Americans, 2005*
- New section: FAQ: Should I Switch to Low-Carb Foods?
- New section: Glycemic Index and Glycemic Load
- New section: FAQ: Should I Take Vitamins?
- New sections: Using the MyPyramid System, with subsections on the key messages of the 2005 Dietary Guidelines
- New section: Nutrition 101: The Eating Habits of College Students
- New section: How Can I Find Snacks That Are Good for Me?

Chapter 7: Taking Control of Your Weight— New to this edition

- The Global Epidemic
- Body Image
- Understanding Weight Problems
- Body Composition
- Health Dangers of Excess Weight
- A Practical Guide to Weight Loss
- The Psychology of Losing Weight
- Your Life Coach: Get a Grip on Emotional Eating
- Treating Severe Obesity
- Unhealthy Eating Behavior
- Eating Disorders
- Learn It/Live It: Managing Your Weight

Chapter 8: Communicating and Relating

- New section: Your Social Health
- New section: Should You Keep Dating?
- New section: Hooking Up

- Your Life Coach: Building Healthy Relationships
- New section: Dysfunctional Relationships
- New section: FAQ: What Is Emotional Abuse?
- Codependency—Revised
- New section: Infatuation
- New section: "Twixters": Transition into Adulthood
- New sections within Committed Relationships:
  - Domestic Partners
  - Long-Term Same-Sex Relationships
  - Same-Sex Marriage
  - The Benefits of Marriage
  - Conflict in Marriage
  - Saving Marriages
- Five new graphs from new book, *The State of Our Unions, 2005,* by Poponoe and Whitehead

Chapter 9: Personal Sexuality

- New section: Sexuality and the Dimensions of Health
- New section: Sexual and Gender Identity
- New section: FAQ: What Are the Benefits and Drawbacks of Circumcision?
- Your Life Coach: Making Responsible Sexual Decisions
- New section: Teen Sexual Behaviors
- Transgenderism—Completely revised
- Nonpenetrative Sexual Activity—Revised
- New section: Other Models of Sexual Response
- Revised section on Safer Sex
- New subsections on Erectile Dysfunction

Chapter 10: Reproductive Choices

- Revised section on Birth Control Basics
- All contraceptive sections revised/updated
- All contraceptive advantages/disadvantages now in easy-to-read bullet lists
- New section: Home Pregnancy Tests
- Updated section: Emergency Contraception
- Updated section: Assisted Reproductive Technology

Chapter 11: Avoiding Addictive Behaviors and Drug Abuse

- New section: Addictive Behaviors and the Dimensions of Health
- New section: Gambling, with subsections:
  - Risk Factors for Problem Gambling
  - What Happens to Problem Gamblers?
- Your Life Coach: Developing Positive Addictions

- Drug Use on Campus updated
- New main section on Medications, with updated subsections on OTC drugs and prescription drugs
- New Savvy Consumer: Avoiding Medication Mistakes
- New table on commonly abused drugs, with column on Potential Health Consequences
- Cannabis updated
- Club Drugs updated (Ecstasy, GHB, Ketamine, and new subsection on Nitrites)
- New section: Methamphetamine, with four subsections: How Users Feel, Risks, The Toll on Society, Withdrawal
- New section: Prescription Stimulants
- New section: Prescription Opioids

Chapter 12: Alcohol Use, Misuse, and Abuse
- New section: Alcohol Poisoning
- New section: Abstinence
- New FAQ section: What Is Moderate Drinking?
- Binge section completely revised
- Drinking on Campus revised
- Your Life Coach: Taking Charge of Alcohol Use

Chapter 13: Tobacco Use, Misuse, and Abuse
- Tobacco Use on Campus revised and updated
- New FAQ section: Is Social Smoking Less Risky?
- Smoking, Race, and Gender revised and updated
- Other Forms of Tobacco updated
- New Savvy Consumer: Are "Safer" Cigarettes Really Safe?
- Your Life Coach: Quitting updated
- New FAQ section: Does Quitting Eliminate the Risks Associated with Smoking?

Chapter 14: Defending Yourself Against Infectious Diseases
- New section: Immunizations for College Students, with new table
- Influenza section updated
- New FAQ section: Are College Students at Higher Risk of Colds and Flu?
- Meningitis section updated
- New subsections of Bioterror Infections: Botulism and Tularemia
- New FAQ section: How Common Are STIs on Campus?
- New section: Risk Factors and Risk Continuums
- Your Life Coach: Safer, Smarter Sex
- STI sections reordered and updated
- HIV and AIDS updated

Chapter 15: Keeping Your Heart Healthy
- Your Life Coach: Making Heart/Healthy Changes
- Under Risk Factors You Can Control:
  - Metabolic Syndrome totally revised and updated with newest criteria
  - Psychosocial Factors updated with new information on depression and Type-D Personality
- New section: Prescription Painkillers
- Updated section: Your Lipoprotein Profile
- New FAQ section: Should I Take a Statin to Prevent Heart Disease?
- Completely revised section: C-Reactive Protein (CRP)
- Completely revised section: Homocysteine
- Atherosclerosis section completely revised to include latest on inflammation
- New section: Cardiopulmonary Resuscitation (CPR) and Defibrillation
- Revised section: Aspirin and the Heart
- New Strategy for Prevention: How to Recognize a Stroke

Chapter 16: Preventing Cancer and Other Illnesses
- Your Life Coach: Lowering Your Cancer Risk
- Updated section: Skin Cancer
- New FAQ section: Are You Addicted to Tanning?
- Updated section: Breast Cancer
- Updated section: Colon and Rectal Cancer
- Diabetes Mellitus section completely revised and expanded
  - New subsections: Types of Diabetes, Diabetes Signs and Symptoms, Detecting Diabetes, Diabetes Management
- New FAQ section: What Should I Do in Case of an Asthma Attack?
- Revised section: Backaches

Chapter 17: Health-Care Consumerism and Complementary/Alternative Medicine
- New section: Safeguarding Your Health
- New table: Screening Tests and Recommendations
- New Strategy for Prevention: When Is LASIK Not for Me?
- CAM: Mind-Body Medicine section expanded
- New FAQ section: How Do I Choose an HMO?
- Updated section: The Uninsured

Chapter 18: Healthy Aging and the Circle of Life
- Your Life Coach: Staying Healthy Longer
- Hormone Therapy section updated, with new Savvy Consumer

- Osteoporosis section updated, with new subsections:

   Risk Factors

   Treating Osteoporosis

- Updated section: How We Die
- Updated section: Grief's Effects on Health

Chapter 19: Staying Safe: Preventing Injury, Violence, and Victimization

- New section: Becoming a Safer Driver
- FAQ section updated: Talking on the Phone While Driving
- New section: Intimate Partner Violence
- New section: Crime and Violence on Campus
- New section: Stalking
- New section: Dating Violence
- Your Life Coach: Preventing Rape

Chapter 20: Working Toward a Healthy Environment

- Global Warming section updated, with new art
- Updated section: Clearing the Air
- Indoor Pollutants: Mercury updated, with FDA warning on mercury in fish
- New FAQ section: Is Listening to Music Through Earbuds Hazardous to My Hearing?
- New section: Chemical Weapons

SUPPLEMENTAL RESOURCES

HealthNow™ Class-tested and student-praised, Health-Now™ offers a variety of features that support course objectives and interactive learning. This online tutorial for students, available with new texts, offers a Personalized Change Plan, pre- and post-tests, a wellness journal, and a variety of activities, all designed to get students involved in their learning progress and to be better prepared for class participation and class quizzes and tests. Students log on to HealthNow by using the access code available with the text.

Instructor's Manual and Test Bank These two essential ancillaries are bound together for your convenience. The Instructor's Manual provides chapter outlines, learning objectives, classroom handouts, discussion questions, a video list, a resource integration guide, and more. The test bank for the new edition contains a variety of questions to test students' understanding and comprehension of the text. It contains at least 75 questions per chapter, with 50 multiple-choice questions, 20 fill-in-the-blank questions, and 5 essay questions.

ExamView® Computerized Testing Create, deliver, and customize the thorough Test Bank in minutes with this easy-to-use assessment and tutorial system. *Exam View* offers both a *Quick Test Wizard* and an *Online Test Wizard* that guide you step-by-step through the process of creating tests, while it allows you to see the test you are creating on the screen exactly as it will print or display online. You can build tests of up to 250 questions using up to 12 question types. Using *Exam View's* complete word-processing capabilities, you can enter an unlimited number of new questions or edit existing questions.

Multimedia Manager for An Invitation to Health: A Microsoft® PowerPoint® Link Tool This dual-platform presentation CD-ROM includes hundreds of Microsoft® PowerPoint® slides featuring text art, an electronic version of the Instructor's Manual and Test Bank, and digital video from our ABC Video Series.

JoinIn®on TurningPoint™ Enhance how your students interact with you, your lecture, and each other using JoinIn™ content for Response Systems tailored to this text. Thomson's exclusive agreement to offer TurningPoint® software lets you pose book-specific questions and display students' answers seamlessly within the Microsoft® PowerPoint® slides of your own lecture, in conjunction with the "clicker" hardware of your choice.

Transparency Acetates More than 100 transparency acetates of art taken from the text enhance lectures and provide visual support in the classroom.

Walk4Life® Elite Model Pedometer This pedometer tracks steps, elapsed time, distance, and includes a calorie counter. Whether to be used as an activity in class or as a tool to encourage students to simply track their steps and walk towards better fitness awareness, this is a valuable item for everyone.

Readings in Healthy Living As a frequent author of health-related articles produced by Parade® Magazine, Dianne Hales has published numerous articles that students will find useful and interesting. This 12-article reader is a collection of key articles, including *Take Your Meds—The Right Way* and *You Can Think Yourself Thin*.

Behavior Change Workbook The Behavior Change Workbook includes a brief discussion of the current theories behind making positive lifestyle changes, along with exercises to help students effect those changes in their everyday lives.

TestWell This online assessment tool allows students to complete a 100-question wellness inventory related to the dimensions of wellness. Students complete the personal assessment to evaluate their personal health status related to nutrition, emotional health, spirituality, sexuality, physical health, self-care, safety, environmental health, occupational health, and intellectual health.

InfoTrac®College Edition with InfoMarks™ This fully searchable online database offers more than 20 years' worth of full-text articles (not abstracts) from almost 5,000 diverse sources. Students log on to InfoTrac College Edition by using the access code available with the text.

InfoTrac College Edition Student Guide for Health This 24-page booklet offers detailed guidance for students on how to use the *Info Trac® College Edition* database. This includes log-in help, a complete search tips "cheat sheet," and a topic list of key word search terms for health, fitness, and wellness. It is available FREE when packaged with the text. The text also features InfoTrac College Edition Activities for each chapter that challenge the student to critically read articles and studies relating to key topics in the chapters. These activities help guide students through the vast database and answer questions relating to specific articles.

Telecourse Study Guide For use with the Dallas County Community College Telecourse, the telecourse guide contains a brief summary of each lesson, followed by learning objectives, study assignments for the text and video, key terms, a list of the experts interviewed with their affiliations, video focus points, individual health plan assignments, enrichment opportunities, and practice tests with page-referenced answers.

Health, Fitness, and Wellness Internet Explorer This handy full-color trifold brochure contains dozens of useful health, fitness, and wellness Internet links.

Health and Wellness Resource Center at *http://www.gale.com/health* Gale's Health and Wellness Resource Center is a new comprehensive website that provides easy-to-find answers to health questions.

Careers in Health, Physical Education, and Sport This is the essential manual for majors who are interested in pursuing a position in their chosen field. It guides them through the complicated process of picking the type of career they want to pursue, suggests how to prepare for the transition into the working world, and offers information about different career paths, education requirements, and reasonable salary expectations. The supplement also describes the differences in credentials found in the field and testing requirements for certain professions.

Integrative Medicine: The Mind-Body Prescription This interesting supplement, written by Dr. John Janowiak from Appalachian State University, explains the relationship between Western medical practice and more traditional therapies. The supplement explains the evolution of integrative medicine, provides a detailed list of Internet resources, a comprehensive list of herbs and their interactions, and more.

Diet Analysis Plus 7.0 *Diet Analysis Plus* is the market-leading diet assessment program used by colleges and universities that allows students to create their own personal profiles based on height, weight, age, sex, and activity level. Its new dynamic interface makes it easy for students to track the types and serving sizes of the foods they consume, from one day to 365 days! Now including even more exciting features, the updated 7.0 version includes a 10,000 food database, nine reports for analysis, a new food recipe fea-

ture, the latest Dietary References, and goals and actual percentages of essential nutrients, vitamins, and minerals. Students can use this information to adjust their diet and gain a better understanding of how nutrition relates to their personal health goals. Thoroughly revised and updated, the software is available online or on a new Windows/Mac® compatible CD-ROM.

http://thomsonedu.com/health When you adopt *An Invitation to Health,* Twelfth Edition, you and your students will have access to a rich array of teaching and learning resources that you won't find anywhere else. This outstanding site features both student resources for the text, including quizzes, web links, suggested online readings, and discussion forums, and instructor resources, including downloadable supplementary resources and multimedia presentation shdes.You will also find an online catalog of Wadsworth's health, fitness, wellness, and physical education books and supplements.

ABC Videos for Health and Wellness These videos allow you to integrate the newsgathering and programming power of the ABC News networks into the classroom to show students the relevance of course topics to their everyday lives. The videos include news clips correlated directly with the text and can help you launch a lecture, spark a discussion, or demonstrate an application. Students can see firsthand how the principles they learn in the course apply to the stories they hear in the news.

Relaxation: A Guide to Personal Stress Management This 30-minute video shows students how to manage their stress and what is a healthy stress level in their life. Experts explain relaxation techniques and guide the student through progressive relaxation, guided imagery, breathing, and physical activity.

Trigger Video Series: Fitness This 60-minute video focuses on changing concepts of fitness, contains five 8–10 minute clips followed by questions for answer or discussion, and material appropriate to the fitness chapters in the text.

ACKNOWLEDGMENTS

One of the joys of writing *An Invitation to Health* is the opportunity to work with a team I consider the very best of the best in textbook publishing.

Nedah Rose, our health editor, has been endlessly supportive and enthusiastic and has made every step of the process of creating this edition go smoothly.

My deepest thanks go to Pat Brewer, the developmental editor on this edition, whose contributions always extend far beyond the demands of duty. I consider her a partner, co-conspirator, and friend. Once again I have come to think of Dusty Friedman of The Book Company as a worker of miracles and other marvels. In hundreds of ways, this edition is a more complete, accurate, and attractive book because of their contributions.

I thank Colin Blake, our editorial assistant, who provided endless help—with endless patience and good humor. Thanks to Andy Marinkovich, Project Manager, for expertly shepherding this edition from conception to production, to John Walker for its vibrant new design, and to Randy Miyake for art. This book, like others I've written, owes much of its vibrant impact to the late Myrna Engler, whose photo selections reflected her creativity and enthusiasm. She was a joy to work with, and our entire team will miss her as a colleague and as a friend. I appreciate the skills and dedication of copy editor Yonie Overton, who takes each edition and makes it better.

My thanks to Jennifer Somerville, Marketing Manager, for her enthusiastic support, to Jessica Perry for her work on the promotional materials, and to Kari Hopperstead, who guides the ancillaries.

To one and all I extend my appreciation and admiration. Finally, I would like to thank the reviewers whose input has been so valuable through these many editions. For the twelfth edition, I thank the following for their comments and helpful assistance:

Robert Dollinger, *Florida International U.*

Rosemarie Monahan, *High Point U.*

Laurie Tucker, *American University*

Sharron Zakus, *City College of San Francisco*

Elaine Bryan, *Georgia Perimeter College*

Jack Gutierrez, *Central C. C.*

Lynne Fitzgerald, *Morehead State U.*

Mary Hunt, *Madonna U.*

John Kowalczyk, *U. of Minnesota–Duluth*

Liz Belyea, *Cosumnes River College*

For their help as reviewers or focus group participants from previous editions, I want to thank the following:

Ghulam Aasef, *Kaskaskia College*

Andrea Abercrombie, *Clemson University*

Judy Baker, *East Carolina University*

Marcia Ball, *James Madison University*

Jeremy Barnes, *Southeast Missouri State University*

Rick Barnes, *East Carolina University*

Lois Beach, *SUNY-Plattsburg*

Betsy Bergen, *Kansas State University*

Nancy Bessette, *Saddleback College*

Carol Biddington, *California University of Pennsylvania*

David Black, *Purdue University*

Jill M. Black, *Cleveland State University*

Cynthia Pike Blocksom, *Cincinnati Health Department*

James Brik, *Willamette University*

Mitchell Brodsky, *York College*

Jodi Broodkins-Fisher, *University of Utah*

James G. Bryant, Jr., *Western Carolina University*

Marsha Campos, *Modesto Junior College*

Richard Capriccioso, *University of Phoenix*

James Lester Carter, *Montana State University*

Peggy L. Chin, *University of Connecticut*

Patti Cost, *Weber State University*

Maxine Davis, *Eastern Washington University*

Lori Dewald, *Shippensburg University of Pennsylvania*

Julie Dietz, *Eastern Illinois University*

Robert Dollinger, *Florida International University*

Gary English, *Ithaca College*

Melinda K. Everman, *The Ohio State University*

Michael Felts, *East Carolina University*

Kathie C. Garbe, *Kennesaw State College*

Gail Gates, *Oklahoma State University*

Dawn Graff-Haight, *Portland State University*

Carolyn Gray, *New Mexico State University*

Mary Gress, *Lorain County Community College*

Janet Grochowski, *University of St. Thomas*

Stephen Haynie, *College of William and Mary*

Ron Heinrichs, *Central Missouri State University*

Michael Hoadley, *University of South Dakota*

Harold Horne, *University of Illinois at Springfield*

Linda L. Howard, *Idaho State University*

Kim Hyatt, *Weber State University*

Dee Jacobsen, *Southeastern Louisiana University*

John Janowiak, *Appalachian State University*

Peggy Jarnigan, *Rollins College*

Jim Johnson, *Northwest Missouri State University*

Chester S. Jones, *University of Arkansas*

Herb Jones, *Ball State University*

Jane Jones, *University of Wisconsin, Stevens Point*

Lorraine J. Jones, *Muncie, Indiana*

Becky Kennedy-Koch, *Ohio State University*

Mark J. Kittleson, *Southern Illinois University*

Darlene Kluka, *University of Central Oklahoma*

Debra A. Krummel, *West Virginia University*

Roland Lamarine, *California State University, Chico*

David Langford, *University of Maryland, Baltimore County*

Terri Langford, *University of Central Florida*

Beth Lanning, *Baylor University*

Norbert Lindskog, *Harold Washington College*

Loretta Liptak, *Youngstown State University*

David G. Lorenzi, *West Liberty State College*

S. Jack Loughton, *Weber State University*

Rick Madson, *Palm Beach Community College*

Ashok Malik, *College of San Mateo*

Michele P. Mannion, *Temple University*

Jerry Mayo, *Hendrix College*

Jessica Middlebrooks, *University of Georgia*

Esther Moe, *Oregon Health Sciences University*

Kris Moline, *Lourdes College*

Richard Morris, *Rollins College*

John W. Munson, *University of Wisconsin–Stevens Point*

Anne O'Donnell, *Santa Rosa Junior College*

Randy M. Page, *University of Idaho*

Carolyn P. Parks, *University of North Carolina*

Anthony V. Parrillo, *East Carolina University*

Miguel Perez, *University of North Texas*

Pamela Pinahs-Schultz, *Carroll College*

Rosanne Poole, *Tallahassee Community College*

Janet Reis, *University of Illinois at Urbana-Champaign*

Pamela Rost, *Buffalo State College*

Sadie Sanders, *University of Florida*

Steven Sansone, *Chemeketa Community College*

Debra Secord, *Coastline College*

Behjat Sharif, *California State University–Los Angeles*

Andrew Shim, *Southwestern College*

Steve Singleton, *Wayne State University*

Larry Smith, *Scottsdale Community College*

Teresa Snow, *Georgia Institute of Technology*

Carl A. Stockton, *Radford University*

Linda Stonecipher, *Western Oregon State College*

Emogene Johnson Vaughn, *Norfolk State University*

David M. White, *East Carolina University*

Sabina White, *University of California—Santa Barbara*

Robert Wilson, *University of Minnesota*

Roy Wohl, *Washburn University*

Martin L. Wood, *Ball State University*

ABOUT THE AUTHOR

Dianne Hales, a contributing editor for *Parade,* has written more than 2,000 articles for national publications. Her trade books include *Think Thin, Be Thin; Just Like a Woman: How Gender Science Is Redefining What Makes Us Female* and the award-winning compendium of mental health information, *Caring for the Mind: The Comprehensive Guide to Mental Health.* Dianne Hales is one of the few journalists to be honored with national awards for excellence in magazine writing by both the American Psychiatric Association and the American Psychological Association. She also has won the EMMA (Exceptional Media Merit Award) for health reporting from the National Women's Political Caucus and Radcliffe College, and numerous writing awards from various organizations, including the Arthritis Foundation, California Psychiatric Society, CHAAD (Children and Adults with Attention-Deficit Disorders), Council for the Advancement of Scientific Education, National Easter Seal Society, and the New York City Public Library.

Taking Charge of Your Health

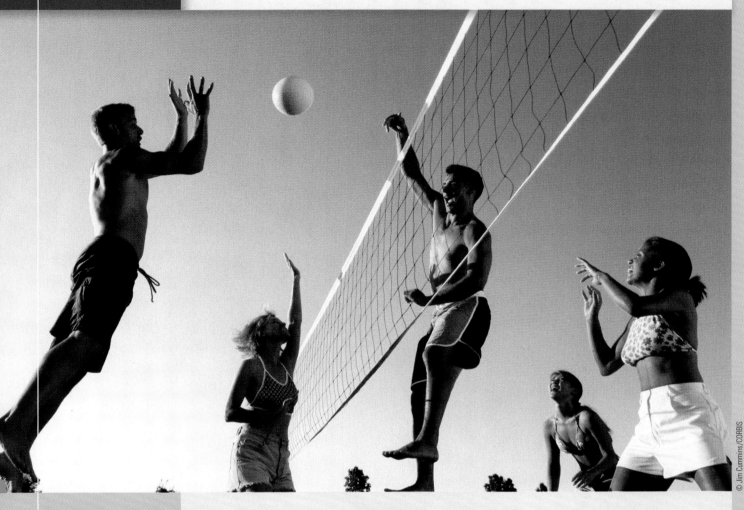

© Jim Cummins/CORBIS

Health may be a science; living is an art. The principles that can help you understand the science and practice the art are simple and timeless and form the basic premise of this book: You have more control over your life and well-being than anything or anyone else does. Through the decisions you make and the habits you develop, you can influence how well—and perhaps how long—you will live. This section defines health and wellness and provides the information you need to take charge of your well-being now and in the years to come.

1 Your Invitation to Health

"How are you?" You may hear that question dozens of times each day. "Fine," you answer, without thinking. But are you *really?* How do you feel about yourself and your life? Are you stressed? Are you eating well and exercising regularly? Do you have close friends? If you choose to be sexually active, what do you do to prevent unwanted pregnancy or sexually transmitted illnesses? Do you drink, smoke, or use drugs? Are you taking steps to prevent major illnesses? Do you get regular checkups? Are you aware of safety and environmental threats to your health? How are you going to make the most of your life? What do you hope to accomplish before you die?

This book asks these questions and many more. It is a book about you: your mind and your body, your spirit and your social ties, your needs and your wants, your past and your potential. It will help you explore options, discover possibilities, and find new ways to make your life worthwhile. If you don't make the most of what you are, you risk never discovering what you might become.

Health involves more than physical well-being. It is a state of body, mind, and spirit that must be viewed within the context of community, society, and environment. By providing the information and understanding you need to take care of your own health, *An Invitation to Health* can help you live more fully, more happily, and more healthfully.

The invitation to health that we extend to every reader is one offer you literally cannot afford to refuse: The quality of your life depends on it.

(FAQ) Frequently Asked Questions

▌ How many Americans practice healthy life-style behaviors? *p. 7*

▌ Does gender matter? *p. 12*

▌ What can I do to improve my health if my racial background puts me at risk? *p. 15*

After studying the material in this chapter, you should be able to:

▌ **Name** the dimensions of health and **describe** how they relate to total wellness.

▌ **Define** and **differentiate** prevention and protection.

▌ **Discuss** ways that your family health history can affect your health.

▌ **Describe** how gender, race, and ethnicity can influence health and access to health care.

HEALTH AND WELLNESS

By simplest definition, **health** means being sound in body, mind, and spirit. The World Health Organization defines health as "not merely the absence of disease or infirmity," but "a state of complete physical, mental, and social well-being."[1] Health is the process of discovering, using, and protecting all the resources within our bodies, minds, spirits, families, communities, and environment.

Health has many dimensions: physical, psychological, spiritual, social, intellectual, and environmental. This book takes a *holistic* approach, one that looks at health and the individual as a whole, rather than part by part. Your own definition of health may include different elements, but chances are you and your classmates agree that it includes at least some of the following:

- A positive, optimistic outlook.
- A sense of control over stress and worries; time to relax.
- Energy and vitality; freedom from pain or serious illness.
- Supportive friends and family and a nurturing intimate relationship with someone you love.
- A personally satisfying job.
- A clean environment.

Wellness can be defined as purposeful, enjoyable living or, more specifically, a deliberate lifestyle choice characterized by personal responsibility and optimal enhancement of physical, mental, and spiritual health. Health professionals use other definitions to encompass this broad, active meaning of wellness:

- As a decision you make to move toward optimal health.
- As a way of life you design to achieve your highest potential.
- As a process of developing awareness that health and happiness are possible in the present moment.
- As the integration of body, mind, and spirit.
- As the belief that everything you do, think, and feel has an impact on your state of health and the health of the world.[2]

"The 'well' person is not necessarily the strong, the brave, the successful, the young, the whole, or even the illness-free being," notes John Travis, M.D., author of *The Wellness Workbook.* "No matter what your current state of health, you can begin to appreciate yourself as a growing, changing person and allow yourself to move toward a happier life and positive health."

Dr. Travis, who created the Wellness Inventory (see Self Survey on page 16) uses the analogy of an iceberg (Figure 1-1) to describe optimal health and wellness. Only about one-tenth of the mass of an iceberg is visible; the rest

is submerged. Your current state of health is like the tip of the iceberg—the part that shows.

"To understand all that creates and supports your current state of health," says Dr. Travis, "you have to look 'underwater.'" The first hidden level—the "lifestyle/behavioral" level—consists of what you eat, how active you are, how

Health is the process of discovering, using, and protecting all the resources within our bodies, minds, spirits, families, communities, and environment.

you manage stress, and how you protect yourself from hazards. Below this dimension is the "cultural/psychological/motivational" level, the often-invisible influences that lead us to choose a certain lifestyle. The foundation of the iceberg is the "spiritual/being/meaning" realm, which encompasses issues such as your reason for being, the meaning of your life, and your place in the universe. "Ultimately," says Dr. Travis, "this realm determines whether the tip of the iceberg, representing your state of health, is one of disease or wellness."[3]

In wellness, health, and sickness, there is considerable overlap of the functions of the mind, body, and spirit. As scientists have shown again and again in recent decades, psychological factors play a major role in enhancing physical well-being and preventing illness, but they also can trigger,

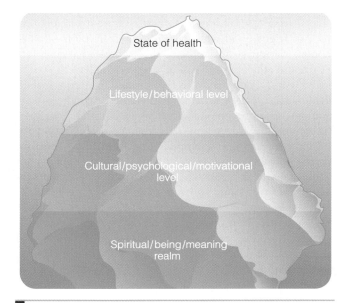

FIGURE 1-1   **Iceberg Model of Wellness**

Like an iceberg, only a small part of your total wellness is visible: your current state of health. Just as important are hidden levels, including lifestyle habits, cultural and psychological factors, and the realm of spiritual meaning and being.

Source: Reprinted with permission, *The Wellness Workbook,* 3rd ed., John W. Travis, M.D., and Regina Sara Ryan, Celestial Arts, Berkeley, CA. © 1981, 1988, 2004 by John W. Travis, www.wellnessbook.com.

worsen, or prolong physical symptoms. Similarly, almost every medical illness affects people psychologically as well as physically.

THE DIMENSIONS OF HEALTH

By learning more about the six dimensions of health, you can explore the hidden levels of the iceberg.

PHYSICAL HEALTH

The various states of health can be viewed as points on a continuum (Figure 1-2). At one end is early and needless death; at the other is optimal wellness, in which you feel and perform at your very best. In the middle, individuals are neither sick enough to need medical attention nor well enough to live each day with zest and vigor.

What matters even more than your place on the continuum is the direction in which you are moving: toward high-level wellness or toward premature death. Individuals in physical good health who are always worrying or not working to develop more fully may be on the right of the neutral point but facing left. Others who may be disabled or have a chronic health problem may have a positive outlook and a network of mutually supportive relationships that keeps them focused toward wellness.[4]

For the sake of optimal physical health, we must take positive steps away from illness and toward well-being. We must feed our bodies nutritiously, exercise them regularly, avoid harmful behaviors and substances, watch out for early signs of sickness, and protect ourselves from accidents.

PSYCHOLOGICAL HEALTH

Like physical well-being, psychological health is more than the absence of problems or illness. Psychological health refers to both our emotional and mental states—that is, to our feelings and our thoughts. It involves awareness and acceptance of a wide range of feelings in oneself and others, the ability to express emotions, to function independently, and to cope with the challenges of daily stressors. (Chapter 3 provides more information on psychological health.)

FIGURE 1-2   **Wellness–Illness Continuum**

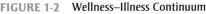

SPIRITUAL HEALTH

Spiritually healthy individuals identify their own basic purpose in life; learn how to experience love, joy, peace, and fulfillment; and help themselves and others achieve their full potential. As they devote themselves to others' needs more than their own, their spiritual development produces a sense of greater meaning in their lives. (See Chapter 3 for an in-depth discussion of spirituality.)

Prayer, a spiritual practice of millions, is the most commonly used form of complementary and alternative medicine. However, only in recent years has science launched rigorous investigations of the healing power of prayer. Dr. Dale Matthews of Georgetown University, author of *The Faith Factor,* estimates that about 75 percent of studies of spirituality have confirmed health benefits.[5]

 According to a UCLA study, college students majoring in the fine arts, education, and the humanities have the highest level of religious commitment. Earning better-than-expected grades in college also is associated with higher levels of religious involvement.[6]

SOCIAL HEALTH

Social health refers to the ability to interact effectively with other people and the social environment, to develop satisfying interpersonal relationships, and to fulfill social roles. It

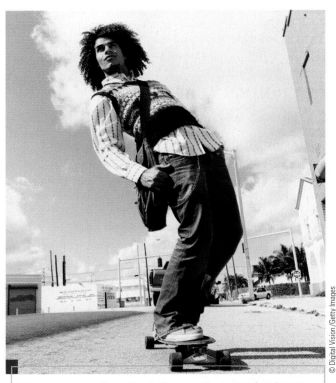

Where are you on the wellness–illness continuum? What direction are you moving?

© Digital Vision/Getty Images

involves participating in and contributing to your community, living in harmony with fellow human beings, developing positive interdependent relationships (discussed in Chapter 8), and practicing healthy sexual behaviors.

In times of crisis, social connections provide comfort and support. Even in tranquil times, social isolation increases the risk of sickness and mortality. In a landmark study of 4,725 men and women in Alameda County, California, death rates were twice as high for loners as for those with strong social ties. In other studies, social isolation greatly increased the risk of dying of a heart attack. Heart attack patients have a better chance of long-term survival if they believe they have adequate help in performing daily tasks from family and friends. People with spouses, friends, and a rich social network may outlive isolated loners by as much as 30 years.

As numerous studies have shown, people function best in socially supportive environments. This is certainly true of college students. Undergraduates who have a support network of friends and who feel supported by their families report fewer physical symptoms than others.[7]

Health educators are placing greater emphasis on social health in its broadest sense as they expand the traditional individualistic concept of health to include the complex interrelationships between one person's health and the health of the community and environment. This change in perspective has given rise to a new emphasis on **health promotion,** which educators define as "any planned combination of educational, political, regulatory, and organizational supports for actions and conditions of living conducive to the health of individuals, groups, or communities."[8] Examples on campus include smoke-free policies for all college buildings, residences, and dining areas, prohibiting tobacco advertising and sponsorship of campus social events, and banning tobacco sales on campus.

INTELLECTUAL HEALTH

Your brain is the only one of your organs capable of self-awareness. Every day you use your mind to gather, process, and act on information; to think through your values; to make decisions, set goals, and figure out how to handle a problem or challenge. Intellectual health refers to your ability to think and learn from life experience, your openness to new ideas, and your capacity to question and evaluate information. Throughout your life, you'll use your critical thinking skills, including your ability to evaluate health information, to safeguard your well-being.

ENVIRONMENTAL HEALTH

You live in a physical and social setting that can affect every aspect of your health. Environmental health refers to the impact your world has on your well-being. It means protecting yourself from dangers in the air, water, and soil, and in products you use—and also working to preserve the environment itself. (Chapter 20 offers a thorough discussion of environmental health.)

HOW HEALTHY ARE AMERICANS?

Americans are living longer and healthier lives than ever before in history. Life expectancy has reached a new high of 77.4 years, increasing for both men and women and blacks and whites. The gender gap between male and female life expectancies has narrowed to 5.2 years. The age-adjusted death rate has hit an all-time low of 847 deaths per 100,000 people, with declines in mortality from stroke, heart disease, cancer, and accidents.[9]

We could be doing much better. How? Making better lifestyle choices and committing ourselves to healthy changes in our behavior could prevent one of every three premature deaths in this country.

(FAQ) HOW MANY AMERICANS PRACTICE HEALTHY LIFESTYLE BEHAVIORS?

Over the years the evidence for the benefits of a healthy lifestyle has grown stronger. Study after study has shown lower risks of heart disease, stroke, diabetes, and cancer in individuals with healthy behaviors. A recent national survey looked at how many Americans are taking such findings to heart and adopting four key health-boosting behaviors:[10]

- **Not smoking.**
- **Controlling weight.**
- **Eating five servings of fruits and vegetables a day.**
- **Exercising 30 minutes or more at moderate intensity five or more times a week.**

In a sample of about 154,000 men and women over age 18, only 3 percent engaged in all these healthy behaviors. However, the majority reported at least one "healthy lifestyle characteristic," or HLC. Three in four did not smoke. Two in five had a healthy weight. About one in four consumed the recommended amount of fruits and vegetables or engaged in regular physical activity.

The Americans most likely to have healthy lifestyles include women, those between ages 18 and 24 years or over age 55, college graduates, those with household incomes higher than $50,000, and individuals who describe their health as very good or excellent.

HEALTHY PEOPLE 2010

Healthy People 2010 is the prevention agenda for the nation. Every decade the federal government identifies the most significant preventable threats to health and creates leading indicators that assess the health of Americans. Its first

goal is to help individuals of all ages increase life expectancy *and* improve their quality of life. Its second goal is to eliminate health disparities among different segments of the population.

Among the specific goals of *Healthy People 2010* are:

- **Reduce the prevalence of cigarette smoking** among adults to 12 percent from the current 21 percent.
- **Reduce the number of new cancer cases** as well as the illnesses, disabilities, and deaths caused by cancer.
- **Promote the health of people with disabilities,** prevent secondary conditions, and eliminate disparities between people with and without disabilities in the U.S. population.
- **Reduce foodborne illnesses.**
- **Reduce the proportion of obese children and adolescents** from 11 percent to 5 percent.
- **Reduce the number of adolescents and adults** using illegal substances.
- **Reduce the number of adults** engaging in binge drinking.[11]

HEALTHY CAMPUS 2010

The American College Health Association has adapted the federal *Healthy People 2010* for college and universities. Its *Healthy Campus 2010* initiative has identified 28 focus areas (and 310 objectives) particularly relevant for students. Schools that participate in the program can compare data on their students to national norms and identify the key targets that would most improve health on their campuses.

As an example, the University of Southern California chose seven goals:

1. The improve access to comprehensive, high-quality health care services by increasing the proportion of students with health insurance.
2. To decrease alcohol and drug use through increased access to information on preventing substance abuse.
3. To decrease unintentional pregnancies.
4. To improve health, fitness, and quality of life through daily physical activity.
5. To increase fruit and vegetable consumption in order to promote health and reduce chronic disease.
6. To decrease sexual assault, including rape, attempted rape, or sexual assault on campus.
7. To decrease depression through increased access to treatment.[12]

Find out if your school is participating in *Healthy Campus 2010*. If it is, what are the target objectives for your campus?

HOW HEALTHY ARE TODAY'S STUDENTS?

The majority of college students are in the physical prime of life. As young, healthy adults, they are statistically less likely to develop life-threatening illnesses than older men and women. But contrary to what they may believe, they are not invincible. College students can and do develop a wide range of illnesses, from allergies (which afflict almost half of undergraduates) to potentially deadly cancers and heart conditions.

The number of college students with disabilities has tripled in the last two decades. According to the National Center for Educational Statistics, about 9 percent of full-time undergraduates report disabilities. The most common involve learning or health.[13]

College itself can seem hazardous to health. Dormitories have proved to be breeding grounds for serious infectious diseases, such as meningitis and Group B streptococcus (discussed in Chapter 14). Secondhand smoke can present a long-term threat to smokers' roommates. Binge drinking imperils not only the drinkers but those in their immediate environment, including anyone on the road if an intoxicated student gets behind the wheel of a car.

However, most students see themselves as healthy. Many health problems on campus stem from unhealthy choices or behaviors, not from underlying illnesses.

A REPORT CARD ON STUDENT HEALTH

According to the U.S. Department of Education, 15.9 million students—86 percent undergraduates—are enrolled in more than 4,000 colleges and universities. Although various agencies survey students about their behaviors, the American College Health Association National College Health Assessment (ACHA-NCHA) provides the most comprehensive view of the state of student health. Among its key findings:

░ More than nine in ten students describe their health as good, very good, or excellent (see Student Snapshot: "Health and Health Problems on Campus").

░ About two-thirds of students—70 percent of women and 58 percent of men—are at healthy weights. One in five—17 percent of women and 29 percent of men—are overweight. Nine percent—8 percent of women and 11 percent of men—are obese.

░ Only 7 percent of students report eating five or more servings of fruits and vegetables every day.

░ 44 percent of students exercise vigorously for at least 20 minutes or moderately for at least 30 minutes three or more days a week. About

You may be in prime health today, but your choices and behaviors during your college years can influence how healthy you will be in the future.

Student Snapshot

HEALTH AND HEALTH PROBLEMS ON CAMPUS

How Students Rate Their Health	
Good, Very Good, or Excellent	92.5%
Fair	6.4%
Poor	0.8%

Most Reported Health Problems	
1. Allergy	45.7%
2. Back pain	44.2%
3. Sinus infection	26.9%
4. Depression	18.8%
5. Strep throat	12.6%

*Based on surveys of 19,497 students on 33 campuses.
Source: American College Health Association. "The American College Health Association National College Health Assessment (ACHA-NCHA), Spring 2003 Reference Group Report." *Journal of American College Health,* March–April 2005, Vol. 53, No. 5, p. 199, www.acha.org.

half exercise to tone or strengthen their muscles at least two days a week.

■ Three in four students report having either no or one sexual partner in the past year—although most believe that other students are having sex with more partners.

■ 96 percent of students having vaginal intercourse report using contraception the last time they had sex. Forty percent relied on birth control pills, 35 percent on condoms, 15 percent on withdrawal (which, as discussed in Chapter 10, is not a reliable form of birth control).

■ 62 percent of students have never smoked; 21 percent smoked in the past month.

■ 18 percent of students never drink alcohol; 68 percent drank at least once in the past month.

■ Almost two-thirds have never used marijuana; 16 percent smoked pot in the previous month.

■ 73 percent of students always wear a seatbelt when riding in a car; 65 percent of those who ride motorcycles always wear helmets, as do 14 percent of bicycle riders.

■ 7 percent of students report being in a physical fight in the previous school year; 4 percent were assaulted.

Asked about their perceptions of how other students behave (see Chapter 2 for a discussion of such "social norms"), students generally overestimate the numbers engaging in risky behavior. For example, only 2 percent think a typical student never uses alcohol, when in fact 18 percent don't drink. Similarly, 7 percent think a typical student doesn't smoke, when in fact 62 percent have never smoked, and 16 percent think a typical student has never used marijuana, when 64 percent have never smoked pot.[14]

How do you compare with the students in this national survey? How do you think your campus compares?

Your Life Coach

Staying Healthy on Campus

The most common health problems that students report are allergies, back pain, sinus and throat infections, and depression.[15] Other health-related impediments also interfere with their academic performance, as shown in Figure 1-3. First and foremost is stress (see Chapter 4 on stress management). Many of the others, such as concerns for troubled friends or relatives and relationship difficulties, are psychological in nature (see Chapter 3 on psychological health). Taking care of yourself to prevent personal or academic problems now can help you perform at your best in college and feel and function your best in the future.

Simply by acquiring more years of schooling you increase your chance of a long and healthful life. Many risk factors for disease—including high blood pressure, elevated cholesterol, and cigarette smoking—decline steadily as education increases, regardless of how much money people make. Education may be good for the body as well as the mind by influencing lifestyle behaviors, problem-solving abilities, and values. People who earn college degrees acquire positive attitudes about the

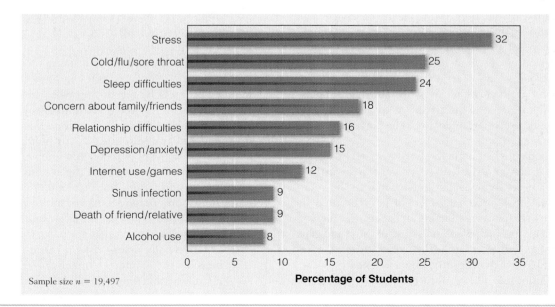

FIGURE 1-3   Health-Related Impediments to Academic Performance

Source: American College Health Association. American College Health Association National College Health Assessment (ACHA-NCHA) Web Summary, June 2004, www.acha.org/projects_programs/ncha_sampledata_public.cfm.

Strategies for Prevention   ::   Smart Steps to Take Now

:: To lower your risk of heart disease, get your blood pressure and cholesterol checked. Don't smoke. Stay at a healthy weight. Exercise regularly. (See Chapters 5, 7, and 15.)

:: To lower your risks of major diseases, get regular checkups. Make sure you are immunized against infectious illnesses. (See Chapter 14.)

:: To lower your risks of substance abuse and related illnesses and injuries, don't drink, or limit how much you drink. Avoid illegal drugs. (See Chapters 11 and 12.)

:: To lower your risk of sexually transmitted infections (STIs) or unwanted pregnancy, abstain from sex. If you decide to engage in potentially risky sexual

activities, protect yourself with contraceptives, condoms, and spermicides. (See Chapter 10.)

:: To prevent car accidents, don't drive when road conditions are hazardous. When you drive, wear a seat belt, and use defensive driving techniques. (See Chapter 19.)

---

benefits of healthy living, learn how to gain access to preventive health services, join peer groups that promote healthy behavior, and develop higher self-esteem and greater control over their lives.

This course in itself may be good for your health. In studies on the impact of health and wellness courses, students reported that they not only learned about the many dimensions of health but made changes to improve their health. Many changed their diet and eating habits, began exercising at a campus gym, developed schedules for better time management, engaged in stress-releasing activities, or altered a dangerous habit, such as smoking or drinking.

PREVENTING HEALTH PROBLEMS

College students often think they are too young to worry about serious health conditions. Yet many chronic problems begin early in life. Two percent of college-age women already have osteoporosis, a bone-weakening disease; another 15 percent have osteopenia, low bone densities that put them at risk of osteoporosis.[16] Many college students have several risk factors for heart disease, including high blood pressure and high cholesterol. Others increase their risk by eating a high-fat diet and not exercising regularly. The time to change is now.

No medical treatment, however successful or sophisticated, can compare with the power of **prevention.** Two out of every three deaths and one in three hospitalizations in the United States could be prevented by changes in six main risk factors: tobacco use, alcohol abuse, accidents, high blood pressure, obesity, and gaps in screening and primary health care. Prevention remains the best weapon against cancer and heart disease.

Prevention can take many forms. Primary, or before-the-fact, prevention efforts might seek to reduce stressors and increase support to prevent problems in healthy people. Consumer education, for instance, provides guidance about how to change our lifestyles to prevent problems and enhance well-being. Other preventive programs identify people at risk and empower them with information and support so they can avoid potential problems. Prevention efforts may target an entire community and try to educate all of its members about the dangers of alcohol abuse or environmental hazards, or they may zero in on a particular group (for instance, seminars on safer sex practices offered to teens) or an individual (such as one-on-one counseling about substance abuse).

PROTECTING YOURSELF

There is a great deal of overlap between prevention and **protection.** Some people might think of immunizations (discussed in Chapter 14) as a way of preventing illness; others see them as a form of protection against dangerous diseases. In many ways, protection picks up where prevention leaves off. You can prevent STIs or unwanted pregnancy by abstaining from sex. But if you decide to engage in potentially risky sexual activities, you can protect yourself with condoms and spermicides (discussed in Chapter 10). Similarly, you can prevent many automobile accidents by not driving when road conditions are hazardous. But if you do have to drive, you can protect yourself by wearing a seat belt and using defensive driving techniques (discussed in Chapter 19).

The very concept of protection implies some degree of risk—immediate and direct (for instance, the risk of intentional injury from an assailant or unintentional harm from a fire) or long-term and indirect (such as the risk of heart disease and cancer as a result of smoking). To know how best to protect yourself, you have to be able to realistically assess risks. (The information on risky behavior in Chapter 2 can help.)

 Colleges and universities take varied steps to protect students' well-being. These range from requiring vaccination against meningitis to banning alcohol at athletic and social events. Find out what your school is doing to protect your health. Would you like to see more programs and policies to safeguard student well-being?

INFORMING YOURSELF

Reliable health information can help you take better care of yourself. In the ACHA-NCHA survey discussed in the previous section, 75 percent of students turned to parents for health-related information. However, parents may not have a realistic sense of the health risks their children face. In a recent study comparing parents' perceptions of their college student children's health and health risk behaviors with the students' own reports, parents tended to be overly optimistic. They rated their children's health higher than the students themselves and underestimated the frequency of their drinking, smoking, marijuana use, and sex-related behaviors. Parents were more accurate in assessing their children's nutrition, exercise, use of seatbelts and bicycle helmets, sun protection, and whether they would ride in a car with someone under the influence of alcohol.[17] Although parents remain an important influence on college students, their misperceptions of risky behaviors may limit the nature and extent of information they provide their children.

Although friends rank second only to parents as a source of information, their credibility is much lower. Only about a quarter of students considered their friends' health advice and information believable. The third most common source of health information is the Internet, which ranked even lower than friends in terms of believability.

In a recent survey at two schools, three in four students reported getting health information online, and

Not all health information is accurate and worthwhile. Get it from a reliable source.

Courtesy of U. of Connecticut Wellness Project

more than 40 percent frequently searched the Internet for health-related materials.[18] As discussed in Chapter 17, you can find reliable, reputable health advice online—if you know where to look and if you remain skeptical about news or breakthroughs that seem too good to be true (see Savvy Consumer: "Too Good to Be True").

About half of students turn to health educators for information—and rank them as the most believable of sources. Health center medical staff rank almost equally as high. Although students regularly turn to flyers, pamphlets, magazines, and television for information, they are less likely to consider these as authoritative, believable sources.

Colleges and universities also provide health-related information to students. The most commonly covered topics are alcohol and drug use prevention, sexual assault/relationship violence prevention, sexually transmitted diseases, physical activity and fitness, HIV/AIDS prevention, and nutrition and dietary behaviors.

Savvy Consumer :: Too Good to Be True?

Almost every week you're likely to come across a commercial or an ad for a new health product that promises better sleep, more energy, clearer skin, firmer muscles, lower weight, brighter moods, longer life—or all of these combined. As the Savvy Consumer throughout this book points out, you can't believe every promise you read or hear. Keep these general guidelines in mind the next time you come across a health claim:

:: If it sounds too good to be true, it probably is. If a magic pill could really trim off excess pounds or banish wrinkles, the world would be filled with thin

people with unlined skin. Look around and you'll realize that's not the case.

:: Look for objective evaluations. If you're watching an infomercial for a treatment or technique, you can be sure that the enthusiastic endorsements have been skillfully scripted and rehearsed. Even ads that claim to be presenting the science behind a new breakthrough are really sales pitches in disguise.

:: Consider the sources. Research findings from carefully controlled scientific studies are reviewed by leading experts in the field and published in scholarly

journals. Just because someone has conducted a study doesn't mean it was a valid scientific investigation.

:: Check credentials. Anyone can claim to be a scientist or a health expert. Find out if advocates of any type of therapy have legitimate degrees from recognized institutions and are fully licensed in their fields.

:: Do your own research. Check with your doctor or with the student health center. Go to the library or do some online research to gather as much information as you can.

HEALTH IN THE TWENTY-FIRST CENTURY

Cloning. Deciphering the human genome. Painless diagnostic tests. Technology that enables the blind to see, the deaf to hear, the paralyzed to walk. Robotic limbs. Bloodless surgery. Once these were the stuff of science fiction. Today they are realities of modern medicine. What will the future bring? Technology is evolving daily, and within decades the current "state-of-the-art" treatments may seem as primitive and old-fashioned as therapies from the turn of the twentieth century.

One of the most exciting scientific frontiers has been genetic research. The completion of the mapping of the human genome sequence in 2001 was a milestone in biological science. So much progress has since been made in the new science of "genomics" that geneticists describe themselves as "swimming in a rapidly rising sea of data." Analysis of that data will point the way to new possibilities in screening, diagnosing, and treating diseases.

In their quest for new cures for deadly or disabling diseases, scientists have ventured into uncharted and highly controversial territory. The ethics of cloning, whether of animals or of human embryos, and the use of embryonic stem cells (which have the potential to grow into any type of cell, such as muscle, bone, or skin) have stirred passionate debate among legislators, scientists, religious leaders, and patient advocacy groups. Gene therapy, which replaces defective genes with normal ones, also has come under attack after the deaths of volunteers in experimental programs. The federal government has restricted funding for certain types of research and has set up a panel of doctors, lawyers, and ethicists to advise the president on stem cells, cloning, and other challenging research issues.

Without doubt, medical advances will touch your life. If injured, you may recover more rapidly because of them. If you develop a serious illness, you may be spared life-threatening complications. Your children will be more likely to be born and to grow up healthy and strong. You may remain active and healthy for decades longer than your great-grandparents. But despite the promise of medical breakthroughs, your future well-being remains in your hands. Your choices, your habits, your lifestyle, your vigilance ultimately will decide how long and how healthfully you will live.

PERSONALIZING YOUR HEALTH CARE

Thanks to advances in genomics (the study of the entire set of human genes), physicians are tailoring tests and treatments to individual patients. "Personalized" medicine can alert your doctor to potential threats that might be prevented, delayed, or detected at an earlier, more treatable stage and,

if you do develop a disease, pinpoint the medications that will do the most good and cause the least harm.

But "personalizing" health care is also a personal responsibility. You can take charge of your own health by compiling a family health history and informing yourself about risks related to your gender, race, and ethnicity.

YOUR FAMILY HEALTH HISTORY

Someday a DNA scan from a single drop of blood may tell you the diseases you're most likely to develop. A family history can do the same—now.

Mapping your family medical history can help identify health risks you may face in the future. One way of charting your health history is to draw a medical family "tree" that includes your parents and siblings (who share half your genes), as well as grandparents, uncles, aunts, and cousins. Depending on how much information you're able to obtain for each relative, your medical family tree can include health issues each family member has faced, including illnesses with a hereditary component, such as high blood pressure, diabetes, some cancers, and certain psychiatric disorders. Although having a relative with a certain disease may increase your risk, your likelihood of ending up with the same condition also depends on your health habits, such as diet and exercise. Knowing now that you're at risk can motivate you to change any unhealthy behaviors.

"Family history is the single greatest risk factor for disease," says Dr. Paula Yoon of the CDC's Family Health Initiative, which is encouraging consumers to complete a family history and discuss it with their doctors. Physicians spend less than 2.5 minutes discussing family history and rarely include a family tree in a patient's file. Yet realizing that you have a relative with, say, colon cancer could mean that you should start screening tests ten years before others because you're at risk of developing a tumor at an earlier age. Says Yoon, "Knowing your family history could save your life."[19]

For guidance on creating a family history, check these websites: **www.mayoclinic.com** or **www.ashg.org/genetics/ashg/educ/007.shtml.**

ⓕⓐⓠ DOES GENDER MATTER?

"Sex does matter. It matters in ways that we did not expect. Undoubtedly, it also matters in ways that we have not begun to imagine." This was the conclusion of the Institute of Medicine Committee on Understanding the Biology of Sex and Gender Differences in the first significant review of the status of sex and gender differences in biomedical research.

Sex, the committee stated, is "a classification, generally as male or female, according to the reproductive organs and functions that derive from the chromosomal complement." *Gender* refers to "a person's self-representation as male or female or how that person is responded to by social institutions on the basis of the individual's gender presentation." Rooted in biology, gender is shaped by environment and experience.

The experience of being male or female in a particular culture and society can and does have an effect on physical and psychological well-being. In fact, sex and gender may have a greater impact than any other variable on how our bodies function, how long we live, and the symptoms, course, and treatment of the diseases that strike us.

This realization is both new and revolutionary. For centuries, scientists based biological theories solely on a male model and viewed women as shorter, smaller, and rounder versions of men. Even modern medicine is based on the assumption that, except for their reproductive organs, both sexes are biologically interchangeable. We now know that this simply isn't so (Figure 1-4). Sex begins in the womb, but sex and gender differences affect behavior, perception, and health throughout life.

Recognition of these gender differences is transforming medical research and practice. *Gender-specific medicine* is replacing one-size-fits-all health care with new definitions of what is normal in both men and women, more complex concepts of disease, more precise diagnostic tests, and more effective treatments.

He:

- averages 12 breaths a minute
- has lower core body temperature
- has a slower heart rate
- has more oxygen-rich hemoglobin in his blood
- is more sensitive to sound
- produces twice as much saliva
- has a 10 percent larger brain
- is 10 times more likely to have attention deficit disorder
- as a teen, has an attention span of 5 minutes
- is more likely to be physically active
- is more prone to lethal diseases, including heart attacks, cancer, and liver failure
- is five times more likely to become an alcoholic
- has a life expectancy of 74.7 years

She:

- averages 9 breaths a minute
- has higher core body temperature
- has a faster heart rate
- has higher levels of protective immunoglobulin in her blood
- is more sensitive to light
- takes twice as long to process food
- has more neurons in certain brain regions
- is twice as likely to have an eating disorder
- as a teen, has an attention span of 20 minutes
- is more likely to be overweight
- is more vulnerable to chronic diseases, like arthritis and autoimmune disorders, and age-related conditions like osteoporosis
- is twice as likely to develop depression
- has a life expectancy of 79.9 years

FIGURE 1-4 Men and Women *Are* Different

DIVERSITY AND HEALTH

 We live in the most diverse nation on Earth, one that is becoming increasingly diverse. For society, this variety can be both enriching and divisive. Tolerance and acceptance of others have always been part of the American creed. By working together, Americans have created a country that remains, to those outside our borders, a symbol of opportunity. Yet members of different ethnic groups still have to struggle against discrimination.

Although the top three causes and seven of the ten leading causes of death are the same for blacks and whites (Table 1-1), the incidence, complications, and death rates of these diseases and injuries are often greater for African Americans and Hispanics than for whites. Black Americans lose substantially more years of potential life to homicide (nine times as many), stroke (three times as many), and diabetes (three times as many) as whites.[20] Hispanics suffer more fatal injuries, chronic liver disease, and cirrhosis of the liver.

How Race Affects Health

 Race and ethnicity affect the health of various minority groups in the United States in many ways.

- The infant mortality rate for African-American babies remains higher than for white babies.
- Life expectancy for African Americans, though increasing, is five years lower than for whites.
- African Americans have higher rates of high blood pressure (hypertension), develop this problem earlier in life, suffer more severe hypertension, and have higher rates of strokes.
- African Americans have higher rates of glaucoma, systemic lupus erythematosus, liver disease, and kidney failure than whites. They also have less access to kidney transplants.[21]
- Overall, black American are more likely to develop cancer than persons of any other racial or ethnic group. Black women have higher rates of colon, pancreatic, and stomach cancer. Black men have higher rates of prostate, lung, colon, and stomach cancer.[22]
- Fewer African-American and Hispanic children are given prescriptions. White children receive more pain medication than black children treated for the same conditions in emergency centers. Fewer psychiatric medications are provided to African-American youths.[23]
- Latinos living in the United States have high rates of eye disease and visual impairment, particularly of diabetic retinopathy, an eye complication of diabetes, and open-angle glaucoma, a disease that damages the optic nerve.[24]

TABLE 1-1 TOP TEN CAUSES OF DEATH FOR BLACKS, WHITES, HISPANICS, AND ASIANS

Blacks	Whites	Hispanics	Asians/Pacific Islanders
1. Heart disease	1. Heart disease	1. Heart disease	1. Cancer
2. Cancer	2. Cancer	2. Cancer	2. Heart disease
3. Stroke	3. Stroke	3. Unintentional injury	3. Stroke
4. Diabetes	4. Chronic lower respiratory disease	4. Stroke	4. Unintentional injury
5. Unintentional injury	5. Unintentional injury	5. Diabetes	5. Diabetes
6. Homicide	6. Influenza & pneumonia	6. Chronic liver disease & cirrhosis	6. Influenza & pneumonia
7. Chronic lower respiratory disease	7. Alzheimer's disease	7. Homicide	7. Chronic lower respiratory disease
8. HIV/AIDS	8. Diabetes	8. Chronic lower respiratory disease	8. Suicide
9. Kidney disease	9. Kidney disease	9. Influenza & pneumonia	9. Kidney disease
10. Septicemia (life-threatening infection)	10. Suicide	10. Birth defects	10. Septicemia

Sources: "Health Disparities Experienced by Black or African Americans—United States." *Morbidity and Mortality Weekly Report*, Vol. 54, No. 1, January 14, 2005, p.1; National Center for Health Statistics, www.cdc.gov/nchs.

▫ Women of Filipino, Hawaiian, Indian, Pakistani, Mexican, South and Central American, and Puerto Rican descent are 20 to 260 percent more likely to be diagnosed with late-stage breast cancer than white women.[25]

▫ Caucasians are prone to osteoporosis (progressive weakening of bone tissue); cystic fibrosis; skin cancer; and phenylketonuria (PKU), a metabolic disorder that can lead to mental retardation.

▫ Asians and Asian Americans metabolize some medications faster than whites and thus require much smaller doses.

▫ Native Americans have the highest rate of diabetes in the world. Among the Pima Indians, half of all adults have diabetes.

▫ Native Hawaiian women have a higher rate of breast cancer than women from other racial and ethnic groups.

▫ Native Americans, including those indigenous to Alaska, are more likely to die young than the population as a whole, primarily as a result of accidental injuries, cirrhosis of the liver, homicide, pneumonia, and the complications of diabetes.

▫ The suicide rate among American Indians and Alaska Natives is 50 percent higher than the national rate. The rates of co-occurring mental illness and substance abuse (especially alcohol) are also higher among Native American youth and adults.

▫ American Indians and Alaska Natives have the poorest survival rate from all cancers combined, when compared with all other racial and ethnic groups.[26]

Are these increased susceptibilities the result of genetics, an unhealthy lifestyle, lack of access to health services, poverty, or the stress of living with discrimination? It is hard to say precisely. Certainly, poverty presents a major barrier to seeking preventive care and getting timely and effective treatment.

In some cases, both genetic and environmental factors may play a role. Take, for example, the high rates of diabetes among the Pima Indians. Until 50 years ago, these Native Americans were not notably obese or prone to diabetes. After World War II, the tribe started trading handmade baskets for lard and flour. Their lifestyle became more sedentary and their diet higher in fats. In addition, researchers have discovered that many Pima Indians have an inherited resistance to insulin that increases their susceptibility to diabetes. The combination of a hereditary predisposition and environmental factors may explain why the Pimas now have epidemic levels of diabetes.

 Ending Health Disparities

In the words of a National Institutes of Health report, minorities have carried "an unequal burden with respect to disease and disability, resulting in a lower life expectancy." Each year minorities in the United States—African Americans, Hispanics, Asian Americans, Pacific Islanders, Native Americans, and other groups—experience as many as 75,000 more deaths than they would if they lived under the same health conditions as the white population.

But race itself isn't the primary reason for the health problems faced by minorities in the United States. Poverty is. Without adequate insurance or the ability to pay, many cannot afford the tests and treatments that could prevent

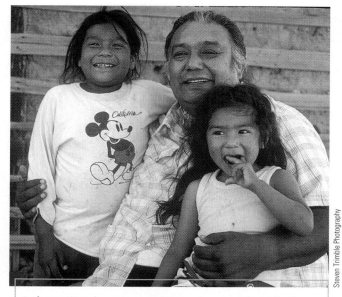

Steven Trimble Photography

Both genetic and environmental factors have contributed to the increase in diabetes among the Pima tribe. Half of all Pima adults have diabetes.

illness or overcome it at the earliest possible stages. One in three Hispanics under age 65 has no health insurance. According to public health experts, low income may account for one-third of the racial differences in death rates for middle-aged African-American adults. High blood pressure, high cholesterol, obesity, diabetes, and smoking are responsible for another third. The final third has been blamed on "unexplained factors," which may well include poor access to health care and the stress of living in a society in which skin color remains a major barrier to equality.

When African Americans receive the same cancer treatments as whites, they are equally likely to survive. In a study of nearly 3,400 colon cancer patients, white and black patients treated with surgery and chemotherapy had virtually the same five-year survival rates. When blacks and whites have equal access to quality health care, perhaps some of the race-based differences in overall health will also be reduced.

The racial gap is closing for many simple, relatively inexpensive medical procedures, such as mammograms and eye exams and blood sugar testing for diabetes. However, disparities continue for more expensive surgical procedures such as heart and back surgeries and total hip replacement.[27]

FAQ What Can I Do to Improve My Health If My Racial Background Puts Me at Risk?

As a risk factor for certain health conditions, race is beyond anyone's control. However, classifications such as "black" or "Hispanic" may be overly broad. Among Hispanics, for instance, Puerto Ricans suffer disproportionately from asthma, HIV/AIDS, and high infant mortality, while Mexican Americans have higher rates for diabetes. If, like many Americans, you come from a racially mixed background, your health profile may be complex.

Awareness of potential risks is the first step to protecting your health. If you do face greater health threats because of your race or ethnicity, it is up to you to educate yourself, take responsibility for the risks within your control, and become a savvy, assertive consumer of health-care services. The federal Office of Minority Health (www.cdc.gov/omh), which provides general information and the latest research and recommendations, is a good place to start.

Certain health risks may be genetic, but behavior influences their impact. If you are African American, for instance, you are significantly more likely to develop high blood pressure, diabetes, and kidney disease. Being overweight or obese adds to the danger. The information in Chapters 5, 6, and 7 can help you lower your risk by keeping in shape, making healthy food choices, and managing your weight.

Because diabetes and high blood pressure run in families, knowing your family history is crucial (see page 12). The National Kidney Disease Education Program has launched an initiative to encourage African Americans, who have a four-times greater risk of kidney disease, to share information about these conditions at holiday gatherings or family reunions.

Hispanics and Latinos have disproportionately high rates of respiratory problems, such as asthma, chronic obstructive lung disease, and tuberculosis. To protect your lungs, stop smoking and avoid secondary smoke. Learn as much as you can about the factors that can trigger or worsen lung diseases.

As discussed earlier in this chapter, research in personalized medicine has led to development of medications tailored to an individual's genetic make-up, including his or her race and ethnicity. Once such drug, BiDil, has been approved to treat heart failure, a potentially life-threatening condition, in black patients. If you or a family member require treatment for a chronic illness, ask your doctor whether any medications have proved particularly effective for your racial or ethnic background.

Health disparities aren't solely the result of genetics or biology. Poverty, lack of health insurance, limited or no access to preventive care, and language and cultural barriers also play a role. Use the information in Chapter 17 to learn about your rights as a health-care consumer and to ensure that you get the best possible care. Here and on page 25 are some suggestions that may help:

■ Know as much as you can about your family's medical history.

■ Ask if you are at risk for any medical conditions or disorders based on your family history, racial, or ethnic background.

Self Survey ⊞ Wellness Inventory

WHAT IS WELLNESS?*

by John W. Travis, M.D.

Health Now™ Go to HealthNow for more activities.

Most of us think in terms of illness and assume that the absence of illness indicates wellness. There are actually many degrees of wellness, just as there are many degrees of illness. The Wellness Inventory is designed to stir up your thinking about many areas of wellness.

While people often lack physical symptoms, they may still be bored, depressed, tense, anxious, or generally unhappy with their lives. Such emotional states often set the stage for physical and mental disease. Even cancer may be brought on through the lowering of the body's resistance from excessive stress. These same emotional states can also lead to abuse of the body through smoking, overdrinking, and overeating. Such behaviors are usually substitutes for other, more basic human needs such as recognition from others, a more stimulating environment, caring and affection from friends, and greater self-acceptance.

Wellness is not a static state. High-level wellness involves giving good care to your physical self, using your mind constructively, expressing your emotions effectively, being creatively involved with those around you, and being concerned about your physical, psychological, and spiritual environments.

Instructions

Set aside a half hour for yourself in a quiet place where you will not be disturbed while taking the Inventory. Record your responses to each statement in the columns to the right where:

2 = Yes, usually
1 = Sometimes, maybe
0 = No, rarely

Select the answer that best indicates how true the statement is for you presently.

* Abridged from the Wellness Index in *The Wellness Workbook*, Travis & Ryan, Ten Speed Press, 1988. Used with the permission of John W. Travis, M.D., www .thewellspring.com.

After you have responded to all the appropriate statements in each section, compute your average score for that section and transfer it to the corresponding box provided around the Wellness Inventory Wheel on page 17. Your completed Wheel will give you a clear presentation of the balance you have given to the many dimensions of your life.

You will find some of the statements are really two in one. We do this to show an important relationship between the two parts—usually an awareness of an issue, combined with an action based on that awareness. Mentally average your score for the two parts of the question.

Each statement describes what we believe to be a wellness attribute. Because much wellness information is subjective and "unprovable" by current scientific methods, you (and possibly other authorities as well) may not agree with our conclusions. Many of the statements have further explanation in a footnote. We ask only that you keep an open mind until you have studied available information, then decide.

This questionnaire was designed to educate more than to test. All statements are worded so that you can easily tell what we think are wellness attributes (which also makes it easy to "cheat" on your score). This means there can be no trick questions to test your honesty or consistency—the higher your score, the greater you believe your wellness to be. Full responsibility is placed on you to answer each statement as honestly as possible. It's not your score but what you learn about yourself that is most important.

If you decide that a statement does not apply to you, or you don't want to answer it, you can skip it and not be penalized in your score.

Transfer your average score from each section to the corresponding box around the Wheel. Then graph your score by drawing a curved line between the "spokes" that define each segment. (Use the scale provided—beginning at the center with 0.0 and reaching 2.0 at the circumference.) Last, fill in the corresponding amount of each wedge-shaped segment, using different colors if possible.

Sample Questions

	Yes, usually	Sometimes, maybe	No, rarely
	2	**1**	**0**
1. I am an adventurous thinker.	✔		
2. I have no expectations, yet look to the future optimistically.		✔	
3. I am a nonsmoker.	✔		
4. I love long, hot baths.			✔

Total points for this section = $\boxed{5}$ __4__ + __1__ + __0__

Divided by __4__ **(number of statements answered)** = __1.3__ **Average score for this section.**

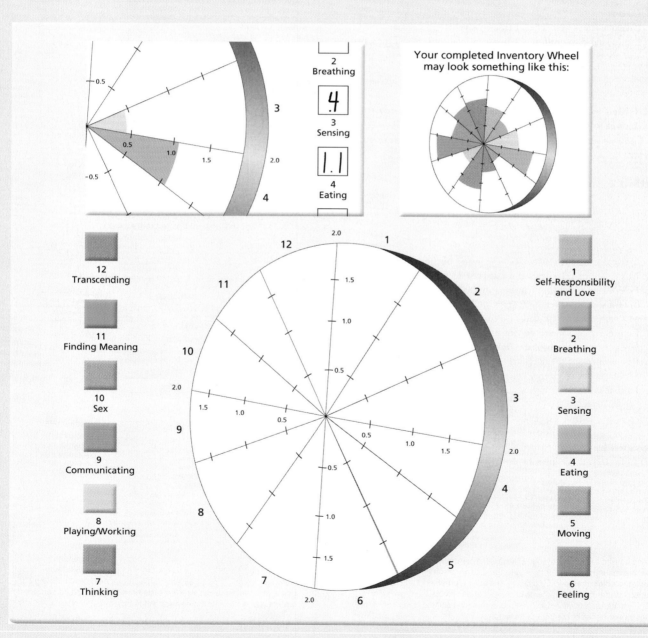

Your completed Inventory Wheel may look something like this:

12 Transcending
11 Finding Meaning
10 Sex
9 Communicating
8 Playing/Working
7 Thinking

1 Self-Responsibility and Love
2 Breathing
3 Sensing
4 Eating
5 Moving
6 Feeling

Section 1 WELLNESS, SELF-RESPONSIBILITY, AND LOVE

	Yes, usually	Sometimes, maybe	No, rarely
	2	1	0
1. I believe how I live my life is an important factor in determining my state of health, and I live it in a manner consistent with that belief.	_____	_____	_____
2. I vote regularly.[1]	_____	_____	_____
3. I feel financially secure.	_____	_____	_____
4. I conserve materials/energy at home and at work.[2]	_____	_____	_____
5. I protect my living area from fire and safety hazards.	_____	_____	_____
6. I use dental floss and a soft toothbrush daily.	_____	_____	_____
7. I am a nonsmoker.	_____	_____	_____
8. I am always sober when driving or operating dangerous machinery.	_____	_____	_____
9. I wear a safety belt when I ride in a vehicle.	_____	_____	_____
10. I understand the difference between blaming myself for a problem and simply taking responsibility (ability to respond) for that problem.	_____	_____	_____

Total points for this section = ☐ _____ + _____ + _____

Divided by _____ **(number of statements answered) =** _____ **Average score for this section.**
(Transfer to the Wellness Inventory Wheel on **p. 17.**)

Section 2 WELLNESS AND BREATHING

	Yes, usually	Sometimes, maybe	No, rarely
	2	1	0
1. I stop during the day to become aware of the way I am breathing.	_____	_____	_____
2. I meditate or relax myself for at least 15 to 20 minutes each day.	_____	_____	_____
3. I can easily touch my hands to my toes when standing with knees straight.[3]	_____	_____	_____
4. In temperatures over 70°F (21°C), my fingers feel warm when I touch my lips.[4]	_____	_____	_____
5. My nails are healthy and I do not bite or pick at them.	_____	_____	_____
6. I enjoy my work and do not find it overly stressful.	_____	_____	_____
7. My personal relationships are satisfying.	_____	_____	_____
8. I take time out for deep breathing several times a day.	_____	_____	_____
9. I have plenty of energy.	_____	_____	_____
10. I am at peace with myself.	_____	_____	_____

Total points for this section = ☐ _____ + _____ + _____

Divided by _____ **(number of statements answered) =** _____ **Average score for this section.**
(Transfer to the Wellness Inventory Wheel on **p. 17.**)

[1] Voting is a simple measure of your willingness to participate in the social system, which ultimately impacts your state of health.

[2] Besides recycling glass, paper, aluminum, and other recyclables, if you purchase products that are reusable rather than disposable, and are packaged with a minimum of material, you will reduce the drain of resources and the toxic load on the environment caused by the disposal of wastes.

[3] A lack of spinal flexibility is usually a symptom of chronic muscle tension as well as indicative of a poor balance of physical activities.

[4] If your hand temperature is below 85°F (30°C) in a warm room, you're cutting off circulation to your hands via an overactive sympathetic nervous system. You can learn to warm your hands with biofeedback and to thereby better relax.

Section 3 WELLNESS AND SENSING

	Yes, usually	Sometimes, maybe	No, rarely
	2	1	0
1. My place of work has mostly natural lighting or full-spectrum fluorescent lighting.[5]	____	____	____
2. I avoid extremely noisy areas or wear protective ear covers.[6]	____	____	____
3. I take long walks, hikes, or other outings to actively explore my surroundings.	____	____	____
4. I give myself presents, treats, or nurture myself in other ways.	____	____	____
5. I enjoy getting, and can acknowledge, compliments and recognition from others.	____	____	____
6. It is easy for me to give sincere compliments and recognition to other people.	____	____	____
7. At times I like to be alone.	____	____	____
8. I enjoy touching or hugging other people.[7]	____	____	____
9. I enjoy being touched or hugged by others.[8]	____	____	____
10. I get and enjoy backrubs or massages.	____	____	____

Total points for this section = ☐ ____ + ____ + ____

Divided by _____ **(number of statements answered)** = ____ **Average score for this section.**
(Transfer to the Wellness Inventory Wheel on **p. 17.**)

Section 4 WELLNESS AND EATING

	Yes, usually	Sometimes, maybe	No, rarely
	2	1	0
1. I am aware of the difference between refined carbohydrates and complex carbohydrates and eat a majority of the latter.[9]	____	____	____
2. I think my diet is well balanced and wholesome.	____	____	____
3. I drink fewer than five alcoholic drinks per week.	____	____	____
4. I drink fewer than two cups of coffee or black (nonherbal) tea per day.[10]	____	____	____
5. I drink fewer than five soft drinks per week.[11]	____	____	____
6. I add little or no salt to my food.[12]	____	____	____
7. I read the labels for the ingredients of all processed foods I buy and I inquire as to the level of toxic chemicals used in production of fresh foods—choosing the purest available to me.	____	____	____
8. I eat at least two raw fruits or vegetables each day.	____	____	____
9. I have a good appetite and am within 15 percent of my ideal weight.	____	____	____
10. I can tell the difference between "stomach hunger" and "mouth hunger," and I don't stuff myself when I am experiencing only "mouth hunger."[13]	____	____	____

Total points for this section = ☐ ____ + ____ + ____

Divided by _____ **(number of statements answered)** = ____ **Average score for this section.**
(Transfer to the Wellness Inventory Wheel on **p. 17.**)

---

[5] Full-spectrum light, like sunlight, contains many different wavelengths. Most eyeglasses, and the glass windows in your home or car, block the "near" ultraviolet light needed by your body. Special bulbs and lenses are available.

[6] Loud noises that leave your ears ringing cause irreversible and cumulative nerve damage over time. Ear plugs/muffs, obtained in sporting goods stores, should be worn around power saws, heavy equipment, and rock concerts!

[7,8] Long recognized by hospitals as therapeutic, touch can be a powerful preventative as well.

[9] Refined carbohydrates (white flour, sugar, white rice, alcohol, and others) are burned up by the body very quickly and contain no minerals or vitamins. Complex carbohydrates (fruits and vegetables) burn evenly and provide the bulk of dietary nutrients.

[10] Coffee and nonherbal teas contain stimulants that, when overused, abuse your body's adrenal glands.

[11] Besides caffeine, the empty calories in these chemical brews may cause a sugar "crash" shortly after drinking. Artificially sweetened ones may be worse. Consider the other nutrients you won't be getting, and the prices!

[12] In addition to having a presumed connection with high blood pressure, the salting of foods during cooking draws out minerals, which are lost when the water is poured off.

[13] Stomach hunger is a signal that your body needs food. Mouth hunger is a signal that it needs something else (attention/acknowledgment), which you are not getting, so it asks for food, a readily available "substitute."

Section 5 WELLNESS AND MOVING

	Yes, usually	Sometimes, maybe	No, rarely
	2	1	0
1. I climb stairs rather than ride elevators.[14]	____	____	____
2. My daily activities include moderate physical effort.[15]	____	____	____
3. My daily activities include vigorous physical effort.[16]	____	____	____
4. I run at least 1 mile three times a week (or do equivalent aerobic exercise).[17]	____	____	____
5. I run at least 3 miles three times a week (or do equivalent aerobic exercise).	____	____	____
6. I do some form of stretching/limbering exercise for 10 to 20 minutes at least three times per week.[18]	____	____	____
7. I do some form of stretching/limbering exercise for 10 to 20 minutes at least six times per week.	____	____	____
8. I enjoy exploring new and effective ways of caring for myself through the movement of my body.	____	____	____
9. I enjoy stretching, moving, and exerting my body.	____	____	____
10. I am aware of and respond to messages from my body about its needs for movement.	____	____	____

Total points for this section = ☐ ____ + ____ + ____

Divided by ____ **(number of statements answered)** = ____ **Average score for this section.**
(Transfer to the Wellness Inventory Wheel on **p. 17**.)

Section 6 WELLNESS AND FEELING

	Yes, usually	Sometimes, maybe	No, rarely
	2	1	0
1. I am able to feel and express my anger in ways that solve problems, rather than swallow anger or store it up.[19]	____	____	____
2. I allow myself to experience a full range of emotions and find constructive ways to express them.	____	____	____
3. I am able to say "no" to people without feeling guilty.	____	____	____
4. I laugh often and easily.	____	____	____
5. I feel OK about crying and allow myself to do so when appropriate.[20]	____	____	____
6. I listen to and consider others' criticisms of me rather than react defensively.	____	____	____
7. I have at least five close friends.	____	____	____
8. I like myself and look forward to the rest of my life.	____	____	____
9. I easily express concern, love, and warmth to those I care about.	____	____	____
10. I can ask for help when needed.	____	____	____

Total points for this section = ☐ ____ + ____ + ____

Divided by ____ **(number of statements answered)** = ____ **Average score for this section.**
(Transfer to the Wellness Inventory Wheel on **p. 17**.)

---

[14] If a long elevator ride is necessary, try getting off five flights below your destination. Urge building managers to keep stair doors unlocked.

[15] Moderate = rearing young children, gardening, scrubbing floors, brisk walking, and so on.

[16] Vigorous = heavy construction work, farming, moving heavy objects by hand, and so on.

[17] An aerobic exercise (like running) should keep your heart rate at about 60 percent of its maximum (120–150 bpm) for 12–20 minutes. Brisk walking for 20 minutes every day can produce effects similar to aerobic exercise.

[18] The stretching of muscles is important for maintaining maximum flexibility of joints and ligaments. It feels good, too.

[19] Learning to take charge of your emotions and using them to solve problems can prevent disease, improve communications, and increase your self-awareness. Suppressing emotions or using them to manipulate others is destructive to all.

[20] Crying over a loss relieves the body of pent-up feelings. In our culture males often have a difficult time allowing themselves to cry, while females may have learned to cry when angry, using tears as a means of manipulation.

Section 7 WELLNESS AND THINKING

	Yes, usually	Sometimes, maybe	No, rarely
	2	1	0
1. I am in charge of the subject matter and the emotional content of my thoughts and am satisfied with what I choose to think about.[21]	_____	_____	_____
2. I am aware that I make judgments wherein I think I am "right" and others are "wrong."[22]	_____	_____	_____
3. It is easy for me to concentrate.	_____	_____	_____
4. I am conscious of changes (such as breathing pattern, muscle tension, skin moisture, and so on) in my body in response to certain thoughts.[23]	_____	_____	_____
5. I notice my perceptions of the world are colored by my thoughts at the time.[24]	_____	_____	_____
6. I am aware that my thoughts are influenced by my environment.	_____	_____	_____
7. I use my thoughts and attitudes to make my reality more life-affirming.[25]	_____	_____	_____
8. Rather than worry about a problem when I can do nothing about it, I temporarily shelve it and get on with the matters at hand.	_____	_____	_____
9. I approach life with the attitude that no problem is too big to confront, and some mysteries aren't meant to be solved.	_____	_____	_____
10. I use my creative powers in many aspects of my life.	_____	_____	_____

Total points for this section = ☐ _____ + _____ + _____

Divided by _____ **(number of statements answered)** = _____ **Average score for this section.**
(Transfer to the Wellness Inventory Wheel on **p. 17.**)

Section 8 WELLNESS AND PLAYING/WORKING

	Yes, usually	Sometimes, maybe	No, rarely
	2	1	0
1. I enjoy expressing myself through art, dance, music, drama, sports, or other activities and make time to do so.	_____	_____	_____
2. I regularly exercise my creativity "muscles."	_____	_____	_____
3. I enjoy spending time without planned or structured activities and make the effort to do so.	_____	_____	_____
4. I can make much of my work into play.	_____	_____	_____
5. At times I allow myself to do nothing.[26]	_____	_____	_____
6. At times I can sleep late without feeling guilty.	_____	_____	_____
7. The work I do is rewarding to me.	_____	_____	_____
8. I am proud of my accomplishments.	_____	_____	_____
9. I am playful and the people around me support my playfulness.	_____	_____	_____
10. I have at least one activity, hobby, or sport that I enjoy regularly but do not feel compelled to do.	_____	_____	_____

Total points for this section = ☐ _____ + _____ + _____

Divided by _____ **(number of statements answered)** = _____ **Average score for this section.**
(Transfer to the Wellness Inventory Wheel on **p. 17.**)

[21] When you are unconscious of the content of your thoughts, they are more likely to control you. Observing them objectively develops self-awareness and strengthens your ability to take charge.

[22] Rather than trying to completely stop yourself from judging, you can observe your judgments as efforts by your ego to avoid getting on with life and hiding behind "right/wrong" game playing.

[23] Both biofeedback and the field of psycho-neuro-immunology have shown the connections between the mind, nervous system, and body. The more you become consciously aware of that connection, the greater responsibility you can take for your health.

[24] Being aware of your internal distortion of perceptions can allow you to step back and reassess a situation more objectively.

[25] Honesty, tempered with care and concern, clears out many negative thoughts that can clutter up your mind, thus making your reality more fun. "Positive thinking" without honesty and truthfulness can backfire by suppressing valid concerns that must be addressed.

[26] Doing "nothing" can give us access to the more creative and nonverbal aspects of our being, so from another perspective, doing nothing becomes doing much more.

Section 9 WELLNESS AND COMMUNICATING

	Yes, usually	Sometimes, maybe	No, rarely
	2	**1**	**0**
1. In conversation I can introduce a difficult topic and stay with it until I've gotten a satisfactory response from the other person.	_____	_____	_____
2. I enjoy silence.	_____	_____	_____
3. I am truthful and caring in my communications with others.	_____	_____	_____
4. I assert myself (in a nonattacking manner) in an effort to be heard, rather than be passively resentful of others with whom I don't agree.[27]	_____	_____	_____
5. I readily acknowledge my mistakes, apologizing for them if appropriate.	_____	_____	_____
6. I am aware of my negative judgments of others and accept them as simply judgments—not necessarily truth.[28]	_____	_____	_____
7. I am a good listener.	_____	_____	_____
8. I am able to listen to people without interrupting them or finishing their sentences for them.	_____	_____	_____
9. I can let go of my mental "labels" (for example, this is good, that is wrong) and judgmental attitudes about events in my life and see them in light of what they offer me.	_____	_____	_____
10. I am aware when I play psychological "games" with those around me and work to be truthful and direct in my communications.[29]	_____	_____	_____

Total points for this section = ☐ _____ + _____ + _____

Divided by _____ **(number of statements answered)** = _____ **Average score for this section.**
(Transfer to the Wellness Inventory Wheel on **p. 17.**)

Section 10 WELLNESS AND SEX

	Yes, usually	Sometimes, maybe	No, rarely
	2	**1**	**0**
1. I feel comfortable touching and exploring my body.	_____	_____	_____
2. I think it's OK to masturbate if one chooses to do so.	_____	_____	_____
3. My sexual education is adequate.	_____	_____	_____
4. I feel good about the degree of closeness I have with men.	_____	_____	_____
5. I feel good about the degree of closeness I have with women.	_____	_____	_____
6. I am content with my level of sexual activity.[30]	_____	_____	_____
7. I fully experience the many stages of lovemaking rather than focus only on orgasm.[31]	_____	_____	_____
8. I desire to grow closer to some other people.	_____	_____	_____
9. I am aware of the difference between needing someone and loving someone.	_____	_____	_____
10. I am able to love others without dominating or being dominated by them.	_____	_____	_____

Total points for this section = ☐ _____ + _____ + _____

Divided by _____ **(number of statements answered)** = _____ **Average score for this section.**
(Transfer to the Wellness Inventory Wheel on **p. 17.**)

---

[27] Attacking others rarely accomplishes your goals in the long run. Persisting in your convictions without using force is more effective and usually solves the problem without creating new ones.

[28] It is important to recognize that our internal judgments of others are based on personal biases that often have little objective basis.

[29] Psychological games, as defined by Eric Berne in *Games People Play*, are complex unconscious manipulations that result in the players getting negative attention and feeling bad about themselves.

[30] Including the choice to have no sexual activity.

[31] A common problem for many people is an overemphasis on performance and orgasm, rather than on enjoying a close sensual feeling with their partner whether or not they experience orgasm.

Section 11   WELLNESS AND FINDING MEANING

	Yes, usually	Sometimes, maybe	No, rarely
	2	1	0
1. I believe my life has direction and meaning.	_____	_____	_____
2. My life is exciting and challenging.	_____	_____	_____
3. I have goals in my life.	_____	_____	_____
4. I am achieving my goals.	_____	_____	_____
5. I look forward to the future as an opportunity for further growth.	_____	_____	_____
6. I am able to talk about the death of someone close to me.	_____	_____	_____
7. I am able to talk about my own death with family and friends.	_____	_____	_____
8. I am prepared for my death.	_____	_____	_____
9. I see my death as a step in my evolution.[32]	_____	_____	_____
10. My daily life is a source of pleasure to me.	_____	_____	_____

Total points for this section = ☐ _____ + _____ + _____

Divided by _____ **(number of statements answered)** = _____ **Average score for this section.**
(Transfer to the Wellness Inventory Wheel on **p. 17.**)

This portion of the Inventory goes beyond the scope of most generally accepted "scientific" principles and expresses the values and beliefs of the authors. It is intended to stimulate interest in these areas. If you have strong beliefs to the contrary, you can skip the questions or make up your own.

Section 12   WELLNESS AND TRANSCENDING

	Yes, usually	Sometimes, maybe	No, rarely
	2	1	0
1. I perceive problems as opportunities for growth.	_____	_____	_____
2. I experience synchronistic events in my life (frequent "coincidences" seeming to have no cause–effect relationship).[33]	_____	_____	_____
3. I believe there are dimensions of reality beyond verbal description or human comprehension.	_____	_____	_____
4. At times I experience confusion and paradox in my search for understanding of the dimensions referred to above.	_____	_____	_____
5. The concept of God has personal definition and meaning to me.	_____	_____	_____
6. I experience a sense of wonder when I contemplate the universe.	_____	_____	_____
7. I have abundant expectancy rather than specific expectations.	_____	_____	_____
8. I allow others their beliefs without pressuring them to accept mine.	_____	_____	_____
9. I use the messages interpreted from my dreams.	_____	_____	_____
10. I enjoy practicing a spiritual discipline or allowing time to sense the presence of a greater force in guiding my passage through life.	_____	_____	_____

Total points for this section = ☐ _____ + _____ + _____

Divided by _____ **(number of statements answered)** = _____ **Average score for this section.**
(Transfer to the Wellness Inventory Wheel on **p. 17.**)

[32] Seeing your death as a stage of growth and preparing yourself consciously is an important part of finding meaning in your life.

[33] Modern physics reveals that the idea of cause and effect may be as limited as Newton's theory of a mechanical universe. It suggests that we must expand our view to see that everything in the universe is connected to everything else. (Synchronicity describes that experience.)

YOUR ACTION PLAN FOR MAXIMUM WELLNESS

When you have completed the Wellness Inventory, study your wheel's shape and balance. How smoothly would it roll? What does it tell you? Are there any surprises in it? How does it feel to you? What don't you like about it? What do you like about it?

We recommend that you use colored pens to go back over the questions, noting the ones on which your scores were low and choosing some areas on which you are interested in working. It is easy to overwhelm yourself by taking on too many areas at once. Ignore, for now, those of lower priority to you. Remember, if you don't enjoy at least some aspects of the changes you are making, they probably won't last.

Here are some guidelines to help you:

▪ Read the following chapter on "Changing Your Life." It will provide you with detailed guidance on formulating and achieving goals.

▪ Get support from friends, but don't expect them to supply all the reinforcement you need. You may join a group of overweight individuals and rely on their encouragement to stick to your diet. That's a great way to get going, but in the long run your own commitment to losing weight has got to be strong enough to help you keep eating right and light.

▪ Focus on the immediate rewards of your new behavior. You may stop smoking so that you'll live longer, but take note of every other benefit it brings you—more stamina, less coughing, more spending money, no more stale tobacco taste in your mouth.

▪ Remind yourself of past successes you've had in making changes. Give yourself pep talks, commending yourself on how well you've done so far and how well you'll continue to do. This will boost your self-confidence.

▪ Reward yourself regularly. Plan a pleasant reward as an incentive for every week you stick to your new behavior—sleeping in on a Saturday morning, going out with some friends, or spending a sunny afternoon outdoors. Small, regular rewards are more effective in keeping up motivation than one big reward that won't come for many months.

▪ Expect and accept some relapses. The greatest rate of relapse occurs in the first few weeks after making a behavior change. During this critical time, get as much support as you can. In addition, work hard on self-motivation, reminding yourself daily of what you have to gain by sticking with your new health habit.

CASE IN POINT

Student: Jamie, 19

Goal: To achieve more balance among the dimensions of life represented in the Wellness Wheel

Action Plan:

▪ To enhance self-responsibility by recycling and riding a bike rather than driving to class.

▪ To enhance serenity by pausing during the day to become aware of breathing and tension.

▪ To enhance feeling by listening to an considering criticisms rather than reacting defensively.

▪ To enhance thinking by shelving problems that temporarily can not be solved and focusing on a task at hand.

▪ To enhance transcending by allowing time for a spiritual practice or quiet sitting every day.

Health Now™ To write goals for balancing your Wellness Wheel, go to the **Wellness Journal at HealthNow** at http://healthnow.brookscole.com.

- Find out if there are tests that could determine your risks. Discuss the advantages and disadvantages of such testing.

- Ask what steps you can take, such as weight loss, that might lower your vulnerability to a disease.

- Bring someone else with you for support and to help you remember what you learn.

Learn It / Live It

Maximum Health

Ultimately you have more control over your health than anyone else. Use this course as an opportunity to zero in on at least one less-than-healthful behavior and improve it. Here are some suggestions for small steps that can have a big payoff:

- **Use seat belts.** In the last decade, seat belts have saved more than 40,000 lives and prevented millions of injuries.

- **Eat an extra fruit or vegetable every day.** Adding more fruit and vegetables to your diet can improve your digestion and lower your risk of several cancers.

- **Get enough sleep.** A good night's rest provides the energy you need to make it through the following day.

- **Take regular stress breaks.** A few quiet minutes spent stretching, looking out the window, or simply letting yourself unwind are good for body and soul.

- **Lose a pound.** If you're overweight, you may not think a pound will make a difference, but it's a step in the right direction.

- **If you're a woman, examine your breasts regularly.** Get in the habit of performing a breast self-examination every month after your period (when breasts are least swollen or tender).

- **If you're a man, examine your testicles regularly.** These simple self-exams can spot the early signs of cancer when they're most likely to be cured.

- **Get physical.** Just a little exercise will do some good. A regular workout schedule will be good for your heart, lungs, muscles, bones—even your mood.

- **Drink more water.** Eight glasses a day are what you need to replenish lost fluids, prevent constipation, and keep your digestive system working efficiently.

- **Do a good deed.** Caring for others is a wonderful way to care for your own soul and connect with others.

Making This Chapter Work for You

Review Questions

1. Wellness is defined as
  a. purposeful, enjoyable living, characterized by personal responsibility and enhancement of physical, mental, and spiritual health.
  b. a state of complete physical, mental, and social well-being.
  c. attitudes and beliefs that contribute to a healthy state of mind.
  d. the absence of physical or mental illness.

2. Which of the following statements about the dimensions of health are true?
  a. Spirituality provides solace and comfort for those who are severely ill, but it has no health benefits.
  b. The people who reflect the highest levels of social health are usually among the most popular individuals in a group and are often thought of as the life of the party.
  c. Intellectual health refers to one's academic abilities.
  d. Optimal physical health requires a nutritious diet, regular exercise, avoidance of harmful behaviors and substances, and self-protection from accidents.

3. The most important dimension of wellness is
  a. physical wellness
  b. spiritual wellness
  c. psychological wellness
  d. trick question—All of the dimensions of wellness are vital to leading a balanced and satisfying life.

4. The goals of the *Healthy People 2010* initiative include all of the following *except*
  a. Reduce the proportion of obese adults and children in the population.
  b. Decrease the number of teens using illegal substances.
  c. Increase the number of adults engaging in daily vigorous physical activity for 30 minutes per occasion.
  d. Reduce the percentage of teens and adults who report smoking cigarettes in the past month.

5. The majority of college students are in the physical prime of their lives. To stay well, you should avoid
  a. binge drinking.
  b. unprotected sex.
  c. smoking.
  d. all of the above.

6. Which statement about today's college students is not true?
  a. Most students are at a healthy weight.
  b. More than 20 percent of students eat five or more servings of fruits and vegetables every day.

c. More than 60 percent of students have never smoked.

d. More than 70 percent of students always wear their seatbelts when riding in a car.

7. Which of these actions should you take to "personalize" your health care?
   a. Write down your family medical history.
   b. Learn more about gene therapy.
   c. Get a mammogram even if you are male.
   d. Be tested for diabetes.

8. A group of students is discussing the differences between the sexes. Whose statement is incorrect?
   a. Matt: "Men breathe faster but have a slower heart rate—and have a larger brain."
   b. Elena: "But women have more neurons in certain brain regions."
   a. Kristin: "And women are less likely to get arthritis."
   d. Rick: "Got me there—Men *are* more likely to have heart attacks and to get cancer."

9. Health risks faced by different ethnic and racial groups include all of the following *except*
   a. Whites have higher rates of hypertension, lupus, liver disease, and kidney failure than African Americans.
   b. Native Americans have a higher rate of diabetes than other racial and ethnic groups.
   c. Infant mortality is higher for African-American babies than for white babies.
   d. Latinos living in the United States have high rates of eye disease.

10. Which of these factors is not responsible for some of the racial and ethnic differences in susceptibility to disease?
    a. genetics
    b. unhealthy lifestyles
    c. Medicare
    d. poverty

Answers to these questions can be found on page 587.

Critical Thinking

1. What is the definition of health according to the text? Does your personal definition differ from this? If so, in what ways? How would you have defined health before reading this chapter?

2. Talk to classmates from different racial or ethnic backgrounds than yours about their culture's health attitudes. Ask them what is considered healthy behavior in their culture. For example, is having a good appetite a sign of health? What kinds of self-care practices did their parents and grandparents use to treat colds, fevers, rashes, and other health problems? What are their attitudes about the health-care system?

3. Where are you on the wellness–illness continuum? What variables might affect your place on the scale? What do you consider your optimum state of health to be?

4. In what ways would you like to change your present lifestyle? What steps could you take to make those changes?

Media Menu

Health Now™

Throughout the chapter, this icon introduces a list of resources on the HealthNow website at http://healthnow.brookscole.com/ith that will:
- Help you evaluate your knowledge of the material.
- Allow you to take an exam-prep quiz.
- Provide a Personalized Learning Plan targeting resources that address areas you should study.
- Coach you through identifying target goals for behavior change and creating and monitoring your personal change plan throughout the semester.

INTERNET CONNECTIONS

Go Ask Alice
www.goaskalice.columbia.edu/index.html
Sponsored by Columbia University, this site offers questions and answers as well as an interactive service on a wide variety of health-related topics.

Lifescan Health Risk Appraisal
http://wellness.uwsp.edu/other/lifescan/lifescan.htm
This site, created by Bill Hettler, M.D., of the National Wellness Institute, helps you identify specific lifestyle factors that can impair your health and longevity. Take the health questionnaire to determine your personal lifestyle risks. Your results provide a score for general results, nutrition results, and height/weight results. Your ranking among the top ten causes of death is provided, as well as suggestions on how to improve.

Healthy People 2010
www.healthypeople.gov
Healthy People 2010 is a statement of national health objectives developed by the Office of Disease Prevention and Health Promotion, U.S. Department of Health and Human Services. This collection of national health objectives is designed to identify the most significant preventable causes of acute and chronic illnesses and accidents and to establish national goals to reduce these threats to health. The goals are aimed at improving the health of all Americans by the year 2010.

InfoTrac College Edition Activity Log on, insert ***Healthy People 2010*** into the Keyword search box, and limit your search to the past year. When you get the results, Mark articles to review, then Select one to read. Summarize three or four key points from the article.

You can find additional readings related to personal

health with InfoTrac College Edition, an online library of more than 900 journals and publications. Follow the instructions for accessing InfoTrac College Edition that were packaged with your textbook; then search for articles using a keyword search.

For additional links, resources, and suggested readings on InfoTrac College Edition, visit our Health and Wellness Resource Center at **http://health .wadsworth.com.**

Key Terms

The terms listed are used on the page indicated. Definitions of the terms are in the Glossary at the end of this book.

health 4
health promotion 6
prevention 10
protection 10
wellness 4

2 Changing for Life

Jessica describes herself as an average college student in almost every way: grades, looks, athletic ability—and health. Yes, she could make better food choices. Yes, she should exercise more consistently. Yes, she gets stressed out and doesn't get enough sleep. Occasionally she drinks too much. She smokes with friends who light up. She knows that heart disease "runs" in her family, but she doesn't understand exactly what that means. Ask Jessica if she'd like to be better than average, and she'll say yes. But she doesn't know where to begin.

Do you want to be and feel and do as well as possible, to live and work at your maximum potential? This chapter can help you begin. Whatever physical shape and psychological state you're in, you can improve your fitness and health. But doing so requires more than reading this book or taking this course. You have to commit yourself to change.

Personal change always begins in the same place: the brain. As decades of research have shown, your thoughts determine how you feel and how you behave. Your thoughts determine every choice that you make. The discovery that thoughts create feelings and drive behavior—one of the most important psychological breakthroughs of the last 50 years—is the foundation of all cognitive and behavioral therapy approaches. These methods emphasize setting goals (defining what you intend to accomplish) and changing the way you think about or interpret a situation.

This chapter is a primer in behavioral change. It describes the factors that influence health behavior and the stages of readiness for change. As you read it, you can immediately apply the information and insights to your own health behaviors. As you do, you will develop goals and begin moving toward them—and lifting your life well above average.

FAQ Frequently Asked Questions

▪ What are the stages of change? *p. 31*
▪ What is an affirmation? *p. 35*
▪ How can I change a bad health habit? *p. 37*

After studying the material in this chapter, you should be able to:

▪ **Define** the three factors that shape health behaviors.

▪ **Name** the three key components of the transtheoretical model of change.

▪ **Describe** the stages of change and give an example of each.

▪ **Name** at least two mental attitudes that can help you successfully make a change.

MAKING HEALTHY CHANGES

Nothing is certain in life except change. Every day ushers in changes large and small, but the changes that matter most are those we make ourselves. In recent decades behavioral scientists have dissected the process of how people change, mapping the stages of change and identifying the components of successful change. The following sections describe some of the steps that can help you make changes for the better.

UNDERSTANDING HEALTH BEHAVIOR

Your choices and behaviors affect how long and how well you live. Nearly half of all deaths in the United States are linked to behaviors such as tobacco use, improper diet, abuse of alcohol and other drugs, use of firearms, motor vehicle accidents, risky sexual practices, and lack of exercise.

If you would like to improve your health behavior, you have to realize that change isn't easy. Between 40 and 80 percent of those who try to kick bad health habits lapse back into their unhealthy ways within six weeks. To make lasting beneficial changes, you have to understand the three types of influences that shape behavior: predisposing, enabling, and reinforcing factors (Figure 2-1).

Predisposing Factors

Predisposing factors include knowledge, attitudes, beliefs, values, and perceptions. Unfortunately, knowledge isn't enough to cause most people to change their behavior; for example, people fully aware of the grim consequences of smoking often continue to puff away. Nor is attitude—one's likes and dislikes—sufficient; an individual may dislike the smell and taste of cigarettes but continue to smoke regardless.

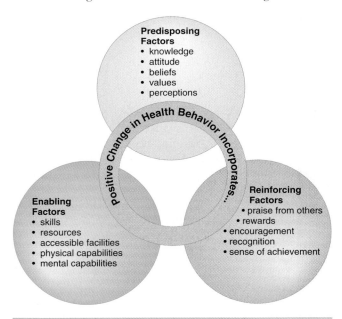

FIGURE 2-1   **Factors that Shape Positive Behavior**

Beliefs are more powerful than knowledge and attitudes, and researchers report that people are most likely to change health behavior if they hold three beliefs:

▪ **Susceptibility.** They acknowledge that they are at risk for the negative consequences of their behavior.

▪ **Severity.** They believe that they may pay a very high price if they don't make a change.

▪ **Benefits.** They believe that the proposed change will be advantageous to their health.

There can be a gap between stated and actual beliefs, however. Young adults may say they recognize the very real dangers of casual, careless sex in this day and age. Yet, rather than act in accordance with these statements, they may impulsively engage in unprotected sex with individuals whose health status and histories they do not know. The reason: Like young people everywhere and in every time, they feel invulnerable, that nothing bad can or will happen to them, that if there were a real danger, they would somehow know it. Often it's not until something happens—a former lover may admit to having a sexually transmitted infection—that their behaviors become consistent with their stated beliefs.

 Young people, especially young men, are the greatest risk takers, a fact reflected in their high rates of auto accidents, binge drinking, drug use, and pathological gambling. The death rates for injuries related to swimming, boating, driving, cycling, and even crossing the street are higher in college-age men than women.

The value or importance we give to health also plays a major role in changing behavior. Many people aren't concerned about their health just for the sake of being healthy. Usually, they want to look or feel better, be more productive or competitive, or behave more independently. They're more likely to change, and to stick with a change, if they can see that the health benefits also enhance other important aspects of their lives.

Perceptions are the way we see things from our unique perspective; they vary greatly with age. As a student, you may not think that living a few hours longer is a significant gain; as you grow older, however, you may prize every additional second.

Enabling Factors

Enabling factors include skills, resources, accessible facilities, and physical and mental capacities. Before you initiate a change, assess the means available to reach your goal. No matter how motivated you are, you'll become frustrated if you keep encountering obstacles. That's why breaking a task or goal down into step-by-step strategies is so important in behavioral change.

Reinforcing Factors

Reinforcing factors may be praise from family and friends, rewards from teachers or parents, or encouragement and recognition for meeting a goal. Although these help a great deal in the short run, lasting change depends not on external rewards but on an internal commitment and sense of

Your *stated* knowledge-based belief may be that unsafe driving can cause accidents, but your *actual* belief is that it won't happen to you. To learn how to change this predisposing factor that influences your behavior, read on.

achievement. To make a difference, reinforcement must come from within.

A decision to change a health behavior should stem from a permanent, personal goal, not from a desire to please or impress someone else. If you lose weight for the homecoming dance, you're almost sure to regain pounds afterward. But if you shed extra pounds because you want to feel better about yourself or get into shape, you're far more likely to keep off the weight.

THE TRANSTHEORETICAL MODEL OF CHANGE

This theoretical model of behavioral change, developed by psychologist James Prochaska and his colleagues, focuses on the individual's decision making rather than on social or biological influences on behavior.[1] It is the foundation of programs for smoking cessation, exercise, healthy food choices,[2] alcohol abuse, weight control, condom use, drug abuse,[3] mammography screening, and stress management. However, conclusive scientific evidence for its usefulness in lifestyle change remains limited.[4]

These key components of the **transtheoretical model of change** are described in the following sections:

▪ **Stages of Change**
▪ **Processes of Change**—cognitive and behavioral activities that facilitate change
▪ **Self-efficacy**—the confidence people have in their ability to cope with challenge

(FAQ) WHAT ARE THE STAGES OF CHANGE?

According to the transtheoretical model of change, individuals progress through a sequence of stages as they make a change (Figure 2-2). No one stage is more important than another, and people often move back and forth between them. Most "spiral" from stage to stage, slipping from maintenance to contemplation or from action to precontemplation before moving forward again.

People usually cycle and recycle through the stages several times. Smokers, for instance, report making three or four serious efforts to quit before they succeed.

The six stages of change are:

1. **Precontemplation.** Whether or not they're aware of a problem behavior, people in this stage have no intention of making a change in the next six months. Busy college students in good health, for instance, might never think about getting more exercise.

2. **Contemplation.** Individuals in this stage are aware they have a problem behavior and are considering changing it within the next six months. However, they may be torn between the positives of the new behavior and the amount of energy, time, and other resources required to change.[5] Students in a health course, for instance, may start thinking about exercising but struggle to balance potential benefits with the effort of getting up early to jog or go to the gym.

3. **Preparation.** People in this stage intend to change a problem behavior within the next month. Some focus on a master plan. For instance, they might look into fitness classes, gyms, or other options for working out. Others might start by making small changes, such as walking to classes rather than taking a campus shuttle bus.

4. **Action.** People in this stage are modifying their behavior according to their plan. For instance, they might be jogging or working out at the gym three times a week.

5. **Maintenance.** In this stage, individuals have continued to work at changing their behavior and have avoided relapse for at least six months. New exercisers are likely to stop during the first three to six months. One reason that researchers have identified: the temptation to not exercise. However, follow-up, whether by mail, e-mail, or phone calls from supportive friends, family, or a counselor, can help maintain physical activity levels.[6]

6. **Termination.** While it may take two to five years, a behavior becomes so deeply ingrained that a person can't imagine abandoning it. More than eight in ten college seniors who exercised regularly remain as active, or even more active, after graduation.

 As research on college students has shown, attitudes and feelings are related to stages of change. Smokers

FIGURE 2-2   The Stages of Change and Some Change Processes
These change processes can help you progress through the stages of change. Each may be most useful at particular stages.

who believe that continuing to smoke would have only a minor or no impact on their health remain in the precontemplation stage; those with respiratory symptoms move on to contemplation and preparation.[7] In a study at Ohio State University, researchers classified student heavy drinkers according to the stages of change: Nearly two-thirds of the "precontemplators" continued to drink heavily and had no intention of changing their behavior. In the maintenance stage, students drank an average of one alcoholic drink a month even though they felt that heavy drinking was the norm on their campus.[8]

THE PROCESSES OF CHANGE

Anything you do to modify your thinking, feeling, or behavior can be called a change process. The nine included in the transtheoretical model are:

Consciousness-raising The most widely used change process involves increasing knowledge about yourself or the nature of your problem. As you learn more, you gain understanding and feedback about your behavior.

Example: Reading Chapter 6 on making healthy food choices.

Social liberation This process takes advantage of alternatives in the external environment that can help you begin or continue your efforts to change.

Example: Spending as much time as possible in non-smoking areas.

Emotional arousal This process, also known as dramatic relief, works on a deeper level than consciousness-raising and is equally important in the early stages of change. Emotional arousal means experiencing and expressing feelings about a problem behavior and its potential solutions.

Example: Resolving never to drink and drive after the death of a friend in a car accident.

Self-reevaluation This process requires a thoughtful reappraisal of your problem, including an assessment of the person you might be once you have changed the behavior.

Example: Recognizing that you have a gambling problem and imagining yourself as a nongambler.

Commitment This process acknowledges—first privately and then publicly—that you are responsible for your behavior and the only one who can change it.

Example: Joining a self-help or support group.

Countering Countering, or counterconditioning, substitutes healthy behaviors for unhealthy ones.

Example: Chewing gum rather than smoking.

Environmental control This action-oriented process restructures your environment so you are less likely to engage in a problem behavior.

Example: Getting rid of your stash of sweets.

Rewards This process reinforces positive behavioral changes with self-praise or small gifts.

Example: Getting a massage after a month of consistent exercise.

Helping relationships This process recruits individuals—family, friends, therapist, coach—to provide support, caring, understanding, and acceptance.

Example: Finding an exercise buddy.

SELF-EFFICACY AND LOCUS OF CONTROL

Do you see yourself as master of your fate, asserting control over your destiny? Or do so many things happen in your life that you just hang on and hope for the best? The answers to

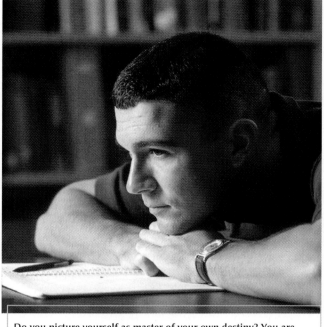

Do you picture yourself as master of your own destiny? You are more likely to achieve your health goals if you do.

these questions reveal two important characteristics that affect your health: your sense of **self-efficacy** (the belief in your ability to change and to reach a goal) and your **locus of control** (the sense of being in control of your life).

Your confidence in your ability to cope with challenge can determine whether you can and will succeed in making a change. In his research on self-efficacy psychologist Albert Bandura of Stanford University found that the individuals most likely to reach a goal are those who believe that they can. The stronger their faith in themselves, the more energy and persistence they put into making a change. The opposite is also true, especially for health behaviors. Among people who begin an exercise program, those with lower self-efficacy are more likely to drop out.

If you believe that your actions will make a difference in your health, your locus of control is internal. If you believe that external forces or factors play a greater role, your locus of control is external. Hundreds of studies have compared people who have these different perceptions of control. "Internals," who believe that their actions largely determine what happens to them, act more independently, enjoy better health, and are more optimistic about their future. "Externals," who perceive that chance or outside forces determine their fate, find it harder to cope with stress and feel increasingly helpless over time. When it comes to weight, for instance, they see themselves as destined to be fat.

HOW YOU CHANGE

Awareness of a negative behavior is always the first step toward changing it. Once you identify what you'd like to change, keep a diary for one or two weeks, noting what you do, when, where, and what you're feeling at the time. If you'd like, enlist the help of friends or family to call attention to your behavior. Sometimes self-observation in itself proves therapeutic: Just the act of keeping a diary can be enough to help you lose weight or kick the smoking habit.

Decisional Balance

In making a change, you have to weigh its potential pluses and minuses. Decisional balance involves consideration of the consequences of change to yourself and others and the reactions of both yourself and others as a result of change. These can be both positive and negative.

For instance, if your target health behavior goal is to stop smoking, you will definitely benefit in many ways, such as breathing more easily and lowering your risk of heart disease and cancer. But you may gain a few pounds or miss the camaraderie of hanging out with fellow smokers. You are more likely to make—and maintain—a health change if you see the pros of the change outweighing the cons. (Take the Self Survey on page 40 to determine your readiness to change a health behavior.)

Self-Management

Once you've identified the situations, moods, thoughts, or people that act as cues for a behavior, identify the most powerful ones and develop a plan to avoid them. For instance, if you snack continuously when studying in your room, try working in the library, where food is forbidden.

Planning ahead is a crucial part of successful change. If you can't avoid certain situations, anticipate how you might cope with the temptation to return to your old behavior. Develop alternatives. Visualize yourself walking past the desserts in the cafeteria or chewing gum instead of lighting a cigarette.

Some people find it helpful to sign a "contract," a written agreement in which they make a commitment to change, with their partner, parent, or health educator. Spelling out what they intend to do, and why, underscores the seriousness of what they're trying to accomplish (see the example on page 42).

Norms

Social and cultural **norms**—behaviors that are expected, accepted, or supported by a group—can work against a person's best intentions. You may resolve to eat less, for instance, yet your mother may keep offering you home-made fudge and brownies because your family's norm is to show love by making and offering delicious treats. Or you might decide to drink less, yet your friends' norm may be to equate drinking with having a good time.

If you're aware of the norms that influence your behavior, you can devise strategies either to change them (by encouraging your friends to dance more and drink less at parties, for example) or adapt to them (having just a bite of your mother's sweets). Another option is to develop relationships with people who share your goals and whose norms can reinforce your behavior.

Strategies for Change ▪ Use the Language of Change

Pay attention both to what you say when you talk or think about a health behavior change and how you say it. Then consciously edit the words in your mind and as you say them.

▪ **Watch out for weasel words.** Are you "planning" to quit smoking? "Hoping" to lose weight? When you use linguistic loopholes like "trying" or "hoping," you give yourself permission to settle for whatever happens. When you speak of goals, use definitive, unequivocal language.

▪ **Trade tenses.** When thinking or talking about bad health habits, switch to the past tense. Instead of saying, "I'm too lazy to exercise," tell yourself, "I used to be too lazy to exercise." This reminds you that you have changed, are changing, or at the least are capable of change.

▪ **Not "if" but "when."** Instead of saying, "If I could exercise more," say to yourself, "When I start exercising more." This simple switch sets the stage for believing that you will be able to change your lifestyle.

▪ **Just "because."** According to social psychology research, using the word "because" when making a request or seeking agreement can boost your compliance as high as 80 to 90 percent. For instance, you might tell yourself: "I won't buy doughnuts *because* I don't want to be tempted."

▪ **Guard against demeaning words and phrases.** When a derogatory statement about yourself forms in your brain, say firmly, "Stop!" or "Delete!"

▪ **Don't focus on what you can't do.** Remind yourself of your strengths every day. Say to yourself, "I can go another five minutes on the treadmill" or "I can stand another half hour without a cigarette."

Self-Talk

Your **self-talk**—the messages you send yourself—also can play a role. In recent decades, mental health professionals have recognized the conscious use of positive self-talk as a powerful force for changing the way individuals think, feel, and behave. "We have a choice about how we think," explains psychologist Martin Seligman, Ph.D., author of *Learned Optimism.* As he notes, by learning to challenge automatic negative thoughts that enter our brains and asserting our own statements of self-worth, we can transform ourselves into optimists who see what's right rather than pessimists forever focusing on what's wrong.[9]

Incentives

Get support from friends, but don't expect them to supply all the motivation you need. You may join a group of overweight individuals and rely on their encouragement to stick to your diet. That's a great way to get going; but in the long run, your own commitment to making a change has got to be strong enough to help you sustain your new behaviors.

Reinforcements—either positive (a reward) or negative (a punishment)—also can play a role. Plan a pleasant reward as an incentive for every week you stick to your new behavior—sleeping in on a Saturday morning, going out with some friends, or spending a sunny afternoon outdoors. Small, regular rewards are more effective in keeping up motivation than one big reward that won't come for many months.

> *Some businesses are offering cash bonuses or rewards such as a weekend at a resort for employees who lose weight or stop smoking. Can such "incentives" lead to permanent behavior change, or are they bribes that will work only in the short term?* **You decide.**

Your Life Coach

Going for Your Goals

Think of goals as road maps that give you both a destination and a planned itinerary for getting there. "To set goals means to set a course for your life," says psychologist James Fadiman, author of *Unlimit Your Life: Setting and Getting Goals.* "Without goals, you remain what you were. With goals, you become what you wish."[10] As studies of performance in students, athletes, and employees have shown, the one single characteristic that separates high- and low-achievers is having a clear, specific goal.[11] (See Student Snapshot: "The Top Goals of Undergraduates.") The following sections describe the most effective strategies for using goals to map your way to the life you want.

SET YOUR SIGHTS ON A DESTINATION OR TARGET

You wouldn't board a bus without knowing where you want to go, but it's easy to drift through life with only a vague sense of where you're heading. Unfortunately, goals that don't lead somewhere—like wanting to be healthy—tend to go nowhere. A specific, focused, realistic goal—like developing your upper body strength or reaching a certain weight—can fast-forward you into the future.

The more vividly that you can see, feel, touch, and taste what you want, the more likely you are to achieve it. The reason, explains psychologist Kenneth W. Christian, author of *Your Own Worst Enemy,* is that a destination goal transforms your brain into a satellite dish picking up the signals that are most relevant to your quest. "You begin to see possibilities that pull you closer to your goal. You meet people who can help you. It can seem magical,

Strategies for Change :: Is Your Goal S.M.A.R.T.?

Many professional coaches use the following questions to help clients set effective goals:

:: **Specific?** Identifying exactly what you want to accomplish helps you plan the steps that lead to your goal.

:: **Measurable?** Your goal should be concrete enough so that both you and others can see the progress you're making.

:: **Attainable?** Set goals that are slightly out of your immediate grasp but not so far that there is no hope of achieving them.

:: **Realistic?** Maybe you dream of being an Olympian, but a realistic goal might be to try out for the rowing team.

:: **Targeted?** A clear objective, such as quitting smoking, encourages laserlike focus.

---

but it's not. Your unconscious mind is working on your goal while you go on with your life."[12]

TAKE A STEP AND A STRETCH

With your target goal in sight, set "step-and-stretch" goals. Think of them like stair steps that lift you out of your comfort zone and keep you moving forward. It doesn't matter how many there are. In some instances, it may be six; in others, sixty. Every goal should be a reach from where you are that will bring you to the next level.

Break down each step goal into projects, and every project into tasks. Ask yourself the following questions, and write down the answers.

- What skills do I need to achieve this?
- What information and knowledge must I acquire?
- What help, assistance, or resources do I need?
- What can block my progress? (For each potential barrier, list solutions.)
- Whom can I turn to for support?
- Who or what is likely to get in my way?
- How am I most likely to sabotage myself?

As you develop your game plan, make sure each goal is within your control. "Other people should not have to change in order for you to meet your goal," emphasizes Fadiman. Don't depend on your roommate to jump on your get-organized bandwagon, or your friends to sizzle with the same enthusiasm for shaping up for a marathon. Focus on the process not the outcome.

(FAQ) WHAT IS AN AFFIRMATION?

Once you've pictured your goal in detail, express it in an **affirmation,** a single positive sentence. As decades of psychological research have shown, affirmations serve as powerful tools for behavioral change. One key to their success is the present tense. "In your mind's inner grammar, the present tense predicts the future while the words 'I will' delays it," says Fadiman, "The impact is subtle but critical when you're setting goals."

In Fadiman's work with smokers, those who repeated the phrase "I am not a smoker" daily—even though they were allowed to continue smoking—typically threw away their cigarettes within a few weeks. "If you are not a smoker, you don't need or want cigarettes," he explains. "If you hold any statement in your conscious mind, there is an effort to bring it into reality. That's why when you change your thoughts and attitudes, your behavior follows." You don't need to tag a deadline onto a destination goal. "If you tell yourself you're going to lose weight by the end of the year, that's how long it will take," says Fadiman. "Why wait?"

Once you've polished your affirmation, put it on paper. By putting it in writing, you become more committed to making your words come true. Some people post their affirmations on their computers and night stands or carry them in their wallets; others scrawl them in big letters across the bathroom mirror. Wherever you jot yours, look at your affirmation often—ideally at least once a day.

VISUALIZE THE HURDLES

During training, many athletes visualize crossing the finish line or scoring the winning point. Gold medal Olympian Edwin Moses used a different technique: He visualized every hurdle in a 400-meter race, calculating the distance between each, and seeing himself clearing each one. Goal-getters do the same. If you think ahead to what might go wrong, you can come up with ways of going over, under, around, or through whatever obstacles you encounter. If you don't anticipate and problem-solve, obstacles turn into excuses.

Remember that you don't have to go it alone. A buddy or accountability partner can help—by checking in every week, joining you if you're going to the gym, or reminding you of why you set your goal in the first place.

GO ALL THE WAY

Despite good intentions and considerable progress, many people give up their goals just before the rainbow's end—and congratulate themselves for getting that far. "Would you ever board a plane for Chicago and say, 'Well, we got three-quarters of the way there!' as if that were good?" asks psychologist Christian, who urges goal-seekers to persist, persevere, and "not settle for almost-there." If you stall on the final stretch, do a quick reality

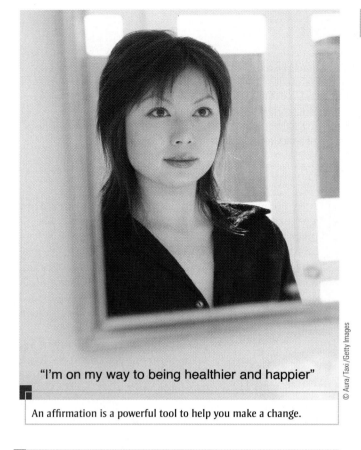

"I'm on my way to being healthier and happier"

An affirmation is a powerful tool to help you make a change.

Student Snapshot

THE TOP GOALS OF UNDERGRADUATES

The percentage of students who say this is a goal

Goal	
Raising a family	75%
Being very well off financially	74%
Helping others who are in difficulty	62%
Becoming an authority in my field	58%
Obtaining recognition from my colleagues for my contributions to my field	52%

Based on a national survey of 289,452 students at 440 colleges and universities. *Source:* Sax, Linda, et al. *The American Freshman: National Norms for Fall 2004.* Los Angeles: UCLA Higher Education Research Institute, 2004.

check. Maybe you need to add some smaller-step goals, seek more support, or simply allow yourself more time.

Set aside a page or section in your Wellness Journal to amend, modify, refine, expand, and extend your goals. Whenever you achieve one, check it off, acknowledge it, tell a friend, or just raise your hands above your head like a runner crossing the finish line. This is what builds your sense of, "I can do it. I AM doing it. Look how far I've come!"

RISKY BEHAVIORS ON CAMPUS

Risky behaviors are not new or unusual on campus, but today's students face different—and often deadlier—risks than undergraduates did a generation ago. Now as then, many students are sexually active, but these days there are more and more serious sexually transmitted infections (STIs) on campus. Despite awareness of these dangers, almost three in four students report that they have engaged in unprotected sex. Of those who have had unprotected sex, about two-thirds said they didn't believe they were at risk of STIs.

Although smoking has declined nationwide, according to the National Household Survey on Drug Abuse, college-age young adults have the highest percentage of smokers. The more and the longer they smoke, the more these young men and women boost their risks of heart disease, respiratory problems, several types of cancer, and a shortened lifespan.

Drinking also has long been part of college life, and despite the efforts across U.S. college campuses to curb alcohol abuse, two out of five students engage in binge drinking—consumption of five or more drinks at a single session for men, four for women. Heavy drinking increases the likelihood of other risky behaviors, such as smoking cigarettes, using drugs, or having multiple sexual partners.

In a survey of substance use on college campuses, about half of undergraduates reported that they had smoked marijuana; approximately one-fifth reported using pot within the previous month.[13] In general, drug use has remained steady in recent years with one exception—a doubling of ecstasy use on campus, although the percentage of students who use ecstasy is small.[14]

Some behaviors are riskier than students realize. "Body art"—piercings and tattoos—may seem harmless, but health officials warn of hidden risks, including Hepatitis B and C infection and transmission of HIV (see Chapter 14). In a survey of undergraduates at a university in New York, almost one in five students who had had a body part pierced reported medical complications.[15]

 College-age men are more likely than women to engage in risk-taking behaviors—to use drugs and alcohol; to engage in risky sexual behaviors, such as having sex while under the influence of alcohol; and to drive dangerously. Men also are more likely to be hospitalized for injuries and to commit suicide. Three-fourths of the deaths in the 15- to 24-year age range are men.

UNHEALTHY HABITS ON CAMPUS

Often on their own for the first time, college students leave behind their family's ways of eating, sleeping, and relaxing and develop new habits and routines—usually not healthier ones. Many simply don't get enough sleep or keep irregular schedules that throw their sleep patterns off. Often it seems that there aren't enough hours in the day for all the things undergraduates need or want to do—study, socialize, pursue extracurricular activities, surf the Internet,

Savvy Consumer :: Assessing Risks

At any age, the greatest health threats stem from high-risk behaviors—smoking, excessive drinking, not getting enough exercise, eating too many high-fat foods, driving recklessly, and not getting regular medical checkups, to name just a few. That's why changing unhealthy habits is the best way to reduce risks and prevent health problems.

Environmental health risks are the subject of newspaper headlines. Every year brings calls of alarm about a new hazard to health: electromagnetic radiation, fluoride in drinking water, hair dyes, silicone implants, radon, lead. Often the public response is panic. Consumers picket and protest. Individuals arrange for elaborate testing. Yet how do we know whether or not alleged health risks are acceptable? Some key factors to consider are:

- **Are there possible benefits?** Advantages—such as the high salary paid for working with toxic chemicals or radioactive materials—may make some risks seem worth taking.

- **Is the risk voluntary?** All of us tend to accept risks that we freely choose to take, such as playing a sport that could lead to injuries, as opposed to risks imposed on us, such as threats of terrorism.

- **Is the risk fair?** The risk of skin cancer affects us all. We may worry about it and take action to protect ourselves and our planet, but we don't resent it the way we resent living with the risk of violence because the only housing we can afford is in a high-crime area.

- **Are there alternatives?** As consumers, we may become upset about cancer-causing pesticides or food additives when we learn about safer chemicals or methods of preservation.

- **Are lives saved or lost?** Our thinking about risks often depends on how they're presented. For instance, if we're told that a new drug may kill 1 out of every 100 people, we react differently than if we're told that it may save the lives of 99 percent of those who use it.

work at part-time jobs, participate in community service. Sleeping less, juggling more, students can quickly end up exhausted—and at greater risk for colds, flus, digestive problems, and other maladies.

Poor sleep can be both a symptom and a cause of stress, which is especially common among freshmen. More undergraduates are seeking psychological counseling to deal with the strain they feel as well as mental disorders such as anxiety and depression.

Students who endure harassment or abuse of any sort are more likely to report health-related symptoms. Those most at risk include minority students as well as gay, lesbian, and bisexual undergraduates.

Nutrition habits also change during college. As discussed in Chapter 6, the majority of freshmen say their diet has changed for the worse. During their first year, students often gain a few pounds (although less than the notorious "freshman 15").

Students also become more sedentary in college, as they log more hours in classes and in front of computers. The combination of a high-fat diet and a sedentary lifestyle in college can set the stage for the development of health problems that include obesity, diabetes, metabolic syndrome, heart disease, and certain cancers.

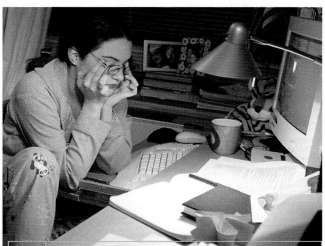

Unhealthy habits often become routine for college students—and may make them more susceptible to health problems both in the short and long term.

© Dex Images/CORBIS

FAQ HOW CAN I CHANGE A BAD HEALTH HABIT?

Change is never easy—even if it's done for the best possible reasons. When you decide to change a behavior, you have to give up something familiar and easy for something new and challenging. Change always involves risk—and the prospect of rewards.

Researchers have identified approaches other than the transtheoretical model that people use to make beneficial changes. In the moral model, you take responsibility for a problem (such as smoking) and its solution; success depends on adequate motivation, while failure is seen as a sign of character weakness. In the enlightenment model, you submit to strict discipline to correct a problem; this is the approach used in Alcoholics Anonymous. The behavioral model involves rewarding yourself when you make positive changes. The medical model sees the behavior as caused by forces beyond your control (a genetic predisposition to being overweight, for example) and employs an expert to provide advice or treatment. For many people, the most effective approach is the compensatory model, which doesn't assign blame but puts responsibility on individuals to acquire whatever skills or power they need to overcome their problems.

Before they reach the stage where they can and do take

TABLE 2-1 STAGES OF LIFESTYLE CHANGE

Stage of Change	Appropriate Change Goal
1. **Precontemplation:** You are not truly convinced about the importance of the lifestyle goal.	Get more information about the value of the lifestyle change goal.
2. **Contemplation:** You have no definite plan for when to begin but would like to change.	Set a date for making the change.
3. **Preparation:** You have set a date to begin the new behavior and are planning the best strategy to carry out the change.	Develop a plan and tell others about the change.
4. **Action:** You are engaged in making changes.	Adjust to new lifestyle and manage unexpected emotional and physical reactions.
5. **Maintenance:** You are working to integrate the lifestyle change into normal day-to-day life.	Continue to pay attention to the behavior and work through any relapse. Help others achieve similar lifestyle goals.
6. **Termination/Moving On:** You have maintained the change for six months to a year and are ready to move on to other lifestyle interests.	Set new health-enhancing goals. Move on from support systems that are focused exclusively on the prior lifestyle goal.

Source: Human Resources Institute, www.healthyculture.com/Articles/mentorarticle.html, reprinted with permission.

action to change, most people go through a process comparable to religious conversion. First, they reach a level of accumulated unhappiness that makes them ready for change. Then they have a moment of truth that makes them want to change. One pregnant woman, for instance, felt her unborn baby quiver when she drank a beer and swore never to drink again. As people change their behavior, they change their lifestyles and identities as well. Ex-smokers, for instance, may start an aggressive exercise program, make new friends at the track or gym, and participate in new types of activities, like racquetball games or fun runs.

Think about the behavior you want to change. Now think about which of the six stages of change you are in with regard to that behavior. Table 2-1 lists some appropriate change goals for each stage. Set your goal and go for it!

RECOVERING FROM A RELAPSE

Once you are ready to change, getting started with an action plan is not the greatest challenge you'll face. That usually comes weeks or months later, when your progress hits a wall or you return to your old, unhealthy habits. Rather than looking for someone or something to help you get back on track, try the following:

- **Gather data.** Keep a detailed log of your behavior for a week, including a weekend. If you're trying to make healthier food choices, record everything you put in your mouth. If your goal is to get into better shape, keep track of how much time you spend on sedentary pursuits, what derails your plans to exercise, the types of activities you most enjoy, and so forth.

- **Reassess your goals.** Are your expectations too high? Is your timetable unrealistic? Have you been derailed by finals, stress, the flu, a family crisis?

- **Check with your doctor.** Various medical conditions, such as infections, depression, diabetes, and medications (including corticosteroids and hormones) can undermine your energy and ability to pursue your wellness goals.

- **Problem-solve your way around the wall.** Ask yourself the following questions, and write down your answers.

  1. What is your biggest challenge right now? Make it specific: For example, I stick to my diet during the week but blow it on weekends. Or I smoke when I play poker with my friends.

  2. List every way you can think of to solve this problem. The more solutions you list, the greater your chance of finding the one that will work best for you. For instance, to avoid weekend overeating, you might volunteer at a hospice or library. Or you might change your poker site to a nonsmoking setting.

  3. Read over your solution list, and put a check by those that make the most sense for your lifestyle. Pick one solution and implement it this week. If after a month, this solution has failed you or you have failed it, read over your list again, and pick the next one on the list.

- **Autopsy setbacks.** If you blow your diet or slide back into couch-potato habits, analyze what went wrong and why. Start with the following questions:

  - What blindsided, distracted, demoralized, or otherwise derailed you?
  - What excuses did you use?
  - Who were the saboteurs who undermined your efforts?
  - How did they sidetrack you?

  Now focus on the future.

  - What potential pitfalls do you anticipate?
  - How will you overcome them?
  - What are your back-up plans in case something or someone unexpectedly tries to sabotage your current efforts to change a health behavior?

Learn It / Live It

Changing for Good

Every day you make decisions that have immediate and long-term effects on your health. You decide what to eat, whether to drink or smoke, when to exercise, and how to cope with a sudden crisis. Beyond these daily matters, you decide when to see a doctor, what kind of doctor, and with what sense of urgency. You decide what to tell your doctor and whether to follow the advice given, whether to keep up your immunizations, whether to have a prescription filled and comply with the medication instructions, and whether to seek further help or a second opinion. The entire process of maintaining or restoring health depends on your decisions; it cannot start or continue without them.

The small decisions of everyday life—what to eat, where to go, when to study—are straightforward choices. Larger decisions—which major to choose, what to do about a dead-end relationship, how to handle an awkward work situation—are more challenging. However, if you think of decision making as a process, you can break down even the most difficult choices into manageable steps:

▪ **Set priorities.** Rather than getting bogged down in details, step back and look at the big picture. What matters most to you? What would you like to accomplish in the next week, month, year? Look at the decision you're about to make in the context of your values and goals.

▪ **Inform yourself.** The more you know—about a person, a position, a place, a project—the better you'll be able to evaluate it. Gathering information may involve formal research, such as an online or library search for relevant data, or informal conversations with teachers, counselors, family members, or friends.

▪ **Consider all your options.** Most complex decisions don't involve simple either/or alternatives. List as many options as you can think of, along with the advantages and disadvantages of each.

▪ **Tune in to your gut feelings.** After you've gotten the facts and analyzed them, listen to your intuition. While it's not infallible, your sixth sense can provide valuable feedback. If something just doesn't feel right, try to figure out why. Are there any fears you haven't dealt with? Do you have doubts about taking a certain path?

▪ **Consider a worst-case scenario.** When you're come close to a final decision, imagine what will happen if everything goes wrong—the workload becomes overwhelming, your partner betrays your trust, your expectations turn out to be unrealistic. If you can live with the worst consequences of a decision, you're probably making the right choice.

Making This Chapter Work for You

Review Questions

1. The development of health behaviors is influenced by all of the following *except*
   a. reinforcing factors, which involve external recognition for achieving a goal.
   b. preexisting health factors, which take into account the individual's current position on the wellness continuum.
   c. predisposing factors, which include knowledge, attitudes, and beliefs.
   d. enabling factors, which are related to an individual's skills and capabilities to make behavior changes.

2. Change processes, cognitive and behavior activities that facilitate change, include all of these *except*
   a. consciousness raising   *c.* health awareness
   b. countering   *d.* helping relationships

3. Dylan decided to learn how to meditate to enhance his spiritual health and signed up for a workshop starting in two weeks. Dylan is in which stage of change?
   a. precontemplation   *c.* preparation
   b. contemplation   *d.* action

4. Bianca almost caused an accident last week when she was weaving between cars on the freeway. The incident scared her so much that she decided to change her driving habits and has stayed at the speed limit all this week. Which stage of change is Bianca in?
   a. contemplation   *c.* action
   b. preparation   *d.* maintenance

5. According to the stages of change in the transtheoretical model of change, which statement is *incorrect?*
   a. In the maintenance stage, individuals have avoided relapse for six months.
   b. In the contemplation stage, individuals are considering changing a problem behavior in the next six months.
   c. In the action stage, individuals are actually modifying their behavior according to their plan.
   d. In the preparation stage, individuals intend to change a problem behavior in the next six months.

6. Michelle has a strong internal locus of control. According to research, she is more likely to
   a. enjoy better health.
   b. get a better job.
   c. become a health-care professional.
   d. be worried about the future.

7. If you want to change unhealthy behavior, which of the following strategies is *least* likely to promote success?
   a. Believe that you can make the change.
   b. Reward yourself regularly.
   c. During self-talks, remind yourself about all your faults.
   d. Accept that you are in control of your health.

8. Which of the following are effective strategies for achieving your wellness goals?
   a. Set "step and stretch" goals.
   b. Write and recite an affirmation using the present tense.
   c. Visualize possible obstacles.
   d. All of the above.

(*continued on p. 43*)

Self Survey ▪▪ Where Are You? The Readiness to Change Ruler

1. On the ruler below, mark where you are now on this line that measures change in behavior. Are you not prepared to change, already changing, or someplace in the middle?

Not prepared   Already
to change   changing

⟵   ⟶

2. Answer the following questions that apply to you.
   - If your mark is on the left side of the line:
     How will you know when it's time to think about changing?
     What signals will tell you to start thinking about changing?
     What qualities in yourself are important to you?
     What connection is there between those qualities and "not considering a change"?
   - If your mark is somewhere in the middle:
     Why did you put your mark there and not farther to the left?
     What might make you put your mark a little farther to the right?
     What are the good things about the way you're currently trying to change?
     What are the not-so-good things?
     What would be the good result of changing?
     What are the barriers to changing?
   - If your mark is on the right side of the line:
     Pick one of the barriers to change and list some things that could help you overcome this barrier.
     Pick one of those things that could help and decide to do it by _____ (write in a specific date).
   - If you've taken a serious step in making a change:
     What made you decide on that particular step?
     What has worked in taking this step?
     What helped it work?
     What could help it work even better?
     What else would help?
     Can you break that helpful step down into smaller pieces?
     Pick one of those pieces and decide to do it by _____ (write in a specific date).
   - If you're changing and trying to maintain that change:
     Congratulations! What's helping you?
     What else would help?
     What are your high-risk situations?
   - If you've "fallen off the wagon":
     What worked for a while?
     Don't kick yourself—long-term change almost always takes a few cycles.
     What did you learn from the experience that will help you when you give it another try?
3. The following are stages people go through in making important changes in their health behaviors. All the stages are important. We learn from each stage.

We go *from* "not thinking about it" *to* "weighing the pros and cons" *to* "making little changes and figuring out how to deal with the really hard parts" *to* "doing it!" *to* "making it part of our lives."

Many people "fall off the wagon" and go through all the stages several times before the change really lasts.

Source: Zimmerman, Gretchen. "A 'Stages of Change' Approach to Helping Patients Change Behavior." American Academy of Family Physician, Vol. 61(5): March 1, 2000. Reprinted with permission. www.aafp.org/afp/20000301/1409.html.

YOUR ACTION PLAN FOR HEALTHY CHANGE

Now that you have a sense of your stage of readiness for change, use the following stage-specific ideas to get you going in the right direction.

Precontemplation (not active and not thinking about becoming active)

- Commit yourself to attending class, reading the textbook, and completing assignments and labs.
- List what you see as the cons of behavioral change. For example, do you fear making a change will be too difficult or will take up too much time? Write down a healthy change that you could make tomorrow that would take fewer than 15 minutes of your time.

Contemplation (not active but thinking about becoming active)

- Think back to activities and experiences you found enjoyable in the past. Did they include playing a sport, taking hikes, singing in a group? Ask friends and coworkers if they can put you in touch with others with the same interest.
- Take a realistic look at your daily schedule and life circumstances. How much time could you carve out for a new healthy behavior? How much money could you invest in it?
- Find an image of the life you'd like to have—from a magazine article or advertisement, for example—and post it where you can see it often.

Preparation (active but not at recommended levels)

- Identify specific barriers that limit your activity. If you live in a dorm, your food choices may be limited. If you have a part-time job, you may feel you're constantly on the run and can't take steps to de-stress your life.
- Set specific daily and weekly goals. Your daily goal might begin with 10 or 15 minutes of exercise or relaxation and increase by 5 minutes every week or two. If you're trying to overcome shyness, your weekly goal might be to strike up a conversation with five strangers or to attend one social event.
- Document your progress. Track what's going right and what's not. Take time to brainstorm every night about what you might do differently the next day.

Action and Maintenance (active at recommended levels for less than six months)

- Reach out for support. If you're dieting, log on to a diet blog. If you're shaping up, join a team that's training for a charity run or an intramural competition.
- Develop new interests and skills that reinforce your goal. If you are quitting smoking, spend more and more time in places where you can't smoke and with people who don't smoke.
- Become a mentor. As you incorporate your healthy new behavior into your identity, reach out to help others who want to do the same. Swap diet strategies with a friend who's just committed to losing weight. Demonstrate some of the more challenging postures and exercises to a newcomer to your Pilates or yoga class.

CASE IN POINT

Student: Nicole, 18

Target Goal: Manage her time better

Action Plan:

- Keep an hourly log of her activities for five days (including a weekend).
- Highlight "lost" hours spent surfing the Internet, watching television, and so on.
- Set aside specific times for homework, studying for tests, exercise, special projects.
- Create a daily to-do list.
- Review each week to monitor how well she did and plan ahead for the coming week.

Health(☺)Now™   If you want to write your own goals for managing your time, go to the **Wellness Journal in HealthNow** at http://healthnow .brookscole.com.

*My Contract For Change**

Note: See your Lab Booklet for a goal-setting activity.

Date: _____

Wellness goal: _____

_____

_____

_____

Change(s) I promise to make to reach this goal:

_____

Plan for making this change: _____

_____

_____

Start date: _____

Short-term goals: _____

_____

_____

_____

If I need help: _____

_____

_____

Target date for reaching goal: _____

Reward for achieving goal: _____

Penalty for failing to achieve goal: _____

_____

Signed: _____

Witnessed by: _____

*Also available on HealthNow

9. Cameron feels good because he has made the decision to get fit. What does Cameron have to do next?
   a. Get more specific about his goal.
   b. Start working out.
   c. Find a friend to work out with.
   d. Jog regularly.

10. Relapses are common (you're human, aren't you?), but don't let them keep you from your goal. Which of these strategies might help you recover from a relapse?
    a. Have a hot fudge sundae.
    b. Decide to think about it after finals.
    c. Analyze what went wrong and why.
    d. Put yourself back into contemplation stage.

Answers to these questions can be found on page 587.

Critical Thinking

1. Think about a behavioral change you have made in your life in the past three years in any of the dimensions of health (physical, psychological, spiritual, social, intellectual, environmental). Can you remember going through each of the six stages of the transtheoretical model of change?

2. Self-control is a basic human trait usually learned as a child. How might feelings of self-control differ between individuals with an internal locus of control and those with an external locus of control? How do you think "internals" and "externals" differ in their approach to personal change?

3. It is normal for people to require several trips through the stages of change to make a lasting change, and relapse is viewed as a normal part of the change process, just as in the learning process. What do we learn from our relapses? And how do they help us focus?

Media Menu

Health Now™

Throughout the chapter, this icon introduces a list of resources on the Health-Now website at http://healthnow.brookscole.com/ith that will:
- Help you evaluate your knowledge of the material.
- Allow you to take an exam-prep quiz.
- Provide a Personalized Learning Plan targeting resources that address areas you should study.
- Coach you through identifying target goals for behavior change and creating and monitoring your personal change plan throughout the semester.

INTERNET CONNECTIONS

The Transtheoretical Model
www.med.usf.edu/~kmbrown/Stages_of_Change_Overview.htm
This site, from the University of South Florida Community and Family Health, describes the historical develop-ment of the Transtheoretical Model and features several useful print references.

Transtheoretical Model—Cancer Prevention Research Center
www.uri.edu/research/cprc/TTM/detailedoverview.htm
This site describes the Transtheoretical Model, including descriptions of effective interventions to promote health behavior change, focusing on the individual's decision-making strategies.

Theories of Behavioral Change
www.csupomona.edu/~jvgrizzell/best_practices/bctheory.html
This very comprehensive site, by the Department of Health Promotion at California Polytechnic University at Pomona, describes all of the theories of behavioral change, including Learning Theories, Transtheoretical Model, Health Belief Model, Relapse Prevention Model, Reasoned Action and Planned Behavior, Social Learning/Social Cognitive Theory, and Social Support.

InfoTrac College Edition Activities Log on, insert **self-efficacy** into the Keyword search box, and limit your search to the past year. When you get the results, Mark articles to review, then Select one to read. Summarize three or four key points from the article.

You can find additional readings related to personal health with InfoTrac College Edition, an online library of more than 900 journals and publications. Follow the instructions for accessing InfoTrac College Edition that were packaged with your textbook; then search for articles using a keyword search.

For additional links, resources, and suggested readings on the InfoTrac College Edition, visit our Health and Wellness Resource Center at http://health.wadsworth.com.

Key Terms

The terms listed are used on the page indicated. Definitions of the terms are in the Glossary at the end of the book.

affirmation 35
enabling factors 30
locus of control 33
norms 33
predisposing factors 30
reinforcement 34
reinforcing factors 30
self-efficacy 33
self-talk 34
transtheoretical model of change 31

Psychological Health

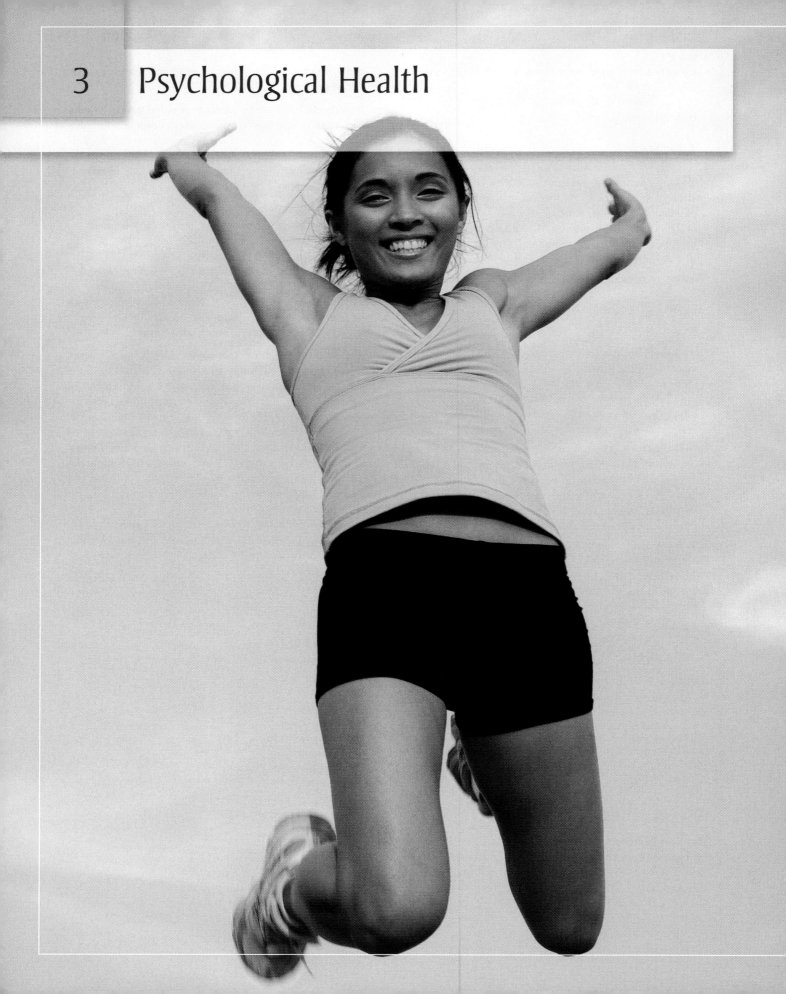

For years, Travis put on his "happy face" around his friends and family. Popular and athletic in high school, he never let anyone know how desperately unhappy he actually felt. "Whatever I was doing during the day, nothing was on my mind more than wanting to die," he recalls. On a perfectly ordinary day in his senior year, Travis tried to kill himself with an overdose of pills. Rushed to a hospital, Travis recovered, resumed his studies, and entered college. By the middle of his freshman year, he was struggling once more with feelings of hopelessness. This time he realized what was happening and sought help from a therapist. "I thought college was supposed to be the happiest time of your life," he said. "What went wrong?"

This is a question many young people might ask. Although youth can seem a golden time, when body and mind glow with potential, the process of becoming an adult is a challenging one in every culture and country. Psychological health can make the difference between facing this challenge with optimism and confidence or feeling overwhelmed by expectations and responsibilities.

This isn't always easy. At some point in life almost half of Americans develop an emotional disorder.[1] Young adulthood—the years from the late teens to the mid-twenties—is a time when many serious disorders, including bipolar illness (manic depression) and schizophrenia, often develop. The saddest fact is not that so many feel so bad, but that so few realize they can feel better. In the course of a year, 60 percent of those with a mental disorder receive no treatment at all.[2] Yet 80 to 90 percent of those treated for psychological problems recover, most within a few months.

By learning about psychological disorders, you may be able to recognize early warning signals in yourself or your loved ones so you can deal with potential difficulties or seek professional help for more serious problems.

After studying the material in this chapter, you should be able to:

- **Identify** the characteristics of emotional, mental, and spiritual health.
- **Describe** the values and other self-esteem components of psychological health.
- **Identify** effective coping strategies that promote positive attitudes and actions.
- **Describe** the effects of spirituality, gratitude, and forgiveness on psychological and physical health.
- **List** the key structures of the brain and **describe** the role of neurons in communication within the brain.
- **Explain** the differences between mental health and mental illness and **list** some effects of mental illness on physical health.
- **Name** the major mental illnesses and their characteristic symptoms.
- **Discuss** some of the factors that may lead to suicide, as well as strategies for prevention.
- **Describe** the treatment options available for those with psychological problems.

WHAT IS PSYCHOLOGICAL HEALTH?

Unlike physical health, psychological well-being cannot be measured, tested, X-rayed, or dissected. Yet psychologically healthy men and women generally share certain characteristics: They value themselves and strive toward happiness and fulfillment. They establish and maintain close relationships with others. They accept the limitations as well as the possibilities that life has to offer. And they feel a sense of meaning and purpose that makes the gestures of living worth the effort required.

Psychological health encompasses both our emotional and mental states—that is, our feelings and our thoughts. **Emotional health** generally refers to feelings and moods, both of which are discussed later in this chapter. Characteristics of emotionally healthy persons, identified in an analysis of major studies of emotional wellness, include the following:

- Determination and effort to be healthy.
- Flexibility and adaptability to a variety of circumstances.
- Development of a sense of meaning and affirmation of life.
- An understanding that the self is not the center of the universe.
- Compassion for others.
- The ability to be unselfish in serving or relating to others.

- Increased depth and satisfaction in intimate relationships.
- A sense of control over the mind and body that enables the person to make health-enhancing choices and decisions.[3]

Mental health describes our ability to perceive reality as it is, to respond to its challenges, and to develop rational strategies for living. The mentally healthy person doesn't try to avoid conflicts and distress but can cope with life's transitions, traumas, and losses in a way that allows for emotional stability and growth. The characteristics of mental health include:

- The ability to function and carry out responsibilities.
- The ability to form relationships.
- Realistic perceptions of the motivations of others.
- Rational, logical thought processes.
- The ability to adapt to change and to cope with adversity.[4]

There is considerable overlap between psychological and **spiritual health,** which involves our ability to identify our basic purpose in life and to experience the fulfillment of achieving our full potential. In one study, more than half of individuals with mental disorders, including depression, turned to spiritual readings or practices to increase calmness, find inner strength and meaning, improve self-awareness, and increase their sense of well-being.[5] Religious support has also been shown to help lower depression and increase life

© Tom Stewart /CORBIS

© Bob Daemmrich Photography

Psychologically healthy people have compassion for others and form strong and deep relationships. They adapt to a variety of circumstances, overcome challenges, and strive to achieve their full potential.

satisfaction beyond the benefits of social support from friends and family.

In addition, **culture** helps to define psychological health. In one culture, men and women may express feelings with great intensity, shouting in joy or wailing in grief, while in another culture such behavior might be considered abnormal or unhealthy. In our diverse society, many cultural influences affect Americans' sense of who they are, where they came from, and what they believe. Cultural rituals help bring people together, strengthen their bonds, reinforce the values and beliefs they share, and provide a sense of belonging, meaning, and purpose.

EMOTIONAL INTELLIGENCE

A person's "IQ"—or intelligence quotient—was once considered the leading predictor of achievement. However, psychologists have determined that another "way of knowing," dubbed **emotional intelligence,** makes an even greater difference in a person's personal and professional success.

"EQ" (for emotional quotient) is the ability to monitor and use emotions to guide thinking and actions. As more than a decade of research has shown, people with high EQ are more productive at work and happier at home. They're also less prone to stress, depression, and anxiety and bounce back quicker from serious illnesses.

According to a recent study of more than 500,000 men and women, most of us remain emotionally clueless. "Seventy percent of people do not handle conflict or stress effectively," says psychologist Travis Bradberry, coauthor of *The Emotional Intelligence Quickbook.*[6]

The good news: While IQ barely budges over a lifetime, you can boost your emotional intelligence. "It's like algebra," says psychologist John Mayer, Ph.D., of the University of New Hampshire, one of the pioneers in EQ research. "Almost anyone can learn emotional intelligence, but you can't expect to figure it out on your own."[7]

Developing emotional awareness requires a conscious effort: Freeze-frame yourself throughout the day, and notice what's going on physically and psychologically. Are you sweating? Is your heart beating fast? Are your muscles tense? All could be signs of anxiety, frustration, or rage. To figure out which, focus on what's running through your mind—dread, doubts, resentments, curses. As you link thoughts with sensations, you'll expand your emotional vocabulary so you can pinpoint whether you're feeling apprehensive about a midterm or irritated by a rude cashier.

SPIRITUAL INTELLIGENCE

Mental health professionals have recognized the power of **spiritual intelligence,** which some define as "the capacity to sense, understand, and tap into the highest parts of ourselves, others, and the world around us." Spiritual intelligence, unlike spirituality, does not center on the worship of a God above, but on the discovery of a wisdom within. All of us are born with the potential to develop spiritual intelligence, but relatively few do. (Spirituality is discussed in depth on page 52.)

THE LESSONS OF POSITIVE PSYCHOLOGY

Psychology, a field that traditionally concentrated on what goes wrong in our lives and in our minds, has shifted its focus to the study of human strengths, virtues, and positive emotions. The three pillars of positive psychology are the study of positive emotions, such as hope and trust; positive traits, such as wisdom and courage; and positive institutions, such as strong families and democracy.

According to psychologist Martin Seligman, Ph.D., the "father" of positive psychology, everyone, regardless of genes or fate, can achieve a happy, gratifying, meaningful life. The goal is not simply to feel good momentarily or to avoid bad experiences, but to build positive strengths and virtues that enable us to find meaning and purpose in life.[8]

"Psychology is not just the study of weakness and damage," Seligman argues, "it is also the study of strength and virtue. Treatment is not just fixing what is broken, it is nurturing what is best within ourselves." The traits that may well protect us from physical and mental illness include courage, optimism, hope, interpersonal skills, a work ethic, responsibility, future-mindedness, honesty, and perseverance.

KNOWING YOUR NEEDS

Newborns are unable to survive on their own. They depend on others for the satisfaction of their physical needs for food, shelter, warmth, and protection, as well as their less tangible emotional needs. In growing to maturity, children take on more responsibility and become more independent. No one, however, becomes totally self-sufficient. As adults, we easily recognize our basic physical needs, but we often fail to acknowledge our emotional needs. Yet they, too, must be met if we are to be as fulfilled as possible.

The humanist theorist Abraham Maslow believed that human needs are the motivating factors in personality development. First, we must satisfy basic physiological needs, such as those for food, shelter, and sleep. Only then can we pursue fulfillment of our higher needs—for safety and security, love and affection, and self-esteem. Few individuals reach the state of **self-actualization,** in which one functions at the highest possible level and derives the greatest possible satisfaction from life (Figure 3-1, page 48).

CLARIFYING YOUR VALUES

Your **values** are the criteria by which you evaluate things, people, events, and yourself; they represent what's most important to you. In a world of almost dizzying complexity, values can provide guidelines for making decisions that are

FIGURE 3-1   The Maslow Pyramid

To attain the highest level of psychological health, you must first satisfy your needs for safety and security, love and affection, and self-esteem.

Source: Maslow, A. *Motivation and Personality,* 3rd ed., © 1997. Reprinted by permission of Pearson Education, Inc.

right for you. If understood and applied, they help give life meaning and structure.

Social psychologist Milton Rokeach distinguished between two types of values. *Instrumental* values represent ways of thinking and acting that we hold important, such as being loving or loyal. *Terminal* values represent goals, achievements, or ideal states that we strive toward, such as happiness. Instrumental and terminal values form the basis for your attitudes and your behavior.

There can be a large discrepancy between what people say they value and what their actions indicate about their values. That's why it's important to clarify your own values, making sure you understand what you believe so that you can live in accordance with your beliefs. To do so, follow these steps:

1. Carefully consider the consequences of each choice.
2. Choose freely from among all the options.
3. Publicly affirm your values by sharing them with others.
4. Act out your values.

Values clarification is not a once-in-a-lifetime task, but an ongoing process of sorting out what matters most to you. If you believe in protecting the environment, do you shut off lights, or walk rather than drive, in order to conserve energy? Do you vote for political candidates who support environmental protection? Do you recycle newspapers, bottles, and cans? Values are more than ideals we'd like to attain; they should be reflected in the way we live day by day.

THE PURSUIT OF SELF-ESTEEM

Each of us wants and needs to feel significant as a human being with unique talents, abilities, and roles in life. A sense of **self-esteem,** of belief or pride in ourselves, gives us confidence to dare to attempt to achieve at school or work and to reach out to others to form friendships and close relationships. Self-esteem is the little voice that whispers, "You're worth it. You can do it. You're okay."

Self-esteem is based, not on external factors like wealth or beauty, but on what you believe about yourself. It's not something you're born with; self-esteem develops over time. It's also not something anyone else can give to you, although those around you can either help boost or diminish your self-esteem.

Strategies for Change   :: Being True to Yourself

:: Take the tombstone test: What would you like to have written on your tombstone? In other words, how would you like to be remembered? Your honest answer should tell you, very succinctly, what you value most.

:: Describe yourself, as you are today, in a brief sentence. Ask friends or family members for their descriptions of you. How would you have to change to become the person you want to be remembered as?

:: Try the adjective test: Choose three adjectives that you'd like to see associated with your reputation. Then list what you've done or can do to earn such descriptions.

Self-esteem, which is based on what you believe about yourself, tends to increase when you experience success.

© 2000 Bob Torrez/Stone/Getty Images

The seeds of self-esteem are planted in childhood when parents provide the assurance and appreciation youngsters need to push themselves toward new accomplishments: crawling, walking, forming words and sentences, learning control over their bladder and bowels.

Adults, too, must consider themselves worthy of love, friendship, and success if they are to be loved, to make friends, and to achieve their goals. Low self-esteem is more common in people who have been abused as children and in those with psychiatric disorders, including depression, anxiety, alcoholism, and drug dependence. Feeling a lack of love and encouragement as a child can also lead to poor self-esteem. Adults with poor self-esteem may unconsciously enter relationships that reinforce their self-perceptions and may prefer and even seek out people who think poorly of them.

One of the most useful techniques for bolstering self-esteem and achieving your goals is developing the habit of positive thinking and talking. While negative observations, such as constant criticisms or reminders of the most minor of faults, can undermine self-image, positive affirmations— compliments, kudos, encouragements—have proved effective in enhancing self-esteem and psychological well-being. Individuals who fight off negative thoughts fare better psychologically than those who collapse when a setback occurs or who rely on others to make them feel better.

 Self-esteem has proved to be one of the best predictors of college adjustment. Students with high self-esteem report better personal, emotional, social, and academic adjustment. However, true self-esteem requires an honest sense of your own worth. In a study of college students, psychology professors followed self-enhancers who began their freshman year with an inflated sense of their own academic ability. These students expected to get much higher college grades than might be predicted based on their high school grades and test scores. While they felt confident and happy for a while, they did no better academically and were no more likely to graduate than their realistic or self-deprecating peers. In fact, the short-term benefits of their self-illusions took a toll over the long term: Their self-esteem and interest in school declined with each passing year.[9]

Your Life Coach

Achieving Your Maximum Potential

Just like physical health, psychological well-being involves more than an absence of problems. By developing your inner strengths and resources, you become the author of your life, capable of confronting challenges and learning from them. As positive psychologists have discovered, you have greater control over how happy, optimistic, upbeat, and lovable you are than anyone or anything else. But only by consciously taking charge of your life can you become all that you have the potential to be.

(FAQ) HOW CAN I FIND HAPPINESS?

A joke, a chocolate, a compliment, or a back rub can make us happy—briefly. The more such happy moments we experience, the more pleasant life feels. But according to positive psychologist Martin Seligman, picture-perfect Hollywood happiness represents the lowest level of gratification. The second category is the good life, which consists of applying core virtues and character strengths daily in relationships, studies, work, and leisure. The third and highest is the meaningful life, in which individuals commit their abilities to the service of some larger purpose.[10]

Many factors influence individual happiness, including genetics. Research on twins raised separately and apart suggests that each of us may have an innate "set point" for happiness. However, you may be able to adjust your happiness thermostat by changing how you think about the past, future, and present. Don't rely on memories of good old days, psychologists caution, because they often weren't as golden as you recall. Expectations also can mislead you because you can't predict what will make you happy. Instead, focus on the moment, and savor the joys every day brings.[11]

 Having an unhappy childhood does not doom anyone to a lifetime of misery, but it does increase the likelihood of unhappiness in adulthood. The risk of having an unhappy adulthood was two-and-a-half times greater for those who'd been unhappy as children.

Life events, such as illness, unemployment, or marriage, can have a temporary impact on happiness. In general, people react to events, whether positive or negative, but quickly adapt back to baseline levels of subjective well-being. Setbacks such as being laid off, achievements such as being promoted, or thrills like winning the lottery lose their impact on happiness levels within a few months. However, a 15-year longitudinal study of the impact of marital transitions on more than 24,000 individuals found significant individual differences. A major loss, such as the death of a loved one, can continue to undermine happiness for several years.[12]

Wealth and health have different and often surprising effects on happiness. Rich people are, on average, only slightly happier than poor ones. Good health is not a prerequisite for happiness. Even seriously ill cancer patients and individuals with serious disabilities differ only slightly from healthier people in life satisfaction. Life satisfaction goes up slightly with age, and emotions become less intense and more stable. Education, intelligence, gender, and race do not matter much for happiness. African Americans and Hispanics have lower rates of depression than white Americans, but they do not report greater happiness. Neither gender is clearly happier, but in different studies women are both happier and sadder than men.

What does make a difference? Love and faith. Married people consistently rank as happier than single or divorced ones. And religious people are usually happier than nonreligious ones. How happy are you? Mark the Satisfaction with Life Scale in Figure 3-2. Relationships are key to happiness among undergraduates. In a survey of 222 college students, psychologists found that the "happiest" 10 percent, as determined by six different rating scales, shared one distinctive characteristic: a rich and fulfilling social life. Almost all were involved in a romantic relationship as well as in rewarding friendships. The happiest students spent the least time alone, and their friends rated them as highest on good relationships.[13]

If you're older than the traditional college student, take heart: You're probably happier. Young people naturally pay more attention to the negative, which may be a way of alerting them to dangers as they encounter novel experiences. Over time, we are increasingly drawn to the familiar, like close friends and relatives. When researchers ask people of different ages if they'd rather have lunch with their favorite author or a close friend, younger people choose the former while older ones opt for the company of someone near and dear.[14]

BECOMING OPTIMISTIC

The dictionary defines **optimism** as "an inclination to anticipate the best possible outcome." For various reasons—because they believe in themselves, because they trust in a higher power, because they feel lucky—optimists expect positive experiences from life. When bad things happen, they tend to see setbacks or losses as specific, temporary incidents. In their eyes, a disappointment is "one of those things" that happens every once in a while, rather than the latest in a long string of disasters. And rather than blaming themselves ("I always mess things up," pessimists might say), optimists look at all the different factors that may have caused the problem.

Individuals aren't born optimistic or pessimistic; in fact, researchers have documented changes over time in

Read the following five statements. Then use a 1-to-7 scale to rate your level of agreement.

1	2	3	4	5	6	7
Not at all true			Moderately true			Absolutely true

1. In most ways my life is close to my ideal.
2. The conditions of my life are excellent.
3. I am satisfied with my life.
4. So far I have gotten the important things I want in life.
5. If I could live my life over, I would change almost nothing.

Total score_____

Scoring: ● 31 to 35: you are extremely satisfied with your life ● 26 to 30: very satisfied ● 21 to 25: slightly satisfied ● 20 is the neutral point ● 15 to 19: slightly dissatisfied ● 10 to 14: dissatisfied ● 5 to 9: extremely dissatisfied

FIGURE 3-2 **Measure Your Happiness**

The Satisfaction with Life Scale was devised in 1980 by University of Illinois psychologist Edward Diener, a founding father of happiness research.

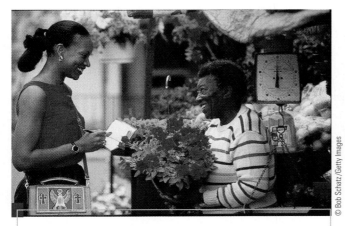

Happiness and optimism go hand in hand. Small rewards can keep spirits high and remind you that you are special.

Giving and getting support from others is fundamental to good psychological health.

the ways that individuals view the world and what they expect to experience in the future. The key is disputing the automatic negative thoughts that flood our brains and choosing to believe in our own possibilities.

Positive psychologist Martin Seligman provides "optimism training" to freshmen at the University of Pennsylvania. According to his follow-up data, those trained to look on the bright side suffered fewer illnesses throughout college than those who were not. Optimism may even help people live longer, healthier lives. On average, people with positive attitudes regarding aging live about 7.5 years longer.[15]

MANAGING YOUR MOODS

Feelings come and go within minutes. A **mood** is a more sustained emotional state that colors our view of the world for hours or days. According to surveys by psychologist Randy Larsen, of the University of Michigan, bad moods descend upon us an average of three out of every ten days. "A few people—about 2 percent—are happy just about every day," he says. "About 5 percent report bad moods four out of every five days."[16]

There are gender differences in mood management: Men typically try to distract themselves (a partially successful strategy) or use alcohol or drugs (an ineffective tactic). Women are more likely to talk to someone (which can help) or to ruminate on why they feel bad (which doesn't help). Learning effective mood-boosting, mood-regulating strategies can help both men and women pull themselves up and out of an emotional slump.

The most effective way to banish a sad or bad mood is by changing what caused it in the first place—if you can figure out what made you upset and why. "Most bad moods are caused by loss or failure in work or intimate relationships," says Larsen. "The questions to ask are: What can I do to fix the failure? What can I do to

remedy the loss? Is there anything under my control that I can change? If there is, take action and solve it." Rewrite the report. Ask to take a makeup exam. Apologize to the friend whose feelings you hurt. Tell your parents you feel bad about the argument you had.

If there's nothing you can do, accept what happened and focus on doing things differently next time. "In our studies, resolving to try harder actually was as effective in improving mood as taking action in the present," says Larsen. You also can try to think about what happened in a different way and put a positive spin on it. This technique, known as *cognitive reappraisal,* or "reframing," helps you look at a setback in a new light: What lessons did it teach you? What would you have done differently? Could there be a silver lining or hidden benefit?

If you can't identify or resolve the problem responsible for your emotional funk, the next-best solution is to concentrate on altering your negative feelings. For example, try setting a quick, achievable goal that can boost your spirits with a small success. Clean out a drawer; sort through the piles of paper on your desk; send an e-mail or instant message to an old friend.

Another good option is to get moving. In studies of mood regulation, exercise consistently ranks as the single most effective strategy for banishing bad feelings. Numerous studies have confirmed that aerobic workouts, such as walking or jogging, significantly improve mood. Even nonaerobic exercise, such as weight lifting, can boost spirits; improve sleep and appetite; reduce

Strategies for Change ▪ How to Be Happy

▪ Make time for yourself. It's impossible to meet the needs of others without recognizing and fulfilling your own.

▪ Invest yourself in closeness. Give your loved ones the gift of your time and caring.

▪ Work hard at what you like. Search for challenges that satisfy your need to do something meaningful.

▪ Be upbeat. If you always look for what's wrong about yourself or your life, you'll find it—and feel even worse.

▪ Organize but stay loose. Be ready to seize an unexpected opportunity to try something different.

---

anxiety, irritability, and anger; and produce feelings of mastery and accomplishment.

LOOKING ON THE LIGHT SIDE

Humor, which enables us to express fears and negative feelings without causing distress to ourselves or others, is one of the healthiest ways of coping with life's ups and downs. Laughter stimulates the heart, alters brain wave patterns and breathing rhythms, reduces perceptions of pain, decreases stress-related hormones, and strengthens the immune system. In psychotherapy, humor helps channel negative emotions toward a positive effect. Even in cases of critical or fatal illnesses, humor can relieve pain and help people live with greater joy until they die.

Joking and laughing are ways of expressing honest emotions, of overcoming dread and doubt, and of connecting with others. They also can defuse rage. After all, it's almost impossible to stay angry when you're laughing. To tickle your funny bone, try keeping a file of favorite cartoons or jokes. Go to a comedy club instead of a movie. If you get an e-mail joke that makes you laugh out loud, don't keep it to yourself—multiply the mirth by sharing it with a friend.

LOVING AND BEING LOVED

"One can live magnificently in this world if one knows how to work and how to love, to work for the person one loves and to love one's work," Leo Tolstoy wrote. You may not think of love as a basic need like food and rest, but it is essential for both physical and psychological well-being.

Mounting evidence suggests that people who lack love and commitment are at high risk for a host of illnesses, including infections, heart disease, and cancer. "Love and intimacy are at the root of what makes us sick and what makes us well," says cardiologist Dean Ornish, author of *Love & Survival: The Scientific Basis for the Healing Power of Intimacy.* "No other factor in medicine—not diet, not smoking, not exercise—has a greater impact."[17]

SPIRITUALITY

Whatever your faith, whether or not you belong to any formal religion, you are more than a body of a certain height and weight occupying space on the planet. You have a mind that equips you to learn and question. And you have a spirit that animates everything you say and do. Spiritual health refers to this breath of life.

Spirituality is a belief in what some call a higher power, in someone or something that transcends the boundaries of self. It gives rise to a strong sense of purpose, values, morals, and ethics. Throughout life you make choices and decide to behave in one way rather than another because your spirituality serves as both a compass and a guide.

The term *religiosity* refers to various spiritual practices. That definition may seem vague, but one thing is clear. According to thousands of studies on the relationship between religious beliefs and practices and health, religious individuals are less depressed, less anxious, and better able to cope with crises such as illness or divorce than nonreligious ones. The more that a believer incorporates spiritual practices, such as prayer, meditation, or attending services, into daily life, the greater their sense of satisfaction with life.

Even when age, health, habits, demographics, and other factors are considered, individuals who pray regularly and attend religious services stay healthier and live longer than those who rarely or never do. In studies at several medical centers, prayer and faith speeded recovery from alcoholism, hip surgery, drug addiction, stroke, rheumatoid arthritis, heart attacks, and bypass surgery.[18]

 In one study, researchers assessed religiosity and symptoms of depression in 104 intercollegiate athletes at a public university in the Southeast. The greater the athletes' intrinsic religiosity, the less likely they were to suffer depressive symptoms.

"Perhaps intrinsic religious beliefs provide a sense of hope and security that protect against distressing events," the researchers speculated. "It may also be that unconditional love by one's God provides a stable sense of self worth" that buffers against stress.[19]

Strategies for Change ■ Enhancing Spiritual Health

■ **If you are religious** Deepen your spiritual commitment through prayer, more frequent church attendance, or joining a prayer group.

■ **If you are not religious** Keep an open mind about the value of religion or spirituality. Consider visiting a church or synagogue. Read the writings of inspired people of deep faith, such as Rabbi Harold Kushner and Rev. Martin Luther King, Jr.

■ **If you are not ready to consider religion** Try nonreligious meditation or relaxation training. In decades of research, Dr. Herbert Benson of Harvard University has shown that focusing the mind on a single sound or image can slow heart rate, respiration, and brain waves; relax muscles; and lower stress-rated hormones—responses similar to those induced by prayer.

FAQ CAN PRAYER KEEP US HEALTHY?

Prayer, a spiritual practice of millions, is the most commonly used form of complementary and alternative medicine. However, only in recent years has science launched rigorous investigations of the healing power of prayer.

Petitionary prayer—praying directly to a higher power—affects both the quality and quantity of life, says Dr. Harold Koenig, director of Duke University's Center for the Study of Religion/Spirituality and Health. "It boosts morale, lowers agitation, loneliness, and life dissatisfaction and enhances ability to cope in men, women, the elderly, the young, the healthy, and the sick."[20]

People who pray regularly have significantly lower blood pressure and stronger immune systems than the less religious, says Dr. Koenig. They're also less prone to alcoholism, less likely to smoke heavily, and are hospitalized less often. Science cannot explain the physiological mechanisms for what happens in human beings when they pray, but in cultures around the world throughout recorded history when people or their loved ones are sick, they pray.

In a national survey, 35 percent of Americans prayed for health concerns, with 75 percent of these praying for wellness and 22 percent praying for alleviation of specific medical conditions, such as chronic headaches, depression, back or neck pain, and digestive problems. Among those who prayed because of a medical condition, 69 percent found prayer very helpful. Only 11 percent of patients using prayer discussed it with their physicians.[21]

Some scientists speculate that prayer may foster a state of peace and calm that could lead to beneficial changes in the cardiovascular and immune systems. Sophisticated brain imaging techniques have shown that prayer and meditation cause changes in blood flow in particular regions of the brain that may lead to lower blood pressure, slower heart rate, decreased anxiety, and an enhanced sense of well-being. Membership in a faith community provides an identity as well as support, although individuals vary in their religious practices and observances.[22]

In recent research, praying for others has not improved their symptoms or recovery. In a study of patients undergoing heart procedures, prayers (whether by Christian, Muslim, Jewish, or Buddhist groups) and other complementary

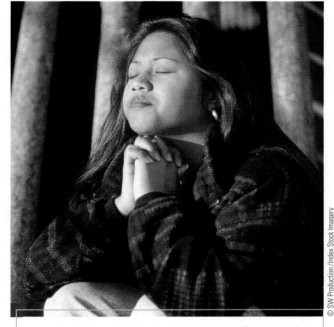

Prayer provides benefits for physical health as well as spiritual well-being.

© SW Production/Index Stock Imagery

bedside therapies, such as imaging and therapeutic touching, did not measurably improve their outcome.[23]

Will science ever be able to prove the power of prayer? No one is certain. "While I personally believe that God heals people in supernatural ways, I don't think science can shape a study to prove it," says Duke's Dr. Koenig. "But we now know enough, based on solid scientific research, to recommend prayer, much like exercise and diet, as one of the best and most cost-effective ways of protecting and enhancing health."

EXPRESSING GRATITUDE

A grateful spirit brightens mood, boosts energy, and infuses daily living with a sense of glad abundance. Although giving thanks is an ancient virtue, only recently have researchers focused on the "trait" of gratitude—appreciation, not just for a special gift, but for everything that makes life a bit better.

"Gratitude is an emotional and intellectual phenomenon that rises out of recognition that someone has treated you benevolently," says psychologist Michael McCullough of Southern Methodist University, a pioneer in gratitude research. "It's not feeling happy because something good happens, but realizing that someone who didn't have to deliberately did something of value to you."[24]

Since gratitude is not just a feeling but a mental outlook, we can consciously become more grateful—with practice. "Volunteers on college campuses who are asked to list things they're grateful for every day report more positive feelings," says McCullough. "They have more energy. They sleep better. They feel richer, regardless of how much money they have. Even their families notice visible, positive changes."

How can you help your gratitude grow? Here are some suggestions:

- Train yourself to pay attention to good things, large and small
- Build a time for thankfulness into your day. Some people write nightly in a gratitude journal or log.
- Develop a "good" memory, one that stores the kindnesses and comforts that have come your way.
- Pass on simple kindnesses. Open the door for a student juggling a backpack and an umbrella. Flash a smile at a server in the cafeteria. Pitch in on a beach or park cleanup. Give others a reason to savor a moment of gratitude.

FORGIVENESS

While "I forgive you" may be three of the most difficult words to say, they are also three of the most powerful—and the most beneficial for the body as well as the soul. Being angry, harboring resentments, or reliving hurts over and over again is bad for your health in general and your heart in particular. The word *forgive* comes from the Greek for letting go, and that's what happens when you forgive: You let go of all the anger and pain that have been demanding your time and wasting your energy.

To some people, forgiveness seems a sign of weakness or submission. People may feel more in control, more powerful, when they're filled with anger, but forgiving instills a much greater sense of power. When you forgive, you reclaim your power to choose. It doesn't matter whether someone deserves to be forgiven; you deserve to be free.

However, forgiveness isn't easy. It's not a one-time thing but a process that takes a lot of time and work. Most people pass through several stages in their journey to forgiveness. The initial response may involve anger, sadness, shame, or other negative feelings. Later, there's a reevaluation of what happened, then reframing to try to make sense of it or to take mitigating circumstances into account. This may lead to a reduction in negative feelings, especially if the initial hurt turns out to be accidental rather than intentional.

DOING GOOD

Altruism—helping or giving to others—enhances self-esteem, relieves physical and mental stress, and protects psychological well-being. Hans Selye, the father of stress research, described cooperation with others for the self's sake as altruistic egotism, whereby we satisfy our own needs while helping others satisfy theirs. This concept is essentially an updated version of the golden rule: Do unto others as you would have them do unto you. The important difference is that you earn your neighbor's love and help by offering them love and help.

 Volunteerism helps those who give as well as those who receive. People involved in community organizations, for instance, consistently report a surge of well-being called *helper's high,* which they describe as a unique sense of calmness, warmth, and enhanced self-worth. College students who provided community service as part of a semester-long course reported changes in attitude (including a decreased tendency to blame people for their misfortunes), self-esteem (primarily a belief that they

---

Strategies for Change ▪ How to Forgive

- Compose an apology letter. Address it to yourself, and write it from someone who's hurt you. This simple task enables you to get a new perspective on a painful experience.
- Leap forward in time. In a visualization exercise imagine that you are very old, meet a person who hurt you long ago, and sit down together on a park bench

on a beautiful spring day. You both talk until everything that needs to be said finally is. This allows you to benefit from the perspective time brings without having to wait for years to achieve it.

- Talk with "safe" people. Vent your anger or disappointment with a trusted friend or a counselor without the danger of saying or doing anything you'll

regret later. And if you can laugh about what happened with a friend, the laughter helps dissolve the rage.

- Forgive the person, not the deed. In themselves, abuse, rape, murder, or betrayal are beyond forgiveness. But you can forgive people who couldn't manage to handle their own suffering, misery, confusion, and desperation.

can make a difference), and behavior (a greater commitment to do more volunteer work).

The options for giving of yourself are limitless: Volunteer to serve a meal at a homeless shelter. Collect donations for a charity auction. Teach in an illiteracy program. Perform the simplest act of charity: Pray for others.

FEELING IN CONTROL

Although no one has absolute control over destiny, we can do a great deal to control how we think, feel, and behave. By assessing our life situations realistically, we can make plans and preparations that allow us to make the most of our circumstances. By doing so, we gain a sense of mastery. In nationwide surveys, Americans who feel in control of their lives report greater psychological well-being than those who do not, as well as extraordinarily positive feelings of happiness.

You may not have complete control over your destiny, but you can control how you respond to challenges.

DEVELOPING AUTONOMY

One goal that many people strive for is **autonomy,** or independence. Both family and society influence our ability to grow toward independence. Autonomous individuals are true to themselves. As they weigh the pros and cons of any decision, whether it's using or refusing drugs or choosing a major or career, they base their judgment on their own values, not those of others. Their ability to draw on internal resources and cope with challenges has a positive impact on both their psychological well-being and their physical health, including recovery from illness.

Those who've achieved autonomy may seek the opinions of others, but they do not allow their decisions to be dictated by external influences. For autonomous individuals, their **locus of control**—that is, where they view control as originating—is *internal* (from within themselves) rather than *external* (from others).

ASSERTING YOURSELF

Being **assertive** means recognizing your feelings and making your needs and desires clear to others. Unlike aggression, a far less healthy means of expression, assertiveness usually works. You can change a situation you don't like by communicating your feelings and thoughts in nonprovocative words, by focusing on specifics, and by making sure you're talking with the person who is directly responsible.

Becoming assertive isn't always easy. Many people have learned to cope by being passive and not communicating their feelings or opinions. Sooner or later they become so irritated, frustrated, or overwhelmed that they explode in an outburst—which they think of as being assertive. However, such behavior is so distasteful to them that they'd rather be passive. But assertiveness doesn't mean screaming or telling someone off. You can communicate your wishes calmly and clearly. Assertiveness is a behavior that respects your rights and the rights of other people even when you disagree.

Even at its mildest, assertiveness can make you feel better about yourself and your life. The reason: When you speak up or take action, you're in the pilot seat. And that's

Strategies for Change :: How to Assert Yourself

:: Use "I" statements to explain your feelings. This allows you to take ownership of your opinions and feelings without putting down others for how they feel and think.

:: Listen to and acknowledge what the other person says. After you speak, find out if the other person understands your position. Ask how he or she feels about what you've said.

:: Be direct and specific. Describe the problem as you see it, using neutral language rather than assigning blame. Also suggest a specific solution, but make it clear that you'd like the lines of communication and negotiation to remain open.

:: Don't think you have to be obnoxious in order to be assertive. It's most effective to state your needs and preferences without any sarcasm or hostility.

always much less stressful than taking a back seat and trying to hang on for dear life.

CONNECTING WITH OTHERS

At every age, people who feel connected to others tend to be healthier physically and psychologically. This is as, if not more, true in college when young adults, often living independently for the first time, need to form new relationships. In a recent study at a large Midwestern university, the students—particularly the women—who felt the greatest sense of belonging reported fewer physical symptoms than those who had not forged close friendships. The research also revealed a gender difference: Female students seek out, forge, and maintain more supportive ties than men, rely on friends more in times of stress, and provide more support than men.[25]

The opposite of *connectedness* is **social isolation,** a major risk factor for illness and early death. Individuals with few social contacts face two to four times the mortality rate of others. The reason may be that their social isolation weakens the body's ability to ward off disease. Medical students with higher-than-average scores on a loneliness scale had lower levels of protective immune cells. The end of a long-term relationship—through separation, divorce, or death—also dampens immunity.

It is part of our nature as mammals and as human beings to crave relationships. But invariably we end up alone at times. Solitude is not without its own quiet joys—time for introspection, self-assessment, learning from the past, and looking toward the future. Each of us can cultivate the joy of our own company, of being alone without crossing the line and becoming lonely.

OVERCOMING LONELINESS

More so than many other countries, we are a nation of loners. Recent trends—longer work hours, busy family schedules, frequent moves, high divorce rates—have created even more lonely people. Only 23 percent of Americans say they're never lonely. Loneliest of all are those who are divorced, separated, or widowed and those who live alone or solely with children. Among single adults who have never been married, 42 percent feel lonely at least sometimes. However, loneliness is most likely to cause emotional distress when it is chronic rather than episodic.

To combat loneliness, people may join groups, fling themselves into projects and activities, or surround themselves with superficial acquaintances. Others avoid the effort of trying to connect, sometimes limiting most of their personal interactions to chat groups on the Internet.

The true keys to overcoming loneliness are developing resources to fulfill our own potential and learning to reach out to others. In this way, loneliness can become a means to personal growth and discovery.

FACING SHYNESS AND SOCIAL ANXIETY

Many people are uncomfortable meeting strangers or speaking or performing in public. In some surveys, as many as 40 percent of people describe themselves as shy or socially anxious. Some shy people—an estimated 10 to 15 percent of children—are born with a predisposition to shyness. Others become shy because they don't learn proper social responses or because they experience rejection or shame.

Some people are "fearfully" shy; that is, they withdraw and avoid contact with others and experience a high degree of anxiety and fear in social situations. Others are "self-consciously" shy. They enjoy the company of others but become highly self-aware and anxious in social situations.[26] In one study of college students, men reported somewhat more shyness than women. African Americans were less shy than either Asian Americans or Caucasians.[27] Students may develop symptoms of shyness or social anxiety when they go to a party or are called on in class. Some experience symptoms when they try to perform any sort of action in the presence of others, even such everyday activities as eating in public, using a public restroom, or writing a check.

About 7 percent of the population could be diagnosed with a severe form of social anxiety, called **social phobia,** in which individuals typically fear and avoid various social situations. Adolescents and young adults with severe social anxiety are at increased risk of major depression. Phobias are discussed later in this chapter. The key difference between these problems and normal shyness and self-consciousness is the degree of distress and impairment that individuals experience.

If you're shy, you can overcome much of your social apprehensiveness on your own, in much the same way as you might set out to stop smoking or lose weight. For example, you can improve your social skills by pushing yourself to introduce yourself to a stranger at a party or to chat about the weather or the food selections with the person next to you in a cafeteria line. Gradually, you'll acquire a sense of social timing and a verbal ease that will take the worry out of close encounters with others. Those with more disabling social anxiety may do best with psychotherapy and medication, which have proved highly effective.

It's time to take a more comprehensive look at how you view your life. Take the Self-Survey on page 76 and read the Health Action Plan for suggestions on improving your psychological health.

THE BRAIN: THE LAST FRONTIER

The brain has intrigued scientists for centuries, but only recently have its explorers made dramatic progress in unraveling its mysteries. Leaders in **neuropsychiatry**—the field that brings together the study of the brain and the mind—remind us that 95 percent of what is known about brain anatomy, chemistry, and physiology has been learned in the last 20 years. These discoveries have reshaped our understanding of the organ that is central to our identity and well-being and have fostered great hope for more effective therapies for the more than 1,000 disorders—psychiatric and neurologic—that affect the brain and nervous system.

INSIDE THE BRAIN

Each human brain contains hundreds of billions of nerve cells, or **neurons,** and support cells called **glia.** Most are present at birth, when the brain weighs less than a pound. In the first six years of life—the period when we acquire more knowledge more rapidly than ever again—the brain reaches its full weight of about 3 pounds (Figure 3-3).

The neurons are the basic working units of the brain. Like snowflakes, no two are exactly the same. Each consists of a cell body containing the **nucleus;** a long fiber, called the **axon,** which can range from less than an inch to several feet in length; an **axon terminal,** or ending; and multiple branching fibers called **dendrites** (Figure 3-4). The glia serve as the scaffolding for the brain, separate the brain from the bloodstream, assist in the growth of neurons, speed up the transmission of nerve impulses, and engulf and digest damaged neurons.

As the master control center for the body, the brain is constantly receiving information from the senses and relaying messages to various parts of the body. Some of these messages travel through the spinal cord, which extends from the neck about two-thirds of the way down the back-bone. Other signals are carried by nerves that connect the brain directly with certain parts of the body.

SEX DIFFERENCES IN THE BRAIN

From birth, male and female brains differ in a variety of ways. Overall, a woman's brain, like her body, is 10 to 15 percent smaller than a man's, yet the regions dedicated to higher cognitive functions such as language are more densely packed with neurons—and women use more of them. When a male puts his mind to work, neurons turn on in highly specific areas. When females set their minds on similar tasks, cells light up all over the brain.

Male and female brains perceive light and sound differently. A man's eyes are more sensitive to bright light and retain their ability to see well at long distances longer in life. A woman hears a much broader range of sounds, and her hearing remains sharper longer.

The female brain responds more intensely to emotion. According to neuroimaging studies, the genders respond differently to emotions, especially sadness, which activates, or turns on, neurons in an area eight times larger in women than men.

Neither gender's brain is "better." Intelligence per se appears equal in both. The greatest gender differences appear both at the top and bottom of the intelligence scales. Men outnumber women both as geniuses and as morons. Nevertheless, more than half the time, regardless of the type of test, most women and men perform more or less equally—

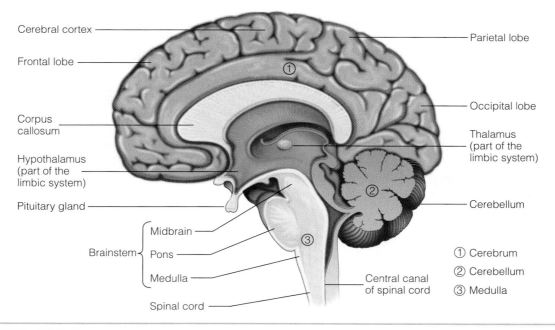

FIGURE 3-3   The Brain

The three major parts of the brain are the cerebrum, cerebellum, and brainstem (medulla). The cerebrum is divided into two hemispheres—the left, which regulates the right side of the body, and the right, which regulates the left side of the body. The cerebellum plays the major role in coordinating movement, balance, and posture. The brainstem contains centers that control breathing, blood pressure, heart rate, and other physiological functions.

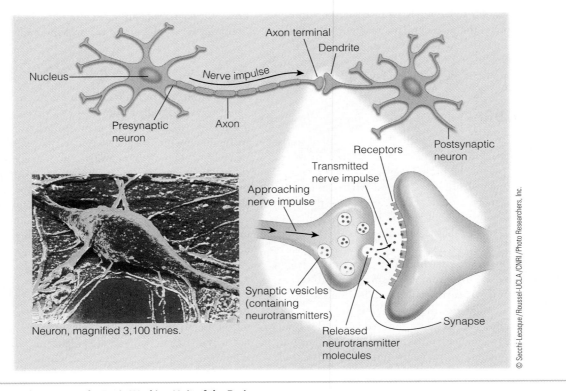

© Secchi-Lecaque/Roussel-UCLA/CNRI/Photo Researchers, Inc.

FIGURE 3-4   **The Neuron, the Basic Working Unit of the Brain**
Neurotransmitters released across the synapse transmit the chemical nerve impulse from one neuron to another.

even though they may well take different routes to arrive at the same answers. Cognitive skills show greater variability both among women and among men than between the genders. The best evaluation may have come from essayist Samuel Johnson. When asked whether women or men are more intelligent, he responded, "Which man? Which woman?"

COMMUNICATION WITHIN THE BRAIN

Neurons "talk" with each other by means of electrical and chemical processes (see Figure 3-4). An electric charge, or impulse, travels along an axon to the terminal, where packets of chemicals called **neurotransmitters** are stored. When released, these messengers flow out of the axon terminal and cross a **synapse,** a specialized site at which the axon terminal of one neuron comes extremely close to a dendrite from another neuron. On the surface of the dendrite are **receptors,** protein molecules designed to bind with neurotransmitters. It takes only about a ten-thousandth of a second for a neurotransmitter and a receptor to come together. Neurotransmitters that do not connect with receptors may remain in the synapse until they are reabsorbed by the cell that produced them—a process called **reuptake**—or broken down by enzymes.

A malfunction in the release of a neurotransmitter, in its reuptake or elimination, or in the receptors or secondary messengers may result in abnormalities in thinking, feeling, or behavior. Some of the most promising and exciting re-

search in neuropsychiatry is focusing on correcting such malfunctions. The neurotransmitter serotonin and its receptors have been shown to affect mood, sleep, behavior, appetite, memory, learning, sexuality, and aggression and to play a role in several mental disorders. The discovery of a possible link between low levels of serotonin and some cases of major depression has led to the development of more precisely targeted **antidepressant** medications that boost serotonin to normal levels. (See "Psychiatric Drugs" later in the chapter.)

THE ROLE OF SLEEP

You stay up late cramming for a final. You drive through the night to visit a friend at another campus. You get up for an early class during the week but stay in bed until noon on weekends. And you wonder: "Why am I so tired?" The answer: You're not getting enough sleep.

Whenever we fail to get adequate sleep, we accumulate what researchers call a *sleep debt*. With each night of too little rest, our body's need for sleep grows until it becomes irresistible. The only solution to sleep debt is the obvious one: paying it back. College students who extended their nightly sleep time were more alert, more productive, and less likely to have accidents.[28] And because sleepy people tend to be irritable and edgy, those who get more rest also tend to be happier, healthier, and easier to get along with.

WHY SLEEP MATTERS

Sleep problems, as medical scientists now recognize, are hazardous to health. Breathing-related sleep disorders, such as chronic snoring and obstructive sleep apnea, increase the risk of high blood pressure, heart attacks, and stroke. Individuals with insomnia, the most common sleep complaint, become irritable and depressed, get into more traffic accidents, develop memory problems, and have difficulties concentrating and doing their jobs. According to recent research, inadequate sleep affects growth hormone secretion, increasing the likelihood of obesity, and impairs the body's ability to use insulin, which can lead to diabetes.[29] Individuals chronically deprived of enough sleep may become more susceptible to certain illnesses, and researchers speculate that disturbed sleep may be the reason why individuals under stress—such as students taking exams or grieving windows and widowers—may have lower levels of certain infection-fighting cells than normal.[30]

 College-age individuals, who often stay up late and sleep in on weekends, may suffer from Sunday night insomnia or may develop chronic problems getting up early. A single all-nighter can lead to lapses of attention and much slower reaction times. Sleep deprivation can increase the risk of physical and psychological symptoms, including depression, in college students.[31]

WHAT HAPPENS WHEN WE SLEEP?

A normal night of sleep consists of several distinct stages of sleep, divided into two major types: an active state, characterized by **rapid eye movement (REM)** and called **REM sleep** (or dream sleep), and a quiet state, referred to as non-REM or NREM sleep, that consists of four stages:

- **In Stage 1,** a twilight zone between full wakefulness and sleep, the brain produces small, irregular, rapid electrical waves. The muscles of the body relax, and breathing is smooth and even.

- **In Stage 2,** brain waves are larger and punctuated with occasional sudden bursts of electrical activity. The eyes are no longer responsive to light. Bodily functions slow still more.

- **Stages 3 and 4** constitute the most profound state of unconsciousness. The brain produces slower, larger waves, and this is sometimes referred to as "delta" or slow-wave sleep (Figure 3-5).

After about an hour in the four stages of non-REM sleep, sleepers enter the time of vivid dreaming called REM sleep, when brain waves resemble those of waking more than those of quiet sleep. The large muscles of the torso, arms, and legs are paralyzed and cannot move—possibly to prevent sleepers from acting out their dreams. The fingers and toes may twitch; breathing is quick and shallow; blood flow through the brain speeds up; men may have partial or full erections.

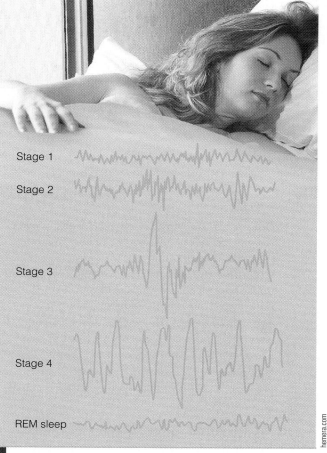

FIGURE 3-5 **Stages of Sleep**
The stages of sleep are defined by these differences in brain wave patterns.

SLEEP DISORDERS

Three of four Americans struggle to get a good night's sleep at least a few nights a week.[32] According to the National Commission on Sleep Disorders Research, 40 million adults suffer from a specific sleep disorder, such as chronic insomnia or sleep apnea; an additional 20 to 30 million have occasional sleep difficulties. [Take the "BEARS" quiz on page 60 to see if you have a sleep disorder.]

Insomnia

Individuals with insomnia—a lack of sleep so severe that it interferes with functioning during the day—may toss and turn for an hour or more when they get into bed, wake frequently in the night, wake up too early, or not be able to sleep long enough to feel alert and energetic the next day.[33] Most often insomnia is transient, typically occurring before or after a major life event, such as a job interview, and lasting for three or four nights. During periods of prolonged stress, such as a breakup, short-term insomnia may continue for several weeks. Chronic or long-term insomnia, which can begin at any age, may persist for months or years.

For about a third of those with chronic insomnia, the underlying problem is a mental disorder, most often depression or an anxiety disorder. Many substances, including alcohol, medications, and drugs of abuse, often disrupt sleep. About 15 percent of those seeking help for chronic insomnia suffer from "learned" or "behavioral" insomnia. While a life crisis may trigger their initial sleep problems, each night they try harder and harder to get to sleep, but they cannot—although they often doze off while reading or watching a movie.

Sleeping pills may be used for a specific, time-limited problem—always with a physician's supervision. In the long term, behavioral approaches, including the following, have proved more effective:

- **Relaxation therapy,** which may involve progressive muscle relaxation, diaphragmatic breathing, hypnosis, or meditation.
- **Cognitive therapy,** which challenges misconceptions about sleep and helps shift a poor sleeper's mind away from anxiety-inducing thoughts.
- **Stimulus control therapy,** in which individuals who do not fall asleep quickly must get up and leave their beds until they are very sleepy.
- **Sleep restriction therapy,** in which sleep times are sharply curtailed in order to improve the quality of sleep.

Breathing Disorders (Snoring and Sleep Apnea)

Although most people snore in certain positions or when they have stuffed-up noses, snoring can be a sign of a serious problem. Caused by the vibration in tissues in the mouth and throat as a sleeper tries to suck air into the lungs, snoring can be so loud that it disrupts a bed partner or others in the same house. In young people, the cause is most likely to be enlarged tonsils or adenoids. In adults, extreme snoring may be a symptom of sleep apnea.

Translated from the Greek words meaning "no" and "breath," apnea is exactly that: the absence of breathing for a brief period. People with sleep apnea may briefly stop breathing dozens or even hundreds of times during the night. As they struggle for breath, they may gasp for air, snore extremely loudly, or thrash about.

Although apnea, which can lead to high blood pressure, stroke, and heart attack, may affect as many as 10 million Americans, most are unaware of the problem. Effective treatments include weight loss (if obesity is contributing to the problem), a nasal mask that provides continuous positive airway pressure (CPAP) to ensure a steady flow of air into the lungs and, in severe cases, surgery to enlarge the upper airway.

Movement Disorders

Restless legs syndrome, which may affect 12 million Americans, is a movement disorder characterized by symptoms that patients describe as pulling, burning, tingling, creepy-crawly, grabbing, buzzing, jitteriness, or gnawing. Many

---

TABLE 3-1   "BEARS": HOW WELL DO YOU SLEEP?
B = Bedtime problems: Do you have any problems falling asleep at bedtime?
E = Excessive daytime sleepiness: Do you feel sleepy a lot during the day? In school? While driving?
A = Awakenings during the night: Do you wake up a lot at night?
R = Regularity and duration of sleep: What time do you usually go to bed on school nights? Weekends? How much sleep do you usually get?
S = Sleep-disordered breathing: Has anyone ever told you that you snore loudly at night?
Your answers to this self-assessment, developed by sleep specialists, may reveal a sleep problem that can interfere with your daytime functioning. If it persists, discuss it with a doctor.

Source: Millman, Richard, et al. "Excessive Sleepiness in Adolescents and Young Adults: Causes, Consequences, and Treatment Strategies." *Pediatrics,* Vol. 115, No. 6, June 2005, p. 1774.

people with these symptoms have difficulty falling or staying asleep but do not realize that the cause is a medical disorder that can be treated with medications.

Circadian Rhythm Sleep Disorders

Problems involving the timing of sleep are called circadian rhythm disorders because they affect the basic circadian ("about a day") rhythm that influences many biological processes. The most common causes are jet lag and shift work. Jet lag generally improves on its own within two to seven days, depending on the length of the trip and the individual's response. Avoiding caffeine and alcohol and immediately switching to the new time zone's schedule can help in overcoming jet lag.

A "shift work" circadian rhythm disorder consists of any inability to sleep when one wants or to stay alert when needed because of frequently changing work shifts. Behavioral strategies and good sleep habits can help. In addition, phototherapy—exposure to bright light for periods ranging from 30 minutes to two hours—has shown promise as an experimental treatment to help shift workers adjust to their changing schedules.

HOW MUCH SLEEP DO I NEED?

Over the last century, we have cut our average nightly sleep time by 20 percent. More than half of us try to get by with fewer than seven hours of shut-eye a night.[34]

College students are no exception. In a recent study of 212 undergraduates, their average sleep time was slightly less than seven hours, with little difference between men and women. Those who slept the least reported the lowest life satisfaction.[35] Short-sleepers also have poorer psychological health, less creativity, and lower academic performance.[36]

No formula can say how long a good night's sleep should be. Normal sleep times range from five to ten hours; the

Strategies for Change :: How to Sleep Like a Baby

:: Keep regular hours for going to bed and getting up in the morning. Stay as close as possible to this schedule on weekends as well as weekdays.

:: Develop a sleep ritual—such as stretching, meditation, yoga, prayer, or reading a not-too-thrilling novel—to ease the transition from wakefulness to sleep.

:: Don't drink coffee late in the day. The effects of caffeine can linger for up to eight hours. And don't smoke. Nicotine is an even more powerful stimulant—and sleep saboteur—than caffeine.

:: Don't rely on alcohol to get to sleep. Alcohol disrupts normal sleep stages, so you won't sleep as deeply or as restfully as you normally would.

:: Don't nap during the day if you're having problems sleeping through the night.

---

average is seven and a half. About one or two people in a hundred can get by with just five hours; another small minority needs twice that amount.[37] Each of us seems to have an innate sleep *appetite* that is as much a part of our genetic programming as hair color and skin tone.

To figure out your sleep needs, keep your wake-up time the same every morning and vary your bedtime. Are you groggy after six hours of shut-eye? Does an extra hour give you more stamina? What about an extra two hours? Since too much sleep can make you feel sluggish, don't assume that more is always better. Listen to your body's signals, and adjust your sleep schedule to suit them.

Are you better off pulling an all-nighter before a big test or closing the books and getting a good night's sleep? According to researchers, that depends on the nature of the exam. If it's a test of facts—Civil War battles, for instance—cramming all night works. However, if you will have to write analytical essays in which you compare, contrast, and make connections, you need to sleep in order to make the most of your reasoning abilities.[38]

UNDERSTANDING MENTAL HEALTH

Mentally healthy individuals value themselves, perceive reality as it is, accept their limitations and possibilities, carry out their responsibilities, establish and maintain close relationships, pursue work that suits their talent and training, and feel a sense of fulfillment that makes the efforts of daily living worthwhile (Figure 3-6).

According to a national report by the Centers for Disease Control (CDC), American adults spend an average of three days a month feeling "sad, blue, or depressed." Individuals who spend more time down in the dumps are more likely to report unhealthy behaviors such as cigarette smoking and physical inactivity.

College-age young adults (18 to 24 years old) report the most days with depressive symptoms. Women had more gloomy days than men (3.5 compared to 2.4). College graduates and those earning more than $50,000 reported half as many sad, bad days as those without a high school diploma or earning less than $15,000.

Regular exercisers had 1.3 fewer days with symptoms of depression than those who did not work out regularly. Those who smoked a pack or more of cigarettes a day had more down days than those who never smoked.[39]

WHAT IS A MENTAL DISORDER?

While lay people may speak of "nervous breakdowns" or "insanity," these are not scientific terms. The U.S. government's official definition states that a serious mental illness is "a diagnosable mental, behavioral, or emotional disorder that interferes with one or more major activities in life, like dressing, eating, or working."

The mental health profession's standard for diagnosing a mental disorder is the pattern of symptoms, or diagnostic criteria, spelled out for the almost 300 disorders in the American Psychiatric Association's *Diagnostic and Statistical*

FIGURE 3-6 The Mentally Healthy Individual
Mental well-being is a combination of many factors.

Manual, 4th edition (DSM-IV). Psychiatrists define a **mental disorder** as "a clinically significant behavioral or psychological syndrome or pattern that occurs in an individual and that is associated with present distress (a painful symptom) or disability (impairment in one or more important areas of functioning) or with a significantly increased risk of suffering death, pain, disability, or an important loss of freedom."[40]

WHO DEVELOPS MENTAL DISORDERS?

In the course of their lifetime, almost half of all Americans—46 percent—will experience a diagnosable psychological problem. In a recent national survey, one in four reported symptoms sufficient for a diagnosis of a disorder requiring treatment during the previous year.[41] The most common problems are anxiety disorders (such as phobias and panic disorder), mood disorders (such as depression and bipolar disorder), impulse control disorders (such as compulsive gambling) and substance abuse disorders (Table 3-2).

Unlike most disabling physical diseases, mental illness starts early in life. Half of all lifetime cases begin by age 14; three-quarters, by age 24. Anxiety disorders often begin in late childhood, mood disorders in late adolescence, and substance abuse in the early twenties. Researchers describe such problems as "the chronic diseases of the young," striking when men and women are in their prime. The prevalence of mental disorders increases from early adulthood (ages 18 to 29) to the next-oldest age group (ages 30 to 44) and then declines. Women have higher rates of depressive and anxiety disorders; men have higher rates of substance abuse and impulse disorders.[42]

About 80 percent of those with mental disorders eventually seek treatment, but many suffer for years, even decades. The median delay for all disorders is nearly 10 years. Those with social phobia and separation anxiety disorders may not get help for more than 20 years. The earlier in life that a disorder begins, the longer that individuals tend to delay treatment.[43]

Without treatment, mental disorders take a toll on every aspect of life, including academics, relationships, careers,

and risk-taking. Symptoms or episodes of a disorder typically become more frequent or severe. Individuals with one mental disorder are at high risk of having a second one (this is called comorbidity).

About 6 percent of Americans have a "severe" mental disorder, one that significantly limits their ability to work or carry out daily activities or that has led to a suicide attempt or psychosis (a gross impairment of a person's perception of reality). On average, they are unable to function for nearly three months of the year.[44]

> *Three-quarters of all mental disorders begin before age 24, yet individuals typically do not seek help for years or even decades. Are they too ashamed or fearful of the stigma of having a mental illness to seek help? Or is access to mental health care too difficult or expensive?* **You decide.**

MENTAL HEALTH ON CAMPUS

About 15 percent of students seek counseling during college.[45] The emotional difficulties of college students have become more complex and more severe than in the past. In one national survey, more than 80 percent of directors of counseling centers reported an increase in the number of students with serious psychological disorders. (Eating disorders, which are common among college students, are discussed in Chapter 7.)

According to the American College Health Association's National College Health Assessment, the incidence of **depression** among college students increased by 4.6 percent over the four-year period from 2000 to 2004. In a survey of 47,202 students from 74 campuses across the country, 15 percent reported ever having been diagnosed with depression, up from 10 percent in 2000. Of those diagnosed with depression, 28 percent were currently in therapy for depression, and 38 percent were taking medication for depression. Roughly 40 percent of men and 50 percent of women reported debilitating incidences of depression.[46] [See Student Snapshot: "Depression on Campus."]

Researchers at the University of Michigan have identified three key contributors to depression in college students: stress, substance abuse, and sleep loss. As they adjust to campus life, undergraduates face the ongoing stress of forging a new identity and finding a place for themselves in various social hierarchies. This triggers the release of the so-called stress hormones (discussed in Chapter 4), which can change brain activity. Drugs and alcohol, widely used on campus, also affect the brain in ways that make stress even harder to manage. Too little sleep adds another ingredient to this dangerous brew. Computers, the Internet, around-the-clock cable television, and the college tradition of pulling all-nighters can conspire to sabotage rest and increase vulnerability to depression.[47]

TABLE 3-2 MENTAL DISORDERS IN THE UNITED STATES

Disorder	18- to 29-Year-Olds	All Adults
Any mental disorder	52%	46%
Anxiety disorders	30%	29%
Impulse control disorders	27%	25%
Mood disorders	21%	21%
Substance abuse disorders	17%	15%

Source: Kessler, Ronald, et al. "Lifetime Prevalence and Age-of-Onset Distributions of *DSM-IV* Disorders in the National Comorbidity Survey Replication." *Archives of General Psychiatry,* Vol. 62, No. 6, June 2005, p. 593.

Student Snapshot

DEPRESSION ON CAMPUS

Felt so depressed it was difficult to function (1 to 10 times)
40.4%
32.8%

Diagnosed with depression
15.7%
8.5%

Treated for depression in last year
6.1%
3.3%

Taking medication for depression
6.6%
3.0%

Currently in therapy
4.4%
2.2%

0   10   20   30   40   50

■ Women   ■ Men

Based on a survey of a random sample of 19,497 students by the American College Health Association.
Source: ACHA–National College Health Assessment, www.acha.org.

According to a Kansas State study of students who sought counseling over a 13-year period, the percentage of students with depression doubled, as did the percentage with suicidal thoughts. Among students who sought counseling at the beginning of the study, trouble with dating and other relationships were reported most frequently. Over the years of the study, stress and anxiety became more common than relationship difficulties.[48]

In a sample of Canadian freshmen, those who maintained or increased their levels of physical activity in their first months of college reported greater levels of vigor and less fatigue and tension than those who exercised less than before.[49]

 The few studies that have looked into ethnic differences in psychological health have yielded conflicting or inconclusive results: Some found no differences; others suggested higher rates of depression among Korean and South Asian students.

THE MIND-BODY CONNECTION

According to a growing number of studies, mental attitude may be just as important a risk factor for certain diseases as age, race, gender, education, habits, and health history.[50] Positive states like happiness and optimism have been linked with longer lifespans as well as lower risk of cardiovascular and lung disease, stroke, diabetes, colds, and upper respiratory infections. Mental disorders, on the other hand,

can undermine physical well-being. **Anxiety** can lead to intensified asthmatic reactions, skin conditions, and digestive disorders. Stress can play a role in hypertension, heart attacks, sudden cardiac death, and immune disorders in the young as well as in older individuals.

Depression has increasingly been recognized as a serious risk factor for physical illness. According to a review of large-scale studies on depression, of more than 36,000 men and women, depressed individuals were up to four times more likely to develop heart problems.[51] In still unknown ways, depression may increase risk factors for heart disease, such as high blood pressure, and for premature death. Together, depression and heart disease worsen a patient's prognosis more than either condition alone. One in five patients hospitalized for a heart attack suffers from major depression, and they are three times more likely to die from a future heart problem.[52]

Major depression is associated with lower bone density in young men, but not in women.[53] A history of depression increases the risk of physical problems such as headache and shoulder and neck pain in women as they reach middle age.[54]

IS EXERCISE A GOOD TREATMENT FOR PSYCHOLOGICAL PROBLEMS?

Imagine a drug so powerful it can alter brain chemistry, so versatile it can help prevent or treat many common mental disorders, so safe that moderate doses cause few, if any, side effects, and so inexpensive that anyone can afford it. This wonder drug, proved in years of research, is exercise.

In addition to its head-to-toe physical benefits, discussed in Chapter 5, exercise may be, as one therapist puts it, the single most effective way to lift a person's spirits and to restore feelings of potency about all aspects of life. People who exercise regularly report a more cheerful mood, higher self-esteem, and less stress. Their sleep and appetite also tend to improve. In clinical studies, exercise has proved effective as a treatment for depression and anxiety disorders.[55] But remember: Although exercise can help prevent and ease problems for many people, it's no substitute for professional treatment of serious psychiatric disorders.

DEPRESSIVE DISORDERS

Depression, the world's most common mental ailment, affects the brain, the mind, and the body in complex ways. An estimated 16.2 percent of adults experience depression at some point in their lives, according to a recent national survey. After a single episode, the risk of a recurrence, or second episode, is about 50 percent. After a third, the risk of a fourth is about 90 percent. Stress-related events may trigger half of all depressive episodes; great trauma in childhood can increase vulnerability to depression later in life.

In a study of young adults ages 18 to 23, those who'd experienced the most adversity were at greatest risk of depression or an anxiety disorder.[56] An estimated 15 to 40 percent of college-age men and women (18- to 24-year-olds) may develop depression. Over a four-year period, depression increased 4.6 percent among college students.[57] Medical students also have higher rates of depression than the general population, but only about a quarter receive treatment.[58]

(FAQ) WHY ARE SO MANY YOUNG PEOPLE DEPRESSED?

Once young people were considered immune to sadness. Now mental health professionals know better. An estimated 5 to 10 percent of American teenagers suffer from a serious depressive disorder; girls are twice as susceptible as boys. Prior to puberty, girls and boys are equally likely to develop depression.

The risks of depression in the young are high. Four in ten depressed adolescents think about killing themselves; two in ten actually try to do so. Every year an estimated 11 to 13 in every 100,000 teens take their own lives, twice as many as the number who die from all natural causes combined.

"Depression is the most common emotional problem in adolescence and the single greatest risk factor for teen suicide," says child psychiatrist Peter Jensen, M.D., director for the Center for the Advancement of Children's Mental Health at Columbia University, who notes that depression rates have been rising over the last half century. "Teens born in the 1980s are more likely to develop depression than those who were born in the 1970s, whose rate of depression is higher than for those born in the 1960s."[59]

No one knows the reason for this steady surge in sadness, but experts point to the breakdown of families, the pressures of the information age, and increased isolation. A family history of depression greatly increases a young person's vulnerability. A mother's anxiety and depression during early childhood can increase the risk that adolescents will develop symptoms of anxiety and depression.[60]

However, the strongest predictor of depression is cigarette smoking. Depressed teens may smoke because they think smoking will make them feel better, but nicotine alters brain chemistry and actually worsens symptoms of depression.

 The link between tobacco and depression continues during college. Students who had been diagnosed with or treated for depression were 7.5 times as likely as other students to use tobacco, possibly because of nicotine's stimulating effects.[61] In another study of college smokers, young women with symptoms of depression and those who did not feel connected with a peer group were more likely to smoke.[62]

Depression can be hard to recognize in the young, who may not look or act sad. Rather than crying, they may snap grouchily at parents or burst into angry tirades. Some turn to alcohol or drugs in hopes of feeling better; others become depressed after they start abusing these substances. As they drop out of activities and pull away from friends, depressed teens spend more time alone. Their schoolwork suffers, and many are labeled as underachievers. Those whose anger explodes in public are branded as troublemakers.

Only in the last decade have researchers in mental health specifically studied treatments for teen depression. They now know that 60 to 75 percent of teenagers—the same percentage as adults—respond to treatment with the medications called SSRIs (a group of antidepressants that includes Prozac and Paxil). The use of these antidepressants in children and teenagers has increased three- to fivefold in recent years, but there is controversy over a potential increase in the risk of suicide (discussed later in this chapter).

According to a landmark study of therapies for depression in adolescents, the most effective treatment is a combination of antidepressant medication and cognitive-behavioral therapy (CBT), which teaches problem-solving skills and ways to change negative thinking (discussed later in this chapter).

GENDER AND DEPRESSION

Female Depression

 Depression is twice as common in women as men, a gender gap found through most of the world.[63] Some have argued that women are simply more willing than men to admit to being depressed or more likely to seek help. But even when these factors are accounted for, the sex difference persists. Others contend that men in distress drown their problems in alcohol rather than becoming sad,

Factors that can contribute to the development of depression in college include stressful events, poor academic performance, loneliness, and relationship problems.

Ranald Mackechnie/The Image Bank/Getty Images

tearful, and hopeless. In studies of the Amish, who prohibit alcohol use, and of Jewish Americans, who also drink less than other groups, women and men are equally likely to develop depression. Yet these data do not mean that fewer women among teetotalers become depressed but that more men do.

Genes may make both men and women more vulnerable to depression. Brain chemistry and sex hormones also may play a role. Women produce less of certain metabolites of serotonin, a messenger chemical that helps regulate mood. Their brains also register sadness much more intensely than men's, and they are more sensitive to changes in light and temperature. Women are at least four times more likely than men to develop seasonal affective disorder (SAD) and to become depressed in the dark winter months. Some women also seem more sensitive to their own hormones or to the changes in them that occur at puberty, during the menstrual cycle, after childbirth, or during perimenopause and menopause.

Childhood abuse also contributes to female vulnerability. In epidemiological studies, 60 percent of women diagnosed with depression—compared with 39 percent of men—were abused as children. In adulthood, relationships may protect women from depression, while a lack of social support increases vulnerability to depression.[64] Women with at least one "confiding relationship," as researchers put it, are physically and psychologically more resilient.

Male Depression

More than six million men in the United States—one in every 14—suffer from this insidious disorder, many without recognizing what's wrong. Experts describe male depression as an "under" disease: underdiscussed, underrecognized, underdiagnosed, and undertreated.

Depression "looks" different in men than women. Rather than becoming sad, men may be irritable or tremendously fatigued. They feel a sense of being dead inside, of worthlessness, hopelessness, helplessness, of losing their life force. Physical symptoms, such as headaches, pain, and insomnia, are common, as are attempts to "self-medicate" with alcohol or drugs.

Genes may make some men more vulnerable, but chronic stress of any sort plays a major role in male depression, possibly by raising levels of cortisol, a stress hormone, and lowering testosterone. Men also are more likely than women to become depressed following divorce, job loss, or a career setback. Whatever its roots, depression alters brain chemistry in potentially deadly ways.

Four times as many men as women kill themselves; depressed men are two to four times more likely to take their own lives than depressed women. "We lose almost twice as many lives to suicide as to homicide—30,000 a year, compared to 18,000 murders," says Thomas Insel, M.D., director of the National Institute of Mental Health. "The unspeakable, relentless agony of untreated depression may make suicide seem the only way out."

MINOR DEPRESSION

Minor depression is a common disorder that is often unrecognized and untreated, affecting about 7.5 percent of Americans during their lifetime. Its symptoms are the same as those of major depression, but less severe and fewer in number. They include either a depressed mood most of the day, nearly every day, or diminished interest or pleasure in daily activities.

Psychotherapy is remarkably effective for mild depression. In more serious cases, antidepressant medication can lead to dramatic improvement in 40 to 80 percent of depressed patients. Exercise also works—several studies have shown that exercise effectively lifts mild to moderate depression.

MAJOR DEPRESSION

The simplest definition of **major depression** is sadness that does not end. The incidence of major depression has soared over the last two decades, especially among young adults. Major depression can destroy a person's joy for living. Food, friends, sex, or any form of pleasure no longer appeals. It is impossible to concentrate on work and responsibilities. Unable to escape a sense of utter hopelessness, depressed individuals may fight back tears throughout the day and toss and turn through long, empty nights. Thoughts of death or suicide may push into their minds.

The characteristic symptoms of major depression include:

- **Feeling depressed,** sad, empty, discouraged, tearful.
- **Loss of interest** or pleasure in once-enjoyable activities.
- **Eating more or less** than usual and either gaining or losing weight.
- **Having trouble sleeping** or sleeping much more than usual.
- **Feeling slowed down** or restless and unable to sit still.
- **Lack of energy.**
- **Feeling helpless,** hopeless, worthless, inadequate.
- **Difficulty concentrating,** forgetfulness.
- **Difficulty thinking clearly** or making decisions.
- **Persistent thoughts of death** or suicide.
- **Withdrawal from others,** lack of interest in sex.
- **Physical symptoms** (headaches, digestive problems, aches and pains).

As many as half of major depressive episodes are not recognized because the symptoms are "masked." Rather than feeling sad or depressed, individuals may experience low energy, insomnia, difficulty concentrating, and physical symptoms. An episode of major depression can trigger a relapse in individuals with substance abuse problems.

TREATING DEPRESSION

Treatment with psychotherapy, medication, or both relieves depression for 80 percent of sufferers—yet only half of those with depression seek help and only 10 to 15 percent get optimal care.

Psychotherapy helps individuals pinpoint the life problems that contribute to their depression, identify negative or distorted thinking patterns, explore behaviors that contribute to depression, and regain a sense of control and pleasure in life. Two specific psychotherapies—cognitive-behavioral therapy and interpersonal therapy (described later in this chapter)—have proved as helpful as antidepressant drugs, although they take longer than medication to achieve results.

Antidepressants help about 70 percent of individuals feel better within six to ten weeks. According to long-term studies, treatment should continue for at least nine months after a single acute episode of depression, longer for chronic or recurrent depression.

When either medication or psychotherapy fails to lift depression, switching from one to the other can be highly effective. Medications have proved effective for patients who did not recover with psychotherapy alone, and psychotherapy can help those who do not benefit from medication alone.[65]

Exercise also has proved beneficial in both the short- and long-term for both men and women. Although walking and jogging have been studied most extensively, all forms of exercise decrease depression to some degree. The greater the length of the exercise program and the larger the total number of sessions, the greater the decrease in depression.

For individuals who cannot take antidepressant medications because of medical problems, or who do not improve with psychotherapy or drugs, *electroconvulsive therapy* (ECT)—the administration of a controlled electrical current through electrodes attached to the scalp—remains the safest and most effective treatment. About 50 percent of depressed individuals who do not get better with antidepressant medication and psychotherapy improve after ECT. Experimental new techniques are using electrical and magnetic stimulation to treat depression.

Even without treatment, depression generally lifts after six to nine months. However, in more than 80 percent of people, it recurs, with each episode lasting longer and becoming more severe and difficult to treat. "All the while the depression goes untreated, it is causing ongoing damage that shrivels important regions of the brain" says John Greden, M.D., director of the University of Michigan Depression Center. "The exciting news is that, as brain scans show, treatment turns the destructive process around and stops depression in its tracks."[66]

If a loved one is depressed:

- **Express your concern,** but don't nag. You might say: "I'm concerned about you. You are struggling right now. We need to find some help."
- **Don't be distracted** by behaviors like drinking or gambling, which can disguise depression in men.

- **Encourage the individual to remain in treatment** until symptoms begin to lift (which takes several weeks).
- **Provide emotional support.** Listen carefully. Offer hope and reassurance that with time and treatment, things will get better.
- **Do not ignore remarks about suicide.** Report them to his or her doctor or, in an emergency, call 911.

(FAQ) ARE ANTIDEPRESSANTS DANGEROUS?

Millions of individuals have benefited from the category of drugs called selective serotonin reuptake inhibitors (SSRIs) over the last two decades. However, like all drugs, they can cause side effects that range from temporary physical symptoms, such as stomach upset and headaches, to more persistent problems, such as sexual dysfunction. The most serious—and controversial—risk is suicide.

Although studies have showed varying results, they generally indicate that, compared with a placebo, all antidepressants, including the SSRIs, seem to double the risk of suicidal thinking, from 1 to 2 percent to 2 to 4 percent in both children and adults.[67] The FDA has issued a "black box" warning about the risk of suicidal thoughts, hostility, and aggression in both children and adults.[68] The danger is greatest just after pill use begins, before depression is really alleviated but when some patients experience more energy and agitation and may be more likely to act on suicidal tendencies.

The debate continues, however, because of the complexity of the problem. Depression itself can be fatal: The lifetime suicide rate for people with major depression is 15 percent, and depression increases the risk of heart disease and other serious illnesses. While the use of SSRIs in adolescents soared in the 1990s, the suicide rate declined. Only 20 percent of teenagers who take their own lives have ever taken an antidepressant.[69]

In every case, physicians have to weigh the potential benefits of antidepressant medication against the possible risks. Both adults and children taking antidepressants should be watched closely for a worsening of depression or an increase in suicidal thoughts, particularly when medications are started for the first time or the dose is changed.

BIPOLAR DISORDER (MANIC DEPRESSION)

Bipolar disorder, or manic depression, consists of mood swings that may take individuals from *manic* states of feeling euphoric and energetic to depressive states of utter despair. In episodes of full mania, they may become so impulsive and out of touch with reality that they endanger their careers, relationships, health, or even survival. One percent of the population—about 2 million American adults—suffer from this serious but treatable disorder. Men tend to develop bipolar disorder earlier in life (between ages 16 to 25), but women have higher rates overall.[70] About 50 percent of patients with bipolar illness have a family history of the disorder.

The characteristic symptoms of bipolar disorder include:

- **Mood swings** (from happy to miserable, optimistic to despairing, and so on).
- **Changes in thinking** (thoughts speeding through one's mind, unrealistic self-confidence, difficulty concentrating, delusions, hallucinations).
- **Changes in behavior** (sudden immersion in plans and projects, talking very rapidly and much more than usual, excessive spending, impaired judgment, impulsive sexual involvement).
- **Changes in physical condition** (less need for sleep, increased energy, fewer health complaints than usual).

During "manic" periods, individuals may make grandiose plans or take dangerous risks. But they often plunge from this highest of highs to a horrible low depressive episode, in which they may feel sad, hopeless, and helpless and develop other symptoms of major depression. The risk of suicide is very real.

Professional therapy is essential in treating bipolar disorders. Mood-stabilizing medications are the keystone of treatment, although psychotherapy plays a critical role in helping individuals understand their illness and rebuild their lives. Most individuals continue taking medication indefinitely after remission of their symptoms because the risk of recurrence is high.

ANXIETY DISORDERS

Anxiety disorders may involve inordinate fears of certain objects or situations (**phobias**), episodes of sudden, inexplicable terror (**panic attacks**), chronic distress (**generalized anxiety disorder, or GAD**), or persistent, disturbing thoughts and behaviors (**obsessive-compulsive disorder**). These disorders can increase the risk of developing depression. Over a lifetime, as many as one in four Americans may experience an anxiety disorder. Only one of every four of these individuals is ever correctly diagnosed and treated. Yet most who do get treatment, even for severe and disabling problems, improve dramatically.[71]

PHOBIAS

Phobias—the most prevalent type of anxiety disorder—are out-of-the-ordinary, irrational, intense, persistent fears of certain objects or situations. About two million Americans develop such acute terror that they go to extremes to avoid whatever it is that they fear, even though they realize that these feelings are excessive or unreasonable. The most common phobias involve animals, particularly dogs, snakes,

insects, and mice; the sight of blood; closed spaces (*claustrophobia*); heights (*acrophobia*); air travel and being in places or situations from which one perceives it would be difficult or embarrassing to escape (*agoraphobia*).

Although various medications have been tried, none is effective by itself in relieving phobias. The best approach is behavioral therapy, which consists of gradual, systematic exposure to the feared object (a process called *systematic desensitization*). Numerous studies have proved that exposure—especially in vivo exposure, in which individuals are exposed to the actual source of their fear rather than simply imagining it—is highly effective. Medical hypnosis—the use of induction of an altered state of consciousness—also can help.[72]

PANIC ATTACKS AND PANIC DISORDER

Individuals who have had panic attacks describe them as the most frightening experiences of their lives. Without reason or warning, their hearts race wildly. They may become light-headed or dizzy. Because they can't catch their breath, they may start breathing rapidly and hyperventilate. Parts of their bodies, such as their fingers or toes, may tingle or feel numb. Worst of all is the terrible sense that something horrible is about to happen: that they will die, lose their minds, or have a heart attack. Most attacks reach peak intensity within ten minutes. Afterward, individuals live in dread of another one. In the course of a lifetime, your risk of having a single panic attack is 7.2 percent.

Panic disorder develops when attacks recur or apprehension about them becomes so intense that individuals cannot function normally. Full-blown panic disorder occurs in about 1.6 percent of all adults in the course of a lifetime and usually develops before age 30. Women are more than twice as likely as men to experience panic attacks, although no one knows why. Parents, siblings, and children of individuals with panic disorders also are more likely to develop them than are others.

The two primary treatments for panic disorder are (1) cognitive-behavioral therapy, which teaches specific strategies for coping with symptoms like rapid breathing, and (2) medication. Treatment helps as many as 90 percent of those with panic disorder either improve significantly or recover completely, usually within six to eight weeks. Individuals who receive cognitive-behavior therapy as well as medication are less likely to suffer relapses than those taking medication alone and often can learn to control their symptoms without drugs.

GENERALIZED ANXIETY DISORDER

About 10 million adults in the United States suffer from a generalized anxiety disorder (GAD), excessive or unrealistic apprehension that causes physical symptoms and lasts for six months or longer. It usually starts when people are in their twenties. Unlike fear, which helps us recognize and avoid real danger, GAD is an irrational or unwarranted response to harmless objects or situations of exaggerated danger. The most common symptoms are faster heart rate, sweating, increased blood pressure, muscle aches, intestinal pains, irritability, sleep problems, and difficulty concentrating.

Chronically anxious individuals worry—not just some of the time, and not just about the stresses and strains of ordinary life—but constantly, about almost everything: their health, families, finances, marriages, potential dangers. Treatment for GAD may consist of a combination of psychotherapy, behavioral therapy, and antianxiety drugs.

OBSESSIVE-COMPULSIVE DISORDER

As many as 1 in 40 Americans has a type of anxiety called obsessive-compulsive disorder (OCD). Some of these individuals suffer only from an *obsession,* a recurring idea, thought, or image that they realize, at least initially, is senseless. The most common obsessions are repetitive thoughts of violence (for example, killing a child), contamination (becoming infected by shaking hands), and doubt (wondering whether one has performed some act, such as having hurt someone in a traffic accident). Most people with OCD also suffer from a compulsion, repetitive behavior performed according to certain rules or in a stereotyped fashion. The most common compulsions involve handwashing, cleaning, hoarding useless items, counting, or checking (for example, making sure dozens of times that a door is locked).

Individuals with OCD realize that their thoughts or behaviors are bizarre, but they cannot resist or control them. Eventually, the obsessions or compulsions consume a great deal of time and significantly interfere with normal routines, job functioning, or usual social activities or relationships with others. A young woman who must follow a very rigid dressing routine may always be late for class, for example; a student who must count each letter of the alphabet as he types may not be able to complete a term paper.

Treatment may consist of cognitive therapy to correct irrational assumptions, behavioral techniques such as progressively limiting the amount of time someone obsessed with cleanliness can spend washing and scrubbing, and medication. About 70 to 80 percent of those with OCD improve with treatment.

ATTENTION DISORDERS

Attention-deficit/hyperactivity disorder (ADHD) is the most common mental disorder in childhood. About 10 percent of boys and 5 percent of girls between ages 5 to 18 suffer from ADHD.[73] Contrary to previous beliefs, most children do not outgrow it. For as many as 65 percent of youngsters, ADHD persists into adolescence and young adulthood. Among adults, 4 to 5 percent may have ADHD.[74]

ADHD looks and feels different in adults. Hyperactivity is more subtle, an internal fidgety feeling rather than a physical restlessness. As youngsters with ADHD mature, academic difficulties become much more of a problem. Students with ADHD may find it hard to concentrate, read, make decisions, complete complex projects, and meet deadlines. Relationships with peers also can become more challenging. Young people with ADHD may become frustrated easily, have a short fuse, and erupt into angry outbursts. Some become more argumentative, negative, and defiant than most other teens. Sleep problems, including sleeping much more or less than normal, are common. The likelihood of developing other emotional problems, including depression and anxiety disorders, is higher. As many as 20 percent of those diagnosed with depression, anxiety, or substance abuse also have ADHD.[75]

The risk of substance use disorders for individuals with ADHD is twice that of the general population. According to several reports, between 15 and 25 percent of adults with substance use disorders have ADHD. In addition, individuals with ADHD start smoking at a younger age and have higher rates of smoking and drinking. (The use of stimulant medication to treat ADHD does not increase the risk of substance abuse.)[76]

The medications most often used for this disorder are stimulants (such as Ritalin), which improve behavior and cognition for about 70 percent of adolescents. Thanks to extended-release preparations, which are longer acting, individuals do not have to take these medications as often as in the past. As discussed in Chapter 11, abuse of prescription stimulants by students without ADHD is a growing problem on college campuses. In one recent report, 8 percent of students reported using prescription stimulants in their lifetime; 5 percent in the last year. Their primary motivations were to stay awake or feel more energetic or to get high.[77]

An alternative nonstimulant treatment is Strattera (atomoxetine), which treats ADHD and co-existing problems such as depression and anxiety. Its effects are more gradual, and it does not seem to have any known potential for abuse. Adverse effects include drowsiness, loss of appetite, nausea, vomiting, and headaches. Its long-term effects are not known.

Psychological therapies have not been studied extensively in adolescents and young adults with ADHD. College health services may provide support for individuals who are enrolled in college, but health insurance coverage for ADHD treatment is limited. Because the median costs of health care for individuals with ADHD are twice those for individuals without this disorder, obtaining private health insurance on their own before they are employed full time is difficult.

 An estimated 1 percent of college students have an attention disorder that can have a significant impact on their academic performance and personal lives. Pediatricians caution undergraduates with ADHD that they are at higher risk of becoming smokers, of abusing alcohol and drugs, and of having automobile accidents. The normal challenges of college, including navigating the complexities of scheduling, course planning, and acquiring study skills, also may be especially daunting. If you have ADHD, check with your student health or counseling center to see if any special services are available.

SCHIZOPHRENIA

Schizophrenia, one of the most debilitating mental disorders, profoundly impairs an individual's sense of reality. As the National Institute of Mental Health (NIMH) puts it, schizophrenia, which is characterized by abnormalities in brain structure and chemistry, destroys "the inner unity of the mind" and weakens "the will and drive that constitute our essential character." It affects every aspect of psychological functioning, including the ways in which people think, feel, view themselves, and relate to others.

The symptoms of schizophrenia include:

- **Hallucinations.**
- **Delusions.**
- **Inability to think** in a logical manner.
- **Talking** in rambling or incoherent ways.
- **Making odd or purposeless movements** or not moving at all.
- **Repeating others' words** or mimicking their gestures.
- **Showing few, if any, feelings;** responding with inappropriate emotions.
- **Lacking will or motivation** to complete a task or accomplish something.
- **Functioning at a much lower level** than in the past at work, in interpersonal relations, or in taking care of themselves.

Individuals with schizophrenia may hear, see, or feel things that do not exist—a voice telling them to jump from a bridge, a statue crying tears of blood, a spaceship beaming a light upon them. Frightened and vulnerable, they may devote all their energy to warding off the demons within. Unable to take care of themselves, they may look messy and disheveled. They often move in unusual ways, such as rocking or pacing, or repeat certain gestures again and again. They may believe that someone or something, such as the devil, is putting thoughts into their heads or controlling their actions. Some think they are reincarnations of Christ or Napoleon. About a third attempt to take their own lives, often in response to a command they hear inside their heads. Researchers have identified early markers of schizophrenia, including impaired social skills, intellectual ability, and capacity for organization.

Schizophrenia is one of the leading causes of disability among young adults. The mean age for schizophrenia to develop is 21.4 years for men and 26.8 years for women. Although symptoms do not occur until then, they are almost certainly the result of a failure in brain development that occurs very early in life. The underlying defect is probably present before birth. Schizophrenia has a strong genetic

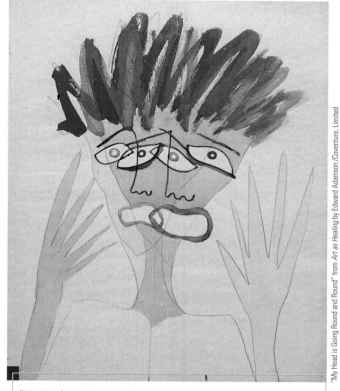

"My Head is Going Round and Round." This drawing by a patient suffering from schizophrenia expresses the anxiety and agitation that may occur with this brain abnormality.

basis and is not the result of upbringing, social conditions, or traumatic experiences.

For the vast majority of individuals with schizophrenia, antipsychotic drugs are the foundation of treatment. They make most people with schizophrenia feel more comfortable and in control of themselves, help organize chaotic thinking, and reduce or eliminate delusions or hallucinations, allowing fuller participation in normal activities. Those who do not improve significantly on medication almost invariably do even worse without it.

SUICIDE

Suicide is not in itself a psychiatric disorder, but it can be the tragic consequence of emotional and psychological problems. Every year 30,000 Americans—among them many young people who seem to have "everything to live for"—commit suicide. An estimated 752,000 attempt to take their own lives; there may be 4.5 million suicide "survivors" in the United States.

 The suicide rate for African-American and Caucasian men peaks between ages 20 and 40. It rises again after age 65 among white men and after age 75 among blacks. In general, whites are at highest risk for suicide, followed by Native Americans, African Americans, Hispanic Americans, and Asian Americans. Internationally,

TABLE 3-3 SUICIDE RISK

	Who attempts suicide?	Who completes suicide?
Sex	Female	Male
Age	Under 35	Under 20 or over 60
Means	Less deadly, such as wrist slashing	More deadly, such as a gun
Circumstances	High chance of rescue	Low chance of rescue

suicide rates are highest in Germany, Scandinavia, Eastern Europe, and Japan, average in the United States, Canada, and Great Britain, and low in Italy, Spain, and Ireland.

At all ages, men *commit* suicide three times more frequently than women, but women *attempt* suicide much more often than men (Table 3-3). Elderly men are ten times more likely to take their own lives than older women.

SUICIDE IN THE YOUNG

Although rates have declined in the last decade, suicide remains the third leading cause of death among children and adolescents 10 to 19 years old in the United States. An estimated 500,000 U.S. teens attempt suicide every year. Almost 2,000 die.[78]

Suicide is also the second-leading cause of death among college-aged Americans.[79] Males in this age group have a suicide rate six times greater than that of females. Participation in sports seems to have a protective effect and decreases the odds of suicide among male and female college students.

One-half of the adolescents who take their own lives suffer from major depression. "In psychological interviews after a teen suicide, we see that the warning signs were there," child psychiatrist Madelyn Gould, M.D., of Columbia University, notes, "but no one realized the underlying problem was depression."[80]

Native American communities have especially high rates of suicide among both young men and women. Young African-American men, historically at low suicide risk, are narrowing the gap with their white peers, while suicide by Hispanic young men has declined. The lowest rates are for Asian Pacific males and African-American females.[81]

Firearms and suffocation (mainly by hanging) are the most common methods of suicide among young people. In recent years, deaths with firearms have decreased, in part because of laws restricting access to guns by youngsters.[82] However, deaths by hanging have increased, particularly among younger teens.

Researchers also have identified factors that protect young people from suicide. Number one for both boys and girls was feeling connected to their parents and family. For girls, emotional well-being was also protective; grade point average was an additional protective factor for boys. High parental expectations for their child's school achievement,

more people living in the household, and religiosity were protective for some of the boys, but not for the girls. Availability of counseling services at school and parental presence at key times during the day were protective for some of the girls, but not for the boys.

Suicide is not inevitable. Appropriate treatment can help as many as 70 to 80 percent of those at risk for suicide. Among young people, early recognition and treatment for depressive disorders and alcohol and drug use could save thousands of lives each year.

(FAQ) WHAT LEADS TO SUICIDE?

Researchers have looked for explanations for suicide by studying everything from phases of the moon to seasons (suicides peak in the spring and early summer) to birth order in the family. They have found no conclusive answers. A constellation of influences—mental disorders, personality traits, biologic and genetic vulnerability, medical illness, and psychosocial stressors—may combine in ways that lower an individual's threshold of vulnerability. The risk of suicide is higher in people who live in cities, are single, have a low income, or are unemployed. No one factor in itself may ever explain fully why a person chooses death.

Mental Disorders More than 95 percent of those who commit suicide have a mental disorder. Two in particular—depression and alcoholism—account for two-thirds of all suicides. Suicide also is a risk for those with other disorders, including schizophrenia, posttraumatic stress disorder, and personality disorders.

Antidepressant Medications As the FDA has warned, antidepressants can increase the risk of suicidal thoughts and attempts. Recent studies have confirmed an increase in suicide attempts in some individuals, including adolescents, during the first four weeks of treatment, especially the first nine days, with various antidepressants, including Prozac and Paxil.[83] Because depression itself increases the danger of suicide, psychiatrists contend that the benefits of treatment outweigh the risk but call for increased monitoring for increased agitation or suicidal thoughts.

Substance Abuse Many of those who commit suicide drink beforehand, and their use of alcohol may lower their inhibitions. Since alcohol itself is a depressant, it can intensify the despondency suicidal individuals are already feeling. Alcoholics who attempt suicide often have other risk factors, including major depression, poor social support, serious medical illness, and unemployment. Drugs of abuse also can alter thinking and lower inhibitions against suicide.

Hopelessness The sense of utter hopelessness and helplessness may be the most common contributing factor in suicide. When hope dies, individuals view every experience in negative terms and come to expect the worst possible outcomes for their problems. Given this way of thinking, suicide often seems a reasonable response to a life seen as not worth living.

Family History One of every four people who attempt suicide has a family member who also tried to commit suicide. While a family history of suicide is not in itself considered a predictor of suicide, two mental disorders that can lead to suicide—depression and bipolar disorder (manic depression)—do run in families.

Physical Illness People who commit suicide are likely to be ill or to believe that they are. About 5 percent actually have a serious physical disorder, such as AIDS or cancer. While suicide may seem to be a decision rationally arrived at in persons with serious or fatal illness, this may not be the case. Depression, not uncommon in such instances, can warp judgment. When the depression is treated, the person may no longer have suicidal intentions.

Brain Chemistry Investigators have found abnormalities in the brain chemistry of individuals who complete suicide, especially low levels of a metabolite of the neurotransmitter serotonin. There are indications that individuals with a deficiency in this substance may have as much as a ten times greater risk of committing suicide than those with higher levels.

Access to Guns For individuals already facing a combination of predisposing factors, access to a means of committing suicide, particularly to guns, can add to the risk. Unlike other methods of suicide, guns almost always work. States with stricter gun-control laws have much lower rates of suicides than states with more lenient laws. Health professionals are urging parents whose children undergo psychological treatment or assessment to remove all weapons from their homes and to make sure their youngsters do not have access to potentially lethal medications or to alcohol.

Other Factors Individuals who kill themselves often have gone through more major life crises—job changes, births, financial reversals, divorce, retirement—in the previous six months, compared with others. Long-standing, intense conflict with family members or other important people may add to the danger. In some cases, suicide may be an act of revenge that offers the person a sense of control—however

temporary or illusory. For example, a husband whose wife has had an affair may rationalize that he can get back at her, and have the final word, by killing himself. Others may feel that, by rejecting life, they are rejecting a partner or parent who abandoned or betrayed them.

SUICIDE PREVENTION

If someone you know has talked about suicide, behaved unpredictably, or suddenly emerged from a severe depression into a calm, settled state of mind, don't rule out the possibility that he or she may attempt suicide.

:: **Encourage your friend to talk.** Ask concerned questions. Listen attentively. Show that you take the person's feelings seriously and truly care.

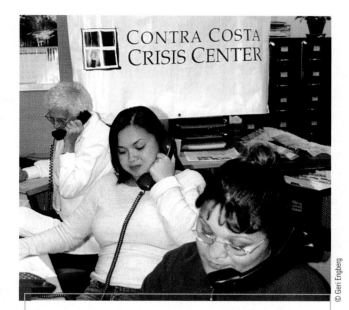

About 20 percent of teenagers seriously consider suicide; a much smaller number actually attempt to take their own lives. Talking to a counselor at a suicide hot line may help a young person deal with feelings of despondency.

Strategies for Prevention :: If You Start Thinking About Suicide

At some point, the thought of ending it all—the disappointments, problems, bad feelings—may cross your mind. This experience isn't unusual. But if the idea of taking your life persists or intensifies, you should respond as you would to other warnings of potential threats to your health—by getting the help you need:

:: Talk to a mental health professional. If you have a therapist, call immediately. If not, call a suicide hot line.

:: Find someone you can trust and talk honestly about what you're feeling. If you suffer from depression or another mental disorder, educate trusted friends or relatives about your condition so they are prepared if called upon to help.

:: Write down your more uplifting thoughts. Even if you are despondent, you can help yourself by taking the time to retrieve some more positive thoughts or memories. A simple record of your hopes for the future and the

people you value in your life can remind you of why your own life is worth continuing.

:: Avoid drugs and alcohol. Most suicides are the results of sudden, uncontrolled impulses, and drugs and alcohol can make it harder to resist these destructive urges.

:: Go to the hospital. Hospitalization can sometimes be the best way to protect your health and safety.

▪ **Don't offer trite reassurances.** List reasons to go on living, try to analyze the person's motives, or try to shock or challenge him or her.

▪ **Suggest solutions or alternatives** to problems. Make plans. Encourage positive action, such as getting away for a while to gain a better perspective on a problem.

▪ **Don't be afraid to ask** whether your friend has considered suicide. The opportunity to talk about thoughts of suicide may be an enormous relief and—contrary to a long-standing myth—will not fix the idea of suicide more firmly in a person's mind.

▪ **Don't think that people who talk** about killing themselves never carry out their threat. Most individuals who commit suicide give definite indications of their intent to die.

OVERCOMING PROBLEMS OF THE MIND

Mental illness costs our society an estimated $150 billion a year in lost work time and productivity, employee turnover, disability payments, and death. Yet many Americans do not have access to mental health services, nor do they have insurance for such services. Despite the fact that treatments for mental disorders have a higher success rate than those for many other diseases, employers often restrict mental health benefits. HMOs and health insurance plans are much more likely to limit psychotherapy visits and psychiatric hospitalizations than treatments for medical illnesses.

Even when cost is not a barrier, many people do not seek treatment because they see psychological problems as a sign of weakness rather than illness. They also may not realize that scientifically proven therapies can bring relief, often in a matter of weeks or months.

According to a national survey, 60 percent of those with a mental disorder got no treatment at all over a one-year period. Primary care or other medical doctors provided care to about 23 percent of those who did seek help; 16 percent saw psychologists, social workers, or other counselors; psychiatrists cared for 12 percent. About 10 percent turned to a nonprofessional counselor or spiritual advisor; 7 percent tried a complementary or alternative source, such as a self-help group.[84]

 Because an individual's perception of a problem is "culture-specific"—that is, influenced by his or her cultural, social, and religious beliefs—immigrants to the United States may treat symptoms of psychological distress in different ways. For instance, Asian-American college students tend to seek medical care for physical symptoms, such as aches, pains, or sleep problems, but forgo counseling for a mental disorder, because it is more appropriate in their native cultures to do so.

WHERE CAN I TURN FOR HELP?

As a student, your best contact for identifying local services may be your health education instructor or department. The health instructors can tell you about general and mental health counseling available on campus, school-based support groups, community-based programs, and special emergency services. On campus, you can also turn to the student health services or the office of the dean of student services or student affairs.

Within the community, you may be able to get help through the city or county health department and neighborhood health centers. Local hospitals often have special clinics and services; and there are usually local branches of national service organizations, such as United Way or Alcoholics Anonymous, other 12-step programs, and various support groups. You can call the psychiatric or psychological association in your city or state for the names of licensed professionals. (Check the telephone directory for listings.) Your primary physician may also be able to help.

The telephone book is also a good resource for special programs, often listed either by the nature of the service, by the name of the neighborhood or city, or by the name of the sponsoring group. In some places, the city's name may precede a listing: the New York City Suicide Hot Line, for instance. In addition to suicide-prevention programs, other listings usually include crisis intervention, violence prevention, and child-abuse prevention programs; drug-treatment information; shelters for battered women; senior citizen centers; and self-help and counseling services. Many services have special hot lines for coping with emergencies. Others provide information as well as counseling over the phone.

An increasing number of mental health professionals—primarily psychologists and marriage and family therapists—are offering "e-therapy" on the Internet. Online

© 2000 Tony Latham/Stone/Getty Images

When choosing a therapist, you should always consider the individual's education, title, and qualifications. Also important are qualities such as compassion and caring.

therapy is convenient, discrete, less costly (some therapists charge for their time or the number of questions a client asks), and may be helpful with relationship or work issues. However, there is no regulation of e-therapists, and mental health professionals warn that online counseling is inadequate for diagnosing or dealing with serious psychological problems.

TYPES OF THERAPISTS

Only professionally trained individuals who have met state licensing requirements are certified as psychiatrists, psychologists, or social workers. Before selecting any of these mental health professionals, be sure to check the person's background and credentials.

Psychiatrists are licensed medical doctors (M.D.) who complete medical school; a year-long internship; and a three-year residency that provides training in various forms of psychotherapy, psychopharmacology, and both outpatient and inpatient treatment of mental disorders. They can prescribe medications and make medical decisions. *Board-certified* psychiatrists have passed oral and written examinations following completion of residency training.

Psychologists complete a graduate program (including clinical training and internships) in human psychology but do not study medicine and cannot prescribe medication. They must be licensed in most states in order to practice independently.

Certified social workers or **licensed clinical social workers (LCSWs)** usually complete a two-year graduate program and have specialized training in helping people with mental problems in addition to conventional social work.

Psychiatric nurses have nursing degrees and have passed a state examination. They usually have special training and experience in mental health care, although no specialty licensing or certification is required.

Marriage and family therapists, licensed in some but not all states, usually have a graduate degree, often in psychology, and at least two years of supervised clinical training in dealing with relationship problems.

Other therapists include pastoral counselors, members of the clergy who offer psychological counseling; hypnotherapists, who use hypnosis for problems such as smoking and obesity; stress-management counselors, who teach relaxation methods; and alcohol and drug counselors, who help individuals with substance abuse problems. Anyone can use these terms to describe themselves professionally, and there are no licensing requirements.

TYPES OF THERAPY

The term **psychotherapy** refers to any type of counseling based on the exchange of words in the context of the unique relationship that develops between a mental health professional and a person seeking help. The process of talking and listening can lead to new insight, relief from distressing psychological symptoms, changes in unhealthy or maladaptive behaviors, and more effective ways of dealing with the world.

Most mental health professionals today are trained in a variety of psychotherapeutic techniques and tailor their approach to the problem, personality, and needs of each person seeking their help. Because skilled therapists may combine different techniques in the course of therapy, the lines between the various approaches often blur.

Because insurance companies and health-care plans often limit the duration of psychotherapy, many mental health professionals are adopting a *time-limited* format in order to make the most of every session, regardless of the length of treatment. Brief or short-term psychotherapy typically focuses on a central theme, problem, or topic and may continue for several weeks to several months. The individuals most likely to benefit are those who are interested in solving immediate problems rather than changing their characters, who can think in psychological terms, and who are motivated to change.

Psychodynamic Psychotherapy

For the most part, today's mental health professionals base their assessment of individuals on a **psychodynamic** understanding that takes into account the role of early experiences and unconscious influences in *actively* shaping behavior. (This is the *dynamic* in psychodynamic.) Psychodynamic treatments work toward the goal of providing greater insight into problems and bringing about behavioral change. Therapy may be brief, consisting of 12 to 25 sessions, or may continue for several years. According to current thinking, psychotherapy can actually rewire the network of neurons within the brain in ways that ease distress and improve functioning in many areas of daily life.

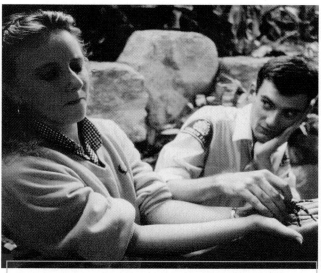

Systematic desensitization is one of the behavior therapies used in the treatment of phobias.

Cognitive-Behavioral Therapy

Cognitive-behavioral therapy (CBT) focuses on inappropriate or inaccurate thoughts or beliefs to help individuals break out of a distorted way of thinking. The techniques of **cognitive therapy** include identification of an individual's beliefs and attitudes, recognition of negative thought patterns, and education in alternative ways of thinking. Individuals with major depression or anxiety disorders are most likely to benefit, usually in 15 to 25 sessions. However, many of the positive messages used in cognitive therapy can help anyone improve a bad mood or negative outlook.

Behavioral therapy strives to substitute healthier ways of behaving for maladaptive patterns used in the past. Its premise is that distressing psychological symptoms, like all behaviors, are learned responses that can be modified or unlearned. Some therapists believe that changing behavior also changes how people think and feel. As they put it, "Change the behavior, and the feelings will follow." Behavior therapies work best for disorders characterized by specific, abnormal patterns of acting—such as alcohol and drug abuse, anxiety disorders, and phobias—and for individuals who want to change bad habits.

Interpersonal Therapy (IPT)

Interpersonal therapy (IPT), originally developed for research into the treatment of major depression, focuses on relationships in order to help individuals deal with unrecognized feelings and needs and improve their communication skills. IPT does not deal with the psychological origins of symptoms but rather concentrates on current problems of getting along with others. The supportive, empathic relationship that is developed with the therapist, who takes an even more active role than in psychodynamic psychotherapy, is the most crucial component of this therapy. The emphasis is on the here and now and on interpersonal—rather than intrapsychic—issues. Individuals with major depression, chronic difficulties developing relationships, chronic mild depression, or bulimia (see Chapter 7 on eating disorders)

are most likely to benefit. IPT usually consists of 12 to 16 sessions.

Psychiatric Drugs

Medications that alter brain chemistry and relieve psychiatric symptoms have brought great hope and help to millions of people. Thanks to the recent development of a new generation of more precise and effective **psychiatric drugs,** success rates for treating many common and disabling disorders—depression, panic disorder, schizophrenia, and others—have soared. Often used in conjunction with psychotherapy, sometimes used as the primary treatment, these medications have revolutionized mental health care.

At some point in their lives, about half of all Americans will take a psychiatric drug. The reason may be depression, anxiety, a sleep difficulty, an eating disorder, alcohol or drug dependence, impaired memory, or another disorder that disrupts the intricate chemistry of the brain. (See Savvy Consumer: "What You Need to Know About Mind-Mood Medications.")

Psychiatric drugs are now among the most widely prescribed drugs in the United States. Serotonin-boosting medications, called SSRIs, have become the drugs of choice in treating depression. They also are effective in treating obsessive compulsive disorder, panic disorder, social phobia, posttraumatic stress disorder, premenstrual dysphoric disorder, and generalized anxiety disorder. New agents, such as Remeron (mirtazapine), a "tetracyclic," stimulate the release of both norepinephrine and serotonin. In patients who don't respond, psychiatrists may add another drug to boost the efficacy of the treatment.

Psychiatric medications affect every aspect of a person's physical, mental, and emotional functioning. Some take effect immediately; others take several weeks to relieve symptoms; a few continue to exert their effects even after an individual discontinues their use. When taken appropriately, psychiatric agents can alleviate tremendous suffering and reduce the financial and personal costs of mental illness by lessening the need for hospitalization and by restoring an

---

Savvy Consumer ▪▪ What You Need to Know About Mind-Mood Medications

Before taking any "psychoactive" drug (one that affects the brain), talk to a qualified health professional. Here are some points to raise:

▪▪ What can this medication do for me? What specific symptoms will it relieve? Are there other possible benefits?

▪▪ When will I notice a difference? How long does it take for the medicine to have an effect?

▪▪ Are there any risks? What about side effects? Do I have to take it before or after eating? Will it affect my ability to study, work, drive, or operate machinery?

▪▪ Is there a risk of increased aggression or suicide? What should I do if I start thinking about taking my own life or of harming others?

▪▪ How will I be able to tell if the medication is working? What are the odds that it will help me?

▪▪ How long will I have to take medication? Is there any danger that I'll become addicted?

▪▪ What if it doesn't help?

▪▪ Is there an herbal or natural alternative? If so, has it been studied? What do you know about its possible risks and side effects?

individual's ability to function normally, to work, and to contribute to society. But they do have side effects and must be used with care.

 According to various studies, 5 to 7 percent of college students take antidepressant medications. Direct-to-consumer advertisements for antidepressant drugs can influence students' perceptions of what is wrong with them. In one study, college women were more likely to rate themselves as having mild-to-moderate depression as a result of reading pharmaceutical company information for popular antidepressants. The researchers cautioned that students should try alternative treatments for mild depression, including simple changes such as reduced class load, increased exercise, and more sleep, before starting medication.[85]

ALTERNATIVE MIND-MOOD PRODUCTS

People with serious mental illnesses, including depression and bipolar disorder, often use at least one alternative health-care practice, such as yoga or meditation. They also are trying "natural" products, such as herbs and enzymes, that claim to have psychological effects. However, because they are not classified as drugs, these products have not undergone the rigorous scientific testing required of psychiatric medications, and little is known about their safety or efficacy. "Natural" doesn't mean risk-free. Opium and cocaine are "natural" substances that have dramatic and potentially deadly effects on the mind.

St. John's wort has been used to treat anxiety and depression in Europe for many years. Data from clinical studies in the United States do not support the efficacy of St. John's wort for moderate to severe depression. In two carefully controlled studies, the herb did not prove more effective than a placebo. However, a German review of more than two-dozen studies found that St. John's wort was similar in efficacy to standard antidepressants.[86] Side effects include dizziness, abdominal pain and bloating, constipation, nausea, fatigue, and dry mouth. St. John's wort should not be taken in combination with other prescription antidepressants. St. John's wort can lower the efficacy of oral contraceptives and increase the risk of an unwanted pregnancy.

Learn It / Live It

Surviving and Thriving

Feeling good does not depend on money, success, recognition, or status. At any age, at any level of education and achievement, regardless of disability or disease, it is possible to find happiness and fulfillment in life. Achieving the highest possible level of psychological well-being, like achieving peak physical well-being, depends primarily on assuming responsibility for yourself.

Like physical health, psychological well-being is not a fixed state of being, but a process. The way you live every day affects how you feel about yourself and your world.

Here are some basic guidelines that you can rely on to make the most of the process of living:

- **Accept yourself.** As a human being, you are, by definition, imperfect. Come to terms with the fact that you are a worthwhile person despite your mistakes.
- **Respect yourself.** Recognize your abilities and talents. Acknowledge your competence and achievements, and take pride in them.
- **Trust yourself.** Learn to listen to the voice within you, and let your intuition be your guide.
- **Love yourself.** Be happy to spend time by yourself. Learn to appreciate your own company and to be glad you're you.
- **Stretch yourself.** Be willing to change and grow, to try something new and dare to be vulnerable.
- **Look at challenges as opportunities for personal growth.** "Every problem brings the possibility of a widening of consciousness," psychologist Carl Jung once noted. Put his words to the test.
- **Think of not only where but also who you want to be a decade from now.** The goals you set, the decisions you make, the values you adopt now will determine how you feel about yourself and your life in the future.

Making This Chapter Work for You

Review Questions

1. Psychological health is influenced by all of the following *except*
   a. spiritual health.
   b. physical agility.
   c. culture.
   d. a firm grasp on reality.

2. Emotional intelligence encompasses which of the following components?
   a. creativity, sense of humor, scholastic achievement
   b. integrity, honesty, and perseverance
   c. piety, tolerance, and self-esteem
   d. empathy, self-awareness, and altruism

3. Which of the following activities can contribute to a lasting sense of personal fulfillment?
   a. becoming a Big Sister or Big Brother to a child from an inner city single-parent home
   b. volunteering at a local soup kitchen on Thanksgiving
   c. being a regular participant in an Internet chat room
   d. going on a shopping spree

4. Individuals who have developed a sense of mastery over their lives are
   a. skilled at controlling the actions of others.
   b. usually passive and silent when faced with a situation they don't like.

(*continued, p. 78*)

Self Survey ▪ Well-Being Scale

Part I

The following questions contain statements and their opposites. Notice that the statements extend from one extreme to the other. Where would you place yourself on this scale? Place a circle on the number that is most true for you at this time. Do not put your circles between numbers.

Life Purpose and Satisfaction

1. During most of the day, my energy level is — very low — 1 2 3 4 5 ⑥ 7 — very high
2. As a whole, my life seems — dull — 1 2 3 4 5 6 ⑦ — vibrant
3. My daily activities are — not a source of satisfaction — 1 2 3 4 5 ⑥ 7 — a source of satisfaction
4. I have come to expect that every day will be — exactly the same — 1 2 3 4 5 6 ⑦ — new and different
5. When I think deeply about life — I do not feel there is any purpose to it — 1 2 3 4 5 ⑥ 7 — I feel there is a purpose to it
6. I feel that my life so far has — not been productive — 1 2 3 4 5 6 ⑦ — been productive
7. I feel that the work* I am doing — is of no value — 1 2 3 4 5 ⑥ 7 — is of great value
8. I wish I were different than who I am. — agree strongly — 1 2 3 4 5 6 ⑦ — disagree strongly
9. At this time, I have — no clearly defined goals for my life — 1 2 3 4 5 ⑥ 7 — clearly defined goals for my life
10. When sad things happen to me or other people — I cannot feel positive about life — 1 2 3 4 5 ⑥ 7 — I continue to feel positive about life
11. When I think about what I have done with my life, I feel — worthless — 1 2 3 4 5 6 ⑦ — worthwhile
12. My present life — does not satisfy me — 1 2 3 4 ⑤ 6 7 — satisfies me
13. I feel joy in my heart — never — 1 2 3 4 5 6 ⑦ — all the time
14. I feel trapped by the circumstances of my life. — agree strongly — 1 2 3 ④ 5 6 7 — disagree strongly
15. When I think about my past — I feel many regrets — 1 2 3 4 5 ⑥ 7 — I feel no regrets
16. Deep inside myself — I do not feel loved — 1 2 3 4 5 ⑥ 7 — I feel loved
17. When I think about the problems that I have — I do not feel hopeful about solving them — 1 2 3 4 5 ⑥ 7 — I feel very hopeful about solving them

*The definition of work is not limited to income-producing jobs. It includes childcare, housework, studies, and volunteer services.

Part II

Self-Confidence During Stress (Answer according to how you feel during stressful times.)

1. When there is a great deal of pressure being placed on me — I get tense — ① 2 3 4 5 6 7 — I remain calm
2. I react to problems and difficulties — with a great deal of frustration — 1 2 3 4 ⑤ 6 7 — with no frustration
3. In a difficult situation, I am confident that I will receive the help that I need. — disagree strongly — 1 2 3 4 5 6 ⑦ — agree strongly
4. I experience anxiety — all the time — 1 ② 3 4 5 6 7 — never
5. When I have made a mistake — I feel extreme dislike for myself — 1 2 3 ④ 5 6 7 — I continue to like myself
6. I find myself worrying that something bad is going to happen to me or those I love — all the time — 1 2 ③ 4 5 6 7 — never
7. In a stressful situation — I cannot concentrate easily — ① 2 3 4 5 6 7 — I can concentrate easily
8. I am fearful — all the time — 1 2 3 4 ⑤ 6 7 — never
9. When I need to stand up for myself — I cannot do it — 1 2 3 4 5 6 ⑦ — I can do it easily
10. I feel less than adequate in most situations — agree strongly — 1 2 3 4 5 ⑥ 7 — disagree strongly
11. During times of stress, I feel isolated and alone. — agree strongly — ① 2 3 4 5 ⑥ 7 — disagree strongly
12. In really difficult situations — I feel unable to respond in positive ways — 1 2 3 4 5 ⑥ 7 — I feel able to respond in positive ways
13. When I need to relax — I experience no peace—only thoughts and worries — 1 2 ③ 4 5 6 7 — I experience a peacefulness—free of thoughts and worries
14. When I am frightened — I panic — 1 ② 3 4 5 6 7 — I remain calm
15. I worry about the future — all the time — 1 2 3 ④ 5 6 7 — never

Scoring

The number you circled is your score for that question. Add your scores in each of the two sections and divide each sum by the number of questions in the section.

- Life Purpose and Satisfaction: 105 ÷ 17 = 6.17
- Self-Confidence During Stress: 102 ÷ 15 = 4.13
- Combined Well-Being:
  (add scores for both) 167 ÷ 32 = 5.22

Each score should range between 1.00 and 7.00 and may include decimals (for example 5.15).

Interpretation:

VERY LOW: 1.00 TO 2.49
MEDIUM LOW: 2.50 TO 3.99
MEDIUM HIGH: 4.00 TO 5.49
VERY HIGH: 5.50 TO 7.00

These scores reflect the strength with which you feel these positive emotions. Do they make sense to you? Review each scale and each question in each scale. Your score on each item gives you information about the emotions and areas in your life where your psychological resources are strong, as well as the areas where strength needs to be developed.

If you notice a large difference between the LPS and SCDS scores, use this information to recognize which central attitudes and aspects of your life most need strengthening. If your scores on both scales are very low, talk with a counselor or a friend about how you are feeling about yourself and your life.

Source: © 1989. Kass, Jared. *Inventory of Positive Psychological Attitudes.* The Well-Being Scale is the self-test version of the Inventory of Positive Psychological Attitudes (IPPA-32) developed by Dr. Jared D. Kass. Reprinted with author's permission. For information, contact: Dr. Jared Kass, Division of Counseling and Psychology, Graduate School of Arts and Social Sciences, Lesley College, Cambridge, MA 02138.

YOUR ACTION PLAN FOR MENTAL HEALTH

Just as you can improve your physical well-being, you can enhance the state of your mind. Here are some suggestions:

- Recognize and express your feelings. Pent-up emotions tend to fester inside, building into anger or depression.
- Don't brood. Rather than merely mulling over a problem, try to find solutions that are positive and useful.
- Take one step at a time. As long as you're taking some action to solve a problem, you can take pride in your ability to cope.
- Spend more time doing those activities you know you do best. For example, if you are a good cook, prepare a meal for someone.
- Separate what you do, especially any mistakes you make, from who you are. Instead of saying, "I'm so stupid," tell yourself, "That wasn't the smartest move I ever made, but I'll learn from it."
- Use affirmations, positive statements that help reinforce the most positive aspects of your personality and experience. Every day, you might say, "I am a loving, caring person," or "I am honest and open in expressing my feelings." Write some affirmations of your own on index cards and flip through them occasionally.
- List the things you would like to have or experience. Construct the statements as if you were already enjoying the situations you list, beginning each sentence with "I am." For example, "I am feeling great about doing well in my classes."
- When your internal critic—the negative inner voice we all have—starts putting you down, force yourself to think of a situation that you handled well.
- Set a limit on self-pity. Tell yourself, "I'm going to feel sorry for myself this morning, but this afternoon, I've got to get on with my life."

- Volunteer. A third of Americans—some 89 million people—give of themselves through volunteer work. By doing the same, you may feel better too.
- Exercise. In various studies around the world, physical exertion ranks as one of the best ways to change a bad mood, raise energy, and reduce tension.

CASE IN POINT: MANAGING MOODS

Student: Tyson, 19
Target Goal: Avoid mood slumps
Action Plan:

- When he gets into a bad mood, do psychological detective work to uncover the possible cause. If at all possible, he will take action to solve or correct the problem. For instance, if he blows up at his roommate, he can apologize for losing his temper rather than just letting the bad feelings fester.
- Reframe negative experiences. If Tyson is beating himself up for losing a lot of money in a poker game, he can learn from the loss and pledge to avoid high-stakes gambling in the future.
- Schedule regular workouts or runs to sweat away tensions.
- Concentrate on a small, achievable task, like washing his car, that gives him a sense of accomplishment.
- Steer clear of trying to drown his frustrations in beer.

Health Now™ If you want to write your own goals for avoiding mood slumps, go to the **Wellness Journal at Health Now http://healthnow.brookscole.com.**

    c. aware that their locus of control is internal, not external.

    d. aware that their locus of control is external, not internal.

5. People who pray regularly
    a. are able to quit smoking more easily.
    b. never get sick.
    c. recover from heart attacks more quickly.
    d. get better grades.

6. A mental disorder can be described as
    a. a condition associated with migraine headaches and narcolepsy.
    b. a condition that is usually caused by severe trauma to the brain.
    c. a behavioral or psychological disorder that impairs an individual's ability to conduct one or more important activities of daily life.
    d. a psychological disorder that is easily controlled with medication and a change in diet.

7. Some characteristic symptoms of major depression are
    a. difficulty concentrating, lack of energy, and eating more than usual.
    b. exaggerated sense of euphoria and energy.
    c. palpitations, sweating, numbness, and tingling sensations.
    d. talking in rambling ways, inability to think in a logical manner, and delusions.

8. Which of the following statements about anxiety disorders is true?
    a. Anxiety disorders are the least prevalent type of mental illness.
    b. An individual suffering from a panic attack may mistake her symptoms for a heart attack.
    c. The primary symptom of obsessive-compulsive disorder is irrational, intense, and persistent fear of a specific object or situation.
    d. Generalized anxiety disorders respond to systematic desensitization behavior therapy.

9. A person may be at higher risk of committing suicide if
    a. he is taking blood pressure medication.
    b. he lives in a rural environment and is married.
    c. he has been diagnosed with hyperactivity disorder.
    d. he has lost his job because of alcoholism.

10. Which of the following statements is true?
    a. Individuals with schizophrenia are most likely to benefit from psychodynamic therapy in combination with nutritional supplements.
    b. Antidepressant medications now require a warning label about the increased risk of suicidal thoughts.
    c. Only children have attention disorders.
    d. Interpersonal therapy focuses on the role of early experiences and unconscious influences in shaping patterns of behavior, such as repeated failed relationships.

Answers to these questions can be found on page 587.

Critical Thinking

1. Would you say that you view life positively or negatively? Would your friends and family agree with your assessment? Ask two of your closest friends for feedback about what they perceive are your typical responses to a problematic situation. Are these indicative of positive attitudes? If not, what could you do to become more psychologically positive?

2. Paula went to a therapist when she was feeling depressed and was given a prescription for an antidepressant called fluoxetine (trade name Prozac). Her therapist recommended the drug because it causes fewer side effects than other medications. However, Paula later read in a news magazine that some patients, claiming that Prozac had made them violent or suicidal, had sued the drug's manufacturers. Their suits didn't win in court, but Paula was less certain about taking the prescribed medication. What do you think she should do? How would you weigh the risks and benefits of taking a psychiatric drug?

3. Research has indicated that many homeless men and women are in need of outpatient psychiatric care, often because they suffer from chronic mental illnesses or alcoholism. Yet government funding for the mentally ill is inadequate, and homelessness itself can make it difficult, if not impossible, for people to gain access to the care they need. How do you feel when you pass homeless individuals who seem disoriented or out of touch with reality? Who should take responsibility for their welfare? Should they be forced to undergo treatment at psychiatric institutions?

Media Menu

Health Now™

Throughout the chapter, this icon introduces a list of resources on the Health-Now website at **http://healthnow.brookscole.com/ith** that will:
- Help you evaluate your knowledge of the material.
- Allow you to take an exam-prep quiz.
- Provide a Personalized Learning Plan targeting resources that address areas you should study.
- Coach you through identifying target goals for behavior change and creating and monitoring your personal change plan throughout the semester.

INTERNET CONNECTIONS

SAVE: Suicide Awareness Voices of Education
www.save.org
This site (formerly American Foundation for Suicide Prevention) offers research, facts, survivor support, and more.

National Institute of Mental Health
www.nimh.nih.gov
The National Institute of Mental Health is a federally sponsored organization that provides useful information on a variety of mental health topics including current mental health research.

American Psychological Association

www.apa.org

The APA is the scientific and professional organization for psychology in the United States. Its website provides up-to-date information on psychological issues and disorders.

National Mental Health Association

www.nmha.org

This site features fact sheets on a variety of mental health topics, including depression screening, college initiative, substance abuse prevention, and information for families. Also available are current mental health articles, an email newsletter, and a bookstore.

InfoTrac College Edition Activities Log on, insert **Psychological Health:** psychological depression into the Keyword search box, and limit your search to the past year. When you get the results, Mark articles to review, then Select one to read. Summarize three or four key points from the article.

You can find additional readings related to personal health with InfoTrac College Edition, an online library of more than 900 journals and publications. Follow the instructions for accessing InfoTrac College Edition that were packaged with your textbook; then search for articles using a keyword search.

For additional links, resources, and suggested readings on the InfoTrac College Edition, visit our Health and Wellness Resource Center at **http://health .wadsworth.com.**

Key Terms

The terms listed are used on the page indicated. Definitions of the terms are in the Glossary at the end of this book.

altruism 54

antidepressant 58

anxiety 63

anxiety disorders 67

assertive 55

attention deficit/hyperactivity disorder (ADHD) 68

autonomy 55

axon 57

axon terminal 57

behavioral therapy 74

bipolar disorder 66

certified social workers 73

cognitive therapy 74

culture 47

dendrites 57

depression 62

emotional health 46

emotional intelligence 47

generalized anxiety disorder (GAD) 67

glia 57

interpersonal therapy (IPT) 74

licensed clinical social workers (LCSW) 73

locus of control 55

major depression 65

marriage and family therapists 73

mental disorder 62

mental health 46

mood 51

neurons 57

neuropsychiatry 56

neurotransmitters 58

nucleus 57

obsessive-compulsive disorder (OCD) 67

optimism 50

panic attacks 67

panic disorder 67

phobias 67

psychiatric drugs 74

psychiatric nurses 73

psychiatrists 73

psychodynamic 73

psychologists 73

psychotherapy 73

rapid-eye-movement (REM) sleep 59

receptors 58

reuptake 58

schizophrenia 69

self-actualization 47

self-esteem 48

social isolation 56

social phobia 56

spiritual health 46

spiritual intelligence 47

synapse 58

values 47

4 Personal Stress Management

Two months into her freshman year, Maria feels as if a tornado has torn through her life. She is living thousands of miles from her family and the friends who share her culture and ethnic background. Her dormmates range from different to downright difficult. Her professors expect her to read and learn more in a week than in an entire month of high school. After blowing her budget decorating her room, she took on a part-time job—only to end up so exhausted that she dozes off in lectures. Stress? Maria considers it a way of life.

Like Maria, you live with stress every day, whether you're studying for exams, meeting people, facing new experiences, or figuring out how to live on a budget. You're not alone. Everyone, regardless of age, gender, race, or income, has to deal with stress—as an individual and as a member of society.

As researchers have demonstrated time and again, stress has profound effects, both immediate and long-term, on our bodies and minds. While stress alone doesn't cause disease, it triggers molecular changes throughout the body that make us more susceptible to many illnesses. Its impact on the mind is no less significant. The burden of chronic stress can undermine one's ability to cope with day-to-day hassles and can exacerbate psychological problems like depression and anxiety disorders.

Yet stress in itself isn't necessarily bad. What matters most is not the stressful situation itself, but an individual's response to it. By learning to anticipate stressful events, to manage day-to-day hassles, and to prevent stress overload, you can find alternatives to running endlessly on a treadmill of alarm, panic, and exhaustion. As you organize your schedule, find ways to release tension, and build up coping skills, you will begin to experience the sense of control and confidence that makes stress a challenge rather than an ordeal.

© Steve Prezant/CORBIS

(FAQ) Frequently Asked Questions

- Is stress hazardous to physical health? *p. 83*
- How can I cope with test stress? *p. 87*
- Why is everyone so angry? *p. 89*
- What can help me relax? *p. 93*
- How can I better manage my time? *p. 98*

After studying the material in this chapter, you should be able to:

- **Define** stress and stressors and **describe** how the body responds to stress according to the general adaptation syndrome theory.

- **List** the physical changes associated with frequent or severe stress and **discuss** how stress can affect the cardiovascular, immune, and digestive systems.

- **Describe** some personal causes of stress, especially those experienced by students, and **discuss** how their effects can be prevented or minimized.

- **Describe** some techniques to help manage stress.

- **Explain** how stressful events can affect psychological health and **describe** the factors contributing to posttraumatic stress disorder.

- **Identify** ways of managing time more efficiently.

WHAT IS STRESS?

People use the word *stress* in different ways: as an external force that causes a person to become tense or upset, as the internal state of arousal, and as the physical response of the body to various demands. Dr. Hans Selye, a pioneer in studying physiological responses to challenge, defined **stress** as "the nonspecific response of the body to any demand made upon it." In other words, the body reacts to **stressors**—the things that upset or excite us—in the same way, regardless of whether they are positive or negative.

Based on nearly 300 studies over four decades, researchers have distinguished five categories of stressors:

▪ **Acute time-limited stressors** include anxiety-provoking situations such as having to give a talk in public or work out a math problem, such as calculating a tip or dividing a bill, under pressure.

▪ **Brief naturalistic stressors** are more serious challenges such as taking SATs or meeting a deadline for a big project.

▪ **Stressful event sequences** are the difficult consequences of a natural disaster or another traumatic occurrence, such as the death of a spouse. The individuals involved recognize that these difficulties will end at some point in the future.

▪ **Chronic stressors** are ongoing demands caused by life-changing circumstances, such as permanent disability following an accident or caregiving for a parent with dementia, that do not have any clear end point.

▪ **Distant stressors** are traumatic experiences that occurred long ago, such as child abuse or combat, yet continue to have an emotional and psychological impact.[1]

Not all stressors are negative. Some of life's happiest moments—births, reunions, weddings—are enormously stressful. We weep with the stress of frustration or loss; we weep, too, with the stress of love and joy. Selye coined the term **eustress** for positive stress in our lives (*eu* is a Greek prefix meaning "good"). Eustress challenges us to grow, adapt, and find creative solutions in our lives. **Distress** refers to the negative effects of stress that can deplete or even destroy life energy. Ideally, the level of stress in our lives should be just high enough to motivate us to satisfy our needs and not so high that it interferes with our ability to reach our fullest potential.

WHAT CAUSES STRESS?

Of the many biological theories of stress, the best known may be the **general adaptation syndrome (GAS),** developed by Hans Selye. He postulated that our bodies constantly strive to maintain a stable and consistent physiological state, called **homeostasis.** Stressors, whether in the form of

© CORBIS

© 2000 PhotoDisc

An automobile accident is an acute negative stressor. Getting married is an example of a positive stressor that triggers both joy and apprehension.

physical illness or a demanding job, disturb this state and trigger a nonspecific physiological response. The body attempts to restore homeostasis by means of an **adaptive response.**

Selye's general adaptation syndrome, which describes the body's response to a stressor—whether threatening or exhilarating—consists of three distinct stages:

1. **Alarm.** When a stressor first occurs, the body responds with changes that temporarily lower resistance. Levels of certain hormones may rise; blood pressure may increase (Figure 4-1). The body quickly makes internal adjustments to cope with the stressor and return to normal activity.

2. **Resistance.** If the stressor continues, the body mobilizes its internal resources to try to sustain

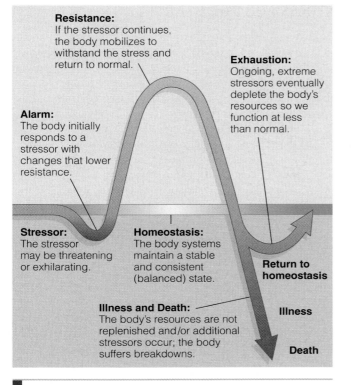

FIGURE 4-1   General Adaptation Syndrome (GAS)
The three stages of Hans Selye's GAS are alarm, resistance, exhaustion.

homeostasis. For example, if a loved one is seriously hurt in an accident, we initially respond intensely and feel great anxiety. During the subsequent stressful period of recuperation, we struggle to carry on as normally as possible, but this requires considerable effort.

3. **Exhaustion.** If the stress continues long enough, we cannot keep up our normal functioning. Even a small amount of additional stress at this point can cause a breakdown.

Among the nonbiological theories is the cognitive-transactional model of stress, developed by Richard Lazarus, which looks at the relation between stress and health. As he sees it, stress can have a powerful impact on health. Conversely, health can affect a person's resistance or coping ability. Stress, according to Lazarus, is "neither an environmental stimulus, a characteristic of the person, nor a response, but a relationship between demands and the power to deal with them without unreasonable or destructive costs."[2] Thus, an event may be stressful for one person but not for another, or it may seem stressful on one occasion but not on another. For instance, one student may think of speaking in front of the class as extremely stressful, while another relishes the chance to do so—except on days when he's not well-prepared.

At any age, some of us are more vulnerable to life changes and crises than are others. The stress of growing up in families troubled by alcoholism, drug dependence, or physical, sexual, or psychological abuse may have a lifelong impact—particularly if these problems are not recognized and dealt with. Other early experiences, positive and negative, also can affect our attitude toward stress—and our resilience to it. Our general outlook on life, whether we're optimistic or pessimistic, can determine whether we expect the worst and feel stressed or anticipate a challenge and feel confident. The when, where, what, how, and why of stressors also affect our reactions. The number and frequency of changes in our lives, along with the time and setting in which they occur, have a great impact on how we'll respond.

"Perceived" stress—an individual's view of how challenging life is—undermines a sense of well-being in people of all ages and circumstances, including urban African-American women and healthy young adults.[3] However, good self-esteem, social support, and internal resources buffer the impact of perceived stress.[4]

Our level of ongoing stress affects our ability to respond to a new day's stressors. Each of us has a breaking point for dealing with stress. A series of too-intense pressures or too-rapid changes can push us closer and closer to that point. That's why it's important to anticipate potential stressors and plan how to deal with them.

Stress experts Thomas Holmes, M.D., and Richard Rahe, M.D., devised a scale to evaluate individual levels of stress and potential for coping, based on *life-change units* that estimate each change's impact. The death of a partner or parent ranks high on the list, but even changing apartments is considered a stressor. People who accumulate more than 300 life-change units in a year are more likely to suffer serious health problems. Scores on the scale, however, represent "potential stress"; the actual impact of the life change depends on the individual's response. (See Self Survey: "Student Stress Scale.")

Holmes has evaluated variations in life events among many groups, including college students, medical students, football players, pregnant women, alcoholics, and heroin addicts. Heroin addicts and alcoholics have the highest totals of life-change units, followed by college students. In general, younger people experience more life changes than do older people; factors such as gender, education, and social class also have a strong impact. Marriage seems to promote greater stability and fewer changes.

If you score high on the Student Stress Scale, think about the reasons your life has been in such turmoil. Of course, some events, such as your parents' divorce or a friend's accident, are beyond your control. Even then, you can respond in ways that may protect you from disease. Review the Action Plan at the end of the Self Survey (p. 101).

(FAQ) IS STRESS HAZARDOUS TO PHYSICAL HEALTH?

While stress alone doesn't cause disease, it triggers molecular changes throughout the body that make us more susceptible to many illnesses. Severe emotional distress—whether caused by a divorce, the loss of a job, or caring for an ill child or parent—can have such a powerful effect on the DNA in body cells that it speeds up aging, adding the equivalent of a decade to biological age.[5] This occurs because of a shortening of structures called telomeres in the chromosomes of cells. An enzyme called telomerase maintains these structures but declines with age. Every time a cell divides, which is a continuous process, the telomeres shorten. The shorter your telomeres, the more likely you are to die.

 In a recent study, scientists studied healthy young women, some caring for healthy children and some under long-term stress because they were caring for a chronically ill child. The longer a woman had been caring for a sick child, the shorter her telomeres and the less active her telomerase became. Tests to determine the women's chronological age showed that those under the greatest stress scored as 10 to 17 years older than those with the lowest stress levels.[6]

Stress also triggers complex changes in the body's endocrine, or hormone-secreting, system. When you confront a stressor, the adrenal glands, two triangle-shaped glands that sit atop the kidneys, respond by producing stress hormones, including catecholamines, cortisol (hydrocortisone), and epinephrine (adrenaline), that speed up heart rate and raise blood pressure and prepare the body to deal with the threat. This "fight-or-flight" response prepares you for quick action: Your heart works harder to pump more blood to your legs and arms. Your muscles tense, your breathing quickens, and your brain becomes extra alert. Because it's nonessential in a crisis, your digestive system practically shuts down (Figure 4-2).

Cortisol speeds the conversion of proteins and fats into carbohydrates, the body's basic fuel, so we have the energy to fight or flee from a threat. However, stress increases the amount of time required to clear triglycerides, a type of fat linked to heart disease, from the bloodstream.

Cortisol can cause excessive central or abdominal fat, which heightens the risk of diseases such as diabetes, high blood pressure, and stroke. Even slender, premenopausal women faced with increased stress and lacking good coping skills are more likely to accumulate excess weight around their waists, thereby increasing their risk of heart disease and other health problems.

 In one study, African-American college students who scored low in coping skills had higher levels of cortisol than those better equipped to cope with stress.[7] Challenges that seem uncontrollable or unpredictable have a greater impact on cortisol than others.[8]

Figure 4-2 illustrates how persistent or repeated increases in the stress hormones can be hazardous throughout the body. In the brain, stress hormones linked to powerful emotions may help create long-lasting memories of events such as the collapse of the World Trade Center towers. But very prolonged or severe stress can damage the brain's ability to remember and can actually cause brain cells, or neurons, to atrophy and die.

STRESS AND THE HEART

Stress may be the most significant inherited risk factor in people who develop heart disease at a young age. According to behavioral researchers, family transmission of emotional and psychosocial stress, specifically anger in males, greatly increases the likelihood of early heart disease.[9] Young adults whose blood pressure spikes in response to stress may be at risk of hypertension as they get older.[10]

In the 1970s, cardiologists Meyer Friedman, M.D., and Ray Rosenman, M.D., compared their patients to individuals of the same age with healthy hearts and developed two general categories of personality: Type A and Type B. Hardworking, aggressive, and competitive, Type As never have time for all they want to accomplish, even though they usually try to do several tasks at once. Type Bs are more relaxed, though not necessarily less ambitious or successful.

The degree of danger associated with Type-A behavior remains controversial. Of all the personality traits linked with Type-A behavior, the most sinister are anger and chronic hostility.[11] People who are always mistrustful, cynical, and suspicious are twice as likely to suffer blockages of their coronary arteries. Social isolation, depression, and stress may be even stronger risk factors for men.[12]

A tragic or shocking event can stun the heart and produce classic heart-attack–like symptoms, including chest pain, shortness of breath, and fluid in the lungs. Triggered by stress hormones, "broken heart syndrome" can cause severe weakness in the heart. Unlike a heart attack, the condition is reversible. Patients typically recover within days and suffer no permanent damage to their hearts.[13]

STRESS AND IMMUNITY

The immune system is the network of organs, tissues, and white blood cells that defend against disease. Impaired immunity makes the body more susceptible to many diseases, including infections (from the common cold to tuberculosis) and disorders of the immune system itself.

A recent "meta-analysis"—a study of studies in peer-reviewed scientific journals—confirmed earlier findings that stress alters immunity, but the effects differ between short-term and long-term stress. In short term, stress "revs up" the immune system, a way of preparing for injury or infection. Acute time-limited stressors, the type that produce a "fight or flight" response, prompt the immune system to ready itself for the possibility of infections resulting from bites, punctures, or other wounds.[14]

However, long-term or chronic stress creates excessive wear and tear, and the system breaks down. Chronic stressors, so profound and persistent that they seem endless and beyond a person's control, suppress immune responses the most. The longer the stress, the more the immune system shifts from potentially adaptive changes to potentially harmful ones, first in cellular immunity and then in broader immune function. Traumatic stress, such as losing a loved one through death or divorce, can impair immunity for as long as a year.

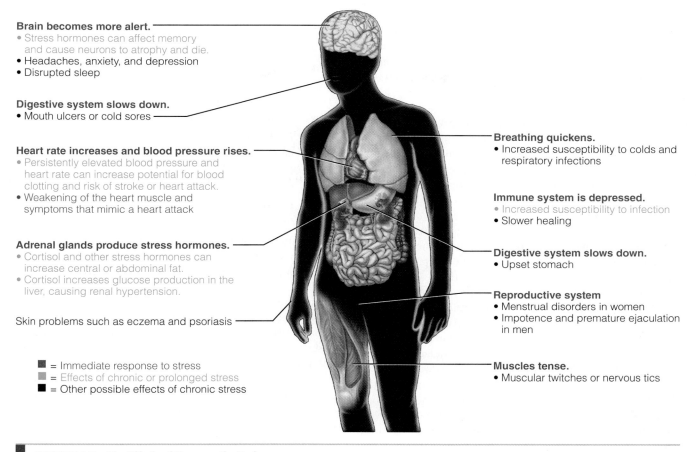

Brain becomes more alert.
• Stress hormones can affect memory and cause neurons to atrophy and die.
• Headaches, anxiety, and depression
• Disrupted sleep

Digestive system slows down.
• Mouth ulcers or cold sores

Heart rate increases and blood pressure rises.
• Persistently elevated blood pressure and heart rate can increase potential for blood clotting and risk of stroke or heart attack.
• Weakening of the heart muscle and symptoms that mimic a heart attack

Adrenal glands produce stress hormones.
• Cortisol and other stress hormones can increase central or abdominal fat.
• Cortisol increases glucose production in the liver, causing renal hypertension.

Skin problems such as eczema and psoriasis

■ = Immediate response to stress
■ = Effects of chronic or prolonged stress
■ = Other possible effects of chronic stress

Breathing quickens.
• Increased susceptibility to colds and respiratory infections

Immune system is depressed.
• Increased susceptibility to infection
• Slower healing

Digestive system slows down.
• Upset stomach

Reproductive system
• Menstrual disorders in women
• Impotence and premature ejaculation in men

Muscles tense.
• Muscular twitches or nervous tics

FIGURE 4-2   The Effects of Stress on the Body

Minor hassles that aren't related to trauma do take a toll. Under exam stress, students experience a dip in immune function and a higher rate of infections. Ohio State University researchers found that during exam periods, there is a significant drop in the immune cells that normally ward off infection and cancer in medical students.

Age and overall health also affect immune response. The immune systems of individuals who are elderly or ill are more vulnerable to acute and chronic stressors, possibly because their bodies find it more difficult to regulate their reactions.

STRESS AND DIGESTION

Do you ever get butterflies in your stomach before giving a speech in class or before a big game? The digestive system is, as one psychologist quips, "an important stop on the tension trail." To avoid problems, pay attention to how you eat; Eating on the run, gulping food, or overeating results in poorly chewed foods, an overworked stomach, and increased abdominal pressure.

Some simple strategies can help you avoid stress-related stomachaches. Many people experience dry mouth or sweat more under stress. By drinking plenty of water, you replenish lost fluids and prevent dehydration. Fiber-rich foods counteract common stress-related problems, such as cramps

and constipation. Do not skip meals. If you do, you're more likely to feel fatigued and irritable.

Good nutrition can help soothe a stressed-out stomach. Complex carbohydrates are an ideal antistress food because they boost the brain's level of the mood-enhancing chemical serotonin. Good sources include broccoli, leafy greens, potatoes, corn, cabbage, spinach, whole-grain breads and pastas, muffins, crackers, and cereals. Leafy vegetables, whole grains, nuts, and seeds also are rich in other important nutrients, including magnesium and vitamin C.

Be wary of overeating under stress. Some people eat more because they scarf down meals too quickly. Others reach for snacks to calm their nerves or comfort themselves. In a study of college women, higher stress increased the risk of binge eating.[15] Watch out for caffeine. Coffee, tea, and cola drinks can make your strained nerves jangle even more. Also avoid sugary snacks. They'll send your blood sugar levels on a roller coaster ride—up one minute, down the next.

OTHER STRESS SYMPTOMS

The first signs of stress include muscle tightness, tension headaches, backaches, upset stomach, and sleep disruptions (caused by stress-altered brain-wave activity). Some people feel fatigued, their hearts may race or beat faster than usual at rest, and they may feel tense all the time, easily frustrated and often irritable. Others feel sad; lose their energy, appetite, or sex drive; and develop psychological problems, including depression anxiety and panic attacks (Chapter 3).

Hundreds of studies over the last 20 years have shown that stress contributes to approximately 80 percent of all major illnesses: cardiovascular disease, cancer, endocrine and metabolic disease, skin rashes, ulcers, ulcerative colitis, emotional disorders, musculoskeletal disease, infectious ailments, premenstrual syndrome (PMS), uterine fibroid cysts, and breast cysts. As many as 75 to 90 percent of visits to physicians are related to stress.

Headaches are one of the most common stress-related conditions. The most common type, tension headache, is caused by involuntary contractions of the scalp, head, and neck muscles. **Migraine headache** is the result of constriction (narrowing), then dilation (widening) of blood vessels within the brain; chemicals leak through the vessel walls, inflame nearby tissues, and send pain signals to the brain. Surveys of college women show that Type-A behavior can trigger both types of headache.

Stress also is closely linked to skin conditions. If you break out the week before an exam, you know firsthand that skin can be extremely sensitive to stress. Skin conditions worsened by stress include acne, psoriasis, herpes, hives, and eczema. With acne, increased touching of the face, perhaps while cramming for a test, may be partly responsible. Other factors, such as temperature, humidity, and cosmetics and toiletries, may also play a role.

STRESS ON CAMPUS

You've probably heard that these are the best years of your life, but being a student—full-time or part-time, in your late teens, early twenties, or later in life—can be extremely stressful. You may feel pressure to perform well to qualify for a good job or graduate school. To meet steep tuition payments, you may have to juggle part-time work and coursework. You may feel stressed about choosing a major, getting along with a difficult roommate, passing a particularly hard course, or living up to your parents' and teachers' expectations. If you're an older student, you may have children, housework, and homework to balance. Your days may seem so busy and your life so full that you worry about coming apart at the seams. One thing is for certain: You're not alone.

After a steady surge upward in the 1990s, the percentage of students who say they are "frequently overwhelmed by all they have to do" has declined from the peak of 30.7 percent in 1999 to 27.4 percent in 2004.[16] However, women are more than twice as likely to report stress as men. (See Student Snapshot: "Stressed Out on Campus.") According to surveys of students at colleges and universities around the country and the world, stressors are remarkably similar. Among the most common are:

▪ **Test pressures.**
▪ **Financial problems.**
▪ **Frustrations,** such as delays in reaching goals.
▪ **Problems in friendships** and dating relationships.
▪ **Daily hassles.**
▪ **Academic failure.**
▪ **Pressures** as a result of competition, deadlines, and the like.
▪ **Changes,** which may be unpleasant, disruptive, or too frequent.
▪ **Losses,** whether caused by the breakup of a relationship or the death of a loved one.

Many students bring complex psychological problems with them to campus, including learning disabilities and mood disorders like depression and anxiety. "Students arrive with the underpinnings of problems that are brought out by the stress of campus life," says one counselor. Some have grown up in broken homes and bear the scars of family troubles. Others fall into the same patterns of alcohol abuse that they observed for years in their families or suffer lingering emotional scars from childhood physical or sexual abuse.

Students aren't the only ones complaining about stress on campus. Professors working toward tenure also report high stress levels—particularly women. The reason for this gender difference may be that women take on more responsibility for mentoring female students and for teaching independent study courses with individual students.[17]

STUDENTS UNDER STRESS

More than a quarter of freshmen feel overwhelmed by all they have to do at the beginning of the academic year; by the year's end, 44 percent feel overwhelmed. In research at three universities, underclassmen were most vulnerable to negative life events, perhaps because they lacked experience in coping with stressful situations. Freshmen had the highest levels of depression; sophomores had the most anger and hostility. Seniors may handle life's challenges better because

Student Snapshot
STRESSED OUT ON CAMPUS

Have You Felt Overwhelmed by All You Had to Do?	
All undergraduates	27%
Men	16%
Women	36%
Four-year colleges	29%
Universities	24%

Source: Sax, Linda, et al. *The American Freshman: National Norms for Fall 2004.* Los Angeles, CA: University of California, Los Angeles Higher Education Research Institute, 2004.

© Purestock/Alamy

they have developed better coping mechanisms. In the study, more seniors reported that they faced problems squarely and took action to resolve them, while younger students were more likely to respond passively, for instance, by trying not to let things bother them.

First-generation college students—those whose parents never experienced at least one full year of college—encounter more difficulties with social adjustment than freshmen whose parents attended college. Second-generation students may have several advantages: more knowledge of college life, greater social support, more preparation for college in high school, a greater focus on college activities, and more financial resources.

The percentage of students seeking psychological help because of stress or anxiety has risen dramatically in the last 15 years (see Chapter 3). Students say they react to stress in various ways: physiologically (by sweating, stuttering, trembling, or developing physical symptoms); emotionally (by becoming anxious, fearful, angry, guilty, or depressed); behaviorally (by crying, eating, smoking, being irritable or abusive); or cognitively (by thinking about and analyzing stressful situations and strategies that might be useful in dealing with them).

A supportive network of friends and family makes a difference. Undergraduates with higher levels of social support and self-efficacy reported feeling less stressed and more satisfied with life than others.

Does stress increase drinking among college students? Many assume so, since life stress is a recognized risk for alcohol use in general. In a recent study of 137 undergraduates, however, the relationship between drinking and stress turned out to be more complex. For some, drinking occasions were times to discuss problems with friends, regardless of the day's stress. On average, students tended to drink more on days when they were feeling good—possibly because of what the researchers called the "celebratory and social" nature of college drinking. Drinking—and positive emotions—also peaked on weekends.[18] (See Chapter 12 for more on student drinking.)

Campuses are providing more frontline services than they have in the past, including career-guidance workshops, telephone hot lines, and special social programs for lonely, homesick freshmen. In one study of 128 undergraduates, those who learned relaxation and stress-reduction techniques in a six-week program reported less stress, anxiety, and psychological distress than a control group of students. The participants—who had described themselves as "extremely stressed" before the intervention—also began to increase health-promoting behaviors.

> *Some campuses are setting up counseling services to help students manage stress. Critics argue that learning to live with stress is a lesson students should master on their own. Should colleges reach out to help students under stress?* **You decide.**

© Bill Aron /PhotoEdit

The first year of college can be overwhelming as you learn your way around the campus, meet new people, and strive to succeed.

(FAQ) HOW CAN I COPE WITH TEST STRESS?

For many students, midterms and final exams are the most stressful times of the year. Studies at various colleges and universities found that the incidence of colds and flu soared during finals. Some students feel the impact of test stress in other ways—headaches, upset stomachs, skin flare-ups, or insomnia.

Because of stress's impact on memory, students with advanced skills may perform worse under exam pressure than their less skilled peers.[19] Sometimes students become so preoccupied with the possibility of failing that they can't concentrate on studying. Others, including many of the best and brightest students, freeze up during tests and can't comprehend multiple-choice questions or write essay answers, even if they know the material.

The students most susceptible to exam stress are those who believe they'll do poorly and who see tests as extremely threatening. Unfortunately, such negative thoughts often become a self-fulfilling prophecy. As they study, these students keep wondering: What good will studying do? I never do well on tests. As their fear increases, they try harder, pulling all-nighters. Fueled by caffeine, munching on sugary snacks, they become edgy and find it harder and harder to concentrate. By the time of the test, they're nervous wrecks, scarcely able to sit still and focus on the exam.

Can you do anything to reduce test stress and feel more in control? Absolutely. One way is to defuse stress through relaxation. Students taught relaxation techniques—such as controlled breathing, meditation, progressive relaxation, and guided imagery (visualization)—a month before finals tend to have higher levels of immune cells during the exam period and feel in better control during their tests.

Strategies for Prevention ■ Defusing Test Stress

■ **Plan ahead.** A month before finals, map out a study schedule for each course. Set aside a small amount of time every day or every other day to review the course materials.

■ **Be positive.** Picture yourself taking your final exam. Imagine yourself walking into the exam room feeling confident, opening up the test booklet, and seeing questions for which you know the answers.

■ **Take regular breaks.** Get up from your desk, breathe deeply, stretch, and visualize a pleasant scene. You'll feel more refreshed than you would if you chugged another cup of coffee.

■ **Practice.** Some teachers are willing to give practice finals to prepare students for test situations, or you and your friends can test each other.

■ **Talk to other students.** Chances are that many of them share your fears

about test taking and may have discovered some helpful techniques of their own. Sometimes talking to your adviser or a counselor can also help.

■ **Be satisfied with doing your best.** You can't expect to ace every test; all you can and should expect is your best effort. Once you've completed the exam, allow yourself the sweet pleasure of relief that it's over.

© Ulrike Welsch

You can take control of your stress responses by practicing relaxation techniques, avoiding cramming, and being positive about your performance on tests.

 ## MINORITIES UNDER STRESS

Regardless of your race or ethnic background, college may bring culture shock. You may never have encountered such a degree of diversity in one setting. You probably will meet students with different values, unfamiliar customs, entirely new ways of looking at the world—experiences you may find both stimulating and stressful.

Mental health professionals have long assumed that minority students may feel a double burden of stress. Many undergraduates experience emotional difficulties (see Chapter 3), and researchers have theorized that students from a racial or ethnic minority would be especially likely to develop psychological symptoms, such as anger, anxiety, and depression, as a result of increased stress.

Racism has indeed been shown to be a source of stress that can affect health and well-being. In the past, some African-American students have described predominately white campuses as hostile, alienating, and socially isolating and have reported greater estrangement from the campus community and heightened estrangement in interactions with faculty and peers. However, the generalization that all minority students are more stressed may not be valid.

A study conducted at a racially diverse university in a large metropolitan area in the Northeast evaluated 595 freshmen. The study group was made up of both genders and students of various racial and ethnic backgrounds, including Asians, African-Americans, and Hispanics.[20] Fewer than 15 percent of these students—whether Asian, African-American, Hispanic, white, or another ethnic minority—reported clincially significant levels of anger, anxiety, and depression, and there was no correlation between these stress-linked symptoms and ethnicity or race.

"Diversity, in and of itself, is unlikely to be related to higher levels of reported psychological symptoms on campus," the researchers concluded, theorizing that minority students "may have developed strengths while growing up within their particular cultures, subcommunities, and families that have often gone unrecognized or unnoted.[21] And some coping mechanisms, especially spirituality, can buffer the negative effects of racism.

All minority students do share some common stressors. In one study of minority freshmen entering a large, competitive university, Asian, Filipino, African-American, and Native American students all felt more sensitive and vulnerable to the college social climate, to interpersonal tensions between themselves and nonminority students and faculty, to experiences of actual or perceived racism, and to racist attitudes and discrimination (discussed later in this chapter). Despite scoring above the national average on the SAT, the minority students in this study did not feel accepted as legitimate students and sensed that others viewed them as unworthy beneficiaries of affirmative action initiatives. While most said that overt racism was rare and relatively easy to deal with, they reported subtle pressures that undermined their academic confidence and their ability to bond with the university. Balancing these stressors, however, was a strong sense of ethnic identity, which helped buffer some stressful effects.

Hispanic students have identified three major types of stressors in their college experiences: academic (related to exam preparation and faculty interaction, social (related to ethnicity and interpersonal competence), and financial (related to their economic situation). Some Asian students who recently immigrated to the United States report feeling ostracized by students of similar ancestry who are second- or third-generation Americans. While they take pride in being truly bicultural and bilingual, the newcomers feel ambivalent about mainstream American culture. "My parents stress the importance of traditions; my friends tell me to get with it and act like an American," says one Asian-born student who has spent five years in the United States. "I feel trapped between cultures."

MEN, WOMEN, AND STRESS

Women, who make up 56 percent of today's college students, also shoulder the majority of the stress load. In a nationwide survey of students in the class of 2008, more women (36.4 percent) described themselves as "overwhelmed by all I have to do," compared with just 16.3 percent of men. More women than men reported feeling depressed, insecure about their physical and mental health, and worried about paying for college. More men—57.1 percent, compared with 45.8 percent of women—considered themselves above average or in the top 10 percent of people their age in terms of emotional health.[22]

Gender differences in lifestyle may help explain why

women feel so stressed. College men, the survey revealed, spend significantly more time doing things that are fun and relaxing: exercising, partying, watching TV, and playing video games. Women, on the other hand, tend to study more, do more volunteer work, and handle more household and child-care chores.

Where can stressed-out college women turn for support? The best source, according to University of California research, is other women. In general, the social support women offer their friends and relatives seems more effective in reducing the blood-pressure response to stress than that provided by men.

At all ages, women and men tend to respond to stress differently. While males (human and those of other species) react with the classic fight-or-flight response, females under attack try to protect their children and seek help from other females—a strategy dubbed *tend and befriend*. When exposed to experimental stress (such as a loud, harsh noise), women show more affection for friends and relatives; men show less. When working mothers studied by psychologists had a bad day, they coped by concentrating on their children when they got home. Stressed-out fathers were more likely to withdraw.

OTHER PERSONAL STRESSORS

At every stage of life, you will encounter challenges and stressors. Among the most common are those related to anger, conflict, work, and illness.

(FAQ) WHY IS EVERYONE SO ANGRY?

In recent years, violent aggressive driving—which some dub *road rage*—has exploded. Sideline rage at amateur and professional sporting events has become so widespread that a Pennsylvania midget football game ended in a brawl involving more than 100 coaches, players, parents, and fans.

No one seems immune. Women fly off the handle just as often as men, although they're less likely to get physical. The young and the infamous, including several rappers and musicians sentenced to anger management classes for violent outbursts, may seem more volatile. However, ordinary senior citizens have erupted into "line rage" and pushed ahead of others simply because they feel they've "waited long enough" in their lives.

"Everyone everywhere seems to be hotter under the collar these days," observes Sybil Evans, a conflict resolution expert who singles out three primary culprits: time, technology, and tension. "Americans are working longer hours than anyone else in the world. The cell phones and pagers that were supposed to make our lives easier have put us on call 24–7–365. Since we're always running, we're tense and low on patience, and the less patience we have, the less we monitor what we say to people and how we treat them."[23]

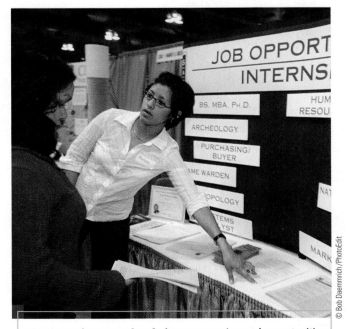

Minority students can often find support services and opportunities to work with others on campus.

Getting a Grip

For years therapists encouraged people to "vent" their anger. However, research now shows that letting anger out only makes it worse. "Catharsis is worse than useless," says psychology professor Brad Bushman of Iowa State University, whose research has shown that letting anger out makes people more aggressive, not less. "Many people think of anger as the psychological equivalent of the steam in a pressure cooker that has to be released or it will explode. That's not true. People who react by hitting, kicking, screaming, and swearing aren't dealing with the underlying cause of their anger. They just feel more angry."[24]

Over time, temper tantrums sabotage physical health as well as psychological equanimity. By churning out stress hormones, chronic anger revs the body into a state of combat readiness, multiplying the risk for stroke and heart attack—even in healthy individuals.

To deal with anger, you have to figure out what's really making you mad. Usually the jammed soda machine is the final straw that unleashes bottled-up fury over a more difficult issue, such as a recent breakup or a domineering parent. Also monitor yourself for early signs of exhaustion and overload. While stress alone doesn't cause a blowup, it makes you more vulnerable to overreacting.

Conflict Resolution

Disagreements are inevitable; disagreeable ways of dealing with them are not. One of the most important skills in any setting—from family room to staff meeting to corporate boardroom—is resolving conflicts. The key is to focus on the problem, not the individual. Try to put aside unconscious biases, such as assuming a person is difficult to deal with, or preconceived notions about what others really want. Rather than planning what you might say, focus your attention on what others are saying.

Professionals recommend the following steps:

■ **Listen.** To work through a conflict, you need to understand the other person's point of view. This demands careful listening in a quiet, private setting, away from activity and background noise. If conflict erupts in a public place, move the discussion elsewhere.

■ **Assimilate.** Rather than taking a position and focusing only on defending it, try not to shut yourself off to other possibilities. Keep open the possibility that no one party is completely right or completely wrong. To get a fresh perspective, consider the situation from the "third person." If you were seeing the conflict from the outside, what would you think about the information? Once you've taken in all available information, ask yourself: What do I know now about the overall situation? Has my opinion changed?

■ **Respond.** Especially if another person is responding in anger, give a calm, well-reasoned response. It will help defuse a highly emotional situation. Try to find a common goal that will benefit you both. Restate the other person's position when both of you are finished speaking so you both know you've been heard and understood.

JOB STRESS

More so than ever, many people find that they are working more and enjoying it less. Many people, including working parents, spend 55 to 60 hours a week on the job. More people are caught up in an exhausting cycle of overwork, which causes stress, which makes work harder, which leads to more stress. Even the workplace itself can contribute to

© Anthony Redpath /CORBIS

How you manage your anger has consequences for your health and for your interactions with others.

Strategies for Change ■ How to Deal with an Angry Person

■ **Become an impartial observer.** Act as if you were watching someone else's two-year-old have a temper tantrum at the supermarket.

■ **Stay calm.** Letting your emotions loose only adds fuel to fury. Talk quietly and slowly; let the person know you understand that he or she is angry.

■ **Refuse to engage.** Step back to avoid invading his or her space. Retreat farther if need be until the person is back in control.

■ **Find something to agree with.** Look for common ground, if only to acknowledge that you're both in a difficult situation.

stress. A noisy, open-office environment can increase levels of stress without workers realizing it.

Yet work in itself is not hazardous to health. Attitudes about work and habits related to how we work are the true threats. In fact, a job—stressful or not, enjoyable or not—can be therapeutic.

People who become obsessed by their work and careers can turn into *workaholics,* so caught up in racing toward the top that they forget what they're racing toward and why. In some cases they throw themselves into their work to mask or avoid painful feelings or difficulties in their own lives. One consequence is **burnout,** a state of physical, emotional, and mental exhaustion brought on by constant or repeated emotional pressure. Particularly in the helping professions, such as social work or nursing, men and women who've dedicated themselves to others may realize they have nothing left in themselves to give.

Early signs of burnout include exhaustion, sleep problems or nightmares, increased anxiety or nervousness, muscular tension (headaches, backaches, and the like), increased use of alcohol or medication, digestive problems, such as nausea, vomiting, or diarrhea, loss of interest in sex, frequent body aches or pain, quarrels with family or friends, negative feelings about everything, problems concentrating, job mistakes and accidents, and feelings of depression, hopelessness, and helplessness.

Age is the one variable most consistently associated with burnout: Younger employees between ages 30 and 40 report the highest rates. Both men and women are susceptible to burnout. Unmarried individuals, particularly men, seem more prone to burnout than married workers. Single employees who've never been married have higher burnout rates than those who are divorced.

ILLNESS AND DISABILITY

Just as the mind can have profound effects on the body, the body can have an enormous impact on our emotions. Whenever we come down with the flu or pull a muscle, we feel under par. When the problem is more serious or persistent—a chronic disease like diabetes, for instance, or a lifelong hearing impairment—the emotional stress of constantly coping with it is even greater.

 A common source of stress for college students is a learning disability, which may affect one of every ten Americans. Most learning-disabled have average or above-average intelligence, but they rarely live up to their ability in school. Some have only one area of difficulty, such as reading or math. Others have problems with attention, writing, communicating, reasoning, coordination, and social skills.

Not all students with learning disabilities experience greater stress. In one in-depth study comparing 34 undergraduates with and without learning disabilities, the learning-disabled (LD) students reported significantly fewer college stressors and demonstrated a higher need for achievement. The LD students also scored significantly higher in resiliency and initiative in solving problems and working toward goals.[25]

SOCIETAL STRESSORS

Not all stressors are personal. Centuries ago the poet John Donne observed that no man is an island. Today, on an increasingly crowded and troubled planet, these words seem truer than ever. Problems such as discrimination and terrorism can no longer be viewed only as economic or political issues. Directly or indirectly, they affect the well-being of all who inhabit the Earth—now and in the future.

The deliberate use of physical force to abuse or injure is a leading killer of young people in the United States—and a potential source of stress in all our lives. Chances are that you or someone you know has been the victim of a violent crime, and awareness of our own vulnerability adds to the stress of daily living.

DISCRIMINATION

Discrimination can take many forms—some as subtle as not being included in a conversation or joke, some as blatant as threats scrawled on a wall, some as violent as brutal beatings and other hate crimes. Because it can be hard to deal with individually, discrimination is a particularly sinister form of stress. By banding together, however, those who experience discrimination can take action to protect themselves, chal-

---

Strategies for Prevention :: Defusing Desk Rage

Desk rage builds in little steps, so you can take it away in little steps. Here are suggestions on how to do so:

:: If you sense a problem, monitor the situation for a week. Write down when you're feeling hungry, tired, overloaded. Try to identify the triggers that might cause you to do something you'll later regret.

:: Get feedback from friends. An objective person who knows you well can provide a fresh take on a troubling situation.

:: If your irritation stems from a coworker, approach him or her in a nonthreatening way. You might say, "Could you hear me out for a few minutes?" To lower the hostility level, start by stating something you have in com-

mon, such as "We both want this project to work."

:: If you fly off the handle, learn from the experience. Do immediate damage control by apologizing to coworkers and explaining that you've been under stress. Plan what you might do differently the next time someone or something sets you off.

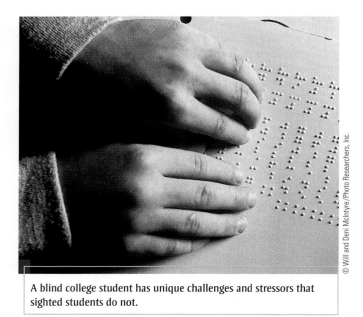

A blind college student has unique challenges and stressors that sighted students do not.

lenge the ignorance and hateful assumptions that fuel bigotry, and promote a healthier environment for all.

In the last decade, there have been reports of increased intolerance among young people and greater tolerance of expressions and acts of hate on college campuses. To counteract this trend, many schools have set up programs and classes to educate students about each other's backgrounds and to acknowledge and celebrate the richness diversity brings to campus life. Educators have called on universities to make campuses less alienating and more culturally and emotionally accessible, with programs and policies targeted not only at minority students but also at the university as a whole.

Your Life Coach

Coping with Stress

The key to coping with stress is realizing that your *perception* of and *response* to a stressor are crucial. Changing the way you interpret events or situations—a skill called *reframing*—makes all the difference. An event, such as a move to a new city, is not stressful in itself. A move becomes stressful if you see it as a traumatic upheaval rather than an exciting beginning of a new chapter in your life.

In times of stress, the following simple exercises can stop the stress buildup inside your body and help you regain a sense of calm and control.

- **Breathing.** Deep breathing relaxes the body and quiets the mind. Draw air deeply into your lungs, allowing your chest to fill with air and your belly to rise and fall. You will feel the muscle tension and stress begin to melt away. When you're feeling extremely stressed, try this calming breath: Sit or lie with your back straight and place the tip of your tongue on the roof of your mouth behind your teeth. Exhale completely through the mouth, then inhale through the nose for 4 seconds. Hold the breath for 7 seconds, then exhale audibly through the mouth for 8 seconds. Repeat four times.

- **Refocusing.** Thinking about a situation you can't change or control only increases the stress you feel. Force your mind to focus on other subjects. If you're stuck in a long line, distract yourself. Check out what other people are buying or imagine what they do for a living. Imagine that you're in a hot shower and a wave of relaxation is washing your stress down the drain.

- **Serenity breaks.** Build moments of tranquility into your day. For instance, while waiting for your computer to start up or a file to download, look at a photograph of someone you love or a poster of a tropical island. If none is available, close your eyes and visualize a soothing scene, such as walking in a meadow or along a beach.

- **Stress signals.** Learn to recognize the first signs that your stress load is getting out of hand: Is your back bothering you? Do you have a headache? Do you find yourself speeding or misplacing things? Whenever you spot these early warnings, force yourself to stop and say, I'm under stress. I need to do something about it.

- **Reality checks.** To put things into proper perspective, ask yourself: Will I remember what's made me so upset a month from now? If I had to rank this problem on a scale of 1 to 10, with worldwide catastrophe as 10, where would it rate?

- **Stress inoculation.** Rehearse everyday situations that you find stressful, such as speaking in class. Think of how you might make the situation less tense, for instance, by breathing deeply before you talk or jotting down notes beforehand. Think of these small "doses" of stress as the psychological equivalent of allergy shots: They immunize you so you feel less stressed when bigger challenges come along.

- **Rx: Laughter.** Humor counters stress by focusing on comic aspects of difficult situations and may, as various studies have shown, lessen harmful effects on the immune system and overall health. However, humor may have different effects on stress in men and women. In a study of 131 undergraduates, humor buffered stress-related physical symptoms in men and women. However, it reduced stress-linked anxiety only in men. The researchers theorized that men may

Shared laughter is a powerful antidote to stress.

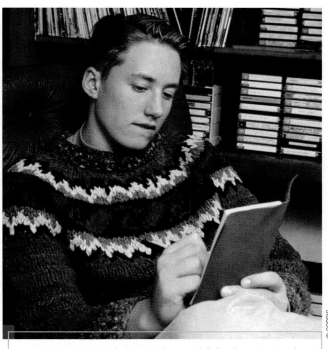

Writing in your journal about feelings and difficulties is a simple and effective way to help control your stress.

prefer humor as a more appropriate way of expressing emotions such as anxiety, whereas women are more likely to use self-disclosure, that is, to confide in friends.

▪ **Spiritual coping.** Saying a prayer under stress is one of the oldest and most effective ways of calming yourself. Other forms of spiritual coping, such as putting trust in God and doing for others (for instance, by volunteering at a shelter for battered women) also can provide a different perspective on daily hassles and stresses.

▪ **Sublimation.** This term refers to the redirection of any drives considered unacceptable into socially acceptable channels. Outdoor activity is one of the best ways to reduce stress through sublimation. For instance, if you're furious with a friend who betrayed your trust or frustrated because your boss rejects all of your proposals, you might go for a long run or hike to sublimate your anger.

▪ **Exercise.** Regular physical activity can relieve stress, boost energy, lift mood, and keep stress under control. Young adults who adopt and continue regular aerobic exercise show less intense cardiovascular responses to stress, which may protect them against coronary heart disease as they age.[26] Strength training may have similar benefits.

 In one study, college students who engaged in an eight-week weight training reported lower stress levels than those who participated in an aerobic dance program.

▪ **Journaling.** One of the simplest, yet most effective, ways to work through stress is by putting your feelings into words that only you will read. The more honest and open you are as you write, the better. College students who wrote in their journals about traumatic events felt much better afterward than those who wrote about superficial topics. Focus on intense emotional experiences and "autopsy" them to try to understand why they affected you the way they did. Rereading and thinking about your notes may reveal the underlying reasons for your response.

DEFENSE MECHANISMS

Sometimes we respond to stress or challenge with self-destructive behaviors, such as drinking or using drugs. These responses can lead to psychological problems, such as anxiety or depression, and physical problems, including psychosomatic illnesses.

Defense mechanisms, such as those described in Table 4-1, are another response to stress. These psychological devices are mental processes that help us cope with personal problems. Such responses also are not the answer to stress—and learning to recognize them in yourself will enable you to deal with your stress in a healthier way.

FAQ **WHAT CAN HELP ME RELAX?**

Relaxation is the physical and mental state opposite that of stress. Rather than gearing up for fight or flight, our bodies and minds grow calmer and work more smoothly. We're less likely to become frazzled and more capable of staying in control. The most effective relaxation tech-

Savvy Consumer ∷ Can Stress-Relief Products Help?

You're stressed out, and you see an ad for a product—an oil, candle, cream, herbal tea, pill, or potion—that promises to make all your cares disappear. Should you soak in an aromatic bath, have a massage, try kava, squeeze foam balls? In most cases, you're probably not doing yourself much harm, but you aren't necessarily doing yourself much good either. Keep these considerations in mind:

∷ Be wary of instant cures. Regardless of the promises on the label, it's unrealistic to expect any magic ingredient or product to make all your problems disappear.

∷ Focus on stress-reducing behavior, rather than a product. An aromatic candle may not bring instant serenity,

but if you light a candle and meditate, you may indeed feel more at peace. A scented pillow may not be a cure for stress, but if it helps you get a good night's sleep, you'll cope better the next day.

∷ Experiment with physical ways to work out stress. Exercise is one of the best ways to lower your stress levels. Try walking, running, swimming, cycling, kickboxing—anything physical that helps you release tension.

∷ Don't make matters worse by smoking (the chemicals in cigarettes increase heart rate, blood pressure, and stress hormones), consuming too much caffeine (it speeds up your system for hours), eating snacks high in sugar

(it produces a quick high followed by a sudden slump), or turning to drugs or alcohol (they can only add to your stress when their effects wear off).

∷ Be cautious when trying "alternative" products. "Natural" products, such as herbs and enzymes, claim to have psychological effects. However, because they are not classified as drugs, these products have not undergone the rigorous scientific testing required of psychiatric medications, and little is known about their safety or efficacy. "Natural" doesn't mean risk-free. Opium and cocaine are "natural" substances that have dramatic and potentially deadly effects on the mind.

TABLE 4-1 COMMON DEFENSE MECHANISMS USED TO ALLEVIATE ANXIETY AND ELIMINATE CONFLICT

Defense Mechanism	Example
Denial: the refusal to accept a painful reality.	You don't accept as true the news that a loved one is seriously ill.
Displacement: the redirection of feelings from their true object to a more acceptable or safer substitute.	Instead of lashing out at a coach or a teacher, you snap at your best friend.
Projection: the attribution of unacceptable feelings or impulses to someone else.	When you want to end a relationship, you project your unhappiness onto your partner.
Rationalization: the substitution of "good," acceptable reasons for the real motivations for our behavior.	You report a classmate who has been mean to you for cheating on an exam and explain that cheating is unfair to other students.
Reaction formation: adopting attitudes and behaviors that are the opposite of what you feel.	You lavishly compliment an acquaintance whom you really despise.
Repression: the way we keep threatening impulses, fantasies, memories, feelings, or wishes from becoming conscious.	You don't "hear" the alarm after a late night, or you "forget" to take out the trash.

niques include progressive relaxation, visualization, meditation, mindfulness, and biofeedback.

Progressive relaxation works by intentionally increasing and then decreasing tension in the muscles. While sitting or lying down in a quiet, comfortable setting, you tense and release various muscles, beginning with those of the hand, for instance, and then proceeding to the arms, shoulders, neck, face, scalp, chest, stomach, buttocks, genitals, and so on, down each leg to the toes. Relaxing the muscles can quiet the mind and restore internal balance.

Visualization, or **guided imagery,** involves creating mental pictures that calm you down and focus your mind. Some people use this technique to promote healing when they are ill (see Chapter 17). Visualization skills require practice and, in some cases, instruction by qualified health professionals.

Meditation has been practiced in many forms over the ages, from the yogic techniques of the Far East to

the Quaker silence of more modern times. Brain scans have shown that meditation activates the sections of the brain in charge of the autonomic nervous system, which governs bodily functions, such as digestion and blood pressure, that we cannot consciously control. Although many studies have documented the benefits of meditation for overall health, it may be particularly helpful for people dealing with stress-related medical conditions such as high blood pressure.

Meditation helps a person reach a state of relaxation, but with the goal of achieving inner peace and harmony. There is no one right way to meditate, and many people have discovered how to meditate on their own, without even knowing what it is they are doing.

 Among college students, meditation has proved especially effective in increasing relaxation. Most forms of meditation have common elements: sitting quietly for 15 to 20 minutes once or twice a day, concentrating on a word or image, and breathing slowly

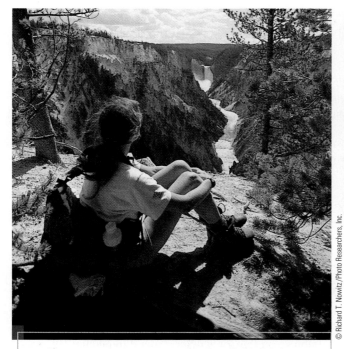

Spending time outdoors is a great way to leave behind daily tensions and gain new perspective.

Biofeedback training uses electronic monitoring devices to teach conscious control over heart rate, body temperature, and muscle tension. Once the technique is learned, the electronic devices are unnecessary.

and rhythmically. If you wish to try meditation, it often helps to have someone guide you through your first sessions. Or try tape recording your own voice (with or without favorite music in the background) and playing it back to yourself, freeing yourself to concentrate on the goal of turning the attention within.

Mindfulness is a modern form of an ancient Asian technique that involves maintaining awareness in the present moment. You tune in to each part of your body, scanning from head to toe, noting the slightest sensation. You allow whatever you experience—an itch, an ache, a feeling of warmth—to enter your awareness. Then you open yourself to focus on all the thoughts, sensations, sounds, and feelings that enter your awareness. Mindfulness keeps you in the here and now, thinking about what is rather than about *what if* or *if only*.

Biofeedback, discussed in Chapter 17, is a method of obtaining feedback, or information, about some physiological activity occurring in the body. An electronic monitoring device attached to the body detects a change in an internal function and communi-

cates it back to the person through a tone, light, or meter. By paying attention to this feedback, most people can gain some control over functions previously thought to be beyond conscious control, such as body temperature, heart rate, muscle tension, and brain waves. Biofeedback training consists of three stages:

1. Developing increased awareness of a body state or function.
2. Gaining control over it.
3. Transferring this control to everyday living without use of the electronic instrument.

The goal of biofeedback for stress reduction is a state of tranquility, usually associated with the brain's production of alpha waves (which are slower and more regular than normal waking waves). After several training sessions, most people can produce alpha waves more or less at will.

STRESS AND PSYCHOLOGICAL HEALTH

Traumatic events (such as a robbery, assault, or sudden death of a loved one) always take a toll on an individual, and it's normal to feel sad, tense, overwhelmed, angry, or

Strategies for Change :: "Mini-Relaxation"

Here is a quick deep-breathing exercise from Harvard psychologist Alice Domar:

:: Sit upright or lie on your back.

:: Place your hand just beneath your navel so you can feel the rise and fall

of your belly as you breathe deeply through your nose.

:: As you inhale, count slowly, saying to yourself, "one, two, three, four." Exhale

slowly, counting back down from four to one.

:: Do this for one minute or longer. [27]

Strategies for Prevention ▪▪ Recognize the Warning Signals of Stress Overload

- Experiencing physical symptoms, including chronic fatigue, headaches, indigestion, diarrhea, and sleep problems.
- Having frequent illness or worrying about illness.
- Self-medicating, including nonprescription drugs.

- Having problems concentrating on studies or work.
- Feeling irritable, anxious, or apathetic.
- Working or studying longer and harder than usual.
- Exaggerating, to yourself and others, the importance of what you do.

- Becoming accident-prone.
- Breaking rules, whether it's a curfew at home or a speed limit on the highway.
- Going to extremes, such as drinking too much, overspending, or gambling.

---

incapable of coping with the ordinary demands of daily living. Usually such feelings and behaviors subside with time. The stressful event fades into the past, and those whose lives it has touched adapt to its lasting impact. But sometimes individuals remain extremely distressed and unable to function as they once did. While the majority of individuals who survive a trauma recover, at least a quarter of such individuals later develop serious psychological symptoms.

Stress can undermine college students' self-esteem and may increase their likelihood of thinking about or attempting suicide. In a study of 88 undergraduates ranging in age from 18 to 34 at a large southern university, 12 percent reported having suicidal thoughts. Both negative stress and low self-esteem increased the likelihood of such thoughts.[28]

POSTTRAUMATIC STRESS DISORDER

In the past, **posttraumatic stress disorder (PTSD)** was viewed as a psychological response to out-of-the-ordinary stressors, such as captivity or combat. However, other experiences can also forever change the way people view themselves and their world. Thousands of individuals experience or witness traumatic events, such as fires or floods. PTSD is widespread, although often not recognized, in inner-city African-American communities.[29] Children, in particular, are likely to develop PTSD symptoms when they live through a traumatic event or witness a loved one or friend being assaulted.

According to research, almost half of car accident victims may develop PTSD. Individuals who were seriously injured are especially vulnerable. The main symptoms are re-experiencing the traumatic event, avoiding the site of the accident, refraining from driving in weather and road conditions similar to those on the day of the accident, and feeling a general increase in distress.

As shown in a recent Canadian study of 65 women over age 18, sexual abuse during childhood or adolescence can increase vulnerability to PTSD later in life.[30] An episode that repeats the abuse, such as a sexual assault or rape, can trigger an intense reaction as individuals "re-experience" the initial trauma.

Childhood abuse—physical, sexual, or emotional—can affect student dropout rates. In one study that followed 210 freshmen (aged 17 to 21 years) for four years, those suffering PTSD symptoms in the second week of their freshman year were less likely to remain enrolled through their senior years. Half of those who'd been sexually abused and 65 percent of those who'd experienced multiple forms of abuse dropped out.[31]

In PTSD, individuals re-experience their terror and helplessness again and again in their dreams or intrusive thoughts. To avoid this psychic pain, they may try to avoid anything associated with the trauma. Some enter a state of emotional numbness and no longer can respond to people and experiences the way they once did, especially when it comes to showing tenderness or affection. Those who've been mugged or raped may be afraid to venture out by themselves.

The sooner trauma survivors receive psychological help, the better they are likely to fare. Often talking about what happened with an empathic person or someone who's shared the experience as soon as possible—preferably before going to sleep on the day of the event—can help an individual begin to deal with what has occurred. Group sessions, ideally beginning soon after the trauma, allow individuals to share views and experiences. Behavioral, cognitive, and psychodynamic therapy (described in Chapter 3) can help individuals suffering PTSD.

RESILIENCE

Adversity—whether in the form of a traumatic event or chronic stress—has different effects on individuals. Some people never recover and continue on a downward slide that may ultimately prove fatal. Others return, though at different rates, to their prior level of functioning. In recent years researchers have focused their attention on a particularly intriguing group: those people who not only survive stressful experiences but also thrive, that is, who actually surpass their previous level of functioning.

Resilience can take many forms. A father whose child is kidnapped and killed may become a nationwide advocate for victims' rights. A student whose roommate dies in a car crash after a party may campaign for tougher laws against drunk driving. A couple whose premature baby spends weeks in a neonatal intensive care unit may find that their marriage has grown closer and stronger. Even though their experiences were painful, the individuals often look back at them as bringing positive changes into their lives.

Trauma survivors can often find support and comfort from those who have shared the experience.

Researchers have studied various factors that enable individuals to thrive in the face of adversity. These include:

- **An optimistic attitude.** Rather than reacting to a stressor simply as a threat, these men and women view stress as a challenge—one they believe they can and will overcome. Researchers have documented that individuals facing various stressors, including serious illness and bereavement, are more likely to report experiencing growth if they have high levels of hope and optimism.
- **Self-efficacy.** A sense of being in control of one's life can boost health, even in times of great stress.
- **Stress inoculation.** People who deal well with adversity often have had previous experiences with stress that toughened them in various ways, such as teaching them skills that enhanced their ability to cope and boosting their confidence in their ability to weather a rough patch.
- **Secure personal relationships.** Individuals who know they can count on the support of their loved ones are more likely to be resilient.
- **Spirituality or religiousness.** Religious coping may be particularly related to growth and resilience. In particular, two types seem most beneficial: spiritually based religious coping (receiving emotional reassurance and guidance from God) and good-deeds coping (living a better, more spiritual life that includes altruistic acts).

Resilience sometimes means developing new skills simply because, in order to get through the stressful experience, people had to learn something they hadn't known how to do before—for instance, wrangling with insurance companies or other bureaucracies. By mastering such skills, they become more fit to deal with an unpredictable world and develop new flexibility in facing the unknown.

Along with new abilities comes the psychological sense of mastery. "I survived this," an individual may say. "I'll be able to deal with other hard things in the future." Such confidence keeps people actively engaged in the effort to cope and is itself a predictor of eventual success. Stress also can make individuals more aware of the fulfilling aspects of life, and they may become more interested in spiritual pursuits. Certain kinds of stressful experiences also have social consequences. If a person experiencing a traumatic event finds that the significant others in his or her life can be counted on, the result can be a strengthening of their relationship.

Focusing on finding meaning in their experience—what some call "cognitive coping"—can help individuals move beyond initial emotional responses such as anxiety, distress, and confusion. Over time, some people may develop what may be the ultimate "gift" of a stressful experience: wisdom.

ORGANIZING YOUR TIME

We live in what some sociologists call hyperculture, a society that moves at warp speed. Information bombards us constantly. The rate of change seems to accelerate every year. Our "time-saving" devices—pagers, cell phones, modems, faxes, palm-sized organizers, laptop computers—have simply extended the boundaries of where and how we work.

As a result, more and more people are suffering from "timesickness," a nerve-racking feeling that life has become little more than an endless to-do list. The best antidote is time management, and hundreds of books, seminars, and experts offer training in making the most of the hours in the day. Yet these well-intentioned methods often fail, and sooner or later most of us find ourselves caught in a time trap.

POOR TIME MANAGEMENT

Every day you make dozens of decisions, and the choices you make about how to use your time directly affect your stress level. If you have a big test on Monday and a term paper due Tuesday, you may plan to study all weekend. Then, when you're invited to a party Saturday night, you go. Although you set the alarm for 7:00 A.M. on Sunday, you don't pull yourself out of bed until noon. By the time you start studying, it's 4:00 P.M., and anxiety is building inside you.

How can you tell if you've lost control of your time? The following are telltale symptoms of poor time management:

- **Rushing.**
- **Chronic inability to make choices or decisions.**
- **Fatigue or listlessness.**
- **Constantly missed deadlines.**
- **Not enough time for rest** or personal relationships.
- **A sense of being overwhelmed** by demands and details and having to do what you don't want to do most of the time.

One of the hard lessons of being on your own is that your choices and your actions have consequences. Stress is just one of them. But by thinking ahead, being realistic about your workload, and sticking to your plans, you can gain better control over your time and your stress levels.

 ## HOW CAN I BETTER MANAGE MY TIME?

Time management involves skills that anyone can learn, but they require commitment and practice to make a difference in your life. It may help to know the techniques that other students have found most useful:

- **Schedule your time.** Use a calendar or planner. Beginning the first week of class, mark down deadlines for each assignment, paper, project, and test scheduled that semester. Develop a daily schedule, listing very specifically what you will do the next day, along with the times. Block out times for working out, eating dinner, calling home, and talking with friends as well as for studying.

- **Develop a game plan.** Allow at least two nights to study for any major exam. Set aside more time for researching and writing papers. Make sure to allow time to revise and print out a paper—and to deal with emergencies like a computer breakdown. Set daily and weekly goals for every class. When working on a big project, don't neglect your other courses. Whenever possible, try to work ahead in all your classes.

- **Identify time robbers.** For several days keep a log of what you do and how much time you spend doing it. You may discover that disorganization is eating away at your time or that you have a problem getting started. (See the following section on Overcoming Procrastination.)

- **Make the most of classes.** Read the assignments before class rather than waiting until just before you have a test. By reading ahead of time, you'll make it easier to understand the lectures. Go to class yourself. Your own notes will be more helpful than a friend's or those from a note-taking service. Read your lecture notes at the end of each day or at least at the end of each week.

- **Develop an efficient study style.** Some experts recommend studying for 50 minutes, then breaking for 10 minutes. Small incentives, such as allowing yourself to call or visit a friend during these 10 minutes, can provide the motivation to keep you at the books longer. When you're reading, don't just highlight passages. Instead, write notes or questions to yourself in the margins, which will help you retain more information. Even if you're racing to start a paper, take a few extra minutes to prepare a workable outline. It will be easier to structure your paper when you start writing.

- **Focus on the task at hand.** Rather than worrying about how you did on yesterday's test or how you'll ever finish next week's project, focus intently on whatever you're doing at any given moment. If your mind starts to wander, use any distraction—the sound of the phone ringing or a noise from the hall—as a reminder to stay in the moment.

- **Turn elephants into hors d'oeuvres.** Cut a huge task into smaller chunks so it seems less enormous. For instance, break down your term paper into a series of steps, such as selecting a topic, identifying sources of research information, taking notes, developing an outline, and so on.

- **Keep your workspace in order.** Even if the rest of your room is a shambles, try to keep your desk clear. Piles of papers are distracting, and you can end up wasting lots of time looking for notes you misplaced or an article you have to read by morning. Try to spend the last ten minutes of the day getting your desk in order so you get a fresh start on the new day.

OVERCOMING PROCRASTINATION

Putting off until tomorrow what should be done today is a habit that creates a great deal of stress for many students. It also takes a surprising toll. In studies with students taking a health psychology course, researchers found that although procrastinating provided short-term benefits, including periods of low stress, the tendency to dawdle had long-term costs, including poorer health and lower grades. Early in the semester, the procrastinators reported less stress and fewer health problems than students who scored low on procrastination. However, by the end of the

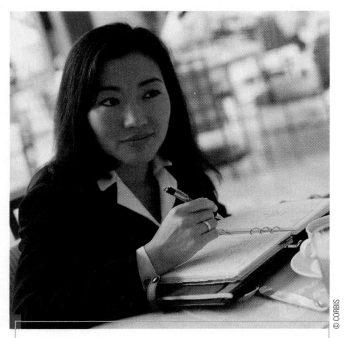

© CORBIS

A calendar or planner is an important tool in time management. You can use it to keep track of assignment due dates, class meetings, and other "to do's."

semester, procrastinators reported more health-related symptoms, more stress, and more visits to health-care professionals than nonprocrastinators. Students who procrastinate also get poorer grades in courses with many deadlines.

The three most common types of procrastination are putting off unpleasant things, putting off difficult tasks, and putting off tough decisions. Procrastinators are most likely to delay by wishing they didn't have to do what they must or by telling themselves they "just can't get started," which means they never do.

To get out of the procrastination trap, keep track of the tasks you're most likely to put off, and try to figure out why you don't want to tackle them. Think of alternative ways to get tasks done. If you put off library readings, for instance, is the problem getting to the library or the reading itself? If it's the trip to the library, arrange to walk over with a friend whose company you enjoy.

Develop daily time-management techniques, such as a to-do list. Rank items according to priorities: A, B, C, and schedule your days to make sure the A's get accomplished. Try not to fixate on half-completed projects. Divide large tasks, such as a term paper, into smaller ones, and reward yourself when you complete a part.

Do what you like least first. Once you have it out of the way, you can concentrate on the tasks you enjoy. Build time into your schedule for interruptions, unforeseen problems, and unexpected events, so you aren't constantly racing around. Establish ground rules for meeting your own needs (including getting enough sleep and making time for friends) before saying yes to any activity. Learn to live according to a three-word motto: Just do it!

Learn It / Live It

De-Stress Your Life

College is a perfect time to learn and practice the art of stress reduction. You can start applying the techniques and concepts outlined in this chapter immediately. You may want to begin by doing some relaxation or awareness exercises. They can give you the peace of mind you need to focus more effectively on larger issues, goals, and decisions.

You needn't see stress as a problem to solve on your own. Reach out to others. As you build friendships and intimate relationships, you may find that some irritating problems are easier to put into perspective. Don't be afraid to laugh at yourself and to look for the comic or absurd aspects of a situation. In addition, you might try some simple approaches that can help boost your stress resistance and resilence, including the following:

- **Focusing.** Take a strain inventory of your body every day to determine where things aren't feeling quite right. Ask yourself, "What's keeping me from feeling terrific today?" Focusing on problem spots, such as stomach knots or neck tightness, increases your sense of control over stress.

- **Reconstructing stressful situations.** Think about a recent episode of distress; then write down three ways it could have gone better and three ways it could have gone worse. This should help you see that the situation wasn't as disastrous as it might have been, and help you find ways to cope better in the future.

- **Self-improvement.** When your life feels out of control, turn to a new challenge. You might try volunteering at a nursing home, going for a long-distance bike trip, or learning a foreign language. As you work toward your new goal, you'll realize that you still can cope and achieve.

If stress continues to be a problem in your life, you may be able to find help through support groups or counseling. Your school may provide counseling services or referrals to mental health professionals; ask your health instructor or the campus health department for this information. Remember that each day of distress robs you of energy, distracts you from life's pleasures, and interferes with achieving your full potential.

Making This Chapter Work for You
Review Questions

1. Stress can be defined as
   a. a negative emotional state related to fatigue and similar to depression.
   b. the physiological and psychological response to any event or situation that either upsets or excites us.
   c. the end result of the general adaptation syndrome.
   d. a motivational strategy for making life changes.

2. According to the general adaptation syndrome theory, how does the body typically respond to an acute stressor?
   a. The heart rate slows, blood pressure declines, and eye movement increases.
   b. The body enters a physical state called eustress and then moves into the physical state referred to as distress.
   c. If the stressor is viewed as a positive event, there are no physical changes.
   d. The body demonstrates three stages of change: alarm, resistance, and exhaustion.

3. Over time, increased levels of stress hormones have been shown to increase a person's risk for which of the following conditions?
   a. diabetes, high blood pressure, memory loss, and skin disorders
   b. stress fractures, male pattern baldness, and hypothyroidism
   c. hemophilia, AIDS, and hay fever
   d. none of the above

Self Survey   ::   Student Stress Scale

The Student Stress Scale, an adaptation of Holmes and Rahe's Life Events Scale for college-age adults, provides a rough indication of stress levels and possible health consequences.

In the Student Stress Scale, each event, such as beginning or ending school, is given a score that represents the amount of readjustment a person has to make as a result of the change. In some studies, using similar scales, people with serious illnesses have been found to have high scores.

To determine your stress score, add up the number of points corresponding to the events you have experienced in the past 12 months.

1.	Death of a close family member	100
2.	Death of a close friend	73
3.	Divorce of parents	65
4.	Jail term	63
5.	Major personal injury or illness	63
6.	Marriage	58
7.	Getting fired from a job	50
8.	Failing an important course	47
9.	Change in the health of a family member	45
10.	Pregnancy	45
11.	Sex problems	44
12.	Serious argument with a close friend	40
13.	Change in financial status	39
14.	Change of academic major	39
15.	Trouble with parents	39
16.	New girlfriend or boyfriend	37
17.	Increase in workload at school	37
18.	Outstanding personal achievement	36
19.	First quarter/semester in college	36
20.	Change in living conditions	31
21.	Serious argument with an instructor	30
22.	Getting lower grades than expected	29
23.	Change in sleeping habits	29
24.	Change in social activities	29
25.	Change in eating habits	28
26.	Chronic car trouble	26
27.	Change in number of family get-togethers	26
28.	Too many missed classes	25

4. Stress levels in college students
   a. may be high due to stressors such as academic pressures, financial concerns, learning disabilities, and relationship problems.
   b. are usually low because students feel empowered living independently of their parents.
   c. are typically highest in seniors because their self-esteem diminishes during the college years.
   d. are lower in minority students because they are used to stressors such as a hostile social climate and actual or perceived discrimination.

5. Which of the following statements about anger is true?
   a. The healthiest way to deal with anger is to express the rage.
   b. When confronted by an angry person, you can usually defuse the situation quickly by explaining that he or she is acting immaturely and inappropriately.
   c. Venting anger can adversely affect one's physical health over time.
   d. Statistics show that anger-related public behaviors such as aggressive driving and workplace outbursts have been on the decrease.

6. Which of the following illustrates the defense mechanism of displacement?
   a. You have a beer in the evening after a tough day.
   b. You act as if nothing has happened after you have been laid off from your job.
   c. You start an argument with your sister after being laid off from your job.
   d. You argue with your boss after he lays you off from your job.

29. Changing colleges	24
30. Dropping more than one class	23
31. Minor traffic violations	20

Total Stress Score 301

Here's how to interpret your score: If your score is 300 or higher, you're at high risk for developing a health problem. If your score is between 150 and 300, you have a 50-50 chance of experiencing a serious health change within two years. If your score is below 150, you have a 1 in 3 chance of a serious health change.

Source: Mullen, Kathleen, and Gerald Costello. *Health Awareness Through Discovery.*

YOUR ACTION PLAN FOR STRESS MANAGEMENT

▪ **Strive for balance.** Review your commitments and plans and, if necessary, scale down.

▪ **Get the facts.** When faced with a change or challenge, seek accurate information, which can bring vague fears down to earth.

▪ **Talk with someone you trust.** A friend or a health professional can offer valuable perspective as well as psychological support.

▪ **Exercise.** Even when your schedule gets jammed, carve out 20 or 30 minutes several times a week to walk, swim, bicycle, jog, or work out at the gym.

▪ **Help others.** One of the most effective ways of dealing with stress is to find people in a worse situation and do something positive for them.

▪ **Cultivate hobbies.** Pursuing a personal pleasure can distract you from the stressors in your life and help you relax.

▪ **Master a form of relaxation.** Whether you choose meditation, yoga, mindfulness, or another technique, practice it regularly.

CASE IN POINT: MANAGING STRESS

Student: Reese, 19
Target Goal: Getting a Grip on Stress
Action Plan:

▪ Draw up a realistic weekly schedule with time blocked out for classes, study, wrestling practice and tournaments, and relaxation.

▪ Learn one stress-reduction technique, such as meditation or yoga, and practice it for 10 to 15 minutes every day.

▪ Develop the habit of stopping every hour or two for a "serenity break," such as looking at a screen saver with a beautiful forest view.

▪ Be on the alert for stress signals, such as upset stomach or headache.

▪ Take deep, mindful breaths during stressful times, such as prior to a wrestling match.

Health ⊗ Now ™   If you want to write your own goals for stress management, go to the **Wellness Journal in HealthNow** at http://healthnow.brookscole.com/ith.

---

7. Which of the following situations is representative of a societal stressor?

   a. Peter has been told that his transfer application has been denied because his transcripts were not sent in by the deadline.

   b. Nia and Kwame find an unsigned note pinned to the door of their new home ordering them to move out or face the consequences.

   c. Kelli's boyfriend drives her car after he had been drinking and has an accident.

   d. Joshua, who is the leading basketball player on his college varsity team, has just been diagnosed with diabetes.

8. If you are stuck in a traffic jam, which of the following actions will help reduce your stress level?

   a. deep slow breathing

   b. honking your horn

   c. berating yourself for not taking a different route

   d. getting on your cell phone to reschedule appointments

9. A relaxed peaceful state of being can be achieved with which of the following activities?

   a. an aerobic exercise class

   b. playing a computer game

   c. meditating for 15 minutes

   d. attending a rap concert

10. A person suffering from posttraumatic stress disorder may experience which of the following symptoms?

   a. procrastination

   b. constant thirst

   c. drowsiness

   d. terror-filled dreams

Answers to these questions can be found on page 587.

Critical Thinking

1. What reasons can you think of to account for high stress levels among college students? Consider possible social, cultural, and economic factors that may play a role.

2. Identify three stressful situations in your life and determine whether they are examples of eustress or distress. Describe both the positive and negative aspects of each situation.

3. Can you think of any ways in which your behavior or attitudes might create stress for others? What changes could you make to avoid doing so?

4. What advice might you give an incoming freshman at your school about managing stress in college? What techniques have been most helpful for you in dealing with stress? Suppose that this student is from a different ethnic group than you. What additional suggestions would you have for this student?

Media Menu

Health Now™

Throughout the chapter, this icon introduces a list of resources on the Health-Now website at **http://healthnow.brookscole.com/ith** that will:

- Help you evaluate your knowledge of the material.
- Allow you to take an exam-prep quiz.
- Provide a Personalized Learning Plan targeting resources that address areas you should study.
- Coach you through identifying target goals for behavior change and creating and monitoring your personal change plan throughout the semester.

INTERNET CONNECTIONS

Stress Management: A Review of Principles

www.unl.edu/stress/mgmt
This is an online series of lectures on stress management presented by Wesley E. Sime, Ph.D., M.P.H., Professor of Health and Human Performance at the University of Nebraska—Lincoln. It features information on the psychobiology of stress and relaxation, as well as the pathophysiology of stress.

How to Survive Unbearable Stress

www.teachhealth.com
This comprehensive website is written specifically for college students by Steven Burns, M.D. It features the following topics: signs of how to recognize stress, two

stress surveys for adults and college students, information on the pathophysiology of stress, the genetics of stress and stress tolerance, and information on how to best manage and even treat stress.

Mind Tools

www.mindtools.com/smpage.html
This site covers a variety of topics on stress management, including recognizing stress, exercise, time management, coping mechanisms, and more. The site also features a free comprehensive personal self-assessment with questions pertaining to work and home stressors, physical and behavioral signs and symptoms, as well as personal coping skills and resources.

InfoTrac College Edition Activities Log on, insert **stress management** into the Keyword search box, and limit your search to the past year. When you get the results, Mark articles to review, then Select one to read. Summarize three or four key points from the article.

You can find additional readings related to personal health with InfoTrac College Edition, an online library of more than 900 journals and publications. Follow the instructions for accessing InfoTrac College Edition that were packaged with your textbook; then search for articles using a keyword search.

For additional links, resources, and suggested readings on the InfoTrac College Edition, visit our Health and Wellness Resource Center at **http://health .wadsworth.com.**

Key Terms

The terms listed are used on the page indicated. Definitions of the terms are in the Glossary at the end of this book.

adaptive response 82	meditation 94
biofeedback 95	migraine headache 86
burnout 91	mindfulness 95
defense mechanisms 93	posttraumatic stress disorder (PTSD) 96
distress 82	
eustress 82	progressive relaxation 94
general adaptation syndrome (GAS) 82	stress 82
	stressors 82
guided imagery 94	visualization 94
homeostasis 82	

Healthy Lifestyles

Y ou have enormous influence over your health and vitality. This section provides information about the tools you have at hand to become healthier and feel more energetic throughout your lifetime. By learning how to eat a balanced and varied diet, how to manage your weight, and how to become physically fit, you can get started on a lifelong journey of becoming all you can be. As you take better care of your body today, you'll build the foundation for feeling your best for many tomorrows to come.

5 The Joy of Fitness

As a boy, Derek never thought about doing anything special to stay physically fit. He loved sports so much that he spent every free moment on a softball field or basketball court. He could sprint faster, jump higher, and hit a ball harder than any of his friends. In high school Derek's life revolved around practices and games. He was a varsity athlete and a regional all-star.

Early in his first year in college, an injury sidelined Derek. Frustrated that he had to sit out the season, he gave up his rigorous training routine. As he became immersed in academics and other activities, Derek stopped going to the gym or working out on his own. Yet he continued to think of himself as an athlete in excellent physical condition. When Derek went home for spring break, he joined his younger brothers on a neighborhood basketball court. While he wasn't surprised that his long shots were off, Derek was amazed by how quickly he got winded. In fifteen minutes, he was panting for breath. "Getting old," one of his brothers joked. "Getting soft," the other teased.

Often the college years represent a turning point in physical fitness. Like Derek, many students, busy with classes and other commitments, devote less time to physical activity. About four in ten undergraduates do not participate in moderate or vigorous physical activity on a regular basis.[1]

The choices you make and the habits you develop now can affect how long and how well you'll live. As you'll see in this chapter, exercise yields immediate rewards: It boosts energy, improves mood, soothes stress, improves sleep, and makes you look and feel better. In the long term, physical activity slows many of the changes associated with chronological aging, such as loss of calcium and bone density, lowers the risk of serious chronic illnesses, and extends the lifespan.

This chapter can help you reap these rewards. It presents the latest activity recommendations, documents the benefits of exercise, describes types of exercise, and provides guidelines for getting into shape and exercising safely.

(FAQ) Frequently Asked Questions

- Do gender and race affect fitness? *p. 107*
- How can I separate fitness facts from fiction? *p. 112*
- How much exercise is enough? *p. 116*
- Does stretching improve athletic performance? *p. 129*
- Can a person be fat and fit? *p. 131*
- How do I buy the right athletic shoe? *p. 132*
- How much water should I drink while exercising? *p. 134*
- How can I prevent injuries? *p. 136*

After studying the material in this chapter, you should be able to:

- **List** the five components of health-related fitness.
- **Discuss** the differences between sedentary and active lifestyles and develop strategies to become more active.
- **Describe** the health benefits of regular physical activity.
- **List** the different forms of cardiorespiratory activities and **describe** their potential health benefits and risks.
- **Explain** the benefits of a muscle training program and **describe** how to design a workout.
- **List** the potential health risks of strength-enhancing drugs and supplements.
- **Define** flexibility and describe the different types of stretching exercises.
- **Describe** the PRICE plan for handling an exercise injury.

You are designed to move. In ways far more complex than the fastest airplane or sleekest car, your body runs, stretches, bends, swims, climbs, glides, and strides—day after day, year after year, decade after decade. While mere machines break down from constant wear and tear, your body thrives on physical activity.

WHAT IS PHYSICAL FITNESS?

The simplest, most practical definition of **physical fitness** is the ability to respond to routine physical demands, with enough reserve energy to cope with a sudden challenge. You can consider yourself fit if you meet your daily energy needs; can handle unexpected extra demands; and are protecting yourself against potential health problems, such as heart disease. Fitness is important both for health and for athletic performance.

HEALTH-RELATED FITNESS

The five health-related components of physical fitness include aerobic or cardiorespiratory endurance, muscular strength, muscular endurance, flexibility, and body composition (the ratio of fat and lean body tissue).

Cardiorespiratory fitness refers to the ability of the heart to pump blood through the body efficiently. It is achieved through **aerobic exercise**—any activity, such as brisk walking or swimming, in which sufficient or excess oxygen is continually supplied to the body. In other words, aerobic exercise involves working out strenuously without pushing to the point of breathlessness.

Muscular strength refers to the force within muscles; it is measured by the absolute maximum weight that you can lift, push, or press in one effort. Strong muscles help keep the skeleton in proper alignment, improve posture, prevent back and leg aches, help in everyday lifting, and enhance athletic performance. Muscle mass increases along with strength, which makes for a healthier body composition and a higher metabolic rate.

Muscular endurance is the ability to perform repeated muscular effort; it is measured by counting how many times you can lift, push, or press a given weight. Important for posture, muscular endurance helps in everyday work as well as in athletics and sports.

Flexibility is the range of motion around specific joints—for example, the stretching you do to touch your toes or twist your torso. Flexibility depends on many factors: your age, gender, and posture; how muscular you are; and how much body fat you have. As children develop, their flexibility increases until adolescence. Then a gradual loss of joint mobility begins and continues throughout adult life. Both muscles and connective tissue, such as tendons and ligaments, shorten and become tighter if not consistently used through their full range of motion.

Body composition refers to the relative amounts of fat and lean tissue (bone, muscle, organs, water) in the body. As discussed in detail in Chapter 7, a high proportion of body fat has serious health implications, including increased incidence of heart disease, high blood pressure, diabetes, stroke, gallbladder problems, back and joint problems, and some forms of cancer.

Physical conditioning (or training) refers to the gradual building up of the body to enhance cardiorespiratory, or aerobic, fitness; muscular strength; muscular endurance; flexibility; and a healthy body composition.

ATHLETIC, OR PERFORMANCE-RELATED, FITNESS

You may jog five miles, work out with weights, and start each day with a stretching routine. This doesn't qualify you for the soccer team. Most sports, such as softball, tennis, and basketball, require additional skills, including:

- **Agility,** the ability to change direction rapidly
- **Balance,** or equilibrium, the ability to maintain a certain body position
- **Coordination,** the ability to integrate the movement of body parts to produce smooth, fluid movements
- **Power,** the product of force and speed
- **Reaction time,** the time required to respond to a stimulus
- **Speed,** or velocity, the ability to move rapidly.

© Lori Adamski Peek/Stone/Getty Images

Fitness can enhance every dimension of your health—improving your mood and your mind as well as your body. Go for the joy!

While many amateur and professional athletes are in superb overall condition, you do not need athletic skills to keep your body operating at maximum capacity throughout life.

FITNESS AND THE DIMENSIONS OF HEALTH

The concept of fitness is evolving. Rather than focusing only on miles run or weight lifted, instructors, coaches, and consumers are pursuing a broader vision of total fitness that encompasses every dimension of health:

▮ **Physical.** As described later in this chapter, becoming fit reduces your risk of major diseases, increases energy and stamina, and may prolong your life.

▮ **Emotional.** Fitness lowers tension and anxiety, lifts depression, relieves stress, improves mood, and promotes a positive self-image.

▮ **Social.** Physical activities provide opportunities to meet new people and to work out with friends or family.

▮ **Intellectual.** Fit individuals report greater alertness, better concentration, more creativity, and improved personal health habits.

▮ **Occupational.** Fit employees miss fewer days of work, are more productive, and incur fewer medical costs.

▮ **Spiritual.** Fitness fosters appreciation for the relationship between body and mind and may lead to greater realization of your potential.

▮ **Environmental.** Fit individuals often become more aware of their need for healthy air and food and develop a deeper appreciation of the physical world.

FAQ ## DO GENDER AND RACE AFFECT FITNESS?

Men and women of all racial backgrounds benefit equally from fitness. However, there are some physiological differences between men and women, many of which are related to size.

 On average, men are 10 to 15 percent bigger than women, with roughly twice the percentage of muscle mass and half the percentage of body fat. They have more sweat glands and a greater maximum oxygen uptake. A man's bigger heart pumps more blood with each beat. His larger lungs take in 10 to 20 percent more oxygen (Figure 5-1). His longer legs cover more distance with each stride. If a man jogs along at 50 percent of his capacity, a woman has to push to 73 percent of hers to keep up.

 Women have a higher percentage of body fat than men, and more is distributed around the hips and thighs; men carry more body fat around the waist and stomach.

College-age men average 15 percent body fat; college-age women, 23 percent. On average, women have 11 percent more body fat and 8 percent less muscle mass than men.[2]

The average woman has a smaller heart and blood volume than a man. Because women have a lower concentration of red blood cells, their bodies are less effective at transporting oxygen to their working muscles during exercise.

Even though training produces the same relative increases for both genders, a woman's maximum oxygen intake remains about 25 to 30 percent lower than that of an equally well-conditioned man. In elite athletes, the gender difference is smaller: 8 to 12 percent. Because the angle of the upper leg bone (femur) to the pelvis is greater in a woman, she is less efficient at running.

In some endurance events, such as ultramarathon running and long-distance swimming, female anatomy and physiology may have some aerobic advantages. The longer a race—on land, water, or ice—the better women perform.

In absolute terms, men are 30 percent stronger, but gender differences in absolute strength do not apply to all muscle groups. Women have about 40 to 60 percent of the upper-body strength of men but 70 to 75 percent of the lower-body strength.

When other measures are used, the strength of men and women is nearly equal. If the amount of lean body mass is taken into consideration, women are about equal in strength to men. When strength is calculated per cross-sectional area of muscle, there are no significant gender differences.

 Racial and ethnic backgrounds also influence fitness. According to recent research, white men perform better than African-American men on exercise stress tests, which evaluate the heart's health. Among women, physical fitness levels are similar between whites and blacks, but obesity is more common among African Americans.[3] These findings suggest that, if you are African American, you may need to place even greater emphasis on improving your overall fitness to reduce your risk of heart disease.[4]

	Female	**Male**
Percent fat	27%	15%
Lean body mass	107.8 pounds	134.2 pounds
Blood volume	4.5–5 liters	5–6 liters
Maximum oxygen consumption	3–3.5 liters per minute	5.5–5.9 liters per minute

FIGURE 5-1 **Physiological Differences Between Men and Women**

THE INACTIVITY EPIDEMIC

One in four Americans reports no physical activity at all, according to the CDC. About half exercise occasionally, but not at the levels recommended by the National Center for Chronic Disease Prevention and Health Promotion. Only one in four adults meets the levels of physical activity recommended by federal health officials.[5]

Many factors affect physical activity levels, including geographic location, gender, education, and income. According to the CDC, city-dwellers are more active than country folks, westerners more active than those in other regions. Men, people with higher education levels, and high-income earners work out more often.

How do Americans spend most of their leisure time? Watching television. We average more than 30 hours a week. Yet the more time spent in front of the TV, the greater the risk of obesity and related chronic diseases. Compared with other sedentary activities, such as reading, writing, or driving, watching TV lowers metabolic rate, so people burn fewer calories.

THE TOLL OF SEDENTARY LIVING

Inactivity increases all causes of mortality, doubles the risk of cardiovascular diseases, diabetes, and obesity, and increases the risk of colon cancer, high blood pressure, osteoporosis, depression, and anxiety. The combination of physical inactivity and being overweight is responsible for more than 300,000 deaths a year.[6] Epidemiologists predict that this deadly duo may soon overtake tobacco as the nation's number-one killer.

The economic impact is equally staggering: an estimated $1 trillion in health-care bills a year. As a risk factor for heart disease, physical inactivity ranks as high as elevated cholesterol, high blood pressure, or cigarette smoking.[7]

WORKING OUT ON CAMPUS: STUDENT BODIES IN MOTION

College students aren't necessarily more active or fit than the general population. In a recent study that followed undergraduates through their first two years of college, about half engaged in regular aerobic exercise; 30 percent did not exercise at all.[8] (See Student Snapshot: "How Much Do Undergraduates Exercise?"). In the most recent American College Health Assessment's National College Health Assessment survey, 44 percent of students reported exercising vigorously for at least 20 minutes and moderately for at least 30 minutes on three or more of the preceding seven days; 51 percent exercised to strengthen or tone their muscles two or more the preceding seven days.[9] Men are consistently more active than women on campus. In one study at a large midwestern university, male students averaged 6.2 hours a week of moderate or vigorous exercise; female students, 5.5 hours. (By comparison, college men spend 12 hours watching TV or DVDs; women, 9.6 hours.)[10]

 Mexican-American students, both male and female, and African-American women report the lowest rates of physical activity. The most physically active men are African American; the most active women, white.[11]

Young adults typically become more sedentary after adolescence. The percentage engaging in regular vigorous physical activity plunges from 70 percent at age 12 to 35 percent at age 21.[12] As freshmen, both men and women report a significant drop in physical activity from high school. But according to a recent study that followed students through their first two years, about seven in ten freshmen and sophomores engaged in some form of exercise, although they shifted from aerobic workouts to strength training and stretching over time.

One factor that influences the exercise levels of undergraduates is the location of an exercise facility. In a recent study of more than 400 students, those who lived closest to a fitness facility (mostly freshmen and sophomores) exercised longer and harder than those (mostly juniors and seniors) who lived farther away.[13] For students living with their families or in off-campus housing, those with home exercise equipment worked out more often and intensely.

Simply enrolling in a health or wellness course can motivate students to get moving. In a study of 1,625 undergraduates enrolled in personal wellness classes, attitudes toward exercise and physical activity improved significantly over the course of a semester. Students who were not active or engaged only in light exercise registered positive changes, as well as the more active ones. The women students, who

---

Student Snapshot

HOW MUCH DO UNDERGRADUATES EXERCISE?

Activity	Freshman Year (Fall Semester)	Sophomore Year (Spring semester)
Aerobic exercise (3–5 days a week)	62%	55%
Strength Training (2–3 days a week)	43%	45%
Stretching (2–3 days a week)	30%	38%
At least one of the above	70%	71%
No exercise	30%	29%

Based on a survey of 764 college students at a midwestern university.
Source: Racette, Susan, et al. "Weight Changes, Exercise, and Dietary Patterns During Freshman and Sophomore Years of College." *Journal of American College Health,* Vol. 53, No. 6, May–June 2005, p. 245.

© Jurgen Reisch/Stone/Getty Images

© MediaImages/Getty Images

Are you ready to become more fit? What would it take? Will this class boost your motivation? Would a better grade?

were generally less active than the males, showed the greatest boost in positive attitudes toward exercise and fitness.[14]

Would you exercise more if your grade in this class depended on it? That's what happened in a University of Texas physical therapy class. Students were told that by reducing their body fat percentage volunteers would earn bonus points toward improving their grades, either on a single exam or for the entire course. The students offered the chance to improve their course grade were more likely to stick with the exercise program and lost more body fat than those offered the lesser reward of improving a single exam grade. The biggest fat losers—and bonus point winners—had also been more physically active prior to the course. Their appreciation of the intangible benefits of regular exercise—stronger muscles, greater stamina, brighter mood, less anxiety and depression—may have served as another form of motivation beyond the academic reward.[15]

Even if grades are a student's only incentive, getting into the exercise habit can have lifelong rewards. Undergraduates who work out regularly tend to stay active—or become even more active—after graduation, while college couch potatoes move even less—and find themselves at greater risk of health problems.[16] In a study that followed men and women between ages 18 and 30 for 15 years, those with the lowest fitness levels were three to six times more likely to develop diabetes, hypertension, and metabolic syndrome (discussed in Chapter 15) than those with higher fitness levels.[17]

PHYSICAL ACTIVITY AND HEALTH

WHY EXERCISE?

If exercise could be packed into a pill, it would be the single most widely prescribed and beneficial medicine in the nation. Why? Because nothing can do more to help your body function at its best—a fact that not all students are aware of. In a recent survey, eight in ten undergraduates realized that physical activity can prevent heart disease and prevent and treat obesity. However, fewer than half knew that it maintains bone density and can help prevent diabetes.[19]

As Figure 5-2 illustrates, exercise provides head-to-toe benefits. With regular activity, your heart muscles become stronger and pump blood more efficiently. Your heart rate and resting pulse slow down. Your blood pressure may drop slightly from its normal level.

Exercise thickens the bones and can slow the loss of calcium that normally occurs with age. Physical activity increases flexibility in the joints and improves digestion and elimination. It speeds up metabolism and builds lean body mass, so the body burns more calories and body fat decreases. It heightens sensitivity to insulin (a great benefit for diabetics) and may lower the risk of developing diabetes. In addition, exercise enhances clot-dissolving substances in the blood, helping to prevent strokes, heart attacks, and pulmonary embolisms (clots in the lungs), and it helps lower the risk of certain cancers. Regular exercise can actually extend your lifespan and sharpen your memory and mind.[20]

Strategies for Change :: Get Moving

:: **Sign up for a fitness class,** such as spinning or step-aerobics, so that exercise is built into your weekly schedule.

:: **Go to the gym with friends.** "Even if it's rainy and cold, I know they're waiting for me so I go," one woman explains.

:: **Find a fun workout.** "I love working out when it's something different—like water aerobics, ice skating, or swing dance," says one student.

:: **Join a team—or root for one.** College sports, whether competitive or informal, can help maintain fitness levels. So can cheerleading, which has become

so physically demanding that college cheerleaders have scored as high a fitness level as college athletes.[18]

:: **Do double-duty.** Some students read class notes while on a Stairmaster or stationary bicycle. Others listen to required reading books as they work out.

Improves your mood, reduces psychological symptoms, and sharpens your thinking.

Increases your respiratory capacity

Reduces your risk of heart disease.

Improves your digestion and your fat metabolism

Lowers your body fat and reduces your weight

Strenghtens your bones and increases joint flexibility.

Increases your muscle strength and tone

Improves your circulation.

FIGURE 5-2 The Benefits of Exercise
Regular physical activity enhances your overall health and helps prevent disease.

Healthier Heart and Lungs

Regular physical activity makes blood less likely to clot and cause a stroke or heart attack. Sedentary people are about twice as likely to die of a heart attack as people who are physically active. (See Chapter 15 for a discussion of heart disease.)

Exercise also lowers levels of one of the indicators of in-

creased risk of heart disease and diabetes (C-reactive protein, which is discussed in Chapter 15).[21] Exercise itself, even without weight loss, may reduce the risk of developing the prediabetic condition called metabolic syndrome, which if untreated can lead to type 2 diabetes and increase the risk of heart disease.[22]

In addition to its effects on the heart, exercise makes the lungs more efficient. The lungs take in more oxygen, and their vital capacity (the maximum amount of air volume the lungs can take in and expel) increases, providing more energy for you to use.

Even in young men, physical fitness is associated with improvements in blood pressure and the makeup of blood fats, including cholesterol and triglycerides.[23] Exercise, along with a healthy weight, keeps blood fats at healthy levels over time. Prolonged, sustained endurance training prevents the stiffening of the heart muscle once thought to be an inevitable consequence of aging.

Protection Against Cancer

As discussed in Chapter 7, fatness increases the risk of several cancers; fitness decreases it. The evidence for exercise's protective effects is strongest for colon and rectal cancer, possibly because it enhances digestion and elimination. Physical activity also lowers the risk of breast cancer in women.[24] Breast cancer patients who perform the equivalent of three to five hours of walking a week live longer and reduce their *risk* of dying.[25]

In a study that followed more than 5,000 men and women for more than 20 years, fitness was a strong predictor of cancer death rates for men, but not for women. The fittest men had the lowest cancer death rates. But for women, body weight, as measured by **body mass index** (**BMI,** discussed in Chapter 7), proved more significant.[26]

Less Risk of Disease

Moderate exercise correlates with a reduced number of sick days. Researchers speculate that exercise may enhance immune function by reducing stress hormones like cortisol that can dampen resistance to disease.

Women who walk briskly for 35 to 45 minutes five days a week experience half the number of sick days with cold symptoms as inactive women. While moderate exercise seems to bolster a person's immune system, heavy training may increase the risk of upper respiratory tract infections for endurance athletes.

Moderate exercise, combined with a balanced diet and weight loss, can cut in half the risk of developing diabetes among those at high risk.[27] For individuals with type 2 (non–insulin-dependent) diabetes, intense aerobic exercise and strength training help control blood sugar levels.[28]

Brighter Mood

Exercise makes people feel good from the inside out. Exercise boosts mood, elevates self-esteem, increases energy, reduces anxiety, improves concentration and alertness, and enables people to handle stress better. During long workouts, some people experience what is called "runner's high," which may be the result of increased levels of mood-elevating brain chemicals called **endorphins.**

Better Mental Health and Functioning

Exercise is an effective—but underused—treatment for mild to moderate depression and may help in treating other mental disorders. Regular, moderate exercise, such as walking, running, or lifting weights, three times a week, has proved helpful for depression and anxiety disorders, including panic attacks.[29] Exercise is as effective as medication in improving mood and also helps prevent relapse.

According to numerous long-term studies, physically fit adults perform better on cognitive tests than their less fit peers.[30] Improving cardiorespiratory fitness reduces the harmful effects of aging on brain structures as well as on memory and other functions.[31] Engaging in a variety of physical activities, such as hiking, dancing, golfing, and gardening, reduces the risk of dementia in older people.[32]

Better Bones

By 2020, one in two Americans over age 50 may suffer **osteoporosis**—a condition in which bones lose their mineral density and become susceptible to injury. Most are unaware that their bone health is in jeopardy. Four times as many men and almost three times as many women actually have osteoporosis than realize they do.[33]

 You may think that weak, brittle bones are a problem only for the elderly. However, 2 percent of college-age women have osteoporosis. According to a recent study, another 15 percent have already sustained significant losses in bone density and are at high risk of osteoporosis. Women who did not participate in high school sports were seven times more likely to have low bone density than were those who had.[34] The college women at greatest risk often were extremely skinny and maintained their low weights and slim looks by dieting and by avoiding exercise so as not to increase their muscle mass. Some had eliminated dairy products, an important source of calcium, from their diets. Depo-Provera, a method of birth control that consists of hormone injections every three months, also was associated with low bone density, especially with long-term use. (See Chapter 10 on contraception.)

 What are the best exercises to boost bone density? According to a study of college women, high-impact aerobics, such as step

TABLE 5-1 RX: HEALTHY BONES

Mode	Intensity	Frequency	Duration
Weight-bearing endurance activities, such as tennis and jogging; activities that involve jumping; and resistance exercise, such as weight lifting	Moderate to high	Weight-bearing activities, 3 to 5 times per week; resistance exercise, 2 or 3 times per week	30 to 60 minutes

Source: "Physical Activity and Bone Health." Position Stand, American College of Sports Medicine, www.acsm-/msse.org.

exercising, "may offer the quickest route to building bone in young women." Resistance exercises such as squats, leg presses, and calf presses strengthened leg muscles but had no effect on bone density.[35] The American College of Sports Medicine recommends moderate- to high-intensity weight-bearing activities to maintain bone mass in adults (Table 5-1).[36]

Lower Weight

For individuals on a diet, exercise provides extra benefits: A combination of dietary change and moderate to high-level intensity exercise leads to greater weight loss than either alone. Dieters who work out lose more fat than lean muscle tissue, which improves their body composition. In one study, college-age men who started exercising lost abdominal fat, which poses the greatest risk to health.[37] (See Chapter 7 for information on exercise and weight control.)

Sexuality

By improving physical endurance, muscle tone, blood flow, and body composition, exercise improves sexual functioning. Simply burning 200 extra calories a day can significantly lower the risk of erectile dysfunction in sedentary men. Exercise also may increase sexual drive, activity, and sexual satisfaction in people of all ages. In a recent study of about 400 students at a southeastern university, college students who exercise frequently and see themselves as physically fit rate themselves higher with regard to sexual performance and sexual desirability than those who exercise less and don't describe themselves as fit. All the men who exercised six to seven days per week rated their sexual desirability as above or much above average.[38]

Benefits for Students

Unlike middle-aged and older individuals, traditional-age college students cite improved fitness as the number-one advantage that exercise offers, followed by improved appearance and muscle tone. Undergraduates who recognize the benefits of exercise are more likely to be physically active than those who focus on barriers to working out.[39]

Will exercise improve your grades? Not necessarily. A study at two Texas universities found that the fittest students didn't necessarily have higher GPAs. However, increasing their level of physical fitness did have a positive impact on the GPAs of the female students.

A More Active Old Age

Exercise slows the changes that are associated with advancing age: loss of lean muscle tissue, increase in body fat, and decrease in work capacity. In addition to lowering the risk of heart disease and stroke, exercise also helps older men and women retain the strength and mobility needed to live independently. Even in old age, exercise boosts strength and stamina, lessens time in wheelchairs, and improves outlook and sense of control.

Longer Life

Capacity for exercise has proved a better predictor of whether a man would die in the next few years than other risk factors, such as high blood pressure, high total cholesterol, or smoking. Formerly sedentary people, even the elderly, who begin to exercise live longer, on average, than those who remain inactive. However, for active people, light to moderate exercise won't do it—only vigorous exercise reduces the risk of dying of heart disease and of premature death from other causes.[40]

EXERCISE GUIDELINES FOR AMERICANS

Because inactivity is so hazardous to our well-being, public health officials have tried many approaches to get Americans moving. Rather than emphasizing vigorous cardiorespiratory or aerobic activity, a landmark report by the Surgeon General in 1996 recommended 30 minutes of moderate intensity exercise—such as brisk walking, bicycling, and gardening—on all or most days of the week.

The most recent federal Dietary Guidelines call for more physical activity for added health benefits:

- *"Engage in regular physical activity and reduce sedentary activities to promote health, psychological well-being, and a healthy body weight.*
  - *To reduce the risk of chronic disease in adulthood: Engage in at least 30 minutes of moderate-intensity physical activity, above usual activity, at work or home on most days of the week.*
  - *For most people, greater health benefits can be obtained by engaging in physical activity of more vigorous intensity or longer duration.*
  - *To help manage body weight and prevent gradual, unhealthy body weight gain in adult-*

hood: Engage in approximately 60 minutes of moderate- to vigorous-intensity activity on most days of the week while not exceeding caloric intake requirements.

- *To sustain weight loss in adulthood: Participate in at least 60 to 90 minutes of daily moderate-intensity physical activity while not exceeding caloric intake requirements. Some people may need to consult with a health-care provider before participating in this level of activity.*
- *Achieve physical fitness by including cardiovascular conditioning, stretching exercises for flexibility, and resistance exercises or calisthenics for muscle strength and endurance."*[41]

(FAQ) ## HOW CAN I SEPARATE FITNESS FACTS FROM FICTION?

No pain, no gain. Strength training makes women bulk up. A gym is the only place for a good workout.

You've probably heard statements like these, but none is true. As noted in Savvy Consumer: "Watch Out for 'Pump Fiction'," there's as much misinformation as information available on fitness. A lot of exercise advice, even if well intentioned, may be outdated or unproven. Here are some common fitness myths—and the facts about them.[42]

- **No pain, no gain.** Some muscle soreness when you start or intensify your exercise program isn't unusual, but you don't have to push yourself to extremes to benefit. Exercise should never hurt. If it does, stop.
- **Women who work with weights look bulky.** Women don't have enough testosterone—the hormone that can develop bulky muscles in men—to start looking like bodybuilders.
- **You need a gym to keep you fit.** Physical activity can take many forms in many places. Ride a bike to class. Hike in the woods. Swim; ski; dance; garden. What matters is moving, not where you do it.
- **All you need is aerobics.** A variety of exercises, including ones for strength and flexibility, keep body and mind at peak performance.
- **Crunches or sit-ups can flatten your stomach.** Although they will strengthen your abdominal muscles, these exercises can't eliminate a pot belly—unless you also lose excess pounds.
- **Once you start working out, you can eat as much as you want.** Unfortunately, you still have to balance the equation between the calories you consume and the calories you burn.

THE PRINCIPLES OF EXERCISE

Your body is literally what you make of it. Superbly designed for multiple uses, it adjusts to meet physical demands. If you need to sprint for a bus, your heart will speed up and pump more blood. Beyond such immediate, short-term adaptations, physical training can produce long-term changes in heart rate, oxygen consumption, and muscle strength and endurance. Although there are limits on the maximum levels of physical fitness and performance that any individual can achieve, regular exercise can produce improvements in everyone's baseline wellness and fitness.

As you begin the process of working toward total fitness, it's important to keep in mind the principles of exercise, discussed next.

OVERLOAD PRINCIPLE

The **overload principle** requires a person exercising to provide a greater stress or demand on the body than it's usually accustomed to handling. For any muscle, including the heart, to get stronger, it must work against a greater-than-normal resistance or challenge. To continue to improve, you need further increases in the demands—but not too much too quickly. **Progressive overloading**—gradually increasing physical challenges—provides the benefits of exercise without the risk of injuries (Figure 5-3).

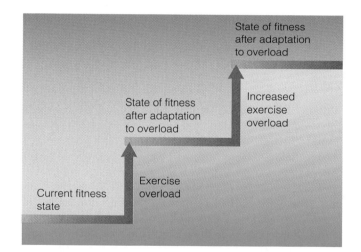

FIGURE 5-3   The Overload Principle
By increasing frequency, intensity, or duration, you will improve your level of fitness. Once your body adapts (becomes comfortable) to the demands, you can again apply the overload principle to achieve a higher level of fitness.

Overloading is specific to each body part and to each component of fitness. Leg exercises develop only the lower limbs; arm exercises, only the upper limbs. This is why you need a comprehensive fitness plan that includes a variety of exercises to develop different parts of the body. If you play a

TABLE 5-2 GUIDELINES FOR PHYSICAL FITNESS: THE FITT PRINCIPLE

	Cardiorespiratory	Strength	Flexibility
Frequency: Most days of the week. Start with three days and gradually increase frequency.	Almost every day	2 to 3 days per week	A minimum of 2 to 3 days per week
Intensity: Start at low to moderate intensity and gradually increase to more vigorous efforts over several weeks.	60 to 85 percent of maximum heart rate	Enough to enhance muscle strength and improve body composition	Enough to develop and maintain a full range of motion
Time: 30 to 60 minutes, using a gradual progression.	20 to 60 minutes	8 to 12 repetitions of 8 to 10 different exercises (minimum)	4 repetitions of 10 to 30 seconds per muscle group (minimum)
Type of activity: Start with low-impact activities (walking, cycling, low-impact aerobics, water exercise); resistance or weight training; flexibility exercises.	Aerobic activity that uses large-muscle groups and can be maintained continuously	Resistance activity that is performed at a controlled speed and through a full range of motion	Stretching activity that uses the major muscle groups

Source: Adapted from American College of Sports Medicine, "Position Stand: The Recommended Quantity and Quality of Exercise for Developing and Maintaining Cardiorespiratory and Muscular Fitness, and Flexibility in Healthy Adults." *Medicine and Science in Sports and Exercise,* Vol. 30, 1998, pp. 975–991; and from Kyle McInnis et al., "Counseling for Physical Activity in Overweight and Obese Patients." *American Family Physician,* Vol. 67, No. 6, March 15, 2003, p. 1254.

particular sport, you also need training to develop sports-specific skills, such as a strong, efficient stroke in swimming.

FITT

Although low-intensity activity can enhance basic health, you need to work harder—that is, at a greater intensity—to improve fitness. Whatever exercise you do, there is a level, or threshold, at which fitness begins to improve; a target zone, where you can achieve maximum benefits; and an upper limit, at which potential risks outweigh any further benefits. The acronym **FITT** sums up the four dimensions of progressive overload: *frequency* (how often you exercise), *intensity* (how hard), *time* (how long), and *type* (specific activity) (Table 5-2).

Frequency

To attain and maintain physical fitness, you need to exercise regularly, but the recommended frequency varies with different types of exercise and with an individual's fitness goals. Health officials urge Americans to engage in moderate-intensity aerobic activity most days and in resistance and flexibility training two or three days a week.

Intensity

Exercise intensity varies with the type of exercise and with personal goals. To improve cardiorespiratory fitness, you need at a minimum to increase your heart rate to a target zone (the level that produces benefits). To develop muscular strength and endurance, you need to increase the amount of weight you lift or the resistance you work against and/or the number of repetitions. For enhanced flexibility, you need to stretch muscles beyond their normal length.

Activities of "moderate" intensity burn 3.5 to 7 calories per minute. They include brisk walking, dancing, bicycling, and mowing the lawn. Activities of "vigorous" intensity—jogging, cycling uphill, swimming continuous laps, and heavy yard work—burn more than 7 calories per minute. The more vigorous an activity is, the less time needed to burn the same number of calories. As Figure 5-4 shows, you can burn 150 calories in just 15 minutes on a stair machine. You would have to shoot hoops for half an hour or play touch football for up to 45 minutes in order to burn the same amount.

Another way to determine how much physical activity a particular exercise provides is by its MET, or metabolic equivalent, a measurement of how much oxygen, or energy, it uses. One MET is the amount of energy you use when you are resting. Two METS is twice resting energy expenditure; three METS is three times, and so on.

Time (Duration)

The amount of time, or duration, of your workouts is also important, particularly for cardiorespiratory exercise. As noted in Table 5-2, the American College of Sports Medicine recommends 30 to 45 minutes of aerobic exercise, preceded by 5 to 10 minutes of warm-up and followed by 5 to 10 min-

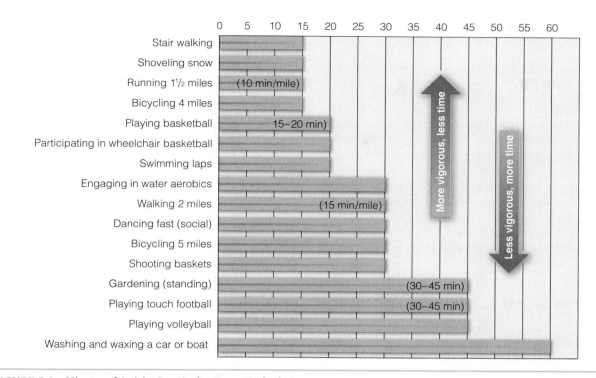

	0	5	10	15	20	25	30	35	40	45	50	55	60

Stair walking
Shoveling snow
Running 1½ miles   (10 min/mile)
Bicycling 4 miles
Playing basketball   15–20 min)
Participating in wheelchair basketball
Swimming laps
Engaging in water aerobics
Walking 2 miles   (15 min/mile)
Dancing fast (social)
Bicycling 5 miles
Shooting baskets
Gardening (standing)   (30–45 min)
Playing touch football   (30–45 min)
Playing volleyball
Washing and waxing a car or boat

More vigorous, less time

Less vigorous, more time

FIGURE 5-4   Minutes of Activity Required to Burn 150 kcalories

Source: Centers for Disease Control and Prevention, www.cdc.gov/accdphp/dnpa/physical/recommendations/adults.htm

utes of stretching. However, experts have found similar health benefits from a single 30-minute session of moderate exercise as from several shorter sessions throughout the day. Duration and intensity are interlinked. If you're exercising at high intensity (biking or running at a brisk pace, for instance), you don't need to exercise as long as when you're working at lower intensity (walking or swimming at a moderate pace). For muscular strength and endurance and for flexibility, duration is defined by the number of sets or repetitions rather than total time.

Type (Specificity)

The **specificity principle** refers to the body's adaptation to a particular type of activity or amount of stress placed upon it. Jogging, for instance, trains the heart and lungs to work more efficiently and strengthens certain leg muscles. However, it does not build upper body strength or enhance flexibility.

REVERSIBILITY PRINCIPLE

The **reversibility principle** is the opposite of the overload principle. Just as the body adapts to greater physical demands, it also adjusts to lower levels. If you stop exercising, you can lose as much as 50 percent of your fitness improvements within two months. If you have to curtail your usual exercise routine because of a busy schedule, you can best maintain your fitness by keeping the intensity constant and reducing frequency or duration. The principle of reversibility is aptly summed up by the phrase, "Use it or lose it."

INDIVIDUALITY

No two bodies are alike, and the same is true of fitness, athletic performance, and sports skills. There are individual limits on each person's adaptability and potential for improvement. Most people can improve their vital capacity— their maximum oxygen intake—by about 15 to 30 percent

The goal of exercise isn't to become a competitive athlete but to improve your well-being and achieve your maximum fitness potential.

through training. This may not be enough to qualify for competitive sports, but it can produce life-long health benefits.

CROSS-TRAINING

Cross-training involves alternating two or more different types of fitness activities. The pioneers of contemporary cross-training were triathletes whose sport combines running, swimming, and cycling. Depending on the specific sports, cross-training can yield various benefits. Alternating aerobic workouts with weight lifting, for example, can increase speed and performance. Alternating running with a low-impact aerobic exercise, such as swimming, lessens the risk of knee, ankle, or shin injuries. Cross-training also offers the pleasures of variety and thus helps exercisers avoid boredom.

(FAQ) HOW MUCH EXERCISE IS ENOUGH?

The answer depends on your reasons for working out. If you want to feel better, boost your energy, tone your muscles, condition your heart, strengthen your bones, protect your heart, and lower your risk of major diseases, leading medical authorities, including the American College of Sports Medicine, the U.S. Surgeon General, and Health Canada's Physical Activity Guide to Healthy Active Living, recommend a minimum of 30 to 60 minutes of moderate activity (such as walking at a speed of three to four miles per hour) most days of the week. According to the most recent research, a minimum of 150 minutes a week of moderate-intensity exercise lifts men and women out of the "low-fitness" category and lowers their risk of cardiovascular disease[43] and diabetes,[44] regardless of weight or body composition.

While half an hour of exercise five days a week is good, according to a recent review of current research, working out more often and more intensely can yield more health dividends, including improved muscular strength and endurance.[45] You may also need to exercise longer and harder to maintain a healthy weight and lose excess pounds. As discussed on page ●●●, the latest Dietary Guidelines for Americans concludes that individuals who've lost weight may need to exercise 60 to 90 minutes a day to keep off the pounds.[46] Vigorous physical activity (such as jogging or spinning) burns calories more rapidly per unit of time than moderate activities like walking. It doesn't matter if your goal is to improve fitness or avoid fatness. The same strategy—regular physical activity—is the key to both.

IMPROVING CARDIORESPIRATORY FITNESS

Cardiorespiratory endurance refers to the ability of the heart, lungs, and circulatory system to deliver oxygen to muscles working rhythmically over an extended period of time. Unlike muscular endurance (discussed later in this chapter), which is specific to individual muscles, cardiorespiratory endurance involves the entire body. **Aerobic exercise,** which improves cardiorespiratory endurance, can take many forms, but all involve working strenuously without pushing to the point of breathlessness. A person who builds up good aerobic capacity can maintain long periods of physical activity without great fatigue.

In **anaerobic exercise,** the amount of oxygen taken in by the body cannot meet the demands of the activity. This quickly creates an oxygen deficit that must be made up later. Anaerobic activities are high in intensity but short in duration, usually lasting only about ten seconds to two minutes. An example is sprinting the quarter-mile, which leaves even the best-trained athletes gasping for air. In *nonaerobic exercise,* such as bowling, softball, or doubles tennis, there is frequent rest between activities. Because the body can take in all the oxygen it needs, the heart and lungs don't get much of a workout.

Aerobic training increases your **maximal oxygen uptake (VO_2 max),** the amount of oxygen you can use during physical activity. Depending on your initial level of fitness, you may be able to increase your maximal oxygen uptake by as much as 30 percent. As a result, you will be able to exercise longer and more intensely before becoming fatigued.

ARE YOU WORKING HARD ENOUGH?

A variety of methods can indicate if you're exercising hard enough to condition your heart and lungs, but not overdoing it. Each of the following methods has both advantages and limitations. Fitness experts advise combining two methods—an objective one like target heart rate, for instance, and a subjective one like the talk test—to assess the intensity of your aerobic workouts.[47]

Target Heart Rate

To use your pulse, or heart rate, as a guide, feel your pulse in the carotid artery in your neck. Slightly tilt your head back and to one side. Use your middle finger or forefinger, or both, to feel for your pulse. (Do not use your thumb; it has a beat of its own.) To determine your heart rate, count the number of pulses you feel for 10 seconds and multiply that number by six, or count for 30 seconds and multiply that number by two. Learn to recognize the pulsing of your heart when you're sitting or lying down. This is your **resting heart rate.**

Start taking your pulse during, or immediately after, exercise, when it's much more pronounced than when you're at rest. Three minutes after heavy exercise, take your pulse again. The closer that reading is to your resting heart rate, the better your condition. If it takes a long time for your pulse to recover and return to its resting level, your body's ability to handle physical stress is poor. As you continue working out, however, your pulse will return to normal much more quickly.

You don't want to push yourself to your maximum heart rate, yet you must exercise at about 60 to 85 percent of that maximum to get cardiorespiratory benefits from your training. This range is called your **target heart rate.** If you don't exercise intensely enough to raise your heart rate at least this high, your heart and lungs won't reap the most benefit from the workout. If you push too hard, and exercise at or near your absolute maximum heart rate, you run the risk of placing too great a burden on your heart. Figure 5-5 shows the target heart rate for various ages and activities. Find your age at the bottom of the figure and move up the grid to find your target heart rate for "aerobic workout."

You can also use the following steps to determine your maximum heart rate and target heart rate (in beats per minute):

1. Maximum heart rate: Subtract your age from 220. So if you are 20, your maximum heart rate is $220 - 20 = 200$ beats per minute.

2. Lower-limit target heart rate: Multiply your maximum heart rate by 0.6. So if you are 20, your lower-limit target heart rate is $200 \times 0.6 = 120$ beats per minute.

3. Upper-limit target heart rate. Multiply your maximum heart rate by 0.85. If you are 20, your upper-limit target heart range is $200 \times 0.85 = 170$.

Your target heart rate range is between your lower and upper limits.

According to the American College of Sports Medicine, for most people, exercising at the lower end of the target heart rate range for a long time is more beneficial than exercising at the higher end of the range for a short time. If your goal is losing weight, exercise at 60 to 70 percent of your maximum heart rate in order to burn fat calories. To improve aerobic endurance and strengthen your heart, work at 70 to 80 percent of your maximum heart rate. Competitive athletes may train at 80 to 100 percent of their maximum heart rate (Figure 5-5).

RATING OF PERCEIVED EXERTION (RPE)

Another option besides heart rate for monitoring your exercise intensity is the **Rating of Perceived Exertion (RPE),** a self-assessment scale that rates symptoms of breathlessness and fatigue. You can use the RPE scale to describe your sensation of effort when exercising and gauge how hard you are working. The American College of Sports Medicine revised the original RPE scale to a range of 0 to 10 (Figure 5-6). Most exercisers should aim for a perceived exertion of "somewhat strong" or "strong," the equivalent of 4 or 5 on the RPE scale.

RPE is considered fairly reliable, but about 10 percent of the population tends to over- or underestimate their exertion. Your health or physical education instructor can help you learn to match what your body is feeling to the RPE scale. By paying attention to how you feel at different exercise intensities, you can learn how to challenge yourself without risking your safety.

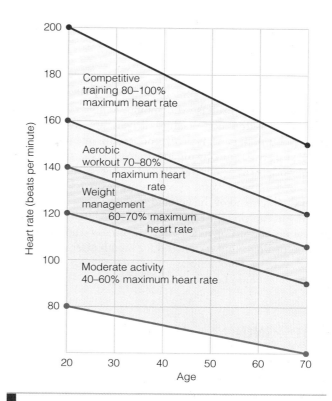

FIGURE 5-5 **Target Heart Rates for Different Ages and Various Levels of Activity**

Your maximum heart rate is 220 minus your age.

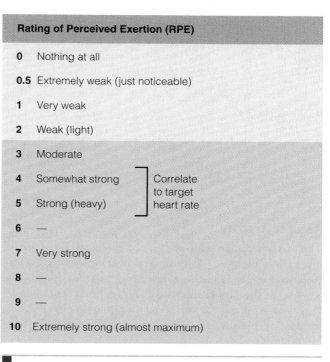

FIGURE 5-6 **Revised Scale for Rating of Perceived Exertion (RPE)**

You can learn to rate your exertion based on this scale.

Source: Original scale from Borg, G. "Psychophysical Bases of Perceived Exertion." *Medicine and Science in Sports and Exercise,* Vol. 14, No. 5, 2003, pp. 377–381.

You can also experiment with other alternative ways for determining exercise intensity. One of the easiest follows.

"TALK TEST"

During "aerobic" exercise you should be able to carry on a somewhat stilted conversation if you are indeed "with oxygen"—which is what the word "aerobic" means.

If you are gasping for air and unable to talk, you are most likely working at or beyond the anaerobic "without oxygen" threshold—a very, very, very hard intensity level at or beyond the high end of the aerobic zone.

If you can sing the entire Star Spangled Banner, you are probably not exerting much effort. If you can sing "Row Row Row Your Boat," but have to take a breath after every other word, you are probably working pretty hard—and just where you should be.

DESIGNING AN AEROBIC WORKOUT

Whatever activity you choose, your aerobic workout should consist of several stages: a warm-up, an aerobic activity, and a cool-down.

Warm-Up

Just as you don't get in your car and immediately gun your engine to 60 miles per hour, you shouldn't do the same with your body. You need to prepare your cardiorespiratory system for a workout, speed up the blood flow to your lungs, and increase the temperature and elasticity of your muscles and connective tissue to avoid injury.

After reviewing more than 350 scientific studies, the American College of Sports Medicine (ACSM) concluded that preparing for sports or exercise should involve a variety of activities and not be limited to stretching alone. They found little to no relationship between stretching and injuries or postexercise pain. A better option, according to the ACSM, is a combination of warm-up, strength training, and balance exercises.[48]

Aerobic Activity

The two key components of this part of your workout are intensity and duration. As described in the previous section, you can use your target heart rate range to make sure you are working at the proper intensity. The current recommendation is to keep moving for 30 to 60 minutes, either in one session or several briefer sessions, each lasting at least 10 minutes.

Cool-Down

After you've pushed your heart rate up to its target level and kept it there for a while, the worst thing you can do is slam on the brakes. If you come to a sudden stop, you put your heart at risk. When you stand or sit immediately after vigorous exercise, blood can pool in your legs. You need to keep moving at a slower pace to ensure an adequate supply of blood to your heart. Ideally, you should walk for 5 to 10 minutes at a comfortable pace before you end your workout session.

YOUR LONG-TERM FITNESS PLAN

One of the most common mistakes people make is to push too hard too fast. Often they end up injured or discouraged and quit entirely. If you are just starting an aerobic program, think of it as a series of phases: beginning, progression, and maintenance:

- **Beginning (4–6 weeks).** Start slow and low (in intensity). If you're walking, monitor your heart rate and aim for 55 percent of your maximum heart rate. Another good rule of thumb to make sure you're moving at the right pace: If you can sing as you walk, you're going too slow; if you can't talk, you're going too fast.
- **Progression (16–20 weeks).** Gradually increase the duration and/or intensity of your workouts. For instance, you might add 5 minutes every two weeks to your walking time. You also can gradually pick up your pace, using your target heart rate as your guide. Keep a log of your workouts so you can chart your progress until you reach your goal.
- **Maintenance (lifelong).** Once you've reached the stage of exercising for an hour every day, you may want to develop a repertoire of aerobic activities you enjoy. Combine or alternate activities to avoid monotony and keep up your enthusiasm (cross-training).

AEROBIC OPTIONS

You have lots of choices for aerobic exercise, so experiment. Focus on one for a few weeks; alternate different activities on different days; try something new every month.

Stepping Out: Walk the Walk

More men and women are taking to their feet. Some are casualties of high-intensity sports and can no longer withstand the wear and tear of rigorous workouts. Others want to shape up, slim down, or ward off heart disease and other health problems. The good news for all is that walking is good exercise. Recent research has demonstrated that walking reduces the risk of cardiorespiratory disease, in some studies, as much as vigorous activity does.[49]

 Why Walk? One major study of women, the Nurses Health Study, found that women who walk briskly three hours a week are as well protected from heart disease as women who spend an hour and a half a week in more vigorous activities, such as aerobics or running. Women engaged in either form of exercise had a rate of heart attacks 30 to 40 percent lower than that of sedentary women.

 Walking also protects men's hearts, whether they're healthy or have had heart problems. Men who regularly engage in light exercise, including walking, have a significantly lower risk of death than their sedentary counterparts.

Walking has proved to be one of the safest and most effective ways of preventing bone and joint disorders in obese individuals.[50]

Can you fit a brisk walk into your weekly schedule? You can reduce your risk of heart disease by walking briskly several times a week.

America on the Move How many steps do you walk every day? The typical adult averages about 5,310 steps; a child from 11,000 to 13,000. According to the American College of Sports Medicine, college students who used a pedometer to count their daily steps took an average of 7,700 steps per day.[51] This falls short of the 10,000 steps recommended as part of the national "America on the Move" program.

How far is 10,000 steps? The average person's stride length is approximately 2.5 feet long. That means it takes just over 2,000 steps to walk 1 mile, and 10,000 steps is close to 5 miles. Wearing a pedometer is an easy way to track your steps each day. Start by wearing the pedometer every day for one week. Put it on when you get up in the morning and wear it until bedtime. Record your daily steps in a log or diary. By the end of the week, you can calculate your average daily steps. To increase your steps, add 500 daily steps every week until you reach 10,000.

Why 10,000 steps? According to researchers' estimates, you take about 5,000 steps just to accomplish your daily tasks. Adding about 2,000 steps brings you to a level that can improve your health and wellness. Another 3,000 steps can help you lose excess pounds and prevent weight gain. People who walk at least 10,000 steps a day are more likely to have healthy weights.[52] In addition, 10,000 steps generally translates into 30 minutes of activity, the minimum recommended by the U.S. Surgeon General.

Counting steps with a pedometer pays off, according to another report by the American College of Sports Medicine.[53] In the study, women who used a pedometer walked substantially more than those who simply tried to take a 30-minute brisk walk on most days.[54]

Treadmills are a good alternative to outdoor walks—and not just in bad weather. They keep you moving at a certain pace, they're easier on the knees, and they allow you to exercise in a climate-controlled, pollution-free environment—a definite plus for many city dwellers. Holding onto the handrails while walking on a treadmill reduces both heart rate and oxygen consumption, so you burn fewer calories. Experts advise slowing the pace if necessary so you can let go of the handrails while working out.

Strategies for Change :: Walk This Way

Here are some guidelines for putting your best foot forward:

:: **Walk very slowly** for 5 minutes, and then do some simple stretches.

:: **Maintain good posture.** Focus your eyes ahead of you, stand erect, and pull in your stomach.

:: **Use the heel-to-toe method** of walking. The heel of your leading foot should touch the ground before the ball or toes of that foot do. When you push off with your trailing foot, bend your knee as you raise your heel. You should be able to feel the action in your calf muscles.

:: **Pump your arms back and forth** to burn 5 to 10 percent more calories and get an upper-body workout as well.

:: **End your walk the way you started it**—let your pace become more leisurely for the last 5 minutes.

Jogging and Running

The difference between jogging and running is speed. You should be able to carry on a conversation with someone on a long jog or run; if you're too breathless to talk, you're pushing too hard.

If your goal is to enhance aerobic fitness, long, slow, distance running is best. If you want to improve your speed, try *interval training*—repeated hard runs over a certain distance, with intervals of relaxed jogging in between. Depending on what suits you and what your training goals are, you can vary the distance, duration, and number of fast runs, as well as the time and activity between them.

If you have been sedentary, it's best to launch a walking program before attempting to jog or run. Start by walking for 15 to 20 minutes three times a week at a comfortable pace. Continue at this same level until you no longer feel sore or unduly fatigued the day after exercising. Then increase your walking time to 20 to 25 minutes, speeding up your pace as well.

When you can handle a brisk 25-minute walk, alternate fast walking with slow jogging. Begin each session walking, and gradually increase the amount of time you spend jogging. If you feel breathless while jogging, slow down and walk. Continue to alternate in this manner until you can jog for 10 minutes without stopping. If you gradually increase your jogging time by 1 or 2 minutes with each workout, you'll slowly build up to 20 or 25 minutes per session. For optimal fitness, you should jog at least three times a week.

Here's how to be sure you're running right:

- **Always take time to warm up** and to stretch. Warm up with jumping jacks or running in place for 3 to 5 minutes. Spend at least one-fourth of the time that you plan to run on stretching exercises.

- **As you run, keep your back straight** and your head up. Run tall, with your buttocks tucked in. Look straight ahead. Hold your arms slightly away from your body. Your elbows should be bent slightly so that your forearms are almost parallel to the ground. Move your arms rhythmically to propel yourself along.

- **Have your heels hit the ground first.** Land on your heel, rock forward, and push off the ball of your foot. If this is difficult, try a more flat-footed style.

- **Avoid running on the balls of your feet;** this produces soreness in the calves because the muscles must contract for a longer time. To avoid shin splints (a dull ache in the lower shins), stretch regularly to strengthen the shin muscles and to develop greater flexibility in your ankles.

- **Avoid running on hard surfaces** and making sudden stops or turns.

Other Aerobic Activities

Because variety is the spice of an active life, many people prefer different forms of aerobic exercise. All can provide many health benefits. Among the popular options:

- **Swimming.** For aerobic conditioning, you have to swim laps using the freestyle, butterfly, breaststroke, or backstroke. (The sidestroke is too easy.) You must also be a good enough swimmer to keep churning through the water for at least 20 minutes. Your heart will beat more slowly in water than on land, so your heart rate while swimming is not an accurate guide to exercise intensity. Try to keep up a steady pace that's fast enough to make you feel pleasantly tired, but not completely exhausted, by the time you get out of the pool.

- **Cycling.** Bicycling, indoors and out, can be an excellent cardiovascular conditioner, as well as an effective way to control weight—provided you aren't just along for the ride. If you coast down too many hills, you'll have to ride longer up hills or on level ground to get a good workout. An 18-speed bike can make pedaling too easy unless you choose gears carefully. To gain aerobic benefits, mountain bikers have to work hard enough to raise their heart rates to their target zone and keep up that intensity for at least 20 minutes.

- **Spinning.**™ Spinning is a cardiovascular workout for the whole body that utilizes a special stationary bicycle. Led by an instructor, a group of bikers listens to music, and modifies their individual bike's resistance and their own pace according to the rhythm. An average spinning class lasts 45 minutes.

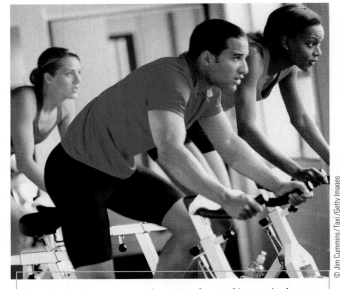

Spinning has become a popular option for aerobic exercise because people of different ages, skills, and fitness levels can participate in the same class.

© Jim Cummins/Taxi/Getty Images

In a recent study, participants at various fitness levels rated their levels of perceived exertion in the high teens through much of a typical spin class. However, the American Council on Exercise cautions that the intensity levels of many spin classes are far beyond what most beginners or part-time exercisers can achieve or maintain. You might want to train on a stationary bike before graduating to high-intensity spinning.[55]

❚ **Cardio kick-boxing.** Also referred to as kick-boxing or boxing aerobics, this hybrid of boxing, martial arts, and aerobics offers an intense cross-training and total-body workout. According to the American Council on Exercise, cardio kick-boxing strengthens body and mind, decreases stress, sharpens reflexes, and increases cardiorespiratory endurance and power. An hour of kick-boxing burns an average of 500 to 800 calories, compared to 300 to 400 calories in a typical step aerobics class.[56]

❚ **Rowing.** Whether on water or a rowing machine, rowing provides excellent aerobic exercise as well as working the upper and lower body. In addition to its benefits for the cardiorespiratory system, rowing tones the shoulders, back, arms, and legs. Correct rowing techniques are important to avoid back injury.

❚ **Skipping rope.** Essentially a form of stationary jogging with some extra arm action thrown in, skipping rope is excellent as both a heart conditioner and a way of losing weight. Always warm up before starting and cool down afterward.

❚ **Aerobic dancing.** This activity combines music with kicking, bending, and jumping. A typical class (you can also dance at home to a video or TV program) consists of stretching exercises and sit-ups, followed by aerobic dances and cool-down exercises. "Soft," or low-impact, aerobic dancing doesn't put as much strain on the joints as "hard," or high-impact, routines.

❚ **Step training, or bench aerobics.** "Stepping" combines step, or bench, climbing with music and choreographed movements. Basic equipment consists of a bench 4 to 12 inches high. The fitter you are, the higher the bench—but the higher the bench, the greater the risk of knee injury.

❚ **Stair-climbing.** You could run up the stairs in an office building or dormitory, but most people use stair-climbing machines available in home models and at gyms and health clubs.

❚ **Inline skating.** Inline skating can increase aerobic endurance and muscular strength and is less stressful on joints and bones than running or high-impact aerobics. Skaters can adjust the intensity of their workout by varying the terrain.

❚ **Tennis.** As with other sports, tennis can be an aerobic activity—depending on the number of players and their skill level. In general, a singles match requires more continuous exertion than playing doubles.

Your Life Coach

Overcoming Exercise Excuses

Why do you work out? Looking better and feeling better are two of the strongest motivators that pull college students to their feet. Studies show that students with a greater sense of self-efficacy and an internal locus of control place greater value on health and fitness, are more conscious about living a healthy lifestyle, and are more likely to be actively involved in activities that maintain or enhance fitness.[57]

The primary motivators for students are a desire to increase their fitness, improve the way their bodies look, enhance muscle tone and strength, and gain a sense of personal accomplishment.

If you don't exercise regularly, why not? As studies have shown, sedentary college students perceive fewer benefits from exercise than their more active peers. They also see more exercise barriers, things that get in the way of even the best intentions. The number-one obstacle for students is lack of time. College women rate the combination of time and effort as the primary barrier to strength training.[58] Feeling tired after exercise, viewing exercise as hard work, and not getting encouragement from family to exercise also discourage students from exercising.

For every excuse not to exercise, there is an excuse buster. Here is a sampling of excuses from an Internet survey of college students—and some effective responses:

Excuse	Excuse-Buster
❚ "Gym membership is too expensive."	You can get all the exercise you need on your own. Invest in a good pair of shoes and start walking or running. Select at-home strength and flexibility exercises from this chapter.
❚ "The school gym is always crowded."	Try different times, for example, early morning or afternoon. Rather than standing in line for machines, work with free weights.
❚ "I don't have time to spend an hour exercising."	Build activity into your day. Walk to classes or

		always take the stairs rather than the elevator in the dorms.
▪	"I mean to exercise, but I get too busy."	Sign up for a fitness "class," such as spinning or cardio kick-boxing, so that exercise is built into your weekly schedule.
▪	"I get to my room and just don't feel like leaving."	Arrange to meet friends at the gym. If you know they're waiting, you'll go out even if it's rainy and cold.
▪	"I get bored."	Find a fun workout. If you hate the treadmill, try spinning, aerobic dance, or inline skating.
▪	"I forget why exercise is important."	Use humor to keep yourself motivated. One student put this sign on the wall: "You think flu season is scary? Wait till bathing suit season hits!"
▪	"Studying takes all my time."	Do double-duty. Some students read class notes while on a stairmaster or stationary bicycle. Others listen to required books through earphones as they work out.

▌ BUILDING MUSCULAR FITNESS

Although aerobic workouts condition your insides (heart, blood vessels, and lungs), they don't exercise many of the muscles that shape your outsides and provide power when you need it. Strength workouts are important because they enable muscles to work more efficiently and reliably. Conditioned muscles function more smoothly and contract somewhat more vigorously and with less effort. With exercise, muscle tissue becomes firmer and can withstand much more strain—the result of toughening the sheath protecting the muscle and developing more connective tissue within it (Figure 5-7).

The two dimensions of muscular fitness are strength and endurance. Muscular **strength** is the maximal force that a muscle or group of muscles can generate for one movement. Muscular **endurance** is the capacity to sustain

repeated muscle actions. Both are important. You need strength to hoist a shovelful of snow—and endurance so you can keep shoveling the entire driveway.

Prolonged exercise prepares the muscles for sustained work by improving the circulation of blood in the tissue. The number of tiny blood vessels, called **capillaries,** increases by as much as 50 percent in regularly exercised muscles, and existing capillaries open wider so that the total circulation increases by as much as 400 percent, thus providing the muscles with a much greater supply of nutrients (Figure 5-7). This increase occurs after about 8 to 12 weeks in young persons, but takes longer in older individuals. Inactivity reverses the process, gradually shutting down the extra capillaries that have developed.

The latest research on fat-burning shows that the best way to reduce your body fat is to add muscle-strengthening exercise to your workouts. Muscle tissue is your very best calorie-burning tissue, and the more you have, the more calories you burn, even when you are resting. You don't have to become a serious body-builder. Using handheld weights (also called *free weights*) two or three times a week is enough. Just be sure you learn how to use them properly, because you can tear or strain muscles if you don't practice the proper weight-lifting techniques. As more people have begun to lift weights, injuries have soared.

A balanced workout regimen of muscle building and aerobic exercise does more for you than just burn fat. It gives you more endurance by promoting better distribution of oxygen to your tissues and increasing the blood flow to your heart.

 Strength training has particular benefits for women: As numerous studies have documented, it makes their muscles stronger, their bodies leaner, and their bones more resistant to falls. In young women, it boosts self-esteem, body image, and emotional well-being. In middle-aged and older women, it enhances self-concept and boosts psychological health.

Yet relatively few women—only an estimated 15 percent—do resistance or strength training. The reason, according to a study of college women at a large eastern university, is not that they aren't aware of the benefits. But those who do not engage in resistance training see more barriers to this type of exercise than women who regularly work their muscles. The number-one barrier: the amount of time and effort required. (As discussed in Your Life Coach: "Overcoming Exercise Excuses," students cite lack of time as the biggest obstacle to working out.)

MUSCLES AT WORK

Your muscles never stay the same. If you don't use them, they atrophy, weaken, or break down. If you use them rigorously and regularly, they grow stronger. The only way to develop muscles is by demanding more of them than you usually do. This is called **overloading.** (Remember the overload principle?) As you train, you have to gradually increase the number of repetitions or the amount of resistance and work

Strength workouts increase circulation

The heart's right half pumps oxygen-poor blood to capillary beds in lungs. There, O_2 diffuses into blood and CO_2 diffuses out. The oxygenated blood flows into the heart's left half where it is then pumped to capillary beds throughout the body.

Strength workouts build muscles

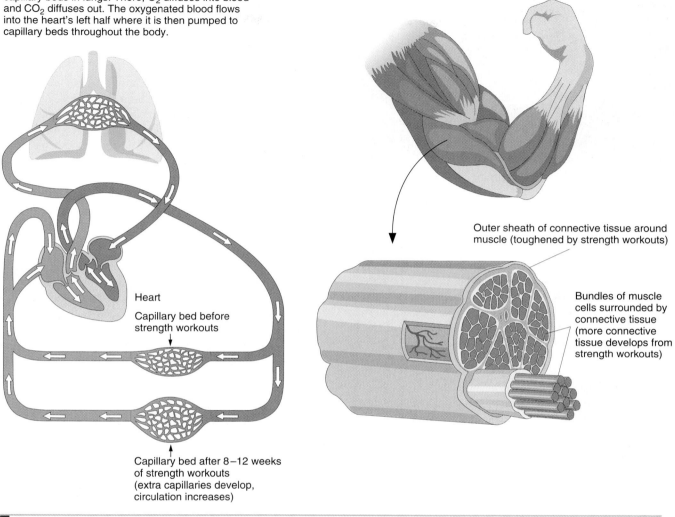

Heart
Capillary bed before strength workouts

Capillary bed after 8–12 weeks of strength workouts (extra capillaries develop, circulation increases)

Outer sheath of connective tissue around muscle (toughened by strength workouts)

Bundles of muscle cells surrounded by connective tissue (more connective tissue develops from strength workouts)

FIGURE 5-7 Benefits of Strength Training on the Body
Strength training increases blood circulation and oxygen supply to body tissues and develops muscles.

the muscle to temporary fatigue. That's why it's important not to quit when your muscles start to tire. Progressive over-load—steadily increasing the stress placed on the body—builds stronger muscles.

You need to exercise differently for strength than for endurance. *To develop strength,* do a few repetitions with heavy loads. As you increase the weight your muscles must move, you increase your strength. *To increase endurance,* you do many more repetitions with lighter loads. If your muscles are weak and you need to gain strength in your upper body, you may have to work for weeks to do a half-dozen regular push-ups. Then you can start building endurance by doing as many push-ups as you can before collapsing in exhaustion.

Muscles can do only two things: contract or relax. As they do so, skeletal muscles either pull on bones or stop pulling on bones. All exercise involves muscles pulling on bones across

a joint. The movement that takes place depends on the struc-ture of the joint and the position of the muscle attachments involved.

In an **isometric** contraction, the muscle applies force while maintaining an equal length. The muscle con-tracts and tries to shorten but cannot overcome the re-sistance. An example is pushing against an immovable object, like a wall, or tightening an abdominal muscle while sitting. The muscle contracts, but there is no movement. Push or pull against the immovable object, with each muscle contraction held for 5 to 8 seconds; repeat five to ten times daily.

An **isotonic** contraction involves movement, but the muscle tension remains the same. In an isotonic ex-ercise, the muscle moves a moderate load several times, as in weight lifting or calisthenics. The best isotonic exercise for producing muscular strength involves

© 2000 PhotoDisc, Inc.

You can build up muscular strength and endurance through various types of weight training.

high resistance and a low number of repetitions. On the other hand, you can develop the greatest flexibility, coordination, and endurance with isotonic exercises that incorporate lower resistance and frequent repetitions.

True **isokinetic** contraction is a constant speed contraction. Isokinetic exercises require special machines that provide resistance to overload muscles throughout the entire range of motion.

DESIGNING A MUSCLE WORKOUT

A workout with weights should exercise your body's primary muscle groups: the *deltoids* (shoulders), *pectorals* (chest), *triceps* and *biceps* (back and front of upper arms), *quadriceps* and *hamstrings* (front and back of thighs), *gluteus maximus* (buttocks), *trapezius* and *rhomboids* (back), and *abdomen* (Figure 5-8). Various machines and free-weight routines focus on each muscle group, but the principle is always the same: Muscles contract as you raise and lower a weight, and you repeat the lift-and-lower routine until the muscle group is tired.

A weight training program is made up of **reps** (the single performance, or **repetition,** of an exercise, such as lifting 50 pounds one time) and **sets** (a *set* number of repetitions of the same movement, such as a set of 20 push-ups). You should allow your breath to return to normal before moving on to each new set. Pushing yourself to the limit builds strength. Although the ideal number of sets in a resistance training program remains controversial, recent evidence suggests that multiple sets lead to additional benefits in short- and long-term training in young and middle-aged adults.

Maintaining proper breathing during weight training is crucial. To breathe correctly, inhale when muscles are relaxed and exhale when you push or lift. Don't ever hold your breath, because oxygen flow helps prevent muscle fatigue and injury.

No one type of equipment—free weight or machine— has a clear advantage in terms of building fat-free body

mass, enhancing strength and endurance, or improving a sport-specific skill. Each type offers benefits but also has drawbacks.

Free weights offer great versatility for strength training. With dumbbells, for example, you can perform a variety of exercises to work specific muscle groups, such as the chest and shoulders. Machines, in contrast, are much more limited; most allow only one exercise.

Strength-training machines have several advantages. They ensure correct movement for a lift, which helps protect against injury and prevent cheating when fatigue sets in. They isolate specific muscles, which is good for rehabilitating an injury or strengthening a specific body part. Because they offer high-tech options like varying resistance during the lifting motion, they can tax muscles in ways that a traditional barbell cannot.

RECOVERY

The American College of Sports Medicine recommends a minimum of eight to ten exercises involving the major muscle groups two to three days a week. Remember that your muscles need sufficient time to recover from a weight-training session. Never work a sore muscle, because soreness may indicate that too-heavy weights have caused tiny tears in the fibers. Allow no less than 48 hours, but no more than 96 hours, between training sessions, so your body can recover from the workout and you avoid overtraining. Workouts on consecutive days do more harm than good because the body can't recover that quickly. Strength training twice a week at greater intensity and for a longer duration can be as effective as working out three times a week. However, your muscles will begin to atrophy if you let more than three or four days pass without exercising them.

FUNCTIONAL STRENGTH EXERCISES

Certain exercises train our bodies in ways that enhance our ability to perform daily functions or tasks, such as lifting, reaching, climbing stairs, or balancing. Three of the simplest and most effective are:

▪ Push-ups, which firm your chest, arms, abdominals, and back. Start with standing push-ups against a wall. Progress to pushing against something lower, such as a kitchen counter or heavy dresser.

▪ Squats or lunges, which strengthen your knees, quadriceps, and hips. Don't let your knees go farther forward than your toes. (This may not be possible if you are extremely tall.)

▪ Lifts, which strengthen your arms. At a gym, use free weights, pulleys, or machines to work the biceps and triceps. At home, lift a heavy grocery bag or laundry basket several times.

Pectoralis minor

Rectus abdominus

Internal oblique

Sartorious

Quadriceps femoris

Trapezius

Deltoid

Pectoralis major

Serratus anterior

Biceps brachii

External oblique

Rhomboid minor

Rhomboid major

Erector spinae

Serratus posterior

Trapezius

Triceps

Latissimus dorsi

Gluteus maximus

Hamstrings

Gastrocnemius

Muscle Group	Exercise
Quadriceps, gluteals	Leg press
Hamstrings	Leg curl
Pectorals	Chest press
Latissimus dorsi	Lat pull down
Deltoids	Lateral raise
Triceps	Triceps press
Biceps	Biceps curl
Abdominals	Curl-up
Erector spinae	Back extension

FIGURE 5-8   Primary Muscle Groups
Different exercises can strengthen and stretch different muscle groups.

Strategies for Prevention   Working with Weights

If you plan to work with free weights, here are some guidelines for using them safely and effectively:

- Don't train alone—for safety's sake. Work with a partner so you can serve as spotters for each other and help motivate each other as well.

- Always warm up before weight training; also be sure to stretch after training.

- Breathe! Holding your breath during exertion can produce a dangerous rise in blood pressure.

- Begin with relatively light weights (50 percent of the maximum you can lift),

and increase the load slowly until you find the weight that will cause muscle failure at anywhere from eight to twelve repetitions. (Muscle failure is the point during a workout at which you can no longer perform or complete a repetition through the entire range of motion.)

- In the beginning, don't work at maximum intensity. Increase your level of exertion gradually over two to six weeks to allow your body to adapt to new stress without soreness.

- Always train your entire body, starting with the larger muscle groups. Don't

focus only on specific areas, although you may want to concentrate on your weakest muscles.

- Always use proper form. Unnecessary twisting, lurching, lunging, or arching can cause serious injury. Remember, quality matters more than quantity. One properly performed set of lifts can produce a greater increase in strength and muscle mass than many sets of improperly performed lifts.

- Work through the full range of motion. Be careful not to hyperextend or overextend.

CORE STRENGTH CONDITIONING

"Core strength," a popular trend in exercise and fitness, refers to the ability of the muscles to support your spine and keep your body stable and balanced. When you have good core stability, the muscles in your pelvis, lower back, hips, and abdomen work in harmony. This improves your posture, breathing, appearance, and performance in sports, while reducing your risk of muscle strain. When your core is weak, you become more susceptible to lower back pain and injury.

The major muscles of your core include the transverse abdominis, the deepest of the abdominal muscles; the external and internal obliques on the side and front of the abdomen around your waist; and the rectus abdominis, a long muscle that extends along the front of the abdomen. Strengthening all of your core muscles provides stability, improves balance, and protects you from injury.

PERFORMANCE-ENHANCING DRUGS

Performance-enhancing substances include any compounds taken to increase strength, power, speed, or endurance (ergogenic) or to change body weight or composition for the sake of boosting athletic performance. Approximately 1 to 3 million people in the United States have used these substances, including an estimated 12 percent of young men and 2 percent of young women.[59]

The discovery that many Major League Baseball players have used drugs to improve their power and performance set off a national scandal. But professional and amateur athletes aren't the only ones turning to drugs to reshape their bodies. Young men use them to look more buff and muscular. Older men try them to fight the effects of aging. All face serious risks to their hearts, liver, reproductive systems, and psychological well-being.

Steroids

Anabolic steroids are synthetic derivatives of the male hormone testosterone that promote the growth of skeletal muscle and increase lean body mass. Taken orally, applied in creams, or injected, anabolic steroids are typically used in cycles of weeks or months, rather than continuously. Users take multiple doses over a specific period of time, stop for a period, and start again. In addition, users frequently combine several different types of steroids to maximize their effectiveness while minimizing their negative effects. This practice is known as stacking.

Anabolic steroids have been reported to increase lean muscle mass, strength, and ability to train longer and harder, but they pose serious health hazards, including liver tumors, jaundice (yellowish pigmentation of skin, tissues, and body fluids), fluid retention, high blood pressure, decreased immune function, and severe acne. Men may experience shrinking of the testicles, reduced sperm count, infertility, baldness, and development of breasts. Women may experience growth of facial hair, acne, changes in or cessation of the menstrual cycle, enlargement of the clitoris, and deepened voice (Table 5-3). In women, these changes are irreversible. In men, side effects may be reversible once abuse stops.[60] In adolescents, steroids may bring about a premature halt in skeletal maturation.

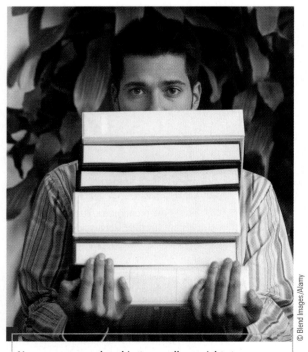

You can use everyday objects as well as weights to strengthen your muscles.

© Blend Images/Alamy

TABLE 5-3 SIDE EFFECTS OF ANABOLIC STEROIDS

Men	Women	Both men and women
Prominent breasts	Deeper voice	Severe acne
Baldness	Enlarged clitoris	High blood pressure
Shrinking of the testicles	Increased facial and body hair	Decreased immune function
Infertility	Hair loss	Liver abnormalities and tumors
	Changes in menstrual cycle	Increased harmful, low-density lipoprotein (LDL) and decreased beneficial, high-density lipoprotein (HDL) cholesterol
		Aggressive behaviors, rage, or violence
		Psychiatric disorders, such as depression

Anabolic steroid abuse may lead to aggression and other psychiatric side effects. Many users report feeling good about themselves while on anabolic steroids, but researchers report that anabolic steroid abuse can cause wild mood swings including manic-like symptoms leading to "'roid rage," or violent, even homicidal, episodes. Researchers have reported that users may suffer from paranoid jealousy, extreme irritability, delusions, and impaired judgment stemming from feelings of invincibility. Stopping the drugs abruptly can lead to depression.

Anabolic steroids are illegal, unless prescribed by a doctor to treat a medical problem. First-time offenders caught with these drugs could be fined and sentenced to up to one year in prison.[61]

Originally marketed as a dietary supplement for enhancing athletic performance, tetrahydrogestrinone (THG) is actually a chemically altered version of an anabolic steroid banned by most sports organizations. THG is referred to as a "designer" steroid because it's undetectable by traditional steroid testing techniques. A new laboratory test, however, now makes its detection possible.[62]

Androstenedione

Androstenedione ("andro") is a testosterone precursor normally produced by the adrenal glands and gonads. Manufacturers claim that androstenedione improves testosterone concentration, increases muscular strength and mass, helps reduce body fat, enhances mood, and improves sexual performances. However, studies have shown that supplemental androstenedione doesn't increase testosterone and muscles don't get stronger with andro use. Andro has been classified as a controlled substance, making its use illegal.[63]

Androstenedione increases concentrations of estrogen, which is associated with breast enlargement and increased risk of cardiovascular disease and pancreatic cancer in men. Androstenedione also raises testosterone above normal levels, which can lead to acne, male pattern baldness, and a decrease in "good" cholesterol. In women, high testosterone levels can also cause increased body hair, deepening of the voice, and other male characteristics.

Creatine

Creatine is an amino acid made by the body and stored predominantly in skeletal muscle. Creatine serves as a reservoir to replenish adenosine triphosphate (ATP), a substance involved in energy production. While some studies show creatine may increase strength and endurance, other effects on the body remain unknown.[64]

Creatine supplements increase muscle stores of the compound, which theoretically allows athletes to work out harder and longer. Athletes typically load up with 20 grams a day for five days and then keep taking 2 grams daily. Some studies have shown that creatine supplements do enhance sports performance and anaerobic power, but only in activities that require repeated short bursts of high-intensity energy, such as sprints and weight lifting, rather than long-distance running or swimming. Side effects, such as water retention and weight gain, may actually hamper performance.

Commercially marketed creatine supplements do not meet the same rigid quality control standards as prescription drugs, so it is difficult to apply efficacy and safety results from published trials to general practice. The dose delivered by a commercially available product may be more or less than that suggested by the labeling. This could influence the effectiveness of the supplement and could lead to unexpected adverse effects.

The Food and Drug Administration has warned consumers to consult a physician before taking creatine supplements. Creatine may cause dehydration and heat-related illnesses, reduced blood volume, and electrolyte imbalances. Some athletes drink large quantities of water hoping to avoid such effects. However, many coaches forbid or discourage creatine use because its long-term effects remain unknown.

Other Ergogenic Aids

Ergogenic aids are substances used to enhance energy and provide athletes with a competitive advantage. By some estimates, more than three of four athletes in some sports use some sort of supplements to enhance their performance and boost energy. These include everyday substances. Caffeine, for instance, may boost alertness in some people but cause jitteriness in others. Baking soda (sodium bicarbonate) is believed to delay fatigue by neutralizing lactic acid in the muscles, but its potential drawbacks include explosive diarrhea, abdominal cramps, bloating, and nausea.

GBL (gamma butyrolactone) is an unapproved drug that is being studied as a treatment for narcolepsy, a disabling sleep disorder. Nevertheless, it is marketed on the Internet and in some professional gyms as a muscle-builder and performance-enhancer. The Food and Drug Administration has warned consumers to avoid any products containing GBL, noting that they have been associated with at least one death and several incidents in which users became comatose or unconscious.

Glycerol is a natural element derived from fats. Some sports-drink manufacturers are testing formulations that include glycerol, which they claim can lower heart rate and stave off exhaustion in marathon events. Glycerol-induced hyperhydration (holding too much water in the blood) can have a negative impact on performance, however, and may be hazardous to health.

> *Some professional and student athletes justify their use of performance-enhancing drugs as another way of winning at any cost. Do they deserve whatever accolades or prizes they win? Or should star athletes caught using drugs to boost their performance be stripped of their titles and records?*
> **You Decide.**

BECOMING MORE FLEXIBLE

Flexibility is the characteristic of body tissues that determines the **range of motion** achievable without injury at a joint or group of joints. There are two types of flexibility: static and dynamic. **Static flexibility**—the type most people think of as flexibility—refers to the ability to assume and maintain an extended position at one end point in a joint's range of motion. **Dynamic flexibility,** by comparison, involves movement. It is the ability to move a joint quickly and fluidly through its entire range of motion with little resistance. The static flexibility in the hip joint determines whether you can do a split; dynamic flexibility is what would enable you to perform a split leap.

Static flexibility depends on many factors, including the structure of a joint and the tightness of the muscles, tendons, and ligaments attached to it. Dynamic flexibility is influenced by static flexibility but also depends on additional factors, such as strength, coordination, and resistance to movement.

Genetics, age, gender, and body composition all influence how flexible you are. Girls and women tend to be more flexible than boys and men, to a certain extent because of hormonal and anatomical differences. The way females and males use their muscles and the activities they engage in can also have an effect. Over time, the natural elasticity of muscles, tendons, and joints decreases in both genders, resulting in stiffness.

THE BENEFITS OF FLEXIBILITY

Just as cardiorespiratory fitness benefits the heart and lungs and muscular fitness builds endurance and strength, a stretching program produces unique benefits, including enhancement of the ability of the respiratory, circulatory, and neuromuscular systems to cope with the stress and demands of our high-pressure world (Figure 5-9). Among the other benefits of flexibility are:

- **Prevention of injuries.** Flexibility training stretches muscles and increases the elasticity of joints. Strong, flexible muscles resist stress better than weak or inflexible ones. Adding flexibility to a training program for sports such as soccer, football, or tennis can reduce the rate of injuries by as much as 75 percent. In one study of competitive runners, weekly stretching sessions significantly reduced the incidence of low-back pain.

- **Relief of muscle strain.** Muscles tighten as a result of stress or prolonged sitting. If you study or work in one position for several hours, you'll often feel stiffness in your back or neck. Stretching helps relieve this tension and enables you to work more effectively.

- **Relaxation.** Flexibility exercises are great stress-busters that reduce mental strain, slow the rate of breathing, and reduce blood pressure.

(a) Foot pull for the groin and thigh muscles

(b) Lateral head tilt

(c) Wall stretch for the Achilles tendon

(d) Triceps stretch for the upper arm and shoulder

(e) Knee-chest pull for lower back muscles

Matthew Farruggio (all)

FIGURE 5-9   Some Simple Stretching Exercises

(a) Sit on the ground and bend your legs so that the soles of your feet touch. Pull your feet closer as you press on your knees with your elbows. Hold for 10 seconds; repeat. **(b)** Gently tilt your head to each side. Repeat several times. **(c)** Stand 3 feet from a wall or post with your feet slightly apart. Keeping your heels on the ground, lean into the wall. Hold for 10 seconds; repeat. **(d)** Place your right hand behind your neck and grasp above the elbow with your left hand. Gently pull the elbow back. Repeat with the left elbow. **(e)** Lying on your back, clasp one knee and pull it toward your chest. Hold for 15–30 seconds; repeat with the other knee.

▪ **Relief of soreness after exercise.** Many people develop delayed-onset muscle soreness (DOMS) one or two days after they work out. This may be the result of damage to the muscle fibers and supporting connective tissue.

▪ **Improved posture.** Bad posture can create tight, stressed muscles. If you slump in your chair, for instance, the muscles in the front of your chest may tighten, causing those in the upper spine to overstretch and become loose.

STRETCHING

When you stretch a muscle, you are primarily stretching the connective tissue. The stretch must be intense enough to increase the length of the connective tissue without tearing it.

Static stretching involves a gradual stretch held for a short time (10 to 30 seconds). A shorter stretch provides little benefit; a longer stretch does not provide additional benefits. Since a slow stretch provokes less of a reaction from the stretch receptors, the muscles can safely stretch farther than usual. Fitness experts most often recommend static stretching because it is both safe and effective. An example of such a stretch is letting your hands slowly slide down the front of your legs (keeping your knees in a soft, unlocked position) until you reach your toes and holding this final position for several seconds before slowly straightening up. You should feel a pull, but not pain, during this stretch.

In **passive stretching,** your own body, a partner, gravity, or a weight serves as an external force or resistance to help your joints move through their range of motion. You can achieve a more intense stretch and a greater range of motion with passive stretching. There is a greater risk of injury, however, because the muscles themselves are not controlling the stretch. If working with a partner, it's very important that you communicate clearly so as not to force a joint outside its normal functional range of motion.

Research on stretching demonstrates a 5 to 20 percent increase in static flexibility within four to six weeks of stretching. Much of this long-term increase in range of motion is due to an increased "stretch tolerance," or ability to tolerate the discomfort of a stretched position.

Active stretching involves stretching a muscle by contracting the opposing muscle (the muscle on the opposite side of the limb). In an active seated hamstring stretch, for example, the stretch occurs by actively contracting the muscles on top of the shin, which produces a reflex that relaxes the hamstring. This method allows the muscle to be stretched farther with a low risk of injury.

The disadvantage of active stretching is that a person may not be able to produce enough of a stretch to increase flexibility only by means of contracting opposing muscle groups. Although active stretching is the safest and most convenient approach, an occasional passive assist can be helpful.

Ballistic stretching is characterized by rapid bouncing movements, such as a series of up-and-down bobs as you try again and again to touch your toes with your hands. These bounces can stretch the muscle fibers too far, causing the muscle to contract rather than stretch. They also can tear ligaments and weaken or rupture tendons, the strong fibrous cords that connect muscles to bones. The heightened activity to stretch receptors caused by the rapid stretches can continue for some time, possibly causing injuries during any physical activities that follow. Because of its potential dangers, fitness experts generally recommend against ballistic stretching.

(FAQ) DOES STRETCHING IMPROVE ATHLETIC PERFORMANCE?

Although conventional wisdom holds that it does, a review of the research finds that this isn't necessarily so.[65] In some cases, acute stretching can impede rather than improve performance in terms of muscle force and jumping height.[66] Passive stretching prior to a sprint—a common practice—also has proved to reduce runners' speed.[67] On the other hand, regular stretching, can improve athletic performance in a variety of sports.[68]

Strategies for Prevention   ▪▪   How to Avoid Stretching Injuries

Before you begin, increase your body temperature by slowly marching or running in place. Sweat signals that you're ready to start stretching.

▪ Don't force body parts beyond their normal range of motion. Stretch to the point of tension, back off, and hold for ten seconds to a minute.

▪ Do a minimum of four repetitions of each stretch, with equal repetitions on each side.

▪ Don't hold your breath. Continue breathing slowly and rhythmically throughout your stretching routine.

▪ Don't attempt to stretch a weak or injured muscle.

▪ Start small. Work the muscles of the smaller joints in the arms and legs first and then work the larger joints like the shoulders and hips.

▪ Stretch individual muscles before you stretch a group of muscles, for instance,

the ankle, knee, and hip before a stretch that works all three.

▪ Don't make any quick, jerky movements while stretching. Stretches should be gentle and smooth.

▪ Certain positions can be harmful to the knees and lower back. In particular, avoid stretches that require deep knee bends or full squats because they can harm your knees and lower back.

For aerobic activities, one of the best times to stretch is after an aerobic workout. Your muscles will be warm, more flexible, and less prone to injury. In addition, stretching after aerobic activity can help a fatigued muscle return to its normal resting length and possibly help reduce delayed muscle soreness.

MIND-BODY APPROACHES

Yoga, Pilates, and t'ai chi, increasingly popular on campuses and throughout the country, can help reduce stress, enhance health and wellness, and improve physical fitness.

Yoga

One of the most ancient of mind-body practices, *yoga* comes from the Sanskrit word meaning "union." Traditionally associated with religion, yoga consists of various breathing and stretching exercises that unite all aspects of a person. According to a national poll, 16.5 million Americans—7.5 percent of the population—practice yoga.[69] The fastest-growing segment are young adults between ages 18 and 34.

Once considered an exotic pursuit, yoga has gained acceptance as part of a comprehensive stress management and fitness program. Scientific studies have demonstrated its benefits, which include:

▪ **Improved flexibility,** which may offer protection from back pain and injuries.

▪ Protection of joints because yoga postures take joints through their full range of motion, providing a fresh supply of nutrients to joint cartilage.

▪ **Stronger, denser bones** from yoga's weight-bearing postures.

▪ Enhanced circulation, which also boosts the supply of oxygen throughout the body.

▪ **Lower blood pressure.**

▪ **Lower levels of the stress hormone cortisol,** which (as discussed in Chapter 4) can affect the immune system, interfere with memory, and increase the risk of depression and osteoporosis.

▪ **Lower blood sugar in people with diabetes,** which reduces the risk of complications.

▪ **Reduced pain** in people with back problems, arthritis, carpal tunnel syndrome, fibromyalgia, and other chronic problems.[70]

The best way to get started is to find a class that appeals to you and learn a few yoga moves and breathing techniques. Once you have mastered these, you can easily integrate yoga into your total fitness program.

The American College of Sports Medicine cautions that yoga should help, not hurt. To prevent injuries to your knees, back, neck, shoulders, wrists, or ankles, avoid forcing your body into difficult postures. Proper technique is essential to safety.

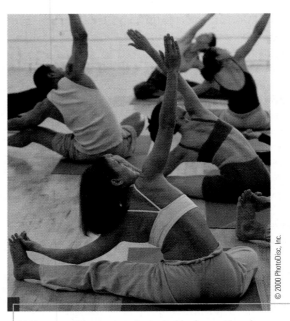

© 2000 PhotoDisc, Inc.

Yoga, one of the most ancient mind-body practices, has many benefits.

Pilates

Used by dancers for deep-body conditioning and injury rehabilitation, Pilates (pronounced Pilah-teez), was developed more than seven decades ago by German immigrant Joseph Pilates. Increasingly used to complement aerobics and weight training, Pilates exercises improve flexibility and joint mobility and strengthen the core by developing pelvic stability and abdominal control.

Pilates-trained instructors offer "mat" or "floor" classes that stress the stabilization and strengthening of the back and abdominal muscles. Fitness centers also may offer training on Pilates equipment, primarily a device called the Reformer, a wooden contraption with various cables, pulleys, springs, and sliding boards attached that is used for a series of progressive, range-of-motion exercises. Instructors typically work one on one or with small groups of two or three participants and tailor exercise sessions to individual flexibility and strength limitations. Unlike exercise techniques that emphasize numerous repetitions in a single direction, Pilates exercises involve very few, but extremely precise, repetitions in several planes of motion.

According to research from the American College of Sports Medicine, Pilates enhances flexibility and muscular endurance, particularly for intermediate and advanced practitioners, but its potential to increase cardiorespiratory fitness and reduce body weight is limited. The intensity of a Pilates workout increases from basic to intermediate to advanced levels, as does the number of calories burned. For intermediate practitioners, a 30-minute session burns 180 calories, with each additional quarter-hour burning another 90 calories. A single weekly session enhances flexibility but has little impact on body composition.[71]

T'ai Chi

This ancient Chinese practice, designed to exercise body, mind, and spirit, gently works muscles, focuses concentration, and improves the flow of "qi" (often spelled "chi"), the vital life energy that sustains health. Popular with all ages, from children to seniors, t'ai chi is easy to learn and perform. Because of its focus on breathing and flowing gestures, t'ai chi is sometimes described as "meditation in motion."

Classes are available on campuses, in fitness centers, community centers, and some martial arts schools. Physicians may recommend t'ai chi for those with musculoskeletal disorders like arthritis to improve flexibility and build muscle strength gently and gradually. As the American College of Sports Medicine reports, t'ai chi has proved effective in reducing falls in the elderly and those with balance disorders.[72]

KEEPING YOUR BACK HEALTHY

The average person has an 80 percent chance of experiencing low-back pain in the course of a lifetime.[73] Back pain strikes slightly more women than men and is most common between the ages of 20 and 55. You are at greater risk if you smoke or if you're overstressed, overweight, or out of shape. Back pain, which accounts for 40 percent of sickness absences, causes more lost workdays and costs the country more than any other malady.

Most severe back pain lasts only a few days, although less severe symptoms may persist for many months, and most patients have intermittent recurrences of back pain. More than 90 percent of individuals with back pain recover within three months.

Once bedrest was the primary treatment for back pain, but now doctors urge patients to avoid it. Even two to seven days of bedrest may provide little, if any, benefit. Acetaminophen (Tylenol) is the first-line therapy for pain relief. If it is not effective, doctors recommend nonsteroidal anti-inflammatory drugs, such as ibuprofen (Motrin or Advil). Muscle relaxants seem to be effective for a spasm in the lower back. The sooner that back patients return to normal activity, the less pain medication they require and the less long-term disability they suffer.[74] Fewer than 1 percent of patients with chronic low-back pain benefit from surgery.

BODY COMPOSITION

A combination of regular exercise and good nutrition is the best way to maintain a healthy body composition. Aerobic exercise helps by burning calories and increasing metabolic rate (the rate at which the body uses calories) for several hours after a workout. Strength training increases the proportion of lean body tissue by building muscle mass, which also increases the metabolic rate.

Experts debate which measure of body composition— BMI, waist circumference, or waist-hip ratio—is the best indicator of central or visceral obesity, which increases the risk of heart disease, metabolic syndrome, diabetes, and other illnesses. (See Chapter 7 for a complete discussion of ways to assess body composition.)

(FAQ) CAN A PERSON BE FAT AND FIT?

Most people assume that fitness comes in only one size: small. That's not necessarily so. There is considerable controversy over how to define a healthy weight. But individuals of every size can improve their physical fitness.

In ten years of research on 25,000 men and 8,000 women, scientists at the Cooper Institute for Aerobics Research in Dallas, Texas, have found that heavier individuals can be just as healthy and physically fit as their leaner counterparts. In their studies, obese people who exercised moderately (30 minutes of daily walking at three or four miles per hour) had half the death rate of those who were slimmer

---

Strategies for Prevention :: Back Talk

:: When standing, shift your weight from one foot to the other. If possible, place one foot on a stool, step, or railing 4 to 6 inches off the ground. Hold in your stomach, tilt your pelvis toward your back, and tuck in your buttocks to provide crucial support for the lower back.

:: Because sitting places more stress on the lower back than standing, try to get up from your seat at least once an hour to stretch or walk around. Whenever possible, sit in a straight chair

with a firm back. Avoid slouching in overstuffed chairs or dangling your legs in midair. When driving, keep the seat forward so that your knees are raised to hip level; your right leg should not be fully extended. A small pillow or towel can help support your lower back.

:: Sleep on a flat, firm mattress. The best sleep position is on your side, with one or both knees bent at right angles to your torso. The pillow should keep your head in line with your body so

that your neck isn't bent forward or to the side.

:: When lifting, bend at the knees, not from the waist. Get close to the load. Tighten your stomach muscles, but don't hold your breath. Let your leg muscles do the work.

:: Don't smoke. Smoking may interfere with circulation to the lower back; and a chronic smoker's cough can be so irritating that it provokes a back spasm.

but more sedentary. Low cardiorespiratory fitness, regardless of an individual's weight, is as great a risk factor for dying of heart disease or other causes such as diabetes, high blood pressure, and other well-recognized threats.

Nonetheless, fitness doesn't completely reverse the increased risks associated with excess weight. If you're obese, even a high level of physical activity does not protect you from premature death. And if you're sedentary, being thin does not cancel out the dangers of inactivity. In the long-term Nurses Health Study, which has followed more than 100,000 women for decades, women who were both obese and inactive were most likely to die. Those who were fit but fat and those who were thin but sedentary also had higher death rates than others.[75]

EVALUATING FITNESS PRODUCTS AND PROGRAMS

As fitness has become a major industry in the United States, consumers have been bombarded with pitches for products that promise to do everything from whittle a waistline to build up biceps. As always, you have to ask questions and do your own research—whether you're buying basic exercise aids or joining a health club. Beware of any promise that sounds too good to be true. And keep in mind that nothing matters more than your own commitment.

EXERCISE EQUIPMENT

Always try out equipment before buying it. If you decide to purchase a stationary bicycle, for instance, read all the product information. Ask someone in your physical education department or at a local gym for recommendations. Try out a bicycle at the gym. Make sure any equipment you purchase is safe and durable.

(FAQ) How Do I Buy the Right Athletic Shoe?

Footwear has come a long way from the days of canvas sneakers. With so many new materials and high-tech options, choosing the right shoe for working out can be confusing. The best shoes aren't necessarily the most expensive but the ones that fit you best. Here are some basic guidelines:

- **Choose the right shoe for your sport.** If you're a walker or runner, you want maximum overall shock absorption for the foot, with extra cushioning in the heel and under the ball of the foot (the metatarsal area) to prevent pain, burning, and tenderness. If you also participate in other types of exercise, consider "cross-trainers," shoes that are flexible enough in the front for running but provide the side-to-side, or lateral, control you need for aerobics or tennis.

- **Check out the shoe.** A "slip-lasted" shoe, made by sewing together the upper like a moccasin and gluing it to the sole, is lightweight and flexible. A "board-lasted" shoe has a leather, nylon mesh, or canvas upper sewn to a cardboardlike material, which provides more support and control. A "combination-last" shoe offers the advantages of both other shoes and works well for a variety of foot types (Figure 5-10).

- **Shop late.** Try on shoes at the end of the day or after a workout, when your foot size is at its maximum (sometimes half a shoe size larger than in the morning). Wear socks similar to those you'll wear for workouts.

Well-padded tongue prevents extensor tendinitis and irritation of dorsum of foot

Laces not too long so they stay tied longer

High, rounded toe box (at least 1½ in. high) prevents subungual hematomas ("black toes")

Studded sole absorbs shock and provides traction in mud and snow

Well-molded Achilles pad prevents irritation of Achilles tendon

Firm heel counter for hindfoot stability

Flared heel for stability and beveled or rounded heel for quick roll-off

Flexible midsole helps prevent Achilles tendon problems

Soft, raised heel wedge to absorb impact at heel strike

Photo by Adidas/Getty Images

FIGURE 5-10 **What to Look for When You Buy Running Shoes**

■ **Give your toes room.** Allow a half-inch, or the width of your index finger, between the end of your longest toe and the tip of the shoe. Try on both shoes. If one foot is larger than the other, buy the larger size.

■ **Check the width.** A shoe should be as wide as possible across the forefoot without allowing the heel to slip. Lace up the shoe completely and walk or jog a few steps to make sure the shoes are comfortable.

■ **Replace shoes when they lose their cushioning.** After about 300 to 500 miles of running or 300 hours of aerobic activity, your shoes are no longer absorbing the pounding and jarring of your sport. Don't put yourself at increased risk of knee and ankle injuries.

Low-Cost Fitness Aids

Not all fitness equipment comes with a big price tag. Here are some affordable ways to expand and enhance a home workout:

■ **Dumbbells.** You can purchase light weights to carry when walking and jogging to build and firm arm muscles. Training with heavier weights increases muscle strength and endurance, improves balance and body composition, and may reverse some bone loss. An adjustable dumbbell set allows you to add more weight as you build strength.

■ **Stability Balls.** A large inflatable rubber ball can be a fun, effective way of building core strength, improving posture, and increasing balance. When performing standard exercises like crunches and abdominal curls, the ball provides an additional challenge: maintaining a stable trunk throughout each exercise. You also can sit on the ball while working with hand weights to build core strength and balance. Introductory videos and DVDs are available for rental or purchase.

■ **Resistance Tubing.** Developed by physical therapists for rehabilitation after injuries, elastic bands and tubing come in different strengths, based on the thickness of the plastic. If you're a beginner, start with a thin band, particularly for the upper body. The lightweight, inexpensive, and easy-to-carry bands aren't particularly risky, but you should check for holes or worn spots, choose a smooth surface, maintain good posture, and perform the exercises in a slow, controlled manner.

FITNESS CENTERS

Begin by checking out the recreational facilities on your own campus. Is there a gym, running track, pool, basketball court, athletic fields? Are they crowded at certain times? Are they convenient? Are classes in spinning or Pilates available?

If you decide to join a private gym or health club, find out exactly what facilities and programs it offers. The club should be located close to home, campus, or work and should be open at convenient hours. Think about your schedule and when you'll have time to work out. Visit the club at the times you're most likely to use it.

A club should have facilities for a complete workout, including both aerobic and muscle workouts: exercycles, rowing machines, treadmills, stair-climbing machines, stationary bicycles, a running track, aerobics classes, a swimming pool, strength-training equipment, and, if it's what you're looking for, racquetball courts and a large gym for basketball and volleyball.

Find out whether all facilities are available to all members at all times. Some clubs reserve the pool for families only or kids' lessons at certain times. Ask if you can try out the club before joining. Find out what the membership includes. Will you end up paying extra for lockers, towels, classes, and the like? Are student discounts offered? Beware of long-term memberships; many clubs go out of business or change ownership often. Do the members seem to be significantly older or younger, or in much better or worse shape, than you are? You're more likely to work out regularly in a place, and with people, you like.

▌ SPORTS NUTRITION

In general, active people need the same basic nutrients as others and should follow the recommendations in Chapter 6. However, athletes in competitive sports—amateur as well as professional—may have increased energy requirements.

Contrary to a common misconception, athletes generally do not need more protein; the exception may be those engaged in intense strength training. Like most Americans, athletes typically consume more than the Recommended Daily Allowance for protein and do not need increased protein. As discussed in Chapter 7, a high-protein diet can be high in fat and low in the nutrients supplied by fruits, vegetables, and grains and can put a strain on the liver and kidneys.

Although complex carbohydrates are essential in an athlete's diet, fat also plays a role. Including the right types of fat in the daily diet can actually improve athletic performance—not just by providing calories, but by replenishing intramuscular fat stores (fat stored within the muscle and used to fuel extended exercise).

Not just *what* you eat but *when* you eat can affect your exercise performance. If you eat immediately prior to a workout, you may feel sluggish or develop nausea, cramping, or diarrhea. If you don't eat, you may feel weak, faint, or tired.

Time your meals so that you exercise three to four hours after a large meal and one to two hours after a small one. Most people can eat a snack right before exercise. After a workout, eat a meal containing both protein and carbohydrates within two hours to help your muscles recover and to replace fuel stores.

(FAQ) HOW MUCH WATER SHOULD I DRINK WHILE EXERCISING?

Water, which we need more than any other nutrient, is even more important during exercise and exertion. Thirst, the body's way of telling you to replace lost fluids, is not a good way for athletes to monitor their fluid needs. Rather than waiting until you're already somewhat dehydrated, you should be fully hydrated when you begin your activity or exercise and, depending on the duration and intensity of your workout, continue to replace fluids both during and afterward.

The American College of Sports Medicine (ACSM) recommends fluid intake before, during, and after exercise to regulate body temperature and replace body fluids lost through sweating. The failure to replace fluids during exercise can lead to dehydration, which can cause muscle fatigue, loss of coordination, heat exhaustion, and an elevation of body-core temperature to dangerously high levels. To avoid this danger, the ACSM advises:

- **Consume a nutritionally balanced diet and drink adequate fluids** in the 24 hours before an exercise event.
- **Drink about 17 ounces of fluid** about two hours before.
- **During exercise, start drinking early** and at regular intervals to replace all the water lost through sweating (i.e., body weight loss).
- **Drink fluids with carbohydrates and/or electrolytes** for exercise lasting more than an hour. For shorter periods, there is little evidence of differences between drinking a carbohydrate–electrolyte drink and plain water.[76]

Too much water during prolonged bouts of exercise, such as a marathon, can lead to *hyponatremia*, or water intoxication. This condition occurs when the body's sodium level falls below normal as a result of salt loss from sweat and dilution of sodium in the bloodstream by overdrinking. Symptoms of hyponatremia include nausea, vomiting, weakness, and in severe cases, seizures, coma, and death.

DIETARY SUPPLEMENTS

Athletes and active individuals of all ages take dietary supplements, sometimes to ensure that they're getting the nutrients they need and sometimes to enhance their performance. Vitamin and mineral supplements, as discussed in Chapter 6, are safe when taken at recommended doses. Excess amounts can contribute to serious health problems. Vitamin supplements marketed for athletes are poorly regulated, and some may be adulterated with banned substances, such as ephedrine. Always look for the USP (United States Pharmacopeias) certification on the label when buying vitamins.

Athletes involved in heavy training may need more of several vitamins, such as thiamin, riboflavin, and B$_6$, which are involved in energy production. The best source, nutritionists advise, is vitamin-rich foods, such as fruits and vegetables.[77]

Mineral deficiencies, such as too little iron in female athletes, can impair athletic performance. Women who exercise rigorously should undergo regular blood testing and, if needed, take iron supplements. In general, calcium, magnesium, iron, zinc, and copper supplements do not enhance sport performance in well-nourished athletes. Chromium, boron, and vanadium have been studied as possible performance-boosters, but researchers have not reported any beneficial effects on body composition or muscular strength and endurance.[78]

ENERGY BARS

Sold as snacks, meal substitutes, or performance enhancers, energy bars come in different forms. High-carbohydrate bars derive more than 70 percent of their calories from carbohydrates (such as corn syrup, grape and pear juice concentrate, oat bran, and brown rice) and are low in protein and fat. Another type gets 40 percent of its energy from carbohydrate, 30 percent from protein, and 30 percent from fat.

Little scientific research has studied the actual benefits of the various types of energy bars, including their effects on blood glucose levels and athletic performance. According to one nutritional analysis, high-carbohydrate energy bars are similar to candy bars in their impact on glucose—even though sugars composed 31 percent of the high-carbohydrate energy bar and 86 percent of the candy bar. In fact, the high-carbohydrate energy bar caused a more rapid peak in blood glucose followed by a sharper decline than did the candy bar. This effect may be desirable for athletes involved in short-duration events who want a quick increase in blood glucose.

Energy bars with a lower carbohydrate level produce a more moderate, sustained increase in blood glucose level, possibly because the protein and fat in a 40–30–30 bar diminish blood glucose response. These bars would be a better choice for athletes involved in endurance events. As an alternative, try fiber-rich whole foods, like nuts and fruit, that provide a steady release of energy.[79]

SAFE AND HEALTHY WORKOUTS

Whenever you work out, you don't want to risk becoming sore or injured. Starting slowly when you begin any new fitness activity is the smartest strategy. Keep a simple diary to record the time and duration of each workout. Get accustomed to an activity first and then begin to work harder or longer. In this way, you strengthen your musculoskeletal system so you're less likely to be injured, you lower the cardiovascular risk, and you build the exercise habit into your schedule.

THINKING OF TEMPERATURE

Prevention is the wisest approach to heat and cold problems. And knowing what can go wrong is part of that preventive approach.

Heat Cramps

These muscle cramps are caused by profuse sweating and the consequent loss of electrolytes (salts). They occur most often during exercise in hot weather. Salty snacks and sports beverages like Gatorade can help, but be aware that sports drinks can be very high in calories. Salt tablets usually aren't necessary except in cases of extreme sweating.

Heat Syndromes

More serious temperature-related conditions include heat exhaustion and heat stroke. These are most likely to occur when both temperature and humidity are high, because sweat does not evaporate as quickly, preventing the body from releasing heat quickly. Other conditions that limit the body's ability to regulate temperature are old age, fever, obesity, dehydration, heart disease, poor circulation, sunburn, and drug and alcohol use. Some medicines that increase the risk include allergy medicines (antihistamines), some cough and cold medicines, blood pressure and heart medicines, diet pills, laxatives, and psychiatric medications.[80]

Heat Exhaustion Heat exhaustion is a mild from of heat-related illness that can be caused by exercise or hot weather. The signs of heat exhaustion are heavy sweating, paleness, muscle cramps, tiredness, weakness, dizziness, headache, nausea or vomiting, and/or fainting. Your pulse rate or heart rate may be fast and weak, and your breathing fast and shallow.

If you think you may have heat exhaustion, get out of the heat quickly. Rest in a cool, shady place and drink plenty of water or other fluids. Do *not* drink alcohol, which can make heat exhaustion worse. If you do not feel better within 30 minutes, see your doctor. If left untreated, heat exhaustion may lead to a heat stroke.

Heat Stroke A heat stroke can occur when the body temperature rises to 106 degrees Fahrenheit or higher within 10 to 15 minutes. A heat stroke is a medical emergency that can be fatal. The warning signs are extremely high temperature; red, hot, and dry skin; rapid, strong pulse; throbbing headache; dizziness; nausea; confusion or unconsciousness.

If you think someone might have heat stroke, you should take him or her to a cool, shady place quickly, and call a doctor. Remove unnecessary clothing and bathe or spray the victim with cool water. People with heat stroke may seem confused. They may have seizures or go into a coma.

The incidence of heat stroke in urban areas of the United States during very warm periods is approximately 20 cases per 100,000 people, and heat stroke accounts for at least 240 deaths in the United States annually.[81]

Coping with Cold

The tips of the toes, fingers, ears, nose, and chin and the cheeks are most vulnerable to exposure to high wind speeds and low temperatures, which can result in **frostnip.**

Because frostnip is painless, you may not even be aware that it is occurring. Watch for a sudden blanching or lightening of your skin. The best early treatment is warming the area by firm, steady pressure with a warm hand; blowing on it with hot breath; holding it against your body; or immersing it in warm (not hot) water. As the skin thaws, it becomes red and starts to tingle. Be careful to protect it from further damage. Don't rub the skin vigorously or with snow, as you could damage the tissue.

More severe is **frostbite.** There are two types of frostbite: *superficial* and *deep.* Superficial frostbite, the freezing of the skin and tissues just below the skin, is characterized by a waxy look and firmness of the skin, although the tissue below is soft. Initial treatment should be to slowly rewarm the area. As the area thaws, it will be numb and bluish or purple, and blisters may form. Cover the area with a dry, sterile dressing, and protect the skin from further exposure to cold. See a doctor for further treatment. Deep frostbite, the freezing of skin, muscle, and even bone, requires medical treatment. It usually involves the tissues of the hands and feet, which appear pale and feel frozen. Keep the victim dry and as warm as possible on the way to a medical facility. Cover the frostbitten area with a dry, sterile dressing.

The center of the body may gradually cool at temperatures above, as well as below, freezing—usually in wet, windy weather. When body temperature falls below 95

▌ Strategies for Prevention ▓▓ Heeding Heat

- Increase your fluid intake during hot temperatures by two to four glasses of cool fluids each hour. Cold beverages can cause stomach cramps; alcoholic beverages can cause you to lose more fluid.

- Cool off with a cool shower or sponge bath.

- Move into an air-conditioned environment.

- Wear lightweight clothing.

- Check weather conditions. The National Weather Service has produced a Heat Index chart that can be accessed online at www.crh.noaa.gov/pub/heat.htm.

Strategies for Prevention ▪ Protecting Yourself from the Cold

▪ Dress appropriately. Choose several layers of loose clothing made of wool, cotton, down, or synthetic down. Make sure your head, feet, and hands are well protected. A pair of cotton socks inside a pair of wool socks will keep your feet warm.

▪ Don't go out in the cold after drinking. Alcohol can make you more susceptible to cold and can impair your judgment and sense of time.

▪ When snowshoeing or cross-country skiing, always let a responsible person know where you're heading and

when you expect to be back. Stick to marked trails.

▪ Carry a small emergency kit that includes waterproof matches, a compass, a map, high-energy food, and water.

▪ Don't eat snow; it could lower your body temperature.

degrees Fahrenheit, the body is incapable of rewarming itself because of the breakdown of the internal system that regulates its temperature. This state is known as **hypothermia.** The first sign of hypothermia is severe shivering. Then the victim becomes uncoordinated, drowsy, listless, and confused and is unable to speak properly. Symptoms become more severe as body temperature continues to drop, and coma or death can result.

Hypothermia requires emergency medical treatment. Try to prevent any further heat loss. Move the victim to a warm place, cover him or her with blankets, remove wet clothing, and replace it with dry garments. If the victim is conscious, administer warm liquids, not alcohol.

Protect yourself in cold weather (or cold indoor gyms) by covering as much of your body as possible, but don't overdress. Wear one layer less than you would if you were outside but not exercising. Don't use warm-up clothes made of waterproof material, because they tend to trap heat and keep perspiration from evaporating. Make sure your clothes are loose enough to allow movement and exercise of the hands, feet, and other body parts, thereby maintaining proper circulation. Choose dark colors that absorb heat. And because 40 percent or more of your body heat is lost through your head and neck, wear a hat, turtleneck, or scarf. Make sure you cover your hands and feet as well; mittens provide more warmth and protection than gloves.

(FAQ) HOW CAN I PREVENT INJURIES?

According to the American Physical Therapy Association, the most common exercise-related injury sites are the knees, feet, back, and shoulders, followed by the ankles and hips. **Acute injuries**—sprains, bruises, and pulled muscles—are the result of sudden trauma, such as a fall or collision. **Overuse injuries,** on the other hand, are the result of overdoing a repetitive activity, such as running. When one particular joint is overstressed—such as a tennis player's elbow or a swimmer's shoulder—tendinitis, an inflammation at the point where the tendon meets the bone, can develop. Other overuse injuries include muscle strains and aches and stress fractures, which are hairline breaks in a bone, usually in the leg or foot.

 Men and women may be vulnerable to different types of injuries. Studies of male and female college basketball and soccer players have shown that gender differences in the neuromuscular control of the knee places female athletes at higher risk for knee injuries.[82] Balance training may reduce the risk.[83]

To prevent exercise-related problems before they happen, use common sense and take appropriate precautions, including the following:

▪ **Get proper instruction** and, if necessary, advanced training from knowledgeable instructors.

▪ **Make sure you have good equipment** and keep it in good condition. Know how to check and do at least basic maintenance on the equipment yourself. Always check your equipment prior to each use (especially if you're renting it).

▪ **Always make sure that stretching** and exercises are preventing, not causing, injuries.

▪ **Use reasonable protective measures,** including wearing a helmet when cycling or skating.

▪ For some sports, such as boating, **always go with a buddy.**

▪ **Take each outing seriously**—even if you've dived into this river a hundred times before, even if you know this mountain like you know your own backyard. Avoid the unknown under adverse conditions (for example, hiking unfamiliar terrain during poor weather or kayaking a new river when water levels are unusually high or low) or when accompanied by a beginner whose skills may not be as strong as yours.

▪ **Never combine alcohol or drugs with any sport.**

BEYOND THE GYM

Many people are trying exhilarating sports that, by their very nature, entail some risk. If you choose these activities, you're responsible for learning how to stay safe as you push to the limit. Here are some sport-specific guidelines:

▪ **Inline skating.** The most common injuries are to the wrists. Skaters should always wear protective gear, including helmet, wrist guards, and knee

Strategies for Prevention :: Avoiding Injury

:: Dress appropriately, and invest in good shoes (see "FAQ: How Do I Buy the Right Athletic Shoe?").

:: Always warm up before and cool down after a workout.

:: Don't push yourself; always build up frequency, intensity, and duration gradually.

:: Keep high-impact exercises to a minimum.

:: Rather than being sedentary all week and then training hard on weekends, try to stay active throughout the week and not overdo on weekends.

pads, and should warm up before strapping on their skates. Learn how to fall: Relax, go down to your knees, and roll to one side.

- **Mountain biking.** Off-road biking requires knowing how to shift your weight to keep a bike stable on rough trails. Know the limits of your endurance and your equipment. Wear a helmet, bicycle gloves, and glasses or goggles to protect your eyes from dirt and overhanging branches. Carry a bike repair kit and a first aid kit if you head for a remote area.

- **Rock climbing.** Rock climbing takes strength, balance, and hand-eye coordination. Training with a qualified instructor is essential to learn proper technique. The best place to learn is indoors, with supervised instruction and controlled conditions.

- **Snowboarding.** Well-fitted snowboarding boots are essential, as is training in how to fall. The most common injuries are to the wrist or thumb, which can fracture if snowboarders put out their palms to break a fall. Sunburn and frostbite are both risks, and snowboarders should wear sunscreen and monitor weather conditions closely.

TAKING CARE OF INJURIES

Sooner or later most active people suffer an injury. Although most are minor, they all require attention. Ignoring a problem or trying to push through the pain can lead to more serious complications.

PRICE

If you develop aches and pains beyond what you might expect from an activity, stop. Never push to the point of fatigue. If you do, you could end up with sprained or torn muscles. Figure 5-11 gives the PRICE prescription for coping with an exercise injury.

- **P**rotect the area with an elastic wrap, a sling, splint, cane, crutches, or an air cast.

- **R**est to promote tissue healing. Avoid activities that cause pain, swelling, or discomfort.

- **I**ce the area immediately, even if you're seeking medical help (don't put the ice pack directly on the

FIGURE 5-11   PRICE: How to Cope with an Exercise Injury

skin). Repeat every two or three hours while you're awake for the first 48 to 72 hours. Cold reduces pain, swelling, and inflammation in injured muscles, joints, and connecting tissues and may slow bleeding if a tear has occurred.

- **C**ompress the area with an elastic bandage until the swelling stops. Begin wrapping at the end farthest from your heart. Loosen the wrap if the pain increases, the area becomes numb, or swelling is occurring below the wrapped area.

- **E**levate the area above your heart, especially at night. Gravity helps reduce swelling by draining excess fluid.

After 48 hours, if the swelling is gone, you may apply warmth or gentle heat, which improves the blood flow and speeds healing.

Overtraining

About half of all people who start an exercise program drop out within six months. One common reason is that they **overtrain,** pushing themselves to work too intensely too frequently. Signs of overdoing it include persistent muscle soreness, frequent injuries, unintended weight loss, nervousness, and an inability to relax. Overtraining for endurance sports like marathon running can damage the lungs and intensify asthma symptoms. You may find yourself unable to complete a normal workout or to recover after a normal workout.

If you develop any of the symptoms of overtraining, reduce or stop your workout sessions temporarily. Make gradual increases in the intensity of your workouts. Allow 24 to 48 hours for recovery between workouts. Make sure you get adequate rest. Check with a physical education instructor, coach, or trainer to make sure your exercise program fits your individual needs.

Exercise Addiction

Excessive exercise can become a form of addiction, and "exercise dependence" is not uncommon among young men and women. Although most physically active college students work out at healthy levels, some exercise to an extent that could signal dependence. In one study of 257 students at an East Coast university (none athletes in training or in season), about one in five exercised more than six hours a week and did so for reasons or in ways that appeared unhealthy. For example, they felt compelled to exercise even when ill or injured and felt guilty if they didn't work out.[84]

Learn It / Live It
Shaping Up

This chapter has given you the basic information you need to launch a fitness program. However, you're more likely to succeed if you create a plan and follow it. These basic steps can help you determine where you are now and how to get to where you want to be.

- **Evaluate your readiness for change.** Use the Self-Survey on page 140 to determine your stage of behavioral change. Don't expect to progress directly from one stage to another just once. Most people "recycle" several times before a change becomes permanent.

- **Consider your fitness goals.** Do you have an overall conditioning goal, such as losing weight? Or do you have a training goal, such as preparing for a 5K race or the tryouts for the volleyball team? Break down your goal into smaller "step" goals that lead you toward it.

- **Think through your personal preferences.** What are your physical strengths and weaknesses? Do you have good upper body strength but easily get winded? Do you have a stiff back? Do your allergies flare up when you exercise outdoors? By paying attention to your needs, likes, and dislikes, you can choose activities you enjoy—and are more likely to continue.

- **Schedule exercise into your daily routine.** If you can, block out a half-hour for working out at the beginning of the day, between classes, or in the evening. Write it into your schedule as if it were a class or doctor's appointment. If you can't find 30 minutes, look for two 15-minute or three 10-minute slots that you can use for "mini-workouts." Once you've worked out a schedule, write it down. A written plan encourages you to stay on track.

- **Assemble your gear.** Make sure you put your athletic shoes in your car or in the locker at the gym. Lay out the clothes you'll need to shoot hoops or play racquetball.

- **Start slowly.** If you are just beginning regular activity or exercise, begin at a low level. If you have an injury, disability, or chronic health problem, be sure you get medical clearance from a physician.

- **Progress gradually.** If you have not been physically active, begin by incorporating a few minutes of physical activity into each day, building up to 30 minutes or more of moderate-intensity activities. If you have been active but not as often or as intensely as recommended, become more consistent. Continue to increase the frequency, intensity, and duration of your workouts.

- **Take stock.** After a few months of leading a more active life, take stock. Think of how much more energy you have at the end of the day. Ask if you're feeling any less stressed, despite the push and pull of daily pressures. Focus on the unanticipated rewards of exercise. Savor the exhilaration of an autumn morning's walk; the thrill of feeling newly toughened muscles bend to your will; or the satisfaction of a long, smooth stretch after a stressful day. Enjoy the pure pleasure of living in the body you deserve.

Making This Chapter Work for You

Review Questions

1. Mary Ann takes a step aerobics class three times a week. Which component of physical fitness does her exercise routine emphasize?
 a. muscular strength and endurance.
 b. flexibility.
 c. cardiorespiratory fitness.
 d. body composition.

2. Which of the following statements is true?
 a. Inactivity does not affect health until middle age.
 b. Total fitness includes emotional and social dimensions of health besides the physical.
 c. Men and women have the same physiological capacities.
 d. Total fitness is one dimension of physical fitness.

3. The benefits of regular physical activity include
 a. decreased bone mass.
 b. lowered risk of shin splints.
 c. enhanced immune response.
 d. altered sleep patterns.

4. To motivate yourself to stick to an exercise program:
 a. Watch professional athletic competitions.
 b. Set a long-term goal, then break it down into short-term goals that can be achieved in a few months.
 c. Keep a detailed record of all the times that you avoided working out.
 d. Join an expensive health club so that you feel pressured to get your money's worth.

5. Michael started a walking program two weeks ago. Which of these workouts would you recommend to him for aerobic exercise?
 a. 5 minutes of brisk walking, 30 minutes of flexibility exercises, 5 minutes of brisk walking
 b. 5 minutes of stretching, 15 minutes of slow walking, 5 minutes of brisk walking, 15 minutes of slow walking
 c. 10 minutes of slow walking, 35 minutes of brisk walking, 5 minutes of slow walking
 d. 10 minutes of stretching, 45 minutes of slow walking

6. The new Exercise Guidelines for Americans recommend all of these *except*
 a. Engage in at least 30 minutes of moderate-intensity physical activity on most days of the week.
 b. Engage in physical activity of more vigorous intensity or longer duration for greater health benefits.
 c. Engage in 60 minutes of moderate- to vigorous-intensity activity on most days of the week to prevent gradual weight gain.
 d. Engage in 120 minutes of vigorous-intensity activity to get really fit.

7. For any muscle to get stronger, it must work against a greater-than-normal resistance. This is called the
 a. reversibility principle.
 b. overload principle.
 c. FITT principle.
 d. principle of compound interest.

8. A regular flexibility program provides which of the following benefits?
 a. stronger heart and lungs
 b. relief of muscle strain and soreness
 c. increased strength and endurance
 d. increased bone mass and leaner muscles

9. Which nutrient is the most important during exercise and exertion?
 a. water
 b. carbohydrates
 c. fat
 d. protein

10. Which of the following precautions could help to prevent a serious sports injury from occurring?
 a. Wear swimming goggles when doing laps to decrease the irritating effects of chlorine.
 b. Wear knee pads when cycling to prevent knee gashes if you fall off your bicycle.
 c. To eliminate persistent muscle soreness, increase the frequency and/or time period of your workout.
 d. Wear a helmet, wrist guards, and knee pads when inline skating to help prevent fractures and head injuries.

Answers to these questions can be found on page 587.

Critical Thinking

1. Allison knows that exercise is good for her health, but she figures she can keep her weight down by dieting and worry about her heart and health when she gets older. "I look good. I feel okay. Why should I bother exercising?" she asks. What would you reply?

2. College athletes have died unexpectedly from heart-related problems. The American Heart Association has identified guidelines to screen competitive athletes. Does your school follow these guidelines? If not, what precautions are taken to protect young athletes?

3. Your younger brother Andre is hoping to get a starting position on his high school football team. Practices began in July. You are aware that a couple of other players have suffered heat-related incidences, but

(*continued, p. 142*)

Self Survey ▪▪ Are You Ready to Become More Active?

Physical Activity Stages of Change Questionnaire

For each of the following questions, please circle Yes or No. Please be sure to read the questions carefully.

Physical activity or exercise includes activities such as walking briskly, jogging, bicycling, swimming, or any other activity in which the exertion is at least as intense as these activities.

1) I am currently physically active.	**NO**	**YES**
2) I intend to become more physically active in the next 6 months.	**NO**	**YES**

For activity to be regular, it must add up to a total of 30 minutes or more per day and be done at least 5 days per week. For example, you could take one 30-minute walk or take three 10-minute walks for a daily total of 30 minutes.

3) I currently engage in regular physical activity.	**NO**	**YES**
4) I have been regularly physically active for the past 6 months.	**NO**	**YES**

Scoring Algorithm:

Precontemplation:	Question One = No
	Question Two = No
Contemplation:	Question One = No
	Question Two = Yes
Preparation:	Question One = Yes and
	Question Three = No
Action:	Question One = Yes
	Question Three = Yes and
	Question Four = No
Maintenance:	Question One = Yes
	Question Three = Yes
	Question Four = Yes

Sources: Marcus, Bess, and Beth Lewis. "Physical Activity and the Stages of Motivational Readiness for Change Model." *President's Council on Physical Fitness and Sports Research Digest,* Series 4, No. 1, March 2003, p. 1. Marcus, H., and L. J. Forsyth. *Motivating People to Be Physically Active.* Champaign, IL: Human Kinetics, 2003. Reprinted, by permission, from B. H. Marcus and L. H. Forsyth, 2003, *Motivating People to be Physically Active* (Champaign, IL: Human Kinetics), p. 21.

YOUR ACTION PLAN FOR PHYSICAL FITNESS

Once you know your stage of motivational readiness, you can employ the cognitive and behavioral strategies most likely to work for you now. As you progress through the stages of change, you can shift to other approaches. Here are some suggestions:

Precontemplation (not active and not thinking about becoming active)

▪ Use this course as an opportunity to learn about the benefits of physical activity, including better mood, lower stress, stronger bones, and a lower risk of cardiovascular disease.

▪ Set a small, reasonable goal that does not involve working up a sweat, such as looking up "exercise, benefits of" in the index of this book and reading the pages cited.

▪ List what you see as the cons of physical activity. For example, do you fear it would take time you need for your studies? Think of small changes that don't require time, for instance, standing rather than sitting when talking on the phone, doing stretches while watching television, or taking a quick walk down the hall or up the stairs while waiting for a friend or a class to begin.

▪ Identify barriers to physical activity, such as lack of money. Take advantage of your student status, and check out facilities, such as the swimming pool at the athletic center, or opportunities, such as an intramural soccer team, available to you free (or almost).

Contemplation (not active but thinking about becoming active)

▪ Think back to activities you found enjoyable in the past. You might consider inline skating to class or around campus, or plan a hike for a weekend or school break.

▪ Determine the types of activity you can realistically fit into your daily schedule. You might join friends for softball every Saturday, or sign up for an evening body-sculpting class.

▪ Visualize success. Focus on the person you want to become: How would you look? What would you do differently? Find an image—from a magazine advertisement, for example—and post it where you can see it often.

▪ Plan your rewards. Use a technique called shaping, which reinforces progress on the way to a goal. For instance, initially you might reward yourself once you engage in physical activity for 15 minutes a day. After a week, you get the reward only after 20 minutes a day. Over time you increase the number of days you are physically active as well as the number of minutes of activity per day.

▪ Reach out for support. Find a friend, family member, or classmate who is willing or able to provide support for being active. Or join an organized martial arts class or an informal team.

Preparation (active but not at recommended levels)

▪ Identify specific barriers that limit your activity. If your daily jogs are rained or snowed out, develop a list of indoor alternatives, such as walking stairs or working out to an exercise video.

▪ Set specific daily and weekly goals. Your daily goal might begin with 10 or 15 minutes of activity. Your weekly goal might be to try a new activity, such as spinning or a dance class.

▪ Divide physical activity over the course of the day with a 10 or 15 minute walk in the morning, another at lunch, and a third at the end of the day.

▪ Document your progress. You could use a monthly calendar to keep track of the number of days you've exercised as well as the length of each workout. Or you can keep a more detailed record, noting the types of exercise you do every day, the intensity you work at, the duration of each workout, and so forth.

Action and Maintenance (active at recommended levels for less than six months)

▪ Identify risk factors that might lead to relapse. If vacations or holiday breaks disrupt your routine, make a plan for alternative ways to remain active before you leave campus.

▪ Stress-proof your fitness program. In crunch times, you may feel you don't have time to spare for exercise. Multiple 10-minute walks during the day may be particularly useful both to keep up your fitness and to relieve stress buildup.

▪ Avoid boredom. Think through ways to vary your exercise routine. Take different routes on your walks. Invite different friends to join you. Alternate working with free weights and resistance machines at the gym.

▪ Set secondary goals. Once you've reached and maintained your goal for physical activity, set goals related to secondary benefits of exercise, for instance, losing weight or changing your body composition.

CASE IN POINT

Student: Yuko, 28

Goal: To build her muscular strength

Action Plan:

▪ Block out 20 to 30 minutes two or three days a week for strength-building exercises.

▪ Find out if her college gym has basic resistance equipment and if trainers are available to explain how to use the machines.

▪ Check out the availability of sculpting or weight-lifting classes at the gym.

▪ Purchase some inexpensive dumbbells she can keep in her room and work out with during study breaks.

▪ Make notes in a computer file or notebook of her baseline muscular fitness, that is, how much weight and how many repetitions she can handle. Monitor her progress on a weekly basis.

Health ☯ Now™ If you want to write your own goals for improved fitness, go to the **Wellness Journal** in HealthNow at http://healthnow.brookscole.com/ith.

according to Andre, these players just weren't tough enough. What can you do to help your brother protect his health?

4. Research is mixed on whether stretching can decrease delayed-onset muscle soreness. Do you think a placebo effect can occur in studies on exercise and training as it does in research on medications? Why?

Media Menu

Health ☙ Now™

Throughout the chapter, this icon introduces a list of resources on the Health-Now website at **http://healthnow.brookscole.com/ith** that will:
- Help you evaluate your knowledge of the material.
- Allow you to take an exam-prep quiz.
- Provide a Personalized Learning Plan targeting resources that address areas you should study.
- Coach you through identifying target goals for behavior change and creating and monitoring your personal change plan throughout the semester.

INTERNET CONNECTIONS

American Council on Exercise

www.acefitness.org

This website features information for the general public as well as for certified fitness trainers. The comprehensive site includes health and fitness news headlines, Fit Facts information sheets, a question and answer site, whole body exercise workouts, daily fitness tips, discussion boards, newsletters, and information on ACE certification.

American Alliance for Health, Physical Education, Recreation and Dance

www.aahperd.org

This organization provides legislative advocacy for healthy lifestyles through high quality programs in health and physical education. The web site features consumer news, career links, listing of graduate programs, research, and a link for the International Electronic Journal of Health Education.

Shape Up America

www.shapeup.org/fitness.html

At this site, you can perform a battery of physical fitness assessments, including activity level, strength, flexibility, and an aerobic fitness test. You get started by entering your weight, height, age, and gender and then take a quick screen test to assess your physical readiness for physical activity. Your final results in each area will be based on your personal data.

Just Move

www.justmove.org

At this website sponsored by the American Heart Association, after a free registration, you can access an interactive exercise diary where you can keep track of your own exercise progress. In addition, an information resource called My Fitness provides recommendations for optimizing your exercise program to match your lifestyle as well as a list of health and fitness resources.

InfoTrac College Edition Activities Log on, insert **cardiorespiratory fitness** into the Keyword search box, and limit your search to the past year. When you get the results, Mark articles to review, then Select one to read. Summarize three or four key points from the article.

You can find additional readings related to personal health with InfoTrac College Edition, an online library of more than 900 journals and publications. Follow the instructions for accessing InfoTrac College Edition that were packaged with your textbook; then search for articles using a keyword search.

For additional links, resources, and suggested readings on the InfoTrac College Edition, visit our Health and Wellness Resource Center at **http://health .wadsworth.com.**

Key Terms

The terms listed are used on the page indicated. Definitions of the terms are in the Glossary at the end of this book.

active stretching 129	ergogenic aids 127
acute injuries 136	FITT 114
aerobic exercise 116	flexibility 106
anabolic steroids 126	frostbite 135
anaerobic exercise 116	frostnip 135
ballistic stretching 129	hypothermia 136
body composition 106	isokinetic 124
body mass index (BMI) 110	isometric 123
capillaries 122	isotonic 123
cardiorespiratory fitness 106	maximal oxygen uptake (VO$_2$ max) 116
cross-training 116	
dynamic flexibility 128	muscular endurance 106
endorphins 111	muscular strength 106
endurance 122	osteoporosis 111

6   Personal Nutrition

The freshmen on the fifth floor of a university dormitory decided to test a dubious premise: that man—and woman—can live on pizza alone. For a month, they vowed to eat nothing but pizza in all its savory varieties—mushroom, pepperoni, sausage, anchovies, extra cheese, thin crust, double crust. In less than a week, most cringed at the very sight of yet another cardboard delivery box. It wasn't just the boredom of having the same meal that got to them. Some felt bloated. Others had stomachaches. A few complained of headaches and fatigue. One was convinced she had scurvy, a vitamin deficiency disease caused by a lack of fruit and vegetables. None of them managed to stick with pizza for an entire month.

As these students discovered, the foods we choose to eat have an enormous impact on how we feel—and not just in the short term. As demonstrated by the science of **nutrition,** the field that explores the connections between our bodies and the foods we eat, our daily diet affects how long and how well we live. Sensible eating can provide energy for our daily tasks, protect us from many chronic illnesses, and may even extend longevity. A high-quality diet also enhances day-to-day vitality, energy, and sense of well-being.

This chapter can help you make better food choices. It translates the latest information on good nutrition, based on the *2005 Dietary Guidelines for Americans,* into specific advice that you can use to nourish yourself as well as enjoy the pleasure of eating well.

FAQ Frequently Asked Questions

- How many calories do I need? *p. 146*
- Should I switch to low-carb foods? *p. 148*
- Do men and women have different nutritional needs? *p. 150*
- Should I take vitamin pills? *p. 155*
- How can I find snacks that are good for me? *p. 161*
- What should I know about vegetarian diets? *p. 163*
- What should I look for on nutrition labels? *p. 164*
- What causes food poisoning? *p. 167*

After studying the material in this chapter, you should be able to:

- **List** the basic nutrients necessary for a healthy body and **describe** their functions.
- **Describe** the key themes of the USDA MyPyramid System.
- **List** five specific nutrition guidelines of the MyPyramid system.
- **Explain** how to interpret the nutritional information provided on food labels.
- **List** the food safety hazards and describe prevention measures.

WHAT YOU NEED TO KNOW ABOUT NUTRIENTS

Every day your body needs certain **essential nutrients** that it cannot manufacture for itself. They provide energy, build and repair body tissues, and regulate body functions. The six classes of essential nutrients, which are discussed in this section, are water, protein, carbohydrates, fats, vitamins, and minerals (Table 6-1).

Water makes up about 60 percent of the body and is essential for health and survival. Besides water, we also need energy to live, and we receive our energy from the carbohydrates, proteins, and fats in the foods we eat. The digestive system (Figure 6-1) breaks down food into these **macronutrients.** They are the nutrients required by the human body in the greatest amounts. The amount of energy that can be derived from the macronutrients is measured in **calories.** There are 9 calories in every gram of fat and 4 calories in every gram of protein or carbohydrate. The other two essential nutrients—the vitamins and minerals—are called **micronutrients** because our bodies need them in only very small amounts.

Your need for macronutrients depends on how much energy you expend. Because fats, carbohydrates, and protein can all serve as sources of energy, they can, to some extent, substitute for one another in providing calories.

Adults, according to federal standards, should get 45 to 65 percent of calories from carbohydrates, 20 to 35 percent from fat, and 10 to 35 percent from protein. Children's fat intake should be slightly higher: 25 to 40 percent of their caloric intake.[1]

To eat well without overeating, choose foods that are "nutrient-dense," that is, foods that provide the most nutritional value. For example, both a cup of nonfat milk and an ounce and a half of cheddar cheese provide about 300 mg of calcium, but the milk offers the same amount of calcium for half the calories. Foods that are extremely low in nutrient density—such as potato chips, candy, and soft drinks—are "empty," delivering only calories with few, if any, nutrients.

(FAQ) HOW MANY CALORIES DO I NEED?

Calories are the measure of the amount of energy that can be derived from food. How many calories you need depends on your gender, age, body-frame size, weight, percentage of body fat, and your **basal metabolic rate (BMR)**—the number of calories needed to sustain your body at rest. Your activity level also affects your calorie requirements. Regardless of whether you consume fat, protein, or carbohydrates, if you take in more calories than required to maintain your size and don't work them off in some sort of physical activity, your body will convert the excess to fat (see Chapter 7).

TABLE 6-1 THE ESSENTIAL NUTRIENTS

	Sources	Functions
Water	Liquids, fruits, and vegetables	Carries nutrients and removes waste; dissolves amino acids, glucose, and minerals; cleans body by removing toxins; regulates body temperature
Proteins	Meat, poultry, fish, eggs, beans, nuts, cheese, tofu, vegetables, some fruits, pastas, breads, cereal, and rice	Help build new tissue to keep hair, skin, and eyesight healthy; build antibodies, enzymes, hormones, and other compounds; provide fuel for body
Carbohydrates	Grains, cereal, pasta, fruits and vegetables, nuts, milk, and sugars	Provide energy
Fats		
Saturated Fats	Red meat, dairy products, egg yolks, and coconut and palm oils; shortening; stick margarine; baked goods	Provide energy; trigger production of cholesterol (see Chapter 15)
Unsaturated Fats	Some fish; avocados; olive, canola, and peanut oils	Also provide energy, but trigger more "good" cholesterol production and less "bad" cholesterol production (see Chapter 15)
Vitamins	Fruits, vegetables, grains, some meat and dairy products	Facilitate use of other nutrients; involved in regulating growth, maintaining tissue, and manufacturing blood cells, hormones, and other body components
Minerals	Many foods	Help build bones and teeth; aid in muscle function and nervous system activity; assist in various body functions including growth and energy production

**Organs That
Aid Digestion**

Salivary Glands
Donate a starch-digesting
enzyme
Donate a trace of
fat-digesting enzyme
(important to infants)

Liver
Manufactures bile, a
detergentlike substance
that facilitates digestion
of fats

Gallbladder
Stores bile until needed

Bile Duct
Conducts bile to
small intestine

Pancreatic Duct
Conducts pancreatic
juice into small intestine

Pancreas
Manufactures enzymes
to digest all energy-
yielding nutrients
Releases bicarbonate
to neutralize stomach
acid that enters
small intestine

**Digestive Tract Organs
That Contain the Food**

Mouth
Chews and mixes food
with saliva

Esophagus
Passes food to stomach

Stomach
Adds acid, enzymes,
and fluid
Churns, mixes, and grinds
food to a liquid mass

Small Intestine
Secretes enzymes that
digest carbohydrate, fat,
and protein
Cells lining intestine absorb
nutrients into blood and
lymph fluids

Large Intestine (Colon)
Reabsorbs water and
minerals
Passes waste (fiber,
bacteria, any unabsorbed
nutrients) and some
water to rectum

Rectum
Stores waste prior
to elimination

Anus
Holds rectum closed
Opens to allow
elimination

FIGURE 6-1 The Digestive System

The organs of the digestive system break down food into nutrients that the body can use.

On average, daily calorie needs are:

❚ Most women, some older adults, children
ages two to six: 1,600

❚ Average adult: 2,000

❚ Most men, active women, teenage girls,
older children: 2,200

❚ Active men, teenage boys: 2,800

WATER

Water, which makes up 85 percent of blood, 70 percent of muscles, and about 75 percent of the brain, performs many essential functions: It carries nutrients, maintains temperature, lubricates joints, helps with digestion, rids the body of waste through urine, and contributes to the production of sweat, which evaporates from the skin to cool the body.

Water is an essential nutrient. Remember: Each day you must replace the amount you use.

Research has correlated high fluid intake with a lower risk of kidney stones, colon cancer, and bladder cancer.

You lose about 64 to 80 ounces of water a day—the equivalent of eight to ten 8-ounce glasses—through perspiration, urination, bowel movements, and normal exhalation. You lose water more rapidly if you exercise, live in a dry climate or at a high altitude, drink a lot of caffeine or alcohol (which increase urination), skip a meal, or become ill. To assure adequate water intake, nutritionists advise drinking a minimum of 64 ounces, enough so that your urine is not dark in color. Healthy individuals can get adequate hydration from beverages other than plain water, including juice and soft drinks.[2]

PROTEIN

Critical for growth and repair, **proteins** form the basic framework for our muscles, bones, blood, hair, and fingernails. Supplying 4 calories per gram, they are made of combinations of 20 **amino acids,** 9 of which we must get from our diet because the human body cannot produce them. These are called *essential amino acids.*

Animal proteins—meat, fish, poultry, and dairy products—are **complete proteins** that provide the nine essential amino acids. Grains, dry beans, and nuts are **incomplete proteins** that may have relatively low levels of one or two essential amino acids but fairly high levels of others. Combining incomplete proteins, such as beans and rice, ensures that the body gets sufficient protein. The recommended level of protein intake is 0.8 gram per kilogram of body weight for adults.

CARBOHYDRATES

Carbohydrates are organic compounds that provide our brains and bodies with *glucose,* their basic fuel. The major sources of carbohydrates are plants—including grains, vegetables, fruits, and beans—and milk. There are two types: *simple carbohydrates* (sugars) and *complex carbohydrates* (starches and fiber). All provide 4 calories per gram. Both adults and children should consume at least 130 grams of carbohydrates each day, the minimum needed to produce enough glucose for the brain to function.

Forms of Carbohydrates

Simple carbohydrates include *natural sugars,* such as the lactose in milk and the fructose in fruit, and *added sugars* that are found in candy, soft drinks, fruit drinks, pastries, and other sweets. Those whose diets are higher in added sugars typically have lower intakes of other essential nutrients.

Complex carbohydrates include grains, cereals, vegetables, beans, and nuts. Americans, however, get most of their complex carbohydrates from refined grains, which have been stripped of fiber and many nutrients.[3]

Far more nutritious are whole grains, which are made up of all components of the grain: the *bran* (or fiber-rich outer layer), the *endosperm* (middle layer), and the *germ* (the nutrient-packed inner layer). Increasing whole-grain consumption has become a public health priority, and the 2005 Dietary Guidelines recommend that Americans increase their consumption of whole-grain foods.[4] Individuals who eat whole-grain products each day have about a 15 to 25 percent reduction in death from all causes, including heart disease and cancer.[5]

FAQ Should I Switch to Low-Carb Foods?

The popularity of diets that restrict carbohydrate intake, such as the Atkins diet discussed in Chapter 7, prompted an explosion in products touted as "low-carb." You can get low-carb versions of everything from beer to bread. However, the Food and Drug Administration (FDA), which regulates health claims on food labels in the United States, hasn't defined what "low-carb" means. Words like "low-carb," "carb-wise," or "carb-free" are marketing terms created by manufacturers to sell their products.

Although many people may buy low-carbohydrate foods because they believe that they're healthier, that isn't necessarily the case. A low-carb nutrition bar, for instance, may be high in saturated fat and calories. Since low-carb food products are relatively new on grocery shelves, no one knows their long-term hazards. Some cause digestive symptoms because food companies often replace the carbohydrates in a cookie or cracker with substances such as the sweetener sorbitol, which can cause diarrhea or stomach cramps.

Dieters often buy low-carb products in order to lose weight. According to proponents of low-carbohydrate diets, if carbohydrates raise blood sugar and insulin levels and cause weight gain, a decrease in carbs should result in lower blood sugar and insulin levels—and weight loss. With limited carbohydrates in the diet, the body would break down fat to provide needed energy.

Some people do lose weight when they switch to low-carb foods, but the reasons are probably that they consume fewer calories, lose water weight, and have decreased appetite because of a buildup of ketones (a by-product of fat metabolism) in the blood. As discussed in Chapter 7, a low-carb diet can lead to fairly rapid weight loss but is no easier to maintain over the long run than any other diet.

Glycemic Index and Glycemic Load

The glycemic index is a ranking of carbohydrates, gram for gram, based on their immediate effect on blood glucose (sugar) levels. Carbohydrates that break down quickly during digestion and trigger a fast, high glucose response have the highest glycemic index rating. Those that break down slowly, releasing glucose gradually into the bloodstream, have low glycemic index ratings. Potatoes, which raise blood sugar higher and faster than apples, for instance, earn a higher glycemic-index rating than apples. Glycemic index does not account for the amount of food you typically eat in a serving.

Glycemic load is a measure of how much a typical serving size of a particular food raises blood glucose. For example, the glycemic index of table sugar is high, but you use so little to sweeten your coffee or tea that its glycemic load is low.[6]

Some diets are based on the theory that high-glycemic-index foods raise blood sugar and insulin levels and cause weight gain, while low-glycemic-index foods lower your blood sugar and insulin levels so you'll lose weight. Although some people do lose weight on low-glycemic diets, this theory has not been scientifically proved. Experts are dubious because many factors play a role in how much blood glucose rises, including age and weight. And people typically don't eat single foods at a meal, but a combination of foods that affect blood sugar differently.

Fiber

Dietary fiber is the nondigestible form of complex carbohydrates occurring naturally in plant foods, such as leaves, stems, skins, seeds, and hulls. **Functional fiber** consists of isolated, nondigestible carbohydrates that may be added to foods and that provide beneficial effects in humans. Total fiber is the sum of both.

The various forms of fiber enhance health in different ways: They slow the emptying of the stomach, which creates a feeling of fullness and aids weight control. They interfere with absorption of dietary fat and cholesterol, which lowers the risk of heart disease and stroke in both middle-aged and elderly individuals.[7] In addition, fiber helps prevent constipation, diverticulosis (a painful inflammation of the bowel), and diabetes.[8] The link between fiber and colon cancer is complex. Some studies have indicated that increased fiber intake reduces risk; a large-scale study of almost 90,000 women found no such correlation.[9]

The Institute of Medicine has set the first-ever recommendations for daily intake levels of total fiber (dietary plus functional fiber): 38 grams of total fiber for men and 25 grams for women. For men and women over 50 years of age, who consume less food, the recommendations are, respectively, 30 and 21 grams. The American Dietetic Association recommends 25 to 35 grams of dietary fiber a day, much more than the amount Americans typically consume.[10]

Good fiber sources include wheat and corn bran (the outer layer); leafy greens; the skins of fruits and root vegetables; oats, beans, and barley; and the pulp, skin, and seeds of many fruits and vegetables, such as apples and strawberries. Because sudden increases in fiber can cause symptoms like bloating and gas, experts recommend gradually adding more fiber to your diet with an additional serving or two of vegetables, fruit, or whole wheat bread.

FATS

Fats carry the fat-soluble vitamins A, D, E, and K; aid in their absorption in the intestine; protect organs from injury; regulate body temperature; and play an important role in growth and development. They provide 9 calories per gram—more than twice the amount in carbohydrates or proteins.

Both high- and low-fat diets can be unhealthy. When people eat very low levels of fat and very high levels of carbohydrates, their levels of high-density lipoprotein, the so-called *good cholesterol*, declines. On the other hand, high-fat diets can lead to obesity and its related health dangers, discussed in Chapter 7.

Forms of Fat

Saturated fats and **unsaturated fats** are distinguished by the type of fatty acids in their chemical structures. Unsaturated fats can be divided into monounsaturated or polyunsaturated, again depending on their chemical structure. All dietary fats are a mix of saturated and unsaturated fats but are predominantly one or the other. Unsaturated fats, like oils, are likely to be liquid at room temperature and saturated fats, like butter, are likely to be solid. In general, vegetable and fish oils are unsaturated, and animal fats are saturated.

Olive, soybean, canola, cottonseed, corn, and other vegetable oils are unsaturated fats. Olive oil is considered a good fat and one of the best vegetable oils for salads and cooking. Used for thousands of years, this staple of the Mediterranean diet, discussed later in this chapter, has been correlated with a lower incidence of heart disease, including strokes and heart attacks.

Fish oils are rich in omega-3 fatty acids, which make molecules such as prostaglandins that enhance cardiovascular health. Fish oils also improve healthy blood lipid levels (fats), prevent blood clots, ward off the age-related vision problem called macular degeneration, and may lower blood pressure, especially in people with hypertension or atherosclerosis.[11]

 However, most college students do not consume the recommended amount of omega-3 fatty acids.[12]

In contrast, saturated fats can increase the risk of heart disease and should be avoided as much as possible. In response to consumer and health professionals' demand for less saturated fat in the food supply, many manufacturers switched to partially hydrogenated oils.

The process of hydrogenation creates unsaturated fatty acids called **trans fat.** They are found in some margarine products and most foods made with partially hydrogenated oils, such as baked goods and fried foods. Even though trans fats are unsaturated, they appear similar to saturated fats in terms of raising cholesterol levels. Epidemiological studies have suggested a possible link between cardiovascular disease risk and high intakes of trans fats, and researchers have concluded that they are, gram for gram, twice as damaging as saturated fat. There is no safe level for trans fats, which occur naturally in meats as well as in foods prepared with partially hydrogenated vegetable oils.

To cut down on both saturated and trans fats, choose soybean, canola, corn, olive, safflower, and sunflower oils, which are naturally free of trans fats and lower in saturated fats. Look for reduced-fat, low-fat, fat-free, and trans fat-free versions of baked goods, snacks, and other processed foods. Table 6-2 compares saturated fat content and calories for some typical foods.

(FAQ)

DO MEN AND WOMEN HAVE DIFFERENT NUTRITIONAL NEEDS?

Men and women do not need to eat different foods, but their nutritional needs are different. Because most men are bigger and taller than most women, they consume more calories. Eating more means it's easier for them to get the nutrients they need, even though many don't make the wisest food choices.

Women, particularly those who restrict their caloric intake or are chronically dieting, are more likely to develop specific deficiencies. Calcium is one example. Women drink less milk than men, and many do not consume the recommended 800 to 1,200 milligrams of calcium daily. This deficiency, combined with a sedentary lifestyle, increases the risk of bone-weakening osteoporosis.[13]

Many women also get too little iron. Even in adolescence, girls are more prone to iron deficiency than boys; some suffer memory and learning impairments as a result. In adult women, menstrual blood loss and poor eating habits can lead to low iron stores, which puts them at risk for anemia. According to U.S. Department of Agriculture research, most women consume only 60 percent of the recommended 15 milligrams of iron per day. (The recommendation for men is 10 milligrams.) Regular blood tests can monitor a woman's iron status.

Here are some gender-specific strategies for better nutrition:

- Men should cut back on fat and meat in their diets, two things they eat too much.

- Women should increase their iron intake by eating meat (iron from animal sources is absorbed better than that from vegetable

TABLE 6-2 COMPARING SATURATED FAT AND CALORIE CONTENT

Food	Saturated Fat Content (grams)	Calories
Cheese (1 oz.)		
Regular cheddar cheese	6.0	114
Low-fat cheddar cheese	1.2	49
Ground Beef (3 oz. cooked)		
Regular ground beef (25% fat)	6.1	236
Extra lean ground beef (5% fat)	2.6	148
Milk (1 cup)		
Whole milk (3.24%)	4.6	146
Low-fat (1%) milk	1.5	102
Breads (1 medium)		
Croissant	6.6	231
Bagel, oat bran (4″)	0.2	227
Frozen desserts (1/2 cup)		
Regular ice cream	4.9	145
Frozen yogurt	2.0	110
Table spreads (1 tsp.)		
Butter	2.4	34
Trans-free soft margarine	0.7	25
Chicken (3 oz. cooked)		
Fried chicken (leg)	3.3	212
Chicken breast	0.9	140
Fish (3 oz.)		
Fried fish	2.8	195
Baked fish	1.5	129

Source: ARS Nutrient Database for Standard Reference, *Dietary Guidelines for Americans 2005,* USDHHS, USDA, www.healthierus.gov/dietary guidelines.

sources) or a combination of meat and vegetable iron sources together (for example, a meat and bean burrito). Those with iron deficiencies should consult a physician. Because large doses of iron can be toxic, iron supplements should be taken only with medical supervision.

- Women should consume more calcium-rich foods, including low-fat and nonfat dairy products, leafy greens, and tofu. Women who cannot get adequate amounts of calcium from their daily diet should take calcium supplements. This is not advised for all men because of a possible connection between calcium and prostate cancer.

- Women who could become pregnant should take a multivitamin with 400 micrograms of **folic acid,** which helps prevent neural tube defects such as spina bifida. Folic acid is also useful to men because it may cut the risk of heart disease, stroke, and colon cancer.

- Both genders should increase their fruit and vegetable intake to ensure that they are getting adequate amounts of vitamins and fiber in their daily diet.

VITAMINS AND MINERALS

Vitamins, which help put proteins, fats, and carbohydrates to use, are essential to regulating growth, maintaining tissue, and releasing energy from foods. Together with the enzymes in the body, they help produce the right chemical reactions at the right times. They're also involved in the manufacture of blood cells, hormones, and other compounds.

The body produces some vitamins, such as vitamin D, which is manufactured in the skin after exposure to sunlight. Other vitamins must be ingested.

Vitamins A, D, E, and K are fat-soluble; they are absorbed through the intestinal membranes and stored in the body.

The B vitamins and vitamin C are water-soluble; they are absorbed directly into the blood and then used up or washed out of the body in urine and sweat. They must be replaced daily. Table 6-3 summarizes key information about the vitamins.

Antioxidants are substances that prevent the harmful effects caused by oxidation within the body. They include vitamins C, E, and beta-carotene (a form of vitamin A), as well as compounds like carotenoids and flavonoids. All share a common enemy: renegade oxygen cells called free radicals released by normal metabolism as well as by pollution, smoking, radiation, and stress.

Diets high in antioxidant-rich fruits and vegetables have been linked with lower rates of esophageal, lung, colon, and stomach cancer. Nevertheless, scientific studies have not proved conclusively that any specific antioxidant, particularly in supplement form, can prevent cancer.

Carbon, oxygen, hydrogen, and nitrogen make up 96 percent of our body weight. The other 4 percent consists of **minerals** that help build bones and teeth, aid in muscle function, and help our nervous systems transmit messages. Every day we need about a tenth of a gram (100 milligrams) or more of the major minerals: sodium, potassium chloride, calcium, phosphorus, magnesium, and sulfur. We also need about a hundredth of a gram (10 milligrams) or less of each of the trace minerals: iron (although premenopausal women need more), zinc, selenium, molybdenum, iodine, copper, manganese, fluoride, and chromium. (See Table 6-4 on page 154 for key information on the minerals.)

Americans get adequate amounts of most nutrients. However, the 2005 Advisory Committee for Dietary Guidelines reported that intakes of several nutrients are low enough to be of concern. Are you getting enough of these nutrients?

- **For adults:** vitamins A, C, and E, calcium, magnesium, potassium, and fiber
- **For children:** vitamin E, calcium, magnesium, potassium, and fiber

Among the groups at highest risk of nutritional deficiencies are:

- **Teenage girls**
- **Women of child-bearing age** (iron and folic acid)

Antioxidants are found in vegetables and fruit. By eating an orange at breakfast and half a carrot for lunch, you will have all the antioxidants you need for the day.

© 2001 PhotoDisc, Inc.

- **Persons over age 50** (vitamin B_{12})
- **The elderly, persons with dark skin,** and those who do not get adequate exposure to sunshine (vitamin D).[14]

Calcium

Calcium, the most abundant mineral in the body, builds strong bone tissue throughout life and plays a vital role in blood clotting and muscle and nerve functioning. Pregnant or nursing women need more calcium to meet the additional needs of their babies' bodies. Calcium may also help control high blood pressure, prevent colon cancer in adults, and promote weight loss.

Adequate calcium intake during childhood, adolescence, and young adulthood is crucial to prevent **osteoporosis,** the bone-weakening disease that strikes one of every four women over the age of 60 (see Chapter 18 for a complete discussion). National health organizations are promoting greater calcium consumption among college students, particularly women, to increase bone density and safeguard against osteoporosis.

In both men and women, bone mass peaks between the ages of 25 and 35. Over the next 10 to 15 years, bone mass remains fairly stable. At about age 40, bone loss equivalent to 0.3 to 0.5 percent per year begins in both men and women. Women may experience greater bone loss, at a rate of 3 to 5 percent, at the time of menopause. This decline continues for approximately five to seven years and is the primary factor leading to postmenopausal osteoporosis.

The higher an individual's peak bone mass, the longer it takes for age- and menopause-related bone loss to increase

TABLE 6-3 KEY INFORMATION ABOUT VITAMINS

Vitamin/Recommended Intake per Day	Significant Sources	Chief Functions	Signs of Severe, Prolonged Deficiency	Signs of Extreme Excess

FAT-SOLUBLE VITAMINS

Vitamin/Recommended Intake per Day	Significant Sources	Chief Functions	Signs of Severe, Prolonged Deficiency	Signs of Extreme Excess
Vitamin A Males 19–50: 900 μg Females 19–50: 700 μg	Fortified milk, cheese, cream, butter, fortified margarine, eggs, liver; spinach and other dark, leafy greens, broccoli, deep orange fruits (apricots, cantaloupes) and vegetables (carrots, sweet potatoes, pumpkins)	Antioxidant; needed for vision, health of cornea, epithelial cells, mucous membranes, skin health, bone and tooth growth, reproduction, immunity	Anemia, painful joints, cracks in teeth, tendency toward tooth decay, diarrhea, depression, frequent infections, night blindness, keratinization, corneal degeneration, rashes, kidney stones	Nosebleeds, bone pain, growth retardation, headaches, abdominal cramps and pain, vomiting, diarrhea, weight loss, overreactive immune system, blurred vision, fatigue, irritability, hair loss, dry skin
Vitamin D Males 19–50: 5 μg Females 19–50: 5 μg	Fortified milk or margarine, eggs, liver, sardines; exposure to sunlight	Mineralization of bones (promotes calcium and phosphorus absorption)	Abnormal growth, misshapen bones (bowing of legs), soft bones, joint pain, malformed teeth	Raised blood calcium, excessive thirst, headaches, irritability, loss of appetite, weakness, nausea, kidney stones, deposits in arteries
Vitamin E Males 19–50: 15 mg Females 19–50: 15 mg	Polyunsaturated plant oils (margarine, salad dressings, shortenings), green and leafy vegetables, wheat germ, whole-grain products, nuts, seeds	Antioxidant; needed for stabilization of cell membranes, regulation of oxidation reactions	Red blood cell breakage, anemia, muscle degeneration, difficulty walking, leg cramps	Augments the effects of anticlotting medication; general discomfort; blurred vision
Vitamin K Males 19–50: 120 μg Females 19–50: 90 μg	Green leafy vegetables, cabbage-type vegetables, soybeans, vegetable oils	Synthesis of blood-clotting proteins and proteins important in bone mineralization	Hemorrhage	Interference with anti-clotting medication; jaundice

WATER-SOLUBLE VITAMINS

Vitamin/Recommended Intake per Day	Significant Sources	Chief Functions	Signs of Severe, Prolonged Deficiency	Signs of Extreme Excess
Vitamin B$_6$ Males 19–50: 1.3 mg Females 19–50: 1.3 mg	Meats, fish, poultry liver, legumes, fruits, whole grains, potatoes, soy products	Part of a coenzyme used in amino acid and fatty acid metabolism, helps make red blood cells	Anemia, depression, abnormal brain wave pattern, convulsions, skin rashes	Impaired memory, irritability, headaches, numbness, damage to nerves, difficulty walking, loss of reflexes
Vitamin B$_{12}$ Males 19–50: 2.4 μg Females 19–50: 2.4 μg	Animal products (meat, fish, poultry milk, cheese, eggs)	Part of a coenzyme used in new cell synthesis, helps maintain nerve cells	Anemia, nervous system degeneration progressing to paralysis, hypersensitivity	None known
Vitamin C Males 19–50: 90 mg Females 19–50: 75 mg	Citrus fruits, cabbage-type vegetables, dark green vegetables, cantaloupe, strawberries, peppers, lettuce, tomatoes, potatoes, papayas, mangoes	Antioxidant, collagen synthesis (strengthens blood vessel walls, forms scar tissue, matrix for bone growth), amino acid metabolism, strengthens resistance to infection, aids iron absorption	Anemia, pinpoint hemorrhages, frequent infections, bleeding gums, loosened teeth, muscle degeneration and pain, joint pain, blotchy bruises, failure of wounds to heal	Nausea, abdominal cramps, diarrhea, excessive urination, headache, fatigue, insomnia, rashes; deficiency symptoms may appear at first on withdrawal of high doses
Thiamin Males 19–50: 1.2 mg Females 19–50: 1.1 mg	Pork, ham, bacon, liver, whole grains, legumes, nuts; occurs in all nutritious foods in moderate amounts	Part of a coenzyme used in energy metabolism, supports normal appetite and nervous system function	Edema, enlarged heart, nervous/muscular system degeneration, difficulty walking, loss of reflexes, mental confusion	None reported

TABLE 6-3 *(continued)*

Vitamin/Recommended Intake per Day	Significant Sources	Chief Functions	Signs of Severe, Prolonged Deficiency	Signs of Extreme Excess
Riboflavin Males 19–50: 1.3 mg Females 19–50: 1.1 mg	Milk, yogurt, cottage cheese, meat, leafy green vegetables, whole-grain or enriched breads and cereals	Part of a coenzyme used in energy metabolism, supports normal vision and skin health	Cracks at corner of mouth, magenta tongue, hyper-sensitivity to light, reddening of cornea, skin rash	None reported
Niacin Males 19–50: 16 mg Females 19–50: 14 mg	Milk, eggs, meat, poultry, fish, whole-grain and enriched breads and cereals, nuts, and all protein-containing foods	Part of a coenzyme used in energy metabolism	Diarrhea, black smooth tongue, irritability, loss of appetite, weakness, dizziness, mental confusion, flaky skin rash on areas exposed to sun	Nausea, vomiting, painful flush and rash, sweating, liver damage
Folate Males 19–50: 400 μg Females 19–50: 400 μg	Leafy green vegetables, legumes, seeds, liver, enriched breads, cereal, pasta, and grains	Part of a coenzyme needed for new cell synthesis	Anemia, heartburn, frequent infections, smooth red tongue, depression, mental confusion	Masks vitamin B_{12} deficiency
Panothenic acid Males 19–50: 5 mg Females 19–50: 5 mg	Widespread in foods	Part of a coenzyme used in energy metabolism	Vomiting, intestinal distress, insomnia, fatigue	Water retention (rare)
Biotin Males 19–50: 30 μg Females 19–50: 30 μg	Widespread in foods	Used in energy metabolism, fat synthesis, amino acid metabolism, and glycogen synthesis	Abnormal heart action, loss of appetite, nausea, depression, muscle pain, drying of facial skin	None reported

Source: Adapted from Sizer, Frances, and Ellie Whitney. *Nutrition: Concepts and Controversies,* 10th ed. Belmont, CA: Wadsworth, 2006.

the risk of fractures. Osteoporosis is less common in groups with higher peak bone mass—men versus women, blacks versus whites. Dietary calcium, according to recent clinical trials, can significantly reduce body fat in obese men and women, even if they are not dieting, and can accelerate weight loss for those on a reduced-calorie diet.[15]

 Calcium is a special concern for African Americans who, as a group, have a higher risk for high blood pressure and obesity than the rest of the population but, on average, consume less than one serving of dairy foods a day. In fact, more than 80 percent of African Americans fail to get their daily recommended amount of calcium.[16]

Recent studies have cast doubt on the usefulness of calcium and vitamin D supplements, which do not prevent fractures when taken by the elderly.[17] Some researchers also question the value of calcium supplementation in childhood and adolescence for long-term bone health. In one study that followed 80 women from ages 12 to 22, only weight-bearing exercise, not calcium intake, was significantly correlated with bone density.[18] Others feel that a combination of regular exercise and dietary calcium is best for building strong bones.

Sodium

Sodium helps maintain proper fluid balance, regulates blood pressure, transmits muscle impulses, and relaxes muscles. Excess sodium isn't a problem for most healthy people, but for those who are sodium-sensitive—as many as 30 percent of the population—too much sodium contributes to high blood pressure.

The National Heart, Lung, and Blood Institute recommends less than 2.4 grams (2,400 milligrams) of sodium a day, the equivalent of about one teaspoon of table salt a day. For someone with high blood pressure, a daily intake of less than 1,500 mg of sodium is better for lowering blood pressure.

Strategies for Change :: Building Stronger Bones

:: Make calcium-rich foods part of your daily diet. These include dairy products, leafy green vegetables, canned fish, and tofu. Also look for products fortified with calcium and vitamin D, which aids in calcium absorption.

:: Avoid cigarette smoking, which has been linked with bone loss.

:: Drink alcohol only in moderation. Prolonged or heavy use of alcohol may decrease bone metabolism.

:: Be wary of high-protein diets. Excess protein intake may increase the rate of calcium loss from the body.

:: Do weight-bearing exercises. Activities such as walking, running, doing push-ups and sit-ups, and lifting weights all contribute to the development and maintenance of bone mass.

TABLE 6-4 KEY INFORMATION ABOUT ESSENTIAL MINERALS

Mineral	Significant Sources	Chief Functions	Signs of Severe, Prolonged Deficiency	Signs of Extreme Excess
MAJOR MINERALS				
Sodium	Salt, soy sauce, processed foods	Needed to maintain fluid balance and acid–base balance in body cells; critical to nerve impulse transmission	Mental apathy, poor appetite, muscle cramps	High blood pressure
Potassium	All whole foods: meats, milk, fruits, vegetables, grains, legumes	Needed to maintain fluid balance and acid–base balance in body cells; needed for muscle and nerve activity	Muscle weakness, mental confusion, paralysis	Irregular heartbeat, heart attack; muscular weakness
Chloride	Salt, soy sauce, processed foods	Aids in digestion; needed to maintain fluid balance and acid–base balance in body cells	Muscle cramps, apathy, poor appetite, growth failure in children	Vomiting
Calcium	Milk and milk products, oysters, small fish (with bones), tofu, greens, legumes	Component of bones and teeth, needed for muscle and nerve activity, blood clotting	Stunted growth in children, adult bone loss (osteoporosis)	Constipation, calcium deposits in kidneys, liver, and other tissues, decreased absorption of other minerals
Phosphorus	All animal tissues	Component of bones and teeth, energy formation, needed to maintain cell membranes	Loss of appetite, muscle weakness, impaired growth	Loss of calcium from bones
Magnesium	Nuts, legumes, whole grains, dark green vegetables, seafoods, chocolate, cocoa	Component of bones and teeth, nerve activity, energy and protein formation	Stunted growth in children, weakness, muscle spasms, personality changes	Diarrhea, dehydration, impaired nerve activity
Sulfur	All protein-containing foods	Component of certain amino acids; stabilizes protein shape	None known; protein deficiency would occur first	Depresses growth in animals
TRACE MINERALS				
Iron	Red meats, fish, poultry, shellfish, eggs, legumes, dried fruits	Aids in transport of oxygen, component of myoglobin, energy formation	Anemia, weakness, fatigue, pale appearance, reduced attention span, developmental delays in children	"Iron poisoning," vomiting, abdominal pain, blue coloration of skin, shock, heart failure, diabetes, decreased zinc absorption
Zinc	Protein-containing foods: fish, shellfish, poultry, grains, vegetables	Protein reproduction, component of insulin	Growth failure, delayed sexual maturation, slow wound healing	Nausea, vomiting, weakness, fatigue, susceptibility to infection, copper deficiency, metallic taste in mouth
Selenium	Meats and seafood, eggs, grains	Acts as an antioxidant in conjunction with vitamin E	Anemia, muscle pain and tenderness, heart failure	Hair and fingernail loss, weakness, liver damage, garlic or metallic breath
Molybdenum	Dried beans, grains, dark green vegetables, liver, milk and milk products	Aids in oxygen transfer from one molecule to another	Rapid heartbeat and breathing, nausea, vomiting, coma	Loss of copper from the body, joint pain, growth failure, anemia, gout
Iodine	Iodized salt, milk and milk products, seaweed, seafood, bread	Component of thyroid hormones that helps regulate energy production and growth	Goiter, cretinism in newborns (mental retardation, hearing loss, growth failure)	Pimples, goiter, decreased thyroid function
Copper	Organ meats, whole grains, nuts and seeds, seafood, drinking water	Component of enzymes involved in the body's utilization of iron and oxygen	Anemia, nerve and bone abnormalities in children, growth retardation	Wilson's disease (excessive accumulation of copper in the liver and kidneys); vomiting, diarrhea, liver disease
Manganese	Whole grains, coffee, tea, dried beans, nuts	Formation of body fat and bone	Weight loss, rash, nausea and vomiting	Infertility in men, disruptions in the nervous system, muscle spasms

TABLE 6-4 (*continued*)

Mineral	Significant Sources	Chief Functions	Signs of Severe, Prolonged Deficiency	Signs of Extreme Excess
Fluoride	Fluoridated water, foods, and beverages; tea; shrimp; crab	Component of bones and teeth (enamel)	Tooth decay and other dental diseases	Fluorosis, brittle bones, mottled teeth, nerve abnormalities
Chromium	Whole grains, liver, meat, beer, wine	Glucose utilization	Poor blood glucose control, weight loss	Kidney and skin damage

Source: Adapted from Brown, Judith E. *Nutrition Now*, 3rd ed. Belmont, CA: Wadsworth, 2002; Sizer, Frances, and Ellie Whitney. *Nutrition: Concepts and Controversies*, 10th ed. Belmont, CA: Wadsworth, 2006.

 Blacks, who have higher rates of high blood pressure and diseases related to hypertension, such as stroke and kidney failure, tend to be more sensitive to salt than nonblacks. African Americans also have lower intakes of calcium and potassium—both of which can protect against heart disease.[19]

PHYTOCHEMICALS

Phytochemicals, compounds that exist naturally in plants, serve many functions, including helping a plant protect itself from bacteria and disease. Some phytochemicals such as solanine, an insect-repelling chemical found in the leaves and stalks of potato plants, are natural toxins, but many are beneficial to humans. Flavonoids, found in apples, strawberries, grapes, onions, green and black tea, and red wine, may decrease atherosclerotic plaque and DNA damage related to cancer development. Phytochemicals are associated with a reduced risk of heart disease, certain cancers, age-related macular degeneration, adult-onset diabetes, stroke, and other diseases. However, in Western societies, research has shown neither an increase nor decrease in breast cancer with consumption of phytochemicals.[20]

FAQ Should I Take Vitamin Pills?

Since vitamins and minerals in food are good for you, you might figure that taking more in the form of dietary supplements would be even better. That's exactly why many people—half of all Americans, by some estimates—have taken vitamin pills, often in high doses, particularly after studies confirmed the benefits of antioxidants in food, particularly vitamins C and E. But recent research indicates that larger-than-recommended doses of vitamins do not reduce the risk of heart disease, cancer, and dementia—and may do more harm than good.

In major trials with nearly 140,000 randomized participants, antioxidant vitamins were essentially of no benefit in preventing cardiovascular disease or cancer. In a 12-year study of nearly 40,000 women, vitamin E failed to show any protective effects against cardiovascular problems or breast, lung, and colon cancer.[21] It is not yet known if it might be beneficial for men.[22] In other studies, antioxidant supplements did not reduce heart disorders or death rates, nor did they help people who already had diabetes or blood vessel disease.[23] Super-high doses of vitamin E also have not helped people with mild cognitive impairment, an early stage of Alzheimer's disease.[24]

High doses of vitamins carry potential risks. Certain antioxidants can interfere with the efficacy of cholesterol-lowering medications. High doses of vitamin E may increase the chances of earlier death. In cancer patients, those taking large doses had an increased risk of a new cancer.[25]

In particular, the fat-soluble vitamins, primarily A and D, can build up in our bodies and cause serious complications, such as damage to the kidneys, liver, or bones. Large doses of water-soluble vitamins, including the B vitamins, may also be harmful. Excessive intake of vitamin B_6 (pyridoxine), often used to relieve premenstrual bloating, can cause neurological damage, such as numbness in the mouth and tingling in the hands. (An excessive amount in this case is 250 to 300 times the recommended dose.) High doses of vitamin C can produce stomachaches and diarrhea. Niacin, often taken in high doses to lower cholesterol, can cause jaundice, liver damage, and irregular heartbeats as well as severe, uncomfortable flushing of the skin.

If you do feel a need for vitamins, choose a multivitamin supplement that does not exceed the recommended doses listed in Tables 6-3 and 6-4.

USING THE MYPYRAMID SYSTEM

Making healthy choices about what and how to eat isn't easy. However, the federal government is trying to help. In its most recent edition of *Nutrition and Your Health: Dietary Guidelines for Americans,* the U.S. Departments of Health and Human Services and of Agriculture provide science-based advice both to promote wellness and to reduce the risk of major chronic diseases. The MyPyramid Food Guidance System (Figure 6-2) translates the guidelines into a personalized, balanced, total diet.

The key themes of MyPyramid are:

- **Variety.** Eating foods from all food groups and subgroups.

- **Proportionality.** Eating more of some foods (fruits, vegetables, whole grains, fat-free or low-fat

FIGURE 6-2 The MyPyramid Food Guidance System

milk products) and less of others (foods high in saturated or trans fats, added sugars, cholesterol, salt, and alcohol). Critics of the new pyramid point out that the guidelines still do not take a hard enough line on the amount of refined starches or red meat in the American diet.[26]

- **Moderation.** Choosing forms of foods that limit intake of saturated or trans fats, added sugars, cholesterol, salt, and alcohol.
- **Activity.** Being physically active every day.
- **Personalization.** To make the most of the new MyPyramid system, you need to go online to www.mypyramid.gov (see Internet Connections, page 172). By filling in your age, gender, and typical level of activity, you will be linked to one of twelve versions of the pyramid, ranging from 1,000 to 3,200 daily calories. You can print out your customized pyramid and use it as a dietary guide. Track what you eat for a week to see how it compares with the recommendations, and go back to the website for specific suggestions.

The following guidelines, based on the MyPyramid system, can help you eat smart—and stay well.

CONSUME A VARIETY OF FOODS

The six colors on the MyPyramid graphic represent the five food groups—grains, vegetables, fruits, milk, and meat and beans—and oils. The greater the variety of colors and of foods you choose, the more likely you are to obtain the nutrients you need—see Table 6-5. In general, the USDA recommends a diet that is high in fruits and vegetables, whole grains, and nonfat or low-fat milk products that provides amounts of nutrients (including potassium and fiber) that can help reduce the risk of chronic disease and is low in saturated fat, cholesterol, added sugars, trans fat, and sodium.

MANAGE YOUR WEIGHT

As discussed in Chapter 7, you must expend as much energy (calories) as you take in to stay at the same weight. Among the best ways to balance this energy equation are limiting portion sizes (discussed later in this chapter), substituting nutrient-rich foods (such as raw vegetables or low-fat soups) for nutrient-poor foods (such as candy and cake), and limiting added sugars, solid fats, and alcoholic beverages.

GET PHYSICAL EVERY DAY

As discussed in Chapter 5, regular physical activity helps maintain a healthy weight and reduces risk for several chronic diseases. While 30 minutes of moderate physical activity (such as walking at a pace of three or four miles an hour) on most days provides important benefits, exercising more often and more intensely yields additional health dividends. Many adults need up to 60 minutes of moderate to vigorous physical activity—the equivalent of 150 to

© Polara Studios Inc.

This cola and bunch of grapes each provide about 150 calories, but the nutrient-rich grapes offer a trace of protein, some vitamins, minerals, and fiber. The cola beverage offers only "empty" calories from sugar without any other nutrients.

200 calories, depending on body size, daily to prevent unhealthy weight gain. Men and women who have lost weight may need 60 to 90 minutes to keep off excess pounds. Children and teenagers require at least 60 minutes of moderate physical activity every day.[27]

INCREASE FOODS FROM CERTAIN FOOD GROUPS

Greater consumption of fruits and vegetables (5 to 13 servings or 2½ to 6½ cups per day, depending on how many calories you burn) may reduce the risk of stroke, certain cancers, and type 2 diabetes (vegetables more so than fruit) as well as helping reach and maintain a healthy weight (Figure 6-3). The more fruits and vegetables men and women consume, the lower their levels of harmful low-density lipoprotein (LDL) cholesterol.[28] Plant-based foods also reduce the risk of rectal cancer in both men and women (Table 6-6).[29]

Among the ways to increase your fruit and vegetable intake:

- **Toss fruit into a green salad** for extra flavor, variety, color, and crunch.
- **Start the day with a daily double:** a glass of juice and a banana or other fruit on cereal.
- **Buy pre-cut vegetables** for snacking or dipping (instead of chips).
- **Make or order sandwiches** with extra tomatoes or other vegetable toppings.

Consuming at least three servings (the equivalent of 3 ounces) of whole grains per day can reduce the risk of

TABLE 6-5 NUTRIENT CONTRIBUTIONS OF EACH FOOD GROUP

Food Group	Major Contribution(s) [1]	Substantial Contribution(s) (>10% of total) [2]		
Fruit Group	Vitamin C	Thiamin Vitamin B_6 Folate	Copper Potassium Carbohydrate	Magnesium Fiber
Vegetable Group	Vitamin A Potassium	Vitamin E Vitamin C Thiamin Niacin Vitamin B_6	Magnesium Iron Zinc Copper Carbohydrate	Folate Calcium Phosphorus Fiber Alpha-linolenic acid
Vegetable Subgroups:				
Dark green vegetables		Vitamin A Vitamin C		
Orange vegetables	Vitamin A			
Legumes		Folate Copper	Fiber	
Starchy vegetables		Vitamin B_6 Copper		
Other vegetables			Vitamin C	
Grain Group	Thiamin Folate Magnesium Iron Copper Carbohydrate Fiber	Vitamin A Riboflavin Niacin Vitamin B_6 Vitamin B_{12} Calcium	Phosphorus Zinc Potassium Protein Linoleic acid Alpha-linolenic acid	
Grain Subgroups:				
Whole grains	Folate (tie) Magnesium Iron Copper Carbohydrate (tie) Fiber	Thiamin Riboflavin Niacin Vitamin B_6	Vitamin B_{12} Phosphorus Zinc Protein	
Enriched grain	Folate (tie) Thiamin Carbohydrate (tie)	Riboflavin Niacin	Iron Copper	
Meat, Poultry, Fish, Eggs, and Nuts Group	Niacin Vitamin B_6 Zinc Protein	Vitamin E Thiamin Riboflavin Vitamin B_{12} Phosphorus	Magnesium Iron Copper Potassium Linoleic acid	
Milk Group	Riboflavin Vitamin B_{12} Calcium Phosphorus	Vitamin A Thiamin Vitamin B_6 Magnesium	Zinc Potassium Carbohydrate Protein	
Oils and Soft Margarines	Vitamin E Linoleic acid Alpha-linolenic acid			

1. *Major contribution* means that the food group or subgroup provides more of the nutrient than any other single food group, averaged over all calorie levels. When two food groups or subgroups provide equal amounts, it is noted as a tie.

2. A *substantial contribution* means that the food group or subgroup provides 10% or more of the total amount of the nutrient in the food patterns, averaged over all calorie levels.

Source: Dietary Guidelines for Americans 2005. USDHHS, USDA, www.healthierus.gov/dietaryguidelines.

FIGURE 6-3 Make Fruits and Vegetables Half Your Plate

TABLE 6-6 WHICH FRUITS AND VEGETABLES[1] PROVIDE THE MOST NUTRIENTS?

Sources of Vitamin A (carotenoids)

Bright orange vegetables like carrots, sweet potatoes, and pumpkin

Dark green leafy vegetables such as spinach, collards, and turnip greens

Bright orange fruits like mango, cantaloupe, and apricots

Sources of Vitamin C

Citrus fruits and juices, kiwi fruit, strawberries, and cantaloupe

Broccoli, peppers, tomatoes, cabbage, and potatoes

Leafy greens such as romaine, turnip greens, and spinach

Sources of Folate

Cooked dried beans and peas

Oranges and orange juice

Deep green leaves like spinach and mustard greens

Sources of Potassium

Baked white or sweet potato, cooked greens (such as spinach), winter (orange) squash

Bananas, plantains, many dried fruits, and orange juice

1. Often, the fruits and vegetables with brighter colors have the higher content of vitamins and minerals.

Source: Dietary Guidelines for Americans 2005, USDHHS, USDA, www.healthierus.gov/dietaryguidelines.

---

diabetes and coronary heart disease and maintain a healthy weight. To increase your intake of grains:

▪ **Check labels of rolls and bread,** and choose those with at least 2 to 3 grams of fiber per slice.

▪ **Add brown rice or barley** to soups.

▪ **Choose whole-grain,** ready-to-eat cereals.

As noted earlier, eating at least three servings of milk, cheese, or yogurt a day may reduce your risk for high blood pressure, obesity, and osteoporosis. Dairy products do not seem to have an effect on breast cancer risk.[30]

To get more dairy products with less fat, try the following:

▪ **Substitute fat-free sour cream** or nonfat, plain yogurt for sour cream.

▪ **Add low-fat milk** instead of water to oatmeal and hot cereals.

▪ **Eat cereals with added calcium** and with milk.

▪ **Top salads or soups with low-fat shredded cheese.**

BE FINICKY ABOUT FATS

Reducing saturated fat, trans fat, and cholesterol can lower harmful LDL cholesterol and your risk of heart disease. You should keep saturated fat below 10 percent of total calories, trans fat as low as possible, and cholesterol intake below 300 mg per day. Your total fat intake should make up no more than 20 to 35 percent of calories. For children ages 2 and 3, recommended minimum fat intake is 30 percent of calories; for those between ages 4 and 18, it is 25 percent.

To keep within these limits:

▪ **Restrict animal fats** (such as those in cheese, milk, butter, ice cream, and other full-fat dairy products, fatty meat, bacon, sausage, poultry skin and fat).

▪ **Cut back** on foods made with partially hydrogenated vegetable oils.

▪ **Limit your intake** of eggs and organ meats.

As noted, other fats, particularly the omega-3 fatty acids found in certain fish, can boost your heart's health and reduce your risk of dying of heart disease. The new guidelines recommend two servings of fish high in omega-3 fatty acids every week. Pregnant or nursing women and children should avoid fish with a high mercury content and limit consumption of fish with a moderate mercury content.

CHOOSE CARBOHYDRATES WISELY

Eating more fruits, vegetables, whole grains, and nonfat or low-fat milk and dairy products is a healthful way to get the carbohydrates you need. Fiber-rich choices—an apple rather than apple juice, for example—have the added benefit of promoting digestive health and reduce the risk of type 2 diabetes and heart disease.

The new guidelines do not include a specific message about sugar but caution against "added" sugars, those added to foods during processing or preparation or at the table. Recent research has implicated sugar-sweetened beverages as a culprit in weight gain.[31] Carbohydrates (including sucrose, glucose, fructose, lactose, and starch) also can increase the risk of dental cavities. Drinking fluoridated water and/or using fluoride-containing dental hygiene products can protect your teeth.

To make sure your grains are whole, choose foods that name one of the following whole-grain ingredients first on the label's ingredient list: brown rice, bulgur, graham flour,

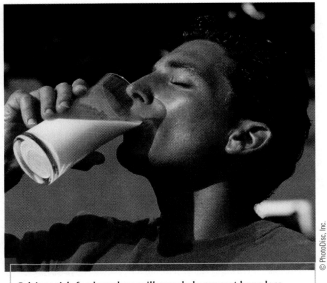

© PhotoDisc, Inc.

Calcium-rich foods such as milk may help prevent bone loss and osteoporosis.

oatmeal, whole-grain corn, whole oats, whole rye, whole wheat, wild rice. Foods labeled multi-grain, stone-ground, 100% wheat, cracked wheat, seven-grain, or bran are usually not whole-grain products.

LIMIT SALT

Reducing salt in your diet is one way to lower your blood pressure and reduce your risk of stroke, heart disease, and kidney disease. Another effective strategy is to eat more foods rich in potassium, which blunts the effects of salt on blood pressure, may decrease bone loss, and reduces the risk of kidney stones.

The guidelines recommend less than 2,300 mg of sodium per day. Many people, including those with hypertension, blacks, and older adults, should reduce their salt intake even more and increase potassium to at least 4,700 mg.

To reduce sodium intake:

- **Look for labels that say "low sodium."** They contain 140 mg or less of sodium per serving.
- **Learn to use spices and herbs rather than salt** to enhance the flavor of food.
- **Go easy on condiments** such as soy sauce, pickles, olives, ketchup, and mustard, which can add a lot of salt to your food.
- **Always check the amount of sodium** in processed foods, such as frozen dinners, packaged mixes, cereals, salad dressings, and sauces. The amount in different types and brands can vary widely.

IF YOU DRINK ALCOHOLIC BEVERAGES, DO SO IN MODERATION

As discussed in Chapter 12, alcohol has different effects on health for different age groups. In middle-aged and older adults, one to two drinks a day seem to lower the risk of

dying, primarily because moderate alcohol consumption protects against heart disease. Compared with nondrinkers, however, women who consume one alcoholic beverage per day appear to have a slightly higher risk of breast cancer. For younger people, alcohol provides little, if any, health benefits and increases the risk of traumatic injury and death. At any age, heavy drinking contributes to automotive accidents and deaths, assaults, liver disease, and other health problems.

MyPyramid includes a category for "discretionary calories," which can be used on fats, added sugar, alcohol, or more food from any food group. However, most people, especially those who are not physically active, "earn" very small discretionary calorie allowances, usually no more than 100 to 300 calories a day.[32]

KEEP FOOD SAFE TO EAT

See page 167 for an in-depth discussion of food safety. The key steps you can take to ensure food safety and prevent a problem with foodborne illnesses are:

- **Thoroughly wash hands,** contact surfaces, and fruits and vegetables (but not meat and poultry).
- **Separate raw, cooked, and ready-to-eat foods** while shopping, preparing, or storing.
- **Cook foods to a safe temperature.**
- **Chill (refrigerate) perishable foods promptly.**

THE WAY WE EAT

Just as there is no one perfect food, there is no one eating pattern that suits all people of all ages and backgrounds at all times. Your ethnic background and family makeup influenced the way you ate as a child. In college, you probably will find yourself eating in different—and not necessarily better—ways. Because the United States is so diverse, you also will have the opportunity to sample the cuisines of many cultures.

 ## NUTRITION 101: THE EATING HABITS OF COLLEGE STUDENTS

Often on their own for the first time, college students typically change their usual eating patterns. In one recent survey, 59 percent of freshmen said their diet had changed since they began college. According to various national samples, many students do not consume adequate amounts of fruits and vegetables and consume too many fried and fast foods. In one study that followed students through their freshman and sophomore years, more than half remained in the precontemplation stage for adopting healthier eating behaviors throughout this time. Only 30 percent of the students consumed at least five fruits and vegetables daily; more than half reported eating high-fat fried or fast foods at least three times during the previous week.[33]

Perhaps because they don't get five daily servings of fruit and vegetables, students also fall short in fiber intake. When 144 undergraduates at a four-year university completed three-day food intake reports, only 19 met the recommended 20 to 35 grams per day of dietary fiber: 13 percent of the women and 16 percent of the men.[34]

The same holds true for consumption of healthful omega-3 polyunsaturated fats, such as fish oils. In a recent study of 51 college-aged women, 84 percent failed to meet the recommended levels for adequate intake. Only the small percentage consuming higher-than-recommended levels for total fat intake met or exceeded the recommended amounts of beneficial fats.[35]

Yet about half of students think they are well informed about nutrition and its impact on health. Seven in ten base their decisions on what to eat on family and friends[36] (see Student Snapshot: "The Way Students Eat"). Some colleges are doing their part to improve student nutrition. Many post nutritional information in dining halls; some have expanded their offerings to include more salads, fewer fried foods, and more ethnic dishes.

Most college students do not calculate portion sizes accurately. One of the best ways to improve such estimates is by using three-dimensional food models. In a study of 380 undergraduates enrolled in an introductory nutrition course, students first estimated the amount of food in three dinners, each with varying portions of five foods (starchy food, cooked vegetables, salad, milk, and meat). After correcting their own estimates, students were asked to estimate portion sizes on a new display with different foods and amounts after one week, and then again after four weeks. Each day between these two tests, different food models were passed around in class. The accuracy of the students' estimates improved significantly afterward.

(FAQ) HOW CAN I FIND SNACKS THAT ARE GOOD FOR ME?

Snacking has become more widespread on campuses, as in other places. College students snack primarily "to satisfy hunger"; the second most common reason is "no time for meals." Other reasons for munching between meals: "for energy," "to be sociable," and "to relieve stress." One-third snack at 9:00 p.m. or later.

In response to consumer demands for smart snack choices, food manufacturers are offering "better-for-you" options that are lower in salt and sugar or free of trans fatty acids and artificial colors.[37] Some new snack items touted as healthy options, such as sugar-free chocolate or organic potato chips, offer little nutritional value. Meat-based snacks, increasingly popular among young men, also can be high in fat and sodium. Read labels carefully, and be sure to check total calories and fat.

A best-for-you option is fruit, such as bananas, apples, or berries, rich in vitamins, low in calories, and packed with fiber. Other nutritious snacks include nuts, trail mix, granola bars, yogurt, sunflower seeds, soy nuts, and dried fruit (such as cranberries). If you enjoy fruit juice, buy 100 percent fruit juice without added sugar. Limit yourself to one serving of these calorie-rich beverages a day.[38]

If you rely on snacks to keep you energized throughout the day, take time to plan in advance so you have choices other than the nearest vending machine. Try to prepare snacks from different food groups: low- or no-fat milk and a few graham crackers, for instance, or celery sticks with peanut butter and raisins. Save part of one meal—half of your breakfast bagel or lunch sandwich—to eat a few hours later. If you're trying to add fiber to your diet, eat high-fiber snacks, such as prunes, popcorn, or sunflower seeds.

Some advocates of healthier eating recommend banning junk food, such as candy bars and chips, from campus vending machines and cafeterias. Others argue that universities should not try to dictate what students can or cannot eat. Should schools take such steps to encourage healthier eating, or should students have the right to make their own food choices? **You decide.**

DIETARY DIVERSITY

Whatever your cultural heritage, you have probably sampled Chinese, Mexican, Indian, Italian, and Japanese foods. If you belong to any of these ethnic groups, you may eat these cuisines regularly. Each type of ethnic cooking has its own nutritional benefits and potential drawbacks.

Student Snapshot

THE WAY STUDENTS EAT

Percentage of Students Who	
Say they have a good understanding of nutrition and how different foods and different nutrients affect health (strongly agree or agree)	56%
Decide what to eat on the basis of:	
information from friends and family	71%
high school health or nutrition class	27%
magazines, books, media	25%
Always use nutrition information on food products	22%
Sometimes use such information	57%

Based on a survey of 1,317 first-year college students who ate in a university dining hall.
Source: Conklin, Martha, et al. "College Students' Use of Point of Selection Nutrition Information." *Topics in Clinical Nutrition,* Vol. 20, No. 2, April–June 2005, p. 97.

Mediterranean Diet

Several years ago epidemiologists noticed something unexpected in the residents of regions along the Mediterranean Sea: a lower incidence of deaths from heart disease. Scientists have identified antioxidants in red wine and olive oil that may account for the beneficial effects on the heart of the Mediterranean diet, which features lots of fruits and vegetables, legumes, nuts, and grains. Meat is used mainly as a condiment rather than as a main course, and fish, yogurt, and low-fat feta cheese are the predominant animal foods. The diet is relatively high in fat, but the main source is olive oil, an unsaturated fat.

Ethnic Cuisines

The cuisine served in Mexico features rice, corn, and beans, which are low in fat and high in nutrients. However, the dishes Americans think of as Mexican are far less healthful. Burritos, especially when topped with cheese and sour cream, are very high in fat. Although guacamole has a high fat content, it contains mostly monounsaturated fatty acids, a better form of fat.

African-American cuisine traces some of its roots to food preferences from west Africa (for example, peanuts, okra, and black-eyed peas), as well as to traditional American foods, such as fish, game, greens, and sweet potatoes. It uses many nutritious vegetables, such as collard greens and sweet potatoes, as well as legumes. However, some dishes include high-fat food products such as peanuts and pecans or involve frying, sometimes in saturated fat.

The mainland Chinese diet, which is plant-based, high in carbohydrates, and low in fats and animal protein, is considered one of the healthiest in the world. However, Chinese restaurants here serve more meat and sauces than are generally eaten in China. According to laboratory tests of typical take-out dishes from Chinese restaurants, many have more fats and cholesterol than hamburger or egg dishes from fast-food outlets.

Traditional French cuisine, which includes rich, high-fat sauces and dishes, has never been considered healthful. Yet, nutritionists have been stumped to explain the so-called French paradox. Despite a diet high in saturated fats, the French have had one of the lowest rates of coronary artery disease in the world. The French diet increasingly resembles the American diet, but French portions tend to be one-third to one-half the size of American portions.

Many Indian dishes highlight healthful ingredients such as vegetables and legumes (beans and peas). However, many also use *ghee* (a form of butter) or coconut oil; both are rich in harmful saturated fats. The best advice in an Indian restaurant is to ask how each dish is prepared. Good choices include *daal* or *dal* (lentils), *karbi* or *karni* (chickpea soup), and *chapati* (tortilla-like bread).

The traditional Japanese diet is very low in fat, which may account for the low incidence of heart disease in Japan. Dietary staples include soybean products, fish, vegetables, noodles, and rice. A variety of fruits and vegetables are also included in many dishes. However, Japanese cuisine is high in salted, smoked, and pickled foods. Watch out for deep-fried dishes such as tempura and salty soups and sauces.

© Corbis

© David Chasey/Photodisc Red/Getty Images

In today's ethnically diverse United States, all-American food ranges from Indian to Japanese. The vegetables and legumes in the Indian diet are healthy and high in protein, but too much saturated fat can cancel some of the benefits. The Japanese diet is high in seafood and rice and low in fats, cheese, and meat.

(FAQ) WHAT SHOULD I KNOW ABOUT VEGETARIAN DIETS?

Not all vegetarians avoid all meats. Some, who call themselves *lacto-ovo-pesco-vegetarians,* eat dairy products, eggs, chicken, and fish but not red meat. **Lacto-vegetarians** eat dairy products as well as grains, fruits, and vegetables; **ovo-lacto-vegetarians** also eat eggs. Pure vegetarians, called **vegans,** eat only plant foods; often they take vitamin B_{12} supplements because that vitamin is normally found only in animal products. If they select their food with care, vegetarians can get sufficient amounts of protein, vitamin B_{12}, iron, and calcium without supplements.

The key to getting sufficient protein from a vegetarian diet is understanding the concept of **complementary proteins.** Meat, poultry, fish, eggs, and dairy products are *complete proteins* that provide the nine essential amino acids—substances that the human body cannot produce itself. *Incomplete proteins,* such as legumes or nuts, may have relatively low levels of one or two essential amino acids but fairly high levels of others. By combining complementary protein sources, you can make sure that your body makes the most of the nonanimal proteins you eat. Many cultures rely heavily on complementary foods for protein. In Middle Eastern cooking, sesame seeds and chickpeas are a popular combination; in Latin American dishes, beans and rice, or beans and tortillas; in Chinese cuisine, soy and rice.

According to the 2005 Dietary Guidelines, vegetarians can best meet their nutrient needs by paying special attention to protein, iron, vitamin B_{12}, calcium, and vitamin D. Instead of a 6-ounce serving of meat, they can substitute one egg, 1.5 ounces of nuts, or two-thirds cup of legumes. Those who avoid milk because of its lactose content may obtain all the nutrients of milk by using lactose-reduced milk or eating other calcium-rich foods, such as broccoli calcium-fortified orange juice, and fortified soy milk.[39]

Vegetarian diets have proven health benefits. Studies show that vegetarians' cholesterol levels are low, and vegetarians are seldom overweight. As a result, they're less apt to be candidates for heart disease than those who consume large quantities of meat. Vegetarians also have lower incidences of breast, colon, and prostate cancer; high blood pressure; and osteoporosis.

FAST FOOD: NUTRITION ON THE RUN

On any given day, about 25 percent of adults in the United States go to a fast-food restaurant. The typical American consumes three hamburgers and four orders of french fries every week.[40] Not all fast foods are junk foods—that is, high in calories, sugar, salt, and fat and low in beneficial nutrients. But while it's not all bad, fast food has definite disadvantages. A meal in a fast-food restaurant may cost twice as much as the same meal prepared at home and may provide half your daily calorie needs. The fat content of many items is extremely high. A Burger King Whopper with cheese contains 723 calories and 48 grams of fat, 18 grams from saturated fat. A McDonald's Sausage McMuffin with egg has 517 calories and 33 grams of fat, 13 grams from saturated fat. Many fast-food chains have switched from beef tallow or lard to unsaturated vegetable oils for frying, but the total fat content of the foods remains the same.

Your Life Coach

Taking Charge of What You Eat

You can't control what you don't know. Because of the Nutrition Labeling and Education Act, food manufacturers must provide information about fat, calories, and ingredients in large type on packaged food labels, and they must show how a food item fits into a daily diet of 2,000 calories. The law also restricts nutritional claims for terms such as *healthy, low-fat,* and *high-fiber.*

 At one university, almost two-thirds of the freshmen reported they were aware of the nutrition labels posted in the dining commons. One-third used them to help make food choices. Female students were significantly more likely to base their food choices on the labels than the men. Students primarily checked overall good/balanced nutrition content of foods, calo-

TABLE 6-7 SUPERSIZING PORTIONS

Food Item	Calories per Portion	
	20 Years Ago	**Today**
Bagel	140 Calories (3-in. diameter)	350 calories (6-in. diameter)
Fast-food cheeseburger	333 calories	590 calories
Spaghetti and meatballs	500 calories (1 cup of spaghetti with sauce and 3 small meatballs)	1,025 calories (2 cups of spaghetti and 3 large meatballs)
Bottle of soda	85 calories (6.5 oz.)	250 calories (20 oz.)
Fast-food French fries	210 calories (2.4 oz.)	610 calories (6.9 oz.)
Turkey sandwich	320 calories	820 calories (10-in. sub)

Source: Dietary Guidelines for Americans 2005, USDHHS, USDA, www.healthierus.gov/dietaryguidelines. Adapted from the Portion Distortion Quiz, National Heart, Lung, and Blood Institute, www.nhlbi.nih.gov.

| 1 medium fruit is about the size of a baseball. | 1 c cooked vegetables is about the size of your fist. | $\frac{1}{2}$ c ice cream is about the size of a racquet ball. | 3 oz. of meat is about the size of a deck of cards. | $1\frac{1}{2}$ oz. cheese is about the size of six stacked dice. | $\frac{1}{4}$ c dried fruit is about the size of a golf ball. | 2 tbs. peanut butter is about the size of a marshmallow. | 4 small cookies are about the size of 4 poker chips. |

FIGURE 6-4   Quick and Easy Estimates of Portion Sizes

ries, fat, saturated fat, and protein. Their top reason for checking labels: to be healthy now.[41]

In evaluating food labels and product claims, keep in mind that while individual foods vary in their nutritional value, what matters is your total diet. If you eat too much of any one food—regardless of what its label states—you may not be getting the variety and balance of nutrients that you need.

PORTIONS AND SERVINGS

Consumers often are confused by what a *serving* actually is, especially since many American restaurants have super-sized the amount of food they put on their customers' plates. The average bagel has doubled in size in the last ten to fifteen years (Table 6-7). A standard fast-food serving of french fries is larger in the United States than in the United Kingdom.

A food-label *serving* is a specific amount of food that contains the quantity of nutrients described on the Nutrition Facts label. A *portion* is the amount of a specific food that an individual eats at one time. Portions can

be bigger or smaller than the servings on food labels. According to nutritionists, "marketplace portions"—the actual amounts served to customers—are two to eight times larger than the standard serving sizes defined by the USDA. In fast-food chains, today's portions are two to five times larger than the original sizes. As studies have shown, people presented with larger portions eat 30 to 50 percent more than they otherwise would.[42]

If you are trying to balance your diet or control your weight, it's important to keep track of the size of your portions so that you do not exceed recommended servings. For instance, a 3-ounce serving of meat is about the size of a pack of playing cards—see Figure 6-4. If you eat a larger amount, count it as more than one serving.

FAQ **WHAT SHOULD I LOOK FOR ON NUTRITION LABELS?**

As Figure 6-5 shows, the Nutrition Facts on food labels present a wealth of information—if you know what to look for. The label focuses on those nutrients most clearly associated with disease risk and health: total fat,

The name and address of the manufacturer, packer, or distributor

The common or usual product name

Approved nutrient claims if the product meets specified criteria

The net contents in weight, measure, or count

Approved health claims stated in terms of the total diet

The serving size and number of servings per container

Calorie information and quantities of nutrients per serving, in actual amounts

Quantities of nutrients as "% Daily Values" based on a 2,000-calorie energy intake

Daily Values reminder for selected nutrients for a 2,000- and a 2,500-calorie diet

Calories per gram reminder

The ingredients in descending order of predominance by weight

Nutrition Facts

| Serving size | ³/₄ cup (28 g) |
| Servings per container | 14 |

Amount per serving

| Calories 110 | Calories from fat 9 |

	% Daily Value*
Total Fat 1 g	2%
Saturated fat 0 g	0%
Trans fat 0 g	0%
Cholesterol 0 mg	0%
Sodium 250 mg	10%
Total Carbohydrate 23 g	8%
Dietary fiber 1.5 g	6%
Sugars 10 g	
3 g	

Vitamin A 25% • Vitamin C 25% • Calcium 2% • Iron 25%

*Percent Daily Values are based on a 2000 calorie diet. Your daily values may be higher or lower depending on your calorie needs.

	Calories:	2000	2500
Total fat	Less than	65 g	80 g
Sat fat	Less than	20 g	25 g
Cholesterol	Less than	300 mg	300 mg
Sodium	Less than	2400 mg	2400 mg
Total Carbohydrate		300 g	375 g
Fiber		25 g	30 g

Calories per gram
Fat 9 • Carbohydrate 4 • Protein 4

INGREDIENTS, listed in descending order of predominance: Corn, Sugar, Salt, Malt flavoring, freshness preserved by BHT. VITAMINS and MINERALS: Vitamin C (Sodium ascorbate), Niacinamide , Iron, Vitamin B₆ (Pyridoxine hydrochloride), Vitamin B₂ (Riboflavin), Vitamin A (Palmitate), Vitamin B₁ (Thiamin hydrochloride), Folic acid, and Vitamin D.

A container with fewer than 40 square inches of surface area can present fewer facts in this format.

Nutrition Facts

Serv.Size ¹/₃ cup (85g)**
Servings 2
Calories 111
Fat Cal. 27
*Percent Daily Values (DV) are based on a 2000 calorie diet.
**Drained solids only

Amount/serving		%DV*	Amount/serving		%DV*
Total Fat	3g	5%	Total Carb.	0g	0%
Sat. Fat	1g	5%	Fiber	0g	0%
Trans Fat	0g				
Cholest.	60mg	20%	Sugars	0g	
Sodium	200mg	8%	Protein	21g	

Vitamin A 0% • Vitamin C 0% • Calcium 0% • Iron 2%

Packages with fewer than 12 square inches of surface area need not carry nutrition information, but they must provide an address or telephone number for obtaining information.

FIGURE 6-5 Understanding Nutrition Labels
The Nutrition Facts label lists the essential nutrient content of packaged food as well as the amount of potentially harmful substances such as fat and sodium.

saturated fat, cholesterol, sodium, total carbohydrate, dietary fiber, sugar, and protein.

■ **Calories.** Calories are the measure of the amount of energy that can be derived from food. Science defines a *calorie* as the amount of energy required to raise the temperature of 1 gram of water by one degree Celsius. In the laboratory, the caloric content of food is measured in 1,000-calorie units called *kilocalories*. The calorie referred to in everyday usage is actually the equivalent of the laboratory kilocalorie.

The Nutrition Facts label lists two numbers for calories: calories per serving and calories from fat per serving. This allows consumers to calculate how many calories they'll consume and to determine the percentage of fat in an item.

■ **Serving size.** Rather than the tiny portions manufacturers sometimes used in the past to keep down the number of calories per serving, the new labels reflect more realistic portions. Serving sizes, which have been defined for approximately 150 food categories, must be the same for similar products (for example, different brands of potato chips) and for similar products within a category (for example, snack foods such as pretzels, potato chips, and popcorn). This makes it easier to compare the nutritional content of foods.

■ **Daily Values (DVs).** DVs refer to the total amount of a nutrient that the average adult should aim to get or not exceed on a daily basis. The DVs for cholesterol, sodium, vitamins, and minerals are the same for all adults. The DVs for total fat, saturated fat, carbohydrate, fiber, and protein are based on a 2,000-calorie daily diet—the amount of food ingested by many American men and active women.

■ **Percent Daily Values (%DVs).** The goal for a full day's diet is to select foods that together add up to 100 percent of the DVs. The %DVs show how a particular food's nutrient content fits into a 2,000-calorie diet. Individuals who consume (or should consume) fewer than 2,000 total calories a day have to lower their DVs for total fat, saturated fat, and carbohydrates. For example, if their caloric intake is 10 percent less than 2,000 calories, they would lower the DV by 10 percent. Similarly, those who consume more than 2,000 calories should adjust the DVs upward.

■ **Calories per gram.** The bottom of the food label lists the number of calories per gram for fat, carbohydrates, and protein.

People zero in on different figures on the food label—for example, calories if they're watching their weight, specific ingredients if they have food allergies. Among the useful items to check are the following:

■ **Calories from fat.** Get into the habit of calculating the percentage of fat calories in a food before buying or eating it.

■ **Total fat.** Since the average person munches on 15 to 20 food items a day, it's easy to overload on fat. Saturated fat and trans fat numbers deserve special attention because of their reported link to several diseases.

■ **Cholesterol.** Cholesterol is made by and contained in products of animal origin only. Many high-fat products, such as potato chips, contain 0 percent cholesterol because they're made from plants and are cooked in vegetable fats. However, if the vegetable fats are hydrogenated, the resulting trans fat is more harmful to the heart than cholesterol.

■ **Sugars.** There is no Daily Value for sugars because health experts have yet to agree on a daily limit. The figure on the label includes naturally present sugars, such as lactose in milk and fructose in fruit, as well as those added to the food, such as table sugar, corn syrup, or dextrose.

■ **Fiber.** A "high-fiber" food has 5 or more grams of fiber per serving. A "good" source of fiber provides at least 2.5 grams. "More" or "added" fiber means at least 2.5 grams more per serving than similar foods—10 percent more of the DV for fiber.

■ **Calcium.** "High" equals 200 milligrams (mg) or more per serving. "Good" means at least 100 mg, while "more" indicates that the food contains at least 100 mg more calcium— 10 percent more of the DV—than the item usually would have.

■ **Sodium.** Most of us routinely get more sodium than we need. Read labels carefully to avoid excess sodium, which can be a health threat.

■ **Vitamins.** A Daily Value of 10 percent of any vitamin makes a food a "good" source; 20 percent qualifies it as "high" in a certain vitamin.

Nutrition labeling for fresh produce, fish, meat, and poultry remains voluntary. Packages too small for a full-sized label must provide an address or phone number so consumers can obtain information from the manufacturer.

FUNCTIONAL FOODS

As the American Dietetic Association has noted, all foods are functional at some physiological level. However, the term *functional* generally applies to a food specifically created to have health-promoting benefits.

The International Food Information Council defines functional foods as those "that provide health benefits beyond basic nutrition."

Some manufacturers are adding biologically active components such as the beta-carotene to food products and promoting them as functional foods. However, the amounts added are often too low to have any effect, and many such foods are high-sugared drinks and snack foods. More research is needed to evaluate their claims of health benefits.[43]

FOOD SAFETY

Foodborne illnesses cause an estimated 76 million illnesses, 325,000 hospitalizations, and 5,000 deaths in the United States every year. Three organisms—*Salmonella, Listeria,* and *Toxoplasma*—are responsible for more than 75 percent of these deaths. Although most foodborne infections cause mild illness, severe infections and serious complications—including death—do occur.

FIGHT BAC!

To improve food safety awareness and practices, government and private agencies have developed the Fight Bac! campaign, which identifies four key culprits in foodborne illness:

- **Improper cooling**
- **Improper hand washing**
- **Inadequate cooking**
- **Failure to avoid cross-contamination.**[44]

FAQ WHAT CAUSES FOOD POISONING?

Salmonella is a bacterium that contaminates many foods, particularly undercooked chicken, eggs, and sometimes processed meat. Eating contaminated food can result in salmonella poisoning, which causes diarrhea and vomiting. The Centers for Disease Control and Prevention (CDC) estimates 40,000 reported cases of salmonella poisoning a year; the actual number of cases could be anywhere from 400,000

to 4 million. The FDA has warned consumers about the dangers of unpasteurized orange juice because of the risk of salmonella contamination.

Another bacterium, *Campylobacter jejuni,* may cause even more stomach infections than salmonella. Found in water, milk, and some foods, campylobacter poisoning causes severe diarrhea and has been implicated in the growth of stomach ulcers.

Bacteria can also cause illness by producing toxins in food. *Staphylococcus aureus* is the most common culprit. When cooked foods are cross-contaminated with the bacteria from raw foods and not stored properly, staph infections can result, causing nausea and abdominal pain anywhere from thirty minutes to eight hours after ingestion.

Even many healthy foods can pose dangers. The FDA has urged consumers to avoid eating raw sprouts because of the risk of getting sick. Sprouts, particularly alfalfa and clover, can be contaminated by salmonella or *E. coli* bacteria, which can cause nausea, diarrhea, and cramping in healthy adults. Children and senior citizens can experience serious symptoms that lead to kidney failure and compromised immune systems. The FDA advises people to either cook sprouts before eating them or request that they be left off sandwiches and other food ordered in restaurants. Homegrown sprouts can also present a risk if they come from contaminated seeds.

An uncommon but sometimes fatal form of food poisoning is **botulism,** caused by the *Clostridium botulinum* organism. Improper home-canning procedures are the most common cause of this potentially fatal problem.

There have been several outbreaks of listeriosis, caused by the bacteria **listeria,** commonly found in deli meats, hot dogs, soft cheeses, raw meat, and unpasteurized milk. Although rare, listeriosis can be life-threatening. At greatest risk are pregnant women, infants, and those with weakened immune systems. You can reduce your risk by cooking meats and leftovers thoroughly and by washing everything that may come into contact with raw meat.

"HAMBURGER DISEASE"/ BARBECUE SYNDROME

Barbecue syndrome is the common name for a type of food poisoning caused by the bacteria *verotoxigenic E. coli,* or VTEC. People who develop this syndrome frequently report

---

Strategies for Prevention :: Protecting Yourself from Food Poisoning

- Always wash your hands with liquid or clean bar soap before handling food. Rub your hands vigorously together for 10 to 15 seconds; the soap combined with the scrubbing action dislodges and removes germs.

- When preparing fresh fruits and vegetables, discard outer leaves, wash under

running water, and when possible, scrub with a clean brush or hands. Do not wash meat or poultry.

- To avoid the spread of bacteria to other foods, utensils, or surfaces, do not allow liquids to touch or drip onto other items. Wipe up all spills immediately.

- Clean out your refrigerator regularly. Throw out any leftovers stored for three or four days.

FIGURE 6-6   Comparing the Food Safety Behavior of Students to the General Public

Source: Data from Morrone, Michele, and Ann Rathbun. "Health Education and Food Safety Behavior in the University Setting." *Journal of Environmental Health,* March 2003, Vol. 65, No. 7, p. 9.

that they ate ground beef hamburgers prior to getting sick. Other kinds of undercooked meat and poultry and drinking unpasteurized milk or unchlorinated water also are culprits.

As shown in Figure 6-6; a higher percentage of students eat pink hamburger meat, while fewer read or remember the labels on raw meat or poultry and change food preparation because of the information on the label.

Symptoms, which can range from mild to life-threatening, usually develop within two to ten days and include severe stomach cramps, vomiting, and a mild fever. Most people recover within seven to ten days. Proper handling and cooking of food can practically eliminate hamburger disease.

PESTICIDES AND IRRADIATION

Plants and animals naturally produce compounds that act as pesticides to aid in their survival. The vast majority of the pesticides we consume are therefore natural, not added by farmers or food processors. *Commercial pesticides* save billions of dollars of valuable crops from pests, but they also may endanger human health and life.

Fearful of potential risks in pesticides, many consumers are purchasing **organic** foods. The term *organic* refers to foods produced without the use of commercial chemicals at any stage. Independent groups now certify foods before they can be labeled organic. Foods that are truly organic are cleaner and have much lower levels of residues than standard commercial produce. There's no guarantee that the organic produce you buy at a grocery or health-food store is more nutritious than other produce. However, buying organic foods is one way in which you can work toward a healthier environment.

Irradiation is the use of radiation, either from radioactive substances or from devices that produce X rays, on food. It doesn't make the food radioactive. Its primary benefit is to prolong the shelf life of food. Like the heat in canning, irradiation can kill all the microorganisms that might grow in a food, and the sterilized food can then be stored for years in sealed containers at room temperature without spoiling. Are irradiated foods safe to eat? The best available answer is a qualified yes, because we don't have complete data yet.

FOOD ALLERGIES

An estimated 12 to 20 percent of adults have some form of food hypersensitivity, an adverse reaction to a particular food. Women are more prone to report hypersensitivity or food allergies than men.[45]

Physicians disagree as to which foods are the most common triggers of food allergies. Cow's milk, eggs, seafood, wheat, soybeans, nuts, seeds, and chocolate have all been identified as culprits. The symptoms they provoke vary. One person might sneeze if exposed to an irritating food; another might vomit or develop diarrhea; others might suffer headaches, dizziness, hives, or a rapid heart-beat. Symptoms may not develop for up to 72 hours, making it hard to pinpoint which food was responsible.

If you suspect that you have a food allergy, see a physician with specialized training in allergy diagnosis. Medical opinion about the merits of many treatments for food allergies is divided. Once you've identified the culprit, the wisest and sometimes simplest course is to avoid it.

NUTRITIONAL QUACKERY

The American Dietetic Association describes nutritional quackery as a growing problem for unsuspecting consumers. Because so much nutritional nonsense is garbed in scientific-sounding terms, it can be hard to recognize bad advice when you get it. One basic rule: If the promises of a nutritional claim sound too good to be true—they probably are (see Savvy Consumer: "Spotting Nutrition Misinformation").

If you seek the advice of a nutrition consultant, carefully check his or her credentials and professional associations. Because licensing isn't required in all states, almost anyone can use the label "nutritionist," regardless of qualifications. Be wary of diplomas from obscure schools and organizations that allow anyone who pays dues to join. (One physician obtained a membership for his dog!) A registered dietitian (R.D.), who has a bachelor's degree and specialized training (including an internship) and who passed a certification examination, is usually a member of the American Dietetic Association (ADA), which sets the standard for quality in diets. A nutrition expert with an M.D. or Ph.D. generally belongs to the ADA, the American Institute of Nutrition, or the American Society of Clinical Nutrition; all have stringent membership requirements.

Savvy Consumer ▪ Spotting Nutrition Misinformation

▪ Don't believe everything you read. A quick way to spot a bad nutrition self-help book is to look in the index for a diet to prevent or treat rheumatoid arthritis (none exists). If you find one, don't buy the book.

▪ Before you try any new nutritional approach, check with your doctor or a registered dietitian or call the American Dietetic Association's consumer hot line, (800)366–1655.

▪ Don't believe ads or advisers basing their nutritional recommendations on hair analysis, which is not accurate in detecting nutritional deficiencies.

▪ Be wary of anyone who recommends megadoses of vitamins or nutritional supplements, which can be dangerous. High doses of vitamin A, which some people take to clear up acne, can be toxic.

▪ Question personal testimonies about the powers of some magical-seeming pill or powder, and be wary of "scientific articles" in journals that aren't reviewed by health professionals.

▪ Be wary of any nutritional supplements sold in health stores or through health and body-building magazines. These products may contain ingredients that have not been tested and proved safe.

Personal testimonials — Hearsay is the weakest form of evidence.

Time-tested — Such findings would be widely publicized and accepted by health professionals.

One product does it all — No one product can possibly treat such a diverse array of conditions. Phony terms hide the lack of scientific proof.

Quick and easy fixes — Even proven treatments take time to be effective.

Meaningless medical jargon

Paranoid accusations — And this product's company doesn't want money? At least the drug company has scientific research proving the safety and effectiveness of its products.

Satisfaction guaranteed — Marketers may make generous promises, but consumers won't be able to collect on them.

Natural — Natural is not necessarily better or safer; any product that is strong enough to be effective is strong enough to cause side effects.

Learn It / Live It

Making Healthy Food Choices

As nutritional knowledge expands and evolves, it's easy to be confused by changing advice on which foods to avoid and which to eat. But even though research may challenge or change thinking on a specific food, some basic principles always apply.

▪ **Eat breakfast.** Easy to prepare breakfasts include cold cereal with fruit and low-fat milk, whole-wheat toast with peanut butter, yogurt with fruit, or whole-grain waffles.

▪ **Don't eat too much of one thing.** Your body needs protein, carbohydrates, fat, and many different vitamins and minerals, such as vitamins C and A, iron, and calcium, from a variety of foods.

▪ **Eat more grains, fruits, and vegetables.** These foods give you carbohydrates for energy, plus vitamins, minerals, and fiber. Try breads such as whole-wheat, bagels, and pita. Spaghetti and oatmeal are also in the grain group.

▪ **Don't ban any food.** Fit in a higher-fat food, like pepperoni pizza, at dinner by choosing lower-fat foods at other meals. And don't forget about moderation. If two pieces of pizza fill you up, don't eat a third.

▪ **Make every calorie count.** Load up on nutrients, not on big portions. Choosing foods that are nutrient dense will help protect against disease and keep you healthy.

Self Survey ▪ How Healthy Is Your Diet?

STEP 1

Keep a food diary for a week, writing down everything you eat and drink for meals and snacks. Include the approximate amount eaten (for example, 1/2 cup, 1 large, 12-oz. can, and so on).

	Mon	Tues	Wed	Thurs	Fri	Sat	Sun
Grains							
Vegetables							
Fruits							
Milk, yogurt, cheese							
Meat, poultry, dry beans, eggs, nuts							
Fats, oil, sweets, cheese							

STEP 2: Are You Getting Enough Vegetables, Fruits, and Grains?

How often do you eat:	Seldom/Never	1–2 times a week	3–5 times a week	Almost daily
At least three servings of vegetables a day?				
Starchy vegetables like potatoes, corn, or peas?				
Foods made with dry beans, lentils, or peas?				
Dark green or deep yellow vegetables (broccoli, spinach, collards, carrots, sweet potatoes, squash)?				
At least two servings of fruit a day?				
Citrus fruits and 100% fruit juices (oranges, grapefruit, tangerines)?				
Whole fruit with skin or seeds (berries, apples, pears)?				
At least six servings of breads, cereals, pasta, or rice a day?				

The best answer for each is "almost daily." Use your food diary to see which foods you should be eating more often.

STEP 3: Are You Getting Too Much Fat?

How often do you eat:	Seldom/Never	1–2 times a week	3–5 times a week	Almost daily
Fried, deep-fat fried, or breaded food?				
Fatty meats, such as sausages, luncheon meat, fatty steaks or roasts?				
Whole milk, high-fat cheeses, ice cream?				
Pies, pastries, rich cakes?				
Rich cream sauces and gravies?				
Oily salad dressings or mayonnaise?				
Butter or margarine on vegetables, rolls, bread, or toast?				

Ideally, you should be eating these foods no more than one or two times a week. If your food diary indicates that you're eating them more frequently, your fat intake may well be too high.

STEP 4: Are You Getting Too Much Sodium?

How often do you eat:	Seldom/Never	1–2 times a week	3–5 times a week	Almost daily
Cured or processed meats, such as ham, sausage, frankfurters, or luncheon meats?				
Canned vegetables or frozen vegetables with sauce?				
Frozen TV dinners, entrees, or canned or dehydrated soups?				
Salted nuts, popcorn, pretzels, corn chips, or potato chips?				
Seasoning mixes or sauces containing salt?				
Processed cheese?				
Salt added to table foods before you taste them?				

Ideally, you should be eating these high-sodium items no more than one or two times a week. If your food diary indicates that you're eating them more frequently, your sodium intake may well be too high.

YOUR ACTION PLAN FOR BETTER NUTRITION

■ **Eat five servings of fruits and vegetables per day.** For breakfast, have 100% fruit juice or add raisins, berries, or sliced fruit to cereal, pancakes, or waffles. For lunch, have vegetable soup or salad with your meal or pile vegetables on your sandwich. For dinner, choose vegetables that are green, orange (such as carrots or squash), and red (such as tomatoes or bell peppers).

■ **Include three servings of whole-grain foods every day.** To identify whole-grain products, check the ingredient list. The first ingredient should be a whole grain, such as "whole-grain oats," "whole-grain wheat," or "whole wheat."

■ **Consume a calcium-rich food at each meal.** Good options include low-fat and nonfat milk; cheese; or yogurt; tofu; broccoli; dried beans; spinach; and fortified soy milk.

■ **Eat less meat.** Rather than making meat the heart of a meal, think of it as a flavoring ingredient.

■ **Avoid high-fat fast foods.** Hot dogs, fried foods, packaged snack foods, and pastries are most likely to be laden with fat.

■ **Check the numbers.** When buying prepared foods, choose items that contain no more than 3 grams of fat per 100 calories.

■ **Think small.** A dinner-size serving of meat should be about the size of a deck of cards; half a cup is the size of a woman's fist; a pancake is the diameter of a CD.

■ **Read labels carefully.** Remember that "cholesterol-free" doesn't necessarily mean fat-free. Avoid products that contain saturated coconut oil, palm oil, lard, or hydrogenated fats.

■ **Switch to low-fat and no-fat dairy products.** Rather than buying whole-fat dairy products, choose skim milk, fat-free sour cream, and low- or nonfat yogurt.

■ **The brighter the better.** When selecting fruits and vegetables, choose the most intense color. A bright orange carrot has more beta-carotene than a pale one. Dark green lettuce leaves have more vitamins than lighter ones. Orange sweet potatoes pack more vitamin A than yellow ones.

CASE IN POINT

Student: Isabella, 23

Goal: Eat more fiber and less fatty food.

Action Plan:

■ Rather than an egg-and-sausage sandwich, eat whole-grain cereal with fruit and low-fat milk.

■ Snack on an apple or raisins instead of a bag of potato chips.

■ At fast-food restaurants, order a plain burger rather than a bacon cheeseburger.

■ In the dining hall, have a salad rather than onion rings or french fries.

■ Eat two vegetables, such as broccoli and corn or green beans and potatoes, at dinner.

Health⊛Now™ If you want to write your own goals for more nutritious choices, go to the **Wellness Journal at HealthNow** http://healthnow.brookscole.com/ith.

Making This Chapter Work for You

Review Questions

1. The classes of essential nutrients include which of the following?
   a. amino acids, antioxidants, fiber, and cholesterol
   b. proteins, calcium, calories, and folic acid
   c. carbohydrates, minerals, fat, and water
   d. iron, whole grains, fruits, and vegetables

2. Which type of fat is *not* considered a threat to heart health?
   a. omega-3 fatty acids
   b. trans fat
   c. triglycerides
   d. saturated fats

3. Antioxidants
   a. are nutrients important in the production of hemoglobin.
   b. are substances added to foods to make them more flavorful or physically appealing.
   c. are suspected triggers of food allergies.
   d. are substances that prevent the harmful effects of free radicals.

4. The MyPyramid system can be personalized to your age, gender, and activity level at www.MyPyramid.gov. Besides personalization, the MyPyramid system has these themes:
   a. variety, proportionality, moderation, and activity
   b. variety, bulimia, activity
   c. variety, moderation, activity, and food safety
   d. variety, moderation, activity, and correct food labeling

5. The MyPyramid system includes this recommendation:
   a. Make half your grains whole.
   b. Go lean with protein.
   c. Focus on fruits.
   d. All of the above.

6. The 2005 Dietary Guidelines for Americans include:
   a. Decrease intake of added sugars.
   b. Increase consumption of olive oil.
   c. Control calorie intake to manage body weight.
   d. Eat dessert no more than three days a week.

7. Food labels on packaged foods include all of the following *except*
   a. total weight of the package.
   b. total amount of nutrients contained in the food.
   c. the percent of nutrient Daily Values provided in the food.
   d. serving size.

8. Since Sam plays poker, it's been easy for him to remember that a recommended serving of 3 ounces of meat means a piece of meat about the size of
   a. one deck of cards.
   b. eight poker chips.
   c. two decks of cards.
   d. a roll of quarters.

9. Some vegetarians may
   a. include chicken and fish in their diets.
   b. avoid vitamin B_{12} supplements if they eat only plant foods.
   c. eat only legumes or nuts because these provide complete proteins.
   d. have high cholesterol levels because of the saturated fats in fruits and vegetables.

10. Common causes of foodborne infections include which of the following?
    a. the influenza virus
    b. *Salmonella* and *E. coli* bacteria
    c. additives
    d. irradiation

Answers to these questions can be found on page 587.

Critical Thinking

1. Which alternative or ethnic diet do you think has the best tasting food? Which is the most healthy? Why?

2. Is it possible to meet nutritional requirements on a limited budget? Have you ever been in this situation? What would you recommend to someone who wanted to eat healthfully on $30 a week?

3. Consider the number of times a week you eat fast food. How much money would you have saved if you had eaten home-prepared meals? Which fast foods could you have selected that would have provided more nutritional value?

Media Menu

Health🏃Now™

Throughout the chapter, this icon introduces a list of resources on the Health-Now website at **http://healthnow.brookscole.com/ith** that will:
- Help you evaluate your knowledge of the material.
- Allow you to take an exam-prep quiz.
- Provide a Personalized Learning Plan targeting resources that address areas you should study.
- Coach you through identifying target goals for behavior change and creating and monitoring your personal change plan throughout the semester.

INTERNET CONNECTIONS

U.S. Food and Nutrition Information Center

www.nal.usda.gov/fnic/

This comprehensive governmental website features reports and scientific studies on a variety of nutrition information, including the 2005 U.S.D.A Dietary Guidelines, an updated Food Guide Pyramid, dietary supplements, dietary assessment, food composition searchable databases, educational brochures, historical food guides, and a topics "A–Z" section.

USDA Center for Nutrition Policy and Promotion

www.usda.gov/cnpp/

This interactive site sponsored by the United States Center for Nutrition Policy and Promotion features the Interactive Health Eating Index, an online dietary assessment that enables you to receive a personalized score on the overall quality of your diet, on a daily basis, based on the recommendations of the Food Guide Pyramid. This tool provides you with information on total fat, cholesterol, sodium, and other nutrients. You can also download a series of brochures featuring dietary guidelines as well as healthy recipes.

Nutrient Analysis Tool

http://nat.crgq.com

This site, provided as a public service by the Food Science and Human Nutrition Department at the University of Illinois, features a free nutrient analysis interactive program that calculates the amount of calories, carbohydrates, protein, fat, vitamins, minerals, and fiber in the foods that make up your daily diet.

Cyberkitchen

www.nhlbi.nih.gov/chd/Tipsheets/cyberkit.htm

This interactive site helps you discover how much you are really eating with an activity on comparing standard serving sizes versus real serving sizes. You also can provide personal information regarding your age, gender, height, weight, and activity level, and the Cyberkitchen will provide you with a healthy diet plan to meet your weight management goals. It's fun and educational.

InfoTrac College Edition Activities Log on, insert **nutrition** into the Keyword search box, and limit your search to the past year. When you get the results, Mark articles to review, then Select one to read. Summarize three or four key points from the article.

You can find additional readings related to personal health with InfoTrac College Edition, an online library of more than 900 journals and publications. Follow the instructions for accessing InfoTrac College Edition that were packaged with your textbook; then search for articles using a keyword search.

For additional links, resources, and suggested readings on the InfoTrac College Edition, visit our Health and Wellness Resource Center at **http://health .wadsworth.com.**

Key Terms

The terms listed are used on the page indicated. Definitions of the terms are in the Glossary at the end of this book.

amino acids 148	listeria 167
antioxidants 151	macronutrients 146
basal metabolic rate (BMR) 146	micronutrients 146
botulism 167	minerals 151
calories 146	nutrition 145
carbohydrates 148	organic 168
complementary proteins 163	osteoporosis 151
complete proteins 148	ovo-lacto-vegetarians 163
complex carbohydrates 148	phytochemicals 155
Daily Values (DVs) 000	proteins 148
dietary fiber 149	saturated fats 149
essential nutrients 146	simple carbohydrates 148
folic acid 150	trans fat 150
functional fiber 149	unsaturated fats 149
incomplete proteins 148	vegans 163
irradiation 168	vitamins 151
lacto-vegetarians 163	

7 Taking Control of Your Weight

eena's mother called it "baby fat." "You'll outgrow it soon enough," she said. Yet Deena's cheeks grew chubbier and her waist wider every year. "Wait for your growth spurt," her mother reassured her. But Deena remained one of the shortest girls in her class—and, she was convinced, the roundest.

Deena went on her first diet in high school. For three days she ate nothing but carrot sticks, cottage cheese, and apples. Then she scarfed down two double cheeseburgers with fries and a chocolate shake. Her other attempts at dieting didn't last much longer. By graduation she was grateful to hide under the flowing black robe as she walked on stage to get her diploma.

When Deena heard about the "freshman 15," the extra pounds many students acquire during their first year at college, she groaned at the prospect of putting on more weight. In her Personal Health class, Deena set one primary goal: not to gain another pound. Rather than going on—and inevitably falling off—one diet after another, she developed a weight management plan that included healthy food choices and regular exercise. Armed with the information and tools provided in this chapter, Deena, for the first time in her life, took charge of her weight.

You can do the same. If you're already at a healthy weight, this chapter can ensure that you remain so in the future. If like two-thirds of Americans, you are overweight, you will find help in these pages. You can choose to lose.

Don't fool yourself into thinking that fat is only a cosmetic problem. Excess weight weakens hearts; raises blood pressure; clogs arteries; strains backs and joints; increases the risk of diabetes, stroke, and certain cancers; and steals years of productive life. The earlier the weight gain, the greater the danger it poses. Obesity at age 20 can cut 20 years off a person's life.[1]

This chapter explains how we grew so big, tells what obesity is and why excess pounds are dangerous, describes current approaches to weight loss, discusses diets that work (and some that don't), offers practical guidelines for exercise and behavioral approaches to losing weight, and examines unhealthy eating patterns and eating disorders. Regardless of your current weight, you will find insights and skills that you will need for healthy weight management throughout your life.

(FAQ) Frequently Asked Questions

After studying the material in this chapter, you should be able to:

▌ **List** the factors besides genetics that have contributed to the global increase in overweight and obesity.

▌ **Define** overweight and obesity, and **describe** the three indicators of weight-related health risks.

▌ **Identify** the main health risks of excess weight.

▌ **Assess** various approaches to weight loss.

▌ **Design** a personal plan for sensible weight management.

▌ **Identify** and **describe** the symptoms and dangers associated with eating disorders.

THE GLOBAL EPIDEMIC

For the first time in history, more than half of the people on the planet are overweight. Obesity, as headlines blare and health experts warn, is emerging as the number-one public health problem of the twenty-first century.

 An estimated 1.1 billion people around the world—seven in ten of the Dutch and Spanish, two in three Americans and Canadians, and one in two Britons, Germans, and Italians—are overweight or obese. In Europe, excess weight ranks as the most common childhood disorder. Since 1980, obesity rates have tripled in parts of Eastern Europe, the Middle East, China, and the Pacific Islands.[2] In many poor countries, obesity is common among city dwellers, while people in rural areas remain underweight and malnourished.

The World Health Organization, in its first global diet, exercise, and health program to combat obesity, recommends that governments promote public knowledge about diet, exercise, and health; offer information that makes healthy choices easier for consumers to make; and require accurate, comprehensible food labels.[3] Although ultimately each individual decides what and how much to eat, policy makers agree that governments also must act to reverse the obesity epidemic.[4]

 Exposure to a Western lifestyle seems to bring out susceptibility to excess weight. Obesity is much more common among the Pima Indians of Arizona compared to Pimas living in Mexico, who have maintained a more traditional lifestyle, with more physical activity and a diet lower in fat and richer in complex carbohydrates. Native Hawaiians who follow a more traditional diet and lifestyle also have lower rates of obesity and cardiovascular disease.[5]

Simply moving to America increases the risk of obesity. In a study of immigrants, the rate of obesity more than doubled within 15 years—from 8 percent among recent immigrants to 19 percent.[6]

SUPERSIZED NATION

Two-thirds of American adults, up from fewer than half 20 years ago, are overweight. About one in every three Americans is obese. Since the 1970s, the obesity rate has doubled for teens and tripled for children between the ages of 6 and 11.[7]

 Although more men than women are overweight, more adult women (38 percent) are obese than men (28 percent). Non-Hispanic black women have the highest obesity rate (50 percent), compared with 40 percent of Hispanic women and 30 percent of white women (Figure 7-1).[8] In some Native American communities, up to 70 percent of all adults are dangerously overweight. Differences in metabolic rates may be one factor.

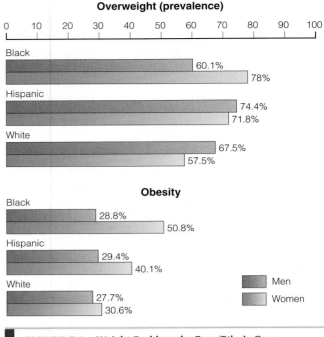

FIGURE 7-1 Weight Problems by Race/Ethnic Group and Gender

Source: "Obesity in Minority Populations," American Obesity Association, www.obesity.org.

Weight problems are starting earlier than ever. One in ten preschoolers and one in five grade schoolers are seriously overweight.[9] According to federal estimates, some 6 million American youngsters are so heavy that their health is in jeopardy. Another 5 million are on the threshold of this danger zone. Not only are more children overweight today, but they're 30 to 50 percent heavier than "fat" kids were a decade ago. The percentage of obese teenagers has tripled in the last 20 years.

Not all Americans are equally likely to be overweight or obese. As Figure 7-2 shows, the southern states have the highest concentration of obese residents. Mississippi is home to the county with the highest percentage of people with a body mass index (BMI) between 30 and 40. (BMI is discussed in a later section—it is defined as the ratio between weight and height that correlates with percentage of body fat.)

States also vary in their efforts to control obesity. According to an ongoing evaluation program at the University of Baltimore, no states deserve an A overall. Only one state—California—earned an A in the report card. For the high grade, the researchers credited the state's legislative package targeted at the nutrition and diets of schoolchildren at risk of becoming obese. Overall, California earned a B for its anti-obesity work for all populations. Five states—Idaho, Nevada, South Dakota, Utah, and Wyoming—received an F on the report card for failing to take any action in combating obesity.[10]

(FAQ) HOW DID WE GET SO FAT?

A variety of factors, ranging from heredity to environment to behavior, played a role in the increase in overweight and obesity. They include:

1. **More calories.** Bombarded by nonstop commercials for taste treats, tempted by foods in every form to munch and crunch, Americans are eating more—some 200 to 400 calories more a day than they did several decades ago. Many of these extra calories come from refined carbohydrates, which can raise levels of heart-damaging blood fats called triglycerides and increase the risk of diabetes as well as obesity.

2. **Bigger portions.** As Table 7-1 shows, the size of many popular restaurant and packaged foods has increased two to five times during the past 20 years.[11] Some foods, like chocolate bars, have grown more than ten times since they were first introduced. Popular 64-ounce sodas can pack a whopping 800 calories. According to studies of appetite and satiety, people presented with larger portions eat up to 30 percent more than they otherwise would.

3. **Fast food.** Young adults who eat frequently at fast-food restaurants gain more weight and develop metabolic abnormalities that increase their risk of

| 15–19% | 20–24% | ≥ 25% |

FIGURE 7-2   Obesity in the United States

This map shows the percentage of people in each state who are obese—they have a body mass index between 30 and 40.

Source: Data from National Center for Chronic Disease Prevention and Health Promotion, 2002.

TABLE 7-1 SUPERSIZED PORTIONS

Food/Beverage	Original Size (year introduced)	Today (largest available)
Budweiser (bottle)	7 oz. (1976)	40 oz.
Nestle's Crunch	1.6 oz. (1938)	5 oz.
Soda (Coca Cola)	6.5 oz. (1916)	34 oz.
French fries (Burger King)	2.6 oz. (1954)	6.9 oz.
Hamburger (McDonald's) (beef only)	1.6 oz. (1955)	8 oz.

Matthew Farruggio (both)

Source: "Are Growing Portion Sizes Leading to Expanding Waistlines?" American Dietetic Association, www.eatright.org.

diabetes in early middle age. In a recent study, those who ate fast food at least twice a week gained an extra 10 pounds and had a two-fold greater increase in insulin resistance, a risk factor for diabetes. The men in the study visited fast-food restaurants more often than the women; blacks did so more frequently than whites.[12]

4. **Physical inactivity.** As Americans eat more, they exercise less. Experts estimate that most adults expend 200 to 300 fewer calories than people did 25 years ago. The most dramatic drop in physical activity often occurs during the college years.[13]

5. **Passive entertainment.** Television is a culprit in an estimated 30 percent of new cases of obesity. TV viewing may increase weight in several ways: It takes up time that otherwise might be spent in physical activities. It increases food intake since people tend to eat more while watching TV. And compared with sewing, reading, driving, or other relatively sedentary pursuits, television watching lowers metabolic rate so viewers burn fewer calories.[14] The combination of watching television (at least two and one-half hours a day) and eating fast food more than twice a week triples the risk of obesity, according to a 15-year study of more than 3,700 white and black young adults.[15]

6. **Modernization.** The growth of industry and technology has led to an abundance of food, less need for physical activity, urbanization, labor-saving devices, and a more sedentary lifestyle. Suburban sprawl directly contributes to obesity, according to a recent study. People who live in neighborhoods where they must drive to get anywhere are significantly more likely to be obese than those who can easily walk to their destinations. Each hour spent in a car was associated with a 6 percent increase in the likelihood of obesity and each half-mile walked per day reduced those odds by nearly 5 percent.[16]

7. **Socioeconomics.** The less money you make, the more likely you are to be overweight. One in four adults below the poverty level is obese, compared with one in six in households earning $67,000 or more. Minorities are at even greater risk. One in three poor African Americans is obese.[17]

8. **Prenatal factors.** A woman's weight before conception and weight gain during pregnancy influence her child's weight. A substantial number of children are prone to gaining weight because their mothers developed gestational diabetes during their pregnancies. Children born to obese women are more than twice as likely to be overweight by age four.[18]

Round-the-clock snacking, fast-food restaurants around every corner, and hours in front of the TV have all contributed to the increase in overweight and obesity.

9. **Childhood development.** Today's children don't necessarily eat more food than in the past, but they eat more high-fat, high-calorie foods and they exercise much, much less. On days when they eat fast food, youngsters consume an average of 187 more calories per day.[19] Fewer than half of grade schoolers participate in daily physical education classes. Many spend five hours or more a day in front of a computer or television screen.[20]

10. **Genetics.** Although scientists have identified genes involved in appetite and metabolism, they have not found a genetic cause for obesity. It may be that various genes contribute a small increase in risk or that rare abnormalities in many genes create a predisposition to weight gain and obesity.[21]

11. **Emotional influences.** Obese people are neither more nor less psychologically troubled than others. Psychological problems, such as irritability, depression, and anxiety, are more likely to be the result of obesity than the cause. As discussed later in this chapter, emotions do play a role in weight problems. Just as some people reach for a drink or a drug when they're upset, others cope by overeating, bingeing, or purging.

BODY IMAGE

Throughout most of history, bigger was better. The great beauties of centuries past, as painted by such artistic masters as Rubens and Renoir, were soft and fleshy, with rounded bellies and dimpled thighs. Culture often shapes views of beauty and health.

 Many developing countries still regard a full figure, rather than a thin one, as the ideal. Fattening huts, in which brides-to-be eat extra food to plump up before marriage, still exist in some African cultures. Among certain Native American tribes of the Southwest, if a girl is thin at puberty, a fat woman places her foot on the girl's back so she will magically gain weight and become more attractive.

Influenced by the media, many Americans are paying more attention to their body images than ever before—and at a younger age (see You Decide). In a study of high school girls, those who regularly read women's health and fitness magazines, which may present unrealistic physical ideals, were more likely to go on low-calorie diets, take pills to suppress their appetites, use laxatives, or force themselves to vomit after eating. In other research, girls who watched a lot of television and expressed concern about slimness and popularity were more dissatisfied with their bodies than girls involved in sports.

Boys' body images also are influenced by media images depicting superstrong, highly muscular males.

> *Some criticize the media for idealizing body shapes, such as extremely thin women and muscular men, that are unrealistic and unhealthy ideals. Others contend that the advertising and entertainment industries are simply reflecting cultural values. Are media images harmful? Or do people use different standards in evaluating their own bodies?*
> **You decide.**

 Being overweight for a long period of time has a cumulative negative impact on body image. In a study of 266 college women, those who described themselves as "always overweight" ranked much lower in current body self-esteem than those with more recent weight problems.[22]

College students of different ethnic and racial backgrounds, including Asians, express as much—and sometimes more—concern about their body shape and weight as whites. In a study of university students, African-American and Caucasian men were similar in their ideals for body size and in their perceptions of their own shapes. As shown in Figure 7-3, both African-American and white women perceived themselves as smaller than they actually were and desired an even smaller body size. However, the African-American women were more accepting of larger size.[23] (BMI, or body mass index, is discussed on page 182.)

MALE AND FEMALE BODY IMAGE

Although women generally report a more negative body image, many men are dissatisfied with their bodies but for different reasons. Often they want either to lose or gain weight or to gain muscle and bulk. Women compare their appearance to others more frequently than men and worry more that others will think negatively about their looks. Yet appearance matters just as much to men, who are just as likely as women to engage in efforts to improve their bodies.[24]

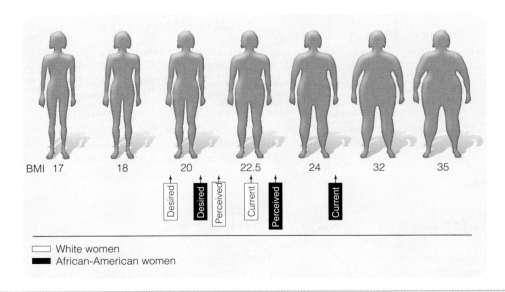

FIGURE 7-3   Body Dissatisfaction in African-American and White Students
In a study of 630 undergraduates, both African-American and white women perceived themselves to be smaller than they actually were—and wished to be even smaller. However, the white students saw themselves and desired to be considerably smaller than did the African-American women. Both African-American and white men rated the silhouette depicting a BMI of 20 as the most desirable.

Source: "Body Dissatisfaction Among College Students," *Nutrition Research Newsletter,* Vol. 21, No. 3, March 2002, p. 9.

Women have long been bombarded by the media with idealized images of female bodies that bear little resemblance to the way most women look. Increasingly, more advertisements and men's magazines are featuring idealized male bodies. Sleek, strong, and sculpted, they too do not resemble the bodies most men inhabit. The gap between reality and ideal is getting bigger for both genders.

In the last decade, numerous studies have shown that women in *Playboy* centerfolds and Miss America pageants weigh less than they did in the 1970s. In one analysis, 29 percent of *Playboy* centerfolds and 17 percent of Miss America pageant winners had BMIs below 17.5, one of the criteria for anorexia nervosa and a definite indication of being severely underweight.

As beauty pageant queens and female models have been shrinking, the men featured in *Playgirl* centerfolds have been bulking up. Their BMIs are higher than in the past, as are the BMIs of a sample of Canadian and American men between the ages of 18 and 24. Researchers do not know if the higher BMIs are the result of an increase in lean body mass or body fat. Their theory: The models have become more muscular over time, accounting for their high BMIs, while real guys may simply have gotten fatter.

When college men and women step on a scale or look in a mirror, they react in different ways. In a study of 525 undergraduates, the women failed to see themselves as underweight, even when they were, and perceived themselves as overweight, even when they were not. Many of the women who considered themselves normal weight nonetheless desired to be thinner. Men in the study generally saw themselves as underweight, even when they were not. Most desired to be heavier, though not obese.

The greater the discrepancy between a woman's current view of her body shape and the ideal she considers most attractive to men, the more likely she is to worry about how others will view her and to doubt her ability to make a desirable impression. Such "social physique anxiety" occurs often in women who feel they do not measure up to what they or others consider most desirable in terms of weight or appearance. Women with high BMIs and greater body-related anxiety may exercise to become thinner or more

How do you decide what your ideal body size is?

© Raoul Minsart/Masterfile

attractive.[25] Those reporting the greatest distress because of body image are at highest risk of disordered eating or actual eating disorders (discussed on page 198).[26]

BODY IMAGE OVER TIME

In early adulthood, body image is linked to self-esteem among women. However, self-esteem is strongly related to overall physical appearance, not just weight. In recent research, women who expressed dissatisfaction with their bodies and those who worried about how they "shaped up" in comparison with others reported relatively few problems in their psychological, social, or sexual functioning, even if their self-esteem was low. Body image had a greater effect

---

Strategies for Change :: How to Boost Your Body Esteem

Whatever your weight or shape, here are some ways to improve your body image:

- Start walking with more bounce in your step.
- Focus on the parts of your body you like. Take pride in your powerful shoulders or large eyes.

:: Treat yourself with the respect you'd like to receive from others. Don't put yourself down or joke about your weight.

:: Work with hand weights. As you build your muscles, your sense of strength and self-confidence also will grow.

:: Don't put off special plans, such as learning to kayak or signing up for an exchange program, until you reach a certain magical weight: Do what you want to do *now*.

:: Pull your shoulders back, suck in your stomach, and stand up straight. You'll look and feel better.

on men between the ages of 30 and 50, even though they usually don't directly express their concerns.[27]

Although concerns about body image are particularly common among college students, they persist throughout life. Both men and women in their thirties and forties are more likely than other age groups to be dissatisfied with their bodies and to attempt to conceal them, for instance, by wearing nonrevealing clothing. Men and women over age 50 remain as negative as younger adults in evaluating their own appearance but they report less concern about what others think of their bodies and compare themselves to others less frequently.

In a study comparing college students, parents, and grandparents, older men and women were more dissatisfied with their appearance than younger people. Women were more concerned with aging than men, but there were no gender differences in overall body dissatisfaction.

But . . .
Calories > Calories = Weight gain
consumed used

Calories < Calories = Weight loss
consumed used

No Weight Change:
$$\frac{\text{Calories}}{\text{consumed}} = \frac{\text{Calories}}{\text{used}}$$

FIGURE 7-4 **Energy Imbalance**
Balancing the calories you eat with the calories you use through physical activity will help you maintain a healthy weight.

UNDERSTANDING WEIGHT PROBLEMS

Weight problems don't develop overnight. Fat accumulates meal by meal, day by day, pound by pound. Ultimately, all weight problems are the result of a prolonged energy imbalance—of consuming too many calories and burning too few in daily activities (Figure 7-4).

How many calories you need depends on your gender, age, body-frame size, weight, percentage of body fat, and your **basal metabolic rate (BMR)**—the number of calories needed to sustain your body at rest. Your activity level also affects your calorie requirements. Regardless of whether you consume fat, protein, or carbohydrates, if you take in more calories than required to maintain your size and don't work them off in some sort of physical activity, your body will convert the excess to fat.

The average American consumes about one million calories a year. Given that number, what difference does an extra 100-calorie soda or 300-calorie brownie make? A lot, because the extra calories that you don't burn every day ac-

cumulate, adding an average of 2 to 4 pounds to your weight every year.

WEIGHT AND THE COLLEGE STUDENT

Obesity rates have increased most rapidly among 18- to 29-year-olds. According to the National College Health Risk Behavior Study, as many as 35 percent of college students may be overweight or obese (see Student Snapshot: "How Students Weigh in on Weight").[28] In other studies, about one in five college students had an unhealthy weight as well as at least one risk factor for metabolic disorder, an important cause of cardiovascular disease (discussed in Chapter 15).[29]

As many students discover, it's easy to gain weight on campuses, which are typically crammed with vending machines, fast-food counters, and cafeterias serving up hearty meals. But the infamous *freshman 15*, the extra pounds acquired in the first year at college, seems to be a myth. Several studies have documented much lower weight gains, ranging from 2.45 to 7 pounds. In one study of changes in both weight and body fat, freshmen estimated that they had

---

Strategies for Prevention :: Holding the Line on College Weight Gain

:: **Plan meals.** Most campus cafeterias post the week's menus in advance. Plan which items you will eat before you see or smell high-fat dishes.

:: **Don't linger.** If you use the cafeteria as a social gathering place, you may end up eating with two or three different groups of people. Set a time limit to eat—then leave.

:: **Plan alternative behaviors.** People who eat when they are stressed or bored need substitute activities ready when they need them. Make a list of things you can do—shower, phone a friend, take a hike—when stress strikes.

:: **Eat at "home."** If the dormitory has a small kitchen, cook some healthful dishes and invite friends to join you.

:: **Take advantage of physical activity programs.** Many college students become less active during their years in college. Aim to maintain or increase the amount of exercise you did in high school. Join a biking club, take a salsa class, learn yoga.

Student Snapshot

HOW STUDENTS WEIGH IN ON WEIGHT

	Total	Women	Men
Percentage of students who described themselves as			
Very underweight	0.7%	0.6%	1.2%
Slightly underweight	10	8	15
About the right weight	53	53	53
Slightly overweight	33	35	28
Very overweight	4	4	3
Percentage who engaged in various weight loss behaviors in the previous 30 days			
Exercised to lose weight	56%	63%	43%
Dieted to lose weight	34	41	21
Vomited or took laxatives	3	4	0.4
Took diet pills	6	7	3

Source: American College Health Association. "The American College Health Association National College Health Assessment (ACHA-NCHA), Spring 2003 Reference Group Report," *Journal of American College Health,* Vol. 53, No. 5, March–April 2005, p. 199.

© SuperStock/Alamy

gained an average of 4.1 pounds. In fact, their weights fluctuated from a gain of 15 pounds to a loss of 15 pounds. Among the 60 percent of freshmen who did put on weight, the average gain was 4.6 pounds.[30]

 Even international students may gain weight and body fat after arriving on American campuses. Ohio University researchers found that after 20 weeks, foreign students, who had incorporated foods high in fat, salt, and sugar into their diets, gained about 3 pounds on average and their percentage of body fat rose by about 5 percent.

FAQ IS MY WEIGHT HEALTHY?

Rather than relying on a range of ideal weights for various heights, as they did in the past, medical experts use various methods to assess body composition and weight. The best indicators of weight-related health risks are Body Mass Index (BMI); waist circumference (WC); and waist-hip ratio (WHR).

If you're a young adult, even mild to moderate overweight poses a threat to your health because it puts you at risk for gaining even more weight—and for facing greater health risks. Obesity has been implicated as a culprit in rising rates of disability among younger Americans as well as a factor in chronic health problems.[31] If you are older than a traditional-aged student, the risks to your health are more immediate.

BODY COMPOSITION

Body composition, the fifth component of fitness mentioned in Chapter 4, can tell you a lot about your risk for cardiovascular disease and diabetes. Here are several methods for assessing body composition.

BODY MASS INDEX (BMI)

Body mass index (BMI), a ratio between weight and height, is a mathematical formula that correlates with body fat. You can determine your BMI from Figure 7-5. A healthy BMI ranges from 18.5 to 24.9.

A BMI of 25 or greater defines **overweight** and marks the point at which excess weight increases the risk of disease. If your BMI is between 25 and 29.9 (23.4 for Asians), your weight is undermining the quality of your life. You suffer more aches and pains. You find it harder to perform everyday tasks. You run a greater risk of serious health problems.

A BMI of 30 or greater defines **obesity** and marks the point at which excess weight increases the risk of death. If your BMI is over 30, you face all the preceding dangers plus one more: dying. The risk of premature death increases even more if your BMI is over 40, a sign of severe or "morbid" obesity.

Doctors use BMI to determine whether a person is at risk for weight-related diseases like diabetes. However, using BMI as an assessment tool has limitations. Muscular individuals, including athletes and body builders, may be miscategorized as overweight or obese because they have greater lean muscle mass. BMI also does not reliably reflect body fat, an independent predictor of health risk, and is not useful for growing children, women who are pregnant or nursing, or the elderly. In addition, BMI, which was developed in Western nations, may not accurately indicate the risk of obesity-related diseases in Asian men and women.

If your BMI is high, you may be at increased risk of developing certain diseases, including hypertension, cardiovascular disease, adult-onset diabetes (type 2), sleep apnea, and osteoarthritis. Although BMIs below 25 are considered healthy, individuals with BMIs between 22 and 24.9 are significantly more likely to develop a weight-related disease, such as high blood pressure, than leaner individuals with BMIs under 22.

WAIST CIRCUMFERENCE

Even if your scale shows that you haven't gained a lot of weight, your waist may widen—particularly if you've been under stress. Because of the physiological impact of stress hormones, fat accumulates around your midsection in times of tension and turmoil.

 A widening waist or "apple" shape is a warning signal. In young women, a wider waist correlates with high levels of harmful blood fats, such as LDL

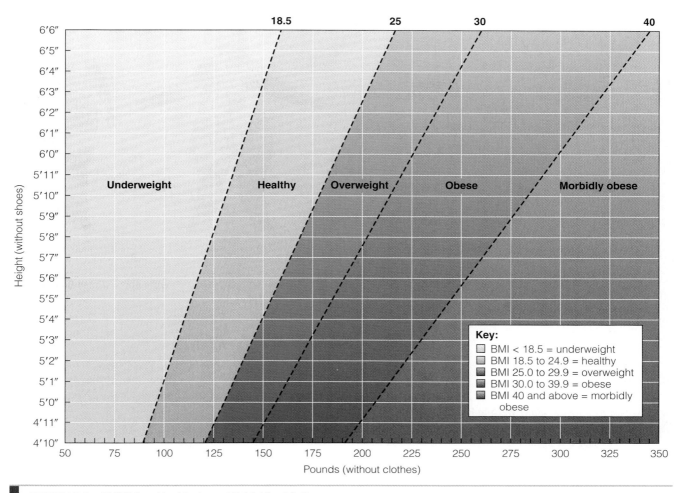

FIGURE 7-5   BMI Values Used to Assess Weight for Adults

cholesterol and triglycerides.[32] In both sexes, abdominal fat, unlike fat in the thighs or hips, increases the risk of high blood pressure, type 2 diabetes, high cholesterol, and metabolic syndrome (a perilous combination of overweight, high blood pressure, and high levels of cholesterol and blood sugar, discussed in Chapter 15).[33]

To measure your waist circumference, place a tape measure around your bare abdomen just above your hip bone. Be sure that the tape is snug but does not compress your skin. Relax, exhale, and measure.

When is a waist too wide? Various studies have produced different results, but the general guideline is that a waist measuring more than 35 inches in a woman or more than 40 inches in a man signals greater health risks. These waist circumferences indicate "central" obesity, which is characterized by fat deposited deep within the central abdominal area of the body. Such "visceral" fat is more dangerous than "subcutaneous" fat just below the skin because it moves more readily into the bloodstream and directly raises levels of harmful cholesterol.

 Body composition varies with race and ethnicity. Asians, for instance, may be more likely and Afri-

can Americans less likely to accumulate visceral fat than Caucasians.[34]

WAIST-TO-HIP RATIO

Another way of determining your health risk is your **waist-to-hip ratio,** or WHR. In addition to measuring your waist, measure your hips at the widest part. Divide your hip measurement into your waist measurement. For women, a ratio of 0.80 or less is considered safe; for men, the recommended ratio is 0.90 or less. For both men and women, a 1.0 or higher is considered "at risk" or in the danger zone for undesirable health consequences, such as heart disease and other ailments associated with being overweight. You can also use Figure 7-6 to determine your WHR.

Men of all ages are more prone to develop the "apple" shape characteristic of central obesity; women in their reproductive years are more likely to accumulate fat around the hips and thighs and acquire a pear shape (Figure 7-7).

 When men and women diet, men lose more visceral fat located around the abdominal area. This weight loss produces more cardiovascular benefits

PEAR
Fat stores around hips predominate

APPLE
Fat stores around waist predominate

FIGURE 7-7   Pear-Shaped Versus Apple-Shaped Bodies

FIGURE 7-6   Determining Waist-to Hip Ratio (WHR)

Use a straightedge to draw a line from your waist circumference (left) to your hip circumference (right). The point at which the line crosses the center column is your waist-to-hip ratio (WHR).

Sources: Data from Gray, G. A., and D. S. Gray. "Obesity: Part I: Pathenogenesis." *Western Journal of Medicine,* Vol. 149, 1988. In Christian, Janet, and Janet Greger, *Nutrition for Living,* 4th ed. Redwood City, CA: Benjamin Cummings, 1994.

for men, including a decrease in triglycerides (fats circulating in the blood) and an increase in the "good" form of cholesterol, high-density lipoprotein (HDL).

MEASURING BODY FAT

Knowing your specific body composition can provide useful information about body fat and health. Ideal body fat percentages for men range from 7 to 25 percent and for women from 16 to 35 percent. Methods of assessing body composition range from skin calipers to more high-tech methods.

Skinfold Measurement

Skinfold measurement is determined using a caliper to measure the amount of skinfold. The usual sites include the chest, abdomen, and thigh for men, and the tricep, hip, and thigh for women. Various equations determine body fat percentage, including calculations that take into account age, gender, race, and other factors. This relatively simple and low-cost method requires considerable technical skill for an accurate reading.

Home Body Fat Analyzers

Handheld devices and stand-on monitors sold online and in specialty stores promise to make measuring your body fat percentage as easy as finding your weight. None has been extensively tested.

Laboratory Methods

▪ **Bioelectrical Impedance Analysis (BIA).** This noninvasive method is based on the principle that electrical current applied to the body meets greater resistance with different types of tissue. Lean tissue, which contains large amounts of water and electrolytes, is a good electrical conductor; fat, which does not, is a poor conductor. In theory, the easier the electrical conduction, the greater an individual's lean body mass.

▪ **Hydrostatic (underwater) weighing.** According to the Archimedes Principle, a body immersed in a fluid is buoyed by a force equal to the weight of the displaced fluid. Since muscle has a higher density than water and fat has a lower density, fat people tend to displace less water than lean people.

▪ **Dual-energy X-ray absorptiometry (DXA).** X rays are used to quantify the skeletal and soft tissue components of body mass. The test requires just 10 to 20 minutes, and radiation dosage is low (800 to 2,000 times lower than a typical chest X ray). Some researchers believe that DXA will supplant hydrostatic testing as the standard for body composition assessment.

▪ **The Bod Pod®.** This large, egg-shaped fiberglass chamber uses an approach based on air displacement plethysmography, that is, the calculation of the relationship between pressure and volume to derive body volume.

Skinfold measure accuracy depends on the technician's skill; laboratory methods such as DXA don't have that subjective component.

(FAQ) I'M TOO THIN: HOW CAN I GAIN WEIGHT?

Being underweight is not an uncommon problem, particularly among adolescent and young adult men as well as among those who diet excessively or suffer from an eating disorder (discussed on page 198). If you lose weight suddenly and don't know the reason, talk to a doctor. Rapid weight loss can be an early symptom of a health problem.

If you're trying to put on pounds, you need to do the opposite of dieters: Consume more calories than you burn. But as with losing weight, you should try to gain weight in healthy ways. Here are some suggestions:

- **Eat more of a variety of foods** rather than more high-fat, high-calorie foods. Get no more than 30 percent of your daily calories from fat. A higher percentage poses a threat to your heart and your health.

- **If your appetite is small, eat more frequently.** Try for five or six smaller meals rather than a big lunch and dinner.

- **Choose some calorie-rich foods,** such as dried fruits rather than fresh ones. Add nuts and cheese to salads and main dishes.

- **Drink juice** rather than regular or diet soda.

- **Try adding a commercial liquid meal** replacement as a snack.

- **Exercise regularly** to build up both appetite and muscle.

HEALTH DANGERS OF EXCESS WEIGHT

The federal government has recognized obesity as a serious, potentially fatal disease. This designation cleared the way for insurance coverage for obesity treatments, rather than just for the medical problems it can cause. The effects of obesity on health are the equivalent of 20 years of aging.[35] They include increased risk of cardiovascular disease, diabetes, and cancer, as well as disability, rheumatoid arthritis, sleep apnea, gout, and liver disease (Figure 7-8). Total medical costs, both direct and indirect, amount to more than $117 billion a year.[36]

THE IMPACT ON THE BODY

The incidence of diabetes, gallstones, hypertension, heart disease, and colon cancer increases with the degree of overweight in both sexes. Those with BMIs of 35 or more are approximately 20 times more likely to develop diabetes. Individuals who are overweight but not obese, with BMIs between 25 and 29.9, are significantly more likely than leaner women to develop gallstones, high blood pressure, high cholesterol, and heart disease. Overweight men and women are at least three times more likely to suffer knee injuries that require surgery to repair.[37]

 Health risks may vary in different races, ethnic groups, and at-risk populations. Even relatively small amounts of excess fat—as little as 5 pounds —can add to the dangers in those already at risk for hypertension and diabetes. According to the National Heart, Lung, and Blood Institute, being overweight, even if not obese, increases the risk of heart failure. Obesity also causes alterations in various measures of immune function and increases the risk of kidney stones and disease.[38]

Overweight young adults have a 70 percent chance of becoming overweight or obese adults.[39] They are two to three times more likely to have high total cholesterol levels and more than 43 times more likely to have cardiovascular disease risk factors such as elevated blood pressure. They also have a higher prevalence of type 2 diabetes.[40]

Major diseases linked to obesity include:

- **Type 2 diabetes.** More than 80 percent of people with type 2 diabetes are overweight. Although the reasons are not known, being overweight may

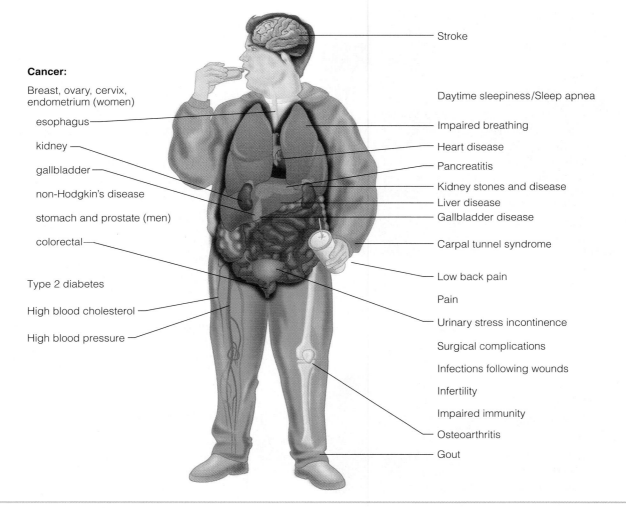

Cancer:

Breast, ovary, cervix, endometrium (women)

esophagus

kidney

gallbladder

non-Hodgkin's disease

stomach and prostate (men)

colorectal

Type 2 diabetes

High blood cholesterol

High blood pressure

Stroke

Daytime sleepiness/Sleep apnea

Impaired breathing

Heart disease

Pancreatitis

Kidney stones and disease

Liver disease

Gallbladder disease

Carpal tunnel syndrome

Low back pain

Pain

Urinary stress incontinence

Surgical complications

Infections following wounds

Infertility

Impaired immunity

Osteoarthritis

Gout

FIGURE 7-8   Health Dangers of Excess Weight

make cells less efficient at using sugar from the blood. This then puts stress on the cells that produce insulin (a hormone that carries sugar from the blood to cells) and makes them gradually fail. You can lower your risk for developing type 2 diabetes by losing weight and increasing the amount of physical activity you do. If you have type 2 diabetes, losing weight and becoming more physically active can help you control your blood sugar levels and may allow you to reduce the amount of diabetes medication you take.

■ **Heart disease and stroke.** People who are overweight are more likely to suffer from high blood pressure, high levels of triglycerides (blood fats) and harmful LDL cholesterol, and low levels of beneficial HDL cholesterol. In addition, people with more body fat have higher blood levels of substances that cause inflammation, which may raise heart disease risk. Losing 5 to 15 percent of your weight can lower your chances for developing heart disease or having a stroke.

People who both smoke and are obese are at especially high risk of cardiovascular disease. Although some smokers have felt that they couldn't lose weight until they stopped smoking, researchers have found that weight loss among smokers is possible and beneficial, leading to a reduction in other risk factors, such as lower blood pressure and lower cholesterol.

■ **Cancer.** According to a study of 900,000 people, the largest ever of its kind, excess weight may account for 14 percent of all cancer deaths in men and 20 percent of those in women. Losing weight, researchers estimate, could prevent as many as one of every six cancer deaths.[41]

While earlier research had linked excess weight to cancers of the breast and uterus, colon and rectum, kidney, esophagus, and gallbladder, this study also linked weight to other cancers, including non-Hodgkin's lymphoma; multiple myeloma; and cancers of the pancreas and liver, the cervix and ovary (in women), and the stomach and prostate (in men). Those with BMIs over 40 had death rates from cancer that were 52 percent higher for men and 62 percent higher for women than those of normal-weight individuals.[42]

 Body size and higher BMI are linked with increased risk of breast cancer in premenopausal women and in postmenopausal women not using hormone replacement therapy.[43]

Too much body fat can influence cancer in several ways: It increases the amount of estrogen in the blood, raising the risk of cancers of the female reproductive system. It raises the levels of insulin, which prompts the body to create a hormone that causes cells to multiply. Acid reflux, which can cause cancer of the esophagus, occurs more frequently in heavy men and women. Obesity also makes cancer harder to diagnose and treat.

Excess pounds affect people around the clock. Overweight and obese individuals sleep less than those with normal weights. Individuals with lower BMIs get an extra 16 minutes of rest a night or two hours a week. (See Chapter 3 for a discussion of sleep.) The lost sleep could add to the risk of medical problems.[44]

LIFE EXPECTANCY

In the past, experts had estimated that obesity might claim more than 300,000 lives a year. However, the CDC recently reported that obesity is becoming less lethal than in the past, possibly as a result of improvements in public health and medical care. Based on BMI, extremely obese individuals are most likely to die. People who are overweight but not obese have a lower risk of death than those of normal weight.[45] The reasons are not clear, although rates of high blood pressure and high cholesterol in the obese have declined in recent decades, to a great extent because of breakthroughs in medications.[46] Since most deaths occur in old age, some researchers theorize that some extra weight might be beneficial in the elderly if it contributes to stronger bones and muscles. Decades of overweight and obesity may take a greater toll on wellness and possibly on lifespan.[47]

THE EMOTIONAL TOLL

In our calorie-conscious and thinness-obsessed society, obesity also affects quality of life, including sense of vitality and physical pain. Many see it as a psychological burden, a sign of failure, laziness, or inadequate willpower. Overweight men and women often blame themselves for becoming heavy and feel guilty and depressed as a result. In fact, the psychological problems once considered the cause of obesity may be its consequence.

A Canadian study found so many overweight and obese individuals (14 percent of the sample) at risk for depression that its authors suggested that all health professionals assess obese patients for depression.[48]

A PRACTICAL GUIDE TO WEIGHT LOSS

Readiness to change is key to successful weight loss (see Self Survey, page 202). However, individuals vary in their readiness to change their diets, increase their physical activity, and seek professional counseling. In one study, participants also varied in specific dietary changes. For instance, some were ready to eat more fruits and vegetables but not to reduce total calories.[49]

One indicator of readiness to change is willingness to talk with a health-care provider about diet or exercise. Unfortunately, only about 40 percent of doctors report counseling patients about weight management.[50] When physicians do provide weight loss counseling, patients are more likely to understand the risks of obesity and the benefits of weight loss and move to a higher stage of readiness.

(FAQ) WHY DO I OVEREAT?

The answer lies not just in the belly but in the brain. Both **hunger,** the physiological drive to consume food, and **appetite,** the psychological desire to eat, influence and control our desire for food. Scientists have discovered appetite receptors within the brain that specifically respond to hunger messengers carried by hormones produced in the digestive tract (Figure 7-9).

Appetite usually begins with the fear of the unpleasant sensation of hunger. We learn to avoid hunger by eating a certain amount of food at certain times of the day, just as dogs in the laboratory learn to avoid electric shocks by jumping at the sound of a warning bell. But appetite is easily led into temptation. In one famous experiment, psychologists bought

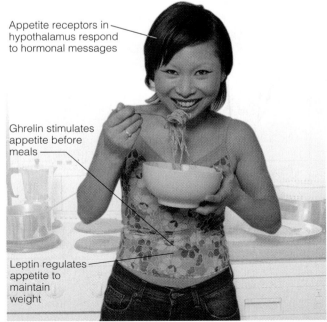

Appetite receptors in hypothalamus respond to hormonal messages

Ghrelin stimulates appetite before meals

Leptin regulates appetite to maintain weight

© Betsie Van der Meer/Stone/Getty Images

FIGURE 7-9 Hormones help regulate our appetites

bags of high-calorie goodies—peanut butter, marshmallows, chocolate-chip cookies, and salami—for their test rats. The animals ate so much on this "supermarket diet" that they gained more weight than any laboratory rats ever had before. The snack-food diet that fattened up these rats was particularly high in fats. Biologists speculate that creamy, buttery, or greasy foods may cause internal changes that increase appetite and, consequently, weight.

A hormone called leptin, produced by fat cells, sends signals to the brain that affect appetite. When leptin levels are normal, people eat just enough to maintain weight. When leptin is low, the brain responds as if fat stores had been depleted and slows down metabolism. This may be one reason why it is so difficult to lose weight by dieting alone.

Other hormones made in the stomach also influence how hungry we feel. One is ghrelin, a natural appetite stimulant. When given shots of ghrelin, people become very hungry and eat 30 percent more than they normally would. Ghrelin typically rises before meals and falls afterward. Dieters tend to have high levels of ghrelin, as if their bodies were trying to stimulate appetite so they regain lost fat.

We stop eating when we feel satisfied; this is called **satiety,** a feeling of fullness and relief from hunger. The neurotransmitter serotonin has been shown to produce feelings of satiety. In addition, several peptides, released from the digestive tract as we ingest food, may signal the brain to stop or restrict eating. However, it takes 20 minutes for the brain to register fullness.

WEIGHT LOSS DIETS

Never before have so many had so much to lose. More than two-thirds of Americans—77 percent of women and 63 percent of men—are either dieting or struggling to maintain their weight. You've probably heard that 95 percent of people who lose weight gain it all back. That widely quoted statistic, based on a small study from 1959, is no longer true, if it ever

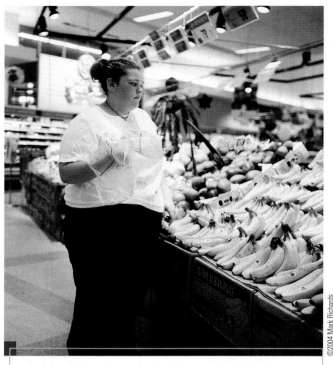

Today's Goal: Have fruit instead of dessert at lunch.

©2004 Mark Richards

was.[52] Diets can and do work. Tens of thousands of dieters have lost excess pounds and maintained lower, healthier weights. Although many regain some weight, most manage to keep off about two-thirds of the weight lost by dieting for at least a year.[53]

Which Weight Loss Diet Works Best?

You've seen the commercials and read the claims that a popular new diet can pare away pounds. Don't believe the hype. According to a review of commercial weight loss programs,

---

Strategies for Prevention ☷ Dietary Guidelines

The 2005 Dietary Guidelines for Americans recommend the following steps for weight management:

- To maintain body weight in a healthy range, balance calories from foods and beverages with calories expended.
- To prevent gradual weight gain over time, make small decreases in food and beverage calories and increase physical activity.

KEY RECOMMENDATIONS FOR SPECIFIC POPULATION GROUPS
- **Those who need to lose weight.** Aim for a slow, steady weight loss by

decreasing calorie intake while maintaining an adequate nutrient intake and increasing physical activity.
- **Overweight children.** Reduce the rate of body weight gain while allowing growth and development. Consult a health-care provider before placing a child on a weight-reduction diet.
- **Pregnant women.** Ensure appropriate weight gain as specified by a health-care provider.
- **Breastfeeding women.** Moderate weight reduction is safe and does not compromise weight gain of the nursing infant.

- **Overweight adults and overweight children with chronic diseases and/or on medication.** Consult a health-care provider about weight loss strategies prior to starting a weight-reduction program to ensure appropriate management of other health conditions.[51]

there is little scientific evidence to back up any claims that popular diets help overweight individuals slim down.[54] In almost any program, people lose weight because they are paying more attention to their food choices and limiting their calories (Table 7-2).[55]

Diets do work—for a while. Low-calorie (1,000 to 1,200 calories daily) and very low-calorie diets produce similar results a year later. Physical activity alone leads to a weight loss of about 2 to 3 percent of initial weight and reduces abdominal fat. A combination of diet and physical activity, particularly along with behavioral therapy, produces greater reductions in weight and abdominal fat than either approach alone. "High-intensity" programs, which provide person-to-person contact more than once a month, are more effective than those with less frequent contact.[56]

In a year-long "battle of the bulge," researchers compared four popular diets: Atkins, Weight Watchers, The Zone, and Ornish. All produced similar results, including a weight loss of about 7 pounds and a lowering of heart disease risk factors—but only in those who stuck with the program. Nearly half of the dieters dropped out before the year was up because the diets were too hard to follow or weren't working. The Atkins and Ornish plans had the highest dropout rates.[57] In another study, Weight Watchers dieters who regularly attended the program lost approximately 5 percent of their body weight in three to six months. Those on very low-calorie diets who finished the program lost up to 25 percent of their initial weight but were at high risk of regaining at least half of it back.[58]

Because of the high relapse rate, researchers are searching for ways to motivate dieters and sustain weight loss for five to ten years. In the meantime, the best treatment of obesity is a "low-fad" approach, with an emphasis on healthy food choices and regular physical activity.[59]

Low-Carbohydrate Diets

An estimated 17 million Americans have tried a low-carb diet in the last year. The diet popularized by the late Dr. Robert Atkins, is high in protein and extremely low in carbohydrates. Followers of the Atkins diet eat unlimited amounts of meat, eggs, and cheese and cut back on bread, pasta, crackers, cakes, cookies, and other carbohydrates. Because they avoid many high-calorie foods and fill up on proteins, which take longer to digest, these dieters typically lose weight without feeling hungry.

Particularly in the initial stages, followers of the Atkins diet may consume 40 percent of their calories in fat, much of it saturated. For years professional groups such as the American Dietetic Association and the American Heart Association warned that low-carb, high-fat weight loss plans like the Atkins diet pose serious health dangers, primarily because the high fat content may increase the risk of heart disease, diabetes, stroke, and kidney and liver disease.

Several studies have challenged these assumptions, at least in the short term. In one six-month trial, participants were more likely to stick with an Atkins-style diet and lost more weight (26 pounds compared with 14 pounds) than

volunteers on a low-fat, low-cholesterol diet. Triglyceride and HDL cholesterol levels improved considerably on the low-carb diet, but its followers reported more negative symptoms, such as constipation, headache, and muscle cramps. "Over six months the diet appears relatively safe, but we need to study the safety for longer durations," said the lead researcher, Dr. Will Yancy, who noted that potential long-term health risks include increases in harmful LDL cholesterol, bone loss, and kidney stones.[60]

In a year-long study, those on a low-carb diet lost more weight in the first six months, but at the end of the year their weight loss was comparable to the participants on a low-fat diet, whose weight declined slowly but steadily. As in the shorter study, the low-carb diet had a more beneficial effect on triglyceride and HDL levels than the low-fat diet.[61]

Diets such as Sugar Busters! and the Glucose Revolution distinguish between "correct" carbs (fruits, vegetables, and whole grains) and "harmful" ones (refined sugars and processed grains). Other popular diets call for specific proportions of nutrients. For instance, the Zone diet advocates meals and snacks that consist of 40 percent carbohydrate, 30 percent fat, and 30 percent protein. Dieters may lose weight because they're paying more attention to what they eat and making better food choices. However, approaches like this generally make smart eating more complicated than it has to be.[62]

Low-Fat Diets

Various diets reduce daily fat intake—some to 25 to 30 percent of calories; others, such as the Dean Ornish program, to less than 10 percent. The Ornish diet has proved effective in reversing atherosclerotic buildup. Low-fat diets also may enhance the immune response.

However, although experts support a decrease in trans and saturated fats for the sake of cardiovascular health, they have challenged the scientific evidence for reducing fat below 30 to 35 percent for the sake of preventing heart disease in healthy individuals. Epidemiological studies have not shown that dietary fat directly increases body fat. "Healthy" fats such as olive oil and fatty acids in fish oils may help control appetite and maintain long-term weight loss.

Low-Calorie Diets

Any diet that restricts calories will lead to weight loss. "There is no substitute for the simple formula that 'calories in must equal calories out' in order to control weight," said the FDA Deputy Commissioner when the agency's Obesity Working Group issued its report in 2004 and called for more focus on calories. The Department of Health and Human Services has launched a public education campaign, similar to earlier stop-smoking initiatives, that emphasizes the simple message, Calories count.

Cutting back 500 to 1,000 calories a day typically leads to a loss of 1 to 2 pounds a week and an average weight loss of about 8 percent of body weight in six months. Expert groups, such as the American Society for Clinical Nutrition, the North American Association for the Study of Obesity,

TABLE 7-2 HOW CONSUMER REPORTS RATES THE DIETS

Better ◉ ◐ ○ ◑ ● Worse

Diet	Price[1]	Overall Score	Nutrition	Weight loss (6 mo.)	Drop-out rate (6 mo.)	Weight loss (1 year)	Drop-out rate (1 year)	Average Daily Calories	Fat	Saturated fat	Carbohydrates	Protein	Grams of fiber/1,000 cal	Fruits & veggies (daily servings)
In performance order:									Percentage of Calories					
1 Weight Watchers	$10–13 per week	◐	◉	○	◐	○	◐	1,450	24	7	56	20	20	11
2 Slim-Fast	$2–3 per day (bars or drinks)	◐	◉	◐	◐	◐	●	1,540	22	6	57	21	21	12
3 Zone (men's menu) (*The Zone*, by Barry Sears Ph.D. with Bill Lawren)[2]	$25.00	◐	◉	○	○	○	◑	1,660	27	7	42	30	21	17
4 Ornish (*Eat More, Weigh Less*, by Dean Ornish M.D.)	$15.00	○	○	○	●	◐	●	1,520	6	1	77	16	31	17
5 Atkins Ongoing Weight Loss (OWL) (*Dr. Atkins' New Diet Revolution*, by Robert C. Atkins M.D.)[3]	$13.95	◑	●	◐	○	○	◑	1,520	60	20	11	29	12	6
6 Atkins Induction (*Dr. Atkins' New Diet Revolution*, by Robert C. Atkins M.D.)	$13.95	◑	●	◐	○	○	◑	1,640	61	19	8	31	8	6
Not Rated: Insufficient Study Data (diets listed in alphabetical order)														
7 eDiets	$12–32 per month	—	◉	—	—	—	—	1,450	23	5	53	24	19	12
8 Jenny Craig	$6–7.65 per week, $11–15 per day (food)	—	◉	—	—	—	—	1,520	18	7	62	20	16	6
9 South Beach Phase One (*The South Beach Diet*, by Arthur Agatston M.D.)	$24.95	—	◑	—	—	—	—	1,530	51	14	15	34	9	12
10 South Beach Phase Two (*The South Beach Diet*, by Arthur Agatston M.D.)	$24.95	—	◐	—	—	—	—	1,340	39	9	38	22	19	13
11 Volumetrics (*The Volumetrics Eating Plan*, by Barbara Rolls Ph.D.)	$25.95	—	◉	—	—	—	—	1,500	23	7	55	22	20	14

[1] Except where noted, price is for the book.

[2] Women's menu similar but about 1,300 calories.

[3] Studies of Atkins used first the induction and then the ongoing diet plans, so our 6-month and 1-year results include both phases.

and the National Heart, Lung, and Blood Institute Obesity Education Initiative, recommend going no lower than 1,000 to 1,200 calories a day for women and 1,200 to 1,600 calories for men.

Very Low-Calorie Diets Very low-calorie diets, which provide fewer than 800 calories a day, lead to rapid weight loss but pose serious, potentially deadly health risks. Whenever people cut back drastically on calories, they immediately lose several pounds because of a loss of fluid. As soon as they return to a more normal way of eating, they regain this weight.

On a very low-calorie diet, as much as 50 percent of the weight you lose may be muscle (so you'll actually look flabbier). Because your heart is a muscle, it may become so weak that it no longer can pump blood through your body. In addition, your blood pressure may plummet, causing dizziness, light-headedness, and fatigue. You may develop nausea and abdominal pain. You may lose hair. If you're a woman, your menstrual cycle may become irregular, or you may stop menstruating altogether. As you lose more water, you also lose essential vitamins, and your metabolism slows down. Even reaction time slows, and crash dieters may not be able to respond as quickly as usual.

Once you go off an extreme diet—as you inevitably must—your metabolism remains slow, even though you're no longer restricting your food intake. The human body appears to alter its energy use to compensate for weight loss. These metabolic changes may make it harder for people to maintain a reduced body weight after dieting.

AVOIDING DIET TRAPS

Whatever your eating style, there are only two effective strategies for losing weight: eating less and exercising more. Unfortunately, most people search for easier alternatives that almost invariably turn into dietary dead ends or unexpected dangers (see Savvy Consumer: "How to Spot a Dubious Diet"). Three common traps to avoid are diet pills, diet foods, and the yo-yo syndrome.

The foods you choose at every meal of every day can affect both your weight and your health.

© Radhika Chalasani /Corbis

Diet Pills

In their search for a quick fix to weight problems, millions of people have tried often risky remedies. In the 1920s, some women swallowed patented weight loss capsules that turned out to be tapeworm eggs. In the 1960s and 1970s, addictive amphetamines were common diet aids. In the 1990s, appetite suppressants known as fen-phen became popular. They were taken off the market after being linked to heart valve problems.

The Food and Drug Administration has warned users of the popular herb ephedra (also identified as ephedrine and ma huang and often combined with caffeine) of heart attacks, strokes, and even death. In a meta-analysis of studies conducted on ephedra products for weight loss, researchers concluded that use of high doses of ephedra or ephedra and caffeine for six months or less does promote weight loss—but also takes a toll on physical and mental well-being. Ephedra products are associated with two to three times the normal risk of psychiatric symptoms, upper gastrointestinal symptoms, and heart palpitations.

Diet Foods

According to the Calorie Control Council, 90 percent of Americans choose some foods labeled "light." But even though these foods keep growing in popularity, Americans' weight keeps rising. There are several reasons: Many people think choosing a food that's lower in calories, fat-free, or light gives them a license to eat as much as they want. What they don't realize is that many foods that are low in fat are still high in sugar and calories. Refined carbohydrates, rapidly absorbed into the bloodstream, raise blood glucose levels. As they fall, appetite increases.

Diet products, including diet sodas and low-fat foods, are a very big business. Many people rely on meal replacements, usually shakes or snack bars, to lose or keep off weight. If used appropriately—as actual replacements rather than supplements to regular meals and snacks—they can be a useful strategy for weight loss. Yet people who use these products often gain weight because they think that they can afford to add high-calorie treats to their diets.

What about the artificial sweeteners and fake fats that appear in many diet products? Nutritionists caution to use them in moderation and not to substitute them for basic foods, such as grains, fruits, and vegetables. Foods made with fat substitutes may have fewer grams of fat, but they don't necessarily have significantly fewer calories. Many people who consume reduced-fat, fat-free, or sugar-free sodas, cookies, chips, and other snacks often cut back on more nutritious foods, such as fruits and vegetables. They also tend to eat more of the low- or no-fat foods so that their daily calorie intake either stays the same or actually increases.

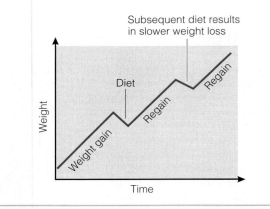

FIGURE 7-10 **Weight-Cycling Effect of Repeated Dieting**
Each round of dieting is typically followed by a rebound leading to a greater weight gain.

The Yo-Yo Syndrome

On-and-off-again dieting, especially by means of very low-calorie diets (under 800 calories a day), can be self-defeating and dangerous. Some studies have shown that weight cycling may make it more difficult to lose weight or keep it off (Figure 7-10). Repeated cycles of rapid weight loss followed by weight gain may even change food preferences. Chronic crash dieters often come to prefer foods that combine sugar and fat, such as cake frosting.

 To avoid the yo-yo syndrome and overcome its negative effects: Exercise. Researchers at the University of Pennsylvania found that when overweight women who also exercised went off a very low-calorie diet, their metabolism did not stay slow but bounced back to the appropriate level for their new, lower body weight. The reason may be exercise's ability to preserve muscle tissue. The more muscle tissue you have, the higher your metabolic rate.

Savvy Consumer ⠿ How to Spot a Dubious Diet

The National Council Against Health Fraud cautions dieters to watch for these warnings of dangerous or fraudulent programs.

⠿ Promises of very rapid weight loss.

⠿ Claims that the diet can eliminate "cellulite" (a term used to describe dimply fatty tissue on the arms and legs).

⠿ "Counselors" who are really salespersons pushing a product or program.

⠿ No mention of any risks associated with the diet.

⠿ Unproven gimmicks, such as body wraps, starch blockers, hormones, diuretics, or "unique" pills or potions.

⠿ No maintenance program.

If you hear about a new diet that promises to melt away fat, don't try it until you get answers to the following questions:

⠿ Does it include a wide variety of nutritious foods?

⠿ Does it provide at least 1,200 calories a day?

⠿ Is it designed to reduce your weight by one-half to two pounds per week?

⠿ Does it emphasize moderate portions?

⠿ Does it use foods that are easy to find and prepare?

⠿ Can you follow it wherever you eat—at home, work, restaurants, or parties?

⠿ Is its cost reasonable?

If the answer to any of these questions is no, don't try the diet; then ask yourself one more question: Is losing weight worth losing your well-being?

If you've been losing (and regaining) the same 5 or 10 pounds for years, try the following suggestions for long-term success:

- **Set a danger zone.** Once you've reached your desired weight, don't let your weight climb more than 3 or 4 pounds higher. Take into account normal fluctuations, but watch out for an upward trend. Once you hit your upper weight limit, take action immediately rather than waiting until you gain 10 pounds.
- **Be patient.** Think of weight loss as a road trip. If you're going across town, you expect to get there in 20 minutes. If your destination is 400 miles away, you know it'll take longer. Give yourself the time you need to lose weight safely and steadily.
- **Try, try again.** Dieters don't usually keep weight off on their first attempt. The people who eventually succeed don't give up. Through trial and error, they find a plan that works for them.

PHYSICAL ACTIVITY

Unplanned daily activity, such as fidgeting or pacing, can make a difference in preventing weight gain. Scientists use the acronym **NEAT**—for **nonexercise activity thermogenesis**—to describe such "nonvolitional" movement and have verified that it can be an effective way of burning calories. In a study of ten lean and ten mildly obese people—all self-confessed couch potatoes—the thinner ones sat an average of two hours less and moved and stood more often than the heavier individuals.[64] Small steps such as taking the stairs for a flight or two or parking farther away can make a difference.[65]

Although physical activity and exercise can prevent weight gain and improve health, usually it does not lead to significant weight loss. However, when combined with diet, exercise ensures that you lose fat rather than muscle and helps keep off excess pounds. Moderate exercise, such as 30 to 60 minutes of daily physical activity, has proved effective in reducing the risk of heart disease and other health threats. Although there are no definitive data, experts generally agree that more exercise—an estimated 60 to 90 minutes daily of moderately intense activity—is necessary to prevent weight gain. Recommending such higher levels of activity to overweight men and women does indeed lead to more exercise—and more lasting weight loss (Table 7-3).

Exercise has other benefits: It increases energy expenditure, builds up muscle tissue, burns off fat stores, and stimulates the immune system. Exercise also may reprogram metabolism so that more calories are burned during and after a workout.

An exercise program designed for both health benefits and weight loss should include both aerobic activity and resistance training. People who start and stick with an exercise program during or after a weight loss program are

TABLE 7-3 CALORIES/HOUR EXPENDED IN SOME COMMON PHYSICAL ACTIVITIES

The second column shows the average number of calories a 154-pound individual will expend by engaging in the activity for 1 hour. The expenditure value encompasses both resting metabolic rate calories and activity expenditure.

Moderate Physical Activity	Approximate Calories/Hr for a 154-lb Person*
Hiking	370
Light gardening/yard work	330
Dancing	330
Golf (walking and carrying clubs)	330
Bicycling (<10 mph)	290
Walking (3.5 mph)	280
Weight lifting (general light workout)	220
Stretching	180

Vigorous Physical Activity	Approximate Calories/Hr for a 154-lb Person*
Running/jogging (5 mph)	590
Bicycling (>10 mph)	590
Swimming (slow freestyle laps)	510
Aerobics	480
Walking (4.5 mph)	460
Heavy yard work (chopping wood)	440
Weight lifting (vigorous effort)	440
Basketball (vigorous)	440

*Calories burned per hour will be higher for persons who weigh more than 154 lb (70 kg) and lower for persons who weigh less.

Source: Adapted from Dietary Guidelines for Americans 2005, USDHHS, USDA, www.healthierus.gov/dietaryguidelines.

consistently more successful in keeping off most of the pounds they've shed.

THE PSYCHOLOGY OF LOSING WEIGHT

Diets change what you eat. Exercise changes body composition, stamina, and strength. But changing your food-related thoughts and behaviors can be the key to lasting weight loss. If you think that you can shed pounds, if you think that you can control what you put in your mouth, if you think that there is a form of exercise that you could enjoy, then you are on your way to reaching your weight loss goals.

WHO'S IN CHARGE?

As discussed in Chapter 2, if you see yourself as having control over your destiny, you have an internal locus of control. And your sense of self-efficacy is the belief in your ability to change and to reach a goal. Feeling in control and self-efficacy go hand in hand. The stronger your faith in yourself, the more energy and persistence you can put into making a change. The opposite is also true, especially for health behaviors.

How do you rate on locus of control and self-efficacy? Read the following questions, and jot down true or false:

1. I am overweight because I eat too much.
2. Weight problems run in my family.
3. Diet pills are my best hope for losing weight.
4. I would keep weight off if I exercised regularly.
5. I wouldn't overeat if I didn't have to cook for my family.
6. Some people are born thin and never have to diet.
7. I lose weight when I eat only diet shakes or prepared foods.
8. I could make time for exercise if I really wanted to.
9. My doctor will make sure I'm at a healthy weight.
10. I'm determined to lose weight, and I know I will.

"True" answers to numbers 1, 4, 8, and 10 indicate that you take responsibility for and see yourself in control of your weight. "True" answers to numbers 2, 3, 5, 6, 7, and 9 suggest that you credit or blame others for your weight. The more that you see external forces as being in charge, the more difficult you will find it to make changes and lose weight permanently.[66]

REACH OUT FOR SUPPORT— REAL AND VIRTUAL

Behind most successful dieters is a friend, spouse, coach, mentor, colleague, support group, or online community. In various studies, dieters with supportive "buddies" were more likely to stick to their diet and workout program and lost more weight.

 If you decide to diet with a roommate, friend, parent, spouse, or coworker, decide on a plan. You might walk or work out together, or check in with each other every evening when you're most prone to overeating. Another alternative is to join a weight loss group, either one that is part of a commercial program or a more informal group that meets on campus or at a church or community center. Support has proved one of the most critical factors in weight management for African-American women.[67]

Every month, an estimated five million Americans log on to commercial websites targeted to dieters. Online dieting is convenient, anonymous, and available around the clock. Some dieters post their weekly weights or before-and-after photos of the way (and weight) they were and how far they've come. Others find support in various blogs and chat groups, where they can commiserate, exchange tales of setbacks and successes, and encourage each other to stay the course. Simply reading diet blogs can help you feel less lonely in your quest.

Although e-dieting is popular, little is known about its usefulness. In a one-year study that compared two groups of women who used either a weight loss manual or eDiets.com, the manual users lost significantly more than those who used the Internet.[68] Other studies suggest that interactive online programs that provide diet and fitness advice are more effective than sites offering support alone.

Your Life Coach

Get a Grip on Emotional Eating

Occasionally all of us seek comfort at the tip of a spoon. However, many people use food as a way of coping with anger, frustration, stress, boredom, or fatigue. Whatever its motivation, emotional eating always involves eating for reasons other than physiological hunger. If you're not sure whether you do this, ask yourself the following questions:

- Do you eat when you're not hungry?
- Do you eat or continue eating even if the food doesn't taste good?
- Do you eat when you can't think of anything else to do?
- Do you eat when you're emotionally vulnerable—tired, frustrated, or worried?
- Do you eat after an argument or stressful situation to calm down?
- Do you eat as one of your favorite ways of enjoying yourself?
- Do you eat to reward yourself?
- Do you keep eating even after you're full?

If you answer yes to more than three of these, you're eating in response to what you feel, not what you need. Diets may work for you, but the extra weight will inevitably creep back unless you confront your hidden motives for overeating. Since neither emotions nor food ever go away, you have to learn to deal with both for as long as you live.

To get a grip on your emotional eating, try this three-step plan:

STEP 1: KNOW YOUR TRIGGERS

Whatever its specific motivation, emotional eating always involves eating for reasons other than physiological hunger. The key to getting it under control is awareness.

What are the feelings that set off an eating binge?

- **Anger?** Many people, especially women, swallow their anger by eating because they're afraid of what might happen if they express it.

- **Guilt?** Some people eat because they feel they're always falling short as children, partners, or parents.

- **Rebellion?** Eating may be the only way some people give themselves permission to take a break from being dutiful.

- **Deprivation?** At the end of a long day, a person may justify turning to food as a well-deserved reward, maybe the first nice thing done for herself or himself all day.

Did any of these possibilities hit home? If so, train yourself to take a step back and ask yourself a series of questions before you take a bite: Are you hungry? If not, what are you feeling? Stressed, tired, bored, anxious, sad, happy? Once you identify your true feeling, push deeper and ask why you feel this way. Try writing down your answers in a notebook. This is an even more effective way to help make sure that every bite you take is a conscious one.

STEP 2: PUT YOUR BODY, NOT YOUR EMOTIONS, IN CHARGE OF WHAT YOU EAT.

To keep mind and body on an even keel, avoid getting so hungry and feeling so deprived that you become desperate and panicky. If you're facing an emotionally intense period—exam week or a visit from an ornery relative—plan your meals and snacks in advance and try, as much as you can, to stick with your program. Rather than swearing off sweets forever, work indulgences into your weekly routine. If you plan to have a brownie for dessert on Friday night, you can look forward to it all week and not waste calories on a candy bar that won't taste as good.

STEP 3: FOCUS ON YOUR FEELINGS

Let yourself feel how you're feeling without eating. Breathe deeply for a minute or two. Focus on the places in your body that feel tense. Rate the intensity of the emotion on a scale from ten (life or death) to one (truly trivial). Ask yourself: What's the worst-case scenario of feeling this way? Is food going to make it better in any way? Will it make it worse?

When you're tempted to eat but aren't hungry, write down the circumstances and try to discern the underlying reasons. If you eat cookies at night, ask, What does it get me? The answer might be that it relaxes you. Once you realize that the cookies are a means to an end, you can figure out something else you can do to get the same emotional benefits.

MAINTAINING WEIGHT LOSS

Surveys of people who lost significant amounts of weight and kept it off for several years show that most did so on their own—without medication, meal substitutes, or membership in an organized weight loss group. When a National Institutes of Health panel reviewed 48 separate weight loss trials, they found that participants lost about 8 percent of their body weight on average and kept it off.

Rather than focusing on why dieters fail, the creators of the National Weight Control Registry study the habits and lifestyles of those who've maintained a weight loss of at least 30 pounds for at least a year. The nearly 4,000 people in the registry have averaged a weight loss of 66 pounds, which they've kept off for 5.5 years.[69]

No one diet or commercial weight loss program helped all these formerly fat individuals. Many, through years of trial and error, eventually came up with a permanent exercise and eating program that worked for them. Despite the immense variety, their customized approaches share certain characteristics:

- **Personal responsibility for change.** Weight loss winners develop an internal locus of control. Rather than blaming others for their weight problem or relying on a doctor or trainer to fix it, they believe that the keys to a healthy weight lie within themselves.

© Rick Gomez / Masterfile

Vigilance helps keep weight off. If the number on the scale creeps upward, take action.

▪ **Exercise.** Registry members report an hour of moderate physical activity almost every day. Their favorite exercise? Three in four say walking, followed by cycling, weight lifting, aerobics, running, and stair climbing. On average, they burn about 2,545 calories per week through physical activity.

▪ **Monitoring.** About 44 percent of registry members count calories, and almost all keep track of their food intake in some way, written or not.

▪ **Vigilance.** Rather than avoiding the scale or telling themselves their jeans shrunk in the wash, successful losers keep tabs on their weight and size. About a third check the scale every week. If the scale notches upward or their waistbands start to pinch, they take action.

▪ **Breakfast.** Your mother probably told you that breakfast is the most important meal of the day, and 40 years of breakfast-related studies, as well as the experience of registry members, have proved her right. A morning meal improves concentration and problem-solving ability, boosts energy levels, and helps control weight. Regular breakfast skippers are four times more likely to be obese than those who eat a morning meal.

TREATING SEVERE OBESITY

The biggest Americans are getting bigger. The prevalence of severe or "morbid" obesity is increasing faster than obesity itself. The number of extremely obese adults—those at least 100 pounds overweight with BMIs over 40—has quadrupled in the last two decades from 1 in 200 to about 1 in every 50 men and women. The number with BMIs greater than 50 has jumped from 1 in 2,000 in the 1980s to 1 in 400.

 Extreme obesity poses extreme danger to health and survival and undermines quality of life. White women report more impairment than men or African-American women, even when they have lower BMIs.[70] Severe obesity also has a profound effect on every aspect of an adolescent's life.

DRUG THERAPY

Obesity medications are recommended only for patients with BMIs equal to or greater than 30 or those with a BMI equal to or greater than 27 with risk factors (like high blood pressure) that increase their risk of disease. Researchers are experimenting with other medications, such as the epilepsy drug zonisamide, to enhance weight loss. Currently, only two weight loss drugs are FDA approved.

Xenical (orlistat) blocks fat absorption by the gut but also inhibits absorption of water and vitamins in some patients and may cause cramping and diarrhea. It produces a weight loss of 2 to 3 percent of initial weight beyond the weight lost by dieting over the course of a year.

Meridia (sibutramine) is in the same chemical class as amphetamines and works by suppressing appetite. It also may increase blood pressure, heart rate, or both. Other side effects include headache, insomnia, dry mouth, and constipation. Patients taking these drugs generally lose less than 10 percent of their body weight, and many regain weight after they stop treatment.

OBESITY SURGERY

Gastric, or bariatric, surgery is recommended only for individuals whose BMIs are higher than 40 or who have BMIs of 35 along with severe health complications. The most common operation uses bands or staples to section off a small portion of the stomach. A small outlet, about the size of a pencil eraser, is left at the bottom of the stomach pouch. Since the outlet is small, food stays in the pouch longer so people feel full for a longer time.

The number of Americans having weight loss surgery has more than quadrupled since 1998.[71] About 80 percent of patients lose some weight; 30 percent reach a normal BMI. The long-term weight loss success rate is 40 to 63 percent of excess body weight over a three-year period and 50 to 60 percent after five years.[72] Besides weight loss, bariatric surgery also eliminates or improves diabetes, high blood pressure, high cholesterol, and obstructive sleep apnea.[73]

Possible complications include leaking of stomach juices into the abdomen, injury to the spleen, slippage or erosion of the band, breakdown of the staple line, and the stomach pouch stretching from overeating. Up to 25 percent of patients may require reoperation within five years. Serious infection or death has been reported in fewer than 1 percent of patients.

UNHEALTHY EATING BEHAVIOR

Unhealthy eating behavior takes many forms, ranging from not eating enough to eating too much too quickly. Its roots are complex. In addition to media and external pressures, family history can play a role. Researchers have linked specific genes to some cases of anorexia nervosa and binge eating, but most believe that a variety of factors, including stress and culture, combine to cause disordered eating.

 About a third of female athletes in every sport show symptoms of disordered eating or eating disorders. Girls and adolescent females who participate regularly in sports are at risk for disordered eating, menstrual dysfunction, and decreased bone mineral density, according to the American Academy of Pediatrics. The combination of these three disorders is known as the *female athlete triad*.

Sooner or later many people don't eat the way they should. They may skip meals, thereby increasing the likelihood that they'll end up with more body fat, a higher weight, and a higher blood cholesterol level. They may live on diet foods, but consume so much of them that they gain weight anyway. Some even engage in more extreme eating behavior: Dissatisfied with almost all aspects of their appearance, they continuously go on and off diets, eat compulsively, or binge on high-fat treats. Such behaviors can be warning signs of potentially serious eating disorders that should not be ignored.

DISORDERED EATING IN COLLEGE STUDENTS

College students—particularly women, including varsity athletes—are at risk for unhealthy eating behaviors. While some college students have full-blown eating disorders, many others develop "partial syndromes" and experience symptoms that are not severe or numerous enough for a diagnosis of anorexia nervosa or bulimia nervosa. Distress over body image increases the risk of all forms of disordered eating in college women.[74]

 In a survey at a large, public, rural university in the mid-Atlantic states, 17 percent of the women were struggling with disordered eating. Younger women (ages 18 to 21) were more likely than older students to have an eating disorder. In this study, eating disorders did not discriminate, equally affecting women of different races (white, Asian, African American, Native American, and Hispanic), religions, athletic involvement, and living arrangements (on or off campus; with roommates, boyfriends, or family). Although the students viewed eating disorders as both mental and physical problems and felt that individual therapy would be most helpful, all said that they would first turn to a friend for help.

In another study of 1,620 students, almost 11 percent of the women and 4 percent of the men were at risk for eating disorders. About 17 percent of the women and 10 percent of the men said concerns about weight interfered with their academic work. Women in sororities were at slightly increased risk of an eating disorder compared with those in dormitories.

In a study of Australian male undergraduates, one in four men worried about shape and weight; one in five displayed attitudes and behaviors characteristic of disordered eating and eating disorders. None ever sought treatment, even if the students recognized they had a problem. The reason, the researchers theorized, may be that the young men hesitated to seek treatment for an illness stigmatized as a problem that affects only women. Some men exercised extremely intensively almost every day, even if ill or injured. None felt they had a problem with excessive exercise.[75]

EXTREME DIETING

About half of girls attempt to control their weight by dieting. In a year-long study of teenagers, both parents and the media had the most influence on the development of weight concerns and weight control practices, including dieting, among adolescents and preadolescents.

Extreme dieters go beyond cutting back on calories or increasing physical activity. They become preoccupied with what they eat and weigh. Although their weight never falls below 85 percent of normal, their weight loss is severe enough to cause uncomfortable physical consequences, such as weakness and sensitivity to cold. Technically, these dieters do not have anorexia nervosa (discussed later in the chapter), but they are at increased risk for it.

Extreme dieters may think they know a great deal about nutrition, yet many of their beliefs about food and weight are misconceptions or myths. For instance, they may eat only protein because they believe complex carbohydrates, including fruits and breads, are fattening.

Sometimes nutritional education alone can help change this eating pattern. However, many avid dieters who deny that they have a problem with food may need counseling (which they usually agree to only at their family's insistence) to correct dangerous eating behavior and prevent further complications.

COMPULSIVE OVEREATING

People who eat compulsively cannot stop putting food in their mouths. They eat fast and they eat a lot. They eat even when they're full. They may eat around the clock rather than at set meal times, often in private because of embarrassment over how much they consume.

Some mental health professionals describe compulsive eating as a food addiction that is much more likely to develop in women. According to Overeaters Anonymous (OA), an international 12-step program, many women who eat compulsively view food as a source of comfort against feelings of inner emptiness, low self-esteem, and fear of abandonment.

The following behaviors may signal a potential problem with compulsive overeating:

- **Turning to food** when depressed or lonely, when feeling rejected, or as a reward
- **A history of failed diets** and anxiety when dieting
- **Thinking about food** throughout the day
- **Eating quickly** and without pleasure
- **Continuing to eat** even when you're no longer hungry
- **Frequently talking about food,** or refusing to talk about food
- **Fear of not being able to stop** eating once you start

Recovery from compulsive eating can be challenging because people with this problem cannot give up entirely the substance they abuse. Like everyone else, they must eat. However, they can learn new eating habits and ways of dealing with underlying emotional problems. An OA survey found that most of its members joined to lose weight but later felt the most important effect was their improved emotional, mental, and physical health. As one woman put it, "I came for vanity but stayed for sanity."

BINGE EATING

Binge eating—the rapid consumption of an abnormally large amount of food in a relatively short time—often occurs in compulsive eaters. The 25 million Americans with a binge-eating disorder typically eat a larger than ordinary amount of food during a relatively brief period, feel a lack of control over eating, and binge at least twice a week for at least a six-month period.[76] During most of these episodes, binge eaters experience at least three of the following:

- **Eating much more rapidly** than usual
- **Eating until they feel uncomfortably full**
- **Eating large amounts of food** when not feeling physically hungry
- **Eating large amounts of food** throughout the day with no planned mealtimes
- **Eating alone** because they are embarrassed by how much they eat and by their eating habits

Binge eaters may spend up to several hours eating, and consume 2,000 or more calories worth of food in a single binge—more than many people eat in a day. After such binges, they usually do not induce vomiting, use laxatives, or rely on other means (such as exercise) to control weight. They simply get fatter. As their weight climbs, they become depressed, anxious, or troubled by other psychological symptoms to a much greater extent than others of comparable weight.

Binge eating is probably the most common eating disorder. An estimated 8 to 19 percent of obese patients in weight loss programs are binge eaters.

EATING DISORDERS

According to the American Psychiatric Association, patients with **eating disorders** display a broad range of symptoms that occur along a continuum between those of anorexia nervosa and those of bulimia nervosa.

As many as 10 percent of teenage girls develop symptoms of or full-blown eating disorders. Among the factors that increase the risk are preoccupation with a thin body; social pressure; and childhood traits such as perfectionism and excessive cautiousness, which can reflect an obsessive-compulsive personality. Teenage girls who diet and have four specific risk factors—a high BMI, menarche (first menstruation) before sixth grade, extreme concern with weight or shape, and teasing by peers—are most likely to have an eating disorder.[77]

The best known eating disorders are anorexia nervosa, which affects fewer than 1 percent of adolescent women, and bulimia nervosa, which strikes 2 to 3 percent. The American Psychiatric Association has developed practice guidelines for the treatment of patients with eating disorders, which include medical, psychological, and behavioral approaches.[78] One of the most scientifically supported is cognitive-behavior therapy.

If you occasionally go on eating binges, use the behavioral technique called *habit reversal,* and replace your bingeing with a competing behavior. For example, every time you're tempted to binge, immediately do something—text-message a friend, play solitaire, check your e-mail—that keeps food out of your mouth.

If you binge twice a week or more for at least a six-month period, you may have binge-eating disorder, which can require professional help. Treatment usually consists of cognitive-behavioral therapy, either individually or in a group setting. As chronic binge eaters recognize their unhealthy behavior and confront the underlying issues, they usually are able to stop bingeing and resume normal eating patterns.

(FAQ) WHO DEVELOPS EATING DISORDERS?

Eating disorders affect an estimated 5 to 10 million women and 1 million men. Despite past evidence that eating disorders were primarily problems for white women, they are increasing among men and members of different ethnic and racial groups.

 In the few studies of eating disorders in minority college students that have been completed, African-American female undergraduates had a slightly lower prevalence of eating disorders than whites. Asian Americans reported fewer symptoms of eating disorders but more body dissatisfaction, concerns about shape, and more intense efforts to lose weight.

In a survey of health-care professionals at the country's largest colleges and universities, 69 percent

---

Strategies for Prevention ▪▪ Do You Have an Eating Disorder?

Physicians have developed a simple screening test for eating disorders, consisting of the following questions:

- Do you make yourself sick because you feel uncomfortably full?
- Do you worry you have lost control over how much you eat?

- Have you recently lost more than 14 pounds in a three-month period?
- Do you believe yourself to be fat when others say you are too thin?
- Would you say that food dominates your life?

Score one point for every "yes." A score of two or more is a likely indication of anorexia nervosa or bulimia nervosa.

Source: Miller, Karl. "Treatment Guideline for Eating Disorders." *American Family Physician,* Vol. 62, No. 1, July 1, 2000.

have professionals on staff who specialize in diagnosing and treating eating disorders. Of all the hurdles to helping students with eating disorders, 39 percent said denial is the biggest, while 24 percent felt it was unwillingness to seek treatment, and 20 percent blamed pressure from peers and the media to stay thin.

 Eating disorders affect every aspect of college students' lives, including dating. Both men and women tend to avoid dating individuals with eating disorders, but men are far less accepting of obesity than women.

Male and female athletes are vulnerable to eating disorders, either because of the pressure to maintain ideal body weight or to achieve a weight that might enhance their performance. Many female athletes, particularly those participating in sports or activities that emphasize leanness (such as gymnastics, distance running, diving, figure skating, and classical ballet) have subclinical eating disorders that could undermine their nutritional status and energy levels. However, there is often little awareness or recognition of their disordered eating.

If someone you know has an eating disorder, let your friend know you're concerned and that you care. Don't criticize or make fun of his or her eating habits. Encourage your friend to talk about other problems and feelings, and suggest that he or she talk to the school counselor or someone at the mental health center, the family doctor, or another trusted adult. Offer to go along if you think that will make a difference.

ANOREXIA NERVOSA

Although *anorexia* means "loss of appetite," most individuals with **anorexia nervosa** are, in fact, hungry all the time. For them, food is an enemy—a threat to their sense of self, identity, and autonomy. In the distorted mirror of their mind's eye, they see themselves as fat or flabby even at a normal or below-normal body weight. Some simply feel fat; others think that they are thin in some places and too fat in others, such as the abdomen, buttocks, or thighs.

The characteristics of anorexia nervosa include:

▪ A refusal to maintain normal body weight (weight loss leading to body weight of less than 85 percent of that expected for age and height).

▪ An intense fear of gaining weight or becoming fat, even though underweight.

▪ A distorted body image so that the person feels fat even when emaciated.

▪ In women, the absence of at least three menstrual cycles.

The incidence of anorexia nervosa has increased in the last three decades in most developed countries. The peak ages for its onset are 14½ and 18 years. According to the American Psychiatric Association's Work Group on Eating Disorders, cases are increasing among males, minorities, women of all ages, and possibly preteens. About 1 percent of American women develop anorexia.[79]

In the *restricting* type of anorexia, individuals lose weight by avoiding any fatty foods, and by dieting, fasting, and exercising. Some start smoking as a way of controlling their weight. In the *binge-eating/purging* type, they engage in binge eating, purging (through self-induced vomiting, laxatives, diuretics, or enemas), or both. Obsessed with an intense fear of fatness, they may weigh themselves several times a day, measure various parts of their body, check mirrors to see if they look fat, and try on different items of clothing to see if they feel tight.

What Causes Anorexia Nervosa?

Many complex factors interact and contribute to this disorder, including biological, psychological, and social ones. Anorexia is more common among close relatives, particularly sisters, than it is in the general population. The relatives of anorexics also have a higher than expected frequency of depressive disorders.

Anorexia is associated with changes within the brain, including abnormalities in the stress-hormone cortisol, the neurotransmitters dopamine, serotonin, and norepinephrine—all of which influence appetite and satiety. Brain chemistry returns to normal after treatment and recovery.[80]

Anorexia also may be a response to a personal loss or a sign of a driven, perfectionist personality. Often young anorexics have above-average grades and an unwarranted fear of failure. Some theorists speculate that young teenage girls may starve themselves because of fear of their budding sexuality. By drastically reducing their weight, they can prevent or stop menstruation and breast development.

Girls who develop anorexia often have little insight or awareness of their feelings, needs, and wants. After years of reacting to the expectations of others, they may feel inadequate as they approach the age of independence. In some ways, starvation may serve as a way of creating an identity and asserting independence.

 In one study that followed 21 college women with eating disorders for six years, 11 got better during their postcollege years, while 10 continued to struggle with disordered eating. The major difference between the two groups revolved around issues of autonomy and relation. Those who could better negotiate the tension between being independent and relating to others had higher self-esteem, a more positive self-concept, and a healthier relationship with food.

About one-third of those with anorexia initially were mildly overweight and cut back on food just to lose a few pounds. Others had normal weights but began to diet to look more attractive or, in the case of male and female athletes and dancers, to gain a performance advantage. Sometimes illness, stress, or surgery triggers weight loss. Often the initial response to their weight loss—from parents, coaches, or friends—is positive. However, starvation seems to take on a life of its own, and anorexics cannot return to a healthy eating pattern. In time, they may place so much

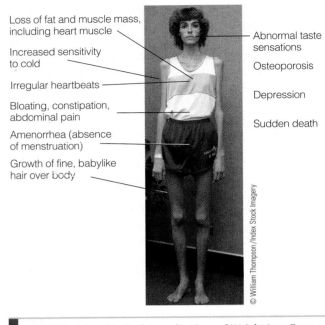

Loss of fat and muscle mass, including heart muscle

Increased sensitivity to cold

Irregular heartbeats

Bloating, constipation, abdominal pain

Amenorrhea (absence of menstruation)

Growth of fine, babylike hair over body

Abnormal taste sensations

Osteoporosis

Depression

Sudden death

© William Thompson /Index Stock Imagery

FIGURE 7-11 Medical Complications of Weight Loss From Anorexia Nervosa.

value on thinness that they cannot recognize the dangers to their health.

Health Dangers and Treatment

The medical consequences of anorexia nervosa are serious (Figure 7-11). Menstrual periods stop in women; testosterone levels decline in men. Adolescents with this disorder do not undergo normal sexual maturation, such as breast development, and may not reach their anticipated height. Even individuals who look and feel reasonably healthy may have subtle or hidden abnormalities, including heart irregularities and arrhythmias that can increase their risk of sudden death. Women who do not menstruate for six months or more may develop osteoporosis and suffer irreversible weakening and thinning of their bones as a result.

Even when they realize that they are jeopardizing their health, people with anorexia tend to fear that treatment will make them worse—that is, fatter. They need repeated reassurance that they will not become overweight and that they can and will find healthier ways of coping with life.

According to current practice guidelines, treatment of anorexia nervosa includes medical therapy (such as "refeeding" to overcome malnutrition) and behavioral, cognitive, psychodynamic, and family therapy. Antidepressant medication sometimes can help, particularly when there is a personal or family history of depression. Most people who get help do return to normal weight, but it can take a long time for their eating behaviors to become normal and for them to deal with troubling body image issues. In a study that followed 95 patients with anorexia, about half—56 percent—had no symptoms of an eating disorder after five years; three had died.

BULIMIA NERVOSA

Individuals with **bulimia nervosa** go on repeated eating binges and rapidly consume large amounts of food, usually sweets, stopping only because of severe abdominal pain or sleep, or because they are interrupted. Those with *purging* bulimia induce vomiting or take large doses of laxatives to relieve guilt and control their weight. In *nonpurging* bulimia, individuals use other means, such as fasting or excessive exercise, to compensate for binges.

The characteristics of bulimia nervosa include:

- Repeated binge eating.
- A feeling of lack of control over eating behavior.
- Regular reliance on self-induced vomiting, laxatives, or diuretics.
- Strict dieting or fasting, or vigorous exercise, to prevent weight gain.
- A minimum average of two bingeing episodes a week for at least three months.
- A preoccupation with body shape and weight.

An estimated 1 to 3 percent of adolescent and young American women develop bulimia. Some experiment with bingeing and purging for a few months and then stop when they change their social or living situation. Others develop longer-term bulimia. Among males, this disorder is about one-tenth as common. The average age for developing bulimia is 18.

What Causes Bulimia Nervosa?

Bulimia usually begins after a rigid diet that lasted from several weeks to a year or more. Strict dieting may affect brain chemistry in such a way as to disrupt the normal mechanisms for appetite and satiety. Semi-starvation eventually sets off a binge; bingeing leads to purging. Once dieters realize that vomiting reduces the anxiety triggered by gorging, they no longer fear overeating. When this happens, bingeing may become more frequent and severe until, in time, it becomes an all-purpose way of coping with stress. However, the driving force in this disorder may not be the overeating but the vomiting or laxative use. If individuals felt they couldn't get rid of food, they might not overeat.

Obesity in adolescence may increase the likelihood of bulimia in adulthood. Extremely obese individuals may lose weight by vomiting and not want to stop because they fear regaining it. Sometimes bulimia develops after recovery from anorexia. Purging becomes an alternative way of staying thin.

As with anorexia, bulimia is associated with changes in brain chemistry, particularly low levels of the peptide cholescystokinin, which produces feelings of satiety. The cycle of bingeing and purging seems to wreak havoc on the biological controls that keep weight at a certain level.

Family conflicts, life stresses such as going away to school, and struggles with the transition to independent adulthood also may play a role. Bulimia also may be a symptom of depression. About 20 to 30 percent of those with this problem are chronically depressed; others have a history of

Abnormal levels of crucial chemicals

Inflammation of the salivary glands

Erosion of the esophagus and stomach

Severe abdominal pain

Erosion and decay of dental enamel, particularly
of front teeth

Fatigue and weakness

Seizures

© Michael Newman/PhotoEdit

FIGURE 7-12 Medical Complications Related to Purging.

depressive episodes. Bulimic individuals also are more likely to experience other problems, including anxiety disorders, substance abuse, and impulse disorders, such as shoplifting (kleptomania) and cutting themselves. A significant percentage of bulimics—from a quarter to a half, by some estimates—may have been victims of incest, sexual molestation, or rape, but this correlation is controversial.

Bulimia may continue for many years, with binges alternating with periods of normal eating. Physiological consequences are cumulative (Figure 7-12). Often dentists are the first to detect bulimia because they notice damage to teeth and gums, including erosion of the enamel from the stomach acids in vomit. Repeated vomiting can lead to other complications as it robs the body of essential nutrients and fluids, causes dehydration and electrolyte imbalances, and impairs the ability of the heart and other muscles to function. Bulimia can trigger cardiac arrhythmias and, occasionally, sudden death.

Cognitive-behavioral therapy (discussed in Chapter 3) has proved more effective than other psychological approaches.[81] Antidepressant medications such as fluoxetine (Prozac) increase levels of the neurotransmitter serotonin and can also help. About 70 percent of those who complete treatment programs reduce their bingeing and purging, although flareups are common in times of stress.

Learn It / Live It

Managing Your Weight

No diet—high-protein, low-fat, or high-carbohydrate—can produce permanent weight loss. Successful weight management, the American Dietetic Association has concluded, "requires a lifelong commitment to healthful lifestyle behaviors emphasizing sustainable and enjoyable eating practices and daily physical activity."[82] Studies have shown that successful dieters are highly motivated, monitor their food intake, increase their activity, set realistic goals, and receive social support from others. Another key to long-term success is tailoring any weight loss program to an individual's gender, lifestyle, and cultural, racial, and ethnic values.

Here are some practical guidelines.

- **Be realistic.** Trying to shrink to an impossibly low weight dooms you to defeat. Start off slowly and make steady progress. If your weight creeps up 5 pounds, go back to the basics of your program. Take into account normal fluctuations, but watch out for an upward trend. If you let your weight continue to creep up, it may not stop until you have a serious weight problem—again.

- **Recognize that there are no quick fixes.** Ultimately, quick-loss diets are very damaging physically and psychologically because when you stop dieting and put the pounds back on, you feel like a failure.

- **Note your progress.** Make a graph, with your initial weight as the base, to indicate your progress. View plateaus or occasional gains as temporary setbacks rather than disasters.

- **Adopt the 90 percent rule.** If you practice eating habits 90 percent of the time, a few cretions won't make a difference. In effe should allow for occasional cheating. don't have to feel guilty about it.

- **Look for joy and meaning b food life.** Make your perso relationships your priorit fuel that allows you to 1

- **Try, try again.** Rem keep weight off on who eventually succee they find the plan that wo

Self Survey ░░ Are You Ready to Lose Weight?

As discussed in Chapter 2, people change the way they behave stage by stage and step by step. The same is true for changing behaviors related to weight. If you need to lose excess pounds, knowing your stage of readiness for change is a crucial first step. Here is a guide to identifying where you are right now.

If you are still in the *precontemplation* stage, you don't think of yourself as having a weight problem, even though others may. If you can't fit into some of your clothes, you blame the dry cleaners. Or you look around and think, "I'm no bigger than anyone else in this class." Unconsciously, you may feel helpless to do anything about your weight. So you deny or dismiss its importance.

In the *contemplation* stage, you would prefer not to have to change, but you can't avoid reality. Your coach or doctor may comment on your weight. You wince at the vacation photos of you in a swimsuit. You look in the mirror, try to suck in your stomach, and say, "I've got to do something about my weight."

In the *preparation* stage, you're gearing up by taking small but necessary steps. You may buy athletic shoes or check out several diet books from the library. Maybe you experiment with some minor changes, such as having fruit instead of cookies for an afternoon snack. Internally, you are getting accustomed to the idea of change.

In the *action* stage of change, you are deliberately working to lose weight. You no longer snack all evening long. You stick to a specific diet and track calories, carbs, or points. You hop on a treadmill or stationary bike for 30 minutes a day. Your resolve is strong, and you know you're on your way to a thinner, healthier you.

In the *maintenance* stage, you strengthen, enhance, and extend the changes you've made. Whether or not you have lost all the weight you want, you've made significant progress. As you continue to watch what you eat and to be physically active, you lock-in healthy new habits.

Where are you right now? Read each of the following statements and decide which best applies to you.

1. I never think about my weight.	Precontemplation Stage
2. I'm trying to zip up a pair of jeans and wondering when was the last time they fit.	Contemplation Stage
3. I'm downloading a food diary to keep track of what I eat.	Preparation Stage
4. I have been following a diet for three weeks and have started working out.	Action Stage
5. I have been sticking to a diet and engaging in regular physical activity for at least six months.	Maintenance Stage

YOUR ACTION PLAN FOR LOSING WEIGHT

Here is a guide to strategies most likely to help you at your particular stage of readiness to change.

Precontemplation (not active and not thinking about becoming active)

▪ **Set a small, reasonable goal** that does not involve working up a sweat, such as standing rather than sitting when blow-drying your hair or doing squats while brushing your teeth.

▪ **Start paying attention** to what, when, where, and why you eat. Take note of the times you eat or continue eating even though you're not hungry.

▌ **List what you see** as the cons of physical activity. For example, do you fear it will take up too much time? Write down three activities you could do if you woke up half an hour earlier.

Contemplation (not active but thinking about becoming active)

▌ **Think back to activities** you found enjoyable in the past. Did you ever try inline skating? Play softball? Row? Ask friends if they can put you in touch with others with the same interest.

▌ **Start drinking more water.** Get used to the idea of ending every meal with water to wash away the taste of what you've eaten and signal that you've stopped putting food in your mouth.

▌ **Determine the types of activity** you can realistically fit into your daily schedule. If you have classes and work most of the day, sign up for an evening body-sculpting or spinning class.

▌ **Find an image of the slimmer body** you'd like to have—from a magazine advertisement, for example—and post it where you can see it often.

Preparation (active but not at recommended levels)

▌ **Record everything you put in your mouth.** List calories and carbs next to each entry. Also describe how you feel as you eat.

▌ **Set specific daily and weekly action-oriented goals.** Your daily goal might begin with 10 or 15 minutes of activity and increase by 5 minutes every week or two. Your weekly goal might be to try a new activity, such as kick-boxing or a dance class.

▌ **Document your progress.** You could use a monthly calendar to keep track of the number of days you've exercised as well as the length of each workout. Or you can keep a more detailed record, noting the types of exercise you do every day, the intensity you work at, the duration of each workout, and so forth.

Action and Maintenance (active at recommended levels for less than six months)

▌ **Find new comfort foods.** Good options include air-popped popcorn, chocolate fruit sundaes (fresh fruit with a spoonful of rich syrup), hot chocolate (with skim milk), and fudgsicles (creamy but low in calories).

▌ **Avoid boredom.** Think through ways to vary your exercise routine. Take different routes on your walks. Invite different friends to join you. Alternate working with free weights with resistance machines at the gym.

▌ **Develop new athletic and sports skills.** Try snowshoeing, kayaking, rock climbing, hiphop dancing. Don't expect instant expertise. It usually takes four to six weeks to feel competent and get in the swing of a new activity.

Don't expect to progress through these stages just once. Most people "recycle" several times before a change becomes permanent. Whether you're moving forward or have temporarily fallen back, remember that change is a journey that happens step by step, meal by meal, day by day, stage by stage.

CASE IN POINT

Student: Evan, 20

Goal: Lose the 13 pounds he's put on since starting college

Action Plan:

▌ Keep a diary of everything he puts in his mouth for a week.

▌ Set a daily goal for being active, starting with 10 or 15 minutes a day.

▌ Start reading the nutrition information on foods served in the dining hall.

▌ Sip on bottled water instead of soda when he studies.

▌ Hang the "skinny" jeans he used to wear in high school where he can see them every day.

Health☯Now™   If you want to write your own goals for weight management, go to the **Wellness Journal** at HealthNow http://healthnow.brookscole .com/ith.

Making This Chapter Work for You

Review Questions

1. Which of the following statements is true?
   a. Obesity is a problem only in industrialized countries.
   b. Obesity is a problem that starts in middle age.
   c. The southern states have the highest percentage of people who are obese.
   d. If you were heavy as a child, you will always be obese.

2. If you are a healthy weight,
   a. you are always hungry.
   b. your BMI is between 18.5 and 24.9.
   c. your waist measurement is 25 to 28 inches.
   d. your waist-to-hip ratio is greater than 1.0.

3. The health dangers of excess weight include all of the following *except*
   a. increased risk of type 2 diabetes, heart disease, and cancer.
   b. increased risk of impaired immunity.
   c. increased risk of auto accidents.
   d. increased risk of dying prematurely.

4. If you have gone online to check out weight-reduction support groups in your area, which stage of readiness for weight behavior change are you in?
   a. precontemplation stage
   b. contemplation stage
   c. preparation stage
   d. action stage

5. Which of the following statements is *incorrect?*
   a. I can lose weight successfully on a low-carbohydrate diet.
   b. I can lose weight successfully on a low-fat diet.
   c. I can lose weight successfully on a low-calorie diet.
   d. I can lose weight successfully by working out once a week.

6. Successful weight management strategies include which of the following?
   a. Learn to distinguish between actual and emotional hunger.
   b. Ask friends for recommendations for methods that helped them to lose weight quickly.
   c. Practice good eating habits 50 percent of the time so that you can balance your cravings with healthy food.
   d. Look at celebrity photos and pick one for a model.

7. Which of the following statements is true?
   a. Very low-calorie diets increase metabolism, which helps burn calories more quickly.
   b. An individual eating low-calorie or fat-free foods can increase the serving sizes.

   c. Low-carbohydrate diets have been shown safe over the short term but long-term studies have not been completed.
   d. Yo-yo dieting works best for long-term weight loss.

8. Which of the following eating behaviors may be a warning sign of a serious eating disorder?
   a. vegetarianism
   b. compulsive food washing
   c. binge eating
   d. weight gain during the first year of college

9. Individuals with anorexia nervosa
   a. believe they are overweight even if they are extremely thin.
   b. typically feel full all the time, which limits their food intake.
   c. usually look overweight, even though their body mass index is normal.
   d. have a reduced risk for heart-related abnormalities.

10. Bulimia nervosa is
   a. characterized by excessive sleeping followed by periods of insomnia.
   b. found primarily in older women who are concerned with the aging process.
   c. associated with the use of laxatives or excessive exercise to control weight.
   d. does not have serious health consequences.

Answers to these questions can be found on page 587.

Critical Thinking

1. In a poll conducted by *Time*/ABC, 87 percent of respondents said that individual Americans bore a "great deal of responsibility" for the nation's obesity problem because of their choice of diet and lack of exercise, while 64 percent identified fast-food restaurants and schools that allow high-calorie snacks and sweets. Where do you think the responsibility lies? Why?

2. Do you think you have a weight problem? If so, what makes you think so? Is your perception based on your actual BMI measurement or on how you believe you look? If you found out that your BMI was within the ideal range, would that change your opinion about your body? Why or why not?

3. Suppose one of your roommates appears to have symptoms of an eating disorder. You have told him or her of your concerns, but your roommate has denied having a problem and brushed off your fears. What can you do to help this individual? Should you contact his or her parent? Why or why not?

Media Menu

Health Now™

Throughout the chapter, this icon introduces a list of resources on the Health-Now website at **http://healthnow.brookscole.com/ith** that will:
- Help you evaluate your knowledge of the material.
- Allow you to take an exam-prep quiz.
- Provide a Personalized Learning Plan targeting resources that address areas you should study.
- Coach you through identifying target goals for behavior change and creating and monitoring your personal change plan throughout the semester.

INTERNET CONNECTIONS

American Obesity Association

www.obesity.org

The American Obesity Association is the leading organization for advocacy and education on the nation's obesity epidemic. This comprehensive website features statistics on overweight and obesity in the United States, research articles, consumer protection links, prevention topics, library resources, fact sheets on a variety of weight management topics, and more.

Weight Control Information Network

http://win.niddk.nih.gov/index.htm

This government-sponsored web site features a variety of publications on nutrition, physical activity and weight control for the general public and for health care professionals in English and Spanish. In addition, there are links for research, a newsletter, statistical data, and a bibliographic collection of journal articles on various aspects of weight management and obesity.

Body Composition Laboratory

www.bcm.edu/bodycomplab/

The Body Composition Laboratory at the Children's Nutrition Research Center in Houston, Texas, sponsors this informative website, which explains the techniques for and applications of body composition measurements in all populations, ranging from low-birth-weight infants to adults. Learn how high-precision instruments are used to measure total body levels of water, minerals, proteins, and fat.

Something Fishy, A Website on Eating Disorders

www.something-fishy.org

This very comprehensive and popular site features the latest news on eating disorders, as well as links regarding signs to watch for, "Recovery Reach-out," treatment finders, doctors and patients, cultural issues, and a support chat.

InfoTrac College Edition Activities Log on, insert **weight control** into the Keyword search box, and limit your search to the past year. When you get the results, Mark articles to review, then Select one to read. Summarize three or four key points from the article.

You can find additional readings related to personal health with InfoTrac College Edition, an online library of more than 900 journals and publications. Follow the instructions for accessing InfoTrac College Edition that were packaged with your textbook; then search for articles using a keyword search.

For additional links, resources, and suggested readings on the InfoTrac College Edition, visit our Health and Wellness Resource Center at **http://health .wadsworth.com.**

Key Terms

The terms listed are used on the page indicated. Definitions of the terms are in the Glossary at the end of the book.

anorexia nervosa 199	hunger 187
appetite 187	hydrostatic weighing 184
basal metabolic rate (BMR) 181	NEAT (nonexercise activity thermogenesis) 000
binge eating 198	
body mass index (BMI) 182	obesity 182
bulimia nervosa 199	overweight 182
dual-energy X-ray absorptiometry (DXA) 184	satiety 188
	skinfold measurement 184
eating disorders 198	waist-to-hip ratio (WHR) 183

Responsible Sexuality

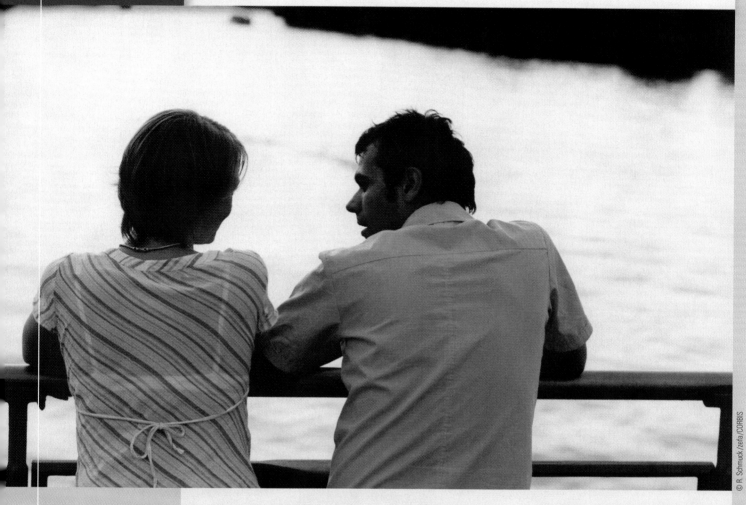

Our most special relationships are those that bring us closer to others—our friends, partners, spouses, parents, and children. Such intimacy is the most rewarding and often the most demanding of human involvements. The giving of ourselves to another—sharing thoughts, feelings, experiences, and sexual pleasure—touches the essence of what it means to be human. This section provides a comprehensive philosophical and practical view of relating to others. Each of the chapters focuses on the unique form of personal responsibility involved in every close relationship: a responsibility that looks beyond the self to those we care for and love.

8 Communicating and Relating

Oona compares the people in her life to threads in a magnificent tapestry. Each brings different tones and textures that complement and contrast with others. Her earliest childhood memories are of loving circles of family and friends that she once thought revolved around only her. Now she sees that she is part of these concentric rings and that the friendship and support she offers others enrich all of their lives.

When she left for a college thousands of miles from her home, Oona worried about the people she was leaving behind and the strangers she would be living among. She wondered if she'd be welcomed or shunned, judged by her looks or her race, invited to join social groups, or excluded from them. What she discovered was that the choice was largely hers. She could reach out to others, smile, and hope that others would smile in return, communicate clearly and honestly, strive to forge connections. Within months of her arrival, Oona was sure she had made friends she would keep forever.

Whether we are shy or outgoing, reserved or exuberant, we all crave human connection. As individuals and as part of society, we need to care about others and to know that others care about us, to feel for others and have others feel for us, to share what we know and to learn from what others know.

Sending clear messages through words, gestures, expressions, and behaviors is the essence of good communication. The more effectively we communicate, the more likely we are to create good relationships built on honesty, understanding, and mutual trust. Such relationships can infuse our lives with a richness no solitary pleasure can match.

This chapter discusses the social needs we all share, the ways some of us respond to those needs, healthy and unhealthy relationships, and the possibilities that exist for coming together from our solitude to warm ourselves in each other's glow.

© Helen Norman/CORBIS

After studying the material in this chapter, you should be able to:

▌ **Describe** the role verbal and nonverbal communication plays in forming and maintaining relationships and **discuss** gender differences in communication.

▌ **Define** friendship and **explain** how friendship grows.

▌ **Discuss** the behavior and emotional expectations for friendship, dating, and intimate relationships.

▌ **Describe** at least three ways to improve a relationship.

▌ **Identify** the behaviors that may result in dysfunctional relationships.

▌ **List** and **describe** the various living arrangements today's adults might choose.

▌ **Identify** the problems likely to affect long-term relationships and **explain** how they can be prevented.

YOUR SOCIAL HEALTH

Your relationships with your family, friends, coworkers, and loved ones may amaze, irritate, exhilarate, frustrate, and delight you. They also may affect your health. As noted in Chapter 1, your ability to communicate, to develop satisfying relationships, and to live in harmony with others is an important dimension of health and wellness.

Recent research has focused on specific qualities in a relationship that affect physical health, particularly *social support*. This term refers to the ways in which we provide information or assistance, show affection, comfort, and confide in others. As mounting evidence shows, people of all ages function best in socially supportive environments.

 This is particularly true of college students, who report more stress and more physical symptoms when they feel a lack of family support. More than any other component of social support, a sense of belonging may have the greatest impact on college students' health. In a recent study of 247 undergraduates, belonging to a social network enhanced women's perceptions of their health and lowered the number of symptoms that men reported. Because college is a transition time, forming new attachments may be especially important—and beneficial to overall health.[1]

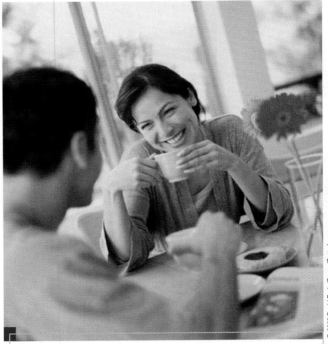

Good communication is essential to a healthy and successful relationship.

© 2000 David Roth/Stone/Getty Images

PERSONAL COMMUNICATION

Getting to know someone is one of life's greatest challenges and pleasures. When you find another person intriguing—as a friend, as a teacher, as a colleague, as a possible partner—you want to find out as much as you can about him or her and to share more and more information about yourself. Roommates may talk for endless hours. Friends may spend years getting to know each other. Partners in committed relationships may delight in learning new things about each other.

Communication stems from a desire to know and a decision to tell. Each of us chooses what information about ourselves we want to disclose and what we want to conceal or keep private. But in opening up to others, we increase our own self-knowledge and understanding.

COMMUNICATING FEELINGS

A great deal of daily communication focuses on facts: on the who, what, where, when, and how. Information is easy to convey and comprehend. Emotions are not. Some people have great difficulty saying "I appreciate you" or "I care about you," even though they are genuinely appreciative and caring. Others find it hard to know what to say in response and how to accept such expressions of affection. Men and women vary in their communication styles.

Some people feel that relationships shouldn't require any effort, that there's no need to talk of responsibility between people who care about each other. Yet responsibility is implicit in our dealings with anyone or anything we value—and what can be more valuable than those with whom we share our lives? Friendships and other intimate relationships always demand an emotional investment, but the rewards they yield are great.

Sometimes people convey strong emotions with a kiss or a hug, a pat or a punch, but such actions aren't precise enough to communicate exact thoughts. Stalking out of a room and slamming the door may be clear signs of anger, but they don't explain what caused the anger or suggest what to do about it. You must learn how to communicate all feelings clearly and appropriately if you hope to become truly close to another person.

As two people build a relationship, they must sharpen their communication skills so that they can discuss all the issues they may confront. They must learn how to communicate anger as well as affection, hurt as well as joy—and they must listen as carefully as they speak.

Listening involves more than waiting for the other person to stop talking. Listening is an active process of trying to understand the other person's feelings and motivation. Effective listeners ask questions when they're not sure they understand the other person and prompt the other person to continue.

NONVERBAL COMMUNICATION

More than 90 percent of communication may be nonverbal. While we speak with our vocal cords, we communicate with our facial expressions, tone of voice, hands, shoulders, legs, torsos, posture. Body language is the building block upon which more advanced verbal forms of communication rest.

Body language can send powerful nonverbal messages about your true state of mind and feelings.

Learning to interpret what people *don't* say can reveal more than what they *do* say. "Understanding nonverbal communication is probably the best tool there is for a good life of communicating, be it personally or professionally," says Marilyn Maple, an educator at the University of Florida. "It's one of the most practical skills you can develop. When you can consciously read what others are saying unconsciously, you can deal with issues before they become problems."[2]

 In a survey of 233 undergraduates at a large southeastern university, those who saw themselves as "involved" daters were more concerned about nonverbal communication than "casual" daters. These individuals were more likely to "work hard" to ensure that their nonverbal behavior backed up the words they said—and to say their partners did the same. Regardless of their dating status, the female students valued nonverbal behavior more than men. They also engaged in more forms of nonverbal communication, such as looking their partners straight in the eye and nodding their heads as their partners spoke.[3]

 Culture has a great deal of influence over body language. In some cultures, for example, establishing eye contact is considered hostile or challenging; in others, it conveys friendliness. A person's sense of personal space—the distance he or she feels most comfortable in keeping from others—varies in different societies.

HOW MEN AND WOMEN COMMUNICATE

Gender differences in communication start early. By age one, boys make less eye contact than girls and pay more attention to moving objects like cars than to human faces.

Both mothers and fathers talk less about feelings (except anger) to sons than daughters, and boys' vocabularies include fewer "feeling" words. In the playground, if not at home, boys learn to choke back tears and show no fear. Their faces—once as openly emotional as girls—become less expressive as they move through the elementary years.

As adults, men use fewer words and talk, at least in public, as a means of putting themselves in a one-up situation—unlike women, who talk to draw others closer. Even with friends, men mainly swap information as they talk shop, sports, cars, computers. "Women talk to clear their heads, but men think before they talk," says psychiatrist Mark Goulston, author of *The 6 Secrets of a Lasting Relationship.* "If they didn't, they'd risk saying something stupid and being humiliated or offending another man and getting beaten up. They're safer not saying anything."[4]

In her insightful studies of language, linguist Deborah Tannen has noted that while men speak more often and for longer periods in public, women speak more in private, usually to build better connections to others. In public and private, women generally are better listeners, facilitating conversation by nodding, asking questions, and signaling interest by saying "uh-huh," or "yes." Men interrupt more, breaking in on another's monologue if they aren't getting the information they need. Women are more likely to wait for the speaker to finish. "There's more than one interpretation for why a woman is less likely to interrupt," says psychologist Judith Hall. "It could show that she's being submissive and not playing the aggressive role. But it also could mean that she is less of a social blunderer and is more adept at reading the other person's signals."[5]

 In social interactions, two white women talking together look into each other's eyes far more often than two men, African-American women are less likely to do so. When a man and a woman are together, the man gazes into the woman's eyes more often than he would a man's, while a woman makes eye contact less often than she would if she were with another woman—a nice exercise in reciprocity. "A man talking with a woman will act more like a woman, and a woman will act more like a man," observes Hall. "It's as if they're adjusting to accommodate each other's cultural norm."

In writing, women use more words overall, more words related to emotion (positive and negative), more idea words, more hearing, feeling, and sensing words, more causal words, such as *because,* and more modal words (*would, should, could*). Men use more numbers, more prepositions, and more articles, such as *an* and *the.*

Gender differences appear online. In general, women tend to write e-mails in much the same way that they talk, using words to build a connection with people. Men's e-mails are briefer and more utilitarian. In chat rooms and online groups, men are more likely to make strong assertions, disagree with others, and to use profanities and sarcasm. Women are more prone to posing questions, making suggestions, and including polite expressions. Communication researchers studying the differences between "he-mails" and "she-mails" have also found that people who are not generally verbally expressive—mainly men—often convey more feelings in e-mails than they do in face-to-face conversations.

FORMING RELATIONSHIPS

We first learn how to relate in our families as children. Our relationships with parents and siblings change dramatically as we grow toward independence. Relationships between friends also change as they move or develop different interests; between lovers, as they come to know more about each other; between spouses, as they pass through life together; and between parents and children, as youngsters develop and mature. But throughout life, close relationships, tested and strengthened by time, allow us to explore the depths of our souls and the heights of our emotions. (See Self Survey on page 230: "How Strong Are the Communication and Affection in Your Relationship?")

I, MYSELF, AND ME

The way each of us perceives himself or herself affects all the ways we reach out and relate to others. If we feel unworthy of love, others may share that opinion. Self-esteem (discussed in Chapter 3) provides a positive foundation for our relationships with others. Self-esteem doesn't mean vanity or preoccupation with our own needs; rather, it is a genuine concern and respect for ourselves so that we remain true to our own feelings and beliefs. We can't know or love or accept others until we know and love and accept ourselves, however imperfect we may be.

Partners with low self-esteem may feel responsible for a partner's unhappiness. In studies of college students, those who scored low on measures of self-esteem were far more likely to feel rejected or hostile if their partners seemed distraught. Regardless of the reason for the distress, insecure, self-doubting individuals may read nonexistent meaning into their partners' ambiguous cues. As a result, they may unwittingly sabotage their relationships. This misreading of cues occurs not just in dating couples, but among long-married partners who still fear that their spouses love them less than they actually do.

FRIENDSHIP

Friendship has been described as "the most holy bond of society." Every culture has prized the ties of respect, tolerance, and loyalty that friendship builds and nurtures. An anonymous writer put it well:

> A friend is one who knows you as you are,
> Understands where you've been,
> Accepts who you've become,
> And still gently invites you to grow.

Friends can be a basic source of happiness, a connection to a larger world, a source of solace in times of trouble.

Although we have different friends throughout life, often the friendships of adolescence and young adulthood are the closest we ever form. They ease the normal break from parents and the transition from childhood to independence.

In the past, many people believed that men and women couldn't become close friends without getting romantically involved. But as the genders have worked together and come to share more interests, this belief has changed. Yet unique obstacles arise in male-female friendships, such as distinguishing between friendship and romantic attraction and dealing with sexual tension. However, men and women who overcome such barriers and become friends benefit from their relationship—but in different ways. For men, a friendship with a woman offers support and nurturance. What they report liking most is talking and relating to women, something they don't do with their male buddies. Women view their friendships with men as more light-hearted and casual, with more joking and less fear of hurt feelings. They especially like getting insight into what guys really think.

Friendship transcends all boundaries of distance and differences and enhances feelings of warmth, trust, love, and affection between two people. It is a common denominator of human existence that cuts across major social categories: In every country, culture, and language, human beings make friends. Friendship is both a universal and a deeply satisfying experience.

"Wishing to be friends," Aristotle wrote, "is quick work, but friendship is a slowly opening fruit." The qualities that make a good friend include honesty, acceptance, dependability, empathy, and loyalty. To sustain a close friendship, both people must be able to see the other's perspective, anticipate each other's needs, and take each other's viewpoint into account. More than anything else, good friends are there when we need them. They see us at our worst but never lose sight of our best. They share our laughter and tears, our triumphs and tragedies.

DATING

A date is any occasion during which two people share their time. It can be a Friday night dance, a bicycle ride, a dinner for two, or a walk in the park. Friends and lovers go on dates; so do complete strangers. Some men date other men; some women date other women. We don't expect to love, or even like, everyone we date. Yet the people you date reveal something about the sort of person you are. Dating peaks among young adults. Nearly 50 percent of 18-year-olds go out at least once a week. By age 32, only about 25 percent date that often.

With more people remaining single longer, the search for a good date has become more complex. Singles bars have become less popular because of the dangers of excessive drinking and casual sex. Cafés, laundromats, health clubs, and bookstores have become more acceptable as places to meet new people. Personal ads and cyberspace are alternative ways to meet potential dates (see Savvy Consumer: "Do's and Don'ts of Online Dating").

Dating can do more than help you meet people. By dating, you can learn how to make conversation, get to know more about others as well as yourself, and share feelings, opinions, and interests. In adolescence and young adulthood, dating also provides an opportunity for exploring your sexual identity. Some people date for months and never share more than a good-night kiss. Others may fall into bed together before they fall in love or even "like."

Separating your emotional feelings about someone you're dating from your sexual desire is often difficult. The first step to making responsible sexual decisions is respecting your sexual values and those of your partner. If you care about the other person—not just his or her body—and the relationship you're creating, sex will be an important, but not the all-important, factor while you're dating.

Dating has potential dangers. As discussed in Chapter 19, approximately one in five female teens is physically and/or sexually abused by a dating partner, though in some cases girls are the aggressors.

Should You Keep Dating?

You've met someone, gone out a few times, and enjoyed yourself. Is it infatuation, "like," or love? Should you keep seeing each other? Here are some positive indications of a relationship worth continuing:

- You feel at ease with your new partner.
- You feel good about your new partner when you're together and when you're not.
- Your partner is open with you about his or her life—past, present, and future.
- You can say no to each other without feeling guilty.

- You feel cared for, appreciated, and accepted as you are.
- Your partner really listens to what you have to say.

Following are some reasons to rethink your relationship:

- You don't feel comfortable together.
- You feel angry or let down when you're together or apart.
- Your partner is very secretive about his or her life.
- You feel your partner isn't attentive to you.
- You don't feel cared for and appreciated.

HOOKING UP

Hooking up refers to a sexual encounter between two people who usually are not seriously dating and who may or may not know each other well. College students use the term to describe a variety of sexual interactions, including petting below the waist, oral sex, and sexual intercourse.

Alcohol often plays a role in hooking up. Under its influence, individuals may engage in sexual activities, including unsafe sex, that they normally would avoid with someone they usually would not choose. Most students surveyed believe that hooking up is more common than it may in fact be and that their peers—particularly men—are more comfortable with hooking up than they are.

Some young people also engage in sexual activities with friends with whom they are not romantically involved. Many "friends with benefits" may have had a sexual relationship in the past. Others have no expectation of any serious involvement.

Savvy Consumer :: Do's and Don'ts of Online Dating

Forget personal ads or singles bars. If you're looking for love in the new millennium, the place more people are turning to is cyberspace. Some estimate that thousands, perhaps millions of people, are using the Internet to find a companion.

E-mail flirtations can be fun, but they also entail some risks, particularly if you decide to go off-line and meet in person. Here are some guidelines:

- Be careful of what you type. Anything you put on the Internet can end up almost anywhere. To avoid embarrassment, don't say anything you wouldn't want to see in newspaper print.
- Don't give out your address, telephone number, or any other identifying information. The people you meet online are strangers, and you should keep your guard up.

- Don't "date" on an office or university computer. You could end up supplying your professors, classmates, or coworkers with unintentional entertainment. Also, many organizations and institutions consider e-mail messages company property.
- Remember that you have no way of verifying if a correspondent is telling the truth about anything—sex, age, occupation, marital status. If your online partner seems insincere or strange in any way, stop corresponding.
- If you do decide to meet, make your first face-to-face encounter a double or group date and make it somewhere public, like a cafe or museum. Don't plan a full-day outing. Coffee or a drink in a crowded place makes the best transition from e-mails.

- Make sure you tell a friend or family member your plans and have your own way of getting home. It's also a good idea to schedule the first meeting in the afternoon or early in the evening rather than later at night.
- Don't let your expectations run wild. Finding Mr. or Ms. Right is no easier in cyberspace than anywhere else, so be realistic about where your relationship might lead.
- Don't rely on the Internet as your only method of meeting people. Continue to get out in the real world and meet potential dates the old-fashioned ways: live and in-person.

Your Life Coach

Building Healthy Relationships

Healthy relationships are built on mutual respect, trust, and consideration. People who've grown up in dysfunctional families or who have had abusive relationships may not have a clear idea of what a healthy relationship is. Here are some of the characteristics to look and strive for:

- **Emotional support and sensitivity**
- **Mutual good will**
- **Respectful asking rather than ordering**
- **Encouragement**
- **Being listened and responded to with courtesy**
- **Acknowledgement and appreciation of your feelings**
- **The right to express your own point of view**
- **Freedom from accusations, blame, criticism, and judgment**
- **Respect for your work and interests**
- **No rage, outbursts of anger, or emotional or physical threats**
- **Sincere apologies for comments or jokes you find offensive**

A healthy relationship requires empathy, the ability to appreciate what another person is experiencing. You may not agree with your roommate's political opinions or your sibling's wardrobe choices, yet you respect their rights to think and dress as the individuals they are.

In an intimate relationship, empathy becomes even more important. You can develop your capacity for empathy by pulling back periodically, particularly in moments of stress or conflict, and asking yourself: "What is my partner or spouse feeling right now? What does he or she need?"

SELF-DISCLOSURE IN RELATIONSHIPS

A key element of relationships—whether friendships or romantic ones—is **self-disclosure,** that is, how much we reveal about ourselves to another person. What you share about yourself is a critical building block that affects the nature and quality of the bonds you establish with others. But both cultural and individual factors can influence self-disclosure.

 In a study of American and Japanese college students, the Japanese undergraduates reported significantly less self-disclosure, whether in passionate love relationships, companionate love relationships, cross-sex friendships, or same-sex friendships. As previous studies have shown,

Talking about your feelings and listening intently move a relationship to a deeper and more meaningful level.

Japanese people talk less about themselves than Americans do and may think that talking about their personal issues would hurt the feelings of people around them. On the other hand, Americans generally strive to express themselves.[6]

Yet both American and Japanese students disclosed more in romantic relationships than in friendships and more in same-sex than in cross-sex friendships. This might be because we talk about more topics with a romantic partner than with a friend. We also may have more in common with people of the same sex so we discuss more with them than with a friend of the other sex.

ASSESSING A RELATIONSHIP

How do you know if you're in a healthy relationship? Ask yourself the following questions:

- **Do you have a clear sense of who you are,** what you believe and value, the goals you want? Such self-knowledge is critical for forming any mature relationship.
- **Do you feel that you can be yourself** when you're with this person? Do you feel good about yourself? Do you get—and give—compliments, support, and praise?
- **Do you share interests and values?** When you have things in common, you have a foundation to expand and build your relationship.
- **Do you respect the other person** and feel respected in return?
- **Do you have differences in values,** politics, religion, age, or race? Can you accept them?
- **Do you still feel like a unique, strong individual** within this relationship?

IMPROVING YOUR RELATIONSHIPS

Being in a relationship should be an opportunity for fun, personal growth, and mutual support, never an excuse for hurting or controlling someone else. The following guidelines can help keep a relationship healthy:

- **Recognize that both people in the relationship have the right to be accepted** as they are, to be treated with respect, to feel safe, to ask for what they want, to say no without feeling guilty, to express themselves, to give and receive affection, and to make some mistakes and be forgiven.

- **Remember that no one in a relationship has the right to force the other to do anything,** to tell the other where or when to speak up or go out, to humiliate the other in public or private, to isolate the other from friends and family, to read personal material without permission, to pressure the other to give up goals or interests, or to abuse the other person verbally or physically.

- **Be willing to open up.** The more you share, the deeper the bond between you and your friend will become.

- **Be sensitive to your friend's or partner's feelings.** Keep in mind that, like you, he or she has unique needs, desires, and dreams.

- **Express appreciation.** Be generous with your compliments. Let your friends and family know you recognize their kindnesses.

- **Know that people will disappoint you from time to time.** We are only human. Accept your loved ones as they are. Admitting their faults need not reduce your respect for them.

- **Talk about your relationship.** If you have any gripes or frustrations, air them.

DYSFUNCTIONAL RELATIONSHIPS

Although they enrich and fulfill us in many ways, our relationships with friends, siblings, parents, or colleagues can also sabotage our health. Mental health professionals define a "toxic" relationship as one in which either person is made to feel worthless or incompetent.

Relationships that don't promote healthy communication, honesty, and intimacy are sometimes called **dysfunctional.** Individuals with addictive behaviors or dependence on drugs or alcohol (see Chapters 11 and 12), and the children or partners of such people, are especially likely to find themselves in such relationships, although they occur in all economic and social groups.

Often partners have magical, unrealistic expectations (e.g., they expect that a relationship with the right person will make their life okay), and one person uses the other almost as if he or she were a mood-altering drug. The partners may compulsively try to get the other to act the way they want. Both persons may not trust or may deceive each other. Often they isolate themselves from others, thus trapping themselves in a recurring cycle of pain.

"Physical symptoms, such as headaches, digestive troubles, tics, and inability to sleep well, can be signs of a destructive relationship," says sociologist Robert Billingham, professor of human development and family studies at Indiana University.[7] Yet, although one person may repeatedly attack, abandon, betray, badger, bully, criticize, deceive, dominate, or demean the other, the responsibility for changing the unhealthy dynamic belongs to both.

"The big question is, 'Do I want or have to keep this relationship going?'" says sociologist Jan Yager, author of *When Friendship Hurts.* "If yes, are you willing to invest time and energy to turn it around?"[8]

(FAQ) WHAT IS EMOTIONAL ABUSE?

Abuse consists of any behavior that uses fear, humiliation, or verbal or physical assaults to control and subjugate another human being. Rather than being physical, emotional abuse

---

Strategies for Change :: Coping with an Unhealthy Relationship

- **Start a dialogue.** Focus on communication, not confrontation. Start with a positive statement, for instance, saying what you really value in the relationship. Volunteer what you might do to make it better, and state what you need from the other person.

- **Distance yourself.** Take a vacation from a toxic friendship. Skip the family reunion or Thanksgiving dinner. When forced into proximity, be polite. If you refuse to engage—not arguing, not getting angry, not trying to make things better—toxic people give up trying to get under your skin.

- **Consult a professional.** A therapist or minister can help people recognize and change toxic behavior patterns.

Changes you make in how you act and react can trigger changes in others.

- **Save yourself.** If you can never get what you need in a relationship, you may need to let it go. Nothing is worth compromising your mental or physical health.

often takes the form of constant berating, belittling, and criticism. Aggressive verbal abuse includes calling names, blaming, threatening, accusing, demeaning, and judging. Trivializing, minimizing, or denying what a person says or feels is a more subtle but equally destructive type of abuse. Even if done for the sake of "teaching" or "helping," emotional abuse wears away at self-confidence, sense of self-worth, and trust and belief in one's self. Because it is more than skin deep, emotional abuse can leave deeper, longer-lasting scars.

In the American College Health Assessment survey, 13 percent of students—15 percent of women and 10 percent of men—reported an emotionally abusive relationship in the last school year. Fewer experienced physical and sexual abuse.[9] (See Student Snapshot: "Abusive Relationships on Campus.")

No one wants to get into an abusive relationship, but often people who were emotionally abused in childhood find themselves in similar circumstances as adults. Dealing with an emotional abuser, regardless of how painful, may feel familiar or even comfortable. Individuals who think very little of themselves also may pick partners who treat them as badly as they believe they deserve.

Abusers also may have grown up with emotional abuse and view it as a way of coping with feelings of fear, hurt, powerlessness, or anger. They may seek partners who see themselves as helpless and who make them feel more powerful. Among the signs of emotional abuse are:

❙ **Attempting to control various aspects of your life,** such as what you say or wear

❙ **Frequently humiliating you** or making you feel badly about yourself

❙ **Making you feel as if you are to blame** for what your partner does

❙ **Wanting to know where you are** and whom you're with at all times

❙ **Becoming jealous or angry** when you spend time with friends

❙ **Threatening to harm you** if you break up

❙ **Trying to coerce you** into unwanted sexual activity with statements such as, "If you loved me, you would. . . ."

If you can never get what you need or if you're afraid, you need to get out of the relationship. Take whatever steps necessary to ensure your safety. Find a trusted adult who can help. Don't isolate yourself from family and friends. This is the time when you need their support and often the support of a counselor, minister, or doctor as well.

CODEPENDENCY

Codependency has expanded its definition to include any maladaptive behaviors learned by family members in order to survive great emotional pain and stress, such as an addiction, chronic mental or physical illness, and abuse. Some

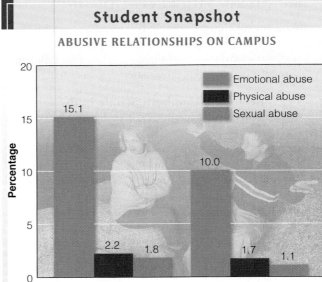

Student Snapshot

ABUSIVE RELATIONSHIPS ON CAMPUS

Legend: ▨ Emotional abuse ▪ Physical abuse ▨ Sexual abuse

Women: 15.1 (Emotional), 2.2 (Physical), 1.8 (Sexual)
Men: 10.0 (Emotional), 1.7 (Physical), 1.1 (Sexual)

Percentage of college students reporting abusive relationships in the last school year.
Source: Reprinted by permission of American College Health Association, www.acha.org/projects_programs/ncha_sampledata_public.cfm.

therapists refer to codependency as a "relationship addiction" because codependent people often form or maintain relationships that are one-sided, emotionally destructive, or abusive. First identified in studies of the relationships in families of alcoholics, codependent behavior can occur in any dysfunctional family.

Codependent individuals, lacking in self-esteem, may develop compulsive behaviors, such as workaholism, or try to feel better by using alcohol or drugs. If they take on a martyr's role, they may sacrifice their own needs and dreams for the sake of helping a parent, child, or spouse. Although codependent people may initially relish being needed, in time they feel overwhelmed and trapped in the relationship, but cannot break away. They come to see themselves as victims and are attracted to that same role in friendships and romantic relationships.

Among the characteristics of codependency are:

❙ **An exaggerated sense of responsibility** for the actions of others

❙ **An attraction to people who need rescuing**

❙ **Always trying to do more than one's share**

❙ **Doing anything to cling to a relationship** and avoid feeling abandoned

❙ **An extreme need for approval and recognition**

❙ **A sense of guilt** about asserting needs and desires

❙ **A compelling need to control others**

❙ **Lack of trust in self and/or others**

❙ **Fear of being alone**

❙ **Difficulty identifying feelings**

- **Rigidity/difficulty** adjusting to change
- **Chronic anger**
- **Lying/dishonesty**
- **Poor communications**
- **Difficulty making decisions**

(FAQ) Am I Codependent?

Check any of these statements that apply to you.

_____ I keep quiet to avoid arguments.

_____ I'm always worried about what other people think of me.

_____ One of my family members has an alcohol or drug problem.

_____ I have had relatives, friends, or partners who abused me verbally or physically.

_____ I always think that the opinions of others are more important than mine.

_____ I find it hard to adjust to changes at work or home.

_____ I feel hurt and rejected when someone close to me spends time with friends.

_____ I am uncomfortable expressing my true feelings.

_____ I feel inadequate and like a "bad person" when I make a mistake.

_____ I have difficulty accepting compliments or gifts.

_____ I think people in my life would fall apart without my constant efforts.

_____ I find it hard to talk to people in authority.

_____ I'm confused about who I am or where I'm going in my life.

_____ I have trouble saying "no" when asked for help and asking for help when I need it.

_____ I am trying to do so many things at once that I can't do any of them well.

If you identify with many of these statements, you may have been or are now in a codependent relationship. Learn as much as you can about it. Turn to the Internet, libraries, drug and alcohol abuse treatment centers, and mental health centers, which often offer educational materials and programs to the public. The more you understand codependency, the better you can cope with its effects.

Overcoming Codependency

Because the roots of codependency run so deep, people don't just "outgrow" this problem or magically find themselves in a healthy relationship. Treatment to resolve childhood hurts and deal with emotional issues may take the form of individual or group therapy, education, or programs such as Codependents Anonymous (www.codependents.org). The goal is to help individuals get in touch with long-buried feelings and build healthier family and relationship dynamics.

Enabling

Experts on the subject of addiction first identified traits of codependency in spouses of alcoholics, who followed a predictable pattern of behavior: While intensely trying to control the drinkers, the codependent mates would act in ways that allowed the drinkers to keep drinking. For example, if an alcoholic found it hard to get up in the morning, his wife would wake him up, pull him out of bed and into the shower, and drop him off at work. If he was late, she made excuses to his boss. The husband was the one with the substance-abuse problem, but without realizing it, his wife was enabling him to continue drinking. In fact, he might not have been able to keep up his habit without her unintentional cooperation.

The different styles or components of **enabling** include the following:

- **Shielding.** Codependents may cover up for abusers, preventing them from experiencing the full impact of the harmful consequences of their behavior—for example, by dropping off a paper or report so that the addicted person can avoid a missed deadline.

- **Controlling.** A codependent may try to control the significant other—for instance, by withholding sex or using sex as a reward for cutting down on an addictive behavior.

- **Taking over responsibilities.** The codependent may take over such household chores as shopping or running errands.

- **Rationalizing.** Codependents try to rationalize their partners' addiction by telling themselves that a compulsive behavior pattern, like workaholism, is making the person more successful, or that drinking helps him or her relax.

- **Cooperating.** Sometimes codependents become involved in the person's compulsion, perhaps placing bets for a gambler or buying alcohol for a drinker.

- **Rescuing.** The codependent may become overprotective—for example, by allowing the user to use drugs at home to avoid the risk of an accident or arrest.

Codependency progresses just as an addiction does, and codependents excuse their own behavior with many of the same defense mechanisms used by addicts, such as rationalization ("I cut class so I could catch up on my reading, not to keep an eye on my partner") and denial ("He likes to gamble, but he never loses more than he can afford"). In time, codependents lose sight of everything but their loved one. They feel that if they can only "fix" this person, everything will be fine.

INTIMATE RELATIONSHIPS

The term **intimacy**—the open, trusting sharing of close, confidential thoughts and feelings—comes from the Latin word for *within*. Intimacy doesn't happen at first sight, or in a day or a week or a number of weeks. Intimacy requires time and nurturing; it is a process of revealing rather than hiding, of wanting to know another and to be known by that other. Although intimacy doesn't require sex, an intimate relationship often includes a sexual relationship, heterosexual or homosexual.

All of our close relationships, whether they're with parents or friends, have a great deal in common. We feel we can count on these people in times of need. We feel that they understand us and we understand them. We give and receive loving emotional support. We care about their happiness and welfare. However, when we choose one person above all others, there is something even deeper and richer—something we call romantic love.

(FAQ) WHAT ATTRACTS TWO PEOPLE TO EACH OTHER?

What draws two people to each other and keeps them together: chemistry or fate, survival instincts or sexual longings? "Probably it's a host of different things," reports sociologist Edward Laumann, coauthor of *Sex in America,* a landmark survey of 3,432 men and women conducted by the National Opinion Research Center at the University of Chicago.[10] "But what's remarkable is that most of us end up with partners much like ourselves—in age, race, ethnicity, socioeconomic class, education."

Why? "You've got to get close for sexual chemistry to occur," says Laumann. "Sparks may fly when you see someone across a crowded room, but you only see a pre-selected group of people—people enough like you to be in the same room in the first place. This makes sense because initiating a sexual relationship is very uncertain. We all have such trepidations about being too fat, too ugly, too undesirable. We try to lower the risk of rejection by looking for people more or less like us."

 Scientists have tried to analyze the combination of factors that attracts two people to each other. In several studies of college students, four predictors ranked as the most important reasons for attraction: warmth and kindness, desirable personality, something specific about the person, and reciprocal liking.[11]

Do opposites attract, or do people find greater happiness with partners who are similar to them? One of the most comprehensive studies ever undertaken on these questions found no evidence that opposites attract. Most people, the researchers found, tend to marry those who are similar in attitudes, religion, and values. However, these similarities have little to do with having a happy marriage. What does matter are similarities in personality, such as being extroverted or conscientious. These take more time to recognize but have a greater impact on how a couple gets along over the long term.[12]

In his cross-cultural research, psychologist David Buss, author of *The Evolution of Desire,* found that men in 37 sample groups drawn from Africa, Asia, Europe, North and

© Daly & Newton/Stone/Getty Images

We tend to be attracted to people who are similar to ourselves in age, race, ethnicity, socioeconomic class, and education.

South America, Australia, and New Zealand rated youth and attractiveness as more important in a possible mate than did women. Women placed greater value on potential mates who were somewhat older, had good financial prospects, and were dependable and hardworking.[13]

Attractive women in different cultures, including the United States, use different mating strategies than less attractive ones, including more "attractiveness enhancement tactics" (such as wearing makeup), flirting with other men to make a date jealous, and acting possessively. Because of what researchers call the "Jennifer Lopez effect," attractive women also may have more opportunities for "trial liaisons" in selecting long-term partners and for replacing a mate who fails to live up to expectations.[14]

INFATUATION

It is tempting to think of love as scenes from a movie script: blazing sunsets and misty nights, fiery glances and passionate embraces, consuming desire and happily-ever-after endings. However, movies only last for 2 hours; ideally, love lasts a lifetime. Infatuation falls somewhere in between.

Certainly, falling in love is an intense, dizzying experience. A person not only enters our life, but also takes possession. We are intrigued, flattered, captivated, delighted—but is this love or a love of loving?

At the time you're experiencing it, there is no difference between infatuation and lasting love. You feel the same giddy, wonderful way. However, if it's infatuation, it won't last. Infatuation refers only to falling in love. People genuinely in love with each other do more than fall: They start building a relationship together.

Infatuation also can be a disguise for something quite different: a strong sex drive, a fear of loneliness, loneliness itself, or a hunger for approval. Sometimes lovers in love with love may become infatuated with someone who doesn't even exist: the projection of their unmet needs for unconditional love.

THE SCIENCE OF ROMANTIC LOVE

We like to think of this powerful force, this source of both danger and delight, as something that defies analysis. However, in recent years, as scientists have attempted to study love objectively, they have provided new perspectives on its nature.

A Psychological View

According to psychologist Robert Sternberg, love can be viewed as a triangle with three faces: passion, intimacy, and commitment (Figure 8-1). Each person brings his or her own triangle to a relationship. If they match well, their relationship is likely to be satisfying.

Sternberg also identified six types of love:

▪ **Liking,** the intimacy friends share
▪ **Infatuation,** the passion that stems from physical and emotional attraction
▪ **Romantic love,** a combination of intimacy and passion

▪ **Companionate love,** a deep emotional bond in a relationship that may have had romantic components
▪ **Fatuous love,** a combination of passion and commitment in two people who lack a deep emotional intimacy
▪ **Consummate love,** which combines passion, intimacy, and commitment over time

An Anthropological View

When you first fall in love, you may be sure that no one else has ever known the same dizzying, wonderful feelings. Yet, while every romance may be unique, romantic love is anything but. Anthropologists have found evidence of romantic love between individuals in most of the cultures they have studied—it seems to be a human universal or, at the least, a near-universal.

Another anthropologist, Helen Fisher, author of *Anatomy of Love: The Natural History of Monogamy, Adultery and Divorce,* describes romantic love "as a very primitive, basic human emotion, as basic as fear, anger or joy." As she explains, it pulled men and women of prehistoric times into the sort of partnerships that were essential to child rearing. But after about four years—just "long enough to rear one child through infancy," says Fisher—romantic love seemed to wane, and primitive couples tended to break up and find new partners. This "four-year itch" may well have endured through the centuries, contends Fisher, who notes that divorce statistics from most of the 62 cultures she has studied still show a pattern of restlessness four years into a marriage.[15]

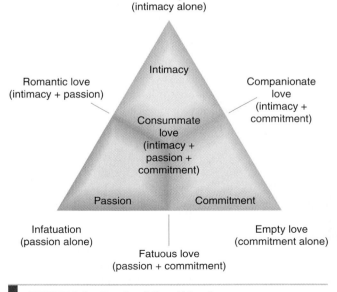

FIGURE 8-1   Sternberg's Love Triangle
The three components of love are intimacy, passion, and commitment. The various kinds of love are composed of different combinations of the three components.

Can romantic love be a matter of chemistry after all? Our neurotransmitters are definitely involved.

© Comstock/PictureQuest

A Biochemical View

The heart is the organ we associate with love, but the brain may be where the action really is. According to research on **neurotransmitters** (messenger chemicals within the brain), love sets off a chemical chain reaction that causes our skin to flush, our palms to sweat, and our lungs to breathe more deeply and rapidly. The "love chemicals" within the brain—dopamine, norepinephrine, and phenylethylamine (PEA)—have effects similar to those of amphetamines, stimulant drugs that intensify physiological reactions (see Chapter 11).

Infatuation may indeed be a natural high, but like other highs, this rush doesn't last—possibly because the body develops tolerance for love-induced chemicals, just as it does with amphetamines. However, as the initial lovers' high fades, other brain chemicals may come into play: the endorphins, morphinelike chemicals that can help produce feelings of well-being, security, and tranquility. These feel-good molecules may increase in partners who develop a deep attachment.

The hormone **oxytocin,** best known for its role in inducing labor during childbirth, seems particularly important in our ability to bond with others. By measuring blood levels of women as they recalled positive and negative relationships, researchers have found that women whose oxytocin levels rose when remembering a positive relationship reported having little difficulty setting appropriate boundaries, being alone, or trying too hard to please others. Women whose oxytocin levels fell in response to remembering a negative emotional relationship reported greater anxiety in close relationships.

MATURE LOVE

Social scientists have distinguished between *passionate love* (characterized by intense feelings of elation, sexual desire, and ecstasy) and *companionate love* (characterized by friendly affection and deep attachment). Often relationships begin with passionate love and evolve into a more companionate love. Sometimes the opposite happens and two people who know each other well discover that their friendship has "caught fire" and the sparks have flamed an unexpected passion.

Mature love is a complex combination of sexual excitement, tenderness, commitment, and—most of all—an overriding passion that sets it apart from all other love relationships in one's life. This passion isn't simply a matter of orgasm but also entails a crossing of the psychological boundaries between oneself and one's lover. You feel as if you're becoming one with your partner while simultaneously retaining a sense of yourself.

WHEN LOVE ENDS

Breaking up is indeed hard to do. Sometimes two people grow apart gradually, and both of them realize that they must go their separate ways. More often, one person falls out of love first. It hurts to be rejected; it also hurts to inflict pain on someone who once meant a great deal to you.

 In a survey of 259 undergraduates, about eight in ten said they knew how to end a relationship, but three in ten reported feeling ambivalent about breaking up. Most students supported getting out of an unsatisfactory dating relationship. About three in four felt that breaking up an unhappy relationship while dating would make for happier marriages in the long term. Non-whites were more likely to end relationships with no future than whites.[16]

 In surveys, college students say it's more difficult to initiate a breakup than to be rejected. Those who decided to end a relationship reported greater feelings of guilt, uncertainty, discomfort, and awkwardness than those with whom they broke up. However, students with high levels of jealousy are likely to feel a desire for vengeance that can lead to aggressive behavior.

Research suggests that people do not end their relationships because of the disappearance of love. Rather a sense of dissatisfaction or unhappiness develops, which may then cause love to stop growing. The fact that love does not dissipate completely may be one of the reasons why breakups are so painful. While the pain does ease over time, it can help both parties if they end their relationship in a way that shows kindness and respect. Your basic guideline should be to think of how you would like to be treated if someone were breaking up with you. Would it hurt more to find out from someone else? Would it be more painful if the person you cared for lied to you or deceived you, rather than admitted

---

Strategies for Change ▪▪ Dealing with Rejection

▪▪ Remind yourself of your own worth. You are no less attractive, intelligent, interesting, or lovable because someone ends his or her relationship with you.

▪▪ Accept the rejection as a statement of the other person's preference rather than trying to debate or defend yourself.

▪▪ Think of other people who value or have valued you, who accept and even see as appealing the same characteristics the rejecting person viewed as undesirable.

▪▪ Don't withdraw from others. Although you may not want to risk further rejection, it's worth the gamble to get involved again. The only individuals who've never been rejected are those who've never reached out to connect with another.

the truth? Saying "I don't feel the way I once did about you; I don't want to continue our relationship" is hard, but it's also honest and direct.

LIVING ARRANGEMENTS

Today's adults have many choices to explore regarding how and with whom they might live: returning to one's primary family, staying single, living with one or more friends, living in a long-term relationship with a lover of the same or opposite sex, or getting married. Increasingly, men and women in their twenties are spending more time considering all their options before committing themselves to an exclusive relationship.

"TWIXTERS": TRANSITION INTO ADULTHOOD

According to the Census Bureau, young adults between the ages of 18 and 24 are more likely to be living in their parents' homes than young people were in the 1970s. Some 18 million Americans between the ages of 18 and 34 are still living with their parents. Of those between ages 19 and 24, 66 percent (including college students) are living at home, compared to 50 percent in 1980.[17] Their reasons include the high cost of housing and the low incomes most men and women earn in their early twenties.

So many young people in their twenties are living with their parents that some have labeled them "twixters." Sociologists debate the benefits and drawbacks of delaying traditional adult milestones, such as supporting themselves and getting their own apartments. Trying different fields or jobs and waiting to commit may help young people make better long-term choices. Yet they also may be ducking responsibility for their own lives.

SINGLE LIFE

In young adulthood, single men outnumber single women; after age 40, however, there are more single women than single men. Perhaps because there are so many singles, more and more Americans are living alone. The number of women living alone has doubled since 1970 and has nearly tripled for men. Approximately one-quarter of the households in the nation are one-person homes.

Among Americans between 25 and 34 years old, about 35 percent (14 million) have never been married. Of African Americans in this age group, 53 percent have never been married. Being single no longer marks a transition phase between living with parents and living with a spouse, but is an accepted, appealing lifestyle for millions of men and women.

The number-one reason people remain single is being unable to find the right person, according to psychologist Florence Kaslow, director of the Florida Couples and Family Institute. For women, the next two reasons for staying single are their careers and independence. For men, independence and resolving personal issues are the second and third reasons for not marrying. Most of the women and all of the men in her study said that they would like to get married—someday. Yet only 5 percent of bachelors over age 40 ever marry.

COHABITATION

Although couples have always shared homes in informal relationships without any official ties, "living together," or **cohabitation,** has become more common. Some 5 million couples are cohabiting in the United States; the vast majority are heterosexual; 40 percent have children.

The number of unmarried couples increased by nearly 1200 percent between 1960 and 2004 (Figure 8-2). About a quarter of unmarried women ages 25 to 39 are currently living with a partner; an additional quarter lived with a partner in the past. Couples live together before more than half of all marriages, a practice that was practically unknown 50 years ago.[18]

 Asians and non-Hispanic white couples are the least likely to cohabit. A higher percentage of Native American, black, and Hispanic couples are unmarried. "Cohabiters" tend to have lower income and education levels. They also are younger—on average, some 12 years younger than married men and women.[19]

According to the Census Bureau, unmarried couples tend to cluster in several zones in the United States, including the western states and the Northeast. In these regions, married couples flock to the suburbs, while unmarried

---

Strategies for Change :: How to Stay Single and Satisfied

- Fill your life with meaningful work, experiences, and people.
- Build a network of supportive friends who care for and about you.
- Be open to new experiences that can expand your feelings about yourself and your world.

- Don't miss out on a special event because you don't have someone to accompany you: Go alone.

- Volunteer to help others less fortunate, or become involved in church and social organizations.

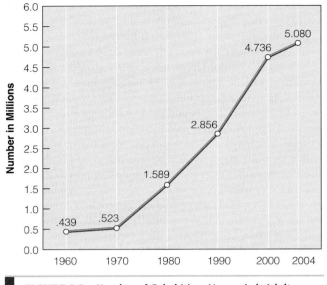

FIGURE 8-2 Number of Cohabiting, Unmarried, Adult Couples of the Opposite Sex (United States)

Source: Poponoe, David, and Barbara Dafoe Whitehead. *The State of Our Union:The Social Health of Marriage in America in 2005.* Copyright 2005 by the National Marriage Project at Rutgers University. Reprinted by permission of the National Marriage Project. http://marriage.rutgers.edu.

couples, especially same-sex ones, are most likely to live in central cities.[20]

Cohabitation can be a prelude to marriage, an alternative to living alone, or an alternative to marriage. Does living together help couples to find out if they get along and avoid a bad marriage? That does not seem to be the case. About half of men and women living together get married within five years; 40 percent break up; 10 percent continue to cohabit for a longer period. Among women cohabiting with a man, one in four says she doesn't ever expect to marry him.[21]

A substantial body of evidence indicates that couples who live together before marriage are more likely to break up after marriage. It's not clear if something about the partners themselves or the actual experience of cohabitation jeopardizes a subsequent marriage.

COMMITTED RELATIONSHIPS

Even though men and women today may have more sexual partners than in the past, most still yearn for an intense, supportive, exclusive relationship, based on mutual commitment and enduring over time. In our society, most such relationships take the form of heterosexual marriages, but partners of the same sex or heterosexual partners who never marry also may sustain long-lasting, deeply committed relationships. These couples are much like married people: They make a home, handle daily chores, cope with problems, celebrate special occasions, plan for the future—all the while knowing that they are not alone, that they are part of a pair that adds up to far more than just the sum of two individual souls.

DOMESTIC PARTNERS

Committed couples, both heterosexual and homosexual, can register as domestic partners in certain areas. This may enable them to qualify for benefits such as health insurance. Employers may require that the couple has lived together for a specified period (generally, at least six months) and are responsible for each other's financial welfare. Recent court rulings have placed domestic partners on the same legal footing as married couples in dealings with businesses.

LONG-TERM SAME-SEX RELATIONSHIPS

Contrary to the stereotype that same-sex relationships tend to be brief, researchers have studied couples who have been together for more than 20 years. Like heterosexual couples, same-sex relationships progress through various stages. The first, blending, is a time of intense passion and romantic love. Gradually the couples move through nesting (starting a home together), to building trust and dependability, to merging assets, to establishing a strong sense of partnership.[22]

Because there are no social norms for same-sex unions, researchers describe these relationships as more egalitarian. Each partner tends to be more self-reliant, and homosexual men and women tend to be more willing to communicate and experiment in terms of sexual behaviors.

Recent studies show that gay and lesbian relationships are comparable to straight relationships in many ways. But same-sex couples have to deal with every day ups-and-downs in a social context of isolation from family, workplace prejudice, and other social barriers. However, gay and lesbian couples are more upbeat in the face of conflict. Compared to straight couples, they use more affection and humor when they bring up a disagreement and remain more positive after a disagreement. They also display less belligerence, domineering, and fear with each other than straight couples do. When they argue, they are better able to soothe each other so they show fewer signs of physiological arousal, such as an elevated heart rate or sweaty palms, than heterosexual couples.[23]

MARRIAGE

Like everything which is not the involuntary result of fleeting emotion but the creation of time and will, any marriage, happy or unhappy, is infinitely more interesting and significant than any romance, however passionate.

W. H. Auden

Contemporary marriage has been described as an institution that everyone on the outside wants to enter and everyone on the inside wants to leave. According to the Census Bureau, nine in ten people marry, but about half of first marriages end in divorce after an average of seven or eight years.

According to the National Marriage Project, marriage rates have slipped nearly 50 percent since 1970 (Figure 8-3). The median age for marriage has risen to 26 for women and 27 for men, compared to 20 for women and 23 for men in 1960.[24]

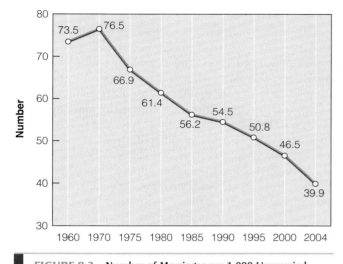

FIGURE 8-3 Number of Marriages per 1,000 Unmarried Women Age 15 and Older (United States)

Source: Poponoe, David, and Barbara Dafoe Whitehead. *The State of Our Union:The Social Health of Marriage in America in 2005.* Copyright 2005 by the National Marriage Project at Rutgers University. Reprinted by permission of the National Marriage Project. http://marriage.rutgers.edu.

Marriage is a formal and legal, lifetime commitment to another person—and a great occasion for celebration!

 Not too long ago, marriage was often a business deal, a contract made by parents for economic or political reasons when the spouses-to-be were still very young. Today, in some countries, it is still culturally acceptable to arrange marriages in this manner. Even in America, certain ethnic groups, such as Asians who have recently immigrated to the United States, plan marriages for their children. In such arrangements, the marriage partners are likely to have similar values and expectations. However, the newlyweds also start out as strangers who may not even know whether they like—let alone love—each other. Sometimes arranged marriages do lead to loving unions; sometimes they trap both partners in loneliness and longing.

Most of today's marriages aren't arranged; most people say they marry for one far-from-simple reason: love.

Preparing for Marriage

With more than half of all marriages ending in divorce, there's little doubt that modern marriages aren't made in heaven. Are some couples doomed to divorce even before they swap "I do's"? Could counseling before a marriage increase its odds of success? According to recent research findings, the answer to both questions is yes.

There have been government attempts to set requirements for couples who want to marry. Some states, such as Arizona and Louisiana, have established "covenant" marriages in which engaged couples are required to get premarital counseling. Utah allows counties to require counseling before issuing marriage licenses to minors and people who have been divorced. Florida requires high school students to take marriage education classes.

Finding Mr. or Ms. Right

Generally, men and women marry people from the geographical area they grew up in and from the same social background. Differences in religion and race can add to the pressures of marriage, but they also can enrich the relationship if they aren't viewed as obstacles. In our culturally diverse society, interracial and crosscultural marriages are becoming more common and widely accepted, although the odds are much greater for partners of the same race to live together or marry.

 In a study of 75,000 couples who lived together and 480,000 married couples in the United States, researchers found that African Americans were 365

Strategies for Prevention ■ Think Twice About Getting Married If:

- You or your partner are constantly asking the other such questions as, "Are you sure you love me?"
- You spend most of your time together disagreeing and quarreling.
- You're both still very young (under the age of 20).

- Your boyfriend or girlfriend has behaviors (such as nonstop talking), traits (such as bossiness), or problems (such as drinking too much) that really bother you and that you're hoping will change after you're married.

- Your partner wants you to stop seeing your friends, quit a job you enjoy, or change your life in some other way that diminishes your overall satisfaction.

times more likely to marry a black than a nonblack spouse and 110 times more likely to live with, or cohabit with, a black partner than someone of another racial group. Asians were 55 times more likely to marry another Asian and 17 times more likely to cohabit with another Asian. Hispanics were 12 times more likely to select a Hispanic spouse and nine times more likely to live with a Hispanic partner. Whites were about eight times more likely to marry another white person and five times more likely to cohabit with someone white rather than nonwhite.[25]

Some of the traits that appeal to us in a date become less important when we select a mate; others become key ingredients in the emotional cement holding two people together. According to psychologist Robert Sternberg of Yale University, the crucial ingredients for commitment are the following:

❙ **Shared values**
❙ **A willingness to change in response to each other**
❙ **A willingness to tolerate flaws**
❙ **A match in religious beliefs**
❙ **The ability to communicate effectively**

The single best predictor of how satisfied one will be in a relationship, according to Sternberg, is not how one feels toward a lover, but the difference between how one would like the lover to feel and how the lover actually feels. Feeling that the partner you've chosen loves too little or too much is, as he puts it, "the best predictor of failure."[26]

Premarital Assessments

There are scientific ways of predicting marital happiness. Some premarital assessment inventories identify strengths and weaknesses in many aspects of a relationship: realistic expectations, personality issues, communication, conflict resolution, financial management, leisure activities, sex, children, family and friends, egalitarian roles, and religious orientation. Couples who become aware of potential conflicts by means of such inventories may be able to resolve them through professional counseling. In some cases, they may want to reconsider or postpone their wedding.

Other common predictors of marital discord, unhappiness, and separation are:

❙ **A high level of arousal during a discussion.**
❙ **Defensive behaviors** such as making excuses and denying responsibility for disagreements.
❙ **A wife's expressions of contempt.**
❙ **A husband's stonewalling** (showing no response when a wife expresses her concerns).

By looking for such behaviors, researchers have been able to predict with better than 90 percent accuracy whether a couple will separate within the first few years of marriage.

Types of Marriage

Sociologists have categorized marriages as traditional or companion-oriented. In **traditional marriages,** the couples assume prescribed societal roles. In **companion-oriented marriages,** the partnership and its rewards—rather than the roles of fathering, mothering, and breadwinning—are primary. In addition, there are **romantic marriages,** in which sexual passion never seems to die, and **rescue marriages,** in which one partner suffered a traumatic childhood and sees marriage as a way of healing. About a fifth of all marriages belong to another category that has grown significantly in recent years: marriages of equally dependent spouses. Each partner in these unions earns between 40 and 59 percent of the total family income. According to research on these marriages, divorces are more common and occur more often at the wife's initiative. Researchers theorize that wives who are not economically dependent on their spouses may be more likely to leave an emotionally unfulfilling relationship. Regardless of type, a marriage can succeed if it fulfills basic tasks, such as providing a sense of intimacy and autonomy and providing a safe haven that is strong enough to absorb inevitable conflicts.

Same-Sex Marriage

In recent years, gay and lesbian couples have formalized their unions by registering as domestic partners in places where allowed and in commitment celebrations. Recognizing this trend, *The New York Times* began covering gay and lesbian unions in the same manner as heterosexual couples who become engaged or wed.

Same-sex marriage has been legalized in several countries, including Spain and Canada. In the United States, advocates have been working for years to change laws to allow gay and lesbian couples to marry. One state, Massachusetts, currently recognizes same-sex marriages. Same-sex couples were able to obtain marriage licenses in San Francisco and in various towns in New Mexico and New York for short intervals of time during 2004. However, none were able to register their marriages.

> *Legalizing marriage between same-sex partners, as other countries have done, has triggered intense controversy and political debate in the United States. Some contend that marriage can only be a union between a man and a woman. Others argue that same-sex couples should have equal economic and civil rights as heterosexual couples and these are only guaranteed by a legally recognized marriage. Should marriage be restricted to heterosexual couples? Or should homosexual couples have the same recognition?* **You decide.**

The Benefits of Marriage

Despite its problems, marriage endures because it is a fulfilling way for two people to live. As researchers have proved, saying "I do" can do wonders for your health. According to a CDC study of more than 127,000 adults, married people are healthier than those who are divorced, widowed, never-married, or live with a partner. The connection between marriage and health was strongest in the youngest group, aged 18 to 44.[27]

Married people are less likely to suffer from health conditions like back pain, headaches, and serious psychological distress. That is true for all ages, ethnicities, and levels of income and education. Married people are less likely to smoke, drink heavily, and be physically inactive.

Marriage does pose one health hazard: weight gain. Married men are more likely to be overweight or obese. Three in four married men aged 45 to 64 are overweight or obese. The slimmest groups are men and women who had never married.

Married men and women also have lower rates of most mental disorders than single or divorced individuals. Both husbands and wives live longer than single or divorced individuals. In one national survey, about 90 percent of husbands and wives survived until at least age 65, compared with only about 60 to 70 percent of divorced and never-married men and women. Although there has not been much research on same-sex committed relationships, most experts believe that gay couples are likely to enjoy similar benefits, as long as they remain together and receive social support for doing so.

For years researchers thought that marriage was especially beneficial to men. Married men have lower rates of alcohol and drug abuse, depression, and risk-taking behavior than divorced men. They also earn more money—possibly because they have more incentive to do so. However, more recent research indicates that marriage boosts mental health and well-being in both spouses.

Issues Couples Confront

No two people can live together in perfect harmony all the time. Some of the issues that crop up in any long-term relationship include expectations, money, sex, and careers.

Unrealistic Expectations Partners may think that their significant others should always be as attractive, charming, and tolerant as they were when they were dating. They may assume that their partners will always agree with them or will automatically see their point of view; or they may believe that their one true love will always be able to meet all their needs. Because no one could ever live up to such expectations, the partners are doomed to disappointment.

Togetherness does not necessarily guarantee happiness. According to one study of more than 2,000 couples, too much time together—particularly doing shopping and chores—may be bad for a marriage.[28]

Fight fair. You can learn to argue effectively, without attacking others or damaging relationships.

© Jon Riley/Stone/Getty Images

Money Money may make the business world go around, but it has the opposite effect on relationships: It knocks them off their tracks, brings them to a halt, twists them upside down. However, even though almost all couples quarrel about money, they rarely fight over how much they have. What matters more—whether they make $10,000 or $100,000 a year—is what money means to both partners. How does each person use money to meet emotional needs? Who decides how the money is spent? Who keeps track? Until they resolve these issues, couples may quarrel over money as long as they're together.

To avoid fighting over money, understand that having different money values or expectations doesn't make one of you right and the other wrong. Recognize the value of unpaid work. A partner who's finishing school or taking care of the children is making an important contribution to the family and its future. It also helps to go over your finances together so that you have a firm basis in reality for what you can and can't afford. Talk about the financial goals you hope to attain five years from now. Set priorities to meet them. Also, set aside money for each of you to spend without asking or answering to the other. Even a small amount can make each partner feel more independent.

Sex Like every other aspect of a relationship, sex evolves and changes over the course of marriage. The red-hot sexual chemistry of the early stages of intimacy invariably cools down. Even so, the happiest couples have sex more often than unhappily married pairs do.

What matters most isn't quantity alone, but the quality of sexual activity and intimacy. Are both partners satisfied with their sexual relationship? Does one partner always initiate sex? Do the partners talk about their preferences and pleasures? Sexuality, like personality, is dynamic and changes throughout life. Do the partners acknowledge and adapt to these changes? Do they feel sufficiently at ease with each other to discuss anxieties about sex? The answers to these questions can determine how sexually gratifying a marriage is for both spouses.

Extramarital Affairs How faithful are American mates? The answer depends on the questions researchers ask and who they ask. In face-to-face interviews, University of Chicago researchers found that 25 percent of men and 15 percent of women had had affairs and that 94 percent of the married subjects had been monogamous in the last year. Another survey of Americans found that one out of six Americans had had an extramarital relationship—19 percent of the men and 15 percent of the women.[29]

High or low, numbers are little comfort when affairs do occur. A husband or wife who learns about a spouse's affair typically feels a devastating sense of betrayal as well as deep feelings of shame, fear of abandonment, depression, and anger. Two crucial questions determine whether a marriage can survive: Do the spouses still feel a serious commitment to each other? And do they love each other and want to grow old together?

Two-Career Couples More than 75 percent of women with children work—a dramatic increase from the 1960s, when only 30 percent of mothers worked outside the home. Two careers can bring pressure to a relationship: Both individuals may come home tired and irritable; both may have to spend a great deal of time on their jobs; both may have to travel or work on weekends. Two-career couples must be able to discuss their problems openly to resolve these pressures.

Couples pursuing individual careers sometimes face difficult choices. What happens, for example, if one of them is offered a promising job in another city? Does the spouse quit his or her job, pack up, and move? Some couples resolve such dilemmas by working in different cities and spending weekends together. Others try to alternate career and home priorities. However imperfect these arrangements may be, they work for some couples.

Do dual careers affect a couple's sex lives? The answers are complex. Some researchers have theorized that long hours and multiple roles would dampen sexual expression in working couples. But that's not necessarily the case. Except for spouses working unusually demanding jobs (more than 54 hours a week), work per se does not cause psychological distress (in women, it actually promotes better mental health), nor does it affect sexual frequency.

In studies comparing homemakers and women working part or full time, there have been no significant differences in frequency of intercourse, sexual satisfaction, or decreased sexual desire. Fatigue does dampen a woman's sex life—but is just as common in homemakers without paid jobs as in employed women.

According to the Bureau of Labor Statistics, 29 percent of wives—an estimated 10.5 million women—outearn their spouses, double the percent with heftier incomes thirty years ago. With more women studying for advanced degrees and charging up corporate ladders, the number of "breadwinner" wives is expected to soar.

How will their marriages fare? Experts once predicted that as a wife's paycheck grew, her marriage would be doomed to discord and divorce. But the few academic studies that have focused on such couples have found not more challenges, but different ones. As they make more money, wives generally report greater marital happiness and well-being.

Conflict in Marriage

While all couples may wish to live happily and peacefully ever after, sooner or later, they argue. Years of research have shown that while conflict is inevitable, the key difference between happy and unhappy couples is the way they fight.

Happier couples interject positive interactions, like a joke or a smile, into their arguments. As long as the ratio of positive to negative interactions remains at least five to one, the relationship remains intact. By comparison, unhappy couples unfurl a barrage of negative words, gestures, criticisms, and hostility at their mates with hardly any positive interactions. Based on observations of couples in conflict, researchers have been able to predict which would divorce with 94 percent accuracy.[30]

Although many assume that women are more nurturing than men, research on married couples at the University of Toledo has found that husbands can be as emotionally sensitive and supportive as wives. However, their timing tends to be off.[31] "Men aren't oblivious," says researcher Lisa Neff, "but wives need to communicate their needs directly to their husbands."

Among the other suggestions therapists offer couples are:

- **Focus on friendship.** If a marriage is not built on a strong friendship, it may be difficult to stay connected over time.
- **Remember what you loved and admired in your partner in the first place.** Focusing on these qualities can foster a much more positive attitude toward him or her.
- **Show respect.** Your spouse deserves the same courtesy and civility that your colleagues do. Without respect, love cannot survive.
- **Compliment what your partner does right.** Noticing the positive can change how both of you feel about each other.
- **Forgive one another.** When your partner hurts your feelings but then reaches out, don't reject his or her attempts to make things better.

Saving Marriages

Fewer than two-thirds of couples—65 percent of husbands and 60 percent of wives—say they are "very happy" in their marriages (Figure 8-4). Each year, hundreds of thousands of couples go into counseling in an effort to make their unions happier. Among the approaches currently in use are marriage education and various forms of couples therapy.

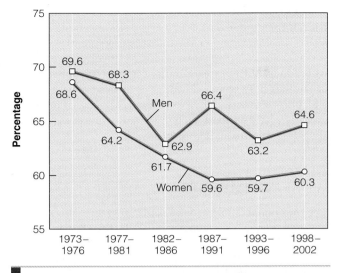

FIGURE 8-4 Percentage of Married Persons Age 18 and Older Who Said Their Marriages Were "Very Happy" (United States)

Source: Poponoe, David, and Barbara Dafoe Whitehead. *The State of Our Union: The Social Health of Marriage in America in 2005.* Copyright 2005 by the National Marriage Project at Rutgers University. Reprinted by permission of the National Marriage Project. http://marriage.rutgers.edu.

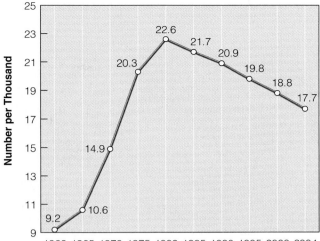

FIGURE 8-5 Number of Divorces per 1,000 Married Women Age 15 and Older (United States)

Source: Poponoe, David, and Barbara Dafoe Whitehead. *The State of Our Union: The Social Health of Marriage in America in 2005.* Copyright 2005 by the National Marriage Project at Rutgers University. Reprinted by permission of the National Marriage Project. http://marriage.rutgers.edu.

Marriage education consists of workshops that teach couples practical skills so they get along better. Some studies indicate that graduates of these programs have a lower divorce rate than unhappy couples who do not enroll in them.

Couples therapy, also called marriage counseling or marriage therapy, uses a variety of psychological techniques to help couples understand and overcome their conflicts. These include:

▪ **Behavioral marital therapy,** which teaches partners to communicate better and to improve their conflict resolution skills.

▪ **Emotionally focused therapy,** which helps couples identify and break free of destructive emotional cycles.

▪ **Insight-oriented marital therapy,** which combines behavioral therapy with techniques for understanding negative behaviors, such as power struggles, within the relationship.

FAQ WHAT IS THE CURRENT DIVORCE RATE?

Like marriage rates, the divorce rate also has fallen—from 22.6 per 1,000 married women 25 years ago to 17.7 per 1,000 married women (Figure 8-5). Your risk of divorce depends on many factors. Simply having some college education improves your odds of a happy marriage. Other factors that do the same are an income higher than $50,000, marrying at age 25 or older, not having a baby during the first seven months after the wedding, coming from an intact family, and having some religious affiliation.[32]

 Race also influences marriage and divorce rates. African-American couples are more likely to break up than white couples, and black divorcées are less likely to marry again. Researchers have found that African Americans place an equally high value on marriage. However, there is a smaller "marriageable pool" of black men for a variety of reasons, including a higher mortality rate.

Children whose parents divorced are less likely to marry and to stay married. However, their adult relationships aren't doomed to fail. "Divorce isn't in the genes," says child psychologist Judith Wallerstein, who has studied divorced families for thirty years. "Divorce is an avoidable human error."

FAMILY TIES

Children have become the exception rather than the rule in American households. A century ago most households contained children under age 18. In 1960, slightly fewer than half did. In 2000, fewer than a third of households included children, and this figure is expected to drop to 28 percent by 2010 (Figure 8-6).

Attitudes also have changed. While many traditionally viewed having children as the primary purpose for getting married, nearly 70 percent of Americans now cite another reason. When young adults—ages 18 to 34—react to the statement, "Those who want children should get married," only about half of men and even fewer women agree.

Fertility has declined in the United States since 1960. At that time, the average woman had about three and one-half children over the course of her life. Today's woman has an average of about two children, which is lower than the "replacement level" of 2.1 children per woman. This is the

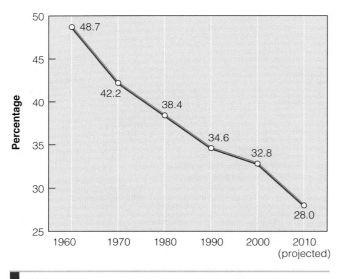

FIGURE 8-6 **Percentage of Households with a Child or Children Under Age 18 (United States)**

Source: Poponoe, David, and Barbara Dafoe Whitehead. *The State of Our Union:The Social Health of Marriage in America in 2005.* Copyright 2005 by the National Marriage Project at Rutgers University. Reprinted by permission of the National Marriage Project. http://marriage.rutgers.edu.

level at which the population would be replaced by births alone. In most European and several Asian countries, fertility has dropped even lower.

DIVERSITY WITHIN FAMILIES

The all-American **family**—as portrayed on television and in movies—is typically white and middle-class. But families of different cultures—Italian to Indian to Indonesian—reflect different traditions, beliefs, and values. Within African-American families, for instance, traditional gender roles are often reversed, with women serving as head of the household, a kinship bond uniting several households, and a strong religious commitment or orientation. In Chinese-American families, both spouses may work and see themselves as breadwinners, but the wife may not have an equal role in decision making. In Hispanic families, wives and mothers are acknowledged and respected as healers and dispensers of wisdom. At the same time, they are expected to defer to their husbands, who see themselves as the strong, protective, dominant head of the family. As time passes and families from different cultures become more integrated into American life, traditional gender roles and decision-making patterns often change, particularly among the youngest family members.

American families are diverse in other ways. *Multigenerational families,* with children, parents, and grandparents, make up 3.7 percent of households. They occur most often in areas where new immigrants live with relatives, where housing shortages or high costs force families to double up their living arrangements, or where high rates of out-of-wedlock childbearing force unwed mothers to live with their children in their parents' home.

Three of every ten households consist of **blended families,** formed when one or both of the partners bring children from a previous union. In the future, social scientists predict, American families will become even more diverse, or pluralistic. But as norms or expectations about the configurations of families have changed, values or ideas about the intents and purposes of families have not. American families of every type still support each other and strive toward values such as commitment and caring.

WORKING PARENTS

The traditional family with a breadwinner and a homemaker has been replaced by what some call "the juggler family." Two working parents or an unmarried working parent head 70 percent of American families with children. As a result, American parents have 22 fewer hours to spend with their children than parents did in 1969.[33] Women, balancing multiple roles as parents, spouses, caregivers, and employees often give their own personal needs the lowest priority.[34]

The Family and Work Institute of New York calculates that American husbands put in 75 percent as much time as wives on workday chores—a dramatic rise from 30 percent in 1977. In actual clocktime, the gender difference in domestic "scutwork" amounts to just 45 minutes a day.

Plenty of sociologists—and lots of weary women still doing the lioness share of chores—doubt whether all men in all income groups are doing as much. However, the trend toward greater husbandly involvement is real—and likely to continue.

SINGLE PARENTS

About 28 percent of all children under age 18 live with just one parent, the majority with their mothers. The number of families headed by single mothers has increased 25 percent since 1990, to more than 7.5 million households. About a third of all babies are born to unmarried women, compared to just 3.8 percent in 1940.

The new breed of single mother doesn't fit the old stereotype of an unwed, minority teenager. The median age for unmarried mothers is the late 20s; the fastest growing group is white women. She may be divorced or unmarried. Forty percent live with men who may be the fathers of one or more of their children.

Single fathers head over two million households. Men now comprise 1 in 6 of the nation's 11.9 million single parents, up from 1 in 7 in 1995 and 1 in 10 in 1980.

The typical single father is 38 years old. One in 9 is under age 25; and 1 in 70 is 60 or older. About 5 of every 6 (83 percent) of the nation's single fathers are white. African Americans and Hispanics together constitute about 13 percent.

Median family income for one-parent families is significantly lower than the median for two-parent families. Twenty percent are poor, compared with 9 percent of two-parent families. Half live in rental housing, compared with one-quarter of two-parent families.

Learn It / Live It
Creating Better Relationships

We are born social. From our first days of life, we reach out to others, struggle to express ourselves, strive to forge connections. The fabric of our lives becomes richer as family and friends weave through it the threads of their experiences. No solitary pleasure can match the gifts that we gain by reaching out and connecting with others.

As with other significant endeavors, good relationships require work—through hard times, despite conflicts, over months and years and decades. As you strive to improve the ties that bind you to others, keep in mind the characteristics of a good relationship. They can serve as the goals you strive to attain:

- **Trust.** Partners are able to confide in each other openly, knowing their confidences will be respected.
- **Togetherness.** In a healthy relationship, two people create a sense of both intimacy and autonomy. They enjoy each other's company but also pursue solitary interests.
- **Expressiveness.** Partners in healthy relationships say what they feel, need, and desire.
- **Staying power.** People in committed relationships keep their bond strong through tough times by proving that they will be there for each other.
- **Security.** Because a good relationship is strong enough to absorb conflict and anger, partners know they can express their feelings honestly. They also are willing to risk vulnerability for the sake of becoming closer.
- **Laughter.** Humor keeps things in perspective—always crucial in any sort of ongoing relationship or enterprise.
- **Support.** Partners in good relationships continually offer each other encouragement, comfort, and acceptance.
- **Physical affection.** Sexual desire may fluctuate or diminish over the years, but partners in loving, long-term relationships usually retain some physical connection.
- **Personal growth.** In the best relationships, partners are committed to bringing out the best in each other and have the other's best interests at heart.
- **Respect.** Caring partners are aware of each other's boundaries, need for personal space, and vulnerabilities. They do not take each other or their relationship for granted.

Making This Chapter Work for You
Review Questions

1. In friendships and other intimate relationships, which of the following is *not* true?
   a. Friends can communicate feelings as well as facts.
   b. Listening is just as important as talking.
   c. Emotional investment is required but the rewards are great.
   d. There is no need to pay attention to nonverbal communication.

2. Which of the following scenarios demonstrates what might be considered gender differences in verbal and nonverbal communication styles?
   a. While Alyssa and Peter are discussing their vacation plans, Alyssa is gazing at the television and Peter is looking at Alyssa.
   b. Good friends Eva and Julia see each other for the first time after Christmas break and greet each other with a nod and a quick "Hi."
   c. New bank manager Alejandro tells the staff that they should consider him "the team coach and the keeper of the playbook."
   d. During an argument, Tony complains to Nicki, "I don't appreciate your crude jokes and constant swearing."

3. Romantic love
   a. is associated with the depletion of the hormone oxytocin.
   b. is an emotional phenomenon between humans that has its roots in prehistoric times and occurs in almost all cultures.
   c. can only occur between people who share interests and goals.
   d. always results in a committed long-term relationship.

4. The characteristics of a good relationship include which of the following?
   a. trust   c. identical interests
   b. financial stability   d. physical attractiveness

5. Which of these is an example of self-disclosure?
   a. Steve tells his friend Twana that he would really like to change jobs sometime in the next year.
   b. Mike and Nicole talk about which cars they prefer.
   c. Maria mentions to Carrie that she and her brother don't get along so he won't be at the picnic.
   d. Angela lets her boyfriend Paul know that she used to be bulimic.

6. Which of the following is more likely a sign of a dysfunctional relationship?
   a. The partners have frequent disagreements about money.

(*continued, p. 232*)

Self Survey ■ How Strong Are the Communication and Affection in Your Relationship?

Effective, caring communication and loving affection markedly enhance a couple's relationship. The following self-test may help you to assess the degree of good communication, love, and respect in your intimate relationship. If you agree or mostly agree with a statement, answer yes. If you disagree or mostly disagree, answer no. You may wish to have your partner respond to this assessment as well. If so, mark your answers on a separate sheet.

1.	My partner seeks out my opinion.	Yes	No
2.	My partner cares about my feelings.	Yes	No
3.	I don't feel ignored very often.	Yes	No
4.	We touch each other a lot.	Yes	No
5.	We listen to each other.	Yes	No
6.	We respect each other's ideas.	Yes	No
7.	We are affectionate toward one another.	Yes	No
8.	I feel my partner takes good care of me.	Yes	No
9.	What I say counts.	Yes	No
10.	I am important in our decisions.	Yes	No
11.	There's lots of love in our relationship.	Yes	No
12.	We are genuinely interested in one another.	Yes	No
13.	I love spending time with my partner.	Yes	No
14.	We are very good friends.	Yes	No
15.	Even during rough times, we can be empathetic.	Yes	No
16.	My partner is considerate of my viewpoint.	Yes	No
17.	My partner finds me physically attractive.	Yes	No
18.	My partner expresses warmth toward me.	Yes	No
19.	I feel included in my partner's life.	Yes	No
20.	My partner admires me.	Yes	No

Scoring:

A preponderance of yes answers indicates that you enjoy a strong relationship characterized by good communication and loving affection. If you answered yes to fewer than seven items, it is likely that you are not feeling loved and respected and that the communication in your relationship is decidedly lacking.

Source: John Gottman, *Why Marriages Succeed or Fail.* New York: Simon & Schuster, 1994.

YOUR ACTION PLAN FOR BETTER COMMUNICATION

Like other skills, communication improves with practice. Here are some suggestions that can enhance your ability to express yourself more precisely and to understand spoken and unspoken messages from others.

- **Tune into your body talk.** Notice details about the way you speak, gesture, and move. If possible, watch yourself on videotape. Analyze the emotions you're feeling at the time and think of how they may be influencing your body language.

- **Learn to establish good eye contact, but don't glare or stare.** If you sense that someone feels uncomfortable with an intense eye grip, shift your focus so that your gaze hits somewhere between the eyes and the chin, rather than pupil-to-pupil.

- **Avoid putting up barriers.** If you fold your arms across your chest, you'll look defensive or uninterested in contact. Crossing your legs or ankles also can seem like a way of keeping your distance.

- **Identify the little things you characteristically do when you're tense.** Some people pat their hair or pick at their ears; others rub their necks, twist a ring or watch, twirl a lock of hair, or play with a pen. Train yourself to become aware of what you're doing (have a friend give your a signal, if necessary) and to control your mannerisms.

- **Use "I" statements.** Describe what's going on with you. Say "I worry about being liked" or "I get frustrated when I can't put my feelings into words." Avoid generalities such as "You never think about my feelings," or "Nobody understands me."

- **Gently ask how the other person feels.** If your friend or partner describes thoughts rather than feelings, ask for more adjectives. Was he or she sad, excited, angry, hurt?

- **Become a very good listener.** When another person talks, don't interrupt, ask why, judge, or challenge. Nod your head. Use your body language and facial expression to show you're eager to hear more.

- **Respect confidences.** Treat a friend's or partner's secrets with the discretion they deserve. Consider them a special gift entrusted to your care.

CASE IN POINT

Student: Selah, 21

Goal: Either improve or end her two-year relationship with an emotionally unavailable man

Action Plan:

- Talk to a trusted friend about why she feels unsatisfied in the relationship.

- Practice "I" statements of her feelings.

- Choose a quiet time and a private setting for a conversation with her boyfriend.

- Communicate without blaming.

- Ask for his feedback, and listen attentively.

Health☺Now™   If you want to write your own goals for enhanced relationship, go to the **Wellness Journal at HealthNow** http://healthnow.brookscole .com/ith.

b. One partner makes all the decisions for the couple and the other partner.

c. Each partner has a demanding career.

d. One partner is much older than the other partner.

7. Partners in successful marital relationships

  a. are generally from the same social and ethnic background.

  b. usually lived together before marrying.

  c. were usually very young at the time of their marriage.

  d. have premarital agreements.

8. Married people

  a. have sex less frequently than unmarried partners.

  b. are more likely to become alcoholics and drug users.

  c. typically have at least one extramarital affair during their marriage.

  d. live longer than single or divorced individuals.

9. Some disagreement is part of every relationship. Here's a good communication method when arguing:

  a. Ignore the subject of the disagreement.

  b. Make fun of your partner's point of view.

  c. Keep your partner's good qualities in mind.

  d. Vent about every misunderstanding over the past two years.

10. Which of the following statements is *false*?

  a. College education increases your chances of a happy marriage.

  b. African-American couples are more likely to divorce than white couples.

  c. Children whose parents divorced are more likely to stay married.

  d. The divorce rate is lower now than it was in 1980.

Answers to these questions can be found on page 587.

Critical Thinking

1. Reread the section on Personal Communication in this chapter, and think about your own communication skills. How does your communication style compare to the patterns for your gender? Do your personal experiences support or contradict the research results?

2. While our society has become more tolerant, marriages between people of different religious and racial groups still face special pressures. What issues might arise if a Christian marries a Jew or Muslim? What about the issues facing partners of different races? How could these issues be resolved? What are your own feelings about mixed marriages? Would you date someone of a different religion or race? Why or why not?

3. What are your personal criteria for a successful relationship? Develop a brief list of factors you consider important, and support your choices with examples or experiences from your own life.

Media Menu

Health⊗Now™

Throughout the chapter, this icon introduces a list of resources on the Health-Now website at **http://healthnow.brookscole.com/ith** that will:

- Help you evaluate your knowledge of the material.
- Allow you to take an exam-prep quiz.
- Provide a Personalized Learning Plan targeting resources that address areas you should study.
- Coach you through identifying target goals for behavior change and creating and monitoring your personal change plan throughout the semester.

INTERNET CONNECTIONS

Go Ask Alice

www.goaskalice.columbia.edu

On this popular site, sponsored by the health education and wellness program of the Columbia University Health Service, educators answer questions on a wide variety of topics, including those related to relationships and marriage and family.

Family and relationship articles from the APA

www.apahelpcenter.org/articles/topic.php?id=2

The American Psychological Association provides a wealth of articles and information on sustaining healthy relationships.

Parenting and Families—information from the University of Minnesota's Children, Youth, and Family Consortium

www.cyfc.umn.edu/family/index.html

This site offers research, programs, publications, and information on all types of parenting, relationships, and family issues.

InfoTrac College Edition Activities Log on, insert **online dating** into the Keyword search box, and limit your search to the past year. When you get the results, Mark articles to review, then Select one to read. Summarize three or four key points from the article.

You can find additional readings related to personal health with InfoTrac College Edition, an online library of more than 900 journals and publications. Follow the instructions for accessing InfoTrac College Edition that were packaged with your textbook; then search for articles using a keyword search.

For additional links, resources, and suggested readings on the InfoTrac College Edition, visit our Health and Wellness Resource Center at **http://health .wadsworth.com.**

Key Terms

The terms listed are used on the page indicated. Definitions of the terms are in the Glossary at the end of this book.

blended families 228

codependency 216

cohabitation 221

companion-oriented
    marriages 224

dysfunctional 215

enabling 217

family 228

intimacy 217

neurotransmitters 220

oxytocin 220

rescue marriages 224

romantic marriages 224

self-disclosure 214

traditional marriages 224

9 Personal Sexuality

Charles, several years older than the typical college freshman, usually doesn't think much about the age difference—until the conversation turns to sex. He understands his younger classmates' seemingly endless fascination with sex, but his perspective is different. As a teenager, he had plunged recklessly into dangerous territory of every type. Sex—casual and sometimes unprotected—was one of them. Looking back, he feels lucky that he didn't, as he puts it, "end up a statistic." But he still regrets the irresponsible ways he acted.

At 28 Charles is a veteran of military service, a married man, and an expectant father. His enjoyment of sex hasn't faded—in many ways, it's deepened and become more gratifying. He now realizes that there is no such thing as casual sex, that sexual choices have consequences and effects on one's own life and on other people. These are the lessons he hopes someday to pass on to his own children.

As Charles learned with time and experience, you are ultimately responsible for your sexual health and behavior. You make decisions that affect how you express your **sexuality,** how you respond sexually, and how you give and get sexual pleasure. Yet most sexual activity involves another person. Therefore, your decisions about sex—more so than those you make about nutrition, drugs, or exercise—have important effects on other people. Recognizing this fact is the key to responsible sexuality.

Human sexuality—the quality of being sexual—is as rich, varied, and complex as life itself. Along with our **sex,** or biological maleness or femaleness, it is an integral part of who we are, how we see ourselves, and how we relate to others. Of all of our involvements with others, sexual **intimacy,** or physical closeness, can be the most rewarding. But while sexual expression and experience can provide intense joy, they also can involve great emotional turmoil.

Sexual responsibility means learning about your body, your partner's body, your sexual development and preferences, and the health risks associated with sexual activity. This chapter is an introduction to your sexual self and an exploration of sexual issues in today's world. It provides the information and insight you can use in making decisions and choosing behaviors that are responsible for all concerned.

Masterfile (RM)/Jon Feingersh

After studying the material in this chapter, you should be able to:

■ **Explain** the roles of hormones in sexual development.

■ **Describe** the male and female reproductive systems and the functions of the individual structures of each system.

■ **Describe** conditions or issues unique to women's and men's sexual health.

■ **Define** sexual health and list behaviors that can contribute to sexually healthy relationships.

■ **Define** sexual orientation and **give examples** of sexual diversity.

■ **List** the range of sexual behaviors practiced by adults.

■ **Describe** the phases of sexual response.

■ **List** the common sexual concerns of men and women.

SEXUALITY AND THE DIMENSIONS OF HEALTH

Our sexuality both affects and is affected by the various dimensions of health. Responsible sexuality and high-level sexual health contribute to the fullest possible functioning of body, mind, spirit, and social relationships. In turn, other aspects of health enhance our sexuality. Here are some examples:

▪ **Physical.** As described in Chapter 14, safer sex practices reduce the risk of sexually transmitted infections that can threaten sexual health, physical health, and even survival. When our bodies are healthy and well, we feel better about how we look and move—which enhances both self-esteem and healthy sexuality.

▪ **Emotional.** By acknowledging and respecting the intimacy of a sexual relationship, responsible sexuality builds trust and commitment. When our emotional health is high, we can better understand and cope with the complex feelings related to being sexual.

▪ **Social.** From dating to mating, we express and fulfill our sexual identities in the context of families, friends, and society as a whole. Having strong friendships, intimate relationships, and caring partnerships enables us to explore our sexuality in safe and healthy ways.

▪ **Intellectual.** Our most fulfilling relationships involve a meeting of minds as well as bodies. High-level intellectual health enables us to acquire and understand sexual information, analyze it critically, and make healthy sexual decisions.

▪ **Spiritual.** At its deepest, most fulfilling level, sexuality uplifts the soul by allowing us to connect to something greater than oneself. Individuals who have developed their spirituality bring to their most intimate relationships an awareness and appreciation that lifts them beyond the physical.

▪ **Environmental.** Responsible sexuality makes people more aware of the impact of their decisions on others. Protecting yourself from sexual threats and creating a supportive environment in which to study and work are crucial to high-level health and to healthy sexuality.

BECOMING MALE OR FEMALE

Physiological maleness or femaleness, or biological sex, is indicated by the sex chromosomes, hormonal balance, and genital anatomy. **Gender** refers to the psychological and sociological, as well as the physical, aspects of being male or female. You are born with a certain *sexual identity* based on your sexual anatomy and appearance; you, your parents, and society mold your *gender identity*.

ARE YOU AN X OR A Y?

Biologically, few absolute differences separate the sexes: Males alone can make sperm and contribute the chromosome that causes embryos to develop as males; females alone are born with sex cells (eggs, or ova), menstruate, give birth, and breast-feed babies. But the process of becoming male or female is a long and complex one.

In the beginning, all human embryos have undifferentiated sex organs. Only after several weeks do the sex organs differentiate, becoming either male or female **gonads** (testes or ovaries), the structures that produce the future reproductive cells of an individual. This initial differentiation process depends on genetic instructions in the form of the sex chromosomes, referred to as X and Y (Figure 9-1). If a Y (or male) chromosome is present in the embryo, about seven weeks after conception, it signals the sex organs to develop into testes. If a Y chromosome isn't present, an embryo begins developing ovaries in the eighth week. From this point on, the sex hormones produced by the gonads, not the chromosomes, play the crucial role in making a male or female.

(FAQ) HOW DO HORMONES WORK?

In Greek, *hormone* means "set into motion"— and that's exactly what our **hormones** do. These chemical messengers, produced by various organs in the body, including the sex organs, and carried to target structures by the

FIGURE 9-1 Genetic Sexual Differentiation
Human cells contain 23 pairs of chromosomes. One of these pairs is the sex chromosomes. A normal female has two X chromosomes and a normal male has an X and a Y chromosome.

© Custom Medical Stock

bloodstream, arouse cells and organs to specific activities and influence the way we look, feel, develop, and behave.

The group of organs that produce hormones is referred to as the **endocrine system.** Except for the sex organs, males and females have identical endocrine systems. Directing the endocrine system is the *hypothalamus,* a pea-sized section of the brain. The pituitary gland, directly beneath the hypothalamus, turns the various glands on and off in response to messages from it.

The ovaries produce the sex hormones most crucial to women, **estrogen** and **progesterone.** The primary sex hormone in men is **testosterone,** which is produced by the testes and the adrenal glands. However, both men and women have small amounts of the hormones of the opposite sex. Estrogen, in fact, is crucial to male fertility and gives sperm what researchers describe as their "reproductive punch."

The sex hormones begin their work early in an embryo's development. As soon as the testes are formed, they start releasing testosterone, which stimulates the development of other structures, such as the penis. The absence of testosterone in an embryo causes female genitals to form. (If the testes of a genetic male don't produce testosterone, the fetus will develop female genitals. Similarly, if a genetic female is exposed to excessive testosterone, the fetus will have ovaries but will also develop male genitals.)

As puberty begins, the pituitary gland initiates the changes that transform boys into men and girls into women (Figure 9-2). When a boy is about 14 years old and a girl about 12, their brains stimulate the hypothalamus to secrete a hormone called *gonadotropin-releasing hormone (GnRH).* This substance causes the pituitary gland to release hormones called **gonadotropins.** These, in turn, stimulate the gonads to make sex hormones.

The gonadotropins are *follicle-stimulating hormone (FSH)* and *luteinizing hormone (LH).* In girls, these hormones travel to the ovary and stimulate the production of estrogen. As estrogen increases, a girl's **secondary sex characteristics** develop. Her breasts become fuller, her external genitals enlarge, and fat is deposited on her hips and buttocks. Estrogen keeps her hair thick and skin smooth. She begins menstruating because she has begun ovulating, the process that prepares her body to conceive and carry a baby.

This process seems to be beginning earlier than in the past. "By eight, 15 percent of white girls and 48 percent of African-American girls show signs of sexual development," says Marcia Herman-Giddens, Ph.D., of the University of North Carolina at Chapel Hill, who analyzed 17,077 growth charts from pediatricians around the country. In her study, the mean ages for breast development were 8.87 years for African-American girls and 9.96 years for white girls. African-American girls reach **menarche**—the term for first menstruation—at a mean age of 12.16 years; white girls, at 12.88 years. By comparison, a hundred years ago girls didn't reach menarche until the relatively ripe age of fifteen.[1]

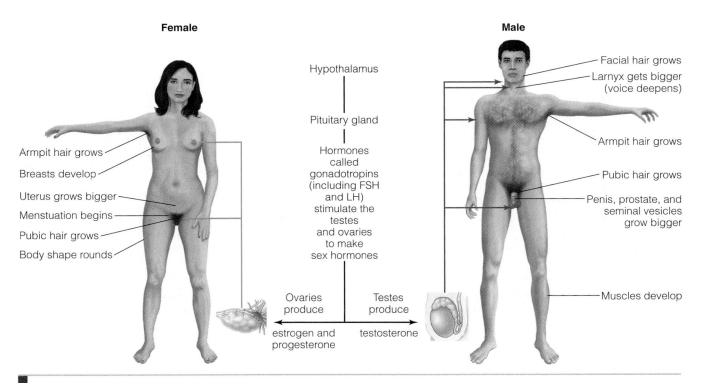

FIGURE 9-2   Puberty

The body's endocrine system produces hormones that trigger body changes, including growth spurts, in boys and girls.

Improved nutrition and good health seem to be the primary factors. Girls today are bigger, taller, better fed, more sedentary, and have a higher percentage of body fat (one of the triggers of sexual maturation). They also grow up amid a host of environmental influences that may further speed development.

 Cultural influences affect a girl's response to menarche. In a cross-cultural study of college students, the most common emotions expressed by American women at menarche were embarrassment, pride, and anxiety. Malaysian women cited fear, embarrassment, and worry. Lithuanian women described themselves as happy or scared, while Sudanese women cited fear, anxiety, embarrassment, and anger. On the positive side, the Lithuanian women reported feeling more valuable and believing they had entered the world of women. American girls worried about whether they could still play sports but felt superior to friends who had not reached menarche and became eager to learn about sex. Malaysians described feeling wise, respected, and mature. Sudanese women felt more beautiful and aware that they could now have children.

In boys, the gonadotropins stimulate the testes to produce testosterone, which triggers the development of male secondary sex characteristics. Their voices deepen, hair grows on their faces and bodies, their penises become thicker and longer, and their muscles become stronger.

The sex hormones released during puberty change the growth pattern of childhood, so that a boy or girl may now spurt up 4 to 6 inches in a single year. The skeleton matures very rapidly until, at the end of puberty (usually around age 18), the growth centers at the ends of the bones close off. Estrogen causes girls' bones to stop growing at an earlier age than boys' bones.

SEXUAL AND GENDER IDENTITY

It's a boy! It's a girl! These statements confer an instant identity on a newborn. However, in recent years, researchers have challenged such either/or distinctions as male or female, masculine or feminine, heterosexual or homosexual. Although most people have the biological characteristics of a male or a female, some possess some degree of both male and female reproductive structures. They are referred to as intersexual.

The continuum for gender identity ranges from extreme stereotypical masculine notions to extreme stereotypical feminine behaviors. Different cultures vary in defining what is masculine or feminine. Individuals who consider themselves androgynous choose not to conform to sexual stereotypes. **Androgyny** includes those who are "positively androgynous," combining positive attributes linked with both sexes, for example, feminine compassion and masculine independence and individuals who are "negatively androgynous" and might show less desirable characteristics of each gender, such as feminine dependency and masculine assertiveness. (Transgenderism is discussed on page 249.)

WOMEN'S SEXUAL HEALTH

Only recently has medical research devoted major scientific investigations to issues in women's health. Until about a decade ago, the National Institutes of Health routinely excluded women from experimental studies because of concerns about menstrual cycles and pregnancy. In clinical settings, women are more likely to have their symptoms dismissed as psychological and not to be referred to a specialist than are men with identical complaints. Some physicians are suggesting the creation of a new medical specialty (distinct from obstetrics and gynecology) that would be devoted to women's health.

FEMALE SEXUAL ANATOMY

As illustrated in Figure 9-3a, the **mons pubis** is the rounded, fleshy area over the junction of the pubic bones. The folds of skin that form the outer lips of a woman's genital area are called the **labia majora.** They cover soft flaps of skin (inner lips) called the **labia minora.** The inner lips join at the top to form a hood over the **clitoris,** a small elongated erectile organ, and the most sensitive spot in the entire female genital area. Below the clitoris is the **urethral opening,** the outer opening of the thin tube that carries urine from the bladder. Below that is a larger opening, the mouth of the **vagina,** the canal that leads to the primary internal organs of reproduction. The **perineum** is the area between the vagina and the anus (the opening to the rectum and large intestine).

At the back of the vagina is the **cervix,** the opening to the womb, or **uterus** (see Figure 9-3b). The uterine walls are lined by a layer of tissue called the **endometrium.** The **ovaries,** about the size and shape of almonds, are located on either side of the uterus and contain egg cells called **ova** (singular, **ovum**). Extending outward and back from the upper uterus are the **fallopian tubes,** the canals that transport ova from the ovaries to the uterus. When an egg is released from an ovary, the fingerlike ends of the adjacent fallopian tube "catch" the egg and direct it into the tube.

Discharge and changes in odor normally occur in a healthy vagina. They typically fluctuate through the menstrual cycle, depending on hormone level. In the past, many women practiced douching, the introduction of a liquid into the vagina, to cleanse the vagina. However, particularly if done frequently, douching may increase the risk of pelvic inflammatory disease (discussed in Chapter 14) and ectopic or out-of-uterus pregnancy. Despite the potential dangers, according to data from a southern university, four in ten female students had douched in the past; half currently douche. African-American women were encouraged to douche by their mothers; white women were more influenced by television advertisements. When advised to stop douching by a doctor or nurse, most students do so.[2]

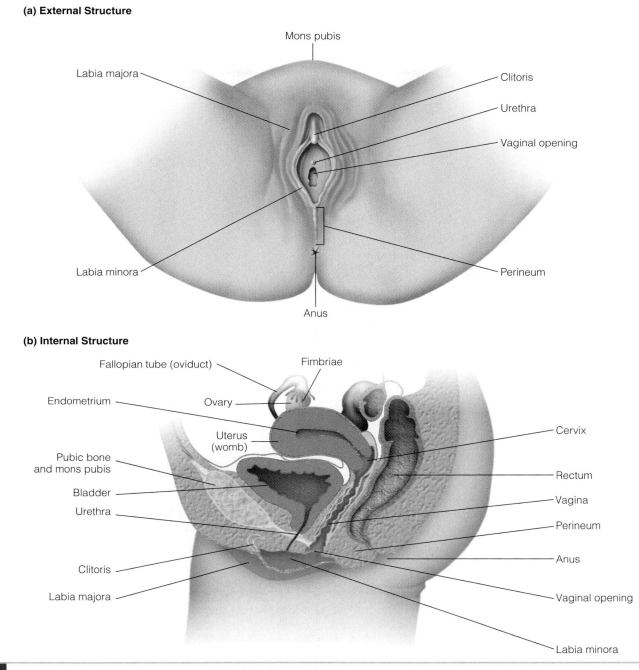

(a) External Structure

- Mons pubis
- Labia majora
- Clitoris
- Urethra
- Vaginal opening
- Perineum
- Labia minora
- Anus

(b) Internal Structure

- Fallopian tube (oviduct)
- Fimbriae
- Endometrium
- Ovary
- Uterus (womb)
- Cervix
- Pubic bone and mons pubis
- Rectum
- Bladder
- Vagina
- Urethra
- Perineum
- Clitoris
- Anus
- Labia majora
- Vaginal opening
- Labia minora

FIGURE 9-3   The Female Sex Organs and Reproductive Structures

THE MENSTRUAL CYCLE

Scientists have discovered that the menstrual cycle actually begins in the brain with the production of gonadotropin-releasing hormone (GnRH). Each month a surge of GnRH sets into motion the sequence of steps that lead to ovulation, the potential for conception, and if conception doesn't occur, menstruation. The hypothalamus monitors hormone levels in the blood and sends messages to the pituitary gland to release follicle-stimulating hormone (FSH) and luteinizing hormone (LH).

As shown in Figure 9-4, in the ovaries, these hormones stimulate the growth of a few of the immature eggs, or ova, stored in follicles in every woman's body. Usually, only one ovum matures completely during each monthly cycle. As it does, it increases its production of the female sex hormone estrogen, which in turn triggers the release of a larger surge of LH.

At midcycle, the increased LH hormone levels trigger **ovulation,** the release of the egg cell, or ovum, from the follicle. Estrogen levels drop, and the remaining cells of the

FIGURE 9-4   Menstrual Cycle

(a) In response to the hypothalamus, the pituitary gland releases the gonadotropins FSH and LH. Levels of FSH and LH stimulate the cycle (and in turn are affected by production of estrogen and progesterone).

(b) FSH does what its name says—it stimulates follicle development in the ovary. The follicle matures and ruptures, releasing an ovum (egg) into the fallopian tube.

(c) The follicle produces estrogen, and the corpus luteum produces estrogen and progesterone. The high level of estrogen at the middle of the cycle produces a surge of LH, which triggers ovulation.

(d) Estrogen and progesterone stimulate the endometrium, which becomes thicker and prepares to receive an implanted, fertilized egg.

If a fertilized egg is deposited in the uterus, pregnancy begins. If the egg is not fertilized, progesterone production decreases, and the endometrium is shed (menstruation). At this point, both estrogen and progesterone levels have dropped, so the pituitary responds by producing FSH, and the cycle begins again.

follicle then enlarge, change character, and form the **corpus luteum,** or yellow body. In the second half of the menstrual cycle, the corpus luteum secretes estrogen and larger amounts of progesterone. The endometrium (uterine lining) is stimulated by progesterone to thicken and become more engorged with blood in preparation for nourishing an implanted, fertilized ovum.

If the ovum is not fertilized, the corpus luteum disintegrates. As the level of progesterone drops, **menstruation** occurs; the uterine lining is shed during the course of a menstrual period. If the egg is fertilized and pregnancy occurs, the cells that eventually develop into the placenta secrete *human chorionic gonadotropin (HCG),* a messenger hormone that signals the pituitary not to start a new cycle. The corpus luteum then steps up its production of progesterone.

A woman's attitudes toward menstruation can affect her sexual attitudes and behaviors. In a Canadian study of 114 romantically involved women, those who had engaged in sex during their periods were significantly more comfortable with menstruation, less sensitive to disgust in general, and more aroused by romantic and unconventional sexual activities.[3]

Many women experience physical or psychological changes, or both, during their monthly cycles. Usually the changes are minor, but more serious problems can occur.

PREMENSTRUAL SYNDROME

Women with **premenstrual syndrome (PMS)** experience bodily discomfort and emotional distress for up to two weeks, from ovulation until the onset of menstruation. Up to 75 percent of menstruating women report one or more premenstrual symptoms; 3 to 9 percent experience disabling, incapacitating symptoms.[4]

Once dismissed as a psychological problem, PMS has been recognized as a very real physiological disorder that may be caused by a hormonal deficiency; abnormal levels of thyroid hormone; an imbalance of estrogen and progesterone; or social and environmental factors, particularly stress. Recent studies indicate that PMS may originate in the brain. Changes in brain receptors during the ovarian cycle may be responsible.[5]

The most common symptoms of PMS are mood changes, anxiety, irritability, difficulty concentrating, forgetfulness, impaired judgment, tearfulness, digestive symptoms (diarrhea, bloating, constipation), hot flashes, palpitations, dizziness, headache, fatigue, changes in appetite, cravings (usually for sweets or salt), water retention, breast tenderness, and insomnia. For a diagnosis to be made, women—using a self-rating symptom scale or calendar—must report troubling premenstrual symptoms in the period before menstruation in at least two successive menstrual cycles.

Treatments for PMS depend on specific symptoms. Diuretics (drugs that speed up fluid elimination) can relieve water retention and bloating. Relaxation techniques have led to a 60 percent reduction in anxiety symptoms. Sleep deprivation, or the use of bright light to adjust a woman's circadian or daily rhythm, also has proven beneficial. Behavioral approaches, such as exercise or charting cycles, help by letting women know when they're vulnerable.

Low doses of medications known as *selective serotonin-reuptake inhibitors* (SSRIs), such as fluoxetine (marketed as Prozac, Sarafem, and in generic forms) provide relief for symptoms such as tension, depression, irritability, and mood swings, even when taken only during the premenstrual phase rather than daily throughout the month. SSRIs are not effective in all women with PMS, and other factors, including a genetic susceptibility, may play a role. Oral contraceptives, though widely prescribed for PMS, have not been shown to be consistently effective.

A diet rich in calcium and vitamin D reduces the risk of PMS. In recent studies that followed women for more than ten years, those whose daily diet included low-fat milk, yogurt, and other good calcium sources lowered their likelihood of PMS symptoms.[6] Other treatments with some reported success include calcium supplements; vitamins; exercise; less caffeine, alcohol, salt and sugar; acupuncture; and stress management techniques such as meditation or relaxation training.

PREMENSTRUAL DYSPHORIC DISORDER (PMDD)

Premenstrual dysphoric disorder (PMDD), which is not related to PMS, occurs in an estimated 3 to 5 percent of all menstruating women. It is characterized by regular symptoms of depression (depressed mood, anxiety, mood swings, diminished interest or pleasure) during the last week of the menstrual cycle. Women with PMDD cannot function as usual at work, school, or home. They feel better a few days after menstruation begins. SSRIs, which are used to treat PMS, also are effective in relieving symptoms of PMDD.

MENSTRUAL CRAMPS

Dysmenorrhea is the medical name for the discomforts—abdominal cramps and pain, back and leg pain, diarrhea, tension, water retention, fatigue, and depression—that can occur during menstruation. About half of all menstruating women suffer from dysmenorrhea. The cause seems to be an overproduction of bodily substances called *prostaglandins,* which typically rise during menstruation. Medications that inhibit prostaglandins can reduce menstrual pain, and exercise can also relieve cramps.

AMENORRHEA

Women may stop menstruating—a condition called **amenorrhea**—for a variety of reasons, including a hormonal disorder, drastic weight loss, strenuous exercise, or change in the environment. "Boarding-school amenorrhea" is common among young women who leave home for school. Distance running and strenuous exercise also can lead to amenorrhea. The reason may be a drop in body fat from the normal range

Strategies for Prevention ▪▪ Reducing Premenstrual Problems

▪▪ Get plenty of exercise. Physically fit women usually have fewer problems both before and during their periods.

▪▪ Eat frequently and nutritiously. In the week before your period, your body doesn't regulate the levels of sugar, or glucose, in your blood as well as it usually does.

▪▪ Swear off salt. If you stop using salt at the table and while cooking, you may gain less weight premenstrually, feel less bloated, and suffer less from headaches and irritability.

▪▪ Cut back on caffeine. Coffee, colas, diet colas, chocolate, and tea can increase breast tenderness and other symptoms.

▪▪ Don't drink or smoke. Some women become so sensitive to alcohol's effects before their periods that a glass of wine hits with the impact of several stiff drinks. Nicotine worsens low blood sugar problems.

▪▪ Watch out for sweets. Premenstrual cravings for sweets are common, but try to resist. Sugar may pick you up, but later you'll feel worse than before.

▪▪ Add more dairy products to your diet. They can lower your risk of problems.

---

of 18 to 22 percent to a range of 9 to 12 percent. To be considered amenorrheic, a woman's menstrual cycle is typically absent for three or more consecutive months. Prolonged amenorrhea can have serious health consequences, including a loss of bone density that may lead to stress fractures or osteoporosis.

Scientists have developed chemical mimics, or analogues, of GnRH—usually administered by nasal spray—that trigger ovulation in women who don't ovulate or menstruate normally.

TOXIC SHOCK SYNDROME

This rare, potentially deadly bacterial infection primarily strikes menstruating women under the age of 30 who use tampons. Both *Staphylococcus aureus* and group A *Streptococcus pyogenes* can produce **toxic shock syndrome (TSS).** Symptoms include a high fever; a rash that leads to peeling of the skin on the fingers, toes, palms, and soles; dizziness; dangerously low blood pressure; and abnormalities in several organ systems (the digestive tract and the kidneys) and in the muscles and blood. Treatment usually consists of antibiotics and intense supportive care; intravenous administration of immunoglobulins that attack the toxins produced by these bacteria also may be beneficial.

MEN'S SEXUAL HEALTH

Because the male reproductive system is simpler in many ways than the female, it's often ignored—especially by healthy young men. However, men should make regular self-exams (including checking their penises and testes, as described in Chapter 16) part of their routine.

MALE SEXUAL ANATOMY

The visible parts of the male sexual anatomy are the **penis** and the **scrotum,** the pouch that contains the **testes** (Figure 9-5). The testes manufacture testosterone, the hormone that stimulates the development of a male's secondary sex characteristics, and **sperm,** the male reproductive cells. Immature sperm are stored in the **epididymis,** a collection of coiled tubes adjacent to each testis.

The penis contains three hollow cylinders loosely covered with skin. The two major cylinders, the *corpora cavernosa,* extend side by side through the length of the penis. The third cylinder, the *corpus spongiosum,* surrounds the **urethra,** the channel for both seminal fluid and urine; see Figure 9-5.

When hanging down loosely, the average penis is about 3¾ inches long. During erection, its internal cylinders fill with so much blood that they become rigid, and the penis stretches to an average length of 6¼ inches. About 90 percent of all men have erect penises measuring between 5 and 7 inches in length. There is no relation, however, between penis size and female sexual satisfaction: A woman's vagina naturally adjusts during intercourse to the size of her partner's penis.

Inside the body are several structures involved in the production of seminal fluid, or **semen,** the liquid in which sperm cells are carried out of the body during ejaculation. The **vas deferens** are two tubes that carry sperm from the epididymis into the urethra. The **seminal vesicles,** which make some of the seminal fluid, join with the vas deferens to form the **ejaculatory ducts.** The **prostate gland** produces some of the seminal fluid, which it secretes into the urethra during ejaculation. The **Cowper's glands** are two pea-sized structures on either side of the urethra (just below where it emerges from the prostate gland) and connected to it via tiny ducts. When a man is sexually aroused, the Cowper's glands often secrete a fluid that appears as a droplet at the tip of the penis. This fluid is not semen, although it occasionally contains sperm.

ⒻⒶ⒬ WHAT ARE THE BENEFITS AND DRAWBACKS OF CIRCUMCISION?

In its natural state, the tip of the penis is covered by a fold of skin called the *foreskin.* About 60 percent of baby boys in the United States undergo **circumcision,** the surgical removal of the foreskin.

A. External structure

B. Internal structure

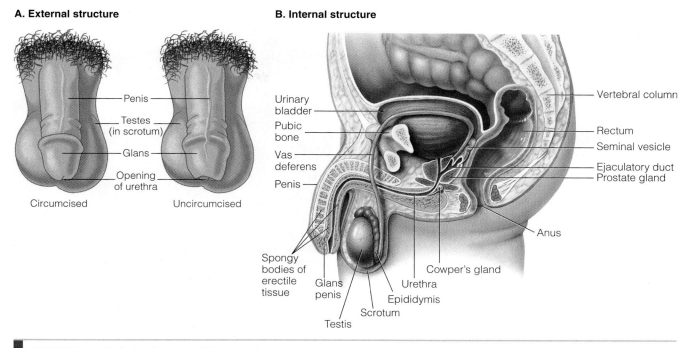

FIGURE 9-5   Male Sex Organs and Reproductive Structures

An estimated 1.2 million newborn males are circumcised in the United States annually for reasons that vary from religious traditions to preventive health measures. Until the last half century, scientific evidence to support or repudiate routine circumcision was limited. The American Academy of Pediatrics (AAP) reviewed 40 years of data and concluded that although there are potential medical benefits, the data were not strong enough to recommend routine neonatal circumcision.[7] However, since this statement, many studies have been published on circumcision and the risks of HIV transmission as well as other diseases.

According to a review of recent scientific evidence, circumcision decreases the incidence of childhood urinary tract infections, the sexual transmission of human papilloma virus (HPV) and HIV, and invasive penile cancer.[8] Studies from sub-Saharan Africa, where rates of HIV infection are extremely high, found that circumcision decreased the risk of acquiring HIV by more than half. Male circumcision may help to prevent the spread of HIV in part because the cells on the foreskin of the penis are more susceptible to HIV infection. Circumcision does not protect against herpes, syphilis, or gonorrhea, suggesting a biological rather than a behavioral explanation for the protective effect of circumcision against HIV.[9]

Boys who are not circumcised are four times as likely to develop urinary tract infections in their first year; however, such infections develop in only 1 percent of circumcised boys. Uncircumcised men are three times as likely to develop penile cancer, but the absolute risk is low. (Only about nine in every million American men ever gets cancer of the penis.)

The drawbacks of circumcision include the risk of complications (which tend to be uncommon and minor) and pain. The AAP recommends that when circumcision is performed, analgesic creams or anesthetic shots be used to minimize discomfort. There is little consensus on what impact the presence or absence of a foreskin has on sexual functioning or satisfaction.

RESPONSIBLE SEXUALITY

The World Health Organization defines **sexual health** as "the integration of the physical, emotional, intellectual, and social aspects of sexual being in ways that are positively enriching, and that enhance personality, communication, and love. . . . Every person has a right to receive sexual information and to consider sexual relationships for pleasure as well as for procreation."

Sexuality education is a lifelong process. Your own knowledge about sex may not be as extensive as you might assume. Most people grow up with a lot of myths and misconceptions about sex. (See Self-Survey: "How Much Do You Know About Sex?" on page 262). Rather than relying on what peers say or what you've always thought was true, find out the facts. This textbook is a good place to start. The student health center and the library can provide additional materials on sexual identity, orientation, behavior, and health, as well as on options for reducing your risk of acquiring sexually transmitted infections (discussed in Chapter 14) or becoming pregnant.

Your Life Coach

Making Responsible Sexual Decisions

Sexual decision making always takes place within the context of an individual's values and perceptions of right and wrong behavior. Making sexually responsible decisions means considering all the possible consequences of sexual behavior for both yourself and your partner. It must always take into account, not just personal preferences and desires, but the very real risks of unwanted pregnancy, sexually transmitted infections (STIs), and long-term medical consequences (such as impaired fertility). You also must consider the emotional consequences of a sexual relationship—not just for yourself but also for your partner.

TALKING ABOUT SEX

Prior to any sexual activity that involves a risk of sexually transmitted infection or pregnancy, both partners should talk about their prior sexual histories (including number of partners and exposure to STIs) and other high-risk behavior, such as the use of injection drugs. They should also discuss the issue of birth control and which methods might be best for them to use. If you know someone well enough to consider having sex with that person, you should be able to talk about such sensitive subjects. If a potential partner is unwilling to talk or hedges on crucial questions, you shouldn't be engaging in sex.

 Styles of communicating vary among white Americans, African Americans, Hispanic Americans, and Asian Americans. While white and African Americans may openly discuss sex with partners, Hispanic-American couples generally do not discuss their sexual relationship. Asian Americans also are less inclined to discuss sex and to value nonverbal, indirect, and intuitive communication over explicit verbal interaction.[10]

Here are some questions to consider as you think and talk about the significance of becoming sexually intimate with a partner:

- **What role do we want relationships and sex to have in our life at this time?**
- **What are my values and my potential partner's values as they pertain to sexual relationships?** Does each of us believe that intercourse should be reserved for a permanent partnership or committed relationship?
- **Will a decision to engage in sex enhance my positive feelings about myself or my partner?** Does either of us have questions about sexual orientation or the kinds of people we are attracted to?

Talking about sex means talking about values, trust, commitment, and responsibility.

© T. Ozonas/Masterfile

- **Do I and my partner both want to have sex?** Is my partner pressuring me in any way? Am I pressuring my partner? Am I making this decision for myself or my partner?
- **Have my partner and I discussed our sexual histories and risk factors?** Have I spoken honestly about any STIs I've had in the past? Am I sure that neither my partner nor I have a sexually transmitted infection?
- **Have we taken precautions against unwanted pregnancy and STIs?**

Whether couples are on a first date or have been married for years, each partner always has the right not to have sex. Unfortunately, "no" sometimes seems to mean different things to men and women.

The following strategies can help you assert yourself when saying no to sex:

- **First of all, recognize** your own values and feelings. If you believe that sex is something to be shared only by people who've already become close in other ways, be true to that belief.
- **Be direct.** Look the person in the eyes, keep your head up, and speak clearly and firmly.
- **Just say no.** Make it clear you're rejecting the offer, not the person. You don't owe anyone an explanation for what you want, but if you want to expand on your reasons, you might say, "I enjoy your company, and I'd like to do something together, but no," or "Thank you. I appreciate your interest, but no."

- **If you're still at a loss for words,** try these responses: "I like you a lot, but I'm not ready to have sex." "You're a great person, but sex isn't something I do to prove I like someone." "I'd like to wait until I'm married to have sex."

- **If you're feeling pressured,** let your date know that you're uncomfortable. Be simple and direct. Watch out for emotional blackmail. If your date says, "If you really like me, you'd want to make love," point out that if he or she really likes you, he or she wouldn't try to force you to do something you don't want to do.

- **If you're a woman, monitor your sexual signals.** Men impute more sexual meaning to gestures (such as casual touching) that women perceive as friendly and innocent.

- **Communicate your feelings** to your date sooner rather than later. It's far easier to say, "I don't want to go to your apartment" than to fight off unwelcome advances once you're there.

- **Remember that if saying no to sex** puts an end to a relationship, it wasn't much of a relationship in the first place.

CREATING A SEXUALLY HEALTHY RELATIONSHIP

A sexually healthy relationship, as defined by the Sexuality Information and Education Council of the United States (SIECUS), is based on shared values and has five characteristics: It is consensual, nonexploitative, honest, mutually pleasurable, and protected against unintended pregnancy and sexually transmitted infections. All individuals also have sexual rights, which include the right to the information, education, skills, support, and services they need to make responsible decisions about their sexuality consistent with their own values, as well as the right to express their sexual orientation without violence or discrimination.

Communication is vital in a sexually healthy relationship, even though these discussions can be awkward. Yet if you have a need or a problem that relates to your partner, it is your responsibility to bring it up. Choose an appropriate time and place for an intimate discussion. In a new relationship, talking in a public place, such as a park bench or a quiet table at a coffee house, can seem safer. If you're in an established relationship, choose a time when you can give each other complete attention and a setting in which you can both relax.

Here are some specific suggestions that can help:

- **Ask open-ended questions** that encourage a dialogue, for instance, "How do you feel about . . . ?" or "What are your thoughts about . . . ?"

- **Listen actively** rather than passively when your partner speaks. Show that you're paying attention by nodding, smiling, and leaning forward. Paraphrase what he or she says to show you understand it fully.

- **Use "I" statements,** such as "I really enjoy making love, but I'm so tired right now that I won't be a responsive partner. Why don't we get the kids to bed early tomorrow so we can enjoy ourselves a little earlier?"

- **Speak up** if something hurts during sex. Be specific.

- **If you would like to try something different, say so.** Practice saying the words first if they embarrass you. If your partner feels uncomfortable, don't force the issue, but do try talking it through.

- **If you want to request changes** or tackle a touchy topic, start with positive statements. Let your partner know how much you enjoy having sex, and then express your desire to enjoy lovemaking more often or in different ways.

- **Encourage small changes.** If you want your partner to be less inhibited, start slowly, perhaps by suggesting sex in a different room or place.

SEXUAL BEHAVIOR

From birth to death, we are sexual beings. Our sexual identities, needs, likes, and dislikes emerge in adolescence and become clearer as we enter adulthood, but we continue to change and evolve throughout our lives. In men, sexual interest is most intense at age 18; in women, it reaches a peak in the 30s. Although age brings changes in sexual responsiveness, we never outgrow our sexuality.

ADOLESCENT SEXUALITY

Early in adolescence, sexual curiosity explodes, and sexual exploration—both alone and with a partner—takes on new meaning and intensity. Sexual education programs can make a difference by helping young people become sexually responsible, enabling them to form satisfying relationships, helping them assess their own attitudes toward sex, and giving them information on sexuality. Good programs can clarify values and enhance communication.

It's not unusual for teenage boys to experience frequent erections during the day and night, including **nocturnal emissions,** or wet dreams, during which ejaculation occurs. **Masturbation** (discussed later in this chapter) is the primary form of sexual expression for many teenagers, especially boys. Self-stimulation helps teens learn about their bodies and their sexual potential and serves as an outlet for

During adolescence, sexuality develops rapidly. Teens explore different social and intimate relationships as they begin to develop a sexual identity.

sexual tension. By the end of adolescence, the majority of teens have masturbated to orgasm.

Other common sexual activities during adolescence include kissing and petting—erotic physical contact that may include holding, touching, manual stimulation of the genitals, and oral sex. As many as 25 percent of teens experience some same-sex attractions. Although many experiment with heterosexual and homosexual sexual experiences, adolescent sexual behavior does not always foretell sexual orientation. Young people, who often feel confused about their sexual identity, may engage in sexual activity with members of the same or the other sex as a way of testing how they really feel.

Teen Sexual Behaviors

For the first time since the federal government started keeping statistics in the early 1970s, fewer American teenagers are becoming sexually active. According to the CDC, the percentage of high school students who had intercourse dropped from 54.1 to 45.6 percent.[11]

According to a national survey of 1,800 teenagers and young adults sponsored by the Kaiser Family Foundation, young people are more concerned about sex and sexual health than any other health issue in their lives. Most—but especially males—report peer pressure to have sex. Three in five respondents described putting off sex as a "nice idea," but something nobody does. One in five reported initial sexual intercourse by age 15. Sexually experienced young teens were far more likely than virgins to engage in other risky behaviors, such as smoking, drinking, and using drugs. Almost a third said they had "done more sexually" because of alcohol or drug use.[12]

One in six young adults and adolescents regard unprotected sex as "not that big a deal." Males are twice as likely as females to feel this way. Pregnancy remains a real concern among young people. Seven in ten college-age young adults have or have had a partner who had a pregnancy test. Nearly two in five reported that they or a partner have been pregnant.[13]

In recent years the popular media have called attention to a rise in casual oral sex among teenagers. In the Kaiser Foundation survey, 42 percent of students in 11th and 12th grade report having had oral sex. In the great majority of cases, girls perform fellatio, rather than boys performing cunnilingus. Experts in human sexuality note that this trend mimics increased acceptance of oral sex in adults in the United States.[14] Teens were less likely to use any form of protection against sexually transmitted infection during oral sex than during intercourse.[15]

(FAQ) HOW SEXUALLY ACTIVE ARE COLLEGE STUDENTS?

According to federal statistics, about two-thirds of never-married 18- to 19-year-olds—69 percent of women and 64 percent of men—have had intercourse.[16] In a recent study of sex, drug use, and binge drinking on campus, more than a third of students reported no sexual intercourse in the previous 12 months. An additional one-third reported sex with only one partner.[17] (See Student Snapshot: "Sex on Campus.")

In a national survey of 1,051 students ages 18 to 24, about 25 percent said they had never engaged in sexual intercourse: 34 percent of men and 18 percent of women. One in four said they had passed on an opportunity to have sex during the previous year. Three in four agreed that sex and contraception should be discussed in advance. The average number of sex partners reported by the students during the previous year was 1.2. Two in three women and one in three men described themselves as being in committed relationships.[18]

Sexual behavior on campus has changed dramatically in the last 25 years. Surveys conducted in the United States and in Canada since 1980 reveal a steady increase in the number of students who have had intercourse and an increase in safer sex practices among sexually active students. Today's undergraduates are more likely to question potential partners about their past, use condoms with a new partner, and maintain fairly long-term monogamous relationships.[19]

College students see sexual activity as normal behavior for their peer group. When researchers at Pennsylvania State University conducted focus groups with undergraduates, most agreed that the majority of college students (80 to 90 percent, in their estimate) are sexually active and that alcohol and drug use make sexual activity more likely.

College students who binge drink or participate in drinking games, which often involve physical skills (such as bouncing a coin into a glass) or word play, increase their odds of sexually risky behavior. Both men and women report being taken advantage of sexually, including someone having sex with them when they were too drunk to give consent, after such games.[20]

Annual spring breaks provide what researchers describe as "ideal conditions for the potentially lethal interaction between alcohol, drugs, and sexual risk-taking."[21] Students typically engage in binge drinking, illicit drug use, and unsafe sexual practices. The likelihood of casual sex depends on several factors, including peer influences, prior experiences with casual sex, alcohol consumption prior to sex, and impulsivity.

 As with other aspects of health, cultural, religious, and personal values affect students' sexual behaviors. Researchers raised concern about young Latina women, who have the highest teen birth rate in the United States (twice the national rate) and are at greater risk of sexually transmitted infections. Although Latinas represent about 10 percent of women over age 21, they account for 20 percent of female AIDS cases. Among college students and other populations, Latinas are more likely to engage in unprotected intercourse than women from other ethnic groups. Sexually active Latina college students also are less likely to use condoms than their peers from other ethnic groups.[22]

Acculturation—the process of adaptation that occurs when immigrants enter a new country—also affects sexual behavior. As Latina immigrants become more acculturated in the United States, some aspects of their sexual behavior become more Americanized; for instance, they become more likely to engage in nonmarital sexual activity and to have multiple partners. In a study of Cuban-American college women, older, less religious, and U.S.-born Latinas were more likely to be sexually active and to engage in risky sexual behavior than other Latinas.[23]

THE SEX LIFE OF AMERICAN ADULTS

The scientific study of Americans' sexual behavior began in 1938, when Alfred Kinsey, Ph.D., a professor of biology at the University of Indiana, and his colleagues asked 5,300 white men and 5,940 white women about their sexual practices. In his landmark studies—*Sexual Behavior in the Human Male,* published in 1948, and *Sexual Behavior in the Human Female,* published in 1953—Kinsey reported that 73 percent of men and 20 percent of women had premarital intercourse by age 20, and 37 percent of men and 17 percent of women had some homosexual experience in their lifetime.

The Janus Report on Sexual Behavior, published in 1993, was based on a survey of 2,765 individuals across the United States. A larger survey, conducted by researchers at the University of Chicago, was based on face-to-face interviews with 3,432 Americans, aged 18 to 59. It became the basis for two books published in 1994: *Sex in America,* aimed at a lay audience, and *The Social Organization of Sexuality,* a more scholarly work. Since then, the researcher's General Social Survey (GSS) database on sexual activity has grown to nearly 10,000 respondents.

The GSS data indicate that overall sexual activity in America is relatively infrequent, with an average of 58 episodes per year, or slightly more than one a week. Yet sexual activity increased compared with earlier decades—even though the population is aging, works longer hours, and can choose among a growing number of distractions. About 15 percent of adults engage in half of all sexual activity; 42 percent of adults engage in 85 percent.[24]

The average adult reports having sex about once a week. However, 1 in 5 Americans has been celibate for at least a year, and 1 in 20 engages in sex at least every other day. Men report more sexual frequency than women—not because men are more boastful about their prowess, the researchers

Student Snapshot

SEX ON CAMPUS

	Men	Women
No sexual intercourse in last 12 months	37%	38%
1 sex partner	36	39
2 to 3 sex partners	20	19
4 to 5 sex partners	7	4
6 to 12 sex partners	0.7	0.5

Source: Duncan, Greg, et al. "Peer Effects in Drug Use and Sex Among College Students." *Journal of Abnormal Child Psychology,* Vol. 33, No. 3, June 2005, p. 375.

© Justin Pumfrey/Taxi/Getty Images

Thinkstock/Getty Images

In a loving, committed relationship, sex serves as an intimate form of communication.

contend, but because the sample of women includes many widows and older women without partners. Among married people, the frequency reports of husbands and wives (not in the same couples) are within one episode per year—58.6 for married men and 57.9 for married women. And if other differences between men and women are statistically controlled (such as sexual preference, age, and educational attainment), married women actually report a slightly higher frequency than men.

Sexual frequency peaks among those with some college education, then decreases among four-year college graduates, and declines even further among those with professional degrees. Americans who have attended graduate school are the least sexually active educational group in the population. These respondents may be more honest than others in reporting sexual activity, or they may be more precise in their definition of what counts as sex.

Does sex make people happier or healthier? Based on their analysis, the researchers concluded that the more sex a person has, the more likely he or she is to report having a happy life and a happy marriage. This connection is stronger among women than men. A second and more important predictor of sexual frequency is the feeling that one's life is exciting rather than routine or dull. "Being excited by life is most strongly associated with being happier," the researchers noted. "It seems that increased sexual activity is one of the many benefits of having a positive attitude."

SEXUAL DIVERSITY

Human beings are diverse in all ways—including sexual preferences and practices. Physiological, psychological, and social factors determine whether we are attracted to members of the same sex or the other sex. This attraction is our **sexual orientation.** Sigmund Freud argued that we all start off **bisexual,** or attracted to both sexes. But by the time we reach adulthood, most males prefer female sexual partners, and most females prefer male partners. **Heterosexual** is the term used for individuals whose primary orientation is toward members of the other sex. In virtually all cultures, some men and women are **homosexuals,** preferring partners of their own sex.

In our society, we tend to view heterosexuality and homosexuality as very different. In reality, these orientations are opposite ends of a spectrum. Sex researcher Alfred Kinsey devised a seven-point continuum representing sexual orientation in American society. At one end of the continuum are those exclusively attracted to members of the other sex; at the opposite end are people exclusively attracted to members of the same sex. In between are varying degrees of homosexual, bisexual, and heterosexual orientation.

According to Kinsey's original data, 4 percent of men and 2 percent of women are exclusively homosexual. More recent studies have found lower numbers. For instance, in the University of Chicago's national survey, 2.8 percent of men and 1.4 percent of women defined themselves as homosexual. However, when asked if they'd had sex with a person of the same gender since age 18, about 5 percent of men and 4 percent of women said yes. When asked if they found members of the same gender sexually attractive, 6 percent of men and 5.5 percent of women said yes.

In a recent survey of lesbian and bisexual women, most reported that their first sexual experience occurred with a man (at the median age of 18) and that sex with a women followed a few years later (at median age 21). Their most frequently reported sexual activities with men were mutual masturbation and vaginal penetration with penis or fingers. Their most common sex practices with women were oral sex, vaginal penetration with fingers, and mutual masturbation.[25]

BISEXUALITY

Bisexuality—sexual attraction to both males and females—can develop at any point in one's life. In some cultures, bisexual activity is considered part of normal sexual experimentation. Among the Sabmia Highlanders in Papua New Guinea, for instance, boys perform oral sex on one another as part of the rites of passage into manhood.[26]

Some people identify themselves as bisexual even if they don't behave bisexually. Some are *serial* bisexuals—that is, they are sexually involved with same-sex partners for a while and then with partners of the other sex, or vice versa. An estimated 7 to 9 million men, about twice the number thought to be exclusively homosexual, could be described as bisexual during some extended period of their lives. The largest group are married, rarely have sexual relations with women other than their wives, and have secret sexual involvements with men.

Fear of HIV infection has sparked great concern about bisexuality, particularly among heterosexual women who worry about becoming involved with a bisexual man. About 20 to 30 percent of women with AIDS were infected by bisexual partners, and health officials fear that bisexual men who hide their homosexual affairs could transmit HIV to many more women.

HOMOSEXUALITY

Homosexuality—social, emotional, and sexual attraction to members of the same sex—exists in almost all cultures. Men and women homosexuals are commonly referred to as *gay;* women homosexuals are also called *lesbians.*

Homosexuality threatens and upsets many people, perhaps because homosexuals are viewed as different, or perhaps because no one understands why some people are heterosexual and others homosexual. *Homophobia* has led to an increase in *gay bashing* (attacking homosexuals) in many communities, including college campuses. Some blame

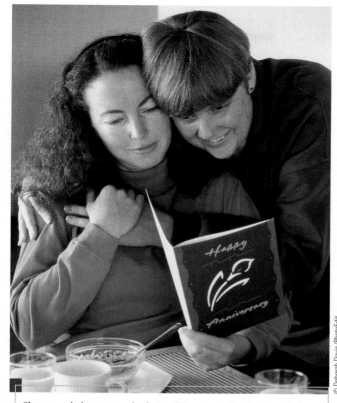

Close-couple homosexual relationships are similar to stable heterosexual relationships.

probably emerges from a complex interaction that includes biological and environmental factors.

For decades, behavioral and medical specialists have debated whether homosexuality is biologically or socially determined. Some say that sexual orientation is genetically determined. However, new research has cast doubt on the existence of a homosexuality gene. Others contend that prenatal hormones influence sexual preference. Today, questions and controversies persist about the roots and nature of sexual orientation.

Homosexuality on Campus

In a study of almost 700 heterosexual students at six small liberal arts colleges, attitudes toward homosexuals and homosexuality varied, depending on students' membership in fraternities or sororities, sex role attitudes, religion and religiosity, and contact with and knowledge of gays, lesbians, and bisexuals. The students most likely to be accepting were those who were women, had less traditional sex-role attitudes, were less religious, attended colleges that did not have Greek social clubs, and had gay, lesbian, and/or bisexual friends.

A survey of 119 colleges and universities found great variation in the resources available to gay, lesbian, and bisexual students. Most (71 percent) have a student organization; 32 percent provide a paid staff member to deal with the students' needs and issues; 40 percent provide a support identification program; 36 percent offered at least one course on gay, lesbian, and bisexual issues.[27]

TRANSGENDERISM

The term **transgender** is used as an umbrella term to describe people who have gender identities, expressions, or behaviors not traditionally associated with their birth sex. Male-to-female transgenders have been assigned a male gender at birth, but identify their gender as female. Female-to-male people were assigned a female gender at birth, but identify their gender as male.

Transgender individuals face varied health risks, including unprotected sex, sexually transmitted diseases, and HIV infection. Violence, including rape, sexual abuse, physical abuse, and suicide, is a major public health issue. In one study the majority of the transgender individuals reported being afraid for their life or physical safety at some point during their lives.[28]

SEXUAL ACTIVITY

Part of learning about your own sexuality is having a clear understanding of human sexual behaviors. Understanding frees us from fear and anxiety so that we can accept ourselves and others as the natural sexual beings we all are.

the emergence of AIDS as a societal danger. However, researchers have found that fear of AIDS has not created new hostility but has simply given bigots an excuse to act out their hatred.

 Different ethnic groups respond to homosexuality in different ways. To a greater extent than white homosexuals, gays and lesbians from ethnic groups tend to stay in the closet longer rather than risk alienation from their families and communities. Often they feel forced to choose between their gay and their ethnic identities.

In general, the African-American community has stronger negative views of homosexuals than whites, possibly because of the influence of strong fundamentalist Christian beliefs. Hispanic culture, with its emphasis on machismo, also has a very negative view of male homosexuality. Asian cultures, which tend to view an individual as a representative of his or her family, tend to view open declarations of sexual orientation as shaming the family and challenging their reputation and future.

Roots of Homosexuality

Most mental health experts agree that nobody knows what causes a person's sexual orientation. Research has discredited theories tracing homosexuality to troubled childhoods or abnormal psychological development. Sexual orientation

CELIBACY

A celibate person does not engage in sexual activity. Complete **celibacy** means that the person doesn't masturbate (stimulate himself or herself sexually) or engage in sexual activity with a partner. In partial celibacy, the person masturbates but doesn't have sexual contact with others. Many people decide to be celibate at certain times of their lives. Some don't have sex because of concerns about pregnancy or STIs; others haven't found a partner for a permanent, monogamous relationship. Many simply have other priorities, such as finishing school or starting a career, and realize that sex outside of a committed relationship is a threat to their physical and psychological well-being.

(FAQ) WHAT DOES IT MEAN TO ABSTAIN?

The CDC defines **abstinence** as "refraining from sexual activities which involve vaginal, anal, and oral intercourse." The definition of abstinence remains a subject of debate and controversy, with some emphasizing positive choices and others avoidance of specific behaviors.[29] In reality abstinence means different things to different people, cultures, and religious groups.

Increasing numbers of adolescents and young adults are choosing to remain virgins and abstain from sexual intercourse until they enter a permanent, committed, monogamous relationship. About 2.5 million teens have taken pledges to abstain from sex. According to a major study, teens who do so are 34 percent less likely to have premarital sex than others and are far older when they finally engage in intercourse. The federal government, which has promoted abstinence as a means of preventing pregnancy and sexually transmitted infections, funded abstinence education programs for two decades. Research on abstinence-only sex education training has found a significant impact at the three-month follow-up, but this disappeared after one year. A program emphasizing safer sex was consistently effective throughout the one-year period.[30]

Many people who were sexually active in the past also are choosing abstinence because the risk of medical complications associated with STIs increases with the number of sexual partners a person has. Abstinence is the safest, healthiest option for many. However, there is confusion about what it means to abstain, and individuals who think they are abstaining may still be engaging in behaviors that put them at risk for HIV and STIs. (See Chapter 10 for more on abstinence as a form of birth control.)

Why abstain? Among the reasons students give are:

❚ **Remaining a virgin until** you meet someone you love and see as a life partner

❚ **Being true to your religious and moral values**

❚ **Getting to know a partner better**

❚ **If you're heterosexual, to avoid pregnancy**

❚ **To be sure you're safe from sexually transmitted infections**

> At some campuses students have organized to promote traditional sexual values, such as abstinence. Supporters feel that these groups enrich the discussion of sexual lifestyles. Others charge that promoters of traditional sexual values are passing moral judgment on those who make other choices. Are they offering a valid alternative? Or are they trying to impose their values on others? **You decide.**

FANTASY

The mind is the most powerful sex organ in the body, and erotic mental images can be sexually stimulating. Sexual fantasies can accompany sexual activity or be pleasurable in themselves. Fantasies generally enhance sexual arousal, reduce anxiety, and boost sexual desire. They're also a way to anticipate and rehearse new sexual experiences, as well as to bolster a person's self-image and feelings of desirability. Part of what makes fantasies exciting is that they provide an opportunity for expressing forbidden desires, such as sex with a different partner or with a past lover.

In the University of Chicago survey, more than half the men (54 percent)—but only 19 percent of the women—said they thought about sex every day or several times a day. Men and women also have different types of sexy thoughts, with men's fantasies containing more explicit genital images and culminating in sexual acts more quickly than women's. In women's fantasies, emotional feelings play a greater role, and there is more kissing and caressing rather than genital contact. For many women, fantasy helps in reaching orgasm during intercourse; a loss of fantasy often is a sign of low sexual desire.

The magic of touch. Thrilling, soothing, stimulating—touch is a powerful way to communicate affection and sexual pleasure.

MASTURBATION

Not everybody masturbates, but most people do. Kinsey estimated that 7 out of 10 women and 19 out of 20 men masturbate (and admit they do). Their reason is simple: It feels good. Masturbation produces the same physical responses as sexual activity with a partner and can be an enjoyable form of sexual release.

Masturbation has been described as immature; unsocial; tiring; frustrating; and a cause of hairy palms, warts, blemishes, and blindness. None of these myths is true. Sex educators recommend masturbation to adolescents as a means of releasing tension and becoming familiar with their sexual organs. Throughout adulthood, masturbation often is the primary sexual activity of individuals not involved in a sexual relationship and can be particularly useful when illness, absence, divorce, or death deprives a person of a partner. In the University of Chicago survey, about 25 percent of men and 9 percent of women said they masturbate at least once a week.

 White men and women have a higher incidence of masturbation than African-American men and women. Latina women have the lowest rate of masturbation, compared with Latino men, white men and women, and black men and women. Individuals with a higher level of education are more likely to masturbate than those with less schooling, and people living with sexual partners masturbate more than those who live alone.

NONPENETRATIVE SEXUAL ACTIVITY (OUTERCOURSE)

Various pleasurable behaviors can lead to orgasm with little risk of pregnancy or sexually transmitted disease. The options for "outercourse" include kissing and hugging but do not involve genital-to-genital, mouth-to-genital, or insertive anal sexual contact.

A kiss is a universal sign of affection. A kiss can be just a kiss—a quick press of the lips—or it can lead to much more. Usually kissing is the first sexual activity that couples engage in, and even after years of sexual experimentation and sharing, it remains an enduring pleasure for partners.

Touching is a silent form of communication between friends and lovers. Although a touch to any part of the body can be thrilling, some areas, such as the breasts and genitals, are especially sensitive. Stimulating these **erogenous** regions can lead to orgasm in both men and women. Though such forms of stimulation often accompany intercourse, more couples are gaining an appreciation of these activities as primary sources of sexual fulfillment—and as safer alternatives to intercourse.

INTERCOURSE

Vaginal **intercourse,** or coitus, refers to the penetration of the vagina by the penis (Figure 9-6). This is the preferred form of sexual intimacy for most heterosexual couples, who may use a wide variety of positions. The most familiar position for intercourse in our society is the so-called missionary position, with the man on top, facing the woman. An alternative is the woman on top, either lying down or sitting upright. Other positions include lying side by side (either face to face or with the man behind the woman, his penis entering her vagina from the rear); lying with the man on top of the woman in a rear-entry position; and kneeling or standing (again, in either a face-to-face or rear-entry position). Many couples move into several different positions for intercourse during a single episode of lovemaking; others may have a personal favorite or may choose different positions at different times.

Sexual activity, including intercourse, is possible throughout a woman's menstrual cycle. However, some women prefer to avoid sex while menstruating because of uncomfortable physical symptoms, such as cramps, or concern about bleeding or messiness. Others use a diaphragm or cervical cap (see Chapter 10) to hold back menstrual flow. Since different cultures have different views on intercourse during a woman's period, partners should discuss their own

---

Savvy Consumer ▓ X-Rated Websites

Sex is the number-one word searched for online. About 15 percent of Americans logging onto the Internet visit sexually oriented sites. Men are the largest consumers of sexually explicit material and outnumber women by a ratio of six to one. However, while men look for visual erotica, women are more likely to visit chat rooms, which offer more interactions. Most people who check out sex sites on the Internet do not suffer any negative impact, but psychologists warn of some potential risks, including the following:

- *Dependence.* Individuals who spend 11 hours or more a week online in sexual pursuits show signs of psychological distress and admit that their behavior interferes with some areas of their lives.
- *Interference with work and study.* While most individuals use their home computers when surfing the Internet for sex-related sites, one in ten has used a school computer. Some universities have strict policies barring such

practices and may take punitive actions against employees who violate the rules.

- *Sexual compulsivity.* A small but significant number of users are at risk of a serious problem as a result of their heavy Internet use.
- *Dishonesty.* Most Internet surfers admit that they occasionally "pretend" about their age on the Internet. Most keep secret how much time they spend on sexual pursuits in cyberspace.

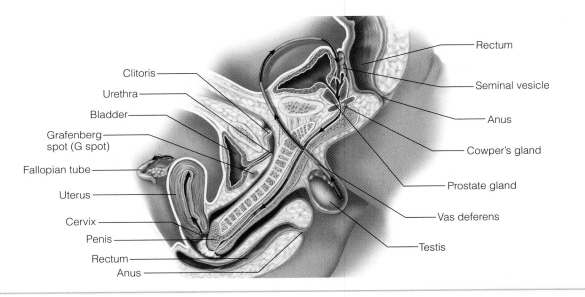

FIGURE 9-6   A Cross-Sectional View of Sexual Intercourse
Sperm are formed in each of the testes and stored in the epididymis. When a man ejaculates, sperm traveling in semen travel up the vas deferens. (The prostate gland and seminal vesicles contribute components of the semen.) The semen is expelled from the penis through the urethra and deposited in the vagina, near the cervix. During sexual excitement and orgasm in a woman, the upper end of the vagina enlarges and the uterus elevates. After orgasm, these organs return to their normal states, and the cervix descends into the pool of semen.

feelings and try to respect each other's views. If they choose not to have intercourse, there are other gratifying forms of sexual activity.

Vaginal intercourse, like other forms of sexual activity involving an exchange of bodily fluids, carries a risk of sexually transmitted infections, including HIV infection. In many other parts of the world, in fact, heterosexual intercourse is the most common means of HIV transmission (See Chapter 14.)

ORAL SEX

Our mouths and genitals give us some of our most intense pleasures. Though it might seem logical to combine the two, some people are very uncomfortable with it. Some people consider oral-genital sex a perversion; it is against the law in some states and a sin in some religions. However, others find it normal and acceptable. (The same comments apply to anal sex as well—see the next section.)

The formal terms for oral sex are **cunnilingus,** which refers to oral stimulation of the woman's genitals, and **fellatio,** oral stimulation of the man's genitals. For many couples, oral sex is a regular part of their lovemaking. For others, it's an occasional experiment. Oral sex with a partner carrying a sexually transmitted infection, such as herpes or HIV infection, can lead to infection, so a condom should be used (with cunnilingus, a condom cut in half to lay flat can be used).

 Different groups of the population have diverse views of oral sex. In one survey, more African-American than white men reported never having performed or received oral sex.[31]

ANAL STIMULATION AND INTERCOURSE

Because the anus has many nerve endings, it can produce intense erotic responses. Stimulation of the anus by the fingers or mouth can be a source of sexual arousal; anal intercourse involves penile penetration of the anus. An estimated 25 percent of adults have experienced anal intercourse at least once. However, anal sex involves important health risks, such as damage to sensitive rectal tissues and the transmission of various intestinal infections, hepatitis, and STIs, including HIV.

CULTURAL VARIATIONS

While the biological mechanisms underlying human sexual arousal and response are essentially universal, the particular sexual stimuli or behaviors that people find arousing are greatly influenced by cultural conditioning. For example, in Western societies, where the emphasis during sexual activity tends to be heavily weighted toward achieving orgasm, genitally focused activities are frequently defined as optimally arousing. In contrast, devotees to Eastern Tantric traditions (where spirituality is interwoven with sexuality) often achieve optimal pleasure by emphasizing the sensual and spiritual aspects of shared intimacy rather than orgasmic release.

Kissing on the mouth, a universal source of sexual arousal in Western society, may be rare or absent in many other parts of the world. Certain North American Eskimo people and inhabitants of the Trobriand Islands would rather rub noses than lips, and among the Thonga of South Africa, kissing is viewed as odious behavior. The Hindu people of India are also disinclined to kiss because they believe such contact symbolically contaminates the act of sexual intercourse. One survey of 190 societies found that mouth kissing was acknowledged in only 21 societies and practiced as a prelude or accompaniment to coitus in only 13.

Oral sex (both cunnilingus and fellatio) is a common source of sexual arousal among island societies of the South Pacific, in industrialized nations of Asia, and in much of the Western world. In contrast, in Africa (with the exception of northern regions), such practices are likely to be viewed as unnatural or disgusting behavior.

Foreplay in general, whether it be oral sex, sensual touching, or passionate kissing, is subject to wide cultural variation. In some societies, most notably those with Eastern traditions, couples may strive to prolong intense states of sexual arousal for several hours. While varied patterns of foreplay are common in Western cultures, these activities often are of short duration as lovers move rapidly toward the "main event" of coitus. In still other societies, foreplay is either sharply curtailed or absent altogether. For example, the Lepcha farmers of the southeastern Himalayas limit foreplay to men briefly caressing their partners' breasts, and among the Irish inhabitants of Inis Beag, precoital sexual activity is reported to be limited to mouth kissing and rough fondling of the woman's lower body by her partner.

SEXUAL RESPONSE

Sexuality involves every part of you: mind and body, muscles and skin, glands and genitals. The pioneers in finding out exactly how human beings respond to sex were William Masters and Virginia Johnson, who first studied more than 800 individuals in their laboratory in the 1950s. They discovered that sexual response is a well-ordered sequence of events, so predictable it could be divided into four phases: excitement, plateau, orgasm, and resolution (Figure 9-7). In real life, individuals don't necessarily follow this well-ordered pattern. But the responses for both sexes are remarkably similar. And sexual response always follows the same sequence, whatever the means of stimulation.

EXCITEMENT

Stimulation is the first step: a touch, a look, a fantasy. In men, sexual stimuli set off a rush of blood to the genitals, filling the blood vessels in the penis. Because these vessels are wrapped in a thick sheath of tissue, the penis becomes erect. The testes lift.

Women respond to stimulation with vaginal lubrication within 10 to 20 seconds of exposure to sexual stimuli. The clitoris becomes larger, as do the vaginal lips (the labia), the

Males

Excitement

Testes enlarge and elevate, penis becomes partially erect

Plateau

Testes are fully elevated; penis reaches full erection, glans swells, drops of fluid are released

Orgasm

Contractions release semen into urethra; urethral sphincter relaxes, penile contractions occur, semen is ejaculated

Resolution

Erection disappears, testes descend

Females

Excitement

Inner vagina expands, clitoris swells, and labia swell

Plateau

Inner vagina becomes fully expanded, outer vagina swells, and clitoris retracts under hood

Orgasm

Anal sphincter contracts, uterus contracts, and outer vagina contracts

Resolution

Uterus lowers, vagina returns to normal

FIGURE 9-7   Human Sexual Response

The four stages of sexual response are excitement, plateau, orgasm, and resolution.

nipples, and later the breasts. The vagina lengthens, and its inner two-thirds increase in size. The uterus lifts, further increasing the free space in the vagina.

PLATEAU

During this stage, the changes begun in the excitement stage continue and intensify. The penis further increases in both length and diameter. The outer one-third of the vagina swells. During intercourse, the vaginal muscles grasp the penis to increase stimulation for both partners. The upper two-thirds of the vagina become wider as the uterus moves up; eventually its diameter is 2½ to 3 inches.

ORGASM

Men and women have remarkably similar **orgasm** experiences. Both men and women typically have 3 to 12 pelvic muscle contractions approximately four-fifths of a second apart and lasting up to 60 seconds. Both undergo contractions and spasms of other muscles, as well as increases in breathing and pulse rates, and blood pressure. Both can sometimes have orgasms simply from kisses, stimulation of the breasts or other parts of the body, or fantasy alone.

The process of **ejaculation** (the discharge of semen by a male) requires two separate events. First, the vas deferens, the seminal vesicles, the prostate, and the upper portion of the urethra contract. The man perceives these subtle contractions deep in his pelvis just before the point of no return—which therapists refer to as the point of "ejaculatory inevitability." Then, seconds later, muscle contractions force semen out of the penis via the urethra.

Female orgasms follow several patterns. Some women experience a series of mini-orgasms—a response sometimes described as "skimming." Another pattern consists of rapid excitement and plateau stages, followed by a prolonged orgasm. This is the most frequent response to stimulation by a vibrator.

Female orgasms are primarily triggered by stimulating the clitoris. When stimulation reaches an adequate level, the vagina responds by contracting. Although it sometimes seems that vaginal stimulation alone can set off an orgasm, the clitoris is usually involved—at least indirectly during the clitoris is usually involved-at least indirectly during full penile penetration.

Some researchers have identified what they call the *Grafenberg* (or G) *spot* (or area) just behind the front wall of the vagina, between the cervix and the back of the public bone (see Figure 9-6). When this region is stimulated, women report various sensations, including slight discomfort, a brief feeling that they need to urinate, and increasing pleasure. Continued stimulation may result in an orgasm of great intensity, accompanied by ejaculation of fluid from the urethra. However, other researchers have failed to confirm the existence and importance of the G spot, and sex therapists disagree about its significance for a woman's sexual satisfaction.

RESOLUTION

The sexual organs of men and women return to their normal, nonexcited state during this final phase of sexual response. Heightened skin color quickly fades after orgasm, and the heart rate, blood pressure, and breathing rate soon return to normal. The clitoris also resumes its normal position and appearance very shortly thereafter, whereas the penis may remain somewhat erect for up to 30 minutes.

After orgasm, men typically enter a **refractory period,** during which they are incapable of another orgasm. The duration of this period varies from minutes to days, depending on age and the frequency of previous sexual activity. If either partner doesn't have an orgasm after becoming highly aroused, resolution may be much slower and may be accompanied by a sense of discomfort.

OTHER MODELS OF SEXUAL RESPONSE

Since Masters and Johnson's pioneering work, other researchers have challenged and expanded their theories. Some argue that their model neglects the importance of desire in sexual response and that the plateau stage is virtually indistinguishable from excitement. Others note that arousal may come before desire, particularly for women who may not have spontaneous feelings of sexual desire.

As many experts have concluded, physiology alone can never explain the complexity of human sexual response. Desire, arousal, pleasure, and satisfaction are highly subjective. Positive feelings like trust and happiness enhance them. Negative emotions like anger and anxiety can undermine them. For women, sexual satisfaction cannot be defined, as it typically is for men, by whether or not they achieved orgasm.

▌SEXUAL CONCERNS

Many sexual concerns stem from myths and misinformation. There is no truth, for instance, behind these misconceptions: men are always capable of erection, sex always involves intercourse, partners should experience simultaneous orgasms, or people who truly love each other always have satisfying sex lives.

Cultural and childhood influences can affect our attitudes toward sex. Even though America's traditionally puritanical values have eased, our society continues to convey mixed messages about sex. Some children, repeatedly warned of the evils of sex, never accept the sexual dimensions of their identity. Others—especially young boys—may be exposed to macho attitudes toward sex and feel a need to prove their virility. Young girls may feel confused by media messages that encourage them to look and act provocatively and a double standard that blames them for leading boys on. In addition, virtually everyone has individual worries. A woman may feel self-conscious about the shape of her breasts; a man may worry about the size of his penis; both partners may fear not pleasing the other.

The concept of sexual normalcy differs greatly in different times, cultures, or racial and ethnic groups. In certain times and places, only sex between a husband and wife has been deemed normal. In other circumstances, "normal" has been applied to any sexual behavior—alone or with others—that does not harm others or produce great anxiety and guilt. The following are some of the most common contemporary sexual concerns.

SAFER SEX

Having sex is never completely safe; the only 100 percent risk-free sexual choice is abstinence. By choosing not to be sexually active with a partner, you can safeguard your physical health, your fertility, and your future.

For men and women who are sexually active, a mutually faithful sexual relationship with just one healthy partner is the safest option. For those not in such relationships, safer-sex practices are essential for reducing risks.

If you are sexually active, condoms can reduce your risk of STIs—if you use them correctly and consistently. Unless you are allergic, always use latex condoms, which block more STI organisms than natural membrane ones. Although condoms do not provide 100 percent protection, they can reduce the risk of transmission of an STI by 50 to 80 percent.[32]

Condoms prevent direct contact between the penis and the vagina, cervix, mouth, or rectum, thereby protecting against lesions, discharges, and infected semen. Condoms are more effective against STIs transmitted by bodily fluids (chlamydia, gonorrhea, trichomoniasis, and HIV) than those transmitted by skin-to-skin contact (herpes, HPV, chancroid, syphilis).

How can you tell if someone you're dating or hope to date has been exposed to an STI? The bad news is you can't. But the good news is it doesn't matter—as long as you avoid sexual activity that could put you at risk of infection. Ideally, before engaging in any such behavior, both of you should talk about your prior sexual history (including number of partners and sexually transmitted infections) and other high-risk behavior, such as the use of injection drugs.

(FAQ) WHY DON'T COLLEGE STUDENTS PRACTICE SAFER SEX?

Decades of education about sexual risks have had an impact. Most young Americans between the ages of 18 and 24 agree that "it's smart to carry condoms," according to a recent national survey. However, their words and actions often differ. Although nine in ten say they take personal responsibility for their sexual health, only half ask potential partners about sexually transmitted infections. Less than half always or often use a condom during sexual activity.[33]

TABLE 9-1 RISKY SEX ON CAMPUS

Men	Percent 1 or 2 partners	3 or more partners
Not using condom (last time)	51	37
Sex with a stranger (ever)	28	72
Active anal intercourse (ever)	27	43
Multiple partners during same act (ever)	12	28
Unwise sex after alcohol/drugs (ever)	45	89

Women	Percent 1 or 2 partners	3 or more partners
Not using condom (last time)	62	46
Sex with a stranger (ever)	16	42
Active anal intercourse (ever)	27	35
Multiple partners during same act (ever)	3	23
Unwise sex after alcohol/drugs (ever)	49	84

Based on a survey of 630 students (247 men and 383 women) at Okanagan University College in British Columbia.

Source: Netting, N. S., and Matthew Burnett. "Twenty Years of Student Sexual Behavior: Subcultural Adaptations to a Changing Health Environment." *Adolescence,* Vol. 39, No. 153, Spring 2004, p. 19.

Heterosexual students—male and female—are more likely to say they always use condoms than gay men. Of those engaging in heterosexual sex, 52 percent of men and 43 percent of women report consistent condom use, compared with 32 percent of men with only male partners.[34]

Researchers explain that the college environment "provides students with a sense of new independence, self-determination, and strong peer pressure to experiment with a variety of sexual behaviors." Yet by engaging in sex with multiple partners and not regularly using condoms, college students put themselves at high risk of contracting HIV and other sexual infections (Table 9-1).

 In a study of African-American undergraduates, male and female students identified barriers to their use of safer sex practices. Negative views of condoms rank first. But the reason men and women don't like condoms is not reduced sensitivity or pleasure, but a sense that not wearing a condom provides a sense of greater intimacy.[35]

 Latino students are less likely to use condoms than African Americans. In a recent analysis, 30 percent of Latino undergraduates reported condom use in the previous three months, compared with 43 percent of African Americans. Those who had ever had a test for HIV following oral sex and who had had anal sex partners of both genders reported more condom use.[36]

Providing information on sexual health does not influence condom use, nor does teaching specific communication skills. In one experiment, 106 heterosexual college students in sexually active relationships were taught specifically how to make direct requests for condom use and how to counter refusals from a partner. Nonetheless, the students did not change their subsequent communication or use condoms more consistently.[37]

Trust is another issue that affects safer sex practices. Men tend to trust a woman as safe and healthy on the basis of the way she looks. Women trust a man because they believe they are in a monogamous relationship after a period of time (one month on average) or number of encounters (twelve). Neither men nor women base their feelings of trust on a discussion with a partner. They simply assume that a partner can be trusted and that condoms are not necessary.

 Race and ethnicity affect risk in the young. Young African-American men, who are more likely to be sexually active and to have more partners than young white men, also have higher STI infection rates. While the chlamydia rate for Hispanics is almost three times that of whites, the rate for blacks is ten times that of whites. The gonorrhea rate for African-American males aged 20 to 24 is 40 times that of whites. Although HIV infection rates have declined for all men, they are falling at a slower rate for African-American men.

SEXUAL DYSFUNCTION

SIECUS defines **sexual dysfunction** as the inability to react emotionally and/or physically to sexual stimulation in a way expected of the average healthy person or according to one's own standards. Sexual dysfunctions, which have a wide range of psychological and physiological origins, can affect different stages in the sexual response cycle. They are not all-or-nothing problems but vary considerably in how severe they are and how frequently they occur. In as many as one-third of people with sexual problems, the partner also has a sexual dysfunction.

Most men and women at one time or another experience some sort of sexual difficulty, but they tend to develop different types. Men are more likely to seek and receive treatment for sexual problems. Nevertheless, they find them very difficult to talk about and may delay or avoid seeking help. In women, the most common sexual dysfunction is loss of desire for sexual activity.

Erectile Dysfunction (ED)

 An NIH consensus conference has defined **erectile dysfunction** (**ED,** also referred to as **impotence**) as the consistent inability to maintain a penile erection sufficient for adequate sexual relations. Virtually all men are occasionally unable to achieve or maintain an erection because of fatigue, stress, alcohol, or drug use, but the incidence of erectile disorders increases with age. Some 30 million American men have ED.[38]

Psychological factors, such as anxiety about performance, may cause erectile dysfunction. But in as many as 80 percent of cases, the problem has physical origins.

Diabetes and reactions to drugs—including an estimated 200 prescription medications—are the most frequent organic causes. Even cigarettes can create erection problems for men sensitive to nicotine.

Preventing Erectile Dysfunction "The way a man lives can affect the way he loves." This was the conclusion of the Harvard's Health Professionals Follow-Up Study, which found that health habits directly affect a man's risk of ED. Here are their key findings:

- **Smoking.** Men who smoke are 2.2 times more likely to develop ED than nonsmokers.
- **Exercise.** Men who exercise for 30 minutes a day are 41 percent less likely to develop erectile dysfunction than sedentary men.
- **Obesity.** Overweight men are more likely to have ED even after age, diabetes, exercise, and other risk factors are taken into account. For example, a man with a 42-inch waist is 50 percent more likely to be impotent than a man with a 32-inch waist.
- **Alcohol.** The effects of alcohol are complex: A man who averages one to two drinks a day is 33 percent less likely to have erectile dysfunction than a nondrinker, but a man who drinks more will increase his risk of sexual dysfunction.[39]

Lifestyle therapy has promise for erectile dysfunction, but men have to make changes early enough to prevent irreversible changes in the arteries and nerves required for normal sexual function.

Treating Erectile Dysfunction Men with erectile dysfunction can get help. If medication for a chronic medical problem is the culprit, a change in treatment may work. Treating underlying diseases, such as diabetes, may also help restore erectile function.

Millions of men have used the "erection pills": Viagra, Levitra, and Cialis. Although simple to take, they cause complex changes. The crucial chemical for erections is nitric oxide, which transmits the impulses of arousal between nerves and also relaxes muscle cells in the penile arteries, causing them to widen and admit more blood. Other chemicals act with nitric oxide to produce an erection. ED pills adjust abnormalities in this system to allow erection.

The three ED medications have similar success rates. In all, about 70 percent of men respond to the drugs but the rates vary according to what is responsible for ED. About half of men with diabetes respond well, while 90 percent of those without an underlying disease benefit.

Because of their effects on the arteries, men with cardiovascular disease should try ED pills only with their doctors' supervision, and some cannot use them under any circumstances. The FDA has warned doctors that some erectile dysfunction drugs, including Viagra, Cialis, and Levitra, could cause vision loss. The FDA is uncertain whether the drugs are directly to blame, or if the problems were caused by high blood pressure or diabetes. Other side effects include headache, facial flushing, nasal congestion, indigestion, and diarrhea.

Men can purchase ED drugs on the Internet, but they are taking a risk in using them without a legitimate medical evaluation. Other men turn to herbal remedies. The FDA warns that "all-natural" supplements may actually contain prescription-strength levels of Viagra that could be life-threatening for men with heart disease.

Erection drugs are not aphrodisiacs, but they can improve the erectile response to erotic stimulation. They correct impotence but do not enhance sexual performance.

Orgasm Problems in Men

About 20 percent of men complain of **premature ejaculation,** which is defined as ejaculating within 30 to 90 seconds of inserting the penis into the vagina, or after 10 to 15 thrusts. Another definition is that a premature ejaculator cannot control or delay his ejaculation long enough to satisfy a responsive partner at least half the time. By this definition, a man may be premature with some women but not with others.[40]

To delay orgasm, men may try to think of baseball or other sports, but this just makes sex boring. Others may masturbate before intercourse, hoping to take advantage of the refractory period, during which they cannot ejaculate again. Others may bite their lips or dig their nails into their palms—although usually this just results in premature ejaculators with bloody lips and scarred palms. Topical anesthetics used to prevent climax dull pleasurable sensations for the woman as well as for the man.

Researchers are studying several medications, including clomipramine, SSRIs, and Viagra, in the treatment of premature ejaculation. The combination of medication and psychological and behavioral counseling seems most effective.[41]

Men can learn to control their ejaculation by concentrating on their sexual responses, rather than by trying to distract themselves or ignore their reactions. Some men find that they have greater control by lying on their backs with their partner on top, by relaxing during intercourse, and by communicating with their partner about when to stop or slow down movements.

Other techniques for delaying ejaculation include *stop-start,* in which a man learns to sense the feelings that precede ejaculation and stop his movements before the point of ejaculatory inevitability, allowing his arousal to subside slightly before restarting sexual activity. In the *squeeze technique,* a man's partner applies strong pressure with her thumb on the frenum (the thin strip of skin that connects the glans to the shaft on the underside of the penis) and her second and third fingers on the top side of the penis, one above and one below the corona (rim of penile glans), until the man loses the urge to ejaculate.

Female Sexual Dysfunction

The American Foundation for Urological Disease classifies female sexual dysfunction into four categories: sexual desire disorders, arousal disorders, orgasmic disorders, and sexual pain disorders.[42] How common are these problems? That's hard to estimate. In an online survey, 40 percent of women reported that they did not seek help from a physician for sexual complaints, even though 5 percent said that they would like to.[43] Some sex therapists have speculated that as many as 43 percent of American women may have some form of sexual dysfunction.

Many health professionals remain dubious about the "medicalization" of various patterns of female sexual response. Scientists at the Kinsey Institute for Research in Sex, Gender, and Reproduction, for instance, caution that a pill, whatever its nature, may not be the solution to many women's sexual concerns. In women, psychology often is as or even more important than physiology, and effective therapy must address psychological problems in a sexual relationship as well as social constraints and inhibitions.[44]

Some forms of female sexual dysfunction do respond to various therapies. These include **dyspareunia,** or pain during intercourse, and **vaginismus,** an extreme form of painful intercourse in which involuntary contractions of the muscles of the outer third of the vagina are so intense that they totally or partially close the vaginal opening. This problem often derives from a fear of being penetrated. Relaxation techniques, such as *Kegel exercises* (alternately tightening and relaxing the muscles of the pelvic floor), or the use of fingers or dilators to gradually open the vagina, can make penetration easier.

The female orgasm has long been a controversial sexual topic. According to recent estimates, about 90 percent of sexually active women have experienced orgasm, but only a much smaller percentage achieve orgasm through intercourse alone. Even fewer reach orgasm if intercourse isn't accompanied by direct stimulation of the clitoris. Is intercourse without orgasm a sexual problem? The best answer is that it is a problem if a woman wants to experience orgasm during intercourse but doesn't.

Many counseling programs urge women who have never had orgasms to masturbate. They are then encouraged to share with their partners what they've learned, communicating with words or gestures what is most pleasing to them. Some women want more than a single orgasm during intercourse. Partners can help by varying positions and experimenting with sexual techniques. However, in sexual response, more is not necessarily better, and the couple should keep in mind that no one else is counting.

SEX THERAPY

Modern sex therapy, pioneered by Masters and Johnson in the 1960s, views sex as a natural, healthy behavior that enhances a couple's relationship. Their approach emphasizes education, communication, reduction of performance anxiety, and sexual exercises that enhance sexual intimacy.

Today most sex therapists, working either alone or with a partner, have modified Masters and Johnson's approach.

Most see couples once a week for eight to ten weeks; the focus of therapy is on correcting dysfunctional behavior, not exploring underlying psychodynamics.

Contrary to common misconceptions, sex therapy does not involve conducting sexual activity in front of therapists. The therapist may review psychological and physiological aspects of sexual functioning and evaluate the couple's sexual attitudes and ability to communicate. The core of the program is the couple's "homework"—a series of exercises, carried out in private, that enhances their sensory awareness and improves nonverbal communication. These techniques have proved effective for couples regardless of their age or general health.

You and your partner should consider consulting a sex therapist if any of the following is true for you:

- **Sex is painful** or physically uncomfortable.
- **You're having sex less** and less frequently.
- **You have a general fear** of, or revulsion toward, sex.
- **Your sexual pleasure is declining.**
- **Your sexual desire is diminishing.**
- **Your sexual problems are increasing** in frequency or persisting for longer periods.

DRUGS AND SEX

Many recreational drugs, such as alcohol and marijuana, are believed to enhance sexual performance. However, none of the popular drugs touted as *aphrodisiacs*—including amphetamines, barbiturates, cantharides ("Spanish fly"), cocaine, LSD and other psychedelics, marijuana, amyl nitrite ("poppers"), and L-dopa (a medication used to treat Parkinson's disease)—is truly a sexual stimulant. In fact, these drugs often interfere with normal sexual response. Researchers are studying one drug that may truly enhance sexual performance: yohimbine hydrochloride, which is derived from the sap of the tropical yohimbe tree that grows in West Africa.

Because many psychiatric problems can lower sexual desire and affect sexual functioning, medications appropriate to the specific disorders can help. In addition, psychiatric drugs may be used as part of therapy. Drugs such as certain antidepressants may be used to prolong sexual response in conditions such as premature ejaculation.

Medications can also cause sexual difficulty. In men, drugs that are used to treat high blood pressure, anxiety, allergies, depression, muscle spasms, obesity, ulcers, irritable colon, and prostate cancer can cause impotence, breast enlargement, testicular swelling, priapism (persistent erection), loss of sexual desire, inability to ejaculate, and reduced sperm count. In women, they can diminish sexual desire, inhibit or delay orgasm, and cause breast swelling or secretions.

ATYPICAL BEHAVIOR

Although sexual desire and response are universal, some individuals develop sexual appetites or engage in activities that are not typical sexual behaviors.

Sexual Addiction

Some men and women can get relief from their feelings of restlessness and worthlessness only through sex (either masturbation or with a partner). Once the sexual high ends, however, they're overwhelmed by the same negative feelings and driven, once more, to have sex.

Some therapists describe this problem as **sexual addiction;** others, as **sexual compulsion.** Professionals continue to debate exactly what this controversial condition is, how to diagnose it, and how to overcome it. However, most agree that for some people, sex is more than a normal pleasure: It is an overwhelming need that must be met, even at the cost of their careers and marriages.

Sex addicts can be heterosexual or homosexual, male or female. Their behaviors include masturbation, phone sex, reading or viewing pornography, attending strip shows, having affairs, engaging in anonymous sex with strangers or prostitutes, exhibitionism, voyeurism, child molestation, incest, and rape. Many were physically and emotionally abused as children or have family members who abuse drugs or alcohol. They typically feel a loss of control and a compulsion for sexual activity, and they continue their unhealthy (and sometimes illegal) sexual behavior despite the dangers, including the risk of contracting STIs. Characteristics exhibited by sex addicts include:

- A preoccupation with sex so intense and chronic that it interferes with a normal sexual relationship with a spouse or lover.
- A compulsion to have sex again and again within a short period of time, and to engage in sexual behavior that results in feelings of anxiety, depression, guilt, or shame.
- A great deal of time spent away from family or work, in order to look for sex partners or engage in sex.
- Use of sex to hide from troubles.

With help, sex addicts can deal with the shame that both triggers and follows sexual activity. Professional therapy may begin with a month of complete sexual abstinence, to break the cycle of compulsive sexual behavior. Several organizations, such as Sexaholics Anonymous and Sexual Addicts Anonymous, offer support from people who share the same problem.

Sexual Deviations

Sexual deviations listed by the American Psychiatric Association include the following:

- **Fetishism:** Obtaining sexual pleasure from an inanimate object or an asexual part of the body, such as the foot.

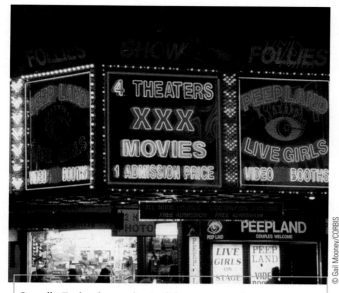

Sex sells. Topless bars and strip clubs are among the businesses that cater to those who enjoy sexual stimulation outside a loving relationship.

- **Transvestitism:** Becoming sexually aroused by wearing the clothing of the opposite sex.
- **Exhibitionism:** Exposing one's genitals to an unwilling observer.
- **Voyeurism:** Obtaining sexual gratification by observing people undressing or involved in sexual activity.
- **Sadism:** Becoming sexually aroused by inflicting physical or psychological pain.
- **Masochism:** Obtaining sexual gratification by suffering physical or psychological pain.

Another, increasingly common sexual variation, hypoxyphilia, involves attempts to enhance the pleasure of orgasm by reducing oxygen intake. Individuals who do so by tying a noose around the neck have accidentally killed themselves.

Psychiatrists distinguish between passive sexual deviancy, which doesn't involve actual contact with another, and aggressive deviancy. Most voyeurs and obscene phone callers don't seek physical contact with the objects of their sexual desire. These behaviors are performed predominantly, but not exclusively, by males.

THE BUSINESS OF SEX

Sex, without affection and individuality, becomes a product to be packaged, marketed, traded, bought, and sold. Two of the billion-dollar industries that treat sex as a commodity are prostitution and pornography.

Prostitution, described as the world's oldest profession, is a nationwide industry grossing more than $1 billion annually. In every state except Nevada (and in all but a few counties there), prostitution is illegal. Besides the threat of jail and fines, prostitutes and their clients face another danger: sexually transmitted infections, including HIV infection and hepatitis B.

Pornography is a multimedia industry—books, magazines, movies, the Internet, phone lines, and computer games are available to those who find sexually explicit material entertaining or exciting. Most laws against pornography are based on the assumption that such materials can set off uncontrollable, dangerous sexual urges, ranging from promiscuity to sexual violence. Research indicates that exposure to scenes of rape or other forms of sexual violence against women, or to scenes of degradation of women, does lead to tolerance of these hostile and brutal acts.

Learn It / Live It
Being Sexually Responsible

We remain sexual beings throughout life. At different ages and stages, sexuality can take on different meanings. As you forge relationships and explore your sexuality, you may encounter difficult situations and unfamiliar feelings. But sex is never just about hormones and body parts. People describe the brain as the sexiest of our organs. Using your brain to make responsible sexual decisions leads to both a smarter and a more fulfilling sex life.

- **Communicate openly.** If you or your partner cannot talk openly and honestly about your sexual histories and contraception, you should avoid having sex. For the sake of protecting your sexual health, you have to be willing to ask—and answer—questions that may seem embarrassing.
- **Share responsibility in a sexual relationship.** Both partners should be involved in protecting themselves and each other from STIs and, if heterosexual, unwanted pregnancy.
- **Respect sexual privacy.** Revealing sexual activities violates the trust between two partners. Bragging about a sexual conquest demeans everyone involved.
- **Do not sexually harass others.** Pinches, pats, sexual comments or jokes, and suggestive gestures are offensive and disrespectful.
- **Be considerate.** A public display of sexual affection can be extremely embarrassing to others. Roommates, in particular, should be sensitive and discrete in their sexual behavior.
- **Be prepared.** If there's any possibility that you may be engaging in sex, be sure you have the means to protect yourself against unwanted pregnancy and sexually transmitted infections.

■ **In sexual situations, always think ahead.** For the sake of safety, think about potential dangers—parking in an isolated area, going into a bedroom with someone you hardly know, and the like—and options to protect yourself.

■ **Be aware of your own and your partner's alcohol and drug intake.** The use of such substances impairs judgment and reduces the ability to say no. While under their influence, you may engage in sexual behavior you'll later regret.

■ **Be sure sexual activity is consensual.** Coercion can take many forms: physical, emotional, and verbal. All cause psychological damage and undermine trust and respect. At any point in a relationship, whether the couple is dating or married, either individual has the right to say no.

Source: Adapted from Hatcher, Robert, et al. *Sexual Etiquette 101 and More.* Atlanta, GA: Emory University School of Medicine, 2002.

Making This Chapter Work for You

Review Questions

1. The hormones that influence the early development of sexual organs.
   a. are released by the ovaries in the female and the testes in the male.
   b. begin to work soon after conception during the embryo's development.
   c. begin to work during puberty, when they stimulate the development of secondary male and female sex characteristics.
   d. determine one's biological sex.

2. Which of the following statements about the menstrual cycle is true?
   a. The pituitary gland releases estrogen and progesterone.
   b. Ovulation occurs at the end of the menstrual cycle.
   c. Premenstrual syndrome is a physiological disorder that usually results in amenorrhea.
   d. The endometrium becomes thicker during the cycle and is shed during menstruation.

3. Which statement about male anatomy is *incorrect?*
   a. The testes manufacture testosterone and sperm.
   b. Sperm cells are carried in the liquid semen.

   c. Cowper's glands secrete semen.
   d. Circumcision is the surgical removal of the foreskin of the penis.

4. Which of the following behaviors is most likely to be a characteristic of sexually healthy and responsible adults?
   a. engages in frequent sexual encounters with many partners
   b. avoids the use of condoms in order to heighten sexual enjoyment for both partners
   c. uses alcohol sparingly and only to help loosen the inhibitions of a resistant partner
   d. engages in sex that is unquestionably consensual

5. Which of the following statements is true about sexual orientation?
   a. Most individuals who identify themselves as bisexual are really homosexual.
   b. Homosexuality is caused by a poor family environment.
   c. Homosexual behavior is found only in affluent and well-educated cultures.
   d. The African-American, Hispanic, and Asian cultures tend to be less accepting of homosexuality than the white community.

6. According to the Centers for Disease Control, abstinence is defined as
   a. refraining from all sexual behaviors that result in arousal.
   b. refraining from all sexual activities that involve vaginal, anal, and oral intercourse.
   c. having sexual intercourse with only one partner exclusively.
   d. refraining from drinking alcohol before sexual activity.

7. Which statement about college students is *not* true?
   a. They consider sexual activity as normal for their peer group.
   b. Most take sex and monogamy seriously.
   c. More than 40 percent do not use condoms.
   d. Women trust a man as safe and healthy on the basis of the way he looks.

8. Which of the following statements about erectile dysfunction (ED) is *false?*
   a. ED is usually caused by physical factors.
   b. A popular treatment for ED is Viagra.
   c. ED is usually caused by psychological factors.
   d. Men who are heavy smokers are at risk for developing ED.

9. Women may experience which of the following problems during intercourse?
   a. vaginismus
   b. excitement

c. vaginal expansion

d. amenorrhea

10. Atypical sexual behaviors include which of the following?

a. masochism

b. sexual desire

c. masturbation

d. celibacy

Answers to these questions can be found on page 587.

Critical Thinking

1. Bill has told his girlfriend, Anita, that he has never taken any sexual risks. But when she suggested that they get tested for STIs, he became furious and refused. Now Anita says she doesn't know what to believe. Could Bill be telling the truth, or is he hiding something? If he is telling the truth, why is Bill so upset? Anita doesn't want to take any risks, but she doesn't want to lose him either. What would you advise her to say or do? What would you advise Bill to say or do?

2. Sex education is always a controversial topic. In SIECUS national surveys, 93 percent of parents of junior high school students and 91 percent of parents of high school students believe it is important to have sexuality education as part of the curriculum. Other parents feel that boys and girls should learn about sex and sexual values in the home. Did you have "sex ed" in junior high or high school? What do you think about such classes—and why?

3. Do you think it is okay to read or look at pornographic books, magazines, websites, and videos? Why or why not?

Media Menu

Health❨⊛❩Now™

Throughout the chapter, this icon introduces a list of resources on the Health-Now website at **http://healthnow.brookscole.com/ith** that will:

- Help you evaluate your knowledge of the material.
- Allow you to take an exam-prep quiz.
- Provide a Personalized Learning Plan targeting resources that address areas you should study.
- Coach you through identifying target goals for behavior change and creating and monitoring your personal change plan throughout the semester.

INTERNET CONNECTIONS

The Sexuality Information and Education Council of the United States (SIECUS)

www.siecus.org

This website is sponsored by SIECUS, a national nonprofit organization that promotes comprehensive education about sexuality and advocates the right of all individuals of all sexual orientations to make responsible sexual choices. The site features a library of fact sheets and articles on a variety of sexuality topics and STIs designed for educators, adults, teens, parents, media, international audiences, and religious organizations.

Youth.org

www.youth.org

This website provides information on gay, lesbian, bisexual, and questioning youth and provides young people with a safe space online to be themselves, to know they are not alone, and to interact with others who have already accepted their sexuality.

Human Rights Campaign

www.hrc.org

The Human Rights Campaign is America's largest gay, lesbian, bisexual, and transgender civil rights organization. Its website features up-to-date information on issues related to gay rights and suggests courses of action to change government policies.

Go Ask Alice

www.goaskalice.columbia.edu/index.html

Sponsored by the health education and wellness program of the Columbia University Health Service, this site features educators' answers to questions on a wide variety of topics of concern to young people, including those related to sexual orientation and healthy sexuality.

InfoTrac College Edition Activities Log on, insert **safe sex** into the Keyword search box, and limit your search to the past year. When you get the results, Mark articles to review, then Select one to read. Summarize three or four key points from the article.

You can find additional readings related to personal health with InfoTrac College Edition, an online library of more than 900 journals and publications. Follow the instructions for accessing InfoTrac College Edition that were packaged with your textbook; then search for articles using a keyword search.

For additional links, resources, and suggested readings on InfoTrac College Edition, visit our Health and Wellness Resource Center at **http://health.wadsworth.com.**

Self Survey ■ How Much Do You Know About Sex?

Mark each of the following statements True or False:

1. Men and women have completely different sex hormones.
2. Premenstrual syndrome (PMS) is primarily a psychological problem.
3. Circumcision diminishes a man's sexual pleasure.
4. Sexual orientation may have a biological basis.
5. Masturbation is a sign of emotional immaturity.
6. Only homosexual men engage in anal intercourse.
7. Despite their awareness of AIDS, many college students do not practice safe sex.
8. After age 60, lovemaking is mainly a fond memory, not a regular pleasure of daily living.
9. Doctors advise against having intercourse during a woman's menstrual period.
10. Only men ejaculate.
11. It is possible to be infected with HIV during a single sexual encounter.
12. Impotence is always a sign of emotional or sexual problems in a relationship.

Answers:

1. False. Men and women have the same hormones, but in different amounts.
2. False. PMS has been recognized as a physiological disorder that may be caused by a hormonal deficiency, abnormal levels of thyroid hormone, or social and environmental factors, such as stress.
3. False. Sex therapists have not been able to document differences in sensitivity to stimulation between circumcised and uncircumcised men.
4. True. Researchers documented structural differences in the brains of homosexual men and women.
5. False. Throughout a person's life, masturbation can be a form of sexual release and pleasure.
6. False. As many as one in every four married couples under age 35 have reported that they occasionally engage in anal intercourse.
7. True. In one recent study, more than a third of college students had engaged in vaginal or anal intercourse at least once in the previous year without using effective protection from conception or sexually transmitted infections (STIs).
8. False. More than a third of American married men and women older than 60 make love at least once a week, as do 10 percent of those older than 70.
9. False. There's no medical reason to avoid intercourse during a woman's menstrual period.
10. False. Stimulation of the Grafenberg spot in a woman's vagina may lead to a release of fluid from her urethra during orgasm.
11. True. Although the risk increases with repeated sexual contact with an infected partner, an individual can contract HIV during a single sexual encounter.
12. False. Many erection difficulties have physical causes.

Key Terms

The terms listed are used on the page indicated. Definitions of the terms are in the Glossary at the end of the book.

abstinence 250
amenorrhea 241
androgyny 238
bisexual 248
celibacy 250
cervix 238
circumcision 242

clitoris 238
corpus luteum 241
Cowper's glands 242
cunnilingus 252
dysmenorrhea 241
dyspareunia 257
ejaculation 254

ejaculatory ducts 242
endocrine system 236
endometrium 238
epididymis 242
erectile dysfunction (ED) 256
erogenous 251
estrogen 236
fallopian tubes 238
fellatio 252
gender 236
gonadotropins 236

gonads 236
heterosexual 248
homosexuals 248
hormones 236
impotence 256
intercourse 251
intimacy 235
labia majora 238
labia minora 238
masturbation 245
menarche 236

YOUR ACTION PLAN FOR RESPONSIBLE SEXUALITY

Your score on the Self Survey may indicate that you know a lot more—or less—about sex than you thought you did. Part of sexual responsibility is being informed about sexuality, including reproductive anatomy, sexual orientation, the range of sexual behaviors, and ways of protecting yourself from sexually transmitted diseases.

The Sexuality Information and Education Council of the United States (SIECUS) has worked with nongovernmental organizations around the world to develop a consensus about the life behaviors of a sexually healthy and responsible adult. These include:

- Appreciating one's own body.
- Seeking information about reproduction as needed.
- Affirming that sexual development may or may not include reproduction or genital sexual experience.
- Interacting with both genders in respectful and appropriate ways.
- Affirming one's own sexual orientation and respecting the sexual orientation of others.
- Expressing love and intimacy in appropriate ways.
- Developing and maintaining meaningful relationships.
- Avoiding exploitative or manipulative relationships.
- Making informed choices about family options and lifestyles.
- Enjoying and expressing one's sexuality throughout life.
- Expressing one's sexuality in ways congruent with one's values.
- Discriminating between life-enhancing sexual behaviors and those that are harmful to oneself and/or others.
- Expressing one's sexuality while respecting the rights of others.
- Seeking new information to enhance one's sexuality.
- Using contraception effectively to avoid unintended pregnancy.
- Preventing sexual abuse.
- Seeking early prenatal care.
- Avoiding contracting or transmitting a sexually transmitted infection, including HIV.

- Practicing health-promoting behaviors, such as regular checkups, breast and testicular self-exam, and early identification of potential problems.
- Demonstrating tolerance for people with different sexual values and lifestyles.
- Exercising democratic responsibility to influence legislation dealing with sexual issues.
- Assessing the impact of family, cultural, religious, media, and societal messages on one's thoughts, feelings, values, and behaviors related to sexuality.
- Promoting the rights of all people to accurate sexuality information.
- Avoiding behaviors that exhibit prejudice and bigotry.
- Rejecting stereotypes about the sexuality of diverse populations.

CASE IN POINT

Student: Tristan, 18

Goal: To resist peer pressure to "hook up" for casual sex

Action Plan:

- Think through his core values and why they matter to him
- Identify the situations in which he is most likely to feel uncomfortable
- Look for friends who share his values
- Plan ahead and arrange to be with people and in places where he doesn't feel any need to compromise his values
- Avoid alcohol or drug use, which often contribute to unwanted sexual experiences

Health✸Now™   If you want to write your own goals for responsible sexual behavior, go to the **Wellness Journal at HealthNow** http://healthnow.brookscole .com/ith.

Reproductive Choices

Jess and Sara, juniors at the same community college, can't remember a time when abortion was illegal, when AIDS wasn't a deadly threat, and when safe sex wasn't a concern of every sexually active individual. Yet even though they were aware of the risks and the realities involved, neither used contraception during every single sexual encounter. Then one of Jess's partners had a pregnancy scare. He decided never again to engage in unprotected sex. Sara had a different reality check: At her regular physical, she learned that she had contracted chlamydia, the most common sexually transmitted infection in the United States.

When Jess and Sara started dating, both of them felt that something was special about their relationship. Despite their mutual attraction, they decided to take every step toward intimacy slowly. Both considered and talked about their personal priorities and concerns. Even though it was awkward, they also discussed their own sexual histories and underwent tests for STIs. Looking toward a continuing committed relationship, they decided on not one but two forms of contraception: the birth control pill and a condom. In the future, they realized that they might switch to other forms of birth control—and might well consider different options, including both marriage and parenthood.

As human beings, we have a unique power: the ability to choose to conceive or not to conceive. No other species on Earth can separate sexual activity and pleasure from reproduction. However, simply not wanting to get pregnant is never enough to prevent conception, nor is wanting to have a child always enough to get pregnant. Both desires require individual decisions and actions.

Anyone who engages in vaginal intercourse must be willing to accept the consequences of that activity—the possibility of pregnancy and responsibility for the child who might be conceived—or take action to avoid those consequences. Although many people are concerned about the risks associated with contraception, using birth control is safer and healthier than not using it. According to the Population Reference Bureau, the use of contraceptives, including oral contraceptives, saves millions of lives each year.

This chapter provides information on conception, birth control, abortion, infertility, adoption, and the processes by which a new human life develops and enters the world.

Masterfile (RM)/Mark Wiens

After studying the material in this chapter, you should be able to:

- **Describe** the process of human conception.

- **List** the major options available for contraception, and **identify** the advantages and disadvantages of each.

- **Describe** the commonly used abortion methods.

- **Discuss** the physiological effects of pregnancy on a woman and **describe** fetal development.

- **Give examples** of prenatal care measures.

- **Describe** the three stages of labor and the birth process.

- **Identify** the options available to infertile couples wanting children.

CONCEPTION

The equation for making a baby is quite simple: One sperm plus one egg equals one fertilized egg, which can develop into an infant. But the processes that affect or permit **conception** are quite complicated. The creation of sperm, or **spermatogenesis,** starts in the male at puberty, and the production of sperm is regulated by hormones. Sperm cells form in the seminiferous tubules of the testes and are passed into the epididymis, where they are stored until ejaculation (Figure 10-1); a single male ejaculation may contain 500 million sperm. Each sperm released into the vagina during intercourse moves on its own, propelling itself toward its target, an ovum.

To reach its goal, the sperm must move through the acidic secretions of the vagina, enter the uterus, travel up the fallopian tube containing the ovum, then fuse with the nucleus of the egg (**fertilization**). Just about every sperm produced by a man in his lifetime fails to accomplish its mission.

There are far fewer human egg cells than there are sperm cells. Each woman is born with her lifetime supply of ova, and between 300 and 500 eggs eventually mature and leave her ovaries during ovulation. As discussed in Chapter 9, every month, one or the other of the woman's ovaries releases an ovum to the nearby fallopian tube. It travels through the fallopian tube until it reaches the uterus, a journey that takes three to four days. An unfertilized egg lives for about 24 to 36 hours, disintegrates, and during menstruation is expelled along with the uterine lining.

Even if a sperm, which can survive in the female reproductive tract for two to five days, meets a ripe egg in a fallopian tube, its success is not assured. A mature ovum releases the chemical allurin, which attracts the sperm. A sperm is able to penetrate the ovum's outer membrane because of a protein called fertilin. The egg then pulls the sperm inside toward its nucleus (Figure 10-2). The fertilized egg travels down the fallopian tube, dividing to form a tiny clump of cells called a **zygote.** When it reaches the uterus, about a week after fertilization, it burrows into the endometrium, the lining of the uterus. This process is called **implantation.**

Conception can be prevented by **contraception.** Some contraceptive methods prevent ovulation or implantation, and others block the sperm from reaching the egg. Some methods are temporary; others permanently alter one's fertility.

BIRTH CONTROL BASICS

Most sexually active women use some form of birth control. According to the Centers for Disease Control and Prevention, more than 98 percent of women between the ages of 15 and 44 who have ever had intercourse have used at least one contraceptive method. Most of the women not using

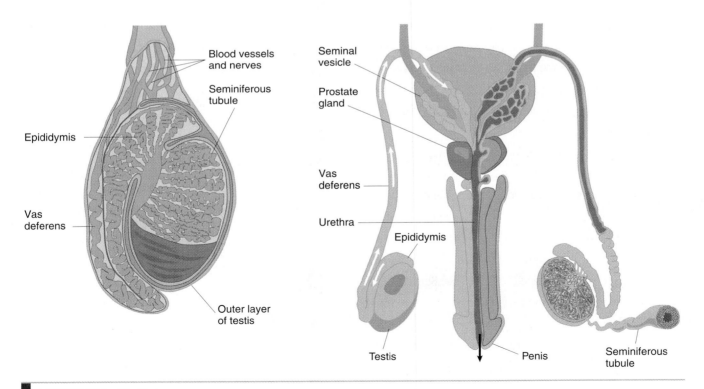

FIGURE 10-1   The Testes

Spermatogenesis takes place in the testes. Sperm cells form in the seminiferous tubules and are stored in the coils of the epididymis. Eventually, the sperm drain into the vas deferens, ready for ejaculation.

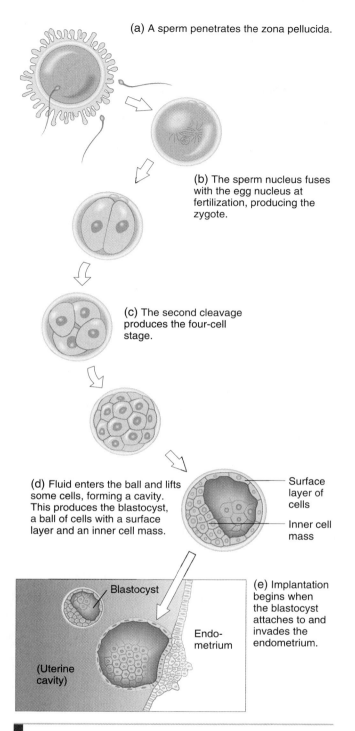

(a) A sperm penetrates the zona pellucida.

(b) The sperm nucleus fuses with the egg nucleus at fertilization, producing the zygote.

(c) The second cleavage produces the four-cell stage.

(d) Fluid enters the ball and lifts some cells, forming a cavity. This produces the blastocyst, a ball of cells with a surface layer and an inner cell mass.

Surface layer of cells

Inner cell mass

Blastocyst

(Uterine cavity)

Endo-metrium

(e) Implantation begins when the blastocyst attaches to and invades the endometrium.

FIGURE 10-2   Fertilization

(a) The efforts of hundreds of sperm may allow one to penetrate the ovum's corona radiata, an outer layer of cells, and then the zona pellucida, a thick inner membrane. (b) The nuclei of the sperm and the egg cells merge, and the male and female chromosomes in the nuclei come together, forming a zygote. (c) The zygote divides into two cells, then four cells, and so on. (d) As fluid enters the ball, cells form a ball of cells called a blastocyst. (e) The blastocyst implants itself in the endometrium.

any form of contraception are pregnant, trying to get pregnant, unable to conceive, or not having intercourse.[1]

The number of couples using contraception the first time they have intercourse has risen to 79 percent, almost double the rate in 1980. Condoms were the contraceptive used by 67 percent of couples for first intercourse.

The leading birth control method is the oral contraceptive pill, followed by female sterilization, and condoms. Other methods, including sponges, intrauterine devices, diaphragms, and foams, have decreased in popularity in the last decade.

If you are engaging in sexual activity that could lead to conception, you have to be realistic about your situation. This may mean assuming full responsibility for your reproductive ability, whether you're a man or a woman. The more you know about contraception, the more likely you are to use birth control.

You also have to recognize the risks associated with various methods of contraception. If you're a woman, the risks are chiefly yours. Various methods of birth control have side effects, but pregnancy and childbirth account for much higher rates of medical complications and deaths than any contraceptive. Although most women never experience any serious complications, it's important to be aware of the potential for long-term risks. Risks that are acceptable to others may not be acceptable to you.

In one study at a western college, undergraduates were more likely to report "almost always" using a reliable, proven method of birth control after completing an introductory health course.[2]

Your Life Coach

Choosing a Birth Control Method

When it comes to deciding which form of birth control to use, there's no one "right" decision. Good decisions are based on sound information. You should consult a physician or family-planning counselor if you have questions or want to know how certain methods might affect existing or familial medical conditions, such as high blood pressure or diabetes.

Table 10-1 presents your contraceptive choices. As the table indicates, contraception doesn't always work. When you evaluate any contraceptive, always consider its *effectiveness* (the likelihood that it will indeed prevent pregnancy). The **failure rate** refers to the number of pregnancies that occur per year for every 100 women using a particular method of birth control.

The reliability of contraceptives in actual, real-life use is much lower than those reported in national surveys or clinical trials. In general, failure rates are highest among cohabiting and other unmarried women, very poor families, black and Hispanic women, adolescents, and women in their twenties.

Some couples use withdrawal or **coitus interruptus,** removal of the penis from the vagina before

TABLE 10-1 OVERVIEW OF CONTRACEPTIVE OPTIONS

Method	Failure Rate— Unintended Pregnancies Within First Year of Use (%)		Women Continuing Use at One Year (%)	Frequency of Use	Protection Against STIs	Cost
	Typical Use	Perfect Use				
None	85	85	–	–	–	–
Spermicide	29	15	42	Each time	No	$0.35 to 12
Withdrawal	27	4	43	Each time	No	None
Periodic abstinence						
Calendar method	25	9	~50	Each time	No	None
Ovulation method	25	3	~50	Each time	No	None
Cervical cap* (women who have not had children)	16	9	57	Each time	No	$30 to 40
Diaphragm*	16	6	57	Each time	Yes	$30 to 40
Female condom	21	5	49	Each time	Yes	$2 to 3 each
Male condom	15	2	53	Each time	Yes	$0.50 to 2 each
The pill	8	0.3	68	Taken daily	No	$20 to 50 per cycle
Contraceptive patch	Unknown	0.3	68	Applied weekly	No	$36 per month
NuvaRing	Unknown	0.3	68	Inserted every 4 weeks	No	$43 per month
Progestin-only pill	3	0.3	56	Given every 12 weeks	No	$30 to 35 every 3 months
Copper-containing IUD	0.8	0.6	78	Inserted every 10 years	No	$250 to 300 every 10 years
Mirena	0.1	0.1	81	Inserted every 5 years	No	$300 to 400 every 5 years
Female sterilization	0.5	0.5	100	Done once	No	$1,200 to 2,500
Male sterilization	0.15	0.10	100	Done once	No	$250 to 1,000

STI = sexually transmitted infection; IUD intrauterine device.

*Used with spermicide.

Source: Adapted from Hatcher, R. A. *A Pocket Guide to Managing Contraception,* 5th ed. Tiger, GA: Bridging the Gap Foundation, Vol. 36, 2000–2003, pp. 44–141.

ejaculation, to prevent pregnancy, even though this is not a reliable form of birth control. About half the men who have tried coitus interruptus find it unsatisfactory, either because they don't know when they're going to ejaculate or because they can't withdraw quickly enough. Also, the Cowper's glands, two pea-sized structures located on each side of the urethra, often produce a fluid that appears as drops at the tip of the penis any time from arousal and erection to orgasm. This fluid can contain active sperm and, in infected men, human immunodeficiency virus (HIV).

As many as 3 million unintentional pregnancies each year in the United States are the result of contraceptive failure, either from problems with the drug or device itself or from improper use. Partners can lower the risk of unwanted pregnancy by using backup methods—that is, more than one form of contraception simultaneously. Emergency or after-intercourse contraception (discussed later in this chapter) could prevent as many as 3 million unwanted pregnancies each year.[3]

Regardless of pregnancy history, about half of adolescents do not use effective contraception. Adolescents who have had previous abortions are three times more likely than never-pregnant adolescents to use hormonal contraception. However, although more likely to use contraceptive injections or implants, adolescent mothers are not more likely than never-pregnant adolescents to use oral contraceptives.

 Even college students aware of the risks associated with unprotected sexual intercourse often do not practice safe-sex behaviors. There are many reasons, ranging from the influence of sex and alcohol to embarrassment about buying condoms. Generally, the ability to talk about a desire to use condoms has been found to be associated with a greater use of condoms.

The bottom line is that it takes two people to conceive a baby, and two people should be involved in deciding not to conceive a baby. In the process, they can also enhance their skills in communication, critical thinking, and negotiating.

Strategies for Prevention   ▪▪   Choosing a Contraceptive

Your contraceptive needs may change throughout your life. To decide which method to use now, you need to know:

▪▪ How well will it fit into your lifestyle?

▪▪ How convenient will it be?

▪▪ How effective will it be?

▪▪ How safe will it be?

▪▪ How affordable will it be?

▪▪ How reversible will it be?

▪▪ Will it protect against sexually transmitted infections?

Source: "Facts About Birth Control." www.plannedparenthood.org.

  In a study of contraceptive decision making among African-American, Hispanic, and European-American women ages 18 to 50, those who made contraceptive decisions alone were older, single, African American, used pregnancy prevention, or had histories of sexually transmitted infections and unintended pregnancies. Older African-American women were more likely to choose no contraception. Among contraceptive users, African Americans used effective methods of pregnancy prevention but not disease prevention. Women who had a history of sexually transmitted infections and younger, more educated women were more likely to use methods that prevent both pregnancy and infections.

ABSTINENCE AND NONPENETRATIVE SEXUAL BEHAVIOR

The contraceptive methods discussed in this chapter are designed to prevent pregnancy as a consequence of vaginal intercourse. Couples who choose abstinence make a very different decision—to abstain from vaginal intercourse and forms of nonpenetrative sexual activity that could result in conception (any in which ejaculation occurs near the vaginal opening).

For many individuals, abstinence represents a deliberate choice regarding their bodies, minds, spirits, and sexuality. People choose abstinence for various reasons, including waiting until they are ready for a sexual relationship or until they find the "right" partner, respecting religious or moral values, enjoying friendships without sexual involvement, recovering from a breakup, or preventing pregnancy and sexually transmitted infection (see Chapter 9).

Abstinence is the only form of birth control that is 100 percent effective and risk-free. It is also an important, increasingly valued lifestyle choice. A growing number of individuals, including some who have been sexually active in the past, are choosing abstinence until they establish a relationship with a long-term partner.

Abstinence offers special health benefits for women. Those who abstain until their twenties and engage in sex with fewer partners during their lifetime are less likely to get sexually transmitted infections, to suffer infertility, or to develop cervical cancer. However, some people find it difficult to abstain for long periods of time. There also is a risk that people will abruptly end their abstinence without being prepared to protect themselves against pregnancy or infection.

Individuals who choose abstinence from vaginal intercourse often engage in activities sometimes called *outercourse,* such as kissing, hugging, sensual touching, and mutual masturbation. Outercourse is nearly 100 percent effective as a contraceptive measure, but pregnancy is possible if there is genital contact. If the man ejaculates near the vaginal opening, sperm can swim up into the vagina and fallopian tubes to fertilize an egg. Except for oral-genital sex, outercourse also may lower the risk of contracting sexually transmitted infections. It is an effective form of safe sex as long as no body fluids are exchanged.

Some couples routinely restrict themselves to outercourse; others temporarily choose such sexual activities when it is inadvisable for them to have vaginal intercourse—for example, after childbirth. Other benefits: Outercourse has no medical or hormonal side effects; it may prolong sex play and enhance orgasm, and it can be used when no other birth control methods are available.

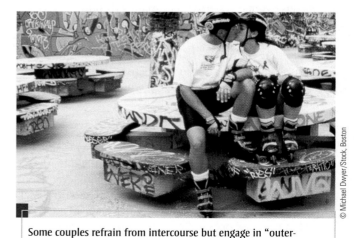

© Michael Dwyer/Stock, Boston

Some couples refrain from intercourse but engage in "outercourse," or intimacy that includes kissing and hugging.

Strategies for Prevention ▪ Is Abstinence the Right Choice for You?

- Think about your values, goals, and priorities. Would abstinence support them?
- Realize that drugs and alcohol could affect your ability to make sexual decisions. Are you prepared to avoid their use to be sure to maintain your abstinence?
- Talk about your feelings before a relationship gets sexual. Can you put your thoughts and feelings about abstinence into words?
- Abstinence does not mean an end to all sexual experiences. What behaviors would you consider acceptable? What limits would you set?

HORMONAL CONTRACEPTIVES

In recent years, birth control methods made with synthetic hormones have become available in a variety of forms. Oral contraceptives have been available for decades, and the birth control pill is one of the most well-researched medications. Other options for hormonal birth control include a skin patch, a vaginal ring, and a monthly or quarterly injection. All are extremely effective when used consistently and conscientiously.

Hormonal contraceptives do not protect against HIV infection and other STIs, so condoms and spermicides should also be used if you need protection against infections.

ORAL CONTRACEPTIVES

The pill—the popular term for **oral contraceptives**—is the method of birth control preferred by unmarried women and by those under age 30, including college students (see Student Snapshot: "Contraception on Campus"). Women 18 to 24 years old are most likely to choose oral contraceptives. In use for 40 years, the pill is one of the most researched, tested, and carefully followed medications in medical history—and one of the most controversial.

Although many women incorrectly think that the risks of the pill are greater than those of pregnancy and childbirth, long-term studies show that oral contraceptive use does not increase mortality rates. Combination oral contraceptives significantly reduce the risk of ovarian and endometrial cancer and produce no increase in breast cancer, diabetes, multiple sclerosis, rheumatoid arthritis, and liver disease.

More than 10 million women in the United States use oral contraceptives to prevent pregnancy. In the first year of use, the failure rate is 6 percent, largely because of incorrect or inconsistent use.[4]

Although research is limited, the use of common antibiotics, including many prescribed for dental procedures or skin conditions, may lower the effectiveness of oral contraceptives, particularly low-dose birth control pills. Always ask a dentist or doctor who prescribes an antibiotic about its potential effect on your oral contraceptive, and check with your gynecologist or primary physician about using an additional nonhormonal means of contraception (such as a condom) to ensure protection against an unwanted pregnancy.

Combination Pills

These pills consist of two hormones, synthetic estrogen and progestin, which play important roles in controlling ovulation and the menstrual cycle. The doses in today's oral contraceptives are much lower—less than one-fourth the amount of estrogen and one-twentieth the progestin in the original pill. This means fewer side effects and lower risk of heart disease and stroke. Stroke risk among women taking newer, low-dose formulations of oral contraceptive pills may be "tenuous at best and perhaps nonexistent," according to a recent meta-analysis of current research.[5]

Monophasic pills release a constant dose of estrogen and progestin throughout a woman's menstrual cycle. **Multiphasic pills** mimic normal hormonal fluctuations of the natural menstrual cycle by providing different levels of estrogen and progesterone at different times of the month.

Student Snapshot

CONTRACEPTION ON CAMPUS

Contraceptive Method	Total	Women	Men
Birth control pills	40%	41%	38%
Condoms (male or female)	35	34	39
Withdrawal	15	15	14
Spermicide	4	3	4
Fertility awareness	3	3	3
Depo-Provera	3	3	2
Diaphragm/cervical cap/sponge	0.3	0.3	0.4
Norplant	0.1	0.1	0.2
Other method	3	3	3
Nothing	4	3	4

Responses of a national sample of students to the question: "If you have had sexual intercourse, what method did you or your partner use to prevent pregnancy the last time?" Because not all respondents answered and they could choose more than one option, the totals do not add up to 100 percent.

Source: American College Health Association. "The American College Health Association-National College Health Assessment, Spring 2003 Reference Group Report." *Journal of American College Health,* Vol. 53, No. 5, March–April 2005, p. 199.

Multiphasic pills reduce total hormonal dose and side effects. Both constant-dose combination and multiphasic pills block the release of hormones that would stimulate the process leading to ovulation. They also thicken and alter the cervical mucus, making it more hostile to sperm, and they make implantation of a fertilized egg in the uterine lining more difficult.

One combination pill, Yasmin, contains a unique progestin that works like a mild diuretic and prevents fluid retention. Researchers have found that it lessens symptoms of premenstrual problems. Women who are taking potassium supplements, daily anti-inflammatory drugs, or heparin, a blood-thinner, should not take Yasmin because of potentially dangerous drug interactions.[6] Other pills offer different benefits, such as clearer skin and reduced facial hair.

Progestin-Only Pills

Progestin-only **"minipills"** contain only a small amount of progestin and no estrogen. They work somewhat differently than combination pills. Women taking **progestin-only pills** probably ovulate, at least occasionally. In those cycles, the pills prevent pregnancy by thickening cervical mucus, making it hard for sperm to penetrate, and by interfering with implantation of a fertilized egg.

The risk of heart disease and stroke is lower with progestin-only pills than with any combination pill. For this reason, they are a good choice for women over age 35 and others who cannot take estrogen-containing pills because of high blood pressure, diabetes, or clotting disorders. Because they do not affect the quality or quantity of breast milk, progestin-only pills often are recommended for nursing mothers, and they are recommended for smokers. Because progestin can affect mood and worsen the symptoms of depression, progestin-only pills are not recommended for women with a history of depression. Anti-seizure medications, such as Dilantin, which accelerate liver metabolism, may make the minipill less effective.

Various types of birth control pills contain different hormones and combinations of hormones.

© Carolyn A. McKeone/Photo Researchers, Inc.

Users of progestin-only pills have to be conscientious about taking these pills, not just every day, but at the same time every day. If you take a progestin-only pill three or more hours later than usual, use a back-up method of contraception, such as a condom, for two days after you resume taking the pill.

Advantages of Oral Contraceptives

- Extremely effective when taken consistently.
- Convenient.
- Moderately priced.
- Do not interrupt sexual activity.
- Reversible within three months of stopping the pill.
- Reduce the risk of benign breast lumps, ovarian cysts, iron-deficiency anemia, pelvic inflammatory disease, endometrial and ovarian cancer.
- May relieve painful menstruation.[7]

Disadvantages of Oral Contraceptives

- Require a prescription.
- Increased risk of cardiovascular problems, primarily for women over age 35 who smoke and those with high blood pressure or other health problems.
- Side effects vary with different brands but include spotting between periods, weight gain or loss, nausea and vomiting, breast tenderness, and decreased sex drive.
- Must be taken at the same time every day (especially critical with low-dose estrogen and progestin-only pills).
- No protection against STIs.
- Must use a secondary form of birth control for the initial seven days of use.

Before Using Oral Contraceptives Before starting on the pill, you should undergo a thorough physical examination that includes the following tests:

- Routine blood pressure test.
- Pelvic exam, including a Pap smear.
- Breast exam.
- Blood test.
- Urine sample.

Let your doctor know about any personal or family incidence of high blood pressure or heart disease, diabetes, liver dysfunction, hepatitis, unusual menstrual history, severe depression, sickle-cell anemia, cancer of the breast, ovaries, or uterus, high cholesterol levels, or migraine headaches. (See Savvy Consumer: "Evaluating the Risks of Contraceptives.")

How to Use Oral Contraceptives The pill usually comes in 28-day packets: 21 of the pills contain the hormones, and 7 are "blanks," included so that the woman can take a pill every day, even during her menstrual period. If a woman

Savvy Consumer ▪▪ Evaluating the Risks of Contraceptives

For individuals with certain medical conditions, specific types of birth control can pose a health risk. To be safe, follow these guidelines:

▪▪ **High blood pressure** (180/110 mmHg or higher): Avoid birth control pills or injectables containing estrogen, which may increase your risk of a heart attack or stroke.

▪▪ **Episodes of depression:** Avoid products that contain progestin, such as Depo-Provera, contraceptive implants, and the minipill. In some women with

depression, progestin may worsen depressive symptoms. Also, check with your doctor if you are taking an antidepressant medication; it may affect or be affected by oral contraceptives and you may require a different dose.

▪▪ **Seizure disorder:** Avoid low-dose birth control pills. Some antiseizure medications, such as Dilantin, accelerate liver metabolism of all substances, including oral contraceptives, and make them less effective.

▪▪ **Ectopic pregnancy:** Avoid IUDs. Although IUDs do not cause ectopic pregnancies, if your fallopian tubes have been scarred by a previous ectopic gestation, you're more likely to have another ectopic if you use an IUD.

▪▪ **Hepatitis:** Avoid birth control pills or injectables containing estrogen, which is metabolized in the liver—an organ damaged by hepatitis.

---

forgets to take one pill, she should take it as soon as she remembers. However, if she forgets during the first week of her cycle or misses more than one pill, she should rely on another form of birth control until her next menstrual period.

Even if you experience no discomfort or side effects while on the pill, see a physician at least once a year for an examination, which should include a blood pressure test, a pelvic, and a breast exam. Notify your doctor at once if you develop severe abdominal pain, chest pain, coughing, shortness of breath, pain or tenderness in the calf or thigh, severe headaches, dizziness, faintness, muscle weakness or numbness, speech disturbance, blurred vision, a sensation of flashing lights, a breast lump, severe depression, or yellowing of your skin.

Generally, when a woman stops taking the pill, her menstrual cycle resumes the next month, but it may be irregular for the next couple of months. However, 2 to 4 percent of pill users experience prolonged delays. Women who become pregnant during the first or second cycle after discontinuing use of the pill may be at greater risk of miscarriage; they also are more likely to conceive twins. Most physicians advise women who want to conceive to change to another method of contraception for three months after they stop taking the pill.

Extended-Use Oral Contraceptives

For years physicians have prescribed prolonged use of birth control pills to lessen the number of menstrual cycles for women with asthma, migraines, rashes, or other conditions that flare up during their periods. Eliminating periods eliminates symptoms, and having fewer cycles also may lower a woman's long-term risk of ovarian cancer. A new package of standard combination birth control pills, called Seasonale, provides pills for 84 days of continuous use so women have four periods a year rather than twelve.

THE PATCH (ORTHO EVRA)

The Ortho Evra birth control patch, the first transdermal (through the skin) contraceptive, works like a combination pill but looks like a bandaid. Embedded in its adhesive layer are two hormones, a low-dose estrogen and a progestin. It prevents pregnancy by delivering continuous levels of estrogen and progestin through the skin into the bloodstream. The hormones in Ortho Evra are slowly released when the patch is applied to the skin. The patch is waterproof and stays on in the shower, swimming pools, or hot tubs.[8]

Ortho-McNeil Pharmaceutical

Advantages of the Patch

▪ Good alternative for women who can't remember, don't like, or have problems swallowing daily pills.

▪ Highly effective when used correctly.

▪ Does not interrupt sexual activity.

▪ Fewer side effects, such as nausea, breakthrough bleeding, and mood swings, than pills.

▪ Fertility returns quickly after you stop using it.

Disadvantages of the Patch

▪ Must apply a new patch every week.

▪ Requires a prescription.

▪ No protection against STIs.

▪ Increased risk of blood clots, heart attack, and stroke particularly for women who smoke or have certain health conditions. About a dozen women, most in their late teens and early 20s, have died of blood clots believed to be related to the patch.

Dozens more have survived strokes and other clot-related problems. The risk of dying or suffering a survivable blood clot while using the patch is estimated to be about three times higher than while using birth control pills.

- Less effective in women who weigh more than 198 pounds.
- Some women report breast tenderness, headaches, upper respiratory infections, or self-consciousness wearing the patch.
- Contact lens wearers may experience vision changes.
- 5 percent of women report that at least one patch slipped off; 2 percent report skin irritation.
- Must use another form of birth control for the initial seven days of use.

How to Use the Patch

A woman applies the 1¾ inch square to her back, upper arm, lower abdomen, or buttocks and changes it every seven days for three weeks. During the patch-free week, she experiences menstrual bleeding. A user should check every day to make sure the patch is still in place. If you don't replace a detached patch within 24 hours, use a backup method of contraception until your next period.

The FDA has warned of counterfeit versions of the birth control patch being marketed on the Internet. The fakes do not provide any protection against pregnancy.[9]

THE NUVARING

The silver-dollar-sized NuvaRing, a 2-inch ring made of flexible, transparent plastic, slowly emits the same hormones as oral contraceptives through the vaginal tissues (Figure 10-3). Smaller than the smallest diaphragm, it contains less estrogen than any pill. As effective as the pill, it provides a steady dose of hormones and causes fewer side effects.[10]

Advantages of NuvaRing

- Under medical supervision, may be safer than birth control pills for women with mild hypertension or diabetes.
- Less likelihood of pill-related side effects, such as nausea, mood swings, spotting, and cramping.
- No need to remember a daily pill or weekly patch.
- Fertility returns quickly when ring is removed.

Disadvantages of NuvaRing

- Some women do not feel comfortable placing and removing something inside their vaginas.
- Possible side effects include vaginal discharge, irritation, and infection.

© ORGANON Communications

▌**FIGURE 10-3** NuvaRing
The NuvaRing releases estrogen and progestin, preventing ovulation. The exact position of NuvaRing in the vagina is not important for it to work.

- Cannot use oil-based vaginal medications for yeast infections while ring is in place.
- No protection against STIs.

How to Use the Ring Unlike a diaphragm, the NuvaRing does not have to be exactly positioned within the vagina or used with a spermicide (sperm-killing foam or jelly). The flexible, plastic 2-inch ring compresses so a woman can easily insert it. Each ring stays in place for three weeks, then is removed for the fourth week of the menstrual cycle.

If a NuvaRing pops out (uncommon but possible), it should be washed, dried, and replaced within three hours. If a longer time passes, users should rely on a backup form of birth control until the ring has been reinserted for a week and the medications have risen to protective levels again.

CONTRACEPTIVE INJECTABLES

Two different hormonal contraceptives are available in the form of "shots" or injections. Lunelle, which consists of the same hormones as combination birth control pills, is administered monthly. Depo-Provera, which contains only progestin, must be given every 12 weeks. Injectable contraceptives provide no protection against HIV and other STIs.

Lunelle

Lunelle is a contraceptive injection of estrogen and progestin, given each month by a health professional (doctor, nurse, or in some places, pharmacist) into the arm, thigh, or buttocks during the first five days of a woman's menstrual cycle. It is considered 99.5 percent effective in preventing pregnancy.[11]

Advantages of Lunelle

■ No risk of user error.

■ No worry about buying, storing, or using contraceptives.

■ No need to think about contraception for four weeks at a time.

Disadvantages of Lunelle

■ Must visit a doctor's office or clinic every month for an injection.

■ Weight gain (average is 4 pounds, but some women gain 10 to 20 pounds).

■ Side effects include nausea, breakthrough bleeding, acne, headache, change in sexual desire, depression, and breast tenderness, particularly during the first few months of use.

■ No protection against STIs.

Depo-Provera

One injection of Depo-Provera, a synthetic version of the natural hormone progesterone, provides three months of contraceptive protection. This long-acting hormonal contraceptive raises levels of progesterone, thereby simulating pregnancy. The pituitary gland doesn't produce FSH and LH, which normally cause egg ripening and release. The endometrial lining of the uterus thins, preventing implantation of a fertilized egg.

Advantages of Depo-Provera

■ Because it contains only progestin, it is safe for women who cannot take combination birth control pills.

■ No risk of user error.

■ No worry about buying, storing, or using contraceptives.

■ No need to think about contraception for three months at a time.

■ Possible protection against endometrial and ovarian cancer.

Disadvantages of Depo-Provera

■ Must visit a doctor or clinic every three months for injection.

■ Menstrual cycles become irregular or cease.

■ Potential side effects include decreased libido, depression, headaches, dizziness, weight gain, frequent urination, and allergic reactions.

■ No protection against STIs.

■ According to recent NIH study, appears to triple risk of acquiring chlamydia and gonorrhea compared to women not using a hormonal contraceptive. Scientists do not know the reason for this increased risk.[12]

■ Delayed return of fertility.

■ Long-term use may significantly reduce bone density.

CONTRACEPTIVE IMPLANTS

Hormonal implants, placed under the skin, deliver a constant low dose of progestin. They work primarily by suppressing ovulation, but they also thicken the cervical mucus (which inhibits sperm migration), inhibit the development and growth of the uterine lining, and limit secretion of progesterone during the second, or luteal, half of the menstrual cycle.

Norplant, consisting of six thin silicone rubber capsules containing a synthetic form of progestin, was the first such implant available in the United States. Approximately 9 million women used this method before it was taken off the market for reasons unrelated to its efficacy. Women with Norplant implants, who include many adolescents and young adults, should consult their doctors. They can safely leave the rods in place for the entire five-year period of contraceptive protection. However, they should discuss all options, including removal of the Norplant rods and switching to an alternative form of contraception.

A newer generation of implants may provide the benefits of long-term pregnancy protection with fewer complications. Implanon, a single Silastic rod that is simpler to insert and remove than Norplant, provides at least three years of contraception. Available in Europe and Australia, it uses a different type of progestin than Norplant and may cause fewer side effects like weight gain or acne. It should be available in the United States soon.

INTRAUTERINE CONTRACEPTIVES: MIRENA

An **intrauterine device (IUD)** is a small piece of molded plastic, with a nylon string attached, that is inserted into the uterus through the cervix. It prevents pregnancy by interfering with implantation. Once widely used, IUDs became less popular after most brands were removed from the market because of serious complications such as pelvic infection and infertility.

A new option is the Mirena intrauterine system, which consists of a T-shaped device inserted in the uterus by a physician, that releases a continuous low dose of progestin and provides five years of protection from pregnancy. Used in Europe, Asia, and Latin America for years, it is 99 percent effective.

Mirena is increasingly being used, not just for contraception, but as an alternative to hysterectomy for extremely heavy menstrual bleeding and as a treatment for problems such as iron-deficiency anemia.

Advantages of Mirena

- Highly effective at preventing pregnancy.
- No need to think about contraception for five years.
- Allows sexual spontaneity; neither partner can feel it.
- Starts working immediately.
- New mothers can breast-feed while using it.
- Periods become shorter and lighter or stop altogether.
- Low incidence of side effects.
- Can be removed at any time.

Disadvantages of Mirena

- Spotting or breakthrough bleeding in first three to six months.
- No protection against STIs.
- Potential side effects include acne, headaches, nausea, breast tenderness, mood changes.
- Increased risk of benign ovarian cysts.
- May take up to a year for fertility to return after discontinuation.

How to Use the Mirena System A physician must insert the Mirena in a woman's uterus. In a five-year clinical trial, about 5 in every 100 women reported that the Mirena had slipped out of the uterus. Users should check for the string that extends from the device through the vagina at least once a month.

BARRIER CONTRACEPTIVES

As their name implies, **barrier contraceptives** block the meeting of egg and sperm by means of a physical barrier (a diaphragm, cervical cap, FemCap, or condom) or a chemical one (vaginal spermicide in jellies, foams, creams, suppositories, or film).

PRESCRIPTION BARRIERS

The prescription barrier contraceptives are used by women: the diaphragm, cervical cap, and FemCap. They are placed in the vagina with a spermicide. They do not protect against HIV infection and most STIs.

Diaphragm

The **diaphragm** is a bowl-like rubber cup with a flexible rim that is inserted into the vagina to cover the cervix and prevent the passage of sperm into the uterus during sexual intercourse (Figure 10-4). When used with a spermicide, the diaphragm is both a physical and a chemical barrier to sperm. The effectiveness of the diaphragm in preventing pregnancy depends on strong motivation (to use it faithfully) and a precise understanding of its use. If diaphragms with spermicide are used consistently and carefully, they can be 95 to 98 percent effective. Without a spermicide, the diaphragm is not effective.

Cervical Cap

Like the diaphragm, the **cervical cap** combined with spermicide serves as both a chemical and physical barrier blocking the path of the sperm to the uterus. The rubber or plastic cap is smaller and thicker than a diaphragm. It resembles a large thimble that fits snugly around the cervix and may work better for some women. It is about as effective as a diaphragm (95 to 98 percent).

© Joel Gordon Photography

FemCap

The FemCap is a nonhormonal, latex-free barrier contraceptive that works with a spermicide (Figure 10-5). The FemCap, designed to conform to the anatomy of the cervix and vagina, comes in three sizes. The smallest usually best suits women who have never been pregnant; the medium size, for women who have been pregnant but have not had a vaginal delivery; the largest, for those who have delivered a full-term baby vaginally.

FIGURE 10-4   Diaphragm
When used correctly and consistently and with a spermicide, the diaphragm is effective in preventing pregnancy. It must be fitted by a health-care professional.

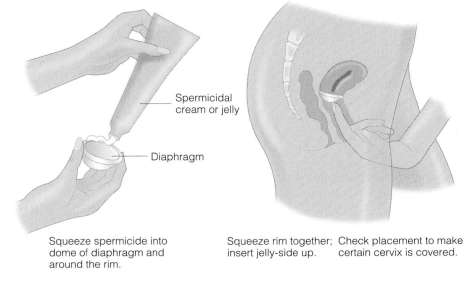

Spermicidal cream or jelly

Diaphragm

Squeeze spermicide into dome of diaphragm and around the rim.

Squeeze rim together; insert jelly-side up.

Check placement to make certain cervix is covered.

FIGURE 10-5 FemCap

The FemCap must be used with spermicide and must be correctly positioned to cover the cervix completely.

Source: Reproduced with permission from FemCap, Inc., and Alfred Shihata, M.D.

Advantages of Prescription Barriers

- Relatively inexpensive.
- Don't interrupt sexual activity; can be inserted hours ahead of time.
- Usually not felt by either partner.
- Can easily be carried in pocket or purse.
- No hormones or side effects.
- Cervical caps are an alternative for women who cannot use diaphragms or find them too messy.

Disadvantages of Prescription Barriers

- Less effective than hormonal contraceptives.
- Available by prescription only.
- Require advance planning or interruption of sexual activity to position the device before intercourse.
- May slip out of place during intercourse.

- May be uncomfortable for some women and their partners.
- Spermicidal foams, creams, and jellies may be messy, cause irritation, and detract from oral-genital sex.
- Some diaphragm users report bladder discomfort, urethral irritation, or recurrent cystitis.
- Some cap users find it more difficult to insert and remove and uncomfortable to wear.

How to Use a Diaphragm Diaphragms are fitted and prescribed by a qualified health-care professional in diameter sizes ranging from 2 to 4 inches (50 to 105 millimeters). The diaphragm's main function is to serve as a container for a spermicidal (sperm-killing) foam or jelly, which is available at pharmacies without a prescription. A diaphragm should remain in the vagina for at least six hours after intercourse to ensure that all sperm are killed. If intercourse occurs again during this period, additional spermicide must be inserted with an applicator tube.

The key to proper use of the diaphragm is having it available. A sexually active woman should keep it in the most accessible place—her purse, bedroom, bathroom. Before every use, a diaphragm should be checked for tiny leaks (hold up to the light or place water in the dome). A health-care provider should check its fit and condition every year when the woman has her annual Pap smear. Oil-based lubricants will deteriorate the latex of the diaphragm and should not be used with one.

How to Use a Cervical Cap Like the diaphragm, the cervical cap is fitted by a qualified health-care professional. For use, the woman fills it one-third to two-thirds full with spermicide and inserts it by holding its edges together and sliding it into the vagina. The cup is then pressed onto the cervix. (Most women find it easiest to do so while squatting or in an upright sitting position.) The cap can be inserted up to 6 hours prior to intercourse and should not be removed for at least 6 hours afterward. It can be left in place up to 24 hours. Pulling on one side of the rim breaks the suction and allows easy removal. Oil-based lubricants should not be used with the cap because they can deteriorate the latex.

How to Use FemCap A prescription is required to purchase FemCap, and the woman selects the appropriate size. Apply spermicide to the bowl of the FemCap (which goes over the cervix), to the outer brim, and to the groove that will face into the vagina. Insert the squeezed, flattened cap into the vagina with the bowl facing upward. The FemCap must be pushed all the way in to cover the cervix completely and left in place at least six hours after intercourse.

NONPRESCRIPTION BARRIERS

The nonprescription barrier contraceptives include the male and female condom, vaginal spermicides, the contraceptive sponge, and vaginal contraceptive film. Both condoms

Pinch or twist the tip of the condom, leaving one-half inch at the tip to catch the semen.

Holding the tip, unroll the condom.

Unroll the condom until it reaches the pubic hairs.

FIGURE 10-6   Male Condom

Condoms effectively reduce the risk of pregnancy as well as STIs if used consistently and correctly.

provide some protection against HIV infection and other STIs; spermicides, sponges, and films do not.

Male Condom

The male **condom** covers the erect penis and catches the ejaculate, thus preventing sperm from entering the woman's reproductive tract (Figure 10-6). Most are made of thin surgical latex or sheep membrane; a new type is made of polyurethane, which is thinner, stronger, more heat sensitive, and more comfortable than latex. In a study of 901 couples over six months, the polyurethane condom was not as effective as the latex condom for pregnancy prevention.[13] Condoms with a spermicidal lubricant (nonoxynol-9) kill most sperm on contact and are thus more effective than other brands.

Although the theoretical effectiveness rate for condoms is 97 percent, the actual rate is only 80 to 85 percent. The condom can be torn during the manufacturing process or during its use; testing by the manufacturer may not be as strenuous as it could or should be. Careless removal can also decrease the effectiveness of condoms. However, the major reason that condoms have such a low actual effectiveness rate is that couples don't use them each and every time they have sex. Users who have little experience with condoms—who are young, single, or childless, or who engage in risky behaviors—are more likely to have condoms break.

Condoms are second only to the pill in popularity among college-age adults (see Student Snapshot: "Contraception on Campus"). Condom use has increased in the last decade. Approximately one in five women ages 15 to 44 who used contraception rely on their partner's use of condoms as their primary method of birth control.[14]

Female Condom

The female condom, made of polyurethane, consists of two rings and a polyurethane sheath, and is inserted into the vagina with a tamponlike applicator (Figure 10-7). Once in place, the device loosely lines the walls of the vagina. Internally, a thickened rubber ring keeps it anchored near the cervix. Externally, another rubber ring, 2 inches in diameter, rests on the labia and resists slippage.

Although not widely used in the West, the female condom is gaining acceptance in Africa, Asia, and Latin America. Properly used, it is believed to be as good or better than the male condom for preventing infections, including HIV, because it is stronger and covers a slightly larger area. However, it is slightly less effective at preventing pregnancy. The efficacy of female condoms does increase with a woman's experience in using them.[15]

Strategies for Prevention   ▓   Seven Steps of Correct Male Condom Use

▓ Use a new condom at each act of intercourse.

▓ Handle the condom carefully to avoid damage from fingernails, teeth, or other sharp objects.

▓ Put on condom after penis is erect and before any genital contact with a partner.

▓ Make sure that air is trapped in the tip of the condom.

▓ Ensure adequate lubrication during intercourse.

▓ Use only water-based lubricants with latex condoms.

▓ Withdraw the penis while it is still erect to prevent slippage. Hold the condom firmly against the base of the penis during withdrawal.

Advantages of Condoms

▪ Effective when used correctly.

▪ Lower a woman's risk of pelvic inflammatory disease (PID) and may protect against some urinary tract and genital infections.

▪ No side effects, unless you're allergic to latex.

▪ No prescription required.

▪ Inexpensive.

▪ The female condom gives women more control in reducing their risk of pregnancy and STIs and does not require a prescription or medical appointment.

Disadvantages of Condoms

▪ Requires consistent and diligent use.

▪ Not 100 percent effective in preventing pregnancy or STIs.

▪ Risk of manufacturing defects, such as pin-size holes, and breaking or slipping off during intercourse.

▪ May inhibit sexual spontaneity.

▪ Users or partners may complain about odor, lubrication (too much or too little), feel, taste, difficulty opening the packages, and disposal.

▪ Some men dislike reduced penile sensitivity or cannot sustain an erection while putting on a condom.

▪ The female condom has a higher failure rate and, because it does not have spermicide on it, provides less protection against STIs. Some women complain that it is difficult to use, squeaks, and looks odd.

How to Use a Male Condom Most physicians recommend prelubricated, spermicide-treated, American-made latex or polyurethane condoms, not membrane condoms ("natural" or "sheepskin"). Before using a condom, check the expiration date and make sure it's soft and pliable. If it's yellow or sticky, throw it out. Don't check for leaks by blowing up a condom before using it; you may weaken or tear it.

The condom should be put on at the beginning of sexual activity, before genital contact occurs (see Figure 10-6). There should be a little space left at the top of the condom to catch the semen. Wait until just before intercourse to apply spermicide. Any vaginal lubricant should be water-based. Petroleum-based creams or jellies (such as Vaseline, baby oil, massage oil, vegetable oils, or oil-based hand lotions) can deteriorate the latex. After ejaculation, the condom should be held firmly against the penis so that it doesn't slip off or leak during withdrawal. Couples engaging in anal intercourse should use a water-based lubricant as well as a condom, but should never assume the condom will provide 100 percent protection from HIV infection or other STIs.

FIGURE 10-7 Female Condom

This device is less effective than the male condom for preventing pregnancy and STIs (since no spermicide is used). Like the male condom, this method does not require a prescription.

How to Use a Female Condom As illustrated in Figure 10-7, a woman removes the condom and applicator from the wrapper and inserts the condom slowly by gently pushing the applicator toward the small of the back. When properly inserted, the outer ring should rest on the folds of skin around the vaginal opening, and the inner ring (the closed end) should fit against the cervix.

The female condom can be washed and reused several times and still meet the standards set by the FDA, according to the study conducted in South Africa in which a sample of women washed, dried, and relubricated female condoms up to seven times.

(FAQ) Do Men and Women Use Condoms for Different Reasons?

The genders have very different motives both for engaging in sex and for using condoms. In focus groups, young women said they engaged in sexual relations because of a desire for physical intimacy and a committed relationship. They generally reported having sex only with men they cared for and deeply trusted and expected that these men would be honest and forthright about their sexual history. This trust played a significant role in their decision whether to insist on condom use.

In contrast, few of the young men said relationships were an important dimension of their sexual involvements. Their primary motivation was a desire for physical and sexual satisfaction. Most said they were not interested in commitment and viewed emotional expectations as a complication of becoming sexually involved with a woman. The young men also admitted to making judgments about types of girls. To them, young women they didn't care about were "sluts" with whom they used a condom for their own protection.

Which partner determined whether a couple would use a condom? In these interviews, the answer was the women— if they chose to do so. Regardless of race or ethnicity, many of the young women were adamant in demanding that their partners use condoms—and many young men said they would not challenge such a demand out of fear of losing the opportunity for sex. Men often expected potential partners to want to use condoms and described themselves as "suspicious" of women who did not.

Both sexes named two primary reasons for using condoms: preventing pregnancy and protecting against sexually transmitted infections. Young women saw an unwanted pregnancy as an occurrence that would be disruptive, expensive, and could "ruin" their lives and their parents' lives. Young men saw condom use as a way of protecting themselves against emotional entanglements and paternity issues.

Vaginal Spermicide

The various forms of **vaginal spermicide** include chemical foams, creams, jellies, vaginal suppositories, and gels. Some creams and jellies are made for use with a diaphragm; others can be used alone. Several vaginal suppositories claim high effectiveness, but no American studies have confirmed these claims. In general, failure rates for vaginal suppositories are as high as 10 to 25 percent.

Vaginal spermicides are available as creams, foams, and jellies. You don't need a prescription, and they have minimal side effects. Spermicides are most effective in preventing pregnancy and STIs when used together with a male condom.

Advantages of Vaginal Spermicide

■ Easy to use.

■ Effective if used with another form of contraception, such as condoms.

■ Reduces the risk of some vaginal infections, PID, and STIs.

■ No effect on fertility.

Disadvantages of Vaginal Spermicide

■ Insertion interrupts sexual spontaneity.

■ May cause irritation.

■ Some people cannot use them because of an allergic reaction.

■ Some users complain that spermicides are messy or interfere with oral-genital contact.

■ Spermicidal suppositories that do not dissolve completely can feel gritty.

How to Use a Vaginal Spermicide The various types of spermicide come with instructions that should be followed carefully for maximum protection. Contraceptive vaginal suppositories take about 20 minutes to dissolve and cover the vaginal walls. Foam, inserted with an applicator, goes into place much more rapidly. You must apply additional spermicide before each additional intercourse. After sex, women should shower rather than bathe to prevent the spermicide from being rinsed out of the vagina, and they should not douche for at least six hours.

Vaginal Contraceptive Film

Available from pharmacies without a prescription, the 2-inch-by-2-inch thin film known as **vaginal contraceptive film (VCF)** is laced with spermicide (Figure 10-8). Once folded and inserted into the vagina, it dissolves into a stay-in-place gel.

The contraceptive sponge works on the same principle as the diaphragm and cervical cap but is available without a prescription.

FIGURE 10-8 **How to Use Vaginal Contraceptive Film (VCF)**

This thin film is laced with spermicide. Its effectiveness is similar to other spermicides and is most effective with a condom.

With one swift movement, place VCF high in your vagina against the cervix. VCF is effective for one hour. One film should be used for each act of intercourse. Follow the instructions in the product leaflet.

Advantages of VCF

▪ Easy to use.

▪ Can be used by people allergic to foams and jellies.

▪ Dissolves gradually and almost unnoticeably.

▪ As effective as most spermicides; almost 100 percent effective paired with a condom.

▪ No effect on fertility.

Disadvantages of VCF

▪ Insertion interrupts sexual spontaneity.

▪ Effective for only one hour and one act of intercourse.

▪ No protection against STIs.

How to Use Vaginal Contraceptive Film Fold one square of VCF in half; place it on your second or third finger; then insert high into the vagina, near the cervix. VCF is effective for one hour. One film should be used for each act of intercourse.

Contraceptive Sponge

The vaginal contraceptive sponge is made of soft polyurethane foam containing the spermicide nonoxynol-9. The Today Sponge was sold as an over-the-counter contraceptive in the United States from 1983 to 1995, when it was withdrawn because of contamina-tion problems at the manufacturing plant. It is now available again.

Advantages of the Contraceptive Sponge

▪ Easy to use.

▪ Can be inserted several hours before intercourse and left in place for 24 hours afterward.

▪ Effective immediately if used correctly.

▪ No effect on fertility.

Disadvantages of the Contraceptive Sponge

▪ May be difficult to remove.

▪ May be less effective in women who have had children.

▪ No reliable protection against STIs.

▪ Requires advance planning to place the sponge.

▪ Side effects include vaginal irritation and allergic reactions.

▪ Should not be used during menstruation.

PERIODIC ABSTINENCE AND FERTILITY AWARENESS METHODS

Awareness of a woman's cyclic fertility can help in both conception and contraception. The different methods of birth control based on a woman's menstrual cycle are sometimes referred to as *natural family planning* or *fertility awareness methods.* They include the calendar method, the basal-body-temperature method, and the cervical mucus method. New fertility monitors that use saliva to determine time of ovulation can improve the accuracy of these methods.

Women's menstrual cycles vary greatly. To use one of the fertility awareness methods, a woman must know and understand her cycle. She should track her cycle for at least eight months—marking day one (the day bleeding begins) on a calendar and counting the length of each cycle. Figure 10-9 shows the days in a 28-day cycle when abstinence or other contraceptive methods would be necessary.

The calendar method, often called the **rhythm method,** is based on counting the woman's safe days based on her individual menstrual cycle. The basal-body temperature method determines the safe days based on the woman's **basal body temperature,** which rises after ovulation. The cervical mucus method, also called the **ovulation method,** is based on observation of changes in the consistency of the woman's vaginal mucus throughout her menstrual cycle. The

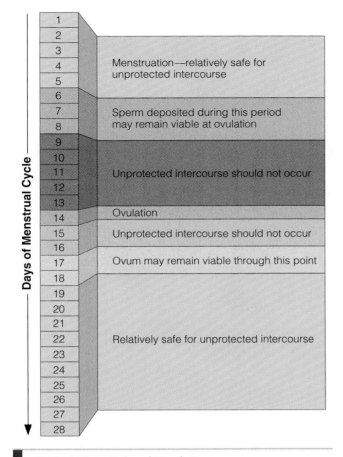

1
2
3
4
5
6
7
8
9
10
11
12
13
14
15
16
17
18
19
20
21
22
23
24
25
26
27
28

Menstruation—relatively safe for unprotected intercourse

Sperm deposited during this period may remain viable at ovulation

Unprotected intercourse should not occur

Ovulation

Unprotected intercourse should not occur

Ovum may remain viable through this point

Relatively safe for unprotected intercourse

FIGURE 10-9   Safe and Unsafe Days
Events in the menstrual cycle determine the relatively safe days for unprotected intercourse.

period of maximum fertility occurs when the mucus is smooth and slippery.

Advantages of Fertility Awareness

- No expense.
- No side effects.
- No need for a prescription, medical visit, or fittings.
- Nothing to insert, swallow, or check.
- No effect on fertility.
- Complies with the teachings of the Roman Catholic Church.

Disadvantages of Fertility Awareness

- Less reliable than other forms of birth control.
- Couples must abstain from vaginal intercourse eight to eleven days a month or use some form of contraception.
- Conscientious planning and scheduling essential.
- May not work for women with irregular menstrual cycles.
- Some women find the mucus or temperature methods difficult to use.

ⒻⒶ⒬ WHAT IS EMERGENCY CONTRACEPTION?

Emergency contraception (EC) is the use of a method of contraception to prevent unintended pregnancy after unprotected intercourse or the failure of another form of contraception, such as a condom breaking or slipping off. Nearly half of all pregnancies in the United States, or about 3 million per year, are unintended. If emergency contraception were widely available and widely used, that number could be cut in half and result in 0.7 million fewer abortions and 22,000 fewer pregnancies due to rape.[16]

Early formulations contained estrogen and progestin and caused severe abdominal cramping. Current pills include only progestin and have a lower incidence of abdominal pain. When either one or both pills are taken within 72 hours of unprotected sex, they reduce the risk of pregnancy to 1 percent.[17] The copper-bearing intrauterine device (IUD) is also an EC option.[18]

Emergency contraception pills (ECPs) stop pregnancy in the same way as other hormonal contraceptives: They delay or inhibit ovulation, inhibit fertilization, or block implantation of a fertilized egg, depending on a woman's phase of the menstrual cycle. They have no effect once a pregnancy has been established.[19]

Most women can safely use ECPs, even if they cannot use birth control pills as their regular method of birth control.[20] (Although ECPs use the same hormones as birth control pills, not all brands of birth control pills can be used for emergency contraception.) Some women may experience spotting or a full menstrual period a few days after taking ECPs, depending on where they were in their cycle when they began therapy. Most women have their next period at the expected time.

 In a national survey of colleges and universities, slightly more than half—52.2 percent—of student health centers offer emergency contraception. Private institutions, as well as those with a high proportion of commuter students, were less likely to do so than large public schools. The primary benefit they cited was pregnancy prevention. Student health centers in the Midwest and South are less likely to offer ECP than those in the Northeast.[21]

The Canadian government has made the morning-after birth control pill more widely available without a prescription. States are moving to improve access to EC, which may become an over-the-counter product available without a prescription to women over age 16.

About two-thirds of women are aware that something can be done to prevent pregnancy after unprotected sex—an increase since 2000. Only 6 percent of women ages 18 to 44 report ever having used ECP. Medical groups are urging physicians to offer advance prescriptions for emergency contraception at regular gynecologic visits to increase its use without downplaying the importance of routine contraception.[22]

STERILIZATION

The most popular method of birth control among married couples in the United States is **sterilization** (surgery to end a person's reproductive capability). Each year an estimated 1 million men and women in the United States undergo sterilization procedures. Fewer than 25 percent ever seek reversal.

MALE STERILIZATION

In men, the cutting of the vas deferens, the tube that carries sperm from one of the testes into the urethra for ejaculation, is called **vasectomy**. During the 15- or 20-minute office procedure, done under a local anesthetic, the doctor makes small incisions in the scrotum, lifts up each vas deferens, cuts them, and ties off the ends to block the flow of sperm (Figure 10-10). Sperm continue to form, but they are broken down and absorbed by the body.

The man usually experiences some local pain, swelling, and discoloration for about a week after the procedure. More serious complications, including the formation of a blood clot in the scrotum (which usually disappears without treatment), infection, and an inflammatory reaction, occur in a small percentage of cases.

Sometimes men want to reverse their vasectomies, usually because they want to have children with a new spouse. Although anyone who chooses to have a vasectomy should consider it permanent, surgical reversal (*vasovasostomy*) is sometimes successful. New microsurgical techniques have led to annual pregnancy rates for the wives of men having undergone vasovasostomies of about 50 percent, depending on such factors as the doctor's expertise and the time elapsed since the vasectomy.

FEMALE STERILIZATION

Eleven million U.S. women ages 15 to 44 rely on tubal sterilization for contraception. An estimated 750,000 tubal sterilization procedures are performed each year in the United States. The average age of sterilization is about 30. Female sterilization procedures modify the fallopian tubes, which each month normally carry an egg from the ovaries to the uterus. The two terms used to describe female sterilization are **tubal ligation** (the cutting or tying of the fallopian tubes) and **tubal occlusion** (the blocking of the tubes). The tubes may be cut or sealed with thread, a clamp, or a clip, or by electrical coagulation to prevent the passage of eggs from the ovaries (Figure 10-11). They also can be blocked with bands of silicone.

One of the common methods of tubal ligation or occlusion uses **laparoscopy**, commonly called *belly-button* or *band-aid surgery*. This procedure is done on an outpatient basis and takes 15 to 30 minutes. A lighted tube called a *laparoscope* is inserted through a half-inch incision made right below the navel, giving the doctor a view of the fallopian tubes. Using surgical instruments that may be inserted

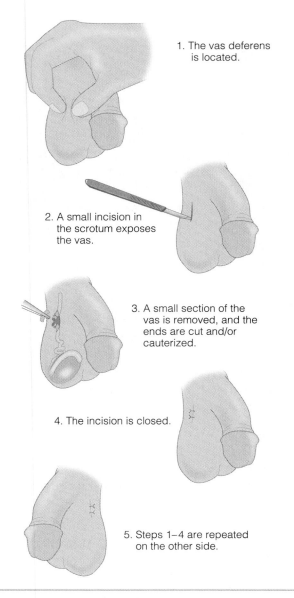

1. The vas deferens is located.

2. A small incision in the scrotum exposes the vas.

3. A small section of the vas is removed, and the ends are cut and/or cauterized.

4. The incision is closed.

5. Steps 1–4 are repeated on the other side.

FIGURE 10-10   Male Sterilization, or Vasectomy

through the laparoscope or through other tiny incisions, the doctor then cuts or seals the tubes, most commonly by electrical coagulation.

The cumulative failure rate of tubal sterilization is about 1.85 percent during a 10-year period. Complications include problems with anesthesia, hemorrhage, organ damage, and mortality.[23]

In a study of 11,232 women ages 18 to 44 who had tubal sterilizations, most expressed no regret after the procedure. However, women 30 years of age and younger at the time of sterilization have an increased probability of expressing regret.[24]

Essure

This new method for permanent sterilization involves placement of small, flexible microcoils into the fallopian tubes via the vagina by a physician. Unlike other methods, it does not

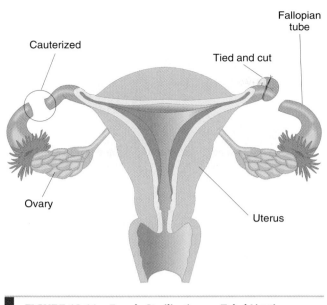

Cauterized

Fallopian tube

Tied and cut

Ovary

Uterus

FIGURE 10-11 Female Sterilization, or Tubal Ligation

require the risks of general anesthesia and surgery. The procedure itself does not require incisions and takes an average of about 35 minutes. Recovery occurs quickly. In clinical trials, about 90 percent of women returned to work within 24 hours. For the first three months after insertion, women should use another form of contraception. An X ray called a hysterosalpingogram must confirm that the inserts are correctly placed and the fallopian tubes are completely blocked.

Like traditional forms of tubal ligation, Essure cannot be reversed. It is recommended only for women who definitely do not want more children and especially for those with medical and health problems (such as diabetes, heart disease, or obesity) that make surgery and anesthesia more dangerous. There is a risk that the microinserts may not be placed correctly at the first attempt (this occurred in 14 percent of women in one study). Because the procedure is new, long-term data on the effectiveness of Essure are not yet available.

Advantages of Sterilization

■ Offers permanent protection against unwanted pregnancy.

■ No effect on sex drive in men or women. Many couples report greater sexual activity and pleasure because they no longer have to worry about pregnancy or deal with contraceptives.

■ Vasectomy and tubal ligation are performed as outpatient procedures, with a quick recovery time.

■ Use of Essure requires no incision, so there's less discomfort and very rapid recovery. Essure may be an option for women with chronic health conditions, such as obesity, diabetes, or heart disease.

Disadvantages of Sterilization

■ All procedures should be considered permanent and used only if both partners are certain they want no more children.

■ No protection against STIs.

■ Must use another form of birth control for first three months.

■ Many long-term risks remain unknown, but there is no evidence of any link between vasectomy and prostate cancer.

ABORTION

More than half of unintended pregnancies end in induced abortions. Abortion rates vary greatly around the world. The U.S. abortion rate, which has declined, still remains higher than that of many Western countries, including Canada, Great Britain, the Netherlands, and Sweden. Although there is no one single or simple explanation for this difference, researchers focus on America's high rate of unintended pregnancies. In many nations with fewer unwanted pregnancies and lower abortion rates, contraceptives are generally easier and cheaper to obtain, and early sex education strongly emphasizes their importance.

No woman in any country ever elects to be in a situation where she has to consider abortion. But if faced with an unwanted pregnancy, many women consider *elective abortion* as an option.

After rising steadily through the 1970s, the number of legal abortions leveled off in the 1980s and declined in the 1990s.[25] According to the most recent data, the U.S. abortion rate is at its lowest in 30 years. The decline is greatest among young women. The reasons include decreased sexual activity among adolescents and increased use of effective contraceptives.[26] Although women of all backgrounds have abortions, abortion in the United States is increasingly likely to occur among single women, racial or ethnic minorities, low-income women, and women who have had at least one child.[27]

Claims that abortion increases the risk of breast cancer, based on retrospective studies that are less accurate because they rely on individuals' recall, have proved false. A recent 12-year study found no correlation between the termination of a pregnancy, whether induced or spontaneous, and increased risk of breast cancer.[28]

THINKING THROUGH THE OPTIONS

A woman faced with an unwanted pregnancy—often alone, unwed, and desperate—can find it extremely difficult to decide what to do. The political debate over the right to life almost always is secondary to practical and emotional matters, such as the quality of her relationship with the baby's father, their capacity to provide for the child, the impact on any children she already has, and other important life issues.

Giving up her child for adoption is an option for women who do not feel abortion is right for them. Because the number of would-be adoptive parents greatly exceeds the number of available newborns, some women considering adoption may feel pressured by offers of money from couples eager to adopt. Others, particularly minority women, may feel cultural pressures to keep a child—regardless of their age, economic situation, or ability to care for an infant. Advocates of adoption reform are pressing for mandatory counseling for all pregnant women considering adoption (available now in agency-arranged, but not private, adoptions) and for extending the period of time during which a new mother can change her mind about giving up her child for adoption.

MEDICAL ABORTION

The term **medical abortion** describes the use of drugs, also called *abortifacients,* to terminate a pregnancy. In 2000, the abortion pill mifepristone (Mifeprex), formerly known as RU-486, became available for use in the United States. Mifepristone, which is 97 percent effective in inducing abortion, blocks progesterone, the hormone that prepares the uterine lining for pregnancy. Two days after taking this compound, a woman takes a prostaglandin to increase uterine contractions. The uterine lining is expelled along with the fertilized egg (Figure 10-12).

Women have compared the discomfort of this experience to severe menstrual cramps. Common side effects include excessive bleeding, nausea, fatigue, abdominal pain, and dizziness. About 1 woman in 100 requires a blood transfusion. The FDA has warned doctors about rare but deadly bloodstream infections in women using mifepristone. The rate of infection is about 1 in 100,000 uses, comparable to infection risks with surgical abortions and childbirth.[29]

Although condemned by right-to-life advocates, abortion medications may in time lower the public profile of pregnancy termination. They are not painless, cheap, or equally available to all, but they do offer women a chance to carry through on their personal choice in greater privacy and safety.

Medical abortion does not require anesthesia and can be performed very early in pregnancy. However, women experience more cramping and bleeding during medical abortion than during surgical abortion, and bleeding lasts for a longer period.

OTHER ABORTION METHODS

About half of all abortions (54 percent) are performed within the first 8 weeks of pregnancy. Only about 1 percent of abortions occur after 20 weeks. Medically, first-trimester abortion is less risky than childbirth. However, the likelihood of complications increases when abortions are performed in the second trimester (the second three-month period) of pregnancy.

The majority of abortions performed in the United States today are surgical. **Suction curettage,** usually done

Step 1. Taken early in pregnancy, mifepristone blocks the action of progesterone and makes the body react as if it weren't pregnant.

Step 2. Prostaglandins, taken two days later, cause the uterus to contract and the cervix to soften and dilate. As a result, the fertilized egg is expelled in 97 percent of cases.

FIGURE 10-12   Medical Abortion
Mifepristone works by blocking the action of progesterone, a hormone produced by the ovaries that is necessary for the implantation and development of a fertilized egg.

from 7 to 13 weeks after the last menstrual period, involves the gradual dilation (opening) of the cervix, often by inserting into the cervix one or more sticks of *laminaria* (a sterilized seaweed that absorbs moisture and expands, thus gradually stretching the cervix). Some women feel pressure or cramping with the laminaria in place. Occasionally, the laminaria itself starts to bring on a miscarriage.

At the time of abortion, the laminaria is removed, and dilators are used to further enlarge the cervical opening, if needed. The physician inserts a suction tip into the cervix, and the uterine contents are drawn out via a vacuum system (Figure 10-13). A *curette* (a spoon-shaped surgical instrument used for scraping) is used to check for complete removal of the contents of the uterus. With suction curettage, the risks of complication are low. Major complications, such as perforation of the uterus, occur in fewer than 1 in 100 cases.

For early second-trimester abortions, physicians generally use a technique called **dilation and evacuation (D and E),** in which they open the cervix and use medical instruments to remove the fetus from the uterus. D and E procedures are performed under local or general anesthesia.

To induce abortion from week 16 to week 20, prostaglandins (natural substances found in most body tissues) are administered as vaginal suppositories or injected

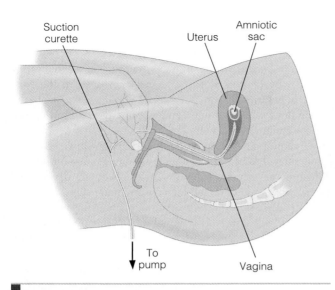

FIGURE 10-13   Suction Curettage
The contents of the uterus are extracted through the cervix with a vacuum apparatus.

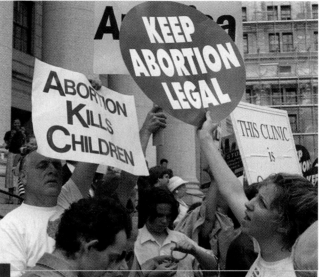

The controversy over abortion has resulted in countless demonstrations and encounters between pro-choice and pro-life supporters.

into the amniotic sac by inserting a needle through the abdominal wall. They induce uterine contractions, and the fetus and placenta are expelled within 24 hours. Injecting saline or urea solutions into the amniotic sac also can terminate the pregnancy by triggering contractions that expel the fetus and placenta. Sometimes vaginal suppositories or drugs that help the uterus contract are used. Complications from abortion techniques that induce labor include nausea, vomiting, diarrhea, tearing of the cervix, excessive bleeding, and possible shock and death.

(FAQ) WHAT IS THE PSYCHOLOGICAL IMPACT OF ABORTION?

Many assume that abortion must be psychologically devastating, that women who abort a fetus sooner or later develop what some have termed *postabortion trauma syndrome*. In her studies at the University of Chicago, psychiatrist Nada Stotland found that there is no such thing. The primary emotion of women who have just had an abortion, she discovered, is relief. Although many women also express feelings of sadness or guilt, their anxiety levels eventually drop until they are lower than they were immediately before the abortion.

Nonetheless, although psychologists consider the mental health risks minimal compared to those of bearing an unwanted child, this does not mean women who have abortions never have regrets. But a feeling—even one as painful as loss, sadness, or guilt—is not a syndrome, and a woman's responses to abortion often change with passing days, weeks, months, or years. Anniversaries—of conception, of the date a woman found out she was pregnant, of the abortion, of the delivery date—can trigger memories and a sense of loss,

but most women deal with these and move on with their lives.

The best predictor of psychological well-being after abortion is a woman's emotional well-being prior to pregnancy. At highest risk are women who have had a psychiatric illness, such as an anxiety disorder or clinical depression, prior to an abortion, and those whose abortions occurred among complicated circumstances (such as a rape, or coercion by parents or a partner). The vast majority of women manage to put the abortion into perspective as one of many life events.

POLITICS OF ABORTION

Abortion is one of the most controversial political, religious, and ethical issues of our time. The issues of when life begins, a woman's right to choose, and an unborn child's right to survival are among the most divisive Americans face. Abortions were legal in the United States until the 1860s. For decades after that, women who decided to terminate unwanted pregnancies did so by attempting to abort on their own or by obtaining illegal abortions—often performed by untrained individuals using unsanitary and unsafe procedures. In the late 1960s, some states changed their laws to make abortions legal. In 1973, the U.S. Supreme Court, following a 1970 ruling on the case of *Roe v. Wade* by the New York Supreme Court, said that an abortion in the first trimester of pregnancy was a decision between a woman and her physician and was protected by privacy laws. The Court further ruled that abortion during the second trimester could be performed on the basis of health risks and that abortion during the final trimester could be performed only for the sake of the mother's health.

The debate over abortion continues to stir passionate emotions, with pro-life supporters arguing that life begins at conception and that abortion is therefore immoral, and pro-choice advocates countering that an individual woman should have the right to make decisions about her body and health. The controversy over abortion has at times become violent: Physicians who performed abortions have been shot and killed; abortion clinics have been bombed, wounding and killing patients and staff members.

Although the majority of Americans continue to support abortion, many feel that it should be more restricted and difficult to obtain. While 61 percent of Americans say abortion should be permitted during the first three months of pregnancy, only 15 percent support second-trimester abortions and 7 percent feel that abortions in the last trimester should be legal.

> *Abortion is one of the most controversial and divisive issues in the United States. Some oppose abortion in any circumstances, even if a woman's life is at risk or if the child was conceived in a rape. Others argue that women, not politicians, should have the right to determine whether to continue a pregnancy. Should the government limit or deny abortions to women who want them? Or should women retain the right to choose?* **You decide.**

Congress has banned partial birth abortion, which is performed in the later stages of pregnancy and involves collapsing the skull to allow a fetus to slip easily from the birth canal. Courts in several states have challenged the ban as "unconstitutional" because it does not provide a "health" exception.

A CROSS-CULTURAL PERSPECTIVE

Throughout the world an estimated 10 to 20 million illegal abortions are performed each year. About 1 in 100 women dies as a result. Women who survive illegal abortions may suffer chronic health problems related to the lack of adequate medical care.

In other countries, abortion laws vary greatly. In Eastern Europe, where abortions were once legal and common, the collapse of communism has led to new restrictions on abortion. By contrast, Spain's supreme court has relaxed legal restrictions on abortions performed on social grounds. In Pakistan, new, more liberal rules on abortion state that abortion is no longer a crime if carried out to provide "necessary treatment." In Latin America, where anti-abortion laws are very strict, Cuba is the only country in which abortion on request is legal in early pregnancy. In other nations of Central and South America, women obtaining abortions and those performing them face criminal penalties, including imprisonment.

CHILDFREE BY CHOICE

In Europe, fertility rates in many nations are at an all-time low. In the United States, one in five women in the baby boom generation has not given birth—many because of a decision not to. More women and men are deliberately choosing to remain "childfree."

According to the limited data available, single childfree women tend to be better educated, more cosmopolitan, less religious, and more professional than those in the general population. In general, childfree women are high achievers, often in demanding careers, who describe their work as exciting and satisfying. Childless couples are predominantly urban, well-educated, and upper middle class, with egalitarian and long-running marriages.

Their reasons for not having children are diverse: a desire to maintain their freedom, more time with their partners, career ambitions, concern about overpopulation and the fate of the Earth. Some women cite the hostile work environment for mothers and the inadequacy of day care. Others say they're disillusioned with the have-it-all hopes of baby boomers and believe in a have-most-of-it philosophy.

Some observers theorize that childfree women will regret their choice after it's too late to do anything about it. However, this doesn't seem to be the case. "Not everybody needs children to have a full life," says Leslie Lafayette, who founded the ChildFree Network (CFN) to create a sense of belonging among people without children.[30]

PREGNANCY

In the last half century, pregnancy rates have generally declined. The average age of mothers in the United States has risen, but about 70 percent of babies are still born to women in their twenties. Mothers are now averaging about two children each.

The number of never-married, college-educated, career women who are becoming single parents has risen dramatically. They want children—with or without an ongoing relationship with a man—and may feel that, because of their age, they can't delay getting pregnant any longer.

PRECONCEPTION CARE

The time *before* a child is conceived can be crucial in assuring that an infant is born healthy, full-size, and full-term. Women who smoke, drink alcohol, take drugs, eat poorly, are too thin or too heavy, suffer from unrecognized infections or illnesses, or are exposed to toxins at work or home may start pregnancy with one or more strikes against them and their unborn babies. The best chance for lowering the infant mortality rate and preventing birth defects is before pregnancy. **Preconception care**—the enhancement of a woman's health and well-being prior to conception in order to ensure a healthy pregnancy and baby—includes risk assessment (evaluation of medical, genetic, and lifestyle risks), health promotion (such as teaching good nutrition), and interventions to reduce risk (such as treatment of infections and other diseases, and assistance in quitting smoking or drug use).

HOME PREGNANCY TESTS

The sooner a woman realizes she is pregnant, the more she can do to take care of herself and her child. Home pregnancy tests detect the presence of human chorionic gonadotropin (hCG), which is secreted as the fertilized egg implants in the uterus. If the concentration of hCG is high enough, a woman will test positive for pregnancy. If the test is done too early, the result will be a false negative. A follow-up test a week later can usually confirm a pregnancy. Although home pregnancy tests are 85 to 95 percent accurate, medical laboratory tests provide definitive confirmation of a pregnancy.

HOW A WOMAN'S BODY CHANGES DURING PREGNANCY

The 40 weeks of pregnancy transform a woman's body. At the beginning of pregnancy, the woman's uterus becomes slightly larger, and the cervix becomes softer and bluish due to increased blood flow. Progesterone and estrogen trigger changes in the milk glands and ducts in the breasts, which increase in size and feel somewhat tender. The pressure of the growing uterus against the bladder causes a more frequent need to urinate. As the pregnancy progresses, the woman's skin stretches as her body shape changes, her center of gravity changes as her abdomen protrudes, and her internal organs shift as the baby grows (Figure 10-14). Pregnancy is typically divided into three-month periods called trimesters.

HOW A BABY GROWS

Silently and invisibly, over a nine-month period, a fertilized egg develops into a human being. When the zygote reaches the uterus, it's still smaller than the head of a pin. Once nestled into the spongy uterine lining, it becomes an **embryo.** The embryo takes on an elongated shape, rounded at one end. A sac called the **amnion** envelops it (see photo on page 289). As water and other small molecules cross the amniotic membrane, the embryo floats freely in the absorbed fluid, cushioned from shocks and bumps. At nine weeks the embryo is called a **fetus.**

A special organ, the **placenta,** forms. Attached to the embryo by the umbilical cord, it supplies the growing baby with fluid and nutrients from the maternal bloodstream and carries waste back to the mother's body for disposal (Figure 10-15).

(FAQ) WHY IS PRENATAL CARE IMPORTANT?

A pregnant woman has to take good care of herself to provide good care for her unborn child. This means regular medical and dental checkups. A woman should have her first prenatal visit as soon as she discovers that she's pregnant. A study group of the American College of Obstetricians and Gynecologists (ACOG) has recommended seven or eight prenatal visits for women with low-risk pregnancies; women at higher risk require more frequent checkups. Many teenage and unmarried pregnant women don't get adequate prenatal care, and some don't see a health-care professional until late in their pregnancy, because they can't afford or don't have access to medical services. Even women who begin prenatal care in the second and third trimesters lower their risk of having a low-birthweight baby.[31]

Age

Risks to the fetus are greater when mothers are older than 35, primarily an increase in fetal birth defects due to chromosomal abnormalities, such as Down syndrome. At age 30, the estimated risk is 2.6 per thousand; the incidence rises to 5.6 per thousand at age 35; 15.8 at age 40; and 53.7 at age 45. However, for healthy women over age 35, pregnancy itself is safe. As discussed later in this chapter, assisted reproductive technologies have enabled women in their forties, fifties, and even sixties to have successful pregnancies.

Nutrition

A well-balanced diet throughout pregnancy is critical for a mother and her fetus both before and at birth. If a woman—regardless of her prepregnancy weight—gains too little weight, the risk to the growing fetus is high. ACOG recommends a weight gain of 22 to 27 pounds during pregnancy. The National Academy of Sciences' Food and Nutrition Board advises a maximum weight gain of 35 pounds, based on findings that weight gain aids fetal growth and lowers the risk of infant mortality and mental retardation.

Substance Use

Smoking endangers two lives: the mother's and the fetus's. The sooner a mother-to-be stops smoking, the better the chances that the fetus will develop normally. Smoking increases the risk of miscarriage, stillbirth, low birthweight, heart defects, and premature birth, and also impairs growth. The fetus's oxygen supply is impaired by the increased levels of carbon monoxide in the smoking mother's bloodstream. Passive smoking (inhaling other people's smoke) can be hazardous for the mother and fetus as well (see Chapter 13).

According to the CDC, more than 8,000 alcohol-damaged babies are born every year. One of every 750 newborns has a cluster of physical and mental defects called **fetal alcohol syndrome (FAS):** low birthweight, smaller-than-normal head circumference, smaller and shorter size, irritability as newborns, and permanent mental impairment as a result of their mothers' alcohol consumption. The milder forms of these problems, particularly impaired intellectual ability and school performance, are called fetal alcohol effects (FAE) (see Chapter 12).

The risk of fetal alcohol syndrome is greatest if a mother drinks 3 ounces or more of pure alcohol (the equivalent of

First Trimester

Increased urination because of hormonal changes and the pressure of the enlarging uterus on the bladder.

Enlarged breasts as milk glands develop.

Darkening of the nipples and the area around them.

Nausea or vomiting, particularly in the morning.

Fatigue.

Increased vaginal secretions.

Pinching of the sciatic nerve, which runs from the buttocks down through the back of the legs, as the pelvic bones widen and begin to separate.

Irregular bowel movements.

Before conception   At 4 months

Second Trimester

Thickening of the waist as the uterus grows.

Weight gain.

Increase in total blood volume.

Slight increase in size and change in position of the heart.

Darkening of the pigment around the nipple and from the navel to the pubic region.

Darkening of the face.

Increased salivation and perspiration.

Secretion of colostrum from the breasts.

Indigestion, constipation, and hemorrhoids.

Varicose veins.

At 7 months

Third Trimester

Increased urination because of pressure from the uterus.

Tightening of the uterine muscles (called Braxton-Hicks contractions).

Shortness of breath because of increased pressure by the uterus on the lungs and diaphragm.

Heartburn and indigestion.

Trouble sleeping because of the baby's movements or the need to urinate.

Descending ("dropping") of the baby's head into the pelvis about two to four weeks before birth.

Navel pushed out.

At 9 months

FIGURE 10-14   Physiological Changes of Pregnancy

six or seven cocktails) a day. However, moderate drinking—one or two cocktails daily—may also have an effect. Even one drink a day has been associated with birth defects; binge drinking (four or more drinks on one occasion) is most toxic. The National Institute on Alcohol Abuse and Alcoholism and the Surgeon General advise pregnant women—and those trying to become pregnant—to abstain from drinking alcohol.

PRENATAL TESTING

All parents worry that their unborn baby might not be normal and healthy. Sophisticated new tests can answer some, but not all, of their questions and can identify more than

250 diseases and defects. Prenatal tests are being performed earlier and with less risk to a fetus than ever before. The most common prenatal tests include the following:

- **Ultrasonography** uses high-frequency sound waves to produce an image of the fetus on a video screen and as a photographic picture. Ultrasound can check fetal age and spot certain birth defects.

- **Alpha-fetoprotein** (*AFP*) *screening,* performed from the 13th to 20th week of pregnancy, measures a substance produced by the baby's kidneys in the mother's blood. Levels that are too high could indicate a neural tube defect; levels that are too low may signal Down syndrome.

Embryo within the amnion.

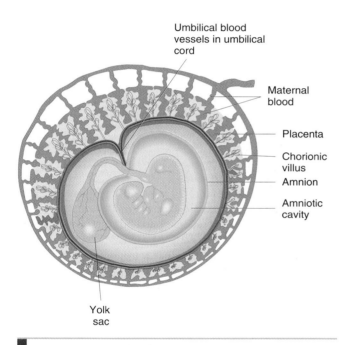

Umbilical blood vessels in umbilical cord

Maternal blood

Placenta

Chorionic villus

Amnion

Amniotic cavity

Yolk sac

FIGURE 10-15 **The Placenta**
The placenta supplies the growing embryo with fluid and nutrients from the maternal bloodstream and carries waste back for disposal.

■ **Chorionic villi sampling** (CVS), performed from the 8th to 10th week of pregnancy, involves suctioning a small sample of the chorionic villi, the tissue surrounding the fetus, for laboratory analysis (Figure 10-16). Results are generally available within a week.

■ **Amniocentesis,** performed from the 14th to 16th week of pregnancy, consists of removing a small amount of the amniotic fluid surrounding the fetus. This fluid contains cells shed by the fetus, which can be grown in tissue culture and then checked for any chromosomal or genetic defects (Figure 10-16).

There are no known risks for ultrasonography and AFP screening. For both amniocentesis and CVS, there is about

Most pregnant women benefit from regular, moderate exercise. For women who were very active before their pregnancies, a higher level of activity is probably fine, but they should consult with their doctors about how long and intensely to exercise.

a 1 percent risk of miscarriage. Some testing centers have reported a higher incidence of both limb defects and miscarriage following CVS than others using this technique. Before choosing a facility for testing, pregnant women should inquire about that facility's experience and complication rate. Prenatal tests are usually recommended only if the mother is over age 35, has had a child with a genetic disorder, or is a known carrier of a detectable genetic disorder.

COMPLICATIONS OF PREGNANCY

In about 10 to 15 percent of all pregnancies, there is increased risk of some problem, such as a baby's failure to grow normally. **Perinatology,** or maternal-fetal medicine, focuses on the special needs of high-risk mothers and their unborn babies. Perinatal centers, with state-of-the-art equipment and 24-hour staffs of specialists in this field, have been set up around the country. Several of the most frequent potential complications of pregnancy are discussed below.

Ectopic Pregnancy

Any woman who is of childbearing age, has had intercourse, and feels abdominal pain with no reasonable cause may have an **ectopic pregnancy.** In this type of pregnancy, the

(a) Chorionic villi sampling

Chorionic villi
Placenta
Catheter
Fetus
(8–10 weeks)

(b) Amniocentesis

Amniotic fluid
withdrawn
Amniotic fluid
Placenta
Cervix
Fetus
(14–16 weeks)

FIGURE 10-16   Prenatal Testing

(A) In chorionic villi sampling (CVS), a tissue sample of the villi is removed from the uterus through either a catheter into the uterus or a needle through the abdominal wall. The tissue sample is then analyzed for chromosomal defects. (B) In amniocentesis, a sample of the amniotic fluid is withdrawn; fetal cells found in that fluid can then be grown in tissue culture and checked for chromosomal defects.

fertilized egg remains in the fallopian tube instead of traveling to the uterus. Ectopic, or tubal, pregnancies have increased dramatically in recent years, now accounting for 2 percent of all reported pregnancies. STIs, particularly chlamydia infections (discussed in Chapter 14), have become a major cause of ectopic pregnancy. Other risk factors include previous pelvic surgery, particularly involving the fallopian tubes; pelvic inflammatory disease; infertility; and use of an IUD.

In an ectopic pregnancy, a misplaced egg develops normally, producing the usual signs of pregnancy, until the cramped amniotic sac bursts, damaging the fallopian tube. The woman will bleed internally and feel lower abdominal pains, or she may feel an aching in her shoulders, as the blood flows upward toward the diaphragm. If the bleeding is substantial, the woman can go into shock, with low blood pressure and a high pulse rate. Symptoms are hot and cold flashes, nausea, dizziness, fainting, pelvic pain, and irregular bleeding.

Treatment for the damaged fallopian tube is usually removal, but microsurgery can often repair the damage. About 50 percent of the women who have had an ectopic pregnancy conceive again; 10 percent have another ectopic pregnancy. Ectopic pregnancies can lead to permanent infertility.

Miscarriage

About 10 to 20 percent of pregnancies end in **miscarriage,** or spontaneous abortion, before the 20th week of gestation. Major genetic disorders may be responsible for 33 to 50 percent of pregnancy losses. The most common cause is an abnormal number of chromosomes. About 0.5 to 1 percent of

women suffer three or more miscarriages, possibly because of genetic, anatomic, hormonal, infectious, or autoimmune factors. An estimated 70 to 90 percent of women who miscarry eventually become pregnant again.

Physicians typically recommend bed rest if a woman begins bleeding or cramping early in pregnancy. In some cases, the cramping stops, and the pregnancy continues normally. In others, the bleeding becomes intense, the cervix widens, and the embryo is expelled. If the miscarriage is complete, the bleeding stops and the uterus returns to its normal state and shape. If it is incomplete, a physician has to remove any bits of tissue remaining in the uterus.

Few medical events are more emotionally devastating than a pregnancy loss. Women often feel the loss in an extremely intense, almost physical way. Many who miscarry had not reached the point in pregnancy where the fetus seems separate from them. Typically, women feel both vulnerable and responsible, as if they did something to cause the loss or should have, could have, done something to prevent it. They try to identify what they did wrong: exercising or not exercising; working or not working; eating too much or not enough. Some women interpret a loss as a punishment for past sins, imagined or real. Such self-inflicted guilt, allowed to fester, can lead to major depression.

Infections

The infectious disease most clearly linked to birth defects is **rubella** (German measles). All women should be vaccinated against this disease at least three months prior to conception, to protect themselves and any children they may bear. (See Chapter 14 for more on immunization.) The most common prenatal infection today is *cytomegalovirus*. This infection produces mild flulike symptoms in adults but can cause brain damage, retardation, liver disease, cerebral palsy, hearing problems, and other malformations in unborn babies.

STIs, such as syphilis, gonorrhea, and genital herpes, can be particularly dangerous during pregnancy if not recognized and treated. If a woman has a herpes outbreak around the date her baby is due, her physician will deliver the baby by caesarean section to prevent infecting the baby. HIV infection endangers both a pregnant woman and her unborn baby, and all pregnant women and new mothers should be aware of the HIV epidemic, the risks to them and their babies, and the availability of anonymous testing.

Premature Labor

Approximately 10 percent of all babies are born too soon (before the 37th week of pregnancy). According to researchers, prematurity is the main underlying cause of stillbirth and infant deaths within the first few weeks after birth. Bed rest, close monitoring, and, if necessary, medications for at-risk women can buy more time in the womb for their babies. But women must recognize the warning signs of **premature labor**—dull, low backache; a feeling of tightness or pressure on the lower abdomen; and intestinal cramps, sometimes with diarrhea. Low-birthweight premature babies face the highest risks, but comprehensive, enriched programs can reduce developmental and health problems.

CHILDBIRTH

A generation ago, delivering a baby was something a doctor did in a hospital. Today parents can choose from many birthing options, including a birth attendant, who can be a physician or a nurse-midwife, and a birthing center, hospital, or home birth.

PREPARING FOR CHILDBIRTH

The most widespread method of childbirth preparation is **psychoprophylaxis,** or the **Lamaze method.** Fernand Lamaze, a French doctor, instructed women to respond to

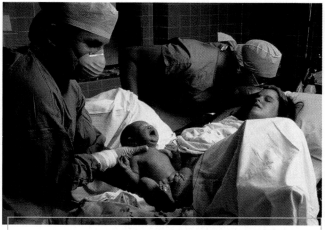

Today's fathers are routinely present at the birth of their children and often act as birth coaches after both parents participate in childbirth preparation classes.

labor contractions with prelearned, controlled breathing techniques. As the intensity of each contraction increases, the laboring woman concentrates on increasing her breathing rate in a prescribed way. Her partner coaches her during each contraction and helps her cope with discomfort.

Women who attend prenatal classes are less likely to undergo Caesarean deliveries and more likely to breast feed.[32] They also tend to have fewer complications and require fewer medications. However, painkillers or anesthesia are always an option if labor is longer or more painful than expected. The lower body can be numbed with an **epidural block,** which involves injecting an anesthetic into the membrane around the spinal cord, or a **spinal block,** in which the injection goes directly into the spinal canal. General anesthesia is usually used only for emergency caesarean births.

(FAQ) WHAT IS CHILDBIRTH LIKE?

There are three stages of **labor.** The first starts with *effacement* (thinning) and *dilation* (opening up) of the cervix. Effacement is measured in percentages, and dilation in centimeters or finger-widths. Around this time, the amniotic

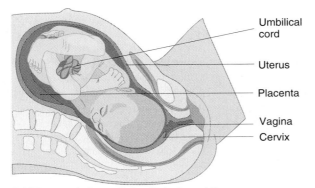

(a) The cervix is partially dilated, and the baby's head has entered the birth canal.

(b) The cervix is nearly completely dilated. The baby's head rotates so that it can move through the birth canal.

(c) The baby's head extends as it reaches the vaginal opening, and the head and the rest of the body pass through the birth canal.

(d) After the baby is born, the placenta detaches from the uterus and is expelled from the woman's body.

FIGURE 10-17 Birth

sac of fluids usually breaks, a sign that the woman should call her doctor or midwife.

The first contractions of the early, or *latent,* phase of labor are usually not uncomfortable; they last 15 to 30 seconds, occur every 15 to 30 minutes, and gradually increase in intensity and frequency. The most difficult contractions come after the cervix is dilated to about 8 centimeters, as the woman feels greater pressure from the fetus. The first stage ends when the cervix is completely dilated to a diameter of 10 centimeters (or five finger-widths) and the baby is ready to come down the birth canal (Figure 10-17). For women having their first baby, this first stage of labor averages 12 to 13 hours. Women having another child often experience shorter first-stage labor.

When the cervix is completely dilated, the second stage of labor occurs, during which the baby moves into the vagina, or birth canal, and out of the mother's body. As this stage begins, women who have gone through childbirth preparation training often feel a sense of relief from the acute pain of the transition phase and at the prospect of giving birth.

This second stage can take up to an hour or more. Strong contractions may last 60 to 90 seconds and occur every two to three minutes. As the baby's head descends, the mother feels an urge to push. By bearing down, she helps the baby complete its passage to the outside.

As the baby's head appears, or *crowns,* the doctor may perform an *episiotomy*—an incision from the lower end of the vagina toward the anus to enlarge the vaginal opening. The purpose of the episiotomy is to prevent the baby's head from causing an irregular tear in the vagina, but routine episiotomies have been criticized as unnecessary. Women may be able to avoid this procedure by trying different birthing positions or having an attendant massage the perineal tissue.

Usually the baby's head emerges first, then its shoulders, then its body. With each contraction, a new part is born. However, the baby can be in a more difficult position, facing up rather than down, or with the feet or buttocks first (a **breech birth**), and a cesarean birth may then be necessary.

In the third stage of labor, the uterus contracts firmly after the birth of the baby and, usually within five minutes, the placenta separates from the uterine wall. The woman may bear down to help expel the placenta, or the doctor may exert gentle external pressure. If an episiotomy has been performed, the doctor sews up the incision. To help the uterus contract and return to its normal size, it may be massaged manually, or the baby may be put to the mother's breast to stimulate contraction of the uterus.

CAESAREAN BIRTH

In a **caesarean delivery** (also referred to as a *caesarean section*), the doctor lifts the baby out of the woman's body through an incision made in the lower abdomen and uterus. The most common reason for caesarean birth is *failure to progress,* a vague term indicating that labor has gone on too long and may put the baby or mother at risk. Other reasons include the baby's position (if feet or buttocks are first) and signs that the fetus is in danger.

Thirty years ago, only 5 percent of babies born in America were delivered by caesarean birth; the current rate is 22.6 percent, substantially higher than in most other industrialized countries. About 36 percent of caesarean sections are performed because the woman has had a previous caesarean birth. However, four of every five women who have had caesarean births can have successful vaginal deliveries in subsequent pregnancies.

Caesarean birth involves abdominal surgery, so many women feel more physical discomfort after a caesarean than a vaginal birth, including nausea, pain, and abdominal gas. Women who have had a caesarean section must refrain from strenuous activity, such as heavy lifting, for several weeks.

AFTER THE BIRTH

Hospital stays for new mothers are shorter than in the past. A primary reason has been pressure to reduce medical costs. Obstetricians have voiced concern that the rush to release new mothers may jeopardize their well-being and the health of their babies, who are more likely to require emergency care for problems such as jaundice. The American College of Obstetricians and Gynecologists and the American Academy of Pediatrics recommend that women remain in the hospital two days after a vaginal delivery and four days after a caesarean birth.

BREAST-FEEDING VERSUS BOTTLE-FEEDING

A generation ago, most middle- and upper-class women bottle-fed their babies. Today, an increasing number of medical professionals state that breast milk is best. Breast-fed babies have fewer illnesses, a much lower hospitalization rate, and a lower mortality rate. Breast milk seems not only to prevent disease but also to help bring infection under control. When breast-fed babies do get sick, they recover more quickly. Breast-feeding women are generally advised not to use contraceptives containing estrogen.

Despite the benefits of breast-feeding, there are valid reasons to choose bottle-feeding. According to the American Council on Science and Health, at least 20 percent of women are unable to breast-feed after their first deliveries, and 50 percent of new mothers encounter significant difficulties nursing. Sometimes the woman's breasts become inflamed, or she must take medications that would endanger her infant; sometimes the infant is unable to suckle vigorously enough to get an adequate milk supply. Another problem is that in certain areas of the country, the levels of pesticides and other chemical contaminants in mother's milk can be high.

 BABIES AT RISK

According to the National Center for Health Statistics, the infant mortality rate in the United States is 7.0 deaths per 1,000 live births. We rank 27th in the world in infant mortality. African-American babies face a much greater risk of dying, primarily because of prematurity and dangerously low birthweight, before their first birthday. Babies of Chinese and Japanese descent have the lowest mortality rates.

In all, more than 1.3 million newborns each year require special care after birth because of prematurity, low birthweight, birth defects, jaundice, respiratory difficulties, or other problems. About 6 percent of newborns—more than 200,000 babies a year—require immediate intensive care for potentially life-threatening problems that developed before, during, or after birth.

Genetic Disorders

In some sense, each of us is a carrier of a genetic problem. Every individual has an estimated four to six defective genes, but the chances of passing them on to a child are slim. Almost all are recessive, which means they are "masked" by a more influential dominant gene. The likelihood of a child inheriting the same faulty recessive gene from both parents is remote—unless the parents are so closely related that they have very similar genetic makeup.

The child of a parent with an abnormal dominant gene has a 50 percent likelihood of inheriting it. The most common of such defects are minor, such as the growth of an extra finger or toe. However, some single-gene defects can be fatal. Huntington's chorea, for example, is a degenerative disease that in the past was usually not diagnosed until midlife.

Genetic tests can identify "carriers" of abnormal recessive genes for diseases such as sickle-cell anemia (the most common genetic disorder among African Americans), beta-thalassemia (found in families of Mediterranean origin), and Tay-Sachs (found in Jews of Eastern European origin). Two carriers of the same abnormal recessive genes can pass such problems on to their children.

The most common genetic disorders include:

- **Cystic fibrosis.** The most common genetic problem among white Americans, this is a disabling abnormality of the respiratory system and sweat and mucous glands.

- **Down syndrome.** This disorder is caused by an extra number 21 chromosome and occurs in one of every 600 to 1,000 births. Infants are born with varying degrees of physical and mental retardation. The chances of a woman delivering an infant with Down syndrome increase with her age. At age 25, the chances are 1 in 1,200; at age 35, they rise to 1 in 365; and at age 40, they are 1 in 100.

- **Sickle-cell anemia.** About 8 to 10 percent of North America's 25 million African Americans carry a gene for sickle-cell anemia, a blood disorder that occurs when hemoglobin, the oxygen-carrying protein of red blood cells, is abnormal and causes red blood cells to assume a crescent (sickle) shape. Unable to provide adequate oxygen to vital organs of the body, sickled cells cause fatigue, loss of interest and appetite, pain, and a host of other symptoms.

- **Phenylketonuria (PKU).** This disease occurs when the liver enzyme needed by the body for the metabolism of the amino acid phenylalanine is absent. If both parents are carriers, there's a one-in-four chance that the child will develop phenylketonuria (PKU). In most states, the law requires testing newborns for PKU. If PKU is detected, an immediate, long-term phenylalanine-free diet can reduce the effects of the disorder. If untreated, the victim becomes severely mentally retarded.

- **Tay-Sachs disease.** Occurring almost exclusively among young children of Eastern European Jewish ancestry, Tay-Sachs disease is caused by an enzyme deficiency. Infants with this disorder appear normal for perhaps nine months, but then gradually deteriorate physically and mentally. Death usually occurs before the fifth birthday. Carriers can be identified by a blood test.

Sudden Infant Death Syndrome (SIDS)

SIDS, or **crib death**—the unexplained death of an apparently healthy baby under one year of age—is the second-leading cause of infant mortality in the United States. Typically, a seemingly healthy infant, usually 1 to 7 months old, is put to bed according to the daily routine. The baby may have some signs of a cold or cough. When the parents return to the crib, they find the child dead. There is no sign of a struggle, nor does the baby suffocate in the blankets. Determining the cause of death often proves impossible. Premature and very small babies are the most vulnerable. A recognized risk factor, based on studies of 20,000 infants during the first week of life, is the "resonance frequency" of each cry—an acoustic measure of a child's cry that cannot be easily determined by listening. Computer analysis found that infants with a high-resonance frequency were more likely to die of SIDS. A screening test based on this factor may be developed to detect newborns at risk.

INFERTILITY

The World Health Organization defines **infertility** as the failure to conceive after one year of unprotected intercourse. Infertility affects one in seven couples. Women between ages 35 and 44 are about twice as likely to have fertility problems as women ages 30 to 34.

Infertility is a problem of the couple, not of the individual man or woman. In 40 percent of cases, infertility is caused by female problems, in 40 percent by male problems, in 10 percent by a combination of male and female problems, and in 10 percent by unexplained causes. A thorough diagnostic workup can reveal a cause for infertility in 90 percent of cases.

In women, the most common causes of subfertility or infertility are age, abnormal menstrual patterns, suppression of ovulation, and blocked fallopian tubes. A woman's fertility peaks between ages 20 and 30 and then drops quickly: by 20 percent after 30, by 50 percent after 35, and by 95 percent after 40. In a survey of 1,168 professional women in the United States, 42 percent of those over 40 were childless—only 14 percent by choice.

Male subfertility or infertility is usually linked to either the quantity or the quality of sperm, which may be inactive, misshapen, or insufficient (less than 20 million sperm per milliliter of semen in an ejaculation of 3 to 5 milliliters). Sometimes the problem is hormonal or a blockage of a sperm duct. Some men suffer from the inability to ejaculate normally, or from retrograde ejaculation, in which some of the semen travels in the wrong direction, back into the body of the male.

Infertility can have an enormous emotional impact.[33] Many women long to experience pregnancy and childbirth and feel great loss if they cannot conceive. Women in their thirties and forties fear that their biological clock is running out of time. Men may be confused and surprised by the intensity of their partner's emotions.

FAQ WHAT ARE THE OPTIONS FOR INFERTILE COUPLES?

The treatment of infertility has become a $2 billion a year enterprise in the United States. The odds of successful pregnancy range from 30 to 70 percent, depending on the specific cause of infertility. One result of successful infertility treatments has been a boom in multiple births, including quintuplets and sextuplets. Multiple births are associated with greater risk, both to the babies—including prematurity, low birthweight, neonatal death, and lifelong disability—and to the mothers, including caesarean section and hemorrhage.

Artificial Insemination

Since the 1960s, **artificial insemination**—the introduction of viable sperm into the vagina by artificial means—has led to an estimated 250,000 births in the United States, primarily in couples in which the husband was infertile. However, some states do not recognize such children as legitimate; others do, but only if the woman's husband gave his consent for the insemination.

Assisted Reproductive Technology

New approaches to infertility include microsurgery, sometimes with lasers, to open destroyed or blocked egg and sperm ducts; new hormone preparations to induce ovulation; and the use of balloons, inserted through the cervix and inflated, to open blocked fallopian tubes (a procedure called *balloon tuboplasty*). More than 35,000 babies are born each year as a result of assisted reproductive technology (ART).

The most common ART procedure is *in vitro fertilization (IVF)*, which involves removing the ova from a woman's ovary and placing the woman's egg and her mate's sperm in a laboratory dish for fertilization. If the fertilized egg cell shows signs of development, within several days it is returned to the woman's uterus, the egg cell implants itself in the lining of the uterus, and the pregnancy continues as normal. The success rate varies but is generally about 25 percent, and the costs are high.

In *gestational surrogacy,* an embryo is conceived in a laboratory dish using a woman's egg and her partner's sperm and then implanted into another woman's (the surrogate's) uterus. Alternatively, the fertilized donor egg can later be transferred to the uterus of the infertile woman, who carries and delivers the developing embryo.

Embryos can be frozen for later implantation in a process (called *cryopreservation*) that is highly controversial because of legal issues concerning the "ownership" of the unborn. Nearly 400,000 embryos are stored in the United States; the majority are targeted for patient use. Some women are considering an experimental technique to freeze some of their eggs at a young age for later use.

More than 40,000 infants are born annually as a result of assisted-reproductive technology. About three in four women undergoing ART use freshly fertilized embryos from their own eggs. Others use thawed embryos from their own eggs, freshly fertilized embryos from donor eggs, or thawed embryos from donor eggs.

About a third of the women using ART succeeded in carrying a baby to term. The odds of a live birth depend on many factors, including age. While 41 percent among women younger than 35 years gave birth, only 7 percent among women older than 42 years did so. The highest success rates also occurred in women who used donor eggs and freshly fertilized embryos.[34]

ADOPTION

Men and women who cannot conceive children biologically can still become parents. **Adoption** matches would-be parents yearning for youngsters to love with infants or children who need loving. Couples interested in adoption can

Adoption matches would-be parents yearning for youngsters to love with infants or children who need loving.

work with either public agencies or private counselors who contact obstetricians directly. Or they can contact organizations that arrange adoptions of children in need from other countries.

Although there are no reliable statistics on the annual number of adoptions in the United States, census records indicate there are currently 1.5 million adopted children in the United States. Each year some 50,000 U.S. children become available for adoption—far fewer than the number of would-be parents looking for youngsters to adopt. By some estimates, only 1 in 30 couples receive a child—and they spend an average of two years and as much as $100,000 on the adoption process.

Not only are the stakes high, but adoption arrangements often are chaotic. Private adoptions are legal in some states, banned in others. In some places, birth mothers sign over all claims to a child within 72 hours of giving birth; in others they have up to a year to change their minds. Sometimes foster parents are encouraged to adopt—particularly if they're African Americans caring for an African-American child. In others, they face a daunting series of bureaucratic barriers. What's needed most, say experts on every side of the issue, are uniform adoption laws in all 50 states.

An increasing number of people support *open adoptions,* which allow for visiting and communication with the biological parents even though the adoptive parents retain legal custody. Even after a *closed adoption,* the biological (or birth) parents may at some point search for their children, if only to explain why they chose to give them up for adoption.

Although fewer than 2 percent of each year's 50,000 adoptions of American children are contested, adoptive parents are nervous and confused.

The best advice for prospective adoptive parents is to learn as much as they can about their state's adoption laws and to prepare for the reality that their plans might not work out.

Learn It / Live It

Protecting Your Reproductive Health

The decisions and choices you make about birth control can affect your current and future reproductive health—and your partner's. Here are some guidelines that can help both prevent pregnancy and protect your reproductive well-being.

- **Abstain.** The only 100 percent safe and effective way to avoid unwanted pregnancy is not to engage in heterosexual intercourse.

- **Limit sexual activity to "outercourse."** You can engage in many sexual activities—kissing, hugging, touching, massage, oral-genital sex—without risking pregnancy.

- **Talk about birth control with any potential sex partner.** If you are considering sexual intimacy with a person, you should feel comfortable enough to talk about contraception.

- **Know what doesn't work—and don't rely on it.** There are many misconceptions about ways to avoid getting pregnant, such as having sex in a standing position or during menstruation. Only the methods described in this chapter are reliable forms of birth control.

- **Talk with a health-care professional.** A great deal of information and advice is available—in writing, from family planning counselors, from physicians on the Internet. Check it out.

- **Choose a contraceptive method that matches your personal habits and preferences.** If you can't remember to take a pill every day, oral contraceptives aren't for you. If you're constantly forgetting where you put things, a diaphragm might not be a good choice.

- **Consider long-term implications.** Since you may well wish to have children in the future, find out about the reversibility of various methods and possible effects on future fertility.

- **Resist having sex without contraceptive protection "just this once."** It only takes once—even the very first time—to get pregnant. Be wary of drugs and alcohol. They can impair your judgment and make you less conscientious about using birth control—or using it properly.

- **Use backup methods.** If there's a possibility that a contraceptive method might not offer adequate protection (for instance, if it's been almost three months since your last injection of Depo-Provera), use an additional form of birth control.

- **Inform yourself about emergency contraception.** Just in case a condom breaks or a diaphragm slips, find out about the availability of forms of after-intercourse contraception.

Making This Chapter Work for You

Review Questions

1. Conception occurs
   a. when a fertilized egg implants in the lining of the uterus.
   b. when sperm is blocked from reaching the egg.
   c. when a sperm fertilizes the egg.
   d. after the uterine lining is discharged during the menstrual cycle.

2. Factors to consider when choosing a contraceptive method include all of the following *except*
   a. cost.
   b. failure rate.
   c. effectiveness in preventing sexually transmitted infections.
   d. preferred sexual position.

3. When used correctly, which is the most effective non-hormonal contraceptive method?
   a. male condom
   b. female condom
   c. spermicide
   d. diaphragm

4. Which of the following contraceptive choices offers the best protection against STIs?
   a. condom alone
   b. condom plus spermicide
   c. abstinence
   d. withdrawal plus spermicide

5. Which statement about prescription contraceptives is *not* true?
   a. Prescription contraceptives do not offer protection against STIs.
   b. Some prescription contraceptives contain estrogen and progestin, and some contain only progestin.
   c. The contraceptive ring must be changed every week.
   d. IUDs prevent pregnancy by preventing or interfering with implantation.

6. Which of the following statements is *true* about sterilization?
   a. In women, the most frequently performed sterilization technique is Essure.
   b. Many couples experience an increase in sexual encounters after sterilization.
   c. Vasectomies are easily reversed with surgery.
   d. Sterilization is recommended for single men and women who are unsure about whether they want children.

7. Which statement about abortion is *false*?
   a. The abortion rate in the United States started declining in the 1990s.
   b. The U.S. abortion rate is higher than the rate in Canada and England.

c. Most women are traumatized by an abortion.

d. Mifepristone is 97 percent effective in inducing abortion.

8. In the third trimester of pregnancy,

a. the woman experiences shortness of breath as the enlarged uterus presses on the lungs and diaphragm.

b. the embryo is now called a fetus.

c. the woman should begin regular prenatal checkups.

d. the woman should increase her activity level to ensure that she is fit for childbirth.

9. During childbirth,

a. breech birth can be prevented by practicing the Lamaze method.

b. the cervix thins and dilates so that the baby can exit the uterus.

c. the intensity of contractions decreases during the second stage of labor.

d. the placenta is expelled immediately before the baby's head appears.

10. Which of the following statements is true about infertility?

a. Infertility is most often caused by female problems.

b. In men, infertility is usually caused by a combination of excess sperm production and an ejaculation problem.

c. In vitro fertilization involves introducing sperm into the vagina with a long needle.

d. In some cases of infertility, no cause can be demonstrated.

Answers to these questions can be found on page 587.

Critical Thinking

1. After reading about the various methods of contraception, which do you think would be most effective for you? What factors enter into your decision (convenience, risks, effectiveness, etc.)?

2. In Wyoming, a pregnant woman went to the police station to report that her husband had beaten her. Instead of charges being brought against him, she was arrested for intoxication and charged with abusing her fetus by drinking. Across the country, other women who use hard drugs or alcohol while pregnant or whose newborns test positive for drugs have been arrested and put on trial for abusing their unborn children. Prosecutors argue that they are defending the innocent victims of substance abuse. Some health officials, on the other hand, argue that addicted women need help, not punishment. What do you think? Why?

3. Suppose that you and your partner were told that your only chance of having a child is by using fertility drugs. After taking the drugs, you and your partner are informed that there are seven fetuses. Would you carry them all to term? What if you knew that the chances of

them all surviving were very slim and that eliminating some of them would improve the odds for the others? What ethical issues do cases like this raise?

Media Menu

Health Now™

Throughout the chapter, this icon introduces a list of resources on the Health-Now website at http://healthnow.brookscole.com/ith that will:
- Help you evaluate your knowledge of the material.
- Allow you to take an exam-prep quiz.
- Provide a Personalized Learning Plan targeting resources that address areas you should study.
- Coach you through identifying target goals for behavior change and creating and monitoring your personal change plan throughout the semester.

INTERNET CONNECTIONS

The Alan Guttmacher Institute
www.agi-usa.org
This site offers excellent resources on teen pregnancy rates and sexual health for teens and young adults, including discussions on contraceptives versus abstinence.

Association of Reproductive Health Professionals
www.arhp.org
ARHP calls their website "the ultimate resource offering comprehensive information and education on all reproductive health topics to healthcare professionals, policymakers, the media, and the public."

National Abortion Rights Action League
www.naral.org
The website of this national organization provides information on the politics of the pro-choice movement.

National Right to Life Committee
www.nrlc.org
The website of this national organization provides information on the politics of the pro-life movement.

Planned Parenthood
www.plannedparenthood.org
The website for the Planned Parenthood Federation of America offers a wealth of information on sexual and reproductive health, reproductive choices, methods of contraception, and reproductive policy.

InfoTrac College Edition Activities Log on, insert **birth control** into the Keyword search box, and limit your search to the past year. When you get the results, Mark articles to review, then Select one to read. Summarize three or four key points from the article.

You can find additional readings related to personal health with InfoTrac College Edition, an online library of more than 900 journals and publications. Follow the instructions for accessing InfoTrac College Edition that

Self Survey :: Which Contraceptive Method Is Best for You?

Answer yes or no to each statement as it applies to you and, if appropriate, your partner.

1. You have high blood pressure or cardiovascular disease.
2. You smoke cigarettes.
3. You have a new sexual partner.
4. An unwanted pregnancy would be devastating to you.
5. You have a good memory.
6. You or your partner have multiple sexual partners.
7. You prefer a method with little or no bother.
8. You have heavy, crampy periods.
9. You need protection against STIs.
10. You are concerned about endometrial and ovarian cancer.
11. You are forgetful.
12. You need a method right away.
13. You're comfortable touching your own and your partner's genitals.
14. You have a cooperative partner.
15. You like a little extra vaginal lubrication.
16. You have sex at unpredictable times and places.
17. You are in a monogamous relationship and have at least one child.

Scoring:

Recommendations are based on Yes answers to the following numbered statements:

The combination pill: 4, 5, 6, 8, 10, 16

The progestin-only pill: 1, 2, 5, 7, 16

The patch: 4, 7, 8, 11, 16

The NuvaRing: 4, 7, 8, 11, 13, 16

Condoms: 1, 2, 3, 6, 9, 12, 13, 14

Depo-Provera: 1, 2, 4, 7, 11, 16

Lunelle: 4, 7, 11, 16

Diaphragm, cervical cap, or FemCap: 1, 2, 13, 14

Mirena IUD: 1, 2, 7, 8, 11, 13, 16, 17

Spermicides: 1, 2, 12, 13, 14, 15

Sponge: 1, 2, 12, 13

were packaged with your textbook; then search for articles using a keyword search.

For additional links, resources, and suggested readings on the InfoTrac College Edition, visit our Health and Wellness Resource Center at **http://health .wadsworth.com.**

Key Terms

The terms listed are used on the page indicated. Definitions of the terms are in the Glossary at the end of this book.

YOUR ACTION PLAN FOR CHOOSING A CONTRACEPTIVE

Your responses may indicate that there's more than one appropriate method of birth control for you. Remember that you may choose different types of birth control at different stages of your life, or switch contraceptives for various reasons. You and your partner should always consider and discuss these factors:

▪ **Effectiveness.** Keep in mind that your own conscientiousness will play an important role. If you forget to take your daily pill, or if you decide not to use a condom "just this once," you'll increase the odds of pregnancy by interfering with effective birth control.

▪ **Suitability.** If you don't have sex very often, a contraceptive with many risks and side effects, such as the pill, may be wrong for you. If you have many sexual partners and are at risk of contracting a sexually transmitted infection, a condom may provide protection against pregnancy and infection, especially if used with a diaphragm or cervical cap.

▪ **Side effects.** Some complications related to contraceptives are serious health threats. Be sure to ask questions and gather as much information as possible about what side effects to expect.

▪ **Safety.** The risks of certain contraceptives, such as the pill, may be too great to allow their use if, for example, you have high blood pressure. Be honest in describing your medical history to your physician.

▪ **Future fertility.** Some women don't return to regular menstrual cycles for six months to a year after discontinuing oral contraceptives. This possibility may or may not be important to you now, but you should try to look ahead.

▪ **Cost.** The only free contraceptive methods are abstinence and rhythm methods. If you're on a tight budget, you might consider the relative costs of a year's prescription of oral contraceptives compared to a year's supply of condoms or spermicidal foam or jelly. You should also think about the long-term costs and consequences.

▪ **Reduced risk of sexually transmitted infections.** Some forms of contraception, in particular barrier contraceptives and spermicides, help reduce the risk of transmission of some STIs. However, none provides complete protection.

CASE IN POINT

Student: Caitlin, 22, and Nic, 25

Goal: To change to a more reliable method of birth control after moving in together

Action Plan:

▪ To continue relying on condoms and spermicide until they make a change

▪ To arrange for a medical examination and consultation with a doctor

▪ To investigate alternatives to daily birth control pills, which Cailtin has found difficult to remember in the past

▪ To research from authoritative websites the advantages and disadvantages of extended-use oral contraceptives or of a vaginal ring

▪ To discuss their long-term plans, including each of their desires to have children some day

Health Now™   If you want to write your own goals for safe and effective contraception, go to **the Wellness HealthNow Journal** at http://healthnow .brookscole.com/ith.

Avoiding Health Risks

We constantly hear messages encouraging us to take risks with our health, to try drugs, to have a drink, to smoke cigarettes. We also live with the consequences of others' drug abuse, alcoholism, and smoking. That's why it's important to know about potentially harmful habits—even if you never rely on drugs to pick you up or bring you down, never smoke, and never drink to excess. This section provides information you can use to avoid or overcome habits that could destroy your health, happiness, and life.

11 Avoiding Addictive Behaviors and Drug Abuse

Justine doesn't do drugs. That's what she says to anyone who asks. Sure, she and her friends occasionally pass a joint around while listening to music. She's tried a tab of ecstasy at a couple of raves. And when she was stressed out after finals, she took some of her roommate's Vicodin. But she thinks of drug users as desperate addicts craving a fix. She's not like that. That's what she tells herself.

Although she doesn't realize it, Justine is at risk of drug-related problems—physical, psychological, and legal—and of developing a substance abuse disorder. Like Justine, the people who try illegal drugs don't think they'll ever lose control. Even regular drug users are convinced that they are smart enough, strong enough, lucky enough not to get caught and not to get hooked. But with continued use, drugs produce changes in an individual's body, mind, and behavior. In time, a person's need for a drug can outweigh everything else, including the values, people, and relationships he or she once held dearest.

Drug abuse takes a huge toll, not just financially, but in terms of lost potential, ruined families, poor health, and unnecessary deaths. But drug use among the young may have peaked.[1] Since 2001, there has been a 17 percent reduction in any drug use among adolescents and an 18 percent drop in marijuana use in the past month.[2] However, the use of inhalants has risen among young teens, and abuse of the prescription drug oxycodone (OxyContin) remains widespread.[3]

Rates of drug use on college campuses are lower than they were several decades ago. Yet more than half of college students report that they have smoked marijuana at least once, and the abuse of club drugs, prescription drugs, and stimulants continues. Nationwide, methamphetamine—a cheap, highly addictive, and life-shattering drug—has surged to the forefront of problem drugs across the United States. Substance abuse remains so widespread that about half of children in America live in homes where a parent or other adult uses tobacco, drinks heavily, or uses illicit drugs.[4]

This chapter provides information on addictive behaviors, the nature and effects of drugs, the impact of drugs, and the drugs Americans most commonly use, misuse, and abuse.

Steve Allen

FAQ Frequently Asked Questions

- What happens to problem gamblers? *p. 306*
- What should I know about over-the-counter drugs? *p. 308*
- What should I know about buying drugs online? *p. 312*
- Is it possible to overdose on caffeine? *p. 313*
- What causes drug dependence and abuse? *p. 315*

After studying the material in this chapter, you should be able to:

- **Name** some of the risk factors for problem gambling.
- **Describe** the different types of drug actions and factors affecting individuals' response to drugs.
- **Give examples** of appropriate and inappropriate use of over-the-counter and prescription medications.
- **Identify** the types of drug dependence, and discuss the factors affecting drug dependence.
- **Describe** the effects and health risks of common drugs of abuse.
- **Describe** the treatment methods available for individuals seeking help for drug dependence.

ADDICTIVE BEHAVIORS AND THE DIMENSIONS OF HEALTH

Substance abuse and other self-destructive behaviors, such as gambling or compulsive eating, can affect every dimension of health. Yet often individuals are unaware of the harmful effects of their unhealthy choices:

- *Physical health.* As shown in this and the following chapters, the abuse of alcohol, tobacco, and drugs takes a toll on every organ system in the body, increasing the likelihood of disease, disability, and premature death.

- *Psychological health.* Sometimes people begin abusing substances or engaging in addictive behavior as a way of "self-medicating" symptoms of anxiety or depression. However, alcohol or drugs provide only temporary relief. As abuse continues, shame and guilt increase, and coping with daily stressors becomes more difficult. Depression and anxiety are as likely to be the consequences as the causes of substance abuse.

- *Spiritual health.* Addictive behavior blocks the pursuit of meaning and inner fulfillment. As they rely more and more on a chemical or behavioral escape, individuals lose their sense of self and of connection with others and with a higher power.

- *Social health.* Addictive behavior strains and, in time, severs the ties that bind an individual to family, friends, colleagues, and classmates. The primary relationship in the life of alcoholics or addicts is with a behavior or a drug. They withdraw from others and become increasingly isolated.

- *Intellectual health.* The brain is one of the targets of alcohol and drugs. Under their influence, logic and reasoning break down. Impulses become more difficult to control. Judgment falters. Certain substances, such as ecstasy, can lead to permanent changes in brain chemistry.

- *Environmental health.* The use of some substances, such as tobacco, directly harms the environment. Abusers of alcohol and drugs also pose indirect threats to others because their behavior can lead to injury and damage.

 ## DRUG USE ON CAMPUS

Drug use on campus has increased since 1993, with the steepest rise in the mid-1990s. Almost half of undergraduates say they have used marijuana; 30 percent report its use in the last year and 17 percent in the last 30 days. Seven percent report that they've used another illicit drug in the last 30 days; 14 percent did so in the last year.

 Drug use has increased most dramatically among minority students, particularly African Americans and Asian–Pacific Islanders. However, white students still have the highest rates of drug use (see Student Snapshot: "Drugs on Campus"). More than 9 in 10 students who used marijuana and other illicit drugs also used other substances, smoked cigarettes, and/or were binge drinkers.

In recent years, ecstasy use more than doubled on campus. The Harvard College Alcohol Study revealed an increase of almost 70 percent in ecstasy use by undergraduates over a two-year period.

There is a large gap between actual drug use on campus and how prevalent students believe drug use to be. When researchers have compared students' self-reports of frequency of drug use with what students perceived to be the frequency of drug use by "the average student," findings show they greatly overestimate the use of a variety of drugs.

Why Students Use Drugs

Various factors influence which students use drugs, including the following:

- **Race/ethnicity.** In general, white students have higher levels of alcohol and drug use than do African-American students. In a comparison of African-American students at predominantly white and predominantly black colleges, those at historically black colleges had lower rates of alcohol and drug use than did either white or African-American students at white schools. The reason, according to the researchers, may be that these colleges provide a greater sense of self-esteem, which helps prevent alcohol and drug use.

- **Perception of risk.** Students seem most likely to try substances they perceive as being "safe," or low

Drug use is a negative addiction; try a "positive" hobby or habit.

© Steve Mercer/Taxi/Getty Images.

Student Snapshot

DRUGS ON CAMPUS

Who Uses Drugs?	Percentage of Students	Days per Week
By sex		
Women	16.5%	3.99
Men	27.5	3.3
By race		
Caucasian	23.9%	3.5
African American	10.7	3.1
Asian	14.6	2.5
By fraternity/sorority membership		
Members	29.2%	3.4
Nonmembers	18.1	3.5

* Based on a study of 740 undergraduates.
Source: Shinew, Kimberly, and Diana Parry. "Examining College Students' Participation in the Leisure Pursuits of Drinking and Illegal Drug Use." *Journal of Leisure Research,* Vol. 37, No. 3, Summer 2005, p. 364(23).

risk. Of these, the top three are caffeine, alcohol, and tobacco; marijuana is listed fourth in terms of perceived safety. Other agents—barbiturates, heroin, cocaine, PCP, speed, LSD, crack, and inhalants—are viewed as more risky and are used much less often.

- **Alcohol use.** Often individuals engage in more than one "risk behavior," and researchers have documented correlations among smoking, drinking, and drug use. Among college students, researchers have found that those who report binge drinking are much more likely than other students to report current or past use of marijuana, cocaine, or other illegal drugs.

- **Environment.** As with alcohol use, students are influenced by their friends, their residence, the general public's attitude toward drug use, and even the Internet. College health officials are realizing that rather than simply trying to change students' substance abuse, they also must change the environment to promote healthier lifestyle choices. One successful innovation is substance-free dorms.

- **Sexual identity.** Gay, lesbian, and bisexual teens may rely on alcohol and marijuana to lessen social anxiety and boost self-confidence when they first come out. However, once they become more involved in the gay community, many are less likely to do so.[5] Nonetheless, self-identified lesbian women are significantly more likely than heterosexual women to use marijuana, ecstasy, and other

drugs.[6] Gay and bisexual men are significantly less likely than heterosexual men to drink heavily but more likely to use some drugs.

- **Gambling.** In a study at four Connecticut universities, one in nine students had a gambling problem significantly connected to a substance-related issue. Problem/pathological gamblers report a higher number of drug and alcohol problems than nongamblers or social gamblers.[7]

GAMBLING

Legal in most states, gambling can take many forms: lottery, scratch cards, casino games, sports betting, Internet gambling, horse and racetrack wagering, videogame betting, and playing cards and dice. In a national survey, about eight in ten adults—and the same percentage of 12- to 17-year-olds—reported they had gambled in the past year.[8]

Although gambling is illegal for anyone under 18 to 21 years of age, depending on individual state law, underage gambling is a significant and growing problem across the country. In a survey of almost 1,000 university students, a majority had gambled—60 percent of the 18-year-olds, 73 percent of the 19-year-olds, 86 percent of the 20-year-olds, and 93 percent of those over 21 years of age—had gambled at least once in a casino.[9]

 College students who gamble do so for fun or excitement, to socialize, to win money, or to "just have something to do"—reasons similar to those for adults who gamble. Simply having access to casino machines, ongoing card games, or Internet gambling sites increases the likelihood that students will gamble.

Although most people who gamble limit the time and money they spend, some cross the line and lose control of their gambling "habit." The term "problem gambling" refers to all individuals with gambling-related problems, including mild or occasional ones. Pathological or compulsive gambling is defined as "persistent and recurrent maladaptive behavior." In one sample of college students, 15 percent of those over 21 and 9 percent of those under 21 were classified as "probable" pathological gamblers.[10]

Risk Factors for Problem Gambling

Adult pathological gamblers are more likely to be male, single, non-Caucasian, and less educated. Women start gambling later than men, but they progress more rapidly to pathological gambling. Genetics and exposure to gambling in childhood are significant influences. More than half of pathological gamblers report at least one first-degree relative with symptoms consistent with gambling problems.[11]

Among young people (ages 16 to 25) the following behaviors indicate increased risk of problem gambling:

- Male sex.
- Gambling at an early age (as young as age eight).

Strategies for Change ▪▪ Do You Have a Gambling Problem?

▪▪ Have you ever felt that your gambling or betting was out of control?

▪▪ Have you ever gotten into a fight with your family or friends because of gambling or betting?

▪▪ Have you ever felt that you lost too much money in gambling or betting?

▪▪ Have you ever felt the need to bet more and more money?

▪▪ Have you ever had to lie to people important to you about how much you gamble?

Even a single yes answer may indicate a problem. Go online or check with

a counselor on campus to find resources, such as a local chapter of Gamblers Anonymous.

- A big win earlier in one's gambling career.
- Consistently chasing losses (betting more to recover money already lost).
- Gambling alone.
- Feeling depressed before gambling.
- Feeling excited and aroused during gambling.
- Behaving irrationally during gambling.
- Poor grades at school.
- Other addictive behaviors (smoking, drinking alcohol, illegal drug use).
- Lower socioeconomic class.
- Parents with a gambling or other addiction problem.
- A history of delinquency or stealing money to fund gambling.
- Skipping class to go gambling.

(FAQ) What Happens to Problem Gamblers?

Gamblers typically progress through various stages. In the winning phase, they feel empowered by their winnings and success. Next comes the losing phase, during which gamblers try to win back their losses. This is followed by the desperation phase, during which a gambler may resort to illegal activity, including stealing, to continue gambling. Some gamblers experience a fourth phase, the giving-up phase, where they desperately try to stay afloat in a game even though they realize they can't win.

As many as three-fourths of adult pathological gamblers suffer from depression. They also are at higher risk of other mood or anxiety disorders, such as panic disorder, phobias, obsessive-compulsive disorder, generalized anxiety, or post-traumatic stress disorder. An estimated 20 percent suffer from attention-deficit/hyperactivity disorder (ADHD). Even more—30 to 50 percent of pathological gamblers—abuse drugs or alcohol.

No standard or proven treatment exists for pathological gambling, but inpatient treatment centers, self-help groups, cognitive-behavioral psychotherapy, and addiction-based psychotherapy can help.

Your Life Coach

Developing Positive Addictions

When you're anxious, bored, restless, or confused, when drugs seem all too appealing as a "quick fix," there are real solutions, "positive addictions" that can help you solve your problems without creating new and bigger ones. A positive addiction—whether it is exercising, mountain-climbing, or listening to music—can produce very real "highs." But there's a crucial difference between this sort of stimulation and drug dependency: one is real, the other is chemical. With one, you're in control; with the other, drugs are.

Here are some examples:

- **If you feel a need for physical relaxation,** if you want more energy or distraction from physical discomforts, you can turn to athletics, exercise (including walking and hiking), dance, or outdoor hobbies.

- **If you want to stimulate your senses,** enhance sexual stimulation, or magnify the sensations of sight, sound, and touch, train yourself to be more sensitive to nature and beauty. Take time to appreciate the sensations you experience when you're walking in the woods or embracing a person you love. Through activities like sailing or sky-diving, you can literally fill up your senses without relying on chemicals.

- **If you have psychological troubles,** if you're anxious or depressed, if you feel inhibited or uptight, if you don't know how to solve complex personal problems and want relief from emotional pain, turn to people who can offer lasting help: in some cases, friends; in others, professional counselors or support groups.

- **If you want peer acceptance,** if you'd like to overcome your shyness, if you want to communicate and relate more effectively, you can join expertly managed sensitivity or encounter groups, enroll in confidence-building seminars, seek counseling, or volunteer in programs in which you can assist others and not focus only on your self-consciousness.

- **If you want to escape mental boredom,** gain new understanding of the world around you, study better, experiment with your levels of awareness, or indulge your intellectual curiosity, challenge your mind through reading, classes, creative games, discussion groups, memory training, or travel.

- **If you want to enhance your creativity** or your appreciation of the arts, pursue training in music, art, singing, gardening, or writing. Sign up for a nongraded course in art history or music appreciation. Attend more concerts, ballets, museum shows.

- **If you want to promote political or social change,** defy the establishment, change drug legislation, or gain power, you can volunteer in political campaigns, work on nonpartisan projects, or join lobbying and political action groups.

- **If you want to find meaning in life,** understand the nature of the universe, or expand your personal awareness, explore various philosophical theories through classes, seminars, and discussion groups. Study different religious orientations, including mysticism, or try yoga and meditation.

- **If you're looking for kicks,** adventure, danger, and excitement, sign up for a wilderness survival course. Take up an adventurous sport, like hang gliding or rock climbing. Set a challenging professional or personal goal and direct your energies to meeting it.

UNDERSTANDING DRUGS AND THEIR EFFECTS

A **drug** is a chemical substance that affects the way you feel and function. In some circumstances, taking a drug can help the body heal or relieve physical and mental distress. In other circumstances, taking a drug can distort reality, undermine well-being, and threaten survival. No drug is completely safe; all drugs have multiple effects that vary greatly in different people at different times. Knowing how drugs affect the brain, body, and behavior is crucial to understanding their impact and making responsible decisions about their use.

Drug misuse is the taking of a drug for a purpose or by a person other than that for which whom it was medically intended. Borrowing a friend's prescription for penicillin when your throat feels scratchy is an example of drug misuse. The World Health Organization defines **drug abuse** as excessive drug use that's inconsistent with accepted medical practice. Taking prescription painkillers to get high is an example of drug abuse.

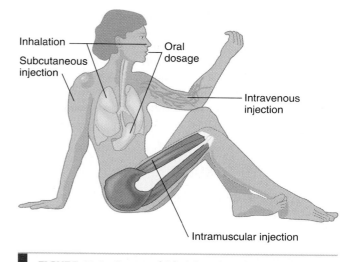

Inhalation
Subcutaneous injection
Oral dosage
Intravenous injection
Intramuscular injection

FIGURE 11-1 Routes of Administration of Drugs

Risks are involved with all forms of drug use. Even medications that help cure illnesses or soothe symptoms have side effects and can be misused. Some substances that millions of people use every day, such as caffeine, pose some health risks. Others—like the most commonly used drugs in our society, alcohol and tobacco—can lead to potentially life-threatening problems. With some illicit drugs, any form of use can be dangerous.

Many factors determine the effects a drug has on an individual. These include how the drug enters the body, the dosage, the drug action, and the presence of other drugs in the body—as well as the physical and psychological makeup of the person taking the drug and the setting in which the drug is used.

ROUTES OF ADMINISTRATION

Drugs can enter the body in a number of ways (Figure 11-1). The most common way of taking a drug is by swallowing a tablet, capsule, or liquid. However, drugs taken orally don't reach the bloodstream as quickly as drugs introduced into the body by other means. A drug taken orally may not have any effect for 30 minutes or more.

Drugs can enter the body through the lungs either by inhaling smoke, for example, from marijuana, or by inhaling gases, aerosol sprays, or fumes from solvents or other compounds that evaporate quickly. Young users of such inhalants, discussed later in this chapter, often soak a rag with fluid and press it over their nose. Or they may place inhalants in a plastic bag, put the bag over their nose and mouth, and take deep breaths—a practice called *huffing* and one that can produce serious, even fatal consequences.

Drugs can also be injected with a syringe subcutaneously (beneath the skin), intramuscularly (into muscle tissue, which is richly supplied with blood vessels), or intravenously (directly into a vein). **Intravenous** (IV) injection gets the drug into the bloodstream immediately (within seconds in most cases); **intramuscular** injection, moderately fast (within a few minutes); and **subcutaneous** injection, more slowly (within ten minutes).

Injecting drugs is extremely dangerous because many diseases, including hepatitis and infection with human immune deficiency virus (HIV), can be transmitted by sharing contaminated needles. Injection-drug users who are HIV-positive are a major source of transmission of HIV among heterosexuals. (See Chapter 14 for more on HIV infection and AIDS.)

DOSAGE AND TOXICITY

The effects of any drug depend on the amount an individual takes. Increasing the dose usually intensifies the effects produced by smaller doses. Also, the kind of effect may change at different dose levels. For example, low doses of barbiturates may relieve anxiety, while higher doses can induce sleep, loss of sensation, even coma and death.

The dosage level at which a drug becomes poisonous to the body, causing either temporary or permanent damage, is called its **toxicity.** In most cases, drugs are eventually broken down in the liver by special body chemicals called *detoxification enzymes.*

INDIVIDUAL DIFFERENCES

Each person responds differently to different drugs, depending on circumstances or setting. The enzymes in the body reduce the levels of drugs in the bloodstream; because there can be 80 variants of each enzyme, every person's body may react differently.

Often drugs intensify the emotional state a person is in. If you're feeling depressed, a drug may make you feel more depressed. A generalized physical problem, such as having the flu, may make your body more vulnerable to the effects of a drug. Genetic differences among individuals also may account for varying reactions.

Personality and psychological attitude also play a role in drug effects. Each user's *mind-set*—his or her expectations or preconceptions about using the drug—affects the experience. Someone who takes a "club drug" (discussed further later in this chapter) to feel more "connected" may feel more sociable simply because that's what he or she expects.

SETTING

The setting for drug use also influences its effects. Passing around a joint of marijuana at a friend's is not a healthy or safe behavior, but the experience of going to a crack house is very different—and entails greater dangers.

TYPES OF ACTION

A drug can act *locally,* as novocaine does to deaden pain in a tooth; *generally,* throughout a body system, as barbiturates do on the central nervous system; or *selectively,* as a drug does when it has a greater effect on one specific organ or system than on others, such as a spinal anesthetic. A drug

that accumulates in the body because it's taken in faster than it can be metabolized and excreted is called *cumulative;* alcohol is such a drug.

Interaction with Other Drugs or Alcohol

A drug can interact with other drugs in four different ways:

▪ **An additive interaction is** one in which the resulting effect is equal to the sum of the effects of the different drugs used.

▪ **A synergistic interaction is** one in which the total effect of the two drugs taken together is greater than the sum of the effects the two drugs would have had if taken by themselves on separate occasions. Mixing barbiturates and alcohol, for example, has up to four times the depressant effect than either drug has alone.

▪ **A drug can be potentiating**—that is, one drug can increase the effect of another. Alcohol, for instance, can increase the drowsiness caused by antihistamines (antiallergy medications).

▪ **Drugs can interact in an antagonistic fashion**—that is, one drug can neutralize or block another drug with opposite effects. Tranquilizers, for example, may counter some of the nervousness and anxiety produced by cocaine.

The danger of mixing alcohol with other drugs cannot be emphasized too strongly. Alcohol and marijuana intensify each other's effects, making driving and many other activities extremely dangerous. Some people have mixed sedatives or tranquilizers with alcohol and never regained consciousness.

▌ MEDICATIONS

As many as half of all patients take the wrong medications, in the wrong doses, at the wrong times, or in the wrong ways. Every year these inadvertent errors lead to an estimated 125,000 deaths and more than $8.5 billion in hospital costs.[12] Mistakes occur among people of all ages, both genders, and every race, occupation, level of education, and personality type. Their number-one cause: not understanding directions (see Savvy Consumer: "Avoiding Medication Mistakes").

(FAQ) WHAT SHOULD I KNOW ABOUT OVER-THE-COUNTER DRUGS?

More than half a million health products—remedies for everything from bad breath to bunions—are readily available without a doctor's prescription. This doesn't mean that they're necessarily safe or effective. Indeed, many widely used **over-the-counter (OTC) drugs** pose unsuspected hazards.

As discussed on page ●●●, federal regulators have issued warnings for many popular painkillers, including over-the-counter pills like Advil and Aleve. Their labels cite risks to

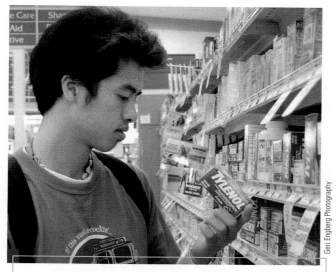

Practically all of these packages have warnings on the back. Read them before using an over-the-counter drug.

the heart, stomach, and skin. Aspirin and Tylenol (acetaminophen) are generally considered safe for people with temporary pain like headaches and muscle aches. However, aspirin can cause stomach irritation and bleeding, and Tylenol should not be taken by anyone who drinks three or more alcoholic beverages a day without consulting a doctor.

A growing number of drugs that once were available only with a doctor's prescription now can be bought over the counter. For consumers, the advantages of this greater availability include lower prices and fewer visits to the doctor. The disadvantages, however, are the risks of misdiagnosing a problem and misusing or overusing medications.

Like other drugs, OTC medications can be used improperly, often simply because of a lack of education about proper use. Among those most often misused are the following:

▪ **Nasal sprays.** Nasal sprays relieve congestion by shrinking blood vessels in the nose. If they are used too often or for too many days in a row, the blood vessels widen instead of contracting, and the surrounding tissues become swollen, causing more congestion. To make the vessels shrink again, many people use more spray more often. The result can be permanent damage to nasal membranes, bleeding, infection, and partial or complete loss of smell.

▪ **Laxatives.** Believing that they must have one bowel movement a day (a common misconception), many people rely on laxatives. Brands that contain phenolphthalein irritate the lining of the intestines and cause muscles to contract or tighten, often making constipation worse rather than better. Bulk laxatives are less dangerous, but regular use is not advised. A high-fiber diet and more exercise are safer and more effective remedies for constipation.

▪ **Eye drops.** Eye drops make the blood vessels of the eye contract. However, as in the case of nasal

sprays, with overuse (several times a day for several weeks), the blood vessels expand, making the eye look redder than before.

▪ **Sleep aids.** Although OTC sleeping pills are widely used, there has been little research on their use and possible risks. A national consensus panel on insomnia concluded that they are not effective and cause side effects such as morning-after grogginess.[13] Medications like Tylenol PM and Excedrin PM combine a pain reliever with a sleep-inducing antihistamine, the same ingredient that people take for hay fever or cold symptoms. Although they make people drowsy, they can leave you feeling groggy the next day, and they dry out the nose and mouth.[14]

▪ **Cough syrup.** Chugging cough syrup (also called *roboing,* after the OTC medication Robitussin) is a growing problem, in part because young people think of dextromethorphan (DXM), a common ingredient in cough medicine, as a "poor man's version" of the popular drug ecstasy.

PRESCRIPTION DRUGS

Both doctors and patients make errors when it comes to prescription drugs. The most frequent mistakes doctors make are over- or under-dosing, omitting information from prescriptions, ordering the wrong dosage form (a pill instead of a liquid, for example), and not recognizing a patient's allergy to a drug.

National attention focused on widely used prescription painkillers after Vioxx and Bextra, two popular medications for pain, were taken off the market. Evidence suggested that these drugs, called COX-2 inhibitors (which block a hormone that promotes inflammation), may double the risk of heart attacks and strokes. Bextra was also linked to serious but rare skin conditions. Celebrex remains on the market but with a black box on the label that warns of possible cardiovascular and gastrointestinal problems.[15] Older pain relievers like ibuprofen (Advil, Motrin, and others) are safe, less expensive, and just as effective in relieving pain.[16]

Abuse

The three classes of prescription drugs that are most commonly abused are:

▪ **Opioids,** which are most often prescribed to treat pain. These include OxyContin, Vicodin, Darvon, Dilaudid, and Demerol.

▪ **Central nervous system (CNS) depressants,** such as Valium, Librium, and Xanax, which treat anxiety, panic attacks, and sleep disorders.

▪ **Stimulants,** which are mainly prescribed for the sleep disorder narcolepsy and attention-deficit hyperactivity disorder (ADHD). These medications include Ritalin, Concerta, Metadate, Adderall, Dexedrine, and Desoxyn.

Savvy Consumer ▪▪ Avoiding Medication Mistakes

- Whenever you get a prescription, be sure to find out from your doctor and pharmacist the name of the drug, what it's supposed to do, and how and when to take it and for how long. Are there foods, drinks, other medications, or activities you should avoid while taking the medication?

- Ask if the drug causes any side effects and what you should do if any occur.

- Keep a record of all your medicines, listing both their brand and generic (chemical) names and the reason you are taking them, and update it regularly. Give a copy of this list to every physician and every pharmacy providing health-care services.

- Inform your doctors of any over-the-counter drugs, vitamins, and herbal products you use regularly. Popular herbal supplements like gingko bilboa and common over-the-counter drugs like aspirin can interact with many prescription drugs to cause

serious problems, such as excessive bleeding.

- Always turn on the lights when you take your medication. Familiarize yourself with the imprint on each tablet or capsule so you can recognize each pill. If a refill looks different, check with your pharmacist or doctor before taking it.

- Don't crush or chew a medicine without checking with your doctor or pharmacist first. Some medications are designed for gradual release rather than all at once and could be harmful if absorbed too quickly.

- Don't use a kitchen spoon to dispense liquid medications. Household teaspoons can hold between 3 and 7 milliliters; a prescription "teaspoon" means 5 milliliters. Either measure the dose in the cup or dropper that came with the medicine or ask the pharmacist for a measuring device.

- Never take someone else's medications. They could interact with your

medications or the dose may be different.

- Always check labels for warnings on interactions with alcohol and instructions on whether or not to take before, with, or after meals.

- Don't take medicine with grapefruit juice, which can interact with more than 200 medications, including cholesterol-lowering statins, sleeping pills, and antianxiety agents.

- Plan ahead to make sure you have adequate amounts of the medications you need.

- Don't leave medicines in a car for prolonged periods. Temperature extremes, along with moisture, light, and oxygen, can affect the potency of many medications.

- Use cues, such as the alarm on your cell phone or Palm Pilot or Post-it notes, to remind you to take your medication on schedule.

Table 11-1 lists the effects of their short- and long-term use. These prescription drugs should not be used with the drugs listed in the last column because of negative drug interactions.

 As discussed later in this chapter, abuse of prescription stimulants and opioids is widespread on college campuses. Various studies have reported that 8 to 17 percent of students abuse stimulants.[17] In a large national survey, 12 percent of undergraduates reported lifetime use of a prescription painkiller for nonmedical reasons; 7 percent had abused painkillers in the previous year.[18]

 Men and women have roughly similar rates of abuse of prescription drugs and are equally likely to become addicted. However, among women and men who abuse a sedative or antianxiety drug, women are almost two times more likely to become addicted than men.

Nonadherence

Many prescribed medications aren't taken the way they should be; millions simply aren't taken at all. As many as 70 percent of adults have trouble understanding dosage information and 30 percent can't read standard labels, according to the FDA, which has called for larger, clearer drug labeling. The dangers of nonadherence (not properly taking prescription drugs) include recurrent infections, serious medical complications, and emergency hospital treatment. The drugs most likely to be taken incorrectly are those that treat problems with no obvious symptoms (such

as high blood pressure), require complex dosage schedules, treat psychiatric disorders, or have unpleasant side effects.

Some people skip prescribed doses or stop taking medications because they fear that any drug can cause tolerance and eventual dependence. Others fail to let doctors know about side effects. For instance, patients may stop taking anti-inflammatory drugs because they irritate their stomach. However, taking the drugs with food can eliminate this problem. The side effects of other drugs may disappear as a person's body becomes accustomed to the drug.

Physical Side Effects

Most medications, taken correctly, cause only minor complications. However, no drug is entirely without side effects for all individuals taking it. Serious complications that may occur include heart failure, heart attack, seizures, kidney and liver failure, severe blood disorders, birth defects, blindness, memory problems, and allergic reactions.

Allergic reactions to drugs are common. The drugs that most often provoke allergic responses are penicillin and other antibiotics (drugs used to treat infection). Aspirin, sulfa drugs, barbiturates, anticonvulsants, insulin, and local anesthetics can also provoke allergic responses. Allergic reactions range from mild rashes or hives to anaphylaxis—a life-threatening constriction of the airways and sudden drop of blood pressure that causes rapid pulse, weakness, paleness, confusion, nausea, vomiting, unconsciousness, and collapse. This extreme response, which is rare, requires

TABLE 11-1 USE AND EFFECTS OF SOME COMMON MEDICATIONS

	Prescribed for	In the Body	Effects of Short-term Use	Effects of Long-term Use	Should Not Be Used with
OPIOIDS					
OxyContin Darvon Vicodin Dilaudid Demerol Lomotil	• Postsurgical pain relief • Management of acute or chronic pain • Relief of coughs and diarrhea	Block the transmission of pain messages to the brain	• Blocked pain messages • Drowsiness • Constipation • Depressed respiration (depending on dose)	Potential for tolerance, physical dependence, and addiction	• Alcohol • Antihistamines • Barbiturates • Benzodiazepines • General anesthetics
CENTRAL NERVOUS SYSTEM DEPRESSANTS					
Valium Librium Xanax Halcion ProSom Mebaral Nembutal	• Anxiety • Tension • Panic attacks • Acute stress reactions • Sleep disorders • Anesthesia (at high doses)	Slow brain activity, producing a calming effect	• "Sleepy" and uncoordinated feeling during the first few days; as the body becomes used to the effects, these feelings diminish	Potential for tolerance, physical dependence and addiction	• Alcohol • Prescription opioid pain medicines • Some OTC cold and allergy medications
STIMULANTS					
Dexedrine Ritalin Meridia	• Narcolepsy • Attention-deficit hyperactivity disorder (ADHD) • Depression that does not respond to other treatments	Enhance brain activity, causing an increase in alertness, attention, and energy	• Elevated blood pressure • Increased heart rate • Increased respiration • Suppressed appetite • Sleep deprivation	Potential for addiction	• OTC cold medicines containing decongestants • Antidepressants, unless supervised by a physician • Some asthma medications

Source: National Institute on Drug Abuse, www.nida.nih.gov/ResearchReports/Prescription/prescription8.html

immediate treatment with an injection of epinephrine (adrenaline) to open the airways and blood vessels.

Psychological Side Effects

Dozens of drugs—both over-the-counter and prescription—can cause changes in the way people think, feel, and behave. Unfortunately, neither patients nor their physicians usually connect such symptoms with medications. Doctors may not even mention potential mental and emotional problems because they don't want to scare patients away from what otherwise may be a very effective treatment. What you don't know about a drug's effects on your mind *can* hurt you.

Among the medications most likely to cause psychiatric side effects are drugs for high blood pressure, heart disease, asthma, epilepsy, arthritis, Parkinson's disease, anxiety, insomnia, and depression. Some drugs—such as the powerful hormones called *corticosteroids,* used for asthma, autoimmune diseases, and cancer—can cause different psychiatric symptoms, depending on dosage and other factors. Other drugs, such as ulcer medications, can cause delirium and disorientation, especially when given in high doses or to elderly patients. More subtle problems, such as forgetfulness or irritability, are common reactions to many drugs that are likely to be ignored or dismissed. The older you are, the sicker you are, and the more medications you're taking, the

greater your risk of developing some psychiatric side effects. Even medications that don't usually cause problems, such as antibiotics, can cause psychiatric side effects in some individuals.

Any medication that slows down bodily systems, as many high blood pressure and cardiac drugs do, can cause depressive symptoms. Estrogen in birth control pills can cause mood changes. As many as 15 percent of women using oral contraceptives have reported feeling depressed or moody. For many people, switching to another medication quickly lifts a drug-induced depression.

Drug Interactions

OTC and prescription drugs can interact in a variety of ways. For example, mixing some cold medications with tranquilizers can cause drowsiness and coordination problems, thus making driving dangerous. Moreover, what you eat or drink can impair or completely wipe out the effectiveness of drugs or lead to unexpected effects on the body. For instance, aspirin takes five to ten times as long to be absorbed when taken with food or shortly after a meal than when taken on an empty stomach. If tetracyclines encounter calcium in the stomach, they bind together and cancel each other out.

To avoid potentially dangerous interactions, check the label(s) for any instructions on how or when to take a medication, such as "with a meal." If the directions say that you should take a drug on an empty stomach, take it at least one hour before eating or two or three hours after eating. Don't drink a hot beverage with a medication; the temperature may interfere with the effectiveness of the drug.

Whenever you take a drug, be especially careful of your intake of alcohol, which can change the rate of metabolism and the effects of many different drugs. Because it dilates the blood vessels, alcohol can add to the dizziness sometimes caused by drugs for high blood pressure, angina, or depression. Also, its irritating effects on the stomach can worsen stomach upset from aspirin, ibuprofen, and other anti-inflammatory drugs.

Generic Drugs

The **generic** name is the chemical name for a drug. A specific drug may appear on the pharmacist's shelf under a variety of brand names, which may cost more than twice the generic equivalent. About 75 percent of all prescriptions specify a brand name, but pharmacists may—and in some states must—switch to a generic drug unless the doctor specifically tells them not to. Prescriptions filled with generic drugs cost 20 to 85 percent less than their brand-name counterparts.

Generic drugs have the same active ingredients as brand-name prescriptions, but their fillers and binders, which can affect the absorption of a drug, may be different. For some serious illnesses, the generics may not be as effective; some experts recommend sticking with brand names for heart medications, psychiatric drugs, and anticonvulsant drugs (for epilepsy and other seizure disorders).

To determine whether you should buy the generic version of a drug, ask your physician whether it matters if you get a brand-name or generic drug. If it does, ask which brand name is best. Also, find out if switching to a generic or from one generic to another might harm your condition in any way.

(FAQ) What Should I Know About Buying Drugs Online?

Millions of people in the United States purchase prescription medications online. Although some websites fill only faxed prescriptions from medical doctors, others ignore or sidestep traditional regulations and safeguards. Cyberspace distributors often ship pills across state lines without requiring a physical examination by a medical doctor. Instead, a "cyberdoc," who may or may not be qualified or up-to-date in a given specialty, reviews information submitted by a "patient." International pharmacies sometimes sell drugs that are not available or approved in the United States. And patients themselves use bulletin boards and other online resources to sell unused or unwanted medications to each other.

Many individuals turn to the Internet for "lifestyle" drugs such as pills for erectile dysfunction, weight control, and smoking cessation. Customers like the convenience and anonymity of buying drugs online. Although many assume drugs cost less on the Internet, shipping costs tend to drive prices up to the same amount or more than the price at a pharmacy.

The dangers of unregulated distribution of medications have alarmed government agencies and medical groups. The American Medical Association has declared it unethical for physicians to write prescriptions for people they've never met. The National Association of Boards of Pharmacy has developed a seal of approval to help customers determine which sites are legitimate. The FDA and other federal agencies, such as the Federal Trade Commission, which regulates advertising, are trying to find ways to impose some controls.

Consumers have to be wary. Ordering a drug like Accutane, an acne treatment, online may seem harmless. However, without close monitoring by a physician, you could develop complications, such as a bad reaction that aggravates hepatitis or inflames the pancreas. Quality control is another concern. Cyberspace pharmacies provide no information on how the drug was stored or whether its expiration date has passed. In addition, since importing medications without a prescription is against the law, you could find yourself in legal trouble.

CAFFEINE AND ITS EFFECTS

Caffeine, which has been drunk, chewed, and swallowed since the Stone Age, is the most widely used **psychotropic** (mind-affecting) drug in the world. Eighty percent of Americans drink coffee, our principal caffeine source—an average of 3.5 cups a day. Coffee contains 100 to 150 milligrams of caffeine per cup; tea, 40 to 100 milligrams; cola, about 45 milligrams. Most medications that contain caffeine are one-third to one-half the strength of a cup of coffee. However, some, such as Excedrin, are very high in caffeine (Table 11-2).

Despite 20 years of reassuring research, many people still avoid caffeinated coffee because they worry about its health effects. In moderation—a few cups a day—coffee is a safe beverage that may offer some health benefits, including lowering the risk for type 2 diabetes.[19] Coffee also may reduce the likelihood of gallstones, Parkinson's disease, and colon cancer.[20]

As a stimulant, caffeine relieves drowsiness, helps in the performance of repetitive tasks, and improves the capacity for work. Caffeine improves performance and endurance during prolonged, exhaustive exercise, and to a lesser degree, enhances short-term, high-intensity athletic performance. Additional benefits include improved concentration, reduced fatigue, and sharpened alertness.

Although doctors have long cautioned against caffeine consumption by people whose hearts "flutter" or beat quickly, recent research has found no evidence for this recommendation.[21] Major sports organizations ban excessive use of caffeine, but these policies remain controversial.

TABLE 11-2 CAFFEINE COUNTS

Substance (typical serving)	Caffeine (milligrams)
No Doz, one pill	200
Coffee (drip), one 5-ounce cup	130
Excedrin, two pills	130
Espresso, one 2-ounce cup	100
Energy drink, one can	80
Instant coffee, one 5-ounce cup	74
Coca-Cola, 12 ounces	46
Tea, one 5-ounce cup	40
Dark chocolate, 1 ounce	20
Milk chocolate, 1 ounce	6
Cocoa, 5 ounces	4
Decaffeinated coffee, one 5-ounce cup	3

 Caffeinated energy drinks such as Red Bull, which typically contain sugar, caffeine, and an amino acid called taurine, are popular on campus. Health experts caution that they should not be mixed with alcohol. Also, do not drink them before intense exercise because of the increased risk of dehydration. In a study of college men and women who normally consumed fewer than three caffeinated beverages per day, caffeine boosted anxiety but did not significantly affect performance on various low-intensity tasks, except for hand-eye coordination, which improved.

You'll stay more alert, particularly if you are fighting sleep deprivation, if you spread your coffee consumption over the course of the day. For instance, rather than drinking two 8-ounce cups in the morning, try consuming smaller servings of an ounce or two during the course of the day.[22]

(FAQ) IS IT POSSIBLE TO OVERDOSE ON CAFFEINE?

Yes, you can overdose on caffeine. The characteristic symptoms of caffeine intoxication are restlessness, nervousness, excitement, insomnia, flushed face, increased urination, digestive complaints, muscle twitching, rambling thoughts and speech, rapid heart rate or arrhythmias, periods of inexhaustibility, and physical restlessness. Some people develop these symptoms after as little as 250 milligrams of caffeine a day; others, only with much larger doses. Higher doses may produce ringing in the ears or flashes of light, grand mal seizures, and potentially fatal respiratory failure.

Caffeine withdrawal for those dependent on this substance can cause headaches and other neurological symptoms. Those who must cut back should taper off gradually. One approach is to mix regular and decaffeinated coffee, gradually decreasing the quantity of the former.

SUBSTANCE USE DISORDERS

People have been using mind-altering, or **psychoactive,** chemicals for centuries. Citizens of ancient Mesopotamia and Egypt used opium. More than 3,000 years ago, Hindus included cannabis products in religious ceremonies. For centuries the Inca in South America have chewed the leaves of the coca bush. Yet while drugs existed in most societies, their use was usually limited to small groups. Today millions of people regularly turn to drugs to pick them up, bring them down, alter perceptions, or ease psychological pain.

After growing significantly in the past half century, the spread of drugs has slowed: 95 percent of the world's people do not use illegal drugs, according to the United Nations. In the last year, fewer than one in every 30 people between ages 15 to 64 used an illicit drug.[23]

In the United States, drug use by young teenagers dropped dramatically in the last decade—from 24 percent to 15 percent.[24] Fewer young people report that they use or have ever used marijuana, ecstasy, amphetamines, methamphetamine, PCP, ketamine, and steroids (discussed in Chapter 5). Among college students, the most widely used drugs are marijuana and "club drugs," including ecstasy, although abuse of prescription stimulant medications has grown.

MEN, WOMEN, AND DRUGS

Beginning at a very early age, males and females show different patterns in drug use. Among 12-year-olds who have been offered drugs, boys are more likely to have received those offers from other males or their parents. Girls

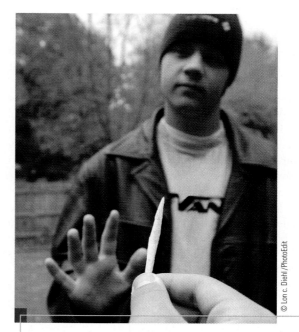

More teenagers are saying no to drugs.

are most likely to have been offered drugs by a female friend or family member. The social setting and nature of drug offers also differ by gender. Boys are more likely to receive offers in a public setting, such as on the street or in a park, and the offers typically emphasize "benefits," such as improved status or self-image. Girls are more likely to receive a straightforward "do you want some?" offer or one that minimizes the risks of drug use. For girls, these offers are usually made in a private setting such as a friend's home.

Men generally encounter more opportunities to use drugs than women, but given an opportunity to use drugs for the first time, both genders are equally likely to do so and to progress from initial use to dependence. Vulnerability to some drugs varies with gender. Both are equally likely to become addicted to or dependent on cocaine, heroin, hallucinogens, tobacco, and inhalants. Women are more likely than men to become addicted to or dependent on sedatives and drugs designed to treat anxiety or sleeplessness and less likely than men to abuse alcohol and marijuana.

Males and females may differ in their biological responses to drugs. In studies of animals given the opportunity to self-administer intravenous doses of cocaine or heroin, females began self-administration sooner than males and administered larger amounts of the drugs. Women may be more sensitive than men to the cardiovascular effects of cocaine. In human studies, women and men given equal doses of cocaine experienced the same cardiovascular response despite the fact that blood concentrations of cocaine did not rise as high in women as in men. Male and female long-term cocaine users showed similar impairment in tests of concentration, memory, and academic achievement following sustained abstinence, even though women in the study had substantially greater exposure to cocaine. Women cocaine users also were less likely than men to exhibit abnormalities of blood flow in the brain's frontal lobes. These findings suggest a gender-related mechanism that may protect women from some of the damage cocaine inflicts on the brain. However, women are more vulnerable to poor nutrition and below-average weight, depression, physical abuse, and if pregnant, preterm labor or early delivery.

Substance abuse compounds the risk of AIDS for women, who may become infected with HIV by sharing needles with other injection-drug users and by engaging in unprotected sex. In all, drug abuse is nearly twice as likely to be directly or indirectly associated with AIDS in women as in men.

There are also differences between men and women who seek treatment for drug abuse. Women in treatment programs are less likely than men to have graduated from high school and to be employed and are more likely than men to have other health problems, to have sought previous drug treatment, to have attempted suicide, and to have suffered sexual abuse or other physical abuse. Traditional drug treatment programs, created for men, have proved to be less effective for women than programs that provide more comprehensive services, including child care, assertiveness training, and parenting training.

UNDERSTANDING SUBSTANCE USE DISORDERS

In early Roman law, *addictus* referred to someone who, because he could not pay his debts, was sentenced into slavery. Indeed, one of the meanings of addiction given by the *Oxford Latin Dictionary* is "enslavement." For much of the twentieth century, addiction to drugs was viewed as a social or criminal problem, and the only people called addicts were "drug-crazed junkies" desperate for a fix. In the 1960s, however, when scientists switched to the *medical model* for understanding addictions, they began to view addictions to chemicals—such as alcohol and psychoactive drugs—as lifelong chronic diseases that affect a person's mind and body.

Today the word **addiction** has moved out of the realm of scientific terminology and into the cultural mainstream. Among laypeople, addiction refers to the habitual use of substances, such as alcohol, psychoactive drugs, and nicotine, and also to compulsive behaviors, such as gambling (see page 305) and overeating (discussed in Chapter 7). Like drugs, these activities can be used repeatedly to numb pain or enhance pleasure; some may alter a person's brain chemistry or create cravings; all can lead to a loss of internal control.

Chemical addiction is now viewed as a lifelong, chronic illness that affects mind, body, and spirit. Its key characteristics are repeated drug use, loss of control over how much or how often a person takes a drug, and continued use despite harmful consequences.

Because addiction is considered too broad and judgmental a term for scientific use, mental health professionals describe drug-related problems in terms of *dependence* and *abuse*. However, they agree that addiction has four characteristic symptoms: compulsion to use the substance, loss of control, negative consequences, and denial (see Self Survey: "Do You Have a Substance Use Disorder?").

DEPENDENCE

Individuals may develop **psychological dependence** and feel a strong craving for a drug because it produces pleasurable feelings or relieves stress and anxiety. **Physical dependence** occurs when a person develops *tolerance* to the effects of a drug and needs larger and larger doses to achieve intoxication or another desired effect. Individuals who are physically dependent and have a high tolerance to a drug may take amounts many times those that would produce intoxication or an overdose in someone who was not a regular user.

Men and women with a substance dependence disorder may use a drug to avoid or relieve withdrawal symptoms, or they may consume larger amounts of a drug or use it over a longer period than they'd originally intended. They may repeatedly try to cut down or control drug use without success; spend a great deal of time obtaining or using drugs or recovering from their effects; give up or reduce important social, occupational, or recreational activities because of their drug use; or continue to use a drug despite knowledge that the drug is likely to cause or worsen a persistent or recurring physical or psychological problem.

Specific symptoms of dependence vary with particular drugs. Some drugs, such as marijuana, hallucinogens, and phencyclidine, do not cause withdrawal symptoms. The degree of dependence also varies. In mild cases, a person may function normally most of the time. In severe cases, the person's entire life may revolve around obtaining, using, and recuperating from the effects of a drug.

Individuals with drug dependence become intoxicated or high on a regular basis—whether every day, every weekend, or several binges a year. They may try repeatedly to stop using a drug and yet fail, even though they realize their drug use is interfering with their health, family life, relationships, and work.

Abuse

Some drug users do not develop the symptoms of tolerance and withdrawal that characterize dependence, yet they use drugs in ways that clearly have a harmful effect on them. These individuals are diagnosed as having a *psychoactive substance abuse disorder.* They continue to use drugs despite their awareness of persistent or repeated social, occupational, psychological, or physical problems related to drug use, or they use drugs in dangerous ways or situations (before driving, for instance).

Intoxication and Withdrawal

Intoxication refers to maladaptive behavioral, psychological, and physiologic changes that occur as a result of substance use. **Withdrawal** is the development of symptoms that cause significant psychological and physical distress when an individual reduces or stops drug use. (Intoxication and withdrawal from specific drugs are discussed later in this chapter.)

Polyabuse

Most users prefer a certain type of drug but also use several others; this behavior is called **polyabuse.** The average user who enters treatment is on five different drugs. The more drugs anyone uses, the greater the chance of side effects, complications, and possibly life-threatening interactions.

Coexisting Conditions

Mental disorders and substance abuse disorders have a great deal of overlap. Most adolescents with substance abuse disorders also have another psychiatric disorder, such as depression.[25] Individuals with such *dual diagnoses* require careful evaluation and appropriate treatment for the complete range of complex and chronic difficulties they face. However, they can benefit from participation in 12-step groups, like Double Trouble in Recovery, that provide treatment for both.[26]

(FAQ) WHAT CAUSES DRUG DEPENDENCE AND ABUSE?

No one fully understands why some people develop drug dependence or abuse disorders, whereas others, who may experiment briefly with drugs, do not. Inherited body chemistry, genetic factors, and sensitivity to drugs may make some individuals more susceptible. These disorders may stem from many complex causes.

The Biology of Dependence

Scientists now view drug dependence as a brain disease triggered by frequent use of drugs that change the biochemistry and anatomy of neurons and alter the way they work. A major breakthrough in understanding dependence has been the discovery that certain mood-altering substances and experiences—a puff of marijuana, a slug of whiskey, a snort of cocaine, a big win at blackjack—trigger a rise in a brain chemical called *dopamine,* which is associated with feelings of satisfaction and euphoria. This brain chemical or neurotransmitter is one of the crucial messengers that links nerve cells in the brain and its level rises during any pleasurable experience, whether it be a loving hug or a taste of chocolate.

The mechanism governing the rise in dopamine levels is not the same for all drugs. Figure 11-2 shows the one for cocaine. Normally, after dopamine is released from the axon terminal of a neuron and activates dopamine receptors on the adjacent neuron, the dopamine is then transported back to its original neuron by "uptake pumps." Cocaine binds to the uptake pumps and prevents them from transporting dopamine back into the neuron terminal. So more dopamine builds up in the synapse and is free to activate more dopamine receptors.[27]

Addictive drugs have such a powerful impact on dopamine and its receptors that they change the pathways within the brain's pleasure centers. Various psychoactive chemicals create a craving for more of the same. According to this hypothesis, addicts do not specifically yearn for heroin,

---

Strategies for Prevention :: Saying No to Drugs

If people offer you a drug, here are some ways to say no.

:: Let them know you're not interested. Change the subject. If the pressure seems threatening, just walk away.

:: Have something else to do: "No, I'm going for a walk now."

:: Be prepared for different types of pressure. If your friends tease you, tease them back.

:: Keep it simple. "No, thanks," "No," or "No way" all get the point across.

:: Hang out with people who won't offer you drugs.

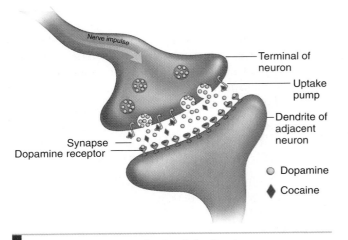

FIGURE 11-2 Dopamine Levels for Cocaine
Within the synapses between adjacent neurons, cocaine binds to the dopamine uptake pumps and thus allows the neurotransmitter dopamine to build up in the synapse and bind to more dopamine receptors.

cocaine, or nicotine but for the rush of dopamine that these drugs produce. Other brain chemicals, including gluta-mate, GABA (gamma-aminobutyric acid), and possibly nor-epinephrine, may also be involved. Some individuals, born with low levels of dopamine, may be particularly susceptible to addiction.

The Psychology of Vulnerability

Although scientists do not believe there is an addictive personality, certain individuals are at greater risk of drug dependence because of psychological factors, including difficulty controlling impulses, a lack of values that might constrain drug use (whether based in religion, family, or so-ciety), low self-esteem, feelings of powerlessness, and de-pression. The one psychological trait most often linked with drug use is denial. Young people in particular are absolutely convinced that they will never lose control or suffer in any way as a result of drug use.

Many diagnosed drug users have at least one mental disorder, particularly depression or anxiety. Disorders that emerge in adolescence, such as bipolar disorder, may in-crease the risk of substance abuse. Many people with psychiatric disorders abuse drugs. Individuals may self-administer drugs to treat psychiatric symptoms; for example, they may take sedating drugs to suppress a panic attack. Contrary to past concerns, treatment of attention deficit/ hyperactivity disorder (ADHD) with stimulant medication does not increase the risk of substance abuse disorders later in life but may in fact decrease their likelihood.[28]

Early Influences

Teen drug abuse has declined in the last decade, but some teens remain more vulnerable. Young people from lower socioeconomic backgrounds are more likely to use drugs than their more affluent peers, possibly because of economic

disadvantage; family instability; a lack of realistic, rewarding alternatives and role models; and increased hopelessness.

 Those whose companions are substance abusers are far more likely to use drugs. Peer pressure to use drugs can be a powerful factor for adolescents, al-though having a drug-using roommate does not increase the odds that a college student will use drugs.[29] The likelihood of drug abuse is also related to family instability, parental re-jection, and divorce.

Parents' own attitudes and drug-use history affect their children's likelihood of using marijuana, according to the Substance Abuse and Mental Health Services Administra-tion. Parents who perceive little risk associated with mari-juana use have children with similar attitudes, and the chil-dren of parents who used marijuana are more likely to try the drug than children whose parents never used the drug.

DRUGS AND DRIVING

About one in three adult drivers ages 21 to 25 have driven under the influence of alcohol or drugs during the past year, according to the Substance Abuse and Mental Health Ser-vices Administration. Older drivers are less likely than youn-ger drivers to drive while under the influence of alcohol or illicit drugs. Among those ages 26 to 34, 24 percent drove while under the influence of alcohol or illicit drugs in the past year, as did 19 percent of those ages 35 to 49.[30]

Different drugs affect driving ability in different ways. Here are the facts from the National Institute on Drug Abuse:

- **Alcohol affects perception, coordination, and judgment,** and increases the sedative effects of tranquilizers and barbiturates.

- **Marijuana affects a wide range of driving skills**—including the ability to track (stay in the lane) through curves, brake quickly, and maintain speed and a safe distance between cars—and slows thinking and reflexes. Normal driving skills remain impaired for four to six hours after smoking a single joint.

- **Sedatives, hypnotics, and antianxiety agents slow reaction time** and interfere with hand–eye coordination and judgment; the greatest impairment is in the first hour after taking the drug. The effects depend on the particular drug: some build up in the body and can impair driving skills the morning after use; others make drivers very sleepy and therefore incapable of driving safely.

- **Amphetamines, after repeated use, impair coordination.** They can also make a driver more edgy and less coordinated and thus more likely to be involved in an accident.

- **Hallucinogens distort judgment** and reality and cause confusion and panic, thus making driving ex-tremely dangerous.

COMMON DRUGS OF ABUSE

Table 11-3 describes the common drugs of abuse within these categories: cannabis, "club drugs," stimulants, depressants, hallucinogens, and inhalants.

CANNABIS

Marijuana (pot) and **hashish** (hash)—the most widely used illegal drugs—are derived from the cannabis plant. The major psychoactive ingredient in both is *THC (delta-9-tetrahydrocannabinol)*. Marijuana is the most widely abused substance, with more than 150 million people reporting they've used it at least once in the last year. Some 12 million Americans use cannabis; more than 1 million cannot control this use.

Teens and young adults who use marijuana are more likely to develop serious mental health problems. According to the National Survey on Drug Use and Health, among individuals age 18 years or older, those who first used marijuana before age 12 were twice as likely to have a serious mental illness as those who first used marijuana at age 18 or older.[31]

 Marijuana use is generally less pervasive than binge-drinking (see Chapter 12) on most campuses, although at some schools as many as a third of students report smoking pot. Students who used marijuana in high school are more likely to do so in college. Roommates have very little impact on drug use. Men who have not used marijuana before college seem if anything, turned off rather than turned on by roommates who have smoked pot. Peers have no clear impact on women's marijuana use.[32]

Different types of marijuana have different percentages of THC. Because of careful cultivation, the strength of today's marijuana is much greater than that used in the 1970s. Today a marijuana joint contains 150 mg of THC, compared to 10 mg in the 1960s.

Usually, marijuana is smoked in a joint (hand-rolled cigarette) or pipe; it may also be eaten as an ingredient in other foods (as when baked in brownies), though with a less predictable effect. The drug high is enhanced by holding the marijuana smoke in the lungs, and experienced smokers learn to hold the smoke for longer periods to increase the amount of drug diffused into the bloodstream. The circumstances in which marijuana is smoked, the communal aspects of its use, and the user's experience all can affect the way a marijuana-induced high feels.

Marijuana has shown some medical benefits, including boosting appetite in patients who are HIV-positive or undergoing chemotherapy, alleviating cancer and neck pain, helping reduce pressure on the eyeball in glaucoma patients, and helping people with spasticity (extreme muscle tension) due to multiple sclerosis or injuries.[33]

Support for the legalization of marijuana for medicinal purposes has grown in recent years, although the majority of Americans still oppose such legislation. Several states allow marijuana to be grown and distributed to people with a doctor's recommendation.

Advocates for the legalization of marijuana contend that making pot legal would reduce the black market and violence associated with its sale and ensure its availability for medicinal purposes. Opponents argue that legalization would increase the number of people who use marijuana and suffer harmful effects such as slowed brain function and lung damage. Should marijuana possession remain a criminal offense? Or should individuals have the right to choose to use this drug? **You decide.**

How Users Feel

In low to moderate doses, marijuana typically creates a mild sense of euphoria, a sense of slowed time (five minutes may feel like an hour), a dreamy sort of self-absorption, and some impairment in thinking and communicating. Users report heightened sensations of color, sound, and other stimuli, relaxation, and increased confidence. The sense of being stoned peaks within half an hour and usually lasts about three hours. Even when alterations in perception seem slight, as noted earlier, it is not safe to drive a car for as long as four to six hours after smoking a single joint.

Some users—particularly those smoking marijuana for the first time or taking a high dose in an unpleasant or unfamiliar setting—experience acute anxiety, which may be accompanied by a panicky fear of losing control. They may believe that their companions are ridiculing or threatening them and experience a panic attack, a state of intense terror.

The immediate physical effects of marijuana include increased pulse rate, bloodshot eyes, dry mouth and throat, slowed reaction times, impaired motor skills, increased appetite, and diminished short-term memory (Figure 11-3). High doses reduce the ability to perceive and to react; all the reactions experienced with low doses are intensified, leading to sensory distortion and, in the case of hashish, vivid hallucinations and LSD-like, psychedelic reactions. The drug remains in the body's fat cells 50 hours or more after use, so people may experience psychoactive effects for several days after use. Drug tests may produce positive results for days or weeks after last use.

Risks

Marijuana produces a range of effects in different bodily systems, such as depression, diminished immune responses, and impaired fertility in men.[34] Other risks include damage to the brain, lungs, and heart, and to babies born to mothers who use marijuana during pregnancy or while nursing (see Figure 11-3).

Brain THC produces changes in the brain that affect learning, memory, and the way the brain integrates sensory experiences with emotions and motivations. Short-term effects include problems with memory and learning; distorted perceptions; difficulty thinking and problem solving; loss of

TABLE 11-3 COMMONLY ABUSED DRUGS

Drug	Street Names	How It's Used	Intoxication Effects / Potential Health Consequences
CANNABIS			
Marijuana	Pot, grass, reefer, weed, blunt, dope, ganja, grass, herb, joints, Mary Jane, sinsemilla, skunk	Smoked, swallowed	Euphoria, slowed thinking and reaction time, confusion, impaired balance and coordination / Cough, frequent respiratory infections; impaired memory and learning; increased heart rate, anxiety; panic attacks; tolerance, addiction
CLUB DRUGS			
MDMA	Ecstasy, E, Eve, X, XTC, clarity, lover's speed, peace, STP	Swallowed	Mild hallucinogenic effects, increased tactile sensitivity, empathic feelings / Impaired memory and learning, hyperthermia, cardiac toxicity, renal failure, liver toxicity
GHB	G, Georgia home boy, grievous bodily harm, liquid ecstasy	Swallowed	Reduced anxiety, feeling of well-being, lowered inhibitions, slowed pulse and breathing, lowered blood pressure, poor concentration / Fatigue; confusion; impaired coordination, memory, judgment; addiction, drowsiness, nausea/vomiting, headache, loss of consciousness, loss of reflexes, seizures, coma, death
Ketamine	Cat, Valiums, K, Special-K, vitamin K	Injected, snorted, smoked	Increased heart rate and blood pressure, impaired motor function / Memory loss; numbness; nausea/vomiting; at high doses, delirium, depression, respiratory depression, and arrest
Nitrites	Poppers	Inhaled	Stimulation, loss of inhibition; headache; nausea/vomiting; slurred speech; loss of motor coordination; wheezing / Unconsciousness, cramps, weight loss, muscle weakness, depression, memory impairment, damage to cardiovascular and nervous systems, sudden death
STIMULANTS			Increased heart rate, blood pressure, metabolism; feelings of exhilaration, energy, increased mental alertness / Rapid or irregular heart beat; reduced appetite, weight loss, heart failure, nervousness, insomnia
Amphetamine	Bennies, black beauties, crosses, hearts, LA turnaround, speed, truck drivers, uppers	Injected, swallowed, smoked, snorted	In addition to preceding: Rapid breathing / Tremor, loss of coordination; irritability, anxiousness, restlessness, delirium, panic, paranoia, impulsive behavior, aggressiveness, tolerance, addiction, psychosis
Methamphetamine	Chalk, crank, crystal, fire, glass, go fast, ice, meth, speed	Injected, swallowed, smoked, snorted	In addition to preceding: Aggression, violence, psychotic behavior / Memory loss, cardiac and neurological damage; impaired memory and learning, tolerance, addiction
Cocaine	Blow, bump, C, candy, Charlie, coke, crack, flake, rock, snow, toot	Injected, smoked, snorted	In addition to preceding: Increased temperature / Chest pain, respiratory failure, nausea, abdominal pain, strokes, seizures, headaches, malnutrition, panic attacks
DEPRESSANTS			Reduced anxiety; feeling of well-being; lowered inhibitions; slowed pulse and breathing; lowered blood pressure; poor concentration / Fatigue; confusion; impaired coordination, memory, judgment; addiction; respiratory depression and arrest, death
Benzodiazepines	Candy, downers, sleeping pills, tranks	Swallowed, injected	In addition to preceding: Sedation, drowsiness / Dizziness
Rohypnol	Forget-me pill, Mexican Valium, R2, Roche, roofies, roofinol, rope, rophies	Swallowed, snorted	Visual and gastrointestinal disturbances, urinary retention, memory loss for the time under the drug's effects
Barbiturates	Barbs, reds, red birds, phennies, tooies, yellows, yellow jackets	Injected, swallowed	In addition to preceding: Sedation, drowsiness / Depression, unusual excitement, fever, irritability, poor judgment, slurred speech, dizziness, life-threatening withdrawal

TABLE 11-3 (*continued*)

Drug	Street Names	How It's Used	Intoxication Effects / Potential Health Consequences
Opioids			Pain relief, euphoria, drowsiness / Nausea, constipation, confusion, sedation, respiratory depression and arrest, tolerance, addiction, unconsciousness, coma, death
Heroin	Brown sugar, dope, H, horse, junk, skag, skunk, smack, white horse	Injected, smoked, snorted	
Morphine	Miss Emma, monkey, white stuff	Injected, swallowed, smoked	
Codeine	Captain Cody, Cody, schoolboy	Injected, swallowed	
OxyContin	Oxy, OC, Killer	Swallowed, snorted, injected	
Vicodin	Vike, Watson-387	Swallowed	
HALLUCINOGENS			Altered states of perception and feeling / Nausea; persisting perception disorder (flashbacks)
LSD	Acid, blotter, boomers, cubes, microdot, yellow sunshines	Swallowed, absorbed through mouth tissues	In addition to preceding: Increased body temperature, heart rate, blood pressure; loss of appetite, sleeplessness, numbness, weakness, tremors, persistent mental disorders
PCP	Angel dust, boat, hog, love boat, peace pill	Injected, swallowed, smoked	Impaired motor function, possible decrease in blood pressure and heart rate, panic, aggression, violence / Memory loss; numbness, nausea/vomiting, loss of appetite, depression
INHALANTS			
Solvents (paint thinners, gasoline, glues) Gases (butane, propane, aerolsol propellants, nitrous oxide)		Inhaled through nose or mouth	Stimulation, loss of inhibition; headache; nausea/vomiting; slurred speech, loss of motor coordination; wheezing / Unconsciousness, cramps, weight loss, muscle weakness, depression, memory impairment, damage to cardiovascular and nervous systems, sudden death

Source: National Institute on Drug Abuse, www.nida.nih.gov/DrugPages/DrugsofAbuse.html

coordination; increased anxiety; and panic attacks. Long-term use produces changes in the brain similar to those seen with other major drugs of abuse.

 According to a study of college students, heavy marijuana use impairs critical skills related to attention, memory, and learning, even 24 hours after its use. Heavy users who smoked marijuana almost every day showed significant difficulty sustaining attention, shifting attention to meet the demands of changes in the environment, and registering, processing, and using information.[35]

Over time, continued heavy marijuana use can interfere with students' ability to learn and perform well in school and in challenging careers. Marijuana contributes significantly to accidental death and injury among adolescents, especially through motor vehicle crashes.

A meta-analysis of 48 long-term studies of the consequences of marijuana use found that teenagers and young adults who used marijuana attained lower levels of education and were more likely to use other illegal drugs than peers who did not smoke pot. However, there was no consistent association between marijuana use and psychological or behavioral problems.[36]

Lungs Smoking cannabis may cause similar effects to smoking tobacco, with many of them appearing at a younger age. They include chronic bronchitis, emphysema, and other lung disorders and increased risk of heart attacks and sudden death.[37] The amount of tar inhaled by marijuana smokers and the level of carbon monoxide absorbed are three to five times greater than among tobacco smokers. The reasons may be that marijuana users inhale more deeply, hold the smoke in the lungs longer, and do not use filters. Smoking a single joint can be as damaging to the lungs as smoking five tobacco cigarettes. Someone who smokes five joints a week may take in as many cancer-causing chemicals as a person who smokes a pack of cigarettes a day.[38]

Heart Otherwise healthy people have suffered heart attacks shortly after smoking marijuana. Experiments have also linked marijuana use to elevated blood pressure and decreased oxygen supply to the heart muscle. The risk of heart attack triples within an hour of smoking pot. Smoking marijuana while shooting cocaine can potentially cause deadly increases in heart rate and blood pressure.

Pregnancy Babies born to mothers who use marijuana during pregnancy are smaller than those born to mothers who did not use the drug, and the babies are more likely to develop health problems. A nursing mother who uses marijuana passes some of the THC to the baby in her breast milk. This may impair the infant's motor development (control of muscle movement).

Withdrawal

Marijuana users can develop a compulsive, often uncontrollable craving for the drug. More than 120,000 people enter treatment every year for marijuana addiction. In addition,

Negative Long-Term Effects

Brain and central nervous system
- Dulls sensory and cognitive skills
- Impairs short-term memory
- Alters motor coordination
- Causes changes in brain chemistry
- Leads to difficulty in concentration, attention to detail, and learning new, complex information
- Increases risk of stroke

Cardiovascular system
- Increases heart rate
- Increases blood pressure
- Decreases blood flow to the limbs, which in extreme cases could require an amputation

Respiratory system
- Damages the lungs (50% more tar than tobacco)
- May cause lung cancer
- May damage throat from inhalation

Reproductive system
- In women, may impair ovulation and cause fetal abnormalities if used during pregnancy
- In men, may suppress sexual functioning and may reduce the number, quality, and motility of sperm, possibly affecting fertility

Positive Short-Term Therapeutic Effects for Patients

Brain and central nervous system
- May help minimize pain from the spread of cancer

Vision
- Reduces intraocular pressure, helping those afflicted with glaucoma

Digestive system
- Combats nausea from chemotherapy and helps minimize vomitting
- Helps restore appetite in people who have lost weight from cancer or AIDS

Muscular system
- May help calm spasms from spinal-cord injury, multiple sclerosis, and possibly epilepsy

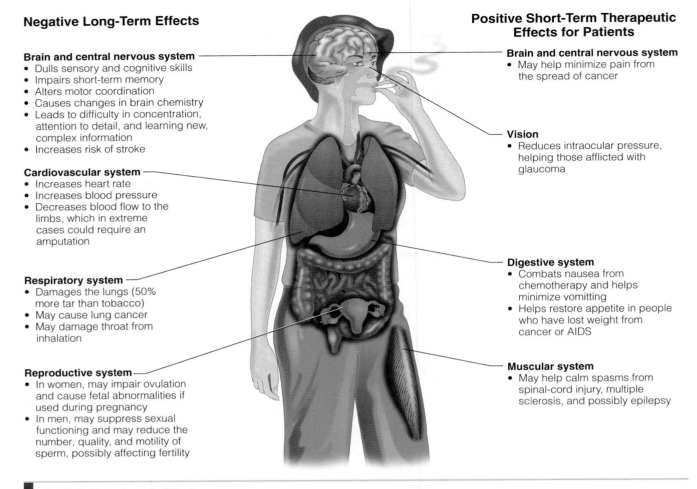

FIGURE 11-3 **Impact of Marijuana**
Marijuana may have positive short-term therapeutic effects for people with cancer, glaucoma, or AIDS, but the long-term effects for healthy users are all negative.

animal studies suggest that marijuana causes physical dependence. Stopping after long-term marijuana use can produce *marijuana withdrawal syndrome,* which is characterized by insomnia, restlessness, loss of appetite, and irritability. People who smoked marijuana daily for many years may become aggressive after they stop using it and may relapse to prevent aggression and other symptoms.

CLUB DRUGS (DESIGNER DRUGS)

The National Institute on Drug Abuse identifies a variety of drugs—alcohol, LSD (acid), MDMA (ecstasy), GHB, GBL, ketamine (Special-K), fentanyl, Rohypnol, and nitrites—as **"club drugs."** They first became popular among teens and young adults at nightclubs, bars, or raves and trances—night-long dances often held in warehouses or other unusual settings. Their use by teenagers has been dropping in recent years.

Young people may take club drugs to relax, energize, and enhance their social interactions, but a large number also experience negative consequences. As many as three in four report side effects such as profuse sweating, hot and cold

flashes, tingling or numbness, blurred vision, trouble sleeping, hallucinations, depression, confusion, anxiety, irritability, paranoia, and loss of libido (sex drive). Some also experience difficulty with their usual daily activities and financial and work troubles.[39]

Ecstasy

Ecstasy (E, XTC, X, hug, beans, love drug) is the most common street name for methylenedioxymethamphetamine (MDMA), a synthetic compound with both stimulant and mildly hallucinogenic properties.

 An estimated 10 to 15 percent of college students report that they've ever used ecstasy. According to earlier studies, students who take ecstasy were more likely to use marijuana, binge-drink, smoke cigarettes, have multiple sexual partners, spend more time socializing with friends and less time studying, and consider parties important and religion as less important. However, researchers who compared students who used ecstasy and other illicit drugs with those who used only marijuana have concluded that undergraduates who use ecstasy may be a subgroup of marijuana users who tend to engage in many risk-taking

Club drugs are often used at raves, even those that are alcohol-free.

behaviors. Ecstasy users also think that their peers smoke more marijuana and use more ecstasy than they actually do.[40]

How It Feels Although it can be smoked, inhaled (snorted), or injected, ecstasy is almost always taken as a pill or tablet. Its effects begin in 45 minutes and last for two to four hours.

MDMA belongs to a family of drugs called *enactogens,* which literally means "touching within." As a mood elevator, it produces a relaxed, euphoric state but does not produce hallucinations. Users of ecstasy often say they feel at peace with themselves and a sense of connectedness with others. In some settings, they reveal intimate details of their lives (which they may later regret); in other settings, they join in collective rejoicing. Like hallucinogenic drugs, MDMA can enhance sensory experience, but it rarely causes visual distortions, sudden mood changes, or psychotic reactions. Regular users may experience depression and anxiety the week after taking MDMA.

Psychologists have experimented with MDMA as a way to enhance self-revelation, self-criticism, and self-exploration and to boost trust between a patient and a therapist. Most clinicians are highly skeptical of its benefits, and there has been no officially sanctioned research on its therapeutic benefits.

Risks Ecstasy poses risks similar to those of cocaine and amphetamines. These include psychological difficulties (confusion, depression, sleep problems, drug craving, severe anxiety, and paranoia) and physical symptoms (muscle tension, involuntary teeth clenching, nausea, blurred vision, rapid eye movement, faintness, chills, sweating, and increases in heart rate and blood pressure that pose a special risk for people with circulatory or heart disease).

Ecstasy can produce nausea, vomiting, and dizziness. When combined with extended physical exertion like dancing, club drugs can lead to hyperthermia (severe overheating), severe dehydration, serious increases in blood pressure, stroke, and heart attack. Without sufficient water, dancers at raves may suffer dehydration and heat stroke, which can be fatal. Individuals with high blood pressure, heart trouble, or liver or kidney disease are in the greatest danger. Several deaths have occurred in teens who suffered brain damage by drinking large amounts of water to counteract the raised body temperature induced by the drug.

MDMA has been implicated in some cases of acute hepatitis, which can lead to liver failure. Even after liver transplantation, the mortality rate for individuals with this condition is 50 percent. Another danger comes from the practice of taking SSRIs (see Chapter 3), which modulate the mood-altering brain chemical serotonin, before ecstasy. This can cause jaw clenching, nausea, tremors, and in extreme cases, potentially fatal elevations in body temperature.

Although not a sexual stimulant (if anything, MDMA has the opposite effect), ecstasy fosters strong feelings of intimacy that may lead to risky sexual behavior. The psychological effects of ecstasy become less intriguing with repeated use, and the physical side effects become more uncomfortable. Ecstasy poses risks to a developing fetus, including a greater likelihood of heart and skeletal abnormalities and long-term learning and memory impairments in children born to women who used MDMA during pregnancy.

Because ecstasy is *neurotoxic* (damaging to brain cells), it depletes the brain of serotonin, a messenger chemical involved with mood, sleep, and appetite, and can lead to depression, anxiety, and impaired thinking and memory. Even short-term use of ecstasy can have long-term neurological consequences that may affect memory and the brain's ability to perform complex thought processes.[41]

According to brain-imaging studies, users, although as mentally alert as nonusers, fared far worse on measures of memory, learning, and general intelligence. The more frequently they took ecstasy, the worse they did, probably because ecstasy alters neuronal function in a brain structure called the hippocampus, which helps create short-term memory. The effect on memory persists for years after discontinuing use.

MDMA pills may contain caffeine, dextromethorphan, heroin, and mescaline. The MDMA-like substance paramethoxyamphetamine (PMA) has been implicated in the deaths of people who mistakenly thought they were taking true MDMA. The deaths were due to complications from hyperthermia.

GHB and GBL

Once sold in health food stores for its muscle-building and alleged fat-burning properties, **gammahydroxybutyrate (GHB,** G, Georgia home boy) was banned because of its effects on the brain and nervous system. The main ingredient is **GBL (gamma butyrolactone),** an industrial solvent often used to strip floors. Once ingested, GBL converts into GHB, an odorless, colorless sedative that can be slipped into a beverage to knock an individual out. Once taken, GHB acts as a sedative while producing feelings of euphoria and heightened sexuality. Because of its amnesic properties, GHB has been used as a "date rape" drug, similar to Rohypnol. Alcohol intensifies its effects.[42]

Larger doses can cause someone to pass out in 15 minutes and fall into a coma within half an hour. Other side effects include nausea, amnesia, hallucinations, decreased heart rate, convulsions, and sometimes blackouts. Long-term use at high doses can lead to a withdrawal reaction: rapid heartbeat, tremor, insomnia, anxiety, and occasionally hallucinations that last a few days to a week.

GHB is addictive. Users who attempt to quit may experience significant withdrawal symptoms, including anxiety, tremors, and insomnia. Most symptoms decrease within one to two weeks of cessation, but severe psychological effects can last for weeks to months.[43]

Ketamine

Ketamine—called K, Special-K, and Vitamin K—is an anesthetic used by veterinarians. When cooked, dried, and ground into a powder for snorting, K blocks chemical messengers in the brain that carry sensory input. As a result, the brain fills the void with hallucinations. Users may report an "out-of-body" experience with distorted perceptions of time and space. The effects typically begin within 30 minutes and last for approximately two hours.

Ketamine has become common in club and rave scenes and has been used as a date rape drug. It can cause anxiety, agitation, paranoia, and vomiting. Higher doses can cause lethal breathing impairments, stroke, and heart attack. Repeated ketamine use can be addictive, and even a single use can occasionally produce audiovisual "flashbacks" similar to those described by phencyclidine (PCP) users, and long-term memory loss.[44]

More than half of emergency department visits for ketamine ingestion involve adolescents and young adults, often after they've taken the drug at a rave.[45]

Nitrites

Nitrites (amyl, butyl, and isobutyl nitrite) are clear, amber-colored liquids that have had a history of abuse for more than three decades, especially in gay and bisexual men. Popular in dance clubs, they are used recreationally for a high feeling, a slowed sense of time, a carefree sense of well-being, and intensified sexual experiences.

Sold in small glass ampules containing individual doses, nitrites are usually inhaled and rapidly absorbed into the bloodstream. Users feel their physiological and psychological impact in seconds. Acute adverse effects include headache, dizziness, a drop in blood pressure, changes in heart rate, increased pressure within the eye, and skin flushing. Some individuals develop respiratory irritation and cough, sneeze, or have difficulty breathing. Chronic use can lead to crusty skin lesions and chemical burns around the nose, mouth, and lips.[46]

Herbal Ecstasy

Herbal ecstasy, also known as herbal bliss, cloud 9, and herbal X, is a mixture of stimulants such as ephedrine, pseudoephedrine, and caffeine. Sold in tablet or capsule form as a "natural" and safe alternative to ecstasy, its ingredients vary greatly. Herbal pills can have dangerous and unpleasant side effects, including stroke, heart attack, and a disfiguring skin condition.

STIMULANTS

Central nervous system **stimulants** are drugs that increase activity in some portion of the brain or spinal cord. Some stimulants increase motor activity and enhance mental alertness, and some combat mental fatigue. Amphetamine, methamphetamine, caffeine, cocaine, and khat are stimulants. Stimulant medications are used to treat conditions such as ADHD.

Amphetamine

Amphetamines trigger the release of epinephrine (adrenaline), which stimulates the central nervous system. They were once widely prescribed for weight control because they suppress appetite, but they have emerged as a global danger. Amphetamines are sold under a variety of names: amphetamine (brand name Benzedrine, streetname bennies), dextroamphetamine (Dexedrine, dex), methamphetamine (Methedrine, meth, speed), and Desoxyn (copilots). Related *uppers* include the prescription drugs methylphenidate (Ritalin), pemoline (Cylert), and phenmetrazine (Preludin). Amphetamines are available in tablet or capsule form.

How Users Feel Amphetamines produce a state of hyperalertness and energy. Users feel confident in their ability to think clearly and to perform any task exceptionally well—although amphetamines do not, in fact, significantly boost performance or thinking. Higher doses make users feel *wired*: talkative, excited, restless, irritable, anxious, moody.

If taken intravenously, amphetamines produce a characteristic rush of elation and confidence, as well as adverse effects, including confusion, rambling or incoherent speech, anxiety, headache, and palpitations. Individuals may become paranoid; be convinced they are having profound thoughts; feel increased sexual interest; and experience unusual perceptions, such as ringing in the ears, a sensation of insects crawling on their skin, or hearing their name called. Crank users may feel high and sleepy or may hallucinate and lose contact with reality.

Risks Dependence on amphetamines can develop with episodic or daily use. Users typically take amphetamines in large doses to prevent crashing. Bingeing—taking high doses over a period of several days—can lead to an extremely intense and unpleasant crash characterized by a craving for the drug, shakiness, irritability, anxiety, and depression. Two or more days are required for recuperation.

Amphetamine intoxication may cause the following symptoms:

- **Feelings of grandiosity,** anxiety, tension, hypervigilance, anger, social hypersensitivity, fighting, jitteriness or agitation, paranoia, and impaired judgment in social or occupational functioning.

▪ **Increased heart rate,** dilated pupils, elevated blood pressure, perspiration or chills, and nausea or vomiting.

▪ **Less frequent effects such as speeding up** or slowing down of physical movement; muscular weakness; impaired breathing, chest pain, heart arrhythmia; confusion, seizures, impaired movements or muscle tone; or even coma.

▪ **In high doses, a rapid or irregular heartbeat,** tremors, loss of coordination, and collapse.

The long-term effects of amphetamine abuse include malnutrition, skin disorders, ulcers, insomnia, depression, vitamin deficiencies, and in some cases, brain damage that results in speech and thought disturbances. Sexual dysfunction and impaired concentration or memory also may occur.

Withdrawal When the immediate effects of amphetamines wear off, users experience a *crash*—they crave the drug and become shaky, irritable, anxious, and depressed. Amphetamine withdrawal usually persists for more than 24 hours after cessation of prolonged, heavy use. Its characteristic features include fatigue, disturbing dreams, much more or less than usual sleep, increased appetite, and speeding up or slowing down of physical movements. Those who are unable to sleep despite their exhaustion often take sedative-hypnotics (discussed later in this chapter) to help them rest and may then become dependent on them in addition to amphetamines. Symptoms usually reach a peak in two to four days, although depression and irritability may persist for months. Suicide is a major risk.

Methamphetamine

Methamphetamine, an addictive stimulant that is less expensive and possibly more addictive than cocaine or heroin, has become America's leading drug problem. More than 12 million Americans have tried methamphetamine, and 1.5 million are regular users, according to federal estimates.[47]

Methamphetamine is chemically related to amphetamine, but its effects on the central nervous system are greater. Made in illegal laboratories, street methamphetamine is referred to by many names, such as speed, meth, and chalk. Methamphetamine hydrochloride, clear chunky crystals resembling ice that can be inhaled by smoking, is called ice, crystal, glass, and tina. Methamphetamine can be snorted, smoked, or injected.

How Users Feel Methamphetamine causes the release of large amounts of dopamine, which creates a sensation of euphoria, increased self-esteem, and alertness. Users also report a marked increase in sexual appetite, which often leads to risky sexual behaviors while under the drug's influence.

Smoking or intravenous injection leads to an intense, pleasurable sensation, called a rush or flash, that lasts only a few minutes. Oral or intranasal use produces a high but not a rush. Users may become addicted quickly, using more methamphetamine more and more frequently. Despair and suicidal thinking can develop when the stimulant effect wears off.

Risks Even small amounts of methamphetamine can increase wakefulness and physical activity, depress appetite, and raise body temperature. Other effects on the central nervous system include irritability, insomnia, confusion, tremors, convulsions, anxiety, paranoia, and aggressiveness.

Methamphetamine increases heart rate and blood pressure and can cause irreversible damage to blood vessels in the brain, producing strokes. Other effects of methamphetamine include respiratory problems, irregular heartbeat, and extreme loss of appetite and weight. During intoxication, the body (and probably brain) temperature rises, sometimes resulting in convulsions. High fevers or collapse of the circulatory system can cause death.

Common psychiatric symptoms are insomnia, irritability, and aggressive behavior. The drug causes intellectual impairment, anxiety, and depression. Chronic users become disorganized and unable to cope with everyday problems. The risk of developing psychotic symptoms—hallucinations and delusions—is very high.

Another side effect is called meth mouth. In short periods of time, sometimes just months, teeth can turn a grayish-brown, twist, begin to fall out, and take on a peculiar texture. This may be the result of methamphetamine's effects on the metabolic system, plus the huge quantities of sugary soft drinks that users consume for the dry mouth caused by the drug.[48]

Meth users engage in more sex, more carelessly. Meth has become popular among gay and bisexual men, and it has been linked to an increase in unsafe sex practices. Methamphetamine use and needle sharing has been linked to a spike in HIV and hepatitis C infections in gay communities.[49]

Methamphetamine causes abnormalities in brain regions associated with selective attention and in those associated with memory.[50] The brain may recover somewhat after months of abstinence, but problems often remain. Former methamphetamine addicts may suffer from chronic apathy and anhedonia (inability to experience pleasure) for years.

Ya-ba/Thai Tabs are a new, powerful form of methamphetamine that tastes sweet like candy.

The Toll on Society Law enforcement officials consider methamphetamine their biggest drug problem. Meth-related arrests have soared. Meth addicts are pouring into prisons and recovery centers at an ever-increasing rate. "Meth babies" are crowding the foster-care system. Meth-making operations have been uncovered in all 50 states, with the greatest number in Missouri. Production releases poisonous gases and results in toxic waste that is often dumped down household drains, in a backyard, or at a roadside. The cost of cleaning up the environment is a growing problem for many communities.

Over-the-counter cold medicines (ephedrine and pseudoephedrine) are commonly used in meth production, which is one reason for federal and state restrictions on their sale. As drug stores and retailers have placed nonprescription cold pills behind the pharmacy counter, meth manufacturing has moved into Mexico, where labs produce hundreds of pounds of meth a year and smuggle it into the United States.

Withdrawal Methamphetamine addiction is difficult to treat. As with cocaine, coming off methamphetamine causes intense distress, so users often seek out the drug to relieve their pain. Treatment usually requires the intervention of the patient's family as well as a substance abuse specialist team experienced in treating methamphetamine addiction. Standard substance abuse treatment methods such as education, behavior therapy, individual and family counseling, and support groups may be effective for some. Methamphetamine abusers often use other illicit drugs as well, a problem that can be addressed as part of a comprehensive program.[51]

Prescription Stimulants

Abuse of stimulants prescribed for treatment of attention deficit/hyperactivity disorder (ADHD), discussed in Chapter 3, has increased among young people. (Individuals with ADHD do not react to these drugs in the same way and are not at greater risk of abusing them.)

In addition to respiratory damage, brain damage, and mental impairment, methamphetamine turns users' teeth from white to grayish-brown. This is how "meth mouth" looks.

Photo by Denise Oda, June 2005

TABLE 11-4 PRESCRIPTION STIMULANT ABUSE ON CAMPUS

Illegal use of prescription stimulants over lifetime	Percentage
All students surveyed	8.1
Women	7.2
Men	9.3
Whites	9.5
Hispanics	8.9
African Americans	2.7
Asians	4.9
Illegal use in last year	**5.4**

*Based on a random sample of 9,161 undergraduates at the University of Michigan.
Source: Teter, Christian, et al. "Prevalence and Motives for Illicit Use of Prescription Stimulants in an Undergraduate Student Sample." *Journal of American College Health,* Vol. 53, No. 6, May–June 2005, p. 253.

In a survey of more than 9,000 undergraduates, 8.1 percent of students—more men than women, more whites and Hispanics than African Americans and Asians—reported that they had illegally used stimulants in the past (Table 11-4).[52] Some studies have found rates of abuse as high as 17 percent in undergraduate men and 11 percent in women.

Abuse of stimulants is much higher among 18- to 25-year-olds than in the general population. Less than 1 percent of Americans over age 12 report illicit use of these drugs. Unique characteristics of the college environment, such as the desire to delay sleep and remain alert during all-nighters, may contribute to stimulant abuse on campus. Undergraduates are most likely to use stimulants during finals weeks, before tests, or when partying.[53] The primary motives that undergraduates give for stimulant abuse are to help with concentration, to increase alertness, and to get more energy.[54] Yet most students who have tried stimulants do not feel that the drugs had a positive effect on their academic performance in the long run.

Cocaine

Cocaine (coke, snow, lady) is a white crystalline powder extracted from the leaves of the South American coca plant. Usually mixed with various sugars and local anesthetics like lidocaine and procaine, cocaine powder is generally inhaled. When sniffed or snorted, cocaine anesthetizes the nerve endings in the nose and relaxes the lung's bronchial muscles.

Cocaine can be dissolved in water and injected intravenously. The drug is rapidly metabolized by the liver, so the high is relatively brief, typically lasting only about 20 minutes. This means that users will commonly inject the drug repeatedly, increasing the risk of infection and damage to their veins. Many intravenous cocaine users prefer the practice of *speedballing,* the intravenous administration of a combination of cocaine and heroin.

Cocaine alkaloid, or *freebase,* is obtained by removing the hydrochloride salt from cocaine powder. *Freebasing* is smoking the fumes of the alkaloid form of cocaine. *Crack,* pharmacologically identical to freebase, is a cheap, easy-to-use, widely available, smokeable, and potent form of cocaine named for the popping sound it makes when burned. Because it is absorbed rapidly into the bloodstream and large doses reach the brain very quickly, it is particularly dangerous. However, its low price and easy availability have made it a common drug of abuse in poor urban areas.

How Users Feel   A powerful stimulant to the central nervous system, cocaine targets several chemical sites in the brain, producing feelings of soaring well-being and boundless energy. Users feel they have enormous physical and mental ability, yet are also restless and anxious. After a brief period of euphoria, users slump into a depression. They often go on cocaine binges, lasting from a few hours to several days, and consume large quantities of cocaine.

With crack, dependence develops quickly. As soon as crack users come down from one high, they want more crack. Whereas heroin addicts may shoot up several times a day, crack addicts need another hit within minutes. Thus, a crack habit can quickly become more expensive than heroin addiction.

Cocaine may cause changes in the brain that affect a user's ability to sense pleasure and may contribute to depression. With continuing use, cocaine users experience less pleasure and more unpleasant effects. Eventually they may reach a point at which they no longer experience euphoric effects and crave the drug simply to alleviate their persistent hunger for it. They constantly think about it, dream about it, spend all their money on it, and borrow, steal, or deal to pay for it. They cannot concentrate on work; they become increasingly irritable and confused. They may also become dependent on alcohol, sedatives, or opioids, which they use to calm down from cocaine's aftereffects.

Risks   Cocaine dependence is an easy habit to acquire. With repeated use, the brain becomes tolerant of the drug's stimulant effects, and users must take more of it to get high. Those who smoke or inject cocaine can develop dependence within weeks. Those who sniff cocaine may not become dependent on the drug for months or years. It is thought that 5 to 20 percent of all coke users—a group as large as the estimated total number of heroin addicts—are dependent on the drug.[55]

The physical effects of acute cocaine intoxication include dilated pupils, elevated or lowered blood pressure, perspiration or chills, nausea or vomiting, speeding up or slowing down of physical activity, muscular weakness, impaired breathing, chest pain, and impaired movements or muscle tone. Prolonged cocaine snorting can result in ulceration of the mucous membrane of the nose and damage to the nasal septum (the membrane between the nostrils) severe enough to cause it to collapse.

Although some users initially try cocaine as a sexual stimulant, it does not enhance sexual performance. At low doses, it may delay orgasm and cause heightened sensory awareness, but men who use cocaine regularly have problems maintaining erections and ejaculating. They also tend to have low sperm counts, less active sperm, and more abnormal sperm than nonusers. Both male and female chronic cocaine users tend to lose interest in sex and have difficulty reaching orgasm.

Cocaine use can cause blood vessels in the brain to clamp shut and can trigger a stroke, bleeding in the brain, and potentially fatal brain seizures. Cocaine users can also develop psychiatric or neurological complications (Figure 11-4). Repeated or high doses of cocaine can lead to impaired judgment, hyperactivity, nonstop babbling, feelings of suspicion and paranoia, and violent behavior. The brain never learns to tolerate cocaine's negative effects; users may become incoherent and paranoid and may experience unusual sensations, such as ringing in their ears, feeling insects crawling on the skin, or hearing their name called.

Cocaine can damage the liver and cause lung damage in freebasers. Smoking crack causes bronchitis as well as lung damage and may promote the transmission of HIV through burned and bleeding lips. Some smokers have died

FIGURE 11-4   Some Effects of Cocaine on the Body

Central nervous system
- Repeated use or high dosages may cause severe psychological problems
- Suppresses desire for food, sex, and sleep
- Can cause strokes, seizures, and neurological damage

Nose
- Damages mucous membrane

Cardiovascular system
- Increases blood pressure by constricting blood vessels
- Causes irregular heartbeat
- Damages heart tissue

Respiratory system
- Freebasing causes lung damage
- Overdose can lead to respiratory arrest

Reproductive system
- In men, affects ability to maintain erections and ejaculate; also causes sperm abnormalities
- In women, may affect ability to carry pregnancy to term

of respiratory complications, such as pulmonary edema (the buildup of fluid in the lungs).

Cocaine causes the heart rate to speed up and blood pressure to rise suddenly. Its use is associated with many cardiac complications, including arrhythmia (disruption of heart rhythm), angina (chest pain), and acute myocardial infarction (heart attack).

The combination of alcohol and cocaine is particularly lethal. Alcohol and cocaine together are second only to the combination of heroin and alcohol in causing deaths related to substance abuse. When people mix cocaine and alcohol, they compound the danger each drug poses. The liver combines the two agents and manufactures cocaethylene, which intensifies cocaine's euphoric effects, while possibly increasing the risk of sudden death.

Cocaine users who inject the drug and share needles put themselves at risk for another potentially lethal problem: HIV infection.

Cocaine is dangerous for pregnant women and their babies, causing miscarriages, developmental disorders, and life-threatening complications during birth. Cocaine can reduce the fetal oxygen supply, possibly interfering with the development of the fetus's nervous system. Infants born to cocaine and crack users can suffer withdrawal and have higher-than-normal rates of respiratory and kidney troubles, visual problems, and developmental retardation, and they may be at greater risk of sudden infant death syndrome.

Withdrawal When addicted individuals stop using cocaine, they often become depressed. This may lead to further cocaine use to alleviate depression. Other symptoms of cocaine withdrawal include fatigue, vivid and disturbing dreams, excessive or too little sleep, irritability, increased appetite, and physical slowing down or speeding up. This initial crash may last one to three days after cutting down or stopping the heavy use of cocaine. Some individuals become violent, paranoid, and suicidal.

Symptoms usually reach a peak in two to four days, although depression, anxiety, irritability, lack of pleasure in usual activities, and low-level cravings may continue for weeks. As memories of the crash fade, the desire for cocaine intensifies. For many weeks after stopping, individuals may feel an intense craving for the drug.

Experimental medical approaches for treating cocaine dependence include antidepressant drugs, anticonvulsant drugs, and the naturally occurring amino acids tryptophan and tyrosine. However, these have only limited benefit. Despite years of research, there is no drug approved in the United States for treating cocaine dependence.[56] Some cocaine abusers fare better with cognitive-behavioral therapy (discussed in Chapter 3); others, with 12-step programs.

Khat (Kat, Catha, Chat, Abyssinian Tea)

For centuries people in East Africa and the Arabian peninsula consumed the fresh young leaves of the *Catha edulis* shrub in ways similar to our drinking coffee. Its active ingredients are two controlled substances, cathinone and cathine.

Chewing alleviates fatigue and reduces appetite. Compulsive use may result in manic behavior, grandiose illusions, paranoia, and hallucinations.

DEPRESSANTS

Depressants depress the central nervous system, reduce activity, and induce relaxation, drowsiness, or sleep. They include the benzodiazepines and the barbiturates, the opioids, and alcohol.

Benzodiazepines and Barbiturates

These depressants are the sedative-hypnotics, also known as anxiolytic or antianxiety drugs. The **benzodiazepines**—the most widely used drugs in this category—are commonly prescribed for tension, muscular strain, sleep problems, anxiety, panic attacks, anesthesia, and in the treatment of alcohol withdrawal. They include such drugs as *chlordiazepoxide* (Librium), *diazepam* (Valium), *oxazepam* (Serax), *lorazepam* (Ativan), *flurazepam* (Dalmane), and *alprazolam* (Xanax). They differ widely in their mechanism of action, absorption rate, and metabolism, but all produce similar intoxication and withdrawal symptoms.

Rohypnol, a trade name for flunitrazepam, is one of the benzodiazepines, and it has been of particular concern for the last few years because of its abuse in date rape. When mixed with alcohol, Rohypnol can incapacitate victims and prevent them from resisting sexual assault. It produces "anterograde amnesia," which means individuals may not remember events they experienced while under the effects of the drug. Rohypnol may be lethal when mixed with alcohol or other depressants.

Benzodiazepine sleeping pills have largely replaced the **barbiturates,** which were used medically in the past for inducing relaxation and sleep, relieving tension, and treating epileptic seizures. These drugs are usually taken by mouth in tablet, capsule, or liquid form. When used as a general anesthetic, they are administered intravenously.

How Users Feel Low doses of these drugs may reduce or relieve tension, but increasing doses can cause a loosening of sexual or aggressive inhibitions. Individuals using this class of drugs may experience rapid mood changes, impaired judgment, and impaired social or occupational functioning.

Young people in their teens or early twenties who have used many illegal substances typically take sedative-hypnotics to obtain a high or a state of euphoria. Some use them in combination with other drugs. Less commonly, individuals may first obtain sedatives, hypnotics, or antianxiety medications by prescription from a physician for insomnia or anxiety and then gradually increase the dose or frequency of use on their own, often by seeking prescriptions from several physicians. While they justify this continued use because of their symptoms, the fact is that they reach a state in which they cannot function normally without the drug.

Risks All sedative-hypnotic drugs can produce physical and psychological dependence within two to four weeks. A complication specific to sedatives is *cross-tolerance* (cross-

Because Rohypnol is colorless, tasteless, and odorless, it can be added to beverages without your knowledge. Never let your drink out of your sight!

addiction), which occurs when users develop tolerance for one sedative or become dependent on it and develop tolerance for other sedatives as well.

Intoxication with these drugs can produce changes in mood or behavior, such as inappropriate sexual or aggressive acts, mood swings, and impaired judgment. Physical signs include slurred speech, poor coordination, unsteady gait, involuntary eye movements, impaired attention or memory, and stupor or coma.

Taken in combination with alcohol, these drugs have a synergistic effect that can be dangerous or even lethal. For example, an individual's driving ability, already impaired by alcohol, will be made even worse, increasing the risk of an accident. Alcohol in combination with sedative-hypnotics leads to respiratory depression and may result in respiratory arrest and death. Regular users of any of these drugs who become physically dependent should not try to cut down or quit on their own. If they try to quit suddenly, they run the risk of seizures, coma, and death.

Withdrawal Withdrawal from sedative-hypnotic drugs may range from relatively mild discomfort to a severe syndrome with grand mal seizures, depending on the degree of dependence. Withdrawal symptoms include malaise or weakness, sweating, rapid pulse, coarse tremors (of the hands, tongue, or eyelids), insomnia, nausea or vomiting, temporary hallucinations or illusions, physical restlessness, anxiety or irritability, and grand mal seizures. Withdrawal may begin within two to three days after stopping drug use, and symptoms may persist for many weeks.

Opioids

The **opioids** include *opium* and its derivatives (*morphine, codeine,* and *heroin*) and synthetic drugs that have similar sleep-inducing and pain-relieving properties. The opioids come from a resin taken from the seedpod of the Asian poppy. Synthetic opioids, such as *meperidine* (Demerol), *methadone,* and *propoxyphene* (Darvon), are synthesized in a chemical laboratory. Whether natural or synthetic, these drugs are powerful *narcotics,* or painkillers.

Heroin (also known as horse, junk, smack, or downtown), the most widely abused opioid, is illegal in this country. In other nations it is used as a potent painkiller for conditions such as terminal cancer. There are an estimated 600,000 heroin addicts in the United States, with men outnumbering women addicts by three to one. Among people aged 18 to 25, the percentage of heroin users who inject the drug has doubled in the last decade. While the number of young heroin users in major cities has dropped by 50 percent, their numbers almost tripled in suburban and rural areas.[57]

Heroin users typically inject the drug into their veins. However, individuals who experiment with recreational drugs often prefer *skin-popping* (subcutaneous injection) rather than *mainlining* (intravenous injection); they also may snort heroin as a powder or dissolve it and inhale the vapors. To try to avoid addiction, some users begin by *chipping,* taking small or intermittent doses. Regardless of the method of administration, tolerance can develop rapidly.

Morphine, used as a painkiller and anesthetic, acts primarily on the central nervous system, eyes, and digestive tract. By producing mental clouding, drowsiness, and euphoria, it does not decrease the physical sensation of pain as much as it alters a person's awareness of the pain; in effect, he or she no longer cares about it.

Prescription Opioids

Two semisynthetic derivatives of morphine are *hydromorphone* (trade name Dilaudid, street name little D), with two to eight times the painkilling effect of morphine, and *oxycodone* (OxyContin, Percocet, Percodan, perkies), similar to codeine but more potent. The synthetic narcotic *meperidine* (Demerol, demies) is now probably second only to morphine for use in relieving pain. It is also used by addicts as a substitute for morphine or heroin.

 Abuse of prescription painkillers, such as OxyContin and Vicodin, is widespread on campuses. In a survey of more than 10,000 students attending 119 colleges, 12 percent of undergraduates reported lifetime use of a prescription painkiller for nonmedical reasons; 7 percent did so in the previous year. Students who are members of fraternities and sororities, enrolled at more competitive schools, earning lower grade point averages, and engaging in substance use and other risky behaviors are more likely to abuse these drugs.[58]

Codeine, a weaker painkiller than morphine, is an ingredient in liquid products prescribed for relieving coughs and in tablet and injectable form for relieving pain. The synthetic narcotic *propoxyphene* (Darvon), a somewhat less potent painkiller than codeine, is no more effective than aspirin in usual doses. It has been one of the most widely prescribed drugs for headaches, dental pain, and menstrual cramps. At higher doses, Darvon produces a euphoric high, which may lead to misuse.

Opioid drugs, made from the Asian poppy, come in both legal and illegal forms. All are highly addictive.

Prescription opioids are taken orally in pill form but can also be injected intravenously. Some individuals first take a medically prescribed opioid for pain relief or cough suppression, then gradually increase the dose and frequency of use on their own, often justifying this because of their symptoms rather than for the sensations the drug induces. They expend increasing efforts to obtain the drug, frequently seeking out several doctors to write prescriptions.

Like other addictions, a prescription drug "habit" is a treatable brain disease. Recovery usually requires carefully supervised detoxification, appropriate medications (similar to those used for opioid dependence), behavior therapy, and ongoing support.

How Users Feel All opioids relax the user. When injected, they can produce an immediate *rush* (high) that lasts 10 to 30 minutes. For two to six hours thereafter, users may feel indifferent, lethargic, and drowsy; they may slur their words and have problems paying attention, remembering, and going about their normal routine. The primary attractions of heroin are the euphoria and pain relief it produces. However, some people experience very unpleasant feelings, such as anxiety and fear. Other effects include a sensation of warmth or heaviness, dry mouth, facial flushing, and nausea and vomiting (particularly in first-time users).

Some addicts report a rush when heroin is injected directly into their veins. Since the effects of heroin do not last long—usually only two to four hours—addicts have to "shoot up" two to five times a day. With large doses, the pupils become smaller, and the skin becomes cold, moist, and bluish. Breathing slows down; the user cannot be awakened and may stop breathing completely.

Risks Addiction is common. Almost all regular users of opioids rapidly develop drug dependence, which can lead to lethargy, weight loss, loss of sex drive, and the continual effort to avoid withdrawal symptoms through repeated drug administration. In addition, they experience anxiety, insomnia, restlessness, and craving for the drug. Users continue taking opioids as much to avoid the discomfort of withdrawal, a classic sign of opioid addiction, as to experience pleasure.

Physical symptoms include constricted pupils (although pupils may dilate from a severe overdose), drowsiness, slurred speech, and impaired attention or memory. Morphine affects blood pressure, heart rate, and blood circulation in the brain. Both morphine and heroin slow down the respiratory system; overdoses can cause fatal respiratory arrest.

Opioid poisoning or overdose causes shock, coma, and depressed respiration and can be fatal. Emergency medical treatment is critical, often with drugs called *narcotic antagonists* that rapidly reverse the effects of opioids when administered intravenously.

Over time, users who inject opioids may develop infections of the heart lining and valves, skin abscesses, and lung congestion. Infections from unsterile solutions, syringes, and shared needles can lead to hepatitis, tetanus, liver disease, and HIV transmission. Depression is common and may be both an antecedent and a risk factor for needle-sharing.

Opioid abuse during pregnancy can cause miscarriage, stillbirth, or low birth weight. Babies born to addicted mothers experience withdrawal symptoms after birth.[59]

Withdrawal If a regular user stops taking an opioid, withdrawal begins within 6 to 12 hours. The intensity of the symptoms depends on the degree of the addiction; they may grow stronger for 24 to 72 hours and gradually subside over a period of 7 to 14 days, though some symptoms, such as insomnia, may persist for several months. Individuals may develop craving for an opioid, irritability, nausea or vomiting, muscle aches, runny nose or eyes, dilated pupils, sweating, diarrhea, yawning, fever, and insomnia. Opioid withdrawal usually is not life-threatening.

Methadone Maintenance

Opioid dependence is a very difficult addiction to overcome. Studies demonstrate that only 10 to 30 percent of heroin users are able to maintain abstinence. This fact contributed to the development of a unique, yet still controversial, treatment for opioid dependence: the use of methadone, a long-acting opioid that users can substitute for heroin or other opioids.

Methadone is used in two basic ways to treat opioid dependence: as an opioid substitute for detoxification, usually with a gradual tapering of methadone over a period of 21 to 180 days, and as a maintenance treatment. Methadone maintenance has been criticized by some as nothing more than the substitution of a legal opioid, methadone, for an illegal opioid, heroin.

Methadone maintenance may be the most thoroughly studied drug treatment. Research has clearly documented several important positive benefits, including decreased use of illicit opioids; decreased criminal behavior; decreased risk of contracting HIV infection (through sharing of infected needles); and improvements in physical health, employment, and other lifestyle factors. Individuals who have been on methadone maintenance for a long time (often

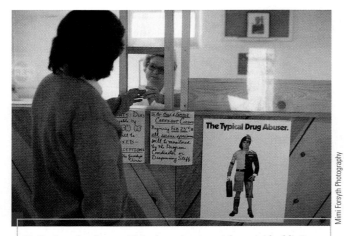

Mimi Forsyth Photography

Methadone has been criticized as a treatment for opioid addiction, but research clearly demonstrates positive benefits. Those who participate in long-term methadone maintenance programs usually move out of the drug culture. Eventually they can leave methadone dependence behind them.

years), have stable relationships and employment, have assimilated themselves into the nondrug culture, and are highly motivated to get off methadone have the best chance for successful detoxification from methadone.

Other medications are used to treat narcotics dependence. Orlam (LAAM, levo alphacetylmethadol) has a longer duration of action than methadone but also has a high abuse potential. Physicians now use buprenorphine, available in sublingual (under the tongue) and injectable forms, as an outpatient treatment for opioid dependence.

HALLUCINOGENS

The drugs known as **hallucinogens** produce vivid and unusual changes in thought, feeling, and perception. Hallucinogens do not produce dependence in the same way as cocaine or heroin. Individuals who have an unpleasant experience after trying a hallucinogen may stop using the drug completely without suffering withdrawal symptoms. Others continue regular or occasional use because they enjoy the effects.

LSD and Mescaline

LSD (*lysergic acid diethylamide,* acid) was initially developed as a tool to explore mental illness. It became popular in the 1960s and resurfaced among teenagers in the 1990s. LSD is taken orally, either blotted onto pieces of paper that are held in the mouth or chewed along with another substance, such as a sugar cube. Peyote (whose active ingredient is *mescaline*) is another hallucinogen, but it is much less commonly used in this country.

The effects of hallucinogens depend greatly on the dose, the individual's expectations and personality, and the setting for drug use. Many users report religious or mystical imagery and thoughts; some feel they are experiencing profound insights. Usually the user realizes that perceptual changes

are caused by the hallucinogen, but some become convinced that they have lost their minds. Drugs sold as hallucinogens are frequently mixed with other drugs, such as PCP and amphetamines, combinations that can produce unexpected and frightening effects.

Individuals having a *bad trip* may blame themselves and feel excessively guilty, tense, and so agitated that they cannot stop talking and have trouble sleeping. They may fear that they have destroyed their brains and will never return to normal. Someone who already is depressed may take a hallucinogen to lift his or her spirits, only to become more depressed. Suicide is a real danger.

Phencyclidine (PCP)

PCP (**phencyclidine,** brand name Sernyl; street names angel dust, peace pill, lovely, and green) is an illicit drug manufactured as a tablet, capsule, liquid, flake, spray, or crystal-like white powder that can be swallowed, smoked, sniffed, or injected. Sometimes it is sprinkled on crack, marijuana, tobacco, or parsley, and smoked. A fine-powdered form of PCP can be snorted or injected. Once PCP was thought to have medicinal value as an anesthetic, but its side effects, including delirium and hallucinations, now make it unacceptable for medical use.

PCP use peaked in the 1970s, but it remains a popular drug of abuse in both inner-city ghettos and suburban high schools. Users often think that the PCP they take together with another illegal psychoactive substance, such as amphetamines, coke, or hallucinogens, is responsible for the highs they feel, so they seek it out specifically.

How Users Feel The effects of PCP are utterly unpredictable. It may trigger violent behavior or irreversible psychosis the first time it is used, or the twentieth time, or never. In low doses, PCP produces changes—from hallucinations or euphoria to feelings of emptiness or numbness—similar to those produced by other psychoactive drugs. Higher doses may produce a stupor that lasts several days, increased heart rate and blood pressure, skin flushing, sweating, dizziness, and numbness.

Risks Some people experience repetitive motor movements (such as facial grimacing), hallucinations, and paranoia. Suicide is a definite risk. Intoxication typically lasts four to six hours, but some effects can linger for several days. Delirium may occur within 24 hours of taking PCP or after recovery from an overdose and can last as much as a week.

INHALANTS

Inhalants or **deleriants** are chemicals that produce vapors with psychoactive effects. The most commonly abused inhalants are solvents, aerosols, model-airplane glue, cleaning fluids, and petroleum products like kerosene and butane. Some anesthetics and nitrous oxide (laughing gas) are also abused.

Young people who have been treated for mental health problems, have a history of foster care, or already abuse other drugs have an increased risk of abusing or becoming dependent on inhalants. In addition, adolescents who first begin using inhalants at an early age are more likely to become dependent on them. Approximately 9 percent of adolescents nationwide report having used inhalants in their lifetime. Teens with inhalant use disorders report coexisting multiple drug abuse and dependence, mental health treatment, and delinquent behaviors.[60]

How Users Feel Inhalants very rapidly reach the lungs, bloodstream, and other parts of the body. At low doses, users may feel slightly stimulated; at higher doses, they may feel less inhibited. Intoxication often occurs within five minutes and can last more than an hour. Inhalant users do not report the intense rush associated with other drugs; nor do they experience the perceptual changes associated with LSD. However, inhalants interfere with thinking and impulse control, so users may act in dangerous or destructive ways.

Often there are visible external signs of use: a rash around the nose and mouth; breath odors; residue on face, hands, and clothing; redness, swelling, and tearing of the eyes; and irritation of throat, lungs, and nose that leads to coughing and gagging. Nausea and headache also may occur.

Risks Regular use of inhalants leads to tolerance, so the sniffer needs more and more to attain the desired effects. Younger children who use inhalants several times a week may develop dependence. Older users who become dependent may use the drugs many times a day.

Although some young people believe inhalants are safe, this is far from true. Inhalation of butane from cigarette lighters displaces oxygen in the lungs, causing suffocation. Users also can suffocate while covering their heads with a plastic bag to inhale the substance or from inhaling vomit into their lungs while high. The effects of inhalants are unpredictable, and even a single episode can trigger asphyxiation or cardiac arrhythmia, leading to disability or death. Abusers also can develop difficulties with memory and abstract reasoning, problems with coordination, and uncontrollable movements of the extremities.

TREATING DRUG DEPENDENCE AND ABUSE

An estimated 6.1 million Americans are in need of drug treatment, but the vast majority—some 5 million—never get treatment.[61] The most difficult step for a drug user is to admit that he or she *is* in fact an addict. If drug abusers are not forced to deal with their problem through some unexpected trauma, such as being fired or going bankrupt, those who care—family, friends, coworkers, doctors—may have to confront them and insist that they do something about their addiction. Often this *intervention* can be the turning point for addicts and their families. Treatment has proven equally successful for young people and for older adults.

Treatment may take place in an outpatient setting, a residential facility, or a hospital. Increasingly, treatment thereafter is tailored to address coexisting or dual diagnoses.

A personal treatment plan may consist of individual psychotherapy, marital and family therapy, medication, and behavior therapy. Once an individual has made the decision to seek help for substance abuse, the first step usually is detoxification, which involves clearing the drug from the body. An exception is methadone maintenance, discussed earlier in this chapter, which does not rely on complete detoxification.

Controlled and supervised withdrawal within a medical or psychiatric hospital may be recommended if an individual has not been able to stop using drugs as an outpatient or in a residential treatment program. Detoxification is most likely to be complicated in a polysubstance abuser, who may require close monitoring and treatment of potentially fatal withdrawal symptoms. Other reasons for inpatient treatment include lack of psychosocial support for maintaining abstinence and the absence of a drug-free living environment. Restrictions on insurance coverage may limit the number of days of inpatient care. Increasingly, once individuals complete detoxification, they continue treatment in residential programs or as outpatients.

Medications are used in detoxification to alleviate withdrawal symptoms and prevent medical and psychiatric complications. Once withdrawal is complete, these medications are discontinued, so the individual is in a drug-free state. However, individuals with mental disorders may require appropriate psychiatric medication to manage their symptoms and reduce the risk of relapse. For example, a person suffering from major depression or panic disorder may require ongoing treatment with antidepressant medication.

The aim of chemical dependence treatment is to help individuals establish and maintain their recovery from alcohol and drugs of abuse. Recovery is a dynamic process of personal growth and healing in which the drug user makes the transition from a lifestyle of active substance use to a drug-free lifestyle.

Whatever their setting, chemical dependence treatment programs initially involve some period of intensive treatment followed by one or two years of continuing aftercare. Most freestanding programs (those not affiliated with a hospital) follow what is known as the *Minnesota model,* a treatment approach developed at Hazelden Recovery Center in Center City, Minnesota, more than 30 years ago. Its key principles include a focus on drug use as the primary problem, not as a symptom of underlying emotional problems; a multidisciplinary approach that addresses the physical, emotional, spiritual, family, and social aspects of the individual; a supportive community; and a goal of abstinence and health.

Outpatient programs for substance abuse, offered by freestanding centers, hospitals, and community mental health centers, often run four or five nights a week for four to eight weeks, or in daily eight-hour sessions for seven to eight days, followed by weekly group therapy. These outpatient programs allow recovering drug users to go on with their daily lives and learn to deal with day-to-day work and family stresses. Mental health professionals in private practice also offer individually structured outpatient treatment.

Many behavioral therapies can help patients achieve and maintain prolonged abstinence. Cognitive behavioral relapse prevention, which teaches new ways of thinking and acting, has proved a lasting therapy for many drug addicted individuals. Contingency management uses a system of rewards and punishments to make abstinence attractive and drug use unattractive.[62]

Therapy groups provide an opportunity for individuals who have often been isolated by their drug use to participate in normal social settings. Small groups with other former drug users can be especially valuable because they all share the experience of drug use. Group members can confront one another with frankness and cut through lies and rationalizations. A professional therapist keeps members of the group from ganging up on one person. After their discharge from inpatient treatment, individuals who became involved in self-help groups are less likely to use drugs, cope better with stress, and develop richer friendship networks.

Based on the Alcoholics Anonymous model, 12-step programs have helped many people overcome addictions. The one requirement for membership is a desire to end a pattern of addictive behavior.

12-STEP PROGRAMS

Since its founding in 1935, Alcoholics Anonymous (AA)—the oldest, largest, and most successful self-help program in the world—has spawned a worldwide movement. As many as 200 different recovery programs are based on the spiritual **12-step program** of AA. Participation in 12-step programs for drug abusers, such as Substance Anonymous, Narcotics Anonymous, and Cocaine Anonymous, is of fundamental importance in promoting and maintaining long-term abstinence.

The basic precept of 12-step programs is that members have been powerless when it comes to controlling their addictive behavior on their own. These programs don't recruit members. The desire to stop must come from the individual, who can call the number of a 12-step program, listed in the telephone book, and find out when and where the next nearby meeting will be held. A representative may offer to send someone to the caller's house to talk about the problem and to escort him or her to the next meeting.

Meetings of various 12-step programs are held daily in almost every city in the country. (Some chapters, whose members often include the disabled or those in remote areas, meet via Internet chat rooms or electronic bulletin boards.) There are no dues or fees for membership. Many individuals belong to several programs because they have several problems, such as alcoholism, substance abuse, and pathological gambling. All have only one requirement for membership: a desire to stop an addictive behavior.

To get the most out of a 12-step program:

- Try out different groups until you find one you like and in which you feel comfortable.

- Once you find a group in which you feel comfortable, go back several times (some recommend a minimum of six meetings) before making a final decision on whether to continue.

- Keep an open mind. Listen to other people's stories and ask yourself if you've had similar feelings or experiences.

- Accept whatever feels right to you and ignore the rest. One common saying in 12-step programs is, "Take what you like and leave the rest."

Strategies for Prevention ■ Relapse-Prevention Planning

The following steps from Terence Gorski and Merlene Miller's *Staying Sober: A Guide for Relapse Prevention,* can lower the likelihood of relapses:

- **Stabilization and self-assessment.** Get control of yourself. Find out what's going on in your head, heart, and life.

- **Education.** Learn about relapse and what to do to prevent it.

- **Warning-sign identification and management.** Make a list of your personal relapse warning signs. Learn how to interrupt them before you lose control.

- **Inventory training.** Learn how to become consciously aware of warning signs as they develop.

- **Review of the recovery program.** Make sure your recovery program is able to help you manage your warning signs of relapse.

- **Involvement of significant others.** Teach them how to help you avoid relapses.

RELAPSE PREVENTION

The most common clinical course for substance abuse disorders involves a pattern of multiple relapses over the course of a lifespan. It is important for individuals with these problems and their families to recognize this fact. When relapses do occur, they should be viewed as neither a mark of defeat nor evidence of moral weakness. While painful, they do not erase the progress that has been achieved and ultimately may strengthen self-understanding. They can serve as reminders of potential pitfalls to avoid in the future.

One key to preventing relapse is learning to avoid obvious cues and associations that can set off intense cravings. This means staying away from the people and places linked with past drug use. Some therapists use conditioning techniques to give former users some sense of control over their urge to use the drug. The theory behind this approach, which is called *extinction* of conditioned behavior, is that with repeated exposure—for example, to videotapes of dealers selling crack cocaine—the arousal and craving will diminish. While this technique by itself cannot ward off relapses, it does seem to enhance the overall effectiveness of other therapies.

Another important lesson that therapists emphasize is that every lapse does not have to lead to a full-blown relapse. Users can turn to the skills acquired in treatment—calling people for support or going to meetings—to avoid a major relapse. Ultimately, users must learn much more than how to avoid temptation; they must examine their entire view of the world and learn new ways to live in it without turning to drugs. This is the underlying goal of the recovery process.

Learn It / Live It

Choosing an Addiction-Free Lifestyle

People with substance abuse disorders and addictive behaviors lose control of their choices and their lives. Their compulsion to gamble or to use a drug seems irresistible. You, in contrast, have a choice. You can create a life and a lifestyle with no need and no room for reliance on a substance or a self-destructive behavior. Here are some ways to go about it:

- **Set goals for yourself.** Think about who you want to become, what you'd like to do, the future you wish for yourself. Focus on what it will take—years of education, perhaps, or specialized training—to achieve these goals. Understand that drugs can only get in the way and diminish your potential.

- **Participate in drug-free activities.** If you're bored or unfocused, drugs may appeal to you simply as something to do. Take charge of your time. Play a sport. Work out at the gym. Join a club. Volunteer. Start a blog.

- **Educate yourself.** Much of the information that young people hear from friends, particularly drug-using friends, is wrong. Drugs that are used as

medicines are not safe for recreational use. The fact that many people at a rave are having fun doesn't mean that some aren't endangering their brains and their lives by taking club drugs. Get the facts for yourself from sites such as those on page 333.

- **Choose friends with a future.** The world of drug users shrinks. Nothing matters more than the next hit, the next high, the next fix. Losing all sense of tomorrow, they focus on getting through the day with the help of drugs. Are these the people you want to spend time with? Choose friends who can broaden your world with new ideas, ambitious plans, and great dreams for tomorrow.

Making This Chapter Work for You

Review Questions

1. Which of the following statements about drugs is *false?*
   a. Toxicity is the dosage level of a prescription.
   b. Drugs can be injected into the body intravenously, intramuscularly, or subcutaneously.
   c. Drug misuse is the taking of a drug for a purpose other than that for which it was medically intended.
   d. An individual's response to a drug can be affected by the setting in which the drug is used.

2. To help ensure that an over-the-counter or prescription drug is safe and effective:
   a. take smaller dosages than indicated in the instructions.
   b. test your response to the drug by borrowing a similar medication from a friend.
   c. ask your doctor or pharmacist about possible interactions with other medications.
   d. buy all of your medications online.

3. Which of the following drugs does *not* cause withdrawal symptoms?
   a. caffeine
   b. marijuana
   c. heroin
   d. aspirin

4. Individuals with substance use disorders
   a. are usually not physically dependent on their drug of choice.
   b. have a compulsion to use one or more addictive substances.
   c. require less and less of the preferred drug to achieve the desired effect.
   d. suffer withdrawal symptoms when they use the drug regularly.

5. Amphetamine is very similar to which of the following in its effects on the central nervous system?

a. marijuana

b. heroin

c. cocaine

d. alcohol

6. Which of the following statements about marijuana is *false?*

   a. People who have used marijuana may experience psychoactive effects for several days after use.

   b. Marijuana has shown some effectiveness in treating chemotherapy-related nausea.

   c. Unlike long-term use of alcohol, regular use of marijuana does not have any long-lasting health consequences.

   d. Depending on the amount of marijuana used, its effects can range from a mild sense of euphoria to extreme panic.

7. Cocaine dependence can result in all of the following *except*

   a. stroke.

   b. paranoia and violent behavior.

   c. heart failure.

   d. enhanced sexual performance.

8. Which of the following statements about club drugs is true?

   a. Club drugs can produce many unwanted effects, including hallucinations and paranoia.

   b. Most club drugs do not pose the same health dangers as "hard" drugs such as heroin.

   c. MDMA is the street name for ecstasy.

   d. When combined with extended physical exertion, club drugs can lead to hypothermia (lowered body temperature).

9. The opioids

   a. are not addictive if used in a prescription form such as codeine or Demerol.

   b. produce an immediate but short-lasting high and feeling of euphoria.

   c. include morphine, which is typically used for cough suppression.

   d. are illegal in the United States, although they are allowed in other countries to help control severe pain.

10. Which of the following statements about drug dependence treatment is *false?*

    a. Chemical dependence treatment programs usually involve medications to alleviate withdrawal symptoms.

    b. Detoxification is usually the first step in a drug treatment program.

    c. Relapses are not uncommon for a person who has undergone drug treatment.

    d. The 12-step recovery program associated with Alcoholics Anonymous has been shown to be ineffective with individuals with drug dependence disorders.

Answers to these questions can be found on p. 587.

Critical Thinking

1. Some state programs send nonviolent drug offenders into drug treatment rather than jail. In one case, about a quarter of those diverted into rehabilitation from prison, including those addicted to methamphetamine, completed their alternative treatment successfully. Would you support more programs like this? Why or why not?

2. Some Web enthusiasts oppose any kind of government regulations on the Internet. Do you agree or disagree? How would you address the problems associated with distributing drugs online?

3. Suppose that a close friend is using amphetamines to keep her energy levels high so that she can continue to attend school full-time and hold down a job to pay her school expenses. You fear that she is developing a substance abuse disorder. What can you do to help her realize the dangers of her behavior? What resources are available at your school or in your community to help her deal with both her drug problem and her financial needs?

Media Menu

Health Now™

Throughout the chapter, this icon introduces a list of resources on the Health-Now website at **http://healthnow.brookscole.com/ith** that will:

- Help you evaluate your knowledge of the material.
- Allow you to take an exam-prep quiz.
- Provide a Personalized Learning Plan targeting resources that address areas you should study.
- Coach you through identifying target goals for behavior change and creating and monitoring your personal change plan throughout the semester.

INTERNET CONNECTIONS

National Institute on Drug Abuse

www.nida.nih.gov

This government site—a virtual clearinghouse of information for students, parents, teachers, researchers, and health professionals—features current treatment and research, as well as a comprehensive database on common drugs of abuse. The science of drug abuse and addictions is discussed with a focus on the major illegal drugs in use, with additional resources on drug testing, treatment research, and trends/statistics.

Partnership for a Drug-Free America

www.drugfree.org

This site features current resources and photographs on a wide spectrum of drugs, including performance-enhancing drugs, club drugs, and commonly abused prescription drugs. The drug guide even allows you to search for a drug using its slang name.

Self Survey ▪▪ Do You Have a Substance Use Disorder?

Check the statements that apply to you.

- Use more of an illegal drug or a prescription medication or use a drug for a longer period of time than you desire or intend. _____
- Try, repeatedly and unsuccessfully, to cut down or control drug use. _____
- Spend a great deal of time doing whatever is necessary in order to get drugs, taking them, or recovering from their use. _____
- Be so high or feel so bad after drug use that you often cannot work or fulfill other responsibilities. _____
- Give up or cut back on important social, work, or recreational activities because of drug use. _____
- Continue to use drugs even though you realize that they are causing or worsening physical or mental problems. _____
- Use a lot more of a drug in order to achieve a "high" or desired effect or feel fewer such effects than in the past. _____
- Use drugs in dangerous ways or situations. _____
- Have repeated drug-related legal problems, such as arrests for possession. _____
- Continue to use drugs, even though the drug causes or worsens social or personal problems, such as arguments with a spouse. _____
- Develop hand tremors or other withdrawal symptoms if you cut down or stop drug use. _____
- Take drugs to relieve or avoid withdrawal symptoms. _____

The more blanks that you (or someone close to you) checks, the more reason you have to be concerned about drug use. The most difficult step for anyone with a substance use disorder is to admit that he or she has a problem. Sometimes a drug-related crisis, such as being arrested or fired, forces individuals to acknowledge the impact of drugs. If not, those who care—family, friends, boss, physician—may have to confront them and insist that they do something about it. This confrontation, planned beforehand, is called an *intervention* and can be the turning point for drug users and their families.

Club Drugs

www.clubdrugs.org

This site is a service of the National Institute of Drug Abuse to provide information on club drugs.

Drug Help

www.drughelp.org

This is a national nonprofit information and referral service providing information on specific drugs and treatment options in addition to referrals to public and private treatment programs, self-help groups, family support groups and crisis centers.

InfoTrac College Edition Activities Log on, insert **drug abuse** into the Keyword search box, and limit your search to the past year. When you get the results, Mark articles to review, then Select one to read. Summarize three or four key points from the article.

You can find additional readings related to personal health with InfoTrac College Edition, an online library of more than 900 journals and publications. Follow the instructions for accessing InfoTrac College Edition that were packaged with your textbook; then search for articles using a keyword search.

For additional links, resources, and suggested readings on the InfoTrac College Edition, visit our Health and Wellness Resourc Center at **http://health .wadsworth.com.**

Key Terms

The terms listed are used on the page indicated. Definitions of the terms are in the Glossary at the end of this book.

addiction 314	deleriants 329
amphetamines 322	drug 307
barbiturates 326	drug abuse 307
benzodiazepines 326	drug misuse 307
club drugs 320	ecstasy (MDMA) 320
cocaine 324	generic 312

YOUR ACTION PLAN FOR RECOGNIZING SUBSTANCE ABUSE

How can you tell if a friend or loved one has a substance use disorder? Look for the following warning signs:

- **An abrupt change in attitude.** Individuals may lose interest in activities they once enjoyed or in being with friends they once valued.

- **Mood swings.** Drug users may often seem withdrawn or "out of it," or they may display unusual temper flareups.

- **A decline in performance.** Students may start skipping classes, stop studying, or not complete assignments; their grades may plummet.

- **Increased sensitivity.** Individuals may react intensely to any criticism or become easily frustrated or angered.

- **Secrecy.** Drug users may make furtive telephone calls or demand greater privacy concerning their personal possessions or their whereabouts.

- **Physical changes.** Individuals using drugs may change their pattern of sleep, spending more time in bed or sleeping at odd hours. They also may change their eating habits and lose weight.

- **Money problems.** Drug users may constantly borrow money, seem short of cash, or begin stealing.

- **Changes in appearance.** As they become more involved with drugs, users often lose regard for their personal appearance and look disheveled.

- **Defiance of restrictions.** Individuals may ignore or deliberately refuse to comply with deadlines, curfews, or other regulations.

- **Changes in relationships.** Drug users may quarrel more frequently with family members or old friends and develop strong allegiances with new acquaintances, including other drug users.

CASE IN POINT

Student: Clay, 18

Goal: Break the habit of using his roommate's ADHD medication when studying for tests

Action Plan:

- Make up a daily and weekly study plan to keep up with reading assignments
- Attend study groups for pre-exam reviews
- Stick to a regular schedule for getting up, working out, and studying during exam weeks
- Avoid overconsumption of caffeinated energy drinks
- Go to bed at a reasonable hour before a test rather than pulling an all-nighter

Health⊗Now™   If you want to write your own goals for avoiding drug misuse, go to the **Wellness Journal at HealthNow** at www.xxxxxx.

12 Alcohol Use, Misuse, and Abuse

It was just another Friday night at the frat house. The drinking started early and usually didn't stop until dawn. One of the brothers, a popular easy-going guy named Ryan—not usually much of a drinker—was celebrating a big birthday: his twenty-first. Egged on by the hooting crowd, Ryan bolted down one drink after another, after another, after another.

By the time Ryan reached twelve, he was slurring his words. As he kept chugging drinks, his face looked flushed; he started sweating heavily. When Ryan lurched to his feet, he swayed unsteadily for a few moments and then collapsed. At first everyone laughed. Then two of his buddies tried to revive him. They couldn't.

"He's not breathing!" one of them shouted. Someone called 911, and paramedics rushed Ryan to the nearest hospital. His blood alcohol concentration was several times above the legal limit. Despite intensive efforts by the medical team, nothing helped. Ryan's twenty-first birthday was his last.

As Ryan's tragic death shows, alcohol, when not used responsibly, can take an enormous toll. No medical conditions, other than heart disease, cause more disability and premature death than alcohol-related problems. No mental or medical disorders touch the lives of more families. No other form of disability costs individuals, employers, and the government more for treatment, injuries, reduced worker productivity, and property damage. The costs in emotional pain and in lost and shattered lives because of irresponsible drinking are beyond measure.

This chapter provides information about alcohol; its impact on the body, brain, behavior, and society; patterns of drinking; drinking on campus; binge drinking; and the recognition, understanding, and treatment of drinking problems and of alcoholism.

© E. Koch /zefa /CORBIS

After studying the material in this chapter, you should be able to:

▌ **Define** a standard drink.

▌ **Describe** the factors affecting a drinker's response to alcohol consumption.

▌ **Describe** the symptoms of alcohol poisoning and state what you should do if someone exhibits any of the symptoms.

▌ **Describe** the impact of alcohol misuse among college students, and **define** binge drinking.

▌ **List** the effects of alcohol on the body systems.

▌ **Define** alcohol abuse, dependence, and alcoholism, and **list** their symptoms.

▌ **List** the negative consequences to individuals, and to our society, from alcohol abuse.

▌ **Explain** the common treatment methods for alcoholism.

YOUR BODY'S RESPONSE TO ALCOHOL

Pure alcohol is a colorless liquid obtained through the fermentation of a liquid containing sugar. **Ethyl alcohol,** or *ethanol,* is the type of alcohol in alcoholic beverages. Another type—methyl, or wood, alcohol—is a poison that should never be drunk. Any liquid containing 0.5 to 80 percent ethyl alcohol by volume is an alcoholic beverage. However, different drinks contain different amounts of alcohol.

 Do you know what a "drink" is? Most students don't. In one experiment undergraduates defined a "drink" as one serving, regardless of how big it was or how much alcohol it contained.[1] In fact, one drink can be any of the following:

- **One bottle or can** (12 ounces) of beer, which is 5 percent alcohol.
- **One glass** (4 ounces) of table wine, such as burgundy, which is 12 percent alcohol.
- **One small glass** (2½ ounces) of fortified wine, which is 20 percent alcohol.
- **One shot** (1 ounce) of distilled spirits (such as whiskey, vodka, or rum), which is 50 percent alcohol.

All of these drinks contain close to the same amount of alcohol—that is, if the number of ounces in each drink is multiplied by the percentage of alcohol, each drink contains the equivalent of approximately ½ ounce of 100 percent ethyl alcohol.

But the words *bottle* and *glass* can be deceiving. Drinking a 16-ounce bottle of malt liquor, which is 6.4 percent alcohol, is not the same as drinking a 12-ounce glass of light beer (3.2% alcohol): The malt liquor contains 1 ounce of alcohol and is the equivalent of two drinks. Two bottles of high-alcohol wines (such as Cisco), packaged to resemble much less powerful wine coolers, can lead to alcohol poisoning, especially in those who weigh less than 150 pounds.

With distilled spirits (such as bourbon, scotch, vodka, gin, and rum), alcohol content is expressed in terms of **proof,** a number that is twice the percentage of alcohol: 100-proof bourbon is 50 percent alcohol; 80-proof gin is 40 percent alcohol. Many mixed drinks are equivalent to one and a half or two standard drinks; for instance, see the margarita in Figure 12-1.

FAQ WHAT IS BLOOD ALCOHOL CONCENTRATION?

The amount of alcohol in your blood at any given time is your **blood-alcohol concentration (BAC).** It is expressed in terms of the percentage of alcohol in the blood and is often measured from breath or urine samples.

Law enforcement officers use BAC to determine whether a driver is legally drunk. All the states have followed the recommendation of the federal Department of Transportation to set 0.08 percent—the BAC that a 150-pound man would have after consuming about three mixed drinks within an hour—as the threshold at which a person can be cited for drunk driving (Figure 12-2).

 Using a formula for blood alcohol concentration developed by highway transportation officials, researchers calculate that when college students drink, their typical BAC is 0.079, dangerously close to the legal limit.[2]

A BAC of 0.05 percent indicates approximately 5 parts alcohol to 10,000 parts other blood components. Most people reach this level after consuming one or two drinks and experience all the positive sensations of drinking—relaxation, euphoria, and well-being—without feeling intoxicated. If they continue to drink past the 0.05 percent BAC level, they start feeling worse rather than better, gradually losing control of speech, balance, and emotions. At a BAC of 0.2 percent, they may pass out. At a BAC of 0.3 percent, they could lapse into a coma; at 0.4 percent, they could die.

Margarita:

1½ oz. tequila (80 proof) = 1.5 oz. × 40 percent alcohol = 0.6 oz. alcohol

¾ oz. triple sec (60 proof) = .75 oz. × 30 percent alcohol = 0.23 oz. alcohol

Splash of sour mix

Dash of lime juice

Salt for the rim

0.83 oz. alcohol = 1½ drinks

Malt liquor:

16 oz. × 6.4 percent alcohol = 1 oz. alcohol = 2 drinks

FIGURE 12-1 How many standard drinks are you drinking?

Men	Approximate blood alcohol percentage								
	Body weight in pounds								
Drinks	100	120	140	160	180	200	220	240	
0	.00	.00	.00	.00	.00	.00	.00	.00	Only safe driving limit
1	.04	.03	.03	.02	.02	.02	.02	.02	Impairment begins
2	.08	.06	.05	.05	.04	.04	.03	.03	Driving skills significantly affected
3	.11	.09	.08	.07	.06	.06	.05	.05	
4	.15	.12	.11	.09	.08	.08	.07	.06	Possible criminal penalties
5	.19	.16	.13	.12	.11	.09	.09	.08	
6	.23	.19	.16	.14	.13	.11	.10	.09	
7	.26	.22	.19	.16	.15	.13	.12	.11	Legally intoxicated
8	.30	.25	.21	.19	.17	.15	.14	.13	
9	.34	.28	.24	.21	.19	.17	.15	.14	Criminal penalties
10	.38	.31	.27	.23	.21	.19	.17	.16	

Subtract 0.01 percent for each 40 minutes of drinking.
One drink is 1.25 oz. of 80 proof liquor, 12 oz. of beer, or 5 oz. of table wine.

Women	Approximate blood alcohol percentage									
	Body weight in pounds									
Drinks	90	100	120	140	160	180	200	220	240	
0	.00	.00	.00	.00	.00	.00	.00	.00	.00	Only safe driving limit
1	.05	.05	.04	.03	.03	.03	.02	.02	.02	Impairment begins
2	.10	.09	.08	.07	.06	.05	.05	.04	.04	Driving skills significantly affected
3	.15	.14	.11	.10	.09	.08	.07	.06	.06	
4	.20	.18	.15	.13	.11	.10	.09	.08	.08	Possible criminal penalties
5	.25	.23	.19	.16	.14	.13	.11	.10	.09	
6	.30	.27	.23	.19	.17	.15	.14	.12	.11	
7	.35	.32	.27	.23	.20	.18	.16	.14	.13	Legally intoxicated
8	.40	.36	.30	.26	.23	.20	.18	.17	.15	
9	.45	.41	.34	.29	.26	.23	.20	.19	.17	Criminal penalties
10	.51	.45	.38	.32	.28	.25	.23	.21	.19	

Subtract 0.01 percent for each 40 minutes of drinking.
One drink is 1.25 oz. of 80 proof liquor, 12 oz. of beer, or 5 oz. of table wine.

FIGURE 12-2   Alcohol Impairment Chart

Source: Adapted from data supplied by the Pennsylvania Liquor Control Board.

Many factors affect an individual's BAC and response to alcohol, including the following:

▪ **How much and how quickly you drink.** The more alcohol you put into your body, the higher your BAC. If you chug drink after drink, your liver, which metabolizes about ½ ounce of alcohol an hour, won't be able to keep up—and your BAC will soar.

▪ **What you're drinking.** The stronger the drink, the faster and harder the alcohol hits. Straight shots of liquor and cocktails such as martinis will get alcohol into your bloodstream faster than beer or table wine. Beer and wine not only contain lower concentrations of alcohol, but they also contain nonalcoholic substances that slow the rate of **absorption** (passage of the alcohol into your body tissues). If the drink contains water, juice, or milk, the rate of absorption will be slowed. However, carbon dioxide—whether in champagne, ginger ale, or a cola—whisks alcohol into your bloodstream. Also, the alcohol in warm drinks—such as a hot rum toddy or warmed sake—moves into your bloodstream more quickly than the alcohol in chilled wine or scotch on the rocks.

- **Your size.** If you're a large person (whether due to fat or to muscle), you'll get drunk more slowly than someone smaller who's drinking the same amount of alcohol at the same rate. Heavier individuals have a larger water volume, which dilutes the alcohol they drink.

- **Your gender.** Women have lower quantities of a stomach enzyme that neutralizes alcohol, so one drink for a woman has the impact that two drinks have for a man. Hormone levels also affect the impact of alcohol. Women are more sensitive to alcohol just before menstruation, and birth control pills and other forms of estrogen can intensify alcohol's impact. (See the section "Alcohol and Gender" later in this chapter.)

- **Your age.** The same amount of alcohol produces higher BACs in older drinkers, who have lower volumes of body water to dilute the alcohol than younger drinkers do.

- **Your race.** Many members of certain ethnic groups, including Asians and Native Americans, are unable to break down alcohol as quickly as Caucasians. This can result in higher BACs, as well as uncomfortable reactions, such as flushing and nausea, when they drink.

- **Other drugs.** Some common medications—including aspirin, acetaminophen (Tylenol), and ulcer medications—can cause blood-alcohol levels to increase more rapidly. Individuals taking these drugs can be over the legal limit for blood-alcohol concentration after as little as a single drink.

- **Family history of alcoholism.** Some children of alcoholics don't develop any of the usual behavioral symptoms that indicate someone is drinking too much. It's not known whether this behavior is genetically caused or is a result of growing up with an alcoholic.

- **Eating.** Food slows the absorption of alcohol by diluting it, by covering some of the membranes through which alcohol would be absorbed, and by prolonging the time the stomach takes to empty.

- **Expectations.** In various experiments, volunteers who believed they were given alcoholic beverages but were actually given nonalcoholic drinks acted as if they were guzzling the real thing and became more talkative, relaxed, and sexually stimulated.

- **Physical tolerance.** If you drink regularly, your brain becomes accustomed to a certain level of alcohol. You may be able to look and behave in a seemingly normal fashion, even though you drink as much as would normally intoxicate someone your size. However, your driving ability and judgment will still be impaired.

Once you develop tolerance, you may drink more to get the desired effects from alcohol. In some people, this can lead to abuse and alcoholism. On the other hand, after years of drinking, some people become exquisitely sensitive to alcohol. Such reverse tolerance means that they can become intoxicated after drinking only a small amount of alcohol.

For some people, even very low blood alcohol concentrations can cause a headache, upset stomach, or dizziness. These reactions often are inborn. People who have suffered brain damage, often as a result of head trauma or encephalitis, may lose all tolerance for alcohol, either temporarily or permanently, and behave abnormally after drinking small amounts. Those who are unusually fatigued or have a debilitating physical illness may also have a low tolerance for alcohol and respond inappropriately to a small amount.

INTOXICATION

If you drink too much, the immediate consequence is that you get drunk—or, more precisely, intoxicated. Alcohol **intoxication,** which can range from mild inebriation to loss of consciousness, is characterized by at least one of the following signs: slurred speech, poor coordination, unsteady gait, abnormal eye movements, impaired attention or memory, stupor, or coma.

Medical risks of intoxication include falls, hypothermia in cold climates, and increased risk of infections because

---

Strategies for Prevention ▪▪ What to Do When Someone Is Intoxicated

- CONTINUALLY MONITOR THE INTOXICATED PERSON.
- CHECK BREATHING, waking the person often to be sure he or she is not unconscious.
- DO NOT force the person to walk or move around.

- DO NOT allow the person to drive a car or ride a bicycle.
- DO NOT give the person food, liquid (including coffee), medicines, or drugs to sober them up.

- DO NOT give the person a cold shower; the shock of the cold could cause unconsciousness.

of suppressed immune function. Time and a protective environment are the recommended treatments for alcohol intoxication.

ALCOHOL POISONING

Every year an estimated 1,700 college students between the ages of 18 and 24 die from an alcohol overdose. Because federal law requires colleges to publish all student deaths, the stories of young lives ended by alcohol poisoning have gained national attention. Yet many students remain unaware that alcohol, in large enough doses, can and does kill.

Alcohol depresses nerves that control involuntary actions, such as breathing and the gag reflex (which prevents choking). A fatal dose of alcohol will eventually suppress these functions. Because alcohol irritates the stomach, people who drink an excessive amount often vomit. If intoxication has led to a loss of consciousness, a drinker is in danger of choking on vomit, which can cause death by asphyxiation. Blood alcohol concentration can rise even after a drinker has passed out because alcohol in the stomach and intestine continues to enter the bloodstream and circulate throughout the body.

How To Tell If Someone Has Alcohol Poisoning

- If the person is breathing less than twelve times per minute or stops breathing for periods of ten seconds or more, **Call 911.**
- If the person is asleep and you are unable to wake him or her up, **Call 911.**
- Look at the person's skin. If it is cold, clammy, pale, bluish in color, **Call 911.**
- Stay with a person who is vomiting! Try to keep him or her sitting up. If the person must lie down, keep him on his side with head turned to the side. Watch for choking; if the person begins to choke, Get help immediately, **Call 911.**

Alcohol poisoning is a medical emergency requiring immediate treatment. Black coffee, a cold shower, or letting a person "sleep it off" does not help. Without medical treatment, breathing slows, becomes irregular, or stops. The heart beats irregularly. Body temperature falls, which can cause cardiac arrest. Blood sugar plummets, which can lead to seizures. Vomiting creates severe dehydration, which can cause seizures, permanent brain damage, or death. Even if the victim lives, an alcohol overdose can result in irreversible brain damage.

Rapid binge drinking is especially dangerous because the victim can ingest a fatal dose before becoming unconscious. If you suspect alcohol poisoning, call 911 for help. Don't try to guess the level of drunkenness. Tell emergency medical technicians the symptoms and, if you know, how much alcohol the victim drank. Prompt action may save a life.

Whenever a student dies of acute alcohol poisoning, blame falls on many different people: fraternities, college officials, campus police, liquor stores that sell to minors, community licensing boards. Is it the responsibility of those in authority to set up and enforce strict alcohol policies that could save students' lives? Or should students and student organizations take personal responsibility for the amount of alcohol they consume or serve? **You decide.**

DRINKING IN AMERICA

According to the most recent statistics available from the National Institute on Alcohol Abuse and Alcoholism, about 60 percent of American adults use alcohol, although they vary in how much and how often they drink. Whites are more likely to be daily or near-daily drinkers than nonwhites. Men tend to drink more and more often than women.

The median age of first alcohol use is 15. Drinking typically accelerates in the late teens, peaks in the early 20s, and decreases as people age.[3] The median age of onset for alcohol-use disorders is 19 to 20.

ABSTINENCE

Because of concern about alcohol's health effects, increasing numbers of Americans are choosing not to drink.

According to the National College Health Assessment, about one in five students (18 percent) reports never using alcohol.[4] With alcohol consumption in the United States at its lowest level in 30 years, nonalcoholic beverages have grown in popularity. They appeal to drivers, boaters, individuals with health problems that could worsen with alcohol, those who are older and can't tolerate alcohol, anyone taking medicines that interact with alcohol (including antibiotics, antidepressants, and muscle relaxers), and everyone interested in limiting alcohol intake. Under federal law, these drinks can contain some alcohol but a much smaller amount than regular beer or wine. Nonalcoholic beers and wines on the market also are lower in calories than alcoholic varieties.

Some people—such as women who are pregnant or trying to conceive; individuals with problems, such as ulcers, that might be aggravated by alcohol; those taking medications such as sleeping pills or anti-depressants; and those driving or operating any motorized equipment—shouldn't drink at all (Figure 12-3).

WHY PEOPLE DRINK

The most common reason people drink alcohol is to relax. Because it depresses the central nervous system, alcohol can make people feel less tense. Some psychologists theorize

Anyone under age 21

Individuals of any age who cannot restrict their drinking to moderate levels. This is a special concern for recovering alcoholics, problem drinkers, and people whose family members have alcohol problems.

Women who may become pregnant or who are pregnant. A safe level of alcohol intake has not been established for women at any time during pregnancy, including the first few weeks. Major birth defects, including fetal alcohol syndrome, can be caused by heavy drinking by the pregnant mother. Other fetal alcohol effects may occur at lower levels.

Individuals who plan to drive, operate machinery, or take part in other activities that require attention, skill, or coordination. Most people retain some alcohol in the blood for up to 2 to 3 hours after a single drink.

Individuals taking prescription or over-the-counter medications that can interact with alcohol. Alcohol alters the effectiveness or toxicity of many medications, and some medications may increase blood alcohol levels. If you take medications, ask your health care provider for advice about alcohol intake.

FIGURE 12-3 **Who Should Not Drink?**

Source: National Council an Alcoholism and Drug Dependence, www.ncadd.org/facts/heath.html

that men engage in *confirmatory drinking;* that is, they drink to reinforce the image of masculinity associated with alcohol consumption. Both genders may engage in *compensatory drinking,* consuming alcohol to heighten their sense of masculinity or femininity.

Here are some other reasons why men, women, or both drink:

▪ **Inherited susceptibility.** In both women and men, genetics accounts for 50 to 60 percent of a person's vulnerability to a serious drinking problem. Female alcoholics are more likely than males to have a parent who abused drugs or alcohol, who had psychiatric problems, or who attempted suicide.

▪ **Childhood traumas.** Female alcoholics often report that they were physically or sexually abused as children or suffered great distress because of poverty or a parent's death.

▪ **Depression.** Women are more likely than men to be depressed prior to drinking and to suffer from both depression and a drinking problem at the same time. Young men who do not drink, as well as those who drink heavily, have high levels of depression and distress.

▪ **Relationship issues.** Single, separated, or divorced men and women drink more and more often than married ones.

▪ **Psychological factors.** Both men and women may drink to compensate for feelings of inadequacy. Women who tend to ruminate or mull over bad feelings may find that alcohol increases this tendency and makes them feel more distressed.

▪ **Self-medication.** More so than men, some women feel it's permissible to use alcohol as if it were a medicine. As long as they're taking it for a reason, it seems acceptable to them, even if they're drifting into a drinking problem.

▪ **Social ease.** When people use alcohol, they may seem bolder, wittier, sexier. At the same time, they become more relaxed and seem to enjoy each other's company more. Because alcohol lowers inhibitions, some people see it as a prelude to seduction.

▪ **Role models.** Athletes, some of the most admired celebrities in our country, have a long history of appearing in commercials for alcohol. Many advertisements feature glamorous women holding or sipping alcoholic beverages.

▪ **Advertising.** Brewers and beer distributors spend $15 to $20 million a year promoting the message: If you want to have fun, have a drink. Adolescents may be especially responsive to such sales pitches.

(FAQ) WHAT IS MODERATE DRINKING?

The federal government's Dietary Guidelines for Americans recommend no more than one drink a day for women and no more than two drinks a day for men (Figure 12-4). The American Heart Association (AHA) advises that alcohol account for no more than 15 percent of the total calories consumed by an individual every day, up to an absolute maximum of 1.75 ounces of alcohol a day—the equivalent of three beers, two mixed drinks, or three and a half glasses of wine. Drinking in moderation may lower the risk of heart disease, mainly among men over age 45 and women over age 55.

The dangers of alcohol increase along with the amount you drink. Heavy drinking destroys the liver, weakens the heart, elevates blood pressure, damages the brain, and increases the risk of cancer. Individuals who drink heavily have a higher mortality rate than those who have two or fewer drinks a day. However, the boundary between safe,

WHAT IS MODERATION?

Women	Men
No more than one drink per day	No more than two drinks per day

This limit is based on differences between the sexes in both weight and metabolism.

COUNT AS A DRINK . . .

Best BEER		
12 oz. of regular beer (150 calories)	5 oz. of wine (100 calories)	1.5 oz. of 80-proof (100 calories)

FIGURE 12-4   What Is Moderation? Recommendations from Dietary Guidelines for Americans

Source: National Council on Alcoholism and Drug Dependence, www.ncadd.org/facts/health.html

Drinking games and binges, which are common on college campuses, are dangerous in themselves and increase the likelihood of other risky behaviors, such as driving while intoxicated.

and moderate drinking and dangerous drinking isn't the same for everyone. For some people, the upper limit of safety is zero: Once they start, they can't stop.

BINGE DRINKING

Binge drinking consists of having five or more drinks in a single sitting for a man or four drinks in a single sitting for a woman. Although this definition is widely used, some criticize it for overlooking body weight and the length of time over which drinking occurs—both factors that influence the effects of alcohol consumption.[5] It also does not take into account alcohol tolerance, metabolism, and medications.

By any measure, drinking multiple drinks at a single setting is common—and hazardous. About half of the alcohol consumed by adults—and 90 percent of alcohol drunk by underage young people—is in the form of binge drinks.[6] Binge drinking accounts for half of alcohol-related deaths and a wide range of serious health and social problems, including motor vehicle accidents, injuries from falls, drowning, hypothermia, and burns; heart attacks; suicide; violence to others; unplanned pregnancy; and sexually transmitted infection.

Recent research shows a strong link between binge drinking and violence, including murders, assaults, robberies, and sexual offenses.

Among high school students who drink, 60 percent report binge-drinking, as do about 40 percent of college students (see page 345). Among adults, about 29 percent of current drinkers report having engaged in a binge in the last months. While the prevalence of binge drinking has remained relatively constant over recent years, the number of binge-drinking episodes by adults has increased 29 percent—up to 1.5 billion.[7]

Binge drinking among women ages 18 to 44 may endanger not only a woman's health but that of her unborn child. Binge drinking during pregnancy, not the total amount of alcohol consumed, doubles the risk of mental retardation and delinquent behavior in children.[8]

Among the solutions public health officials have suggested to halt binge drinking are increased taxes to raise the price of alcohol, enforcing strict restrictions on sales to underage minors, and screening and brief counseling for individuals identified as binge drinkers. But taking personal responsibility also is critical to ending binge drinking and preventing its harmful consequences (see "You Decide").

DRINKING AND DRIVING

Drunk driving is the most frequently committed crime in the United States. Alcohol impairs driving-related skills regardless of the age of the driver or the time of day it is consumed. However, younger drinkers and drivers are at greatest risk. Underage drinkers are more likely to drive after drinking, to ride with intoxicated drivers, and to be injured after drinking—at least in part because they believe that people can drive safely and legally after drinking.

Strategies for Prevention ▪▪ How to Prevent Drunk Driving

- When going out in a group, always designate one person who won't drink at all to serve as the driver.
- Never get behind the wheel if you've had more than two drinks within two hours, especially if you haven't eaten.
- Never let intoxicated friends drive home. Call a taxi, drive them yourself, or arrange for them to spend the night in a safe place.

Public awareness campaigns like this one for designated drivers can help prevent the high incidence of fatalities caused by drunk drivers.

The number of alcohol-related fatalities on American highways has dropped in recent years, but more than 42,000 people still die on the nation's highways each year. Safety groups attribute the decline in alcohol-related deaths to enforcement tools like sobriety checkpoints and to the states' adoption of a uniform drunken-driving standard of a BAC of 0.08 percent.

However, among college students ages 18 to 24, deaths from alcohol-related accidents and other unintentional injuries have increased to more than 1,700 a year.[9] In a recent survey, 29 percent of college students drove after drinking some alcohol; 10 percent after five or more drinks; 23 percent rode in a car with a driver who was high or drunk. The rates of drinking and driving are higher at larger schools and schools in the southern and north-central regions.[10]

In the last two decades, families of the victims of drunk drivers have organized to change the way the nation treats its drunk drivers. Because of the efforts of MADD (Mothers Against Drunk Driving), SADD (Students Against Destructive Decisions), and other lobbying groups, cities, counties, and states are cracking down on drivers who drink. Since courts have held establishments that serve alcohol liable for the consequences of allowing drunk customers to drive, many bars and restaurants have joined the campaign against drunk driving. Many communities also provide free rides home on holidays and weekends for people who've had too much to drink. Designated drivers can help save lives—if they refrain from drinking.

DRINKING ON CAMPUS

College students drink more, more often, and more dangerously than young people of the same age not attending college.[11] About eight in ten undergraduates drink, at least occasionally, although this figure varies on different campuses. College men drink more, more often, and more intensely than women. Caucasians drink more than African Americans or Asians, fraternity and sorority members also use more alcohol more often than non-Greeks.[12] (See "Student Snapshot: Drinking on Campus.)

For most, alcohol usually does not interfere with their school and work responsibilities. However, an increasing number—about two in five—engage in the dangerous practice of binge drinking. A single binge, combined with poor judgment or bad luck, can lead to life-altering and sometimes life-threatening consequences.

When asked how many drinks they had the last time they partied, about 20 percent of students said none, while 42 percent of the women and 25 percent of the men had one to four. An equal percentage of men and women—28 percent—had five to eight drinks. Almost twice as many men as women—28 versus 15 percent—reported more than nine drinks.[13]

According to the National College Health Assessment, 18 percent of students report never using alcohol.[14] Students who don't drink give various reasons for their choice, including not having access to alcohol, parental or peer pressure, being underage, costs, religious reasons, and not liking the taste.[15]

African-American students are more likely than white undergraduates to abstain and to report never having had an alcoholic drink and not having a drink in the past 30 days. They also drink less frequently and consume fewer drinks per occasion than whites. Black undergraduates experience fewer negative consequences of drinking and more regularly use strategies to prevent problem drinking, such as eating before drinking and keeping track of how many drinks they consume.[16]

Students typically overestimate the social norms (discussed in Chapter 2) for drinking, that is, how much other students drink. Although about one in five students never drink alcohol, only 2 percent of students believe that a typical student doesn't drink.[17]

Student Snapshot

DRINKING ON CAMPUS

Who Drinks?	Percentage of Students	Days per Week	Drinks per Occasion
By sex			
Women	79%	2.2%	4.3%
Men	87	2.7	6.7
By race			
Caucasian	89%	2.6%	5.95%
African American	55	1.6	3.4
Asian	62	2.2	4.7
By fraternity/sorority membership			
Members	93%	2.98%	6.2%
Nonmembers	78	2.2	5.4

*Based on a study of 740 undergraduates.
Source: Shinew, Kimberly, and Diana Parry. "Examining College Students' Participation in the Leisure Pursuits of Drinking and Illegal Drug Use." *Journal of Leisure Research,* Vol. 37, No. 3, Summer 2005, p. 364.

Do you drink at sports events? Why?

WHY COLLEGE STUDENTS DRINK

Most college students drink for the same reasons undergraduates have always turned to alcohol: Away from home, often for the first time, many are excited by and apprehensive about their newfound independence. When new pressures seem overwhelming, when they feel awkward or insecure, when they just want to let loose and have a good time, they reach for a drink. In one recent survey, peer pressure was the top-rated reason students gave for drinking. Other motives include to escape, for the effects, to reduce stress, to relax, and for social reasons.[18]

Freshmen may be especially vulnerable to dangerous drinking as they struggle to adapt to an often bewildering new world. Many who were nondrinkers as high school seniors start to drink in college. They are less likely to do so if friends discourage them from drinking. The heaviest drinking occurs among male freshmen and at the beginning of each academic year. By senior year, drinking moderates.

About half of college men and a third of college women report drinking to excess. Male athletes drink more often, consume more alcohol, and drink to intoxication more than other students, while female athletes consume the lowest quantities of alcohol. Of all students, male athletes are the most likely to drink for social reasons and to drink to get high. College women (athletes or not) and men who are not athletes are more likely to drink as a way of coping, for instance, to feel better or "get through it."[19]

College sports events intensify heavy drinking. In one study, drinking before and after a men's National College Athletic Association basketball championship increased. Collegiate sporting events appear to be a particularly heavy-drinking context; sports-related alcohol use can occur in many places (for example, at home, at a bar, at the stadium) and celebratory drinking is a frequently endorsed reason for drinking. College students who are sports fans are more likely to drink heavily and experience more alcohol-related negative consequences compared with those who are not sports fans.[20]

Students drink more at certain colleges, such as those located along the Mexican border,[21] and in certain locations, such as off-campus parties and bars and fraternity and sorority parties. Heavy drinking is most likely to occur at events where many people become intoxicated, illicit drugs are available, and drinking games are played.

On average, students tend to drink more on days when they are feeling good—possibly because of what researchers call the "celebratory and social" nature of college drinking. Drinking—and positive emotions—also peak on weekends.[22]

About 5 percent of college students are experiencing depression or poor mental health at any given time, and they are more vulnerable to alcohol abuse. Depressed young women are at the highest risk. About eight in ten students who report poor mental health or depression drink alcohol. They are more likely to drink to get drunk and to report high levels of harm from alcohol.[23]

BINGE DRINKING ON CAMPUS

Binge drinking—is the leading cause of preventable death among undergraduates and the most serious threat to their intellectual, physical, and psychological development. In spite of great efforts across U.S. college campuses to decrease binge drinking, the national average—two out of five students report binging—remained steady for 20 years.

According to the National College Health Assessment,

Binge drinkers can get into—and cause—trouble. Dangerously large amounts of alcohol can lead to death, and heavy party drinking often results in violence and accidents.

FIGURE 12-5 Who Does Heavy Episodic Drinking on Campus?

Note: Spring 2003, Sample size *n* = 19,497

Source: American College Health Association, www.acha.org

most students—67 percent of women and 49 percent of men—reported no binges in the previous two weeks. However, about a quarter of men had five or more drinks at one sitting at least once in the previous two weeks (Figure 12-5).

Frequent binge drinkers account for almost 70 percent of all alcohol consumed by college students. Students in four-year colleges are more likely to binge than those in two-year colleges.

 Binge drinkers are most likely to be white, fraternity and sorority members, under 24 years of age, involved in athletics, and frequent socializers. White males binge-drink the most; African-American women, the least. Students who study a great deal or are involved in community service or the arts are less likely to binge-drink.

Student binge-drinking rates are higher in states where adults also binge-drink. This may depend on how stringent state alcohol policies are or how rigorously they are enforced.[24]

 More women now binge. At coed schools, 41 percent report at least one binge within the previous two weeks; 17 percent are frequent bingers. At all-female colleges, binge drinking has jumped from one in four to almost one in three: In one recent study, women who reported binge-drinking were more likely to have greater weight concerns than those who did not binge, and the women who were more physically active binged more than those who were the least active. Women who thought their peers drank frequently engaged in more binge drinking episodes than others.[25]

Unplanned sexual activities, date rape, and sexual assault are 150 percent more likely among women who drink than among those who do not. Sophomore, junior, and senior women are much less likely to engage in heavy episodic drinking than freshman women.

Surveys consistently show that students who engage in binge drinking, particularly those who do so more than once a week, experience a far higher rate of problems than other students. Frequent binge drinkers are likely to miss classes, vandalize property, and drive after drinking. Frequent binge drinkers are also more likely to experience five or more different alcohol-related problems and to use other substances, including nicotine, marijuana, cocaine, and LSD.

FAQ **WHY DO STUDENTS BINGE?**

Young people who came from, socialized within, or were exposed to "wet" environments—settings in which alcohol is cheap and accessible and drinking is prevalent—are more likely to engage in binge drinking. Students who report drinking at least once a month during their final year of high school are over three times more likely to binge-drink in college than those who drank less frequently in high school.

The factors that most influence students to binge-drink are:

- **Low price** for alcohol.
- **Easy access to alcohol.** In one study, the density of alcohol outlets (such as bars) near campus affected the drinking of students.
- **Attending a school** or living in a residence with many binge drinkers.

▮ **Belief** that close friends were likely to binge.

▮ **Drinking games**—such as tongue twisters or drinking whenever a certain phrase is mentioned in a song or on a TV program—are dangerous because they can result in high levels of intoxication in a short period of time.

▮ **Parents who drank** or did not disapprove of their children drinking.

▮ **Recreational drinking** before age 16.

Some educators view binging as a product of the college environment. More students binge-drink at the beginning of the school year and then cut back as the semester progresses and academic demands increase. Binge drinking also peaks following exam times, during home football weekends, and during spring break. Many new students engage in binge drinking for the first time very soon after they arrive on campus. Binges become less common in their subsequent years at school and almost always end with education. Real life, one educator notes, is "a strong disincentive" to this type of drinking.

Colleges and health authorities are trying innovative approaches to prevent or stop binge drinking. One school has found that four weekly electronic "newsletters" are as likely to reach students as print ones.[26] The Internet may be a particularly appealing means of communication because of its anonymity, nonjudgmental nature, and 24-7 availability. The myStudentBody website, which includes an interactive intervention for binge drinkers, has helped reduce drinking in women, persistent drinkers, and those who were not highly motivated to change their behavior.[27]

UNDERAGE DRINKING ON CAMPUS

Students under age 21 drink less often than older students, but tend to drink more heavily and to experience more negative alcohol-related consequences. More underage students report drinking "to get drunk" and drinking at binge levels when they consumed alcohol.

Underage college students are most likely to drink if they can easily obtain cheap alcohol, especially beer. They tend to drink in private settings, such as dorms and fraternity parties, and are more likely than students of legal age to experience a host of negative drinking-related consequences, including doing something they regretted; forgetting where they were or what they did; causing property damage; getting into trouble with police; and being hurt or injured. The drinking behavior of underage students also depends on their living arrangements. Those in controlled settings, such as their parents' home or a substance-free dorm, are less likely to binge-drink. Students living in fraternities or sororities were most likely to binge-drink, regardless of age.

Students under age 21 in states with tough laws against underage drinking are less likely to drink than those in states with fewer restrictions. When they drink, underage students are more likely to drink to excess than older ones—possibly because they feel greater pressure to drink quickly before

some authority cuts off their alcohol supply or they get caught.

THE TOLL OF COLLEGE DRINKING

According to research summarized in a College Task Force report to the National Institute on Alcohol Abuse and Alcoholism (NIAAA), the consequences of excessive drinking by college students are more significant, more destructive, and more costly than many students or parents realize. These consequences affect students whether or not they drink. Drinking by college students aged 18 to 24 contributes to an estimated 1,700 student deaths, 599,000 injuries, and 97,000 cases of sexual assault or date rape each year (Table 12-1).[28]

According to the Commission on Substance Abuse at Colleges and Universities, alcohol is involved in two-thirds of college student suicides, nine of ten rapes, and 95 percent of violent crimes on campus. A national survey released by the Higher Education Center for Alcohol and Other Drug Prevention reported that 75 to 90 percent of all violence on college campuses is alcohol-related.

Each year some 2.8 million college students aged 18 to 24 drive after drinking; even more ride in motor vehicles with drinking drivers.[29] About 300,000 of today's college students will eventually die from alcohol-related causes, including drunk-driving accidents, cirrhosis of the liver, various cancers, and heart disease, estimates the Core Institute, an organization that studies college drinking.

According to the National Institute on Alcohol Abuse and Alcoholism, 25 percent of college students report having suffered academic consequences for their drinking habits. In one study at a large public university, nearly 55 percent of college women had experienced at least one alcohol-related problem in the previous 12 months. The most common were doing something they later regretted, forgetting where they were or what they did, physically injuring themselves, and having unprotected sex (Figure 12-6). About two-thirds of college men reported one or more alcohol-linked problems in the same time period. In addition to the same negative

TABLE 12-1 THE CONSEQUENCES OF COLLEGE DRINKING

Consequence	Number of Students per Year
Assault by another student	600,000
Unintentional injury	599,000
Unprotected sex after drinking	400,000
Arrest for alcohol-related violations	110,000
Sexual assault or date rape	97,000
Death	1,700

Source: www.collegedrinkingprevention.gov

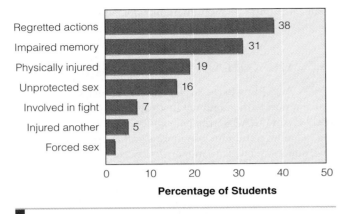

FIGURE 12-6 Reported Consequences After Alcohol Consumption* (Last School Year)

*Nondrinkers omitted from analysis, Spring 2000, Sample size $n = 16,024$
Source: www.acha.org

consequences as the women, more men developed academic difficulties.[30]

Heavy drinking has been correlated with increased casual sex without condoms, an increased number of sex partners, and sexual attacks on women. Alcohol and drug use can lead to earlier sexual initiation, unprotected sexual intercourse, multiple sex partners, and increased risk of sexually transmitted infections.

"SECONDHAND" DRINKING PROBLEMS

Heavy alcohol use can endanger both drinkers and others. Secondhand problems caused by other's alcohol use include loss of sleep, interruption of studies, assaults, vandalism, and unwanted sexual advances. Students living on campuses with high rates of binge drinking are two or more times as likely to experience these secondhand effects as those living on campuses with low rates.

In one study, nearly three-quarters of campus rapes happened when the victims were so intoxicated that they were unable to consent or refuse. Women from colleges with medium and high binge-drinking rates had more than a 1.5-fold increased chance of being raped while intoxicated than those from schools with low binge-drinking rates.[31]

Your Life Coach

Taking Charge of Alcohol Use

Drinking, like other behaviors, is a choice. You—and no one else but you—have the right to decide not to drink, and you owe no one an explanation if you say no to alcohol. As with other risk-taking behaviors, never let anyone intimidate you into doing anything that violates your values.

HOW STUDENTS PROTECT THEMSELVES FROM UNSAFE DRINKING

Smart choices can help you avoid many of the negative consequences of drinking. Various "self-protective" behaviors, such as designating a driver, eating before or during drinking, and keeping track of the number of drinks consumed, have proved effective in reducing alcohol-related problems. Women employ these strategies more often when partying or socializing than men; black students use them more often than white men. The students who used these strategies most often had the fewest problem behaviors.[32]

How do you compare with the students surveyed by the National College Health Assessment?

Behavior	Students Who Always or Usually Use the Strategy
Eat before and/or during drinking	76%
Use a designated driver	77%
Keep track of how many drinks they're having	64%
Avoid drinking games	40%
Decide in advance how many drinks to have	34%
Have a friend let you know when you've had enough	31%
Choose not to drink	27%
Pace yourself to no more than one drink an hour	26%
Alternate alcoholic and nonalcoholic beverages	25%[33]

STAYING IN CONTROL OF YOUR DRINKING

If you do drink, take responsibility for how much and how often you drink. Here are some guidelines that can help:

▪ **Keep a diary.** Write down how much you drink each day. This can make you more aware of exactly how much you drink.

▪ **Pace yourself.** Try having a "spacer," a nonalcoholic drink every second or third drink.

▪ **Stay busy.** You will drink less if you play pool or dance rather than just sitting and drinking.

▪ **Try low-alcohol alternatives,** such as light beers and low- or no-alcohol wines

▪ **Have alcohol-free days.** Don't drink at all at least two days a week.

▪ **Start with a soft drink.** You will drink much faster if you are thirsty, so have a nonalcoholic drink to quench your thirst before you start drinking alcohol.

You can share in the fun and toast a happy occasion with non-alcoholic or alcoholic beverages.

- **Use standard drinks.** Monitor how much alcohol you drink. By converting what you drink into standard drinks, it is easier to keep track.
- **Drink slowly.** Take sips and not gulps. Put your glass down between sips.
- **Avoid salty snacks.** Salty food like chips or nuts make you thirsty so you drink more.
- **Have one drink at a time.** Don't let people top up your drinks. It makes it harder to keep track of how much alcohol you're consuming.
- **Be assertive.** Don't be pressured into drinking more than you want or intend to. Say "Thanks, but no thanks."
- **Pay attention.** Watch as your drink is poured. Don't let your drink out of your sight.
- **Never leave a party with someone you don't know.** This is especially true if you've been drinking and are feeling somewhat intoxicated.
- **Abstain for 48 hours** if you do have an episode of heavy drinking to let your body recover.
- **When you throw a party, be a responsible host.** Collect car keys from your guests. Serve high-protein food like pepperoni pizza, shrimp, or spareribs. Serve nonalcoholic beverages. Do not force drinks on your guests or rush to refill their glasses when empty. Stop serving alcohol about two hours before the party is over.

STAGES OF PERSONAL CHANGE

In a study at Ohio State University, researchers classified student heavy drinkers according to four stages of change:

1. **Precontemplation.** Nearly two-thirds of the students continued to drink heavily and had no intention of changing their behavior. These students drank an average of 12.5 alcoholic beverages a week.
2. **Contemplation.** 12 percent of the students were still drinking heavily but considering changing their drinking behavior.
3. **Action.** 14 percent of the students had stopped their pattern of heavy drinking.
4. **Maintenance.** 9 percent of the students had avoided heavy alcohol use for at least six months. They drank an average of one alcoholic drink a month. These students no longer drank heavily, even though they felt that such drinking was the norm on their campus. However, they saw more risks and fewer benefits associated with alcohol use.

Such change is not unusual, even among students who continued heavy drinking throughout their college years. Despite their heavy drinking as undergraduates, within three years of graduation, students who had been members of fraternities and sororities drink no more than students who did not join Greek houses. Heavy drinking may be the result of students' perceptions that excessive alcohol use is normal in Greek houses, along with the encouragement of peers.

COLLEGE ALCOHOL POLICIES

The majority of college administrators describe students' alcohol use as a problem or a major problem on their campus. All schools report some action to manage campus drinking, although policies vary greatly.

University alcohol policies include campus alcohol bans, no alcohol at university-sponsored events, prohibition of beer kegs, limits on the maximum number of drinks served per student, and dry rushing activities (Table 12-2). Studies suggest that student who attend schools that ban alcohol are less likely to engage in heavy binge drinking, more likely to abstain from using

TABLE 12-2 RESTRICTING ALCOHOL ON CAMPUS

Schools That Prohibit:

Alcohol use on campus	32%
Alcohol possession	38%
Beer kegs	78%
Use at sporting events	14%
Use at home games	85%
Greek alcohol use	25%

Based on a survey of 73 colleges in Minnesota and Wisconsin.

Source: Mitchell, Rebecca, et al. "Alcohol Policies on College Campuses." *Journal of American College Health*, Vol. 53, No. 4, January–February 2005, p. 149.

alcohol, and less likely to experience the secondhand effects of drinking.

Most colleges and universities offer some type of alcohol education program for students, yet in a survey of black colleges, about half of the students were either unaware of or didn't know the specifics of their school's alcohol policy.[34] Some schools post their policies online, but in many cases they are difficult to find among all of the other information on a school's website. Can you find the policy for your school?

A recent survey found that 32 percent of colleges—mostly urban, public, and large institutions—routinely screen students for alcohol use. Other schools screen only about 10 percent of students. When screening reveals a potential drinking problem, schools are most likely to refer students to a campus counseling center, a substance abuse treatment provider in the community, or a 12-step program. In one study at a large northeastern university, only 15 percent of college drinkers reported that a health-care professional had ever asked them about their drinking. But nine in ten of student drinkers said they would cut down on alcohol consumption if a physician advised them to do so.[35]

Fewer than 10 percent of frequent binge drinkers experience any disciplinary action as a result of their drinking. Support for tougher campus restrictions has grown among students, particularly those who do not binge-drink and who have experienced the negative consequences of others' drinking, such as violence and vandalism. According to studies of schools that have lowered binge-drinking rates, a combination of social and environmental approaches has the greatest impact on reducing binge drinking.[36] Key elements are involvement of students and development of alternatives, such as alcohol-free parties and events.

The U.S. Department of Education has begun highlighting innovative antidrinking practices on campus; Mothers Against Drunk Driving (MADD) is planning to rank colleges based on how well they curb student drinking. There has been an increase in on-campus chapters of national support groups such as AA, Al-Anon, Adult Children of Alcoholics, and a peer-education program called BACCHUS: Boost Alcohol Consciousness Concerning the Health of University Students.

THE IMPACT OF ALCOHOL

Unlike food or drugs in tablet form, alcohol is directly and quickly absorbed into the bloodstream through the stomach walls and upper intestine. The alcohol in a typical drink reaches the bloodstream in 15 minutes and rises to its peak concentration in about an hour. The bloodstream carries the alcohol to the liver, heart, and brain (Figure 12-7).

Most of the alcohol you drink can leave your body only after metabolism by the liver, which converts about 95 percent of the alcohol to carbon dioxide and water. The other 5 percent is excreted unchanged, mainly through urination, respiration, and perspiration.

Alcohol is a diuretic, a drug that speeds up the elimination of fluid from the body, so drink water when you drink alcohol to maintain your fluid balance. And alcohol lowers body temperature, so you should never drink to get or stay warm.

DIGESTIVE SYSTEM

Alcohol reaches the stomach first, where it is partially broken down. The remaining alcohol is absorbed easily through the stomach tissue into the bloodstream. In the stomach, alcohol triggers the secretion of acids, which irritate the stomach lining. Excessive drinking at one sitting may result in nausea; chronic drinking may result in peptic ulcers (breaks in the stomach lining) and bleeding from the stomach lining.

The alcohol in the bloodstream eventually reaches the liver. The liver, which bears the major responsibility of fat metabolism in the body, converts this excess alcohol to fat. After a few weeks of four or five drinks a day, liver cells start to accumulate fat. Alcohol also stimulates liver cells to attract white blood cells, which normally travel throughout the bloodstream engulfing harmful substances and wastes. If white blood cells begin to invade body tissue, such as the liver, they can cause irreversible damage.

WEIGHT AND WAISTS

At 7 calories per gram, alcohol has nearly as many calories as fat (9 calories per gram) and significantly more than carbohydrates or protein (which have 4 calories per gram). Since a standard drink contains 12–15 grams of alcohol, the alcohol in a single drink adds about 100 calories to your daily intake. A glass of wine contains as many calories as some candy bars; you would have to walk a mile to burn them off. In addition to being a calorie-dense food, alcohol stimulates the appetite so you're likely to eat more.

"Beer bellies" earn their name. In a study of men and women over age 20 in Copenhagen, those who drank the most beer or spirits had wider waists on a ten-year follow-up. Wine did not have a similar impact. In another study of the waist-hip ratio and body mass index of French adults who consumed varying amounts of alcohol, drinking was linked to an increase in both waist circumference and waist-to-hip ratio in both men and women.[37]

CARDIOVASCULAR SYSTEM

Alcohol gets mixed reviews regarding its effects on the cardiovascular system. As several studies have shown, people who drink moderate amounts of alcohol have lower mortality rates after a heart attack, as well as a lower risk of heart attack compared to abstainers and heavy drinkers.

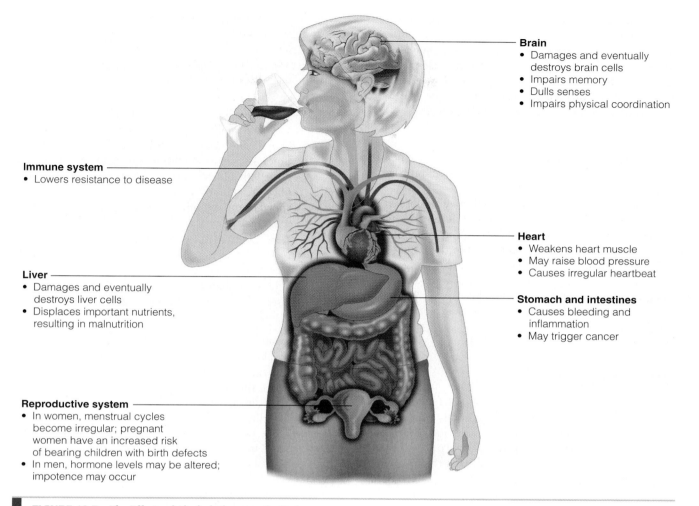

Brain
- Damages and eventually destroys brain cells
- Impairs memory
- Dulls senses
- Impairs physical coordination

Immune system
- Lowers resistance to disease

Liver
- Damages and eventually destroys liver cells
- Displaces important nutrients, resulting in malnutrition

Heart
- Weakens heart muscle
- May raise blood pressure
- Causes irregular heartbeat

Stomach and intestines
- Causes bleeding and inflammation
- May trigger cancer

Reproductive system
- In women, menstrual cycles become irregular; pregnant women have an increased risk of bearing children with birth defects
- In men, hormone levels may be altered; impotence may occur

FIGURE 12-7   The Effects of Alcohol Abuse on the Body
Alcohol has a major effect on the brain, damaging brain cells, impairing judgment and perceptions, and often leading to accidents and altercations. Alcohol also damages the digestive system, especially the liver.

In one of the most recent studies of alcohol and cardiovascular health, men in Harvard's long-term Health Professionals Follow-Up Study who consumed moderate amounts of alcohol (less than two 12-ounce bottles of beer, three 4-ounce glasses of wine, or two shots of liquor) three or more days a week were about a third less likely to have heart attacks over a 12-year period than men who never drank. Unlike in earlier French studies, heart attack protection was most strongly associated with beer and liquor consumption and most weakly linked to red wine.[38]

How does alcohol enhance heart health? Researchers believe that it boosts beneficial high-density lipoproteins (HDL), lowers the risk of blood clots, and also may have an anti-inflammatory effect. According to recent studies, alcohol may lower two blood components, C-reactive protein and fibrinogen, that indicate increased heart disease risk (discussed in Chapter 15).

Some cardiologists contend that the benefits of moderate drinking may be overstated, especially because of alcohol's contribution to the epidemic of obesity around the world. Heavy or abusive drinking accounts for more than 100,000 deaths in the United States each year.[39] Heavier drinking triggers the release of harmful oxygen molecules called free radicals, which can increase the risk of heart disease, stroke, and cirrhosis of the liver. Alcohol use can weaken the heart muscle directly, causing a disorder called cardiomyopathy. The combined use of alcohol and other drugs, including tobacco and cocaine, greatly increases the likelihood of damage to the heart.

BREAST CANCER

According to analysis of data from many large studies, women who take two or more drinks per day are 40 percent more likely to develop breast cancer than women who don't drink at all. The risk occurs with all forms of alcohol—beer, wine, and spirits—and increases the more women drink.

In the Nurses' Health Study, breast cancer rates rose slightly even in women who took as little as half a drink per day. A single daily drink of 1 ounce of spirits, such as whiskey, gin, or vodka, or 3 ounces of wine increases a woman's breast cancer risk slightly—perhaps 3 or 4 percent. Every additional daily drink increases the risk by 7 percent. By four drinks a day, a woman's risk increases 30 percent.[40]

A nondrinking woman's lifetime risk of breast cancer by age 80 is 1 in 11. A heavy drinker has about a 1 in 7 chance of developing breast cancer by age 80, regardless of her race, education, family history, use of hormone replacement therapy, or other risk factors.[41]

Scientists don't know how alcohol increases breast cancer risk. In some studies, alcohol raised levels of estrogen, perhaps by decreasing the body's ability to metabolize the hormone or by promoting its release into the bloodstream. But other studies have not shown increased estrogen levels in women who drink. Alcohol may also interact with carcinogens (cancer-causing agents), perhaps inhibiting the body's capacity to detoxify carcinogens or activating carcinogens directly.[42]

IMMUNE SYSTEM

Chronic alcohol use can inhibit the production of both white blood cells, which fight off infections, and red blood cells, which carry oxygen to all the organs and tissues of the body. Alcohol may increase the risk of infection with human immunodeficiency virus (HIV), by altering the judgment of users so that they more readily engage in activities, such as unsafe sexual practices, that put them in danger. If you drink when you have a cold or the flu, alcohol interferes with the body's ability to recover. It also increases the chance of bacterial pneumonia in flu sufferers.

BRAIN AND BEHAVIOR

At first, when you drink, you feel up. In low dosages, alcohol affects the regions of the brain that inhibit or control behavior, so you feel looser and act in ways you might not otherwise. However, you also experience losses of concentration, memory, judgment, and fine motor control; and you have mood swings and emotional outbursts.

Moderate amounts of alcohol can have disturbing effects on perception and judgment, including the following:

▪ **Impaired perceptions.** You're less able to adjust your eyes to bright lights because glare bothers you more. Although you can still hear sounds, you can't distinguish between them or judge their direction well.

▪ **Dulled smell and taste.** Alcohol itself may cause some vitamin deficiencies, and the poor eating habits of heavy drinkers result in further nutrition problems.

▪ **Diminished sensation.** On a freezing winter night, you may walk outside without a coat and not feel the cold.

▪ **Altered sense of space.** You may not realize, for instance, that you have been in one place for several hours.

▪ **Impaired motor skills.** Writing, typing, driving, and other abilities involving your muscles are impaired. This is why law enforcement officers sometimes ask suspected drunk drivers to touch their nose with a finger or to walk a straight line. Drinking large amounts of alcohol impairs reaction time, speed, accuracy, and consistency, as well as judgment.

▪ **Impaired sexual performance.** While drinking may increase your interest in sex, it may also impair sexual response, especially a man's ability to achieve or maintain an erection. As Shakespeare wrote, "It provokes the desire, but it takes away the performance."

Moderate and heavy drinkers show signs of impaired intelligence, slowed-down reflexes, and difficulty remembering. Because alcohol is a central nervous system depressant, it slows down the activity of the neurons in the brain, gradually dulling the responses of the brain and nervous system. One or two drinks act as a tranquilizer or relaxant. Additional drinks result in a progressive reduction in central nervous system activity, leading to sleep, general anesthesia, coma, and even death.

Heavy alcohol use may pose special dangers to the brains of drinkers at both ends of the age spectrum. Adolescents who drink regularly show impairments in their neurological and cognitive functioning. Elderly people who drink heavily appear to have more brain shrinkage, or atrophy, than those who drink lightly or not at all. In general, moderate drinkers have healthier brains and a lower risk of dementia than those who don't drink and those who drink to excess.[43]

INCREASED RISK OF DYING

Alcohol kills. Alcohol is responsible for 100,000 deaths each year and is the third leading cause of death after tobacco and improper diet and lack of exercise. The leading alcohol-related cause of death is injury. Alcohol plays a role in almost half of all traffic fatalities, half of all homicides, and a quarter of all suicides. The second leading cause of alcohol-related deaths is cirrhosis of the liver, a chronic disease that causes extensive scarring and irreversible damage. In addition, as many as half of patients admitted to hospitals and 15 percent of those making office visits seek or need medical care because of the direct or indirect effects of alcohol.

Young drinkers—teens and those in their early twenties—are at highest risk of dying from injuries, mostly car accidents. Older drinkers over age 50 face the greatest danger of premature death from cirrhosis of the liver, hepatitis, and other alcohol-linked illnesses.

Alcohol plays a role in 40 percent of motor vehicle fatalities.

Most studies of the relationship between alcohol consumption and death from all causes show that moderate drinkers—those who consume approximately seven drinks per week—have a lower risk of death than abstainers, while heavy drinkers have a higher risk than either group. In one ten-year study, never-drinkers showed no elevated risk of dying, while consistent heavier drinkers were at higher risk of dying of any cause than other men.

FETAL ALCOHOL EFFECTS AND SYNDROME

An estimated 15 percent of women drink alcohol while pregnant, most having one drink or less per day. Even light consumption of alcohol can lead to **Fetal Alcohol Effects (FAE):** low birthweight, irritability as newborns, and permanent mental impairment.

The babies of women who consume three or more ounces of alcohol (the equivalent of six or seven cocktails) are at risk of more severe problems. One of every 750 newborns has a cluster of physical and mental defects called **Fetal Alcohol Syndrome (FAS):** small head, abnormal facial features, jitters, poor muscle tone, sleep disorders, sluggish motor development, failure to thrive, short stature, delayed speech, mental retardation, and hyperactivity.[44]

INTERACTION WITH OTHER DRUGS

Alcohol can interact with other drugs—prescription and nonprescription, legal and illegal. Of the 100 most frequently prescribed drugs, more than half contain at least one ingredient that interacts adversely with alcohol. Because alcohol and other psychoactive drugs may work on the same areas of the brain, their combination can produce an effect much greater than that expected of either drug by itself. The consequences of this synergistic interaction can be fatal (see Savvy Consumer: "Alcohol and Drug Interactions"). Alcohol is particularly dangerous when combined with other depressants and antianxiety medications.

Savvy Consumer ▪ Alcohol and Drug Interactions

Drug	Possible Effects of Interaction
Analgesics (painkillers) Narcotic (Codeine, Demerol, Percodan)	Increase in central nervous system depression, possibly leading to respiratory failure and death.
Nonnarcotic (aspirin, acetaminophen)	Irritation of stomach resulting in bleeding and increased susceptibility to liver damage.
Antabuse (disulfiram; an aid to quit drinking)	Nausea, vomiting, headache, high blood pressure, and erratic heartbeat.
Antianxiety drugs (Valium, Librium)	Increase in central nervous system depression; decreased alertness and impaired judgment.
Antidepressants (Prozac, Zoloft)	Increase in central nervous system depression; certain antidepressants in combination with red wine could cause a sudden increase in blood pressure.
Antihistamines (Actifed, Dimetap, and other cold medications)	Increase in drowsiness; driving more dangerous.
Antibiotics	Nausea, vomiting, headache; some medications rendered less effective.
Central nervous system stimulants (caffeine, Dexedrine, Ritalin)	Stimulant effects of these drugs may reverse depressant effect of alcohol but do not decrease its intoxicating effects.
Diuretics (Diuril, Lasix)	Reduction in blood pressure resulting in dizziness upon rising.
Sedatives (Dalmane, Nembutal, Quaalude)	Increase in central nervous system depression, possibly leading to coma, respiratory failure, and death.

ALCOHOL AND GENDER

According to conventional gender stereotypes, drinking is a symbol of manliness. In the past, far more men than women drank. In the United States today, both genders are likely to consume alcohol. However, there are well-documented differences in how often and how much men and women drink. In general, men drink more frequently, consume a larger quantity of alcohol per drinking occasion, and report more problems related to drinking. More than half of women drink: Of these, 45 percent are light drinkers; 3 percent, moderate drinkers; 2 percent, heavy drinkers; and 21 percent, binge drinkers.

The bodies of men and women respond to alcohol in different ways. Because they have a far smaller quantity of a protective enzyme in the stomach to break down alcohol before it's absorbed into the bloodstream, women absorb about 30 percent more alcohol into their bloodstream than men. The alcohol travels through the blood to the brain, so women become intoxicated much more quickly. And because there's more alcohol in the bloodstream to break down, the liver may also be adversely affected. In alcoholic women, the stomach seems to completely stop digesting alcohol, which may explain why women alcoholics are more likely to suffer liver damage than men.

Both men and women experience blackouts after heavy drinking, but women black out after consuming half as much alcohol as men. Women also may be more susceptible to alcohol-induced memory problems when given comparable amounts of alcohol. In addition, they are at greater risk of engaging in risky behavior, including unprotected sex, than men.

Alcohol interferes with male sexual function and fertility through direct effects on testosterone and the testicles. In half of alcoholic men, increased levels of female hormones lead to breast enlargement and a feminine pubic hair pattern. Damage to the nerves in the penis by heavy drinking can lead to impotence. In women who drink heavily, a drop in female hormone production may cause menstrual irregularity and infertility.

As women age, their risk of osteoporosis, a condition characterized by calcium loss and bone thinning, increases. Alcohol can block the absorption of many nutrients, including calcium, and heavy drinking may worsen the deterioration of bone tissue.

ALCOHOL AND RACE

Experts in alcohol treatment are increasingly recognizing racial and ethnic differences in risk factors for drinking problems, patterns of drinking, and most effective types of treatment. Increases in drinking have been traced to stresses related to immigration, acculturation, poverty, racial discrimination, and powerlessness. Environmental factors, such as aggressive marketing and advertising of alcoholic beverages in minority neighborhoods, also play a role. On campus white students report the highest rates of heavy drinking; black students, the lowest. Hispanic students are intermediate.

AFRICAN-AMERICAN COMMUNITY

Overall, African Americans consume less alcohol per person than whites, yet twice as many blacks die of cirrhosis of the liver each year. In some cities, the rate of cirrhosis is ten times higher among African-American than white men. Alcohol also contributes to high rates of hypertension, esophageal cancer, and homicide among African-American men.

Drinking patterns among African Americans are more extreme than those of white drinkers, with more abstinence, but also more occasions of heavy drinking. Both African-American men and women drink more during a single occasion compared to their white counterparts.[45]

HISPANIC COMMUNITY

The various Hispanic cultures tend to discourage any drinking by women but encourage heavy drinking by men as part of machismo, or feelings of manhood. Hispanic men have higher rates of alcohol use and abuse than the general population and suffer a high rate of cirrhosis. Moreover, American-born Hispanic men drink more than those born in other countries.

Few Hispanics enter treatment, partly because of a lack of information, language barriers, and poor community-based services. Hispanic families generally try to resolve problems themselves, and their cultural values discourage the sharing of intimate personal stories, which characterizes Alcoholics Anonymous and other support groups. Churches often provide the most effective forms of help.

NATIVE AMERICAN COMMUNITY

European settlers introduced alcohol to Native Americans. Because of the societal and physical problems resulting from excessive drinking, at the request of tribal leaders, the U.S. Congress in 1832 prohibited the use of alcohol by Native Americans. Many reservations still ban alcohol use, so Native Americans who want to drink may have to travel long distances to obtain alcohol, which may contribute to the high death rate from hypothermia and pedestrian and motor-vehicle accidents among Native Americans. (Injuries are the leading cause of death among this group.)

Certainly, not all Native Americans drink, and not all who drink do so to excess. However, they have three times the general population's rate of alcohol-related injury and illness. Cirrhosis of the liver is the fourth-leading cause of

Navajo Vikki Shirley speaks to parents at Rough Rocks Elementary School in Rough Rocks, Ariz. Shirley, who lost her daughter in an alcohol-related crash, travels to remote Navajo Nation villages to speak to parents throughout Arizona, New Mexico, Utah, and Colorado.

© Ben Chrisman /AP Photo

death among this cultural group. While many Native American women don't drink, those who do have high rates of alcohol-related problems, which affect both them and their children. Their rate of cirrhosis of the liver is 36 times that of white women. In some tribes, 10.5 out of every 1,000 newborns have fetal alcohol syndrome, compared with 1 to 3 out of 1,000 in the general population.

ASIAN-AMERICAN COMMUNITY

Asian Americans tend to drink very little or not at all, in part because of an inborn physiological reaction to alcohol that causes facial flushing, rapid heart rate, lowered blood pressure, nausea, vomiting, and other symptoms. A very high percentage of women of all Asian-American nationalities abstain completely. Some sociologists have expressed concern, however, that as Asian Americans become more assimilated into American culture, they'll drink more—and possibly suffer very adverse effects from alcohol.

ALCOHOL PROBLEMS

By the simplest definition, problem drinking is the use of alcohol in any way that creates difficulties, potential difficulties, or health risks for an individual. Like alcoholics, problem drinkers are individuals whose lives are in some way impaired by their drinking. The only difference is one of degree. Alcohol becomes a problem, and a person becomes an alcoholic, when the drinker can't "take it or leave it." He or she spends more and more time anticipating the next drink, planning when and where to get it, buying and hiding alcohol, and covering up secret drinking. As many as one in six adults in the United States may have a problem with drinking.

Alcohol abuse involves continued use of alcohol despite awareness of social, occupational, psychological, or physical problems related to drinking, or drinking in dangerous ways or situations (before driving, for instance). A diagnosis of alcohol abuse is based on one or more of the following occurring at any time during a 12-month period:

- **A failure to fulfill major role obligations** at work, school, or home (such as missing work or school).
- **The use of alcohol in situations in which it is physically hazardous** (such as before driving).
- **Alcohol-related legal problems** (such as drunk-driving arrests).
- **Continued alcohol use despite persistent or recurring social or interpersonal problems** caused or exacerbated by alcohol (such as fighting while drunk).

Alcohol dependence is a separate disorder in which individuals develop a strong craving for alcohol because it produces pleasurable feelings or relieves stress or anxiety. Over time they experience physiological changes that lead to *tolerance* of its effects; this means that they must consume larger and larger amounts to achieve intoxication. If they abruptly stop drinking, they suffer *withdrawal*, a state of acute physical and psychological discomfort. A diagnosis of

---

Strategies for Prevention :: How to Recognize the Warning Signs of Alcoholism

- :: Experiencing the following symptoms after drinking: frequent headaches, nausea, stomach pain, heartburn, gas, fatigue, weakness, muscle cramps, irregular or rapid heartbeats.
- :: Needing a drink in the morning to start the day.

- :: Denying any problem with alcohol.
- :: Doing things while drinking that are regretted afterward.
- :: Dramatic mood swings, from anger to laughter to anxiety.
- :: Sleep problems.

- :: Depression and paranoia.
- :: Forgetting what happened during a drinking episode.
- :: Changing brands or going on the wagon to control drinking.
- :: Having five or more drinks a day.

alcohol dependence is based on three or more of the following symptoms occurring during any 12-month period:

- **Tolerance,** as defined by either a need for markedly increased amounts of alcohol to achieve intoxication or desired effect, or a markedly diminished effect with continued drinking of the same amount of alcohol as in the past.
- **Withdrawal,** including at least two of the following symptoms: sweating, rapid pulse, or other signs of autonomic hyperactivity; increased hand tremor; insomnia; nausea or vomiting; temporary hallucinations or illusions; physical agitation or restlessness; anxiety; or grand mal seizures.
- **Drinking to avoid** or relieve the symptoms of withdrawal.
- **Consuming larger amounts of alcohol,** or drinking over a longer period than was intended.
- **Persistent desire** or unsuccessful efforts to cut down or control drinking.
- **A great deal of time spent** in activities necessary to obtain alcohol, drink it, or recover from its effects.
- **Important social, occupational, or recreational activities given up** or reduced because of alcohol use.

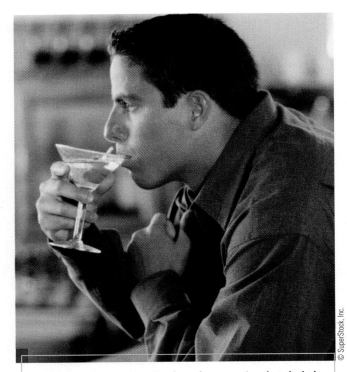

Alcohol dependence may spring from the perception that alcohol relieves stress or creates a pleasant feeling. Daytime drinking and drinking alone can be signs of a serious problem, even though the drinker may otherwise appear to be in control.

- **Continued alcohol use** despite knowledge that alcohol is likely to cause or exacerbate a persistent or recurring physical or psychological problem.

 According to a survey of more than 14,000 undergraduates at four-year colleges, 6 percent of college students met criteria for a diagnosis of alcohol dependence or alcoholism, 31 percent for alcohol abuse. More than two of every five students reported at least one symptom of these conditions and were at increased risk of developing a true alcohol disorder. Few reported seeking treatment since coming to college.

Alcoholism, as defined by the National Council on Alcoholism and Drug Dependence and the American Society of Addiction, is a primary, chronic disease in which genetic, psychosocial, and environmental factors influence its development and manifestations. The disease is often progressive and fatal. Its characteristics include an inability to control drinking, a preoccupation with alcohol, continued use of alcohol despite adverse consequences, and distorted thinking, most notably denial. Like other diseases, alcoholism is not simply a matter of insufficient willpower but a complex problem that causes many symptoms, can have serious consequences, yet can improve with treatment.

A lack of obvious signs of alcoholism can be deceiving. A person who doesn't drink in the morning but feels that he or she must always have a drink at a certain time of the day may have lost control over his or her drinking. A person who never drinks alone but always drinks socially with others may be camouflaging loss of control. A person who is holding a job or taking care of the family may still spend every waking hour thinking about that first drink at the end of the day (preoccupation).

(FAQ) WHAT CAUSES ALCOHOL DEPENDENCE AND ABUSE?

Although the exact cause of alcohol dependence and abuse is not known, certain factors—including biochemical imbalances in the brain, heredity, cultural acceptability, and stress—all seem to play a role. They include the following:

- **Genetics.** Scientists who are working toward mapping the genes responsible for addictive disorders have not yet identified conclusively a specific gene that puts people at risk for alcoholism. However, epidemiological studies have shown evidence of heredity's role. Studies of twins—identical, who share the same genes, and fraternal, who like other siblings share about half their genes—suggest that heredity accounts for two-thirds of the risk of becoming alcoholic in both men and women. Genes also may play a role in successful recovery from alcohol and tobacco addiction.
- **Stress and traumatic experiences.** Many people start drinking heavily as a way of coping

with psychological problems. About half of all individuals who abuse or are dependent on alcohol also have another mental disorder.

▪ **Parental alcoholism.** According to researchers, alcoholism is four to five times more common among the children of alcoholics, who may be influenced by the behavior they see in their parents. The sons and daughters of alcoholics share certain characteristics, including early onset of problem drinking with severe social consequences, an unstable family, poor academic and social performance in school, and antisocial behavior. By some estimates, one of five college students comes from an alcoholic home and may be at increased risk of developing a drinking problem.

▪ **Drug abuse.** Alcoholism is also associated with the abuse of other psychoactive drugs, including marijuana, cocaine, heroin, amphetamines, and various antianxiety medications. Adults under age 30 and adolescents are most likely to use alcohol plus several drugs of abuse, such as marijuana and cocaine.

MEDICAL COMPLICATIONS OF ALCOHOL ABUSE AND DEPENDENCE

Excessive alcohol use adversely affects virtually every organ system in the body, including the brain, the digestive tract, the heart, muscles, blood, and hormones (look back at Figure 12-7, page 351). In addition, because alcohol interacts with many drugs, it can increase the risk of potentially lethal overdoses and harmful interactions. Among the major risks and complications are:

▪ **Liver disease.** Because the liver is the organ that breaks down and metabolizes alcohol, it is especially vulnerable to its effects. Chronic heavy drinking can lead to alcoholic hepatitis (inflammation and destruction of liver cells) and in the 15 percent of people who continue drinking beyond this stage, cirrhosis (irreversible scarring and destruction of liver cells). The liver eventually may fail completely, resulting in coma and death.

▪ **Cardiovascular disease.** Heavy drinking can weaken the heart muscle (causing cardiac myopathy), elevate blood pressure, and increase the risk of stroke. The combined use of alcohol and tobacco greatly increases the likelihood of damage to the heart.

▪ **Cancer.** Heavy alcohol use may contribute to cancer of the liver, stomach, and colon, as well as malignant melanoma, a deadly form of skin cancer. Alcohol in combination with tobacco use also increases the risk of cancer of the mouth, tongue, larynx, and esophagus. Regular drinkers significantly

Mark Nielsen (both)

A normal liver (top) compared to one with cirrhosis.

increase their risk of rectal cancer, but that risk is reduced if wine makes up a third or more of weekly consumption.

▪ **Brain damage.** Chronic brain damage resulting from alcohol consumption is second only to Alzheimer's disease as a cause of cognitive deterioration in adults. Long-term heavy drinkers may suffer memory loss and be unable to think abstractly, recall names of common objects, and follow simple instructions.

▪ **Vitamin deficiencies.** Alcoholics often tend to have very poor nutrition. Alcoholism is associated with vitamin deficiencies, especially of thiamin (B_1), which may be responsible for certain diseases of the neurological, digestive, muscular, and cardiovascular systems. Lack of thiamin may result in Wernicke-Korsakoff syndrome, which is characterized by disorientation, memory failure, hallucinations, and jerky eye movements, and can be disabling enough to require life-long custodial care.

▪ **Digestive problems.** Alcohol triggers the secretion of acids in the stomach that irritate the mucous lining and cause gastritis. Chronic drinking may result in peptic ulcers (breaks in the stomach lining) and bleeding from the stomach lining.

▪ **Accidents and injuries.** Alcohol may contribute to almost half of the deaths caused by car accidents, burns, falls, and choking. Nearly half of those convicted and jailed for criminal acts committed these crimes while under the influence of alcohol.

▪ **Higher mortality.** As discussed earlier, the mortality rate for alcoholics is two to three times higher than that for nonalcoholics of the same age. Injury is the leading alcohol-related cause of death, chiefly in auto accidents involving a drunk driver. Digestive disease, most notably cirrhosis of the liver, is second. Alcohol is a factor in about 30 percent of all suicides. Alcoholics who attempt suicide may have other risk factors, including major depression, poor social support, serious medical illness, and unemployment.

ALCOHOLISM TREATMENTS

Almost 600,000 Americans undergo treatment for alcohol-related problems every year. Until recent years, the only options for professional alcohol treatment were, as one expert puts it, "intensive, extensive, and expensive," such as residential programs at hospitals or specialized treatment centers. Today individuals whose drinking could be hazardous to their health may choose from a variety of approaches. Treatment that works well for one person may not work for another. As research into the outcomes of alcohol treatments has grown, more attempts have been made to match individuals to approaches tailored to their needs and more likely to help them overcome their alcohol problems.

Men and women who have seriously remained sober for more than a decade credit a variety of approaches, including Alcoholics Anonymous (AA), individual psychotherapy, and other groups, such as Women for Sobriety. There is no one sure path to sobriety—a wide variety of treatments may offer help and hope to those with alcohol-related problems.

DETOXIFICATION

The first phase of treatment for alcohol dependence focuses on **detoxification,** the gradual withdrawal of alcohol from the body. For 90 to 95 percent of alcoholics, withdrawal symptoms are mild to moderate. They include sweating; rapid pulse; elevated blood pressure; hand tremor; insomnia; nausea or vomiting; malaise or weakness; anxiety; depressed mood or irritability; headache; and temporary hallucinations or illusions. Withdrawal can be life-threatening when accompanied by medical problems, such as grand mal seizures, pneumonia, liver failure, or gastrointestinal bleeding. The standard treatment is a safer sedative, such as Valium or Ativan, with a gradual reduction in the dose.[46]

Alcohol withdrawal delirium, commonly known as **delirium tremens,** or **DTs,** is most common in chronic heavy drinkers who also suffer from a physical illness, fatigue, depression, or malnutrition. Delirium tremens are characterized by agitated behavior, delusions, rapid heart rate, sweating, vivid hallucinations, trembling hands, and fever. The symptoms usually appear over several days after heavy drinking stops. Individuals frequently report terrifying visual hallucinations, such as seeing insects all over their bodies. With treatment, most cases subside after several days, although delirium tremens has been known to last as long as four or five weeks. In some cases, complications such as infections or heart arrhythmias prove fatal.

(FAQ) ARE THERE MEDICATIONS THAT TREAT ALCOHOLISM?

Antianxiety and antidepressive drugs are sometimes used in early treatment for alcoholism, especially for those with underlying mental disorders. Three drugs—naltrexone, acamprosate, and topiramate—are approved to reduce the persistent craving for alcohol.[47] Vitamin supplements, especially thiamin and folic acid, can help overcome some of the nutritional deficiencies linked with alcoholism.

The drug disulfiram (Antabuse), given to deter drinking, causes individuals to become nauseated and acutely ill when they consume alcohol. Antabuse interrupts the removal of acetaldehye by the liver, so this toxic substance accumulates and causes nausea or vomiting. If individuals taking Antabuse drink at all or consume foods with alcoholic content, they become extremely ill. They must avoid foods cooked or marinated in wine and cough syrup preparations containing alcohol. Some individuals have reactions to the alcohol in after-shave lotion. A large amount of alcohol can make them dangerously ill; fatalities have occurred. Side effects are usually mild and include drowsiness, bad breath, skin rash, and temporary impotence. Because Antabuse does not reduce cravings for alcohol, psychotherapy and support groups remain a necessary part of treatment.

INPATIENT OR RESIDENTIAL TREATMENT

In the past, 28-day treatment programs in a medical or psychiatric hospital or a residential facility were the cornerstone of early recovery treatment. According to outcome studies, inpatient treatment was effective, with as many as 70 percent of "graduates" remaining abstinent or stable, nonproblem drinkers for five years after. However, because of cost pressures from the insurance industry, the length of stay has been reduced, and there's been increasing emphasis on outpatient care.

OUTPATIENT TREATMENT

Outpatient treatment may involve group therapy, individual supportive therapy, marital or family therapy, regular attendance at Alcoholics Anonymous (AA) or another support group, brief interventions, and relapse prevention. According to outcome studies, intensive outpatient treatment at a day hospital (with individuals returning home every evening) are as effective as inpatient care. Outpatient therapy continues for at least a year, but many individuals continue to participate in outpatient programs for the rest of their lives.

Brief Interventions

These methods include individual counseling, group therapy, and training in specific skills—such as assertiveness—all packed into a six- to eight-week period. Offered at a growing number of centers, brief interventions may be most helpful for problem drinkers who are not physically dependent on alcohol. They have proved effective in reducing alcohol consumption up to one year compared with no intervention or standard care. However, at ten years, there is no difference in alcohol consumption among those who had a brief intervention and those who did not. This indicates the need for follow-up advice and counseling.

Moderation Training

Highly controversial, this approach uses cognitive-behavioral techniques, such as keeping a diary to chart drinking patterns and learning "consumption management" techniques, such as never having more than one drink an hour.

Treatment programs in other countries, such as Great Britain and Canada, have long offered moderation training for problem drinkers who consume too much alcohol. However, most experts agree that the best—and perhaps only—hope for recovery for chronic alcoholics who are physically dependent on alcohol is complete abstinence.

Self-Help Programs

The best-known and most commonly used self-help program for alcohol problems is Alcoholics Anonymous (AA), which was founded more than 60 years ago and which has grown into an international organization that includes 2 million members and 185,000 groups worldwide. Acknowledging the power of alcohol, AA offers support from others struggling with the same illness, from a sponsor available at any time of the day or night, and from fellowship meetings that are held every day of the year. Because anonymity is a key part of AA, it has been difficult for researchers to study its success, but it is generally believed to be a highly effective means of overcoming alcoholism and maintaining abstinence. Its 12 steps, which emphasize honesty, sobriety, and acknowlegment of a "higher power," have become the model for self-help groups for other addictive behaviors, including drug abuse (discussed in Chapter 11) and compulsive eating.

The average age of entry into AA is 30; about 60 percent of the members are men. Members encompass a wide range of ages, occupations, nationalities, and socioeconomic classes. People generally attend 12-step meetings every day when they first begin recovery; most programs recommend 90 meetings in 90 days. Many people taper off to one or two meetings a week as their recovery progresses. No one knows exactly how 12-step programs help people break out of addictions. Some individuals stop their drinking, or other destructive behavior, simply on the basis of the information they get at meetings. Others bond to the group and use it as a social support and refuge while they explore and release their inner feelings—a process similar to what happens in psychotherapy.

Alternatives to AA

Secular Organizations for Sobriety (SOS) was founded in 1986 as an alternative for people who couldn't accept the spirituality of AA. Like AA, SOS holds confidential meetings, celebrates sobriety anniversaries, and views recovery as a one-day-at-a-time process.

Rational Recovery, which also emphasizes anonymity and total abstinence, focuses on the self rather than spirituality. Members use reason instead of prayer and learn to control the impulse to drink by learning how to control the emotions that lead them to drink.

One of the most effective programs for women is Women for Sobriety, founded in 1975 by sociologist Jean Kirkpatrick, Ph.D. Its meetings focus on building self-esteem, self-confidence, and responsibility. "AA was started by men, and its message is very disempowering for women," said Kirkpatrick. "We view members as competent women who are struggling with issues that all women must face. Women don't need to recall the painful process of becoming alcoholics. They need to put the past behind them and move on, upward and onward."[48]

RECOVERY

Recovery from alcoholism is a lifelong process of personal growth and healing. The first two years are the most difficult, and relapses are extremely common. By some estimates, more than 90 percent of those recovering from substance use will use alcohol or drugs in any one 12-month period after treatment. However, approximately 70 percent of those who get formal treatment stop drinking for prolonged periods. Even without treatment, 30 percent of alcoholics are able to stop drinking for long periods. Those most likely to remain sober after treatment have the most to lose by continuing to drink: they tend to be employed, married, and upper-middle class. Recovering alcoholics who help other alcoholics stay sober are better able to maintain their own sobriety.[49]

Most recovering alcoholics experience urges to drink, especially during early recovery when they are likely to feel considerable stress. These urges are a natural consequence of years of drinking and diminish with time. Mood swings are common during recovery, and individuals typically describe themselves as alternately feeling relieved or elated and then discouraged or tearful. Such disconcerting ups and downs also decrease over time. Patience—learning to take "one day at a time"—is crucial.

Increasingly, treatment programs focus on **relapse prevention,** which includes the development of coping strategies and learning techniques that make it easier to live with alcohol cravings and rehearsal of various ways of saying "no" to offers of a drink. According to outcomes research, social skills training—a combination of stress management therapy, assertiveness and communication skills training, behavioral self-control training, and behavioral marital therapy—has proved effective in decreasing the duration and severity of relapses after one year in a group of alcoholics.

Strategies for Change ∷ If Someone Close to You Drinks Too Much

∷ Try to remain calm, unemotional, and factually honest in speaking about the drinker's behavior. Include the drinker in family life.

∷ Discuss the situation with someone you trust: a member of the clergy, social worker, friend, or someone who has experienced alcoholism directly.

∷ Never cover up or make excuses for the drinker, or shield him or her from the consequences of drinking. Assuming the drinker's responsibilities undermines his or her dignity and sense of importance.

∷ Refuse to ride with the drinker if he or she is driving while intoxicated.

∷ Encourage new interests and participate in leisure-time activities that the drinker enjoys.

∷ Try to accept setbacks and relapses calmly.

ALCOHOLISM'S IMPACT ON RELATIONSHIPS

Alcoholism shatters families and creates unhealthy patterns of communicating and relating. Separation and divorce rates are high among alcoholics.

GROWING UP WITH AN ALCOHOLIC PARENT

An estimated 28 million children in the United States (or one of every four) are living in a household with an alcoholic adult. Parental alcoholism increases the likelihood of childhood ADHD, conduct disorder, and anxiety disorders. The experience often leads youngsters to play certain roles: The adjuster or "lost child" does whatever the parent says. The responsible child, or "family hero," typically takes over many household tasks and responsibilities. The acting-out child, or "scapegoat," shows his or her anger early in life by causing problems at home or in school and taking on the role of troublemaker. The "mascot" disrupts tense situations by focusing attention on himself or herself, often by clowning. Regardless of which roles they assume, the children of alcoholics are prone to learning disabilities, eating disorders, and addictive behavior.

Numerous studies have linked child abuse and neglect to parental drinking. Children of women who are problem drinkers have twice the risk of serious injury as children of mothers who don't drink. Children with two parents who are problem drinkers are at even higher risk. As teenagers, children of alcoholics are more likely to report early sexual intercourse and face a greater risk of adolescent pregnancy.

ADULT CHILDREN OF ALCOHOLICS

Growing up with an alcoholic parent can have a long-lasting effect. Adult children of alcoholics are at risk for many problems. Some try to fill the emptiness inside with alcohol, drugs, or addictive habits. Others find themselves caught up in destructive relationships that repeat the patterns of their childhood. They are likely to have difficulty solving problems, identifying and expressing their feelings, trusting others, and being intimate. In addition to their own increased risk of addictive behavior, they are likely to marry individuals with some form of addiction and keep on playing out the roles of their childhood. They may feel inadequate, not know how to set limits or recognize normal behavior, be perfectionistic, and want to control all aspects of their lives. However, not all adult children are alike or necessarily suffer from psychological problems or face an increased risk of substance abuse themselves.

Because the impact of alcoholism can be so enduring, support groups—such as Adult Children of Alcoholics, Children of Alcoholics, and Adult Children of Dysfunctional Families—have spread throughout the country in the last decade. These organizations provide adult children of alcoholics a mutually supportive group setting to discuss their childhood experiences with alcoholic parents and the emotional consequences they carry into adult life. Through such groups or other forms of therapy, individuals may learn to move beyond anger and blame, see the part they themselves play in their current state of unhappiness, and create a future that is healthier and happier than their past.

Learn It / Live It

Responsible Drinking

Problems with drinking aren't just the serious ones such as drunk driving and alcoholism. They can start with minor problems, such as missing classes and term paper deadlines. Or they can start with the belief that a party is no fun unless there is a bottle or a six-pack.

As you decide about the role alcohol should play in your life, you might want to follow these guidelines, proposed by BACCHUS, a volunteer college student organization that promotes responsible alcohol-related behavior:

▌ Set a limit on how many drinks you're going to have ahead of time—and stick to it.

- When you're mixing a drink, measure the alcohol.

- Alternate nonalcoholic and alcoholic drinks.

- Drink slowly; don't guzzle.

- Eat before and while drinking.

- Develop alternatives to drinking so you don't turn to alcohol whenever you're depressed or upset. Exercise is a wonderful release for tension; meditation or relaxation techniques can also help you cope.

- Avoid performing tasks that require skilled reactions during or after drinking.

- Don't encourage or reinforce others' irresponsible behavior.

Above all, keep in mind that drinking should not be the primary focus of any activity. Responsible drinking is a matter of you controlling your drinking rather than the drinking controlling you.

Making This Chapter Work for You

Review Questions

1. Which of these is a standard drink?
   a. A margarita
   b. A 12-oz. regular beer
   c. A double martini
   d. A 16-oz. can of malt liquor

2. An individual's response to alcohol depends on all of the following *except*
   a. the rate at which the drink is absorbed into the body's tissues.
   b. the blood alcohol concentration.
   c. socioeconomic status.
   d. gender and race.

3. Responsible drinking includes which of the following behaviors?
   a. Avoiding eating while drinking because eating speeds up absorption of alcohol
   b. Limiting alcohol intake to no more than four drinks in an hour
   c. Taking aspirin while drinking to lower your risk of a heart attack
   d. Socializing with individuals who limit their alcohol intake

4. Which of the following statements about drinking on college campuses is true?
   a. The percentage of students who abstain from alcohol has increased.
   b. The number of women who binge drink has decreased.
   c. Because of peer pressure, students in fraternities and sororities tend to drink less than students in dormitories.
   d. Students who live in substance-free dormitories tend to binge-drink when alcohol is available.

5. Which of the following statements about the effects of alcohol on the body systems is true?
   a. In most individuals, alcohol sharpens the responses of the brain and nervous system, enhancing sensation and perception.
   b. Moderate drinking may have a positive effect on the cardiovascular system.
   c. French researchers have found that drinking red wine with meals may have a positive effect on the digestive system.
   d. The leading alcohol-related cause of death is liver damage.

6. Racial and ethnic patterns related to alcohol use include which of the following?
   a. Asian-American women tend to have higher rates of alcoholism than Asian-American men.
   b. Socioeconomic conditions increase the likelihood of alcohol problems in African Americans and Native Americans.
   c. White Americans tend to have higher rates of cirrhosis of the liver than African Americans or Native Americans.
   d. The Latino culture discourages men from drinking because heavy drinking indicates a lack of machismo.

7. Alcoholism
   a. is considered a chronic disease with genetic, psychosocial, and environment components.
   b. is characterized by a persistent lack of willpower.
   c. may be classified as either Type A, which affects people who are high-strung, or Type B, which affects people who are more mild mannered.
   d. is easily controlled by avoiding exposure to social situations where drinking is common.

8. Which of the following statements about alcohol abuse and dependence is *false?*
   a. Alcohol dependence involves a persistent craving for and an increased tolerance to alcohol.
   b. An individual may have a genetic predisposition for developing alcoholism.
   c. Alcoholics often abuse other psychoactive drugs.
   d. Alcohol abuse and alcohol dependence are different names for the same problem.

9. Health risks of alcoholism include all of the following *except*
   a. hypertension.   *c.* peptic ulcers.
   b. lung cancer.   *d.* hepatitis.

(continued on p. 364)

Self Survey ▪▪ Do You Have a Drinking Problem?

This self-assessment, the Michigan Alcoholism Screening Test (MAST), is widely used to identify potential problems. This test screens for the major psychological, sociological, and physiological consequences of alcoholism.

To complete it, simply answer Yes or No to the following questions, and add up the points shown in the right column for your answers.

	Yes	No	Points
1. Do you enjoy a drink now and then?	___	___	(0 for either)
2. Do you think that you're a normal drinker? (By normal, we mean that you drink less than or as much as most other people.)	___	___	(2 for no)
3. Have you ever awakened the morning after some drinking the night before and found that you couldn't remember part of the evening?	___	___	(2 for yes)
4. Does your wife, husband, a parent, or other near relative ever worry or complain about your drinking?	___	___	(1 for yes)
5. Can you stop drinking without a struggle after one or two drinks?	___	___	(2 for no)
6. Do you ever feel guilty about your drinking?	___	___	(1 for yes)
7. Do friends or relatives think that you're a normal drinker?	___	___	(2 for no)
8. Do you ever try to limit your drinking to certain times of the day or to certain places?	___	___	(0 for either)
9. Have you ever attended a meeting of Alcoholics Anonymous?	___	___	(2 for yes)
10. Have you ever gotten into physical fights when drinking?	___	___	(1 for yes)
11. Has your drinking ever created problems for you and your wife, husband, a parent, or other relative?	___	___	(2 for yes)
12. Have your wife, husband, or other family members ever gone to anyone for help about your drinking?	___	___	(2 for yes)
13. Have you ever lost friends because of your drinking?	___	___	(2 for yes)
14. Have you ever gotten into trouble at work or school because of your drinking?	___	___	(2 for yes)
15. Have you ever lost a job because of your drinking?	___	___	(2 for yes)
16. Have you ever neglected your obligations, your family, or your work for two or more days in a row because of drinking?	___	___	(2 for yes)
17. Do you drink before noon fairly often?	___	___	(1 for yes)
18. Have you ever been told you have liver trouble? Cirrhosis?	___	___	(2 for yes)
19. After heavy drinking, have you ever had delirium tremens (DTs) or severe shaking, or heard voices or seen things that weren't actually there?	___	___	(2 for yes*)
20. Have you ever gone to anyone for help about your drinking?	___	___	(5 for yes)
21. Have you ever been in a hospital because of your drinking?	___	___	(5 for yes)
22. Have you ever been a patient in a psychiatric hospital or on a psychiatric ward of a general hospital where drinking was part of the problem that resulted in hospitalization?	___	___	(2 for yes)
23. Have you ever been seen at a psychiatric or mental health clinic or gone to any doctor, social worker, or clergyman for help with any emotional problem where drinking was part of the problem?	___	___	(2 for yes)
24. Have you ever been arrested for drunk driving, driving while intoxicated, or driving under the influence of alcoholic beverages?	___	___	(2 for yes)
25. Have you ever been arrested, or taken into custody, even for a few hours, because of drunken behavior?	___	___	(2 for yes)
(If Yes, how many times?	___**)		

*Five points for delirium tremens
**Two points for each arrest

Scoring

In general, five or more points places you in an alcoholic category; four points suggests alcoholism; while three or fewer points indicates that you're *not* alcoholic.

YOUR ACTION PLAN FOR AVOIDING DESTRUCTIVE DECISIONS

Students Against Destructive Decisions (originally founded as Students Against Driving Drunk) developed the following statement and contract for college students to discuss and sign. Use it as your health action plan for making responsible decisions about alcohol, drugs, and other behaviors that could put your health at risk:

Despite increased public and legislative awareness, the abuse of legal and illegal alcohol and other drugs is rampant in our society. The consequences of alcohol abuse and drug addiction are devastating and pose a major threat to young people in our society. No age group is more vulnerable to the tragic consequences of this abuse and addiction than are college students and other young adults.

College students across the nation have begun to band together to fight the substance abuse problems affecting their campuses. Innovative SADD programs have highlighted the power of college students to effectively deal with critical problems. The SADD College Contract for Life is designed to facilitate communication between college friends about potentially destructive decisions related to alcohol, drug use, HIV/AIDS, sexuality, date rape, impaired driving, and many more challenges. The Contract provides a practical tool for opening discussion, raising awareness, and demonstrating the desire to help friends find any assistance they need.[50]

Source: http://www.sadd.org/contract.htm#collegecfl

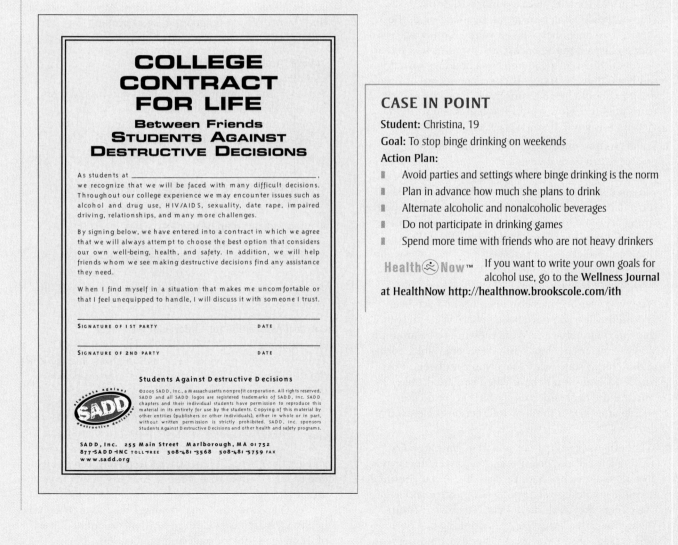

CASE IN POINT

Student: Christina, 19

Goal: To stop binge drinking on weekends

Action Plan:

- Avoid parties and settings where binge drinking is the norm
- Plan in advance how much she plans to drink
- Alternate alcoholic and nonalcoholic beverages
- Do not participate in drinking games
- Spend more time with friends who are not heavy drinkers

Health⊗Now™ If you want to write your own goals for alcohol use, go to the **Wellness Journal** at **HealthNow** http://healthnow.brookscole.com/ith

10. Which of the following statements about alcoholism treatment is true?

   a. Inpatient treatment has been shown to be more effective than outpatient treatment.

   b. Alcoholism can be cured by detoxifying or ridding the body of all traces of alcohol.

   c. Antabuse is a medication given to alcoholics with underlying mental disorders.

   d. A combination of medical, behavioral, and self-help approaches may be necessary to treat alcohol abuse and dependence.

Answers to these questions can be found on page 587.

Critical Thinking

1. Driving home from his high school graduation party, 18-year-old Rick has had too much to drink. As he crosses the dividing line on the two-lane road, the driver of an oncoming car—a young mother with two young children in the backseat—swerves to avoid an accident. She hits a concrete wall and dies instantly, but her children survive. Rick has no record of drunk driving. Should he go to prison? Is he guilty of manslaughter? How would you feel if you were the victim's husband? If you were Rick's friend?

2. Some groups concerned about alcohol abuse advocate greater restrictions on availability, such as prohibiting the sale of alcoholic beverages in supermarkets, convenience stores, and gas stations. They would like to see a ban on advertisements, especially those aimed at young people. Opponents argue that laws have never been effective in controlling alcohol abuse. Do you think our society is too permissive in the way we allow alcohol to be promoted or sold? Would you support anti-alcohol laws? Why or why not?

3. Have you ever been around people who have been intoxicated when you have been sober? What did you think of their behavior? Were they fun to be around? Was the experience not particularly enjoyable, boring, or difficult in some way? Have you ever been intoxicated? How do you behave when you are drunk? Do you find the experience enjoyable? What do the people around you think of your actions when you are drunk?

4. What effects has alcohol use had in your life? Try making a list of the positive and negative effects your own alcohol use has had. Be specific. If you continue to drink at your current rate, what positive and negative effects do you think it will have on your future? What effects has other people's drinking had on your life? List family members and friends who drink regularly and how their drinking has affected you.

Media Menu

Health Now™

Throughout the chapter, this icon introduces a list of resources on the Health-Now website at **http://healthnow.brookscole.com/ith** that will:

- Help you evaluate your knowledge of the material.
- Allow you to take an exam-prep quiz.
- Provide a Personalized Learning Plan targeting resources that address areas you should study.
- Coach you through identifying target goals for behavior change and creating and monitoring your personal change plan throughout the semester.

INTERNET CONNECTIONS

Facts on Tap: Alcohol and Your College Experience
www.factsontap.org
This excellent site is geared to college students. It features links to the following topics and more: "Risky Relationship: Alcohol and Sex," "College Experience: Alcohol and Student Life," "The Naked Truth: Alcohol and Your Body," and "When Someone Else's Drinking Gives You a Hangover."

College Drinking: Changing the Culture
www.collegedrinkingprevention.gov
This website, sponsored by the National Institute of Alcohol Abuse and Alcoholism, focuses on the college alcohol culture with information for students, parents, college health administrators, and more. In addition, the site features information about alcohol prevention, college alcohol policies, research topics, and factual information about the consequences of alcohol abuse and alcoholism.

Al-Anon Family Group Headquarters
www.al-anon.alateen.org
This site provides information and referrals to local Al-Anon and Alateen groups. It also includes a self-quiz to determine if you are affected by someone who has an alcohol problem.

National Association for Children of Alcoholics
www.nacoa.org
This association provides information about and for children of alcoholics. Their website contains numerous links to relevant support groups.

InfoTrac College Edition Activities Log on, insert **alcohol abuse** into the Keyword search box, and limit your search to the past year. When you get the results, Mark articles to review, then Select one to read. Summarize three or four key points from the article.

You can find additional readings related to personal health with InfoTrac College Edition, an online library of more than 900 journals and publications. Follow the instructions for accessing InfoTrac College Edition that were packaged with your textbook; then search for articles using a keyword search.

For additional links, resources, and suggested readings on InfoTrac College Edition, visit our Health and Wellness Resource Center at **http://health.wadsworth .com.**

Key Terms

The terms listed are used on the page indicated. Definitions of the terms are in the Glossary at the end of this book.

absorption 339

alcohol abuse 355

alcohol dependence 355

alcoholism 356

binge drinking 343

blood-alcohol concentration (BAC) 338

delirium tremens (DTs) 358

detoxification 358

ethyl alcohol 338

fetal alcohol effects (FAE) 353

fetal alcohol syndrome (FAS) 353

intoxication 340

proof 338

relapse prevention 359

13 Tobacco Use, Misuse, and Abuse

Andrea didn't really want her first cigarette. Her tent mate at camp had snatched one from a counselor's pack, and the two of them had climbed to a remote rock to share it. Andrea hated everything about her first drag: the taste, the smell, the horrible burning in her throat and lungs. But she loved feeling more grown-up and sophisticated than other seventh graders. By the time she reached high school, Andrea would sneak off to smoke with friends at least once a week. By graduation, she was smoking daily.

As a college freshmen, Andrea discovered that she was part of an unpopular minority. Even though her dorm didn't ban smoking, her roommate declared their room a smoke-free zone. Her college didn't allow smoking in any classrooms or public areas. And many of her new friends reacted as if smoking was a sign of impaired intelligence. Andrea has decided to quit, but she's discovered that nicotine dependence is very difficult to overcome. "I just wish I'd never started smoking in the first place," she says.

According to the Centers for Disease Control and Prevention (CDC), 20.9 percent of American adults—some 44.5 million people—smoke.[1] The more and the longer they smoke, the greater their risks of heart disease, respiratory problems, several types of cancer, and a shortened lifespan.

Despite widespread awareness of the dangers of tobacco, smoking continues to kill more people than AIDS, alcohol, drug abuse, car crashes, murders, suicides, and fires combined. The worldwide death toll is 5 million people a year.[2]

This chapter discusses smoking in America and on campus, the effects of tobacco on the body, tobacco dependence, quitting smoking, smokeless tobacco, and environmental tobacco smoke. The information it provides may help you to breathe easier today—and may help ensure cleaner air for others to breathe tomorrow.

FAQ Frequently Asked Questions

- Why do people start smoking? *p. 369*
- Is social smoking less risky? *p. 371*
- What are bidis? *p. 377*
- Does quitting eliminate the risks associated with smoking? *p. 381*

After studying the material in this chapter, you should be able to:

- **Describe** today's tobacco smokers and the common reasons why they smoke.

- **Describe** some of the tobacco-control policies on college campuses.

- **List** the health effects of smoking tobacco or using smokeless tobacco.

- **Discuss** the health problems that can be prevented by quitting smoking.

- **Identify** the different types of tobacco products.

- **Describe** the health effects of environmental, or secondhand, tobacco smoke.

- **Discuss** several recommended ways to quit smoking.

SMOKING IN AMERICA

Americans are snuffing out cigarettes. The prevalence of smoking in the United States has declined more than 40 percent in recent decades. According to federal surveys, slightly more than one in five Americans smokes. Of these, about eight in ten smoke every day. As Table 13-1 indicates, more men (24.1 percent) than women (19.2 percent) are current smokers. American Indians have the highest smoking rates, while Asians and Hispanics have the lowest. Individuals with undergraduate and graduate degrees are least likely to smoke.[3]

The drop in smoking in the overall population still falls short of the national health objective of reducing cigarette smoking among adults to 12 percent by 2010. However, some groups have met this goal. They include women with undergraduate or graduate degrees, men with graduate degrees, Hispanic and Asian women, and people over age 65. Among all women, smoking has fallen below 20 percent (to 19.2 percent) for the first time since the National Health Interview Survey began collecting data on women in 1965.

Another big drop has occurred in young adults between ages 18 and 24. This was the only age group in which smoking increased from 1993 to 2002, when 28.5 percent of college-age Americans reported smoking. This rate has since fallen to 23.9 percent, higher than the national average but lower than it has been in more than a decade. The National College Health Assessment found a somewhat lower rate of 21.1 percent, which is in line with national averages.[4]

Despite the improvement, smoking still accounts for an estimated 438,000 premature deaths each year in the United States. Roughly one in every three deaths among people ages 35 to 70 is related to tobacco use.[5] Smoking deaths cost the nation $92 billion in lost productivity annually.[6]

Canadians have made even greater progress. Higher tobacco taxes, constant health warnings, and laws that restrict smoking areas have worked effectively to reduce the smoking rate in Canada to 20 percent, compared with 30 percent during the 1990s.

TABLE 13-1 WHO SMOKES IN AMERICA?

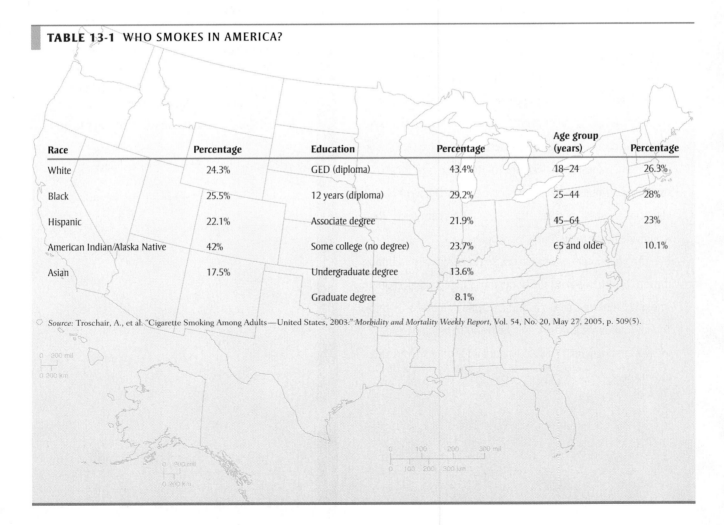

Race	Percentage	Education	Percentage	Age group (years)	Percentage
White	24.3%	GED (diploma)	43.4%	18–24	26.3%
Black	25.5%	12 years (diploma)	29.2%	25–44	28%
Hispanic	22.1%	Associate degree	21.9%	45–64	23%
American Indian/Alaska Native	42%	Some college (no degree)	23.7%	65 and older	10.1%
Asian	17.5%	Undergraduate degree	13.6%		
		Graduate degree	8.1%		

Source: Troschair, A., et al. "Cigarette Smoking Among Adults—United States, 2003." *Morbidity and Mortality Weekly Report*, Vol. 54, No. 20, May 27, 2005, p. 509(5).

ⓕⓐⓠ WHY DO PEOPLE START SMOKING?

Most people are aware that an enormous health risk is associated with smoking, but many don't know exactly what that risk is or how it might affect them.

The two main factors linked with the onset of a smoking habit are age and education. The vast majority of white men with less than a high school education are current or former daily cigarette smokers. White women with a similar educational background are also very likely to smoke or to have smoked every day. Hispanic men and women without a high school education are less likely to be or become daily smokers. Other factors associated with the reasons for smoking are discussed in the following sections.

Genetics

Researchers speculate that genes may account for about 50 percent of smoking behavior, with environment playing an equally important role. Studies have shown that identical twins, who have the same genes, are more likely to have matching smoking profiles than fraternal twins. If one identical twin is a heavy smoker, the other is also likely to be; if one smokes only occasionally, so does the other.

 According to NIDA research, genetic factors play a more significant role for initiation of smoking in women than men, but they play a less significant role in smoking persistence for women.

Parental Role Models

Children who start smoking are 50 percent more likely than youngsters who don't smoke to have at least one smoker in their family. A mother who smokes seems a particularly strong influence on making smoking seem acceptable. The majority of youngsters who smoke say that their parents also smoke and are aware of their own tobacco use.

Adolescents are more likely to smoke, express an intention to smoke, or smoke longer if their parents smoke.

Adolescent Experimentation and Rebellion

For teenagers, smoking may be a coping mechanism for dealing with boredom and frustration; a marker of the transition into high school or college; a bid for adult status; a way of gaining admission to a peer group; or a way to have fun, reduce stress, or boost energy. The teenagers most likely to begin smoking are those least likely to seek help when their emotional needs are not met. They might smoke as a means of gaining social acceptance or to self-medicate when they feel helpless, lonely, or depressed. Depressed teens are more susceptible to cigarette ads than their counterparts. For example, they are more likely to have a favorite cigarette ad or own clothing with cigarette logos.

Teens often misjudge the addictive power of cigarettes. Many, sure that they'll be able to quit any time they want, figure that smoking for a year or two won't hurt them. More than one-half of adolescent smokers smoke "light" cigarettes, which they mistakenly think are less risky and less addictive.[7] But when they try to quit, they can't. Like older smokers, most young people who smoke have tried to quit at least once.

Mental Disorders

The percentage of smokers jumps to more than 90 percent among those with alcoholism and other addictions, 85 percent among schizophrenia patients, and 80 percent among depressed patients. The relationship between depression and smoking is complex. Smokers are more likely to be depressed, while adults who are depressed are 40 to 50 percent more likely to smoke than adults who are not depressed. Research has identified biological connections between smoking and depression, suggesting a biological similarity between substance use and depressive disorders.

Limited Education

People who have graduated from college are much less likely to smoke than high school graduates; those with fewer than 12 years of education are more likely to smoke. An individual with 8 years or less of education is 11 times more likely to smoke than someone with postgraduate training.

Weight Control

Concern about weight is a significant risk factor for smoking among young women. Daily smokers are two to four times more likely to fast, use diet pills, and purge to control their weight than nonsmokers. Although black girls smoke at substantially lower rates than white girls, the common factor in predicting daily smoking among all girls, regardless of race, is concern with weight.

Aggressive Marketing

Cigarette companies spend billions of dollars each year on advertisements and promotional campaigns, with manufacturers targeting ads especially at women, teens, minorities, and the poor. Most controversial are cigarette advertisements in magazines and media aimed at teenagers and even younger children.

Stress

In studies that have analyzed the impact of life stressors, depression, emotional support, marital status, and income, researchers have concluded that an individual with a high stress level is approximately 15 times more likely to be a smoker than a person with low stress. About half of smokers identify workplace stress as a key factor in their smoking behavior.

Addiction

Nicotine addiction is as strong or stronger than addiction to drugs such as cocaine and heroin. The first symptoms of nicotine addiction can begin within a few days of starting to smoke and after just a few cigarettes, particularly in teenagers. Smoking a single cigarette before age 11 increases the

Your peer group can influence your decision to start smoking.

odds of becoming dependent on nicotine.[8] In general, adolescents become addicted to cigarettes more readily than adults.[9]

WHY PEOPLE KEEP SMOKING

Whatever the reasons for lighting up that first cigarette, very different factors keep cigarettes burning pack after pack, year after year. In national polls, seven in ten smokers say that they want to quit but can't. The reason isn't a lack of willpower. Medical scientists have recognized tobacco dependence as an addictive disorder that may be more powerful than heroin dependence and that may affect more than 90 percent of all smokers.

Pleasure

According to the American Cancer Society, nine in ten regular smokers find smoking pleasurable. Nicotine—the addictive ingredient in tobacco—is the reason. Researchers have shown that nicotine reinforces and strengthens the desire to smoke by acting on brain chemicals that influence feelings of well-being. This drug also can improve memory, help in performing certain tasks, reduce anxiety, dampen hunger, and increase pain tolerance.

Mental Disorders

Individuals with mental disorders are twice as likely to smoke as others, and people with mental illness may account for nearly one-half of the tobacco market in the United States. Heavy smoking also is linked with an almost elevenfold risk of anxiety disorders in early adulthood.

Smokers with a history of depression are about half as likely to quit as others. Even after a recovery from major depression, smokers often continue to report some symptoms of depression. Smokers who are depressed tend to smoke

more cigarettes than other smokers, are less successful in their efforts to stop smoking, and are more prone to depression after quitting. The longer people smoke, the more likely they are to develop symptoms of depression and anxiety.[10]

Fear of Weight Gain

Smokers burn up an extra 100 calories a day—the equivalent of walking a mile—probably because nicotine increases metabolic rate. Once they start smoking, many individuals say they cannot quit because they fear they'll gain weight. The CDC estimates that women who stop smoking gain an average of 8 pounds, while men put on an average of 6 pounds. One in eight women and one in ten men who stop smoking put on 29 pounds or more. The reasons for this weight gain include nicotine's effects on metabolism as well as emotional and behavioral factors, such as the habit of frequently putting something into one's mouth. Yet as a health risk, smoking a pack and a half to two packs a day is a greater danger than carrying 60 pounds of extra weight.

Weight gain for smokers who quit is not inevitable. Aerobic exercise helps increase metabolic rate, and limiting alcohol and foods high in sugar and fat can help smokers control their weight as they give up cigarettes.

Dependence

Nicotine has a much more powerful hold on smokers than alcohol does on drinkers. Whereas about 10 percent of alcohol users lose control of their intake of alcohol and become alcoholics, as many as 80 percent of all heavy smokers have tried to cut down on or quit smoking but cannot overcome their dependence.

Nicotine causes dependence by at least three means:

■ It provides a strong sensation of pleasure.

■ It leads to fairly severe discomfort during withdrawal.

■ It stimulates cravings long after obvious withdrawal symptoms have passed.

Few drugs act as quickly on the brain as nicotine does. It travels through the bloodstream to the brain in seven seconds—half the time it takes for heroin injected into a blood vessel to reach the brain. And a pack-a-day smoker gets 200 hits of nicotine a day—73,000 a year.

After a few years of smoking, the most powerful incentive for continuing to smoke is to avoid the discomfort of withdrawal. Generally, ten cigarettes a day will prevent withdrawal effects. For many who smoke heavily, signs of withdrawal, including changes in mood and performance, occur within two hours after smoking their last cigarette. Smokeless tobacco users also get constant doses of nicotine. However, absorption of nicotine by the lungs is more likely to lead to dependence than absorption through the linings of the nose and mouth. As with other drugs of abuse, continued nicotine intake results in tolerance (the need for more of a drug to maintain the same effect), which is why only 2 percent of all smokers smoke just a few cigarettes a day, or smoke only occasionally. (See Self Survey: "Are You Addicted to Nicotine?")

Use of Other Substances

Many smokers also drink or use drugs. According to the Addiction Research Foundation in Canada, tobacco smokers say cigarettes are harder to abandon than other drugs, even when they find them less pleasurable than their preferred drug of abuse. Individuals who drink excessively also find their cigarette habit a hard one to break.

TOBACCO USE ON CAMPUS

After increasing for several years, smoking has dropped in college-age adults, but about one in every four to five students currently smoke. According to the National College Health Assessment survey, about 21 percent of students smoked in the last month (see Student Snapshot: "Tobacco Use on Campus"). A small percentage of undergraduates—about 5 percent—reported smoking every day. About 10 percent smoked fewer than 10 days a month.[11]

 In a survey of more than 17,000 college students from 140 schools, fewer men involved in athletics were current smokers: 15 percent of those who participated in athletics every day, compared with 20 percent of those who were less involved and 26 percent of men not involved in athletics.[12]

Smoking is more common in students who live in housing where smoking is permitted, and in students with a lower psychological sense of well-being.[13] Marijuana and alcohol use and weekend exposure to smoke increase the likelihood of being a tobacco user.[14]

College students smoke for many reasons, including defiance of their parents and relaxed smoking standards in their dorms. Many students who had never tried smoking may experiment with cigarettes in colleges. Students who were occasional smokers in high school are more likely to become more frequent, heavier smokers once in college.

Many college students say they smoke as a way of managing depression or stress. Studies consistently link smoking with depression and low life satisfaction. Smokers are significantly more likely to have higher levels of perceived stress than nonsmokers. In one study, students who had been diagnosed or treated for depression were seven times as likely as other students to use tobacco.[15]

 Male students who smoke are more likely to say that smoking makes them feel more masculine and less anxious. More than half of female smokers feel that smoking helps them control their weight. Overweight female students are more likely to smoke to lose weight and to see weight gain as a barrier to quitting.

The tobacco industry regularly targets college students with marketing strategies such as providing free samples of cigarettes at campus parties or in bars or clubs. This

Student Snapshot
TOBACCO USE ON CAMPUS

	Cigarettes	Cigars	Smokeless Tobacco
Have never used	61.8%	76.3%	90.6%
Not used in last month	17.1	18.9	6.4
Used every day last month	5.4	0.1	0.5

Source: American College Health Association. "The American College Health Association's National College Health Assessment (ACHA-NCHA), Spring 2003 Reference Group Report." *Journal of American College Health*, Vol. 53, No. 5, March–April 2005, p. 199.

approach seems to have a particularly strong effect on nonsmokers. In a group of about 8,500 students who did not smoke prior to college, one in four of those who attended a promotional event became a smoker, twice the rate of those who did not attend such events.[16]

(FAQ) IS SOCIAL SMOKING LESS RISKY?

About half of college students who smoke say they are "social smokers" who average less than one cigarette a day and smoke mainly in the company of

Social smoking has negative health effects and can lead to dependence addiction.

others.[17] On the positive side, social smokers smoke less often and less intensely than other smokers and are less dependent on tobacco. However, they are still jeopardizing their health. The more they smoke, the greater the health risks they face. Even smokers who don't inhale or nonsmokers who breathe in secondhand smoke are at increased risk for negative health effects.

In research studies, smoking less than a pack a week of cigarettes has proved to damage the lining of blood vessels and to increase the risk of heart disease as well as of cancer. In women taking birth control pills, even a few cigarettes a week can increase the likelihood of heart disease, blood clots, stroke, liver cancer, and gallbladder disease. Pregnant women who smoke only occasionally still run a higher risk of giving birth to unhealthy babies. Another risk is addiction. Social smokers are less motivated to quit and make fewer attempts to do so. Many end up smoking more cigarettes for many more years than they intended.

COLLEGE TOBACCO-CONTROL POLICIES

Other than religious institutions, colleges and universities have traditionally had few smoking restrictions. This has changed. Several national health organizations, including the American College Health Association and National Center on Addiction and Substance Abuse, have recommended that colleges ban smoking in and around all campus buildings, including student housing, and prohibit the sale, advertisement, and promotion of tobacco products on campus. Although some schools, particularly large public universities, have made progress in adopting such policies, most still fall short of the national recommendations.

A growing number of public and private schools provide completely smoke-free student housing, a dramatic increase from a decade ago. Two-thirds do not allow tobacco sales on campus; a third of student newspapers do not allow tobacco advertising. None have specifically banned tobacco industry sponsorships and promotions on college property. In general, schools in the West have done the most to implement tobacco policies. Those in the South, particularly in the major tobacco-growing states, have done the least.

An estimated 44 percent of students live in smoke-free dorms, while another 29 percent who don't would like to move into one. Freshmen who did not smoke regularly in high school and who live in smoke-free dorms are 40 percent less likely to take up smoking than those in unrestricted housing, according to a study of the smoking behavior of 4,495 students at 101 schools.[18]

Despite concern about student smoking, more than 40 percent of schools do not offer smoking cessation programs to students who want to quit. Those that do primarily refer students to campus support groups or community-based programs like Nicotine Anonymous; they report little student demand for these options.

SMOKING, RACE, AND GENDER

Cigarette smoking is a major cause of disease and death in all population groups. However, tobacco use varies within and among racial and ethnic minority groups. Among adults, Native Americans and Alaska Natives have the highest rates of tobacco use. African-American and Southeast Asian men also have a high smoking rate. Asian-American and Hispanic women have the lowest rates of smoking. Tobacco use is significantly higher among white college students than among Hispanic, African-American, and Asian students.

Tobacco is the substance most abused by Hispanic youth, whose smoking rates have soared in the last ten years. In general, smoking rates among Hispanic adults increase as they adopt the values, beliefs, and norms of American culture. Recent declines in the prevalence of smoking have been greater among Hispanic men with at least a high school education than among those with less education.

On average, girls who begin smoking during adolescence continue smoking for 20 years, four years longer than boys. Women are at greater risk for developing smoking-related illnesses compared with men who smoke the same amount. Lung cancer now claims more women's lives than breast cancer. In men, cigarette smoking increases the risk of aggressive prostate cancer.

Smoking is a risk factor for developing rheumatoid arthritis for men, but not for women. Women who smoke are more likely to develop osteoporosis, a bone-weakening disease.

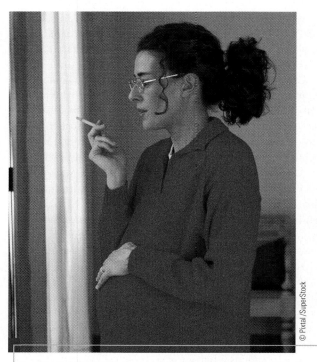

© Pixtal /SuperStock

Smoking late in pregnancy can endanger the physical and intellectual development of the fetus.

According to the U.S. Surgeon General, women account for 39 percent of smoking-related deaths each year, a proportion that has doubled since 1965. Each year, American women lose an estimated 2.1 million years of life due to premature deaths attributable to smoking. If she smokes, a woman's annual risk of dying more than doubles after age 45 compared with a woman who has never smoked.

 High nicotine intake may affect male hormones, including testosterone. Smoking also can reduce blood flow to the penis, impairing a man's sexual performance and increasing the likelihood of erectile dysfunction.[19]

Smoking directly affects women's reproductive organs and processes. Women who smoke are less fertile and experience menopause one or two years earlier than women who don't smoke. Smoking also greatly increases the possible risks associated with taking oral contraceptives.

Women who smoke during pregnancy increase their risk of miscarriage and pregnancy complications, including bleeding, premature delivery, and birth defects such as cleft lip or palate. Smoking during the third trimester affects both physical and intellectual development. In one study, the more cigarettes a mother smoked, the lower her son's birth weight and IQ as he matured.[20]

 Older women who smoke are weaker, have poorer balance, and are at greater risk of physical disability than nonsmokers.

TOBACCO'S IMMEDIATE EFFECTS

Tobacco, an herb that can be smoked or chewed, directly affects the brain. While its primary active ingredient is nicotine, tobacco smoke contains almost 400 other compounds and chemicals, including gases, liquids, particles, tar, carbon monoxide, cadmium, pyridine, nitrogen dioxide, ammonia, benzene, phenol, acrolein, hydrogen cyanide, formaldehyde, and hydrogen sulfide.

HOW NICOTINE WORKS

A colorless, oily compound, **nicotine** is poisonous in concentrated amounts. If you inhale while smoking, 90 percent of the nicotine in the smoke is absorbed into your body. Even if you draw smoke only into your mouth and not into your lungs, you still absorb 25 to 30 percent of the nicotine. The FDA has concluded that nicotine is a dangerous, addictive drug that should be regulated.

Faster than an injection, smoking speeds nicotine to the brain in seconds (Figure 13-1). Nicotine affects the brain in much the same way as cocaine, opiates, and amphetamines, triggering the release of dopamine, a neurotransmitter associated with pleasure and addiction, as well as other messenger chemicals. Because nicotine acts on some of the

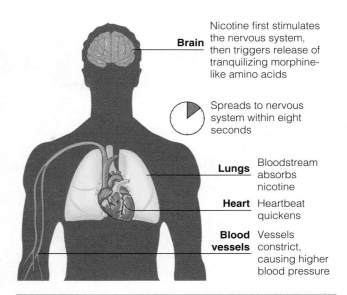

FIGURE 13-1   The Immediate Effects of Nicotine on the Body
The primary active ingredient in tobacco is nicotine, a fast-acting and potent drug.
Source: American Cancer Society, National Cancer Institute.

same brain regions stimulated by interactions with loved ones, smokers come to regard cigarettes as a friend that they turn to when they're stressed, sad, or mad.

Nicotine may enhance smokers' performance on some tasks but leaves other mental skills unchanged. Nicotine also acts as a sedative. How often you smoke and how you smoke determine nicotine's effect on you. If you're a regular smoker, nicotine will generally stimulate you at first, then tranquilize you. Shallow puffs tend to increase alertness because low doses of nicotine facilitate the release of the neurotransmitter *acetylcholine,* which makes the smoker feel alert. Deep drags, on the other hand, relax the smoker because high doses of nicotine block the flow of acetylcholine.

Nicotine stimulates the adrenal glands to produce adrenaline, a hormone that increases blood pressure, speeds up the heart rate by 15 to 20 beats a minute, and constricts blood vessels (especially in the skin). Nicotine also inhibits the formation of urine, dampens hunger, irritates the membranes in the mouth and throat, and dulls the taste buds so foods don't taste as good as they would otherwise.

Nicotine withdrawal usually begins within hours. Symptoms include craving, irritability, anxiety, restlessness, and increased appetite.[21]

TAR AND CARBON MONOXIDE

As it burns, tobacco produces **tar,** a thick, sticky dark fluid made up of several hundred different chemicals—many of them poisonous, some of them *carcinogenic* (enhancing the growth of cancerous cells). As you inhale tobacco smoke, tar and other particles settle in the forks of the branchlike bronchial tubes in your lungs, where precancerous changes are

Negative Long-Term Effects

Brain and central nervous system
- Dulls sensory and cognitive skills
- Impairs short-term memory
- Alters motor coordination
- Causes changes in brain chemistry
- Leads to difficulty in concentration, attention to detail, and learning new complex information
- Increased risk of stroke

Cardiovascular system
- Increases heart rate
- Increases blood pressure
- Decreases blood flow to the limbs

Respiratory system
- Damages the lungs (50% more tar than tobacco)
- May cause lung cancer
- May damage throat from inhalation

Reproductive system
- In women, may impair ovulation and cause fetal abnormalities if used during pregnancy
- In men, may suppress sexual functioning and may reduce the number, quality, and motility of sperm, possibly affecting fertility

Positive Short-Term Therapeutic Effects for Patients

Brain and central nervous system
- May help minimize pain from the spread of cancer

Vision
- Reduces intraocular pressure, helping those afflicted with glaucoma

Digestive system
- Combats nausea from chemotherapy and helps minimize vomiting
- Helps restore appetite in people who have lost weight from cancer or AIDS

Muscular system
- May help calm spasms from spinal-cord injuries, multiple sclerosis. and possible epilepsy

FIGURE 13-2   Some Effects of Smoking on the Body
Smoking harms the respiratory system and the cardiovascular system. The leading cause of death for smokers is heart attack.

apt to occur. In addition, tar and smoke damage the mucus and the cilia in the bronchial tubes, which normally remove irritating foreign materials from your lungs.

Smoke from cigarettes, cigars, and pipes also contains **carbon monoxide,** the deadly gas that comes out of the exhaust pipes of cars, in levels 400 times those considered safe in industry. Carbon monoxide interferes with the ability of the hemoglobin in the blood to carry oxygen, impairs normal functioning of the nervous system, and is at least partly responsible for the increased risk of heart attacks and strokes in smokers.

HEALTH EFFECTS OF CIGARETTE SMOKING

Figure 13-2 shows a summary of the physiological effects of tobacco and the other chemicals in tobacco smoke. If you're a smoker who inhales deeply and started smoking before the age of 15, you're trading a minute of future life for every minute you now spend smoking. On average, smokers die nearly seven years earlier than nonsmokers. Smoking not only eventually kills, it also ages you: Smokers get more wrinkles than nonsmokers.

But the effects of smoking are far more than skin-deep. A cigarette smoker is 10 times more likely to develop lung cancer than a nonsmoker and 20 times more likely to have a heart attack. Daily smokers also are more likely to have suicidal thoughts or attempt suicide, although the reasons are not clear [22] (see Chapter 4).

HEART DISEASE AND STROKE

The toxic chemicals in tobacco signal the heart to beat faster and harder. Blood vessels constrict, forcing blood to travel through a narrower space. Blood pressure increases— temporarily at first. Over time, smokers develop chronic high blood pressure. Smoking increases harmful cholesterol (LDL) and lowers beneficial cholesterol (HDL). It also leads to the buildup of plaques, or fatty deposits within the arteries, hardening of the arteries, and greater risk of blood clots.[23]

Although a great deal of publicity has been given to the link between cigarettes and lung cancer, heart attack is actually the leading cause of deaths for smokers. Smoking doubles the risk of heart disease and increases the risk of sudden death two to four times. The effect of smoking on risk of heart attack is greater in younger smokers.[24]

Smokers who suffer heart attacks have only a 50 percent chance of recovering. Smokers have a 70 percent higher death rate from heart disease than nonsmokers, and those who smoke heavily have a 200 percent higher death rate.

The federal Office of the Surgeon General blames cigarettes for one of every ten deaths attributable to heart disease. Smoking is more dangerous than the two most notorious risk factors for heart disease: high blood pressure and high cholesterol. If smoking is combined with one of these, the chances of heart attack are four times greater. Women who smoke and use oral contraceptives have a ten times higher risk of suffering heart attacks than women who do neither.

In addition to contributing to heart attacks, cigarette smoking increases the risk of stroke two to three times in men and women, even after other risk factors are taken into account.

Even people who have smoked for decades can reduce their risk of heart attack if they quit smoking. However, studies indicate some irreversible damage to blood vessels. Progression of atherosclerosis (hardening of the arteries) among former smokers continues at a faster pace than among those who never smoked.

CANCER

Smoking is linked to at least ten different cancers and accounts for 30 percent of all deaths from cancer. It is the cause of more than 80 percent of all cases of lung cancer. The more people smoke, the longer they smoke, and the earlier they start smoking, the more likely they are to develop lung cancer.

Smoking causes about 130,000 lung cancer deaths each year. Smokers of two or more packs a day have lung cancer mortality rates 15 to 25 times greater than nonsmokers. If smokers stop smoking before cancer has started, their lung tissue tends to repair itself, even if there were already precancerous changes.

Chemicals in cigarette smoke and other environmental pollutants switch on a particular gene in the lung cells of some individuals. This gene produces an enzyme that helps manufacture powerful carcinogens, which set the stage for cancer. The gene seems more likely to be activated in some people than others, and people with this gene are at much higher risk of developing lung cancer. However, smokers without the gene still remain at risk, because other chemicals and genes also may be involved in the development of lung cancer.

Smokers who are depressed are more likely to get cancer than nondepressed smokers. Although researchers don't know exactly how smoking and depression may work together to increase the risk of cancer, one possibility is that stress and depression cause biological changes that lower immunity, such as a decline in natural killer cells that fight off tumors.

RESPIRATORY DISEASES

Smoking quickly impairs the respiratory system, including the cough reflex, a vital protective response. Even some teenage smokers show signs of respiratory difficulty—breathlessness, chronic cough, excess phlegm production—when compared with nonsmokers of the same age. Cigarette smokers are up to 18 times more likely than nonsmokers to die of noncancerous diseases of the lungs.

Cigarette smoking is the major cause of chronic obstructive lung disease (COLD), which includes emphysema and chronic bronchitis. COLD is characterized by progressive limitation of the flow of air into and out of the lungs. In emphysema, the limitation of air flow is the result of disease changes in the lung tissue, affecting the bronchioles (the smallest air passages) and the walls of the alveoli (the tiny air sacs of the lung). Eventually, many of the air sacs are destroyed, and the lungs become much less able to bring in oxygen and remove carbon dioxide. As a result, the heart has to work harder to deliver oxygen to all organs of the body.

In chronic bronchitis, the bronchial tubes in the lungs become inflamed, thickening the walls of the bronchi, and the production of mucus increases. The result is a narrowing of the air passages. Smoking is more dangerous than any form of air pollution, at least for most Americans, but exposure to both air pollution and cigarettes is particularly harmful.

Healthy nonsmoker's lung (left) and smoker's lung (right). Healthy lungs are pink, with a smooth but porous texture. Smoker's lungs show obvious signs of impairment—bronchial tubes are inflamed, air passages are constricted, and tar coats the bronchial tubes.

© Arthur Glauberman/PhotoResearchers, Inc.

Strategies for Prevention ▪ Why Not to Light Up

Before you start smoking—before you ever face the challenge of quitting—think of what you have to gain by not smoking:

▪ A significantly reduced risk of cancer of the lungs, larynx, mouth, esophagus, pancreas, and bladder.

▪ Half the risk of heart disease that smokers face.

▪ A lower risk of stroke, chronic obstructive lung disease (COLD), influenza, ulcers, and pneumonia.

▪ A lower risk of having a low-birthweight baby and of harming your child's long-term physical and intellectual development.

▪ A longer lifespan.

▪ Potential savings of tens of thousands of dollars that you would otherwise spend on tobacco products and medical care.

OTHER SMOKING-RELATED PROBLEMS

Smokers are more likely than nonsmokers to develop gum disease, and they lose significantly more teeth. Even those who quit have worse gum problems than people who never smoked at all. Smoking may also contribute to the loss of teeth and teeth supporting bone, even in individuals with good oral hygiene.

Cigarette smoking is associated with stomach and duodenal ulcers; mouth, throat, and other types of cancer; and cirrhosis of the liver. Smoking may worsen the symptoms or complications of allergies, diabetes, hypertension, peptic ulcers, and disorders of the lungs or blood vessels. Some men who smoke ten cigarettes or more a day may experience erectile dysfunction.[25] Cigarette smokers also tend to miss work one-third more often than nonsmokers, primarily because of respiratory illnesses. In addition, each year cigarette-ignited fires claim thousands of lives.

Smoking is an independent risk factor for high-frequency hearing loss and also adds to the danger of hearing loss for those exposed to noise (Chapter 20). Cigarette smoking also may increase the likelihood of anxiety, panic attacks, and social phobias.

SMOKING AND MEDICATION

Smokers use more medications—aspirin, painkillers, sleeping pills, tranquilizers, antihistamines, cough medicines, stomach medicines, laxatives, diuretics, and antibiotics—than nonsmokers do. According to the American Pharmaceutical Association, nicotine and other tobacco ingredients speed up the process by which the body uses and eliminates drugs, so they may not be able to do what they're intended to do. As a result, smokers may have to take a medication more frequently than do nonsmokers. If you smoke, let your physician know so that he or she can adjust any prescriptions, if necessary.

OTHER FORMS OF TOBACCO

Some 10.7 million Americans smoke cigars; 7.6 million use smokeless tobacco, and 2.1 million smoke pipes. Ingesting tobacco may be less deadly than smoking cigarettes, but it is dangerous. Smoking cigars, clove cigarettes, and pipes and chewing or sucking on smokeless tobacco all put the user at risk of cancer of the lip, tongue, mouth, and throat, as well as other diseases and ailments.

CIGARS

Cigar use has declined in the last few years. However, after cigarettes, cigars are the tobacco product most widely used by college students.

Cigar smoking is as dangerous as cigarette smoking even though cigar smokers do not inhale. Cigars can cause cancer of the lung and the digestive tract. The risk of death related to cigars approaches that of cigarettes, depending on the number of cigars smoked and the amount of cigar smoke inhaled (Figure 13-3). Cigar smoking can lead to nicotine addiction, even if the smoke is not inhaled. The nicotine in the smoke from a single cigar can vary from an amount roughly equivalent to that in a single cigarette to that in a pack or more of cigarettes.

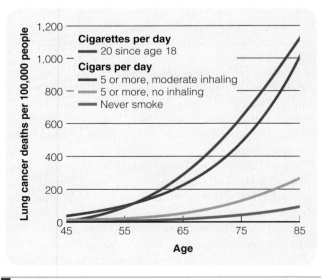

FIGURE 13-3 The Dangers of Cigarettes Versus Cigars

Sources: American Cancer Society, National Cancer Institute.

CLOVE CIGARETTES

Sweeteners have long been mixed with tobacco, and clove, a spice, is the latest ingredient to be added to the recipe for cigarettes. Clove cigarettes typically contain two-thirds tobacco and one-third clove. Consumers of these cigarettes are primarily teenagers and young adults.

Many users believe that clove cigarettes are safer because they contain less tobacco, but this isn't necessarily the case. The CDC reports that people who smoke clove cigarettes may be at risk of serious lung injury. Smoking clove cigarettes during a mild upper respiratory tract illness can lead to severe breathing difficulty. And clove cigarette smokers, like other cigarette smokers, can become addicted to the tobacco.

Clove cigarettes deliver twice as much nicotine, tar, and carbon monoxide as moderate-tar American brands. Eugenol, the active ingredient in cloves (which dentists have used as an anesthetic for years), deadens sensation in the throat, allowing smokers to inhale more deeply and hold smoke in their lungs for a longer time. Chemical relatives of eugenol can produce the kind of damage to cells that may lead to cancer.

(FAQ) WHAT ARE BIDIS?

Skinny, sweet-flavored cigarettes called **bidis** (pronounced "beedees") have become a smoking fad among teens and young adults. For centuries, bidis were popular in India, where they are known as the poor man's cigarette and sell for less than five cents a pack. They look strikingly like clove cigarettes or marijuana joints and are available in flavors like grape, strawberry, and mandarin orange. Bidis are legal for adults and even minors in some states and are sold on the Internet as well as in stores.

Although bidis contain less tobacco than regular cigarettes, their unprocessed tobacco is more potent. Smoke from bidis has about three times as much nicotine and carbon monoxide and five times as much tar as smoke from regular filtered cigarettes. Because bidis are wrapped in nonporous brownish leaves, they don't burn as easily as cigarettes, and smokers have to inhale harder and more often to keep them lit. In one study, smoking a single bidi required 28 puffs, compared to 9 puffs for cigarettes.

PIPES

Many cigarette smokers switch to pipes to reduce their risk of health problems. But former cigarette smokers may continue to inhale, even though pipe smoke is more irritating to the respiratory system than cigarette smoke. People who have smoked only pipes and who do not inhale are much less likely to develop lung and heart disease than cigarette smokers. However, they are as likely as cigarette smokers to develop—and die of—cancer of the mouth, larynx, throat, and esophagus.

SMOKELESS TOBACCO

The consumption of smokeless tobacco products (sometimes called "spit") is rising, particularly among young males. These substances include snuff, finely ground tobacco that can be sniffed or placed inside the cheek and sucked, and chewing tobacco, tobacco leaves mixed with flavoring agents such as molasses. With both, nicotine is absorbed through the mucous membranes of the nose or mouth.

Smokeless tobacco causes a user's heart rate, blood pressure, and epinephrine (adrenaline) levels to jump.[26] In addition, it can cause cancer and noncancerous oral conditions and lead to nicotine addiction and dependence. Smokeless tobacco users are more likely than nonusers to become cigarette smokers.

Powerful carcinogens in smokeless tobacco include nitrosamines, polycyclic aromatic hydrocarbons, and radiation-emitting polonium. Its use can lead to the development of

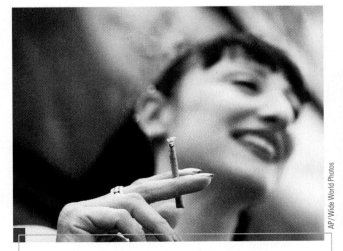

The smoke produced by bidis—skinny, flavored cigarettes—can contain higher concentrations of toxic chemicals than the smoke from regular cigarettes.

Chewing smokeless tobacco can damage the tissues of the mouth and lead to cancer of the lip, pharynx, larynx, esophagus, kidney, pancreas, and bladder.

Savvy Consumer ▓ Are "Safer" Cigarettes Really Safe?

Tobacco companies are producing "lower-risk" cigarettes that they claim reduce secondhand smoke and have fewer carcinogens and less nicotine. For example, Eclipse cigarettes heat rather than burn tobacco inside a cigarette-like tube to reduce the release of carbon monoxide, a big contributor to heart disease. Users of another product, Accord, insert special cigarettes into a small electronic device about the size of a pager that ignites the cigarette when the smoker puffs and sucks up secondhand smoke. Other brands claim to use genetic engineering or a chemical process to remove major carcinogens.

Are these products truly safer? The answer is no. So-called safer cigarettes may actually lead to increased addiction. In one

experiment, smokers puffed on their own brand and then on a so-called safer cigarette brand called Advance. While Advance cigarettes supposedly contain less of a type of cancer-causing substance called nitrosamines, they delivered 25 percent more nicotine, the addictive substance in cigarettes, into the blood than the smokers' own brands.

Accord cigarettes deliver less nicotine and boost smokers' heart rates and carbon monoxide levels less than traditional cigarettes. However, they aren't as satisfying to smokers, who may smoke more of them to reduce withdrawal symptoms such as anxiety, restlessness, and irritability.

Eclipse cigarettes suppress withdrawal symptoms about as well as conventional cigarettes. However, they deliver about 30 percent more carbon monoxide, which has been linked to heart disease, than regular cigarettes.

The bottom line: "Safer" cigarettes may reduce some toxins that are associated with smoking-related diseases, but they may increase levels of other dangerous substances and boost the likelihood of addiction. Don't think that you're protecting your health by switching to a "safe" cigarette. There is no such thing. The only proven way to avoid smoking-related risks of disease and death is to stop smoking.

---

white patches on the mucous membranes of the mouth, particularly on the site where the tobacco is placed. Most lesions of the mouth lining that result from the use of smokeless tobacco dissipate six weeks after the use of the tobacco products is stopped, according to a U.S. Air Force study. However, when first found, about 5 percent of these lesions are cancerous or exhibit changes that progress to cancer within ten years if not properly treated. Cancers of the lip, pharynx, larynx, and esophagus have all been linked to smokeless tobacco.

More than 7 million people, many of them young, use snuff and chewing tobacco. The lowest percentage of users is in the northeast, the highest in the south-central region.

Nicotine replacement with gum or patches (discussed on page 380) decreases cravings for smokeless tobacco and helps with short-term abstinence. However, it does not improve long-term abstinence. Behavioral approaches are more effective for long-term quitting.[27]

Your Life Coach

Quitting

Smoking is a remarkably difficult habit to kick. However, half of all Americans who ever smoked have quit.[28] Half of current smokers try to quit each year, but only 7 percent succeed on their first attempt.[29]

 About half of whites who have smoked were able to kick the habit, compared with 45 percent of Asian Americans, 43 percent of Hispanics, and 37 percent of African Americans. Men and women with college and graduate degrees were much more likely to quit successfully than high school dropouts.[30]

 Compared with men, women seem to have a higher behavioral dependence on cigarettes. For them, wearing a nicotine patch or chewing nicotine gum does not substitute for the "hand-to-mouth" behaviors associated with smoking, such as lighting a cigarette, inhaling, and handling the cigarette. Some investigators have found that women are more likely to quit successfully when they receive a combination of nicotine replacement and the use of a device like a nicotine inhaler to substitute for smoking behaviors.

 Although a large proportion of students have made an attempt to quit, only a minority succeed.

Among current smokers, 59 percent report ever making an attempt to quit. Among those who ever smoked daily, 82 percent have tried to quit, while 75 percent are still smokers. The barriers to quitting in college include fears of weight gain, inability to manage stress without nicotine, and denial of nicotine addition.[31]

One campus-based program that employed peer facilitators to help smokers quit and avoid relapse reported a success rate of 88 percent. Being "in the group" was the single most powerful contributor to quitting, and participants said their sense of connectedness helped them quit and stay smoke-free.[32]

Nicotine withdrawal symptoms can behave like characters in a bad horror flick: Just when you think you've killed them, they're back with a vengeance. In recent studies, some people who tried to quit smoking reported a small improvement in withdrawal symptoms over two weeks, but then their symptoms leveled off and persisted. Others found that their symptoms intensified rather than lessened over time. For reasons scientists cannot yet explain, former smokers who start smoking again put their lungs at even greater jeopardy than smokers who never quit.

FIGURE 13-4   How to Quit

Combining one of the four nicotine replacement therapies (or bupropion/Zyban) with counseling is the most effective strategy to quit smoking.

Once a former smoker takes a single puff, the odds of a relapse are 80 to 85 percent. Smokers are most likely to quit in the third, fourth, or fifth attempt. But thanks to new products and programs, it may be easier now than ever before to become an ex-smoker.

QUITTING ON YOUR OWN

More than 90 percent of former smokers quit on their own—by throwing away all their cigarettes, by gradually cutting down, or by first switching to a less potent brand. One characteristic of successful quitters is that they see themselves as active participants in health maintenance and take personal responsibility for their own health. Often they experiment with a variety of strategies, such as learning relaxation techniques. In women, exercise has proved especially effective for quitting and avoiding weight gain. Making a home a smoke-free zone also increases a smoker's likelihood of successfully quitting.

STOP-SMOKING GROUPS

Joining a support group doubles your chances of quitting for good. The American Cancer Society's FreshStart program runs about 1,500 stop-smoking clinics, each with about 8 to 18 members meeting for eight two-hour sessions over four weeks. Instructors explain the risks of smoking, encourage individuals to think about why they smoke, and suggest ways of unlearning their smoking habit. A quitting day is set for the third or fourth session.

The American Lung Association's Freedom from Smoking program consists of eight one- to two-hour sessions over seven weeks. The approach is similar to the American Cancer Society's, but smokers keep diaries and team up with buddies. Ex-smokers serve as advisers on quitting day. Both groups estimate that 27 or 28 percent of their participants successfully stop smoking.

Stop-smoking classes are also available through science departments and student health services on many college campuses, as well as through community public health departments. The Seventh-Day Adventists sponsor a four-week Breathe Free Plan, in which smokers commit themselves to clean living (no smoking, alcohol, tea, or coffee, along with a balanced diet and regular exercise).

Many businesses sponsor smoking-cessation programs for employees, which generally follow the approaches of professional groups. Motivation may be even higher in these programs than in programs outside the workplace because some companies offer attractive incentives to participants, such as lower rates on their health insurance.

Some smoking-cessation programs rely primarily on **aversion therapy,** which provides a negative experience every time a smoker has a cigarette. This may involve taking drugs that make tobacco smoke taste unpleasant, undergoing electric shocks, having smoke blown at you, or rapid smoking (the inhaling of smoke every six seconds until you're dizzy or nauseated).

Nicotine Anonymous, a nonprofit organization based on the 12 steps to recovery developed by Alcoholics Anonymous (see Chapter 12), acknowledges the power of nicotine and provides support to help smokers, chewers, and dippers live free of nicotine. New members are encouraged to abstain from using nicotine "one day at a time" and to attend meetings regularly. In addition to local meetings, NicA offers online support and networking, which puts people in touch with others in their region who share their desire to quit using nicotine.

Telephone-counseling "quit lines," which advise smokers on how to restructure their lives and deal with urges, are helpful because people can get counseling without leaving their homes. The quality of online smoking cessation websites is not consistent, and information is often hard to find, incomplete, or not based on research.[33]

NICOTINE REPLACEMENT THERAPY (NRT)

This approach uses a variety of products that supply low doses of nicotine in a way that allows smokers to taper off gradually over a period of months. Nicotine replacement therapies include nonprescription products (nicotine gum and nicotine patches) and prescription products (nicotine nasal spray and nicotine inhaler). The nasal spray, dispensed from a pump bottle, delivers nicotine to the nasal membranes and reaches the bloodstream faster than any other nicotine replacement therapy product. The inhaler delivers nicotine into the mouth and enters the bloodstream much more slowly than the nicotine in cigarettes.

Smokers who use NRT are 1.5 to 2 times more likely to quit.[34] Because nicotine is a powerful, addictive substance, using nicotine replacements for a prolonged period is not advised. Pregnant women and individuals with heart disease shouldn't use them.

The most effective approaches combine medication—nicotine patches or Zyban, for instance—with psychological intervention. Each doubles a person's chance of quitting successfully.[35]

 Nicotine replacement therapy, which supplies ex-smokers with lower levels of nicotine in the form of a gum or patch, has proved more beneficial for men than women—particularly with higher doses of nicotine. Men who receive more nicotine achieve a higher quit rate than men getting lower doses. For women, the nicotine "dose" does not have an impact on successful quitting. They are no more likely to stop smoking with high doses than with lower ones, indicating that they may be less dependent on nicotine than men.

Nicotine Gum

Nicotine gum, sold as Nicorette, contains a nicotine resin that's gradually released as the gum is chewed. Absorbed through the mucous membrane of the mouth, the nicotine doesn't produce the same rush as a deeply inhaled drag on a cigarette. However, the gum maintains enough nicotine in the blood to diminish withdrawal symptoms. A month's supply of Nicorette costs roughly $45.

Although this gum is lightly spiced to mask nicotine's bitterness, many users say that it takes several days to become accustomed to its unusual taste. Its side effects include mild indigestion, sore jaws, nausea, heartburn, and stomachache. Also, because Nicorette is heavier than regular chewing gum, it may loosen fillings or cause problems with dentures. Drinking coffee or other beverages may block absorption of the nicotine in the gum; individuals trying to quit smoking shouldn't ingest any substance immediately before or while chewing nicotine gum. You have to chew nicotine gum until you get a tingling sensation, and then place it between the cheek and gum.

Most people use nicotine gum as a temporary crutch and gradually taper off until they can stop chewing it relatively painlessly. However, 5 to 10 percent of users transfer their dependence from cigarettes to the

Nicorette gum, when chewed, gradually releases a nicotine resin and helps some smokers break their habit. Nicorette is available without a prescription.

gum. When they stop using Nicorette, they experience withdrawal symptoms, although the symptoms tend to be milder than those prompted by quitting cigarettes. Intensive counseling to teach smokers coping methods can greatly increase success rates.

Nicotine Patches

Nicotine transdermal delivery system products, or patches, provide nicotine, their only active ingredient, via a patch attached to the skin by an adhesive. Like nicotine gum, the nicotine patch minimizes withdrawal symptoms, such as intense craving for cigarettes. Nicotine patches help nearly 20 percent of smokers quit entirely after six weeks, compared with 7 percent on a placebo patch. Some insurance programs pay for patch therapy. Nicotine patches, which cost between $3.25 and $4 each, are replaced daily during therapy programs that run between 6 and 16 weeks. There is no evidence that continuing their use for more than 8 weeks provides added benefit.

Some patches deliver nicotine around the clock and others for just 16 hours (during waking hours). Those most likely to benefit from nicotine patch therapy are people who smoke more than a pack a day, are highly motivated to quit, and participate in counseling programs. While using the patch, 37 to 77 percent of people are able to abstain from smoking. When combined with counseling, the patch can be about twice as effective as a placebo, enabling 26 percent of smokers to abstain for six months.

Patch wearers who smoke or use more than one patch at a time can experience a nicotine overdose; some users have even suffered heart attacks. Occasional side effects include redness, itching, or swelling at the site of the patch application; insomnia; dry mouth; and nervousness.

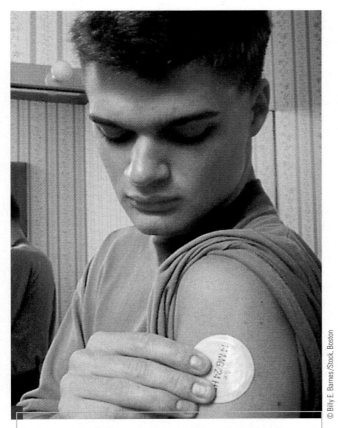

A nicotine patch releases nicotine transdermally (through the skin) in measured amounts, which are gradually decreased over time.

© Billy E. Barnes/Stock, Boston

Nicotrol Inhaler

Available only by prescription, the Nicotrol Inhaler consists of a mouthpiece and a cartridge containing a nicotine-impregnated plug. The smoker inhales through the mouthpiece, using either shallow or deep puffs. The inhaled air becomes saturated with nicotine, which is absorbed mainly through the tissues of the mouth. The Inhaler releases less nicotine per puff than a cigarette and does not contain a cigarette's harmful tars, carbon monoxide, and smoke. Treatment is recommended for three months with a gradual reduction over the next six to twelve weeks. Total treatment should not exceed six months.[36]

BUPROPION (ZYBAN)

An alternative to the patch is **bupropion,** a drug initially developed to treat depression, that is marketed in a slow-release form for nicotine addiction as Zyban. In studies that have combined Zyban with nicotine replacement and counseling, 40 to 60 percent of those treated have remained smoke-free for at least a year after completing the program. This success rate is much higher than the 10 to 26 percent reported among smokers who try to quit by using nicotine replacement alone. The combination

of Zyban and nicotine replacement also prevented the initial weight gain that often accompanies quitting. Other medications used to treat nicotine addiction are clonidine, mecamylamine, and buspirone.

OTHER WAYS TO QUIT

Hypnosis may help some people quit smoking. Hypnotherapists use their techniques to create an atmosphere of strict attention and give smokers in a mild trance positive suggestions for breaking their cigarette habit.

Acupuncture, in which a circular needle or staple is inserted in the flap in front of the opening to the ear, has also had some success. When smokers feel withdrawal symptoms, they gently move the needle or staple, which may increase the production of calming chemicals in the brain.

Since 1976, a November day has been set aside in the United States for the annual Great American Smoke-Out, an idea promoted by the American Cancer Society to encourage smokers to give up cigarettes for 24 hours. As many as 36 percent of American smokers have given up cigarettes on Smoke-Out Day; about 5 to 6 percent have quit permanently; 15 percent reduced smoking for extended periods. In addition, the World Health Organization has established World No-Tobacco Days in May to call on nations to urge tobacco users to abstain for at least one day and perhaps quit for good.

FAQ DOES QUITTING ELIMINATE THE RISKS ASSOCIATED WITH SMOKING?

Not smoking another cigarette is a gift to your body and your life. It is not a guarantee that there will be no consequences of the cigarettes you've already smoked.

Within a year of quitting, an ex-smoker's risk of heart disease drops to half that of active smokers. After 15 years, it approaches that of people who've never smoked. This is great news because the risk of dying prematurely from heart disease is far greater than that of dying from cancer.

The risk of lung cancer from smoking fades more slowly, perhaps because of permanent DNA damage to lung cells. Even 10 to 15 years after quitting, an ex-smoker is several times more likely to die of lung cancer than someone who has never smoked. Former smokers are also more vulnerable to the effects of secondhand smoke in the workplace, even if they haven't lit up for the last ten years.[37]

Does the lung cancer risk ever go away? That may depend partly on how old you are when you quit. Women who quit before age 30 are no more likely to die from lung cancer than those who never smoked. However, a study of American veterans started in the 1950s showed that, even 40 years later, former smokers had a

50 percent greater chance of dying from lung cancer than lifetime nonsmokers.

While quitting sooner is better than later, later is better than never. Even smokers who quit in their sixties significantly reduce their lung cancer risk—and add several years to their life expectancy.

ENVIRONMENTAL TOBACCO SMOKE

Maybe you don't smoke—never have, never will. That doesn't mean you don't have to worry about the dangers of smoking, especially if you live or work with people who smoke. **Environmental tobacco smoke,** or secondhand cigarette smoke, the most hazardous form of indoor air pollution, ranks behind cigarette smoking and alcohol as the third-leading preventable cause of death.

On average, a smoker inhales what is known as **mainstream smoke** eight or nine times with each cigarette, for a total of about 24 seconds. However, the cigarette burns for about 12 minutes, and everyone in the room (including the smoker) breathes in what is known as **sidestream smoke.**

According to the American Lung Association, incomplete combustion from the lower temperatures of a smoldering cigarette makes sidestream smoke dirtier and chemically different from mainstream smoke. It has twice as much tar and nicotine, five times as much carbon monoxide, and 50 times as much ammonia. And because the particles in sidestream smoke are small, this mixture of irritating gases and carcinogenic tar reaches deeper into the lungs. If you're a nonsmoker sitting next to someone smoking seven cigarettes an hour, even in a ventilated room, you'll take in almost twice the maximum amount of carbon monoxide set for air pollution in industry—and it will take hours for the carbon monoxide to leave your body.

Secondhand smoke is the most common and hazardous form of indoor air pollution.

THE RISKS OF SECONDHAND SMOKE

Even a little secondhand smoke is dangerous. According to the CDC, every year environmental tobacco smoke causes about 35,000 deaths from heart disease and 3,000 deaths from lung cancer.[38] As a cancer-causing agent, secondhand smoke may be twice as dangerous as radon gas and more than a hundred times more hazardous than outdoor pollutants regulated by federal law. Secondhand smoke also increases the sick leave rates among employees.

Numerous epidemiological and autopsy studies have linked environmental tobacco smoke with lung cancer and other disorders. The nonsmoking spouses of smokers, for instance, are 30 percent more likely to die of heart disease than other nonsmokers.

Prenatal exposure to tobacco can have significant effects that may extend from infancy into adulthood. Smoking during pregnancy affects a child's growth, cognitive development, and behavior both before and after birth. Birthweight decreases in direct proportion to the number of cigarettes smoked. The babies of teenage mothers who smoke have lower birthweight, length, head circumference, and chest circumference. As they grow, children of smokers tend to be shorter and weigh less than children of nonsmokers.

A mother's smoking during pregnancy may have cognitive and behavioral effects as well. These include abnormal neurological responses, such as more tremors and startles. Among older children, researchers have found deficits in language and reading abilities and poorer visual perception. Youngsters whose mothers smoked during pregnancy also tend to have problems with hyperactivity, inattention, and impulsivity. Some of these behavior problems persist through the teenage years and even into adulthood. At ages 16 to 18, children exposed to prenatal smoking have higher rates of conduct disorder, substance use, and depression than others.

Even if their mothers don't smoke, children exposed to secondhand smoke before birth also are likely to weigh less and to perform more poorly on tests of speech, language skills, intelligence, and visual-spatial abilities and to develop behavior problems. These youngsters perform at a level between that of children of active smokers and children of nonsmokers.

Exposure to smoke after birth increases the risk of sudden infant death syndrome (SIDS) and is associated with lower IQ scores and deficits in cognitive development.

Children who breathe environmental tobacco smoke suffer from more asthma, wheezing, and bronchitis than children in smoke-free homes. They also face increased risk of lung cancer, heart disease, and stroke.

 The negative effects of early exposure to environmental tobacco smoke persist even after youngsters leave home. In recent research at Ohio State University, college students who grew up in a smoking household had higher resting heart rates and blood pressure at rest and during psychological stress than those who grew up in smoke-free homes. Teen exposure to cigarette smoke increases the risk of metabolic syndrome (discussed in Chapter 15).[39]

Felicia Martinez / PhotoEdit

THE POLITICS OF TOBACCO

More than three decades after U.S. government health authorities began to warn of the dangers of cigarette smoking, tobacco remains a politically hot topic. However, a majority of people support tobacco control strategies, including creation of smoke-free environments, an increase in cigarette excise taxes, more funds to prevent people from smoking and to help smokers quit, and restriction of youth access to tobacco.

"BIG TOBACCO"

After many years of difficult negotiations, the tobacco industry and attorneys general from nearly 40 states reached a historic settlement. Major tobacco companies have agreed to pay more than $200 billion to settle smoking-related lawsuits filed by 46 states, to finance antismoking campaigns, to restrict marketing, to permit federal regulation of tobacco, and to pay fines if tobacco use by minors does not decline.

The funds from the U.S. state tobacco settlement, won in 1998, were supposed to support antismoking programs, but the majority of that funding is not being spent on anything related to smoking. Most of the money has gone to make up for budget shortfalls.[40]

Increasing the price of cigarettes by 10 percent reduces the number of smokers by about 2 percent. Many states have raised taxes on cigarettes; some now charge more than a dollar a pack. Although personal health warnings are not particularly effective, new in-your-face warning labels are grabbing smokers' attention; for example, extra-large Canadian cigarette labels show rotting lungs and decaying teeth. According to a Canadian Cancer Society study, the gory warnings have increased smokers' motivation to quit.

THE FIGHT FOR CLEAN AIR

Nonsmokers, realizing that their health is being jeopardized by environmental tobacco smoke, have increasingly turned to legislative and administrative measures to clear the air and protect their rights (Figure 13-5). Most states now have some restrictions on smoking in bars, restaurants, and work-

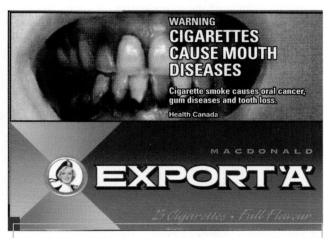

Graphic warning labels on cigarette packages in Canada have discouraged smoking.

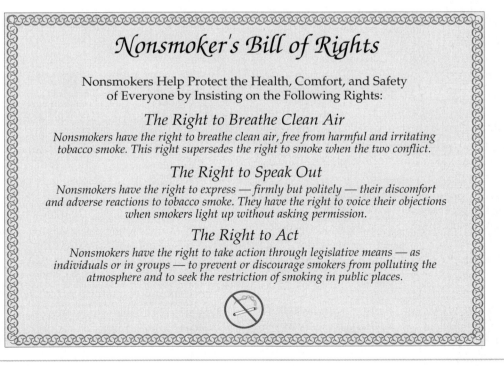

Nonsmoker's Bill of Rights

Nonsmokers Help Protect the Health, Comfort, and Safety of Everyone by Insisting on the Following Rights:

The Right to Breathe Clean Air

Nonsmokers have the right to breathe clean air, free from harmful and irritating tobacco smoke. This right supersedes the right to smoke when the two conflict.

The Right to Speak Out

Nonsmokers have the right to express — firmly but politely — their discomfort and adverse reactions to tobacco smoke. They have the right to voice their objections when smokers light up without asking permission.

The Right to Act

Nonsmokers have the right to take action through legislative means — as individuals or in groups — to prevent or discourage smokers from polluting the atmosphere and to seek the restriction of smoking in public places.

FIGURE 13-5   NONSMOKER'S BILL OF RIGHTS

Strategies for Prevention ⠿ Clearing the Air

⠿ Let people know your feelings in advance by putting up "No Smoking" signs in your office, home, or car. If you're in a car and someone pulls out a cigarette, ask politely if the smoker can hold off until you reach your destination or stop for a break.

⠿ If you're about to participate in a long meeting or class, find out if there are smoking restrictions. If there are, ask that they be enforced. If not, ask for a voluntary moratorium on smoking.

⠿ At restaurants, always ask for a table in the nonsmoking section or, if there is

none, one in a well-ventilated part of the restaurant.

⠿ If someone's smoke is bothering you, speak up. Be polite, not pushy. Say something like, "Excuse me, but smoke bothers me."

---

places.[41] Nationally, the airlines have banned smoking on domestic flights. Many institutions, including medical centers and some universities, no longer allow smoking on their premises.

> State and federal civil rights laws prevent discrimination based on age, race, color, gender, marital status, national origin, weight, height, and religion. Yet smokers argue that they are discriminated against by no-smoking bans in public and private places. Are smokers denied the right to light up victims of discrimination? Or is their habit a threat to public health that should be controlled? **You decide.**

Learn It / Live It

Becoming Smoke-Free

If you smoke—even just a few cigarettes a few times a week—you are at risk of nicotine addiction. Here is how to get back into control:

⠿ **Use delaying tactics.** Have your first cigarette of the day 15 minutes later than usual, then 15 minutes later than that the next day, and so on.

⠿ **Distract yourself.** When you feel a craving for a cigarette, talk to someone, drink a glass of water, or get up and move around.

⠿ **Establish nonsmoking hours.** Instead of lighting up at the end of a meal, for instance, get up immediately, brush your teeth, wash your hands, or take a walk.

⠿ **Never smoke two packs of the same brand in a row.** Buy cigarettes only by the pack, not by the carton.

⠿ **Make it harder to get to your cigarettes.** Lock them in a drawer, wrap them in paper, or leave them in your coat or car.

⠿ **Change the way you smoke.** Smoke with the hand you don't usually use. Smoke only half of each cigarette.

⠿ **Stop completely for just one day at a time.** Promise yourself 24 hours of freedom from cigarettes; when the day's over, make the same commitment for one more day. At the end of any 24-hour period, you can go back to smoking and not feel guilty.

⠿ **Spend more time in places where you can't smoke.** Take up bike-riding or swimming. Shower often. Go to movies or other places where smoking isn't allowed.

⠿ **Go cold turkey.** If you're a heavily addicted smoker, try a decisive and complete break. Smokers who quit completely are less likely to light up again than those who gradually decrease their daily cigarette consumption, switch to low-tar and low-nicotine brands, or use special filters and holders.

Making This Chapter Work for You

Review Questions

1. Which of the following statements about smoking is *false?*
   a. Smoking behavior may have a genetic component.
   b. People who graduate college are less likely to smoke than those who complete only high school.
   c. Most regular smokers enjoy smoking.
   d. Nicotine addiction doesn't take hold until six months after a person starts smoking.

2. Tobacco use on college campuses
   a. is higher among male athletes.
   b. continues to increase despite no-smoking policies by all schools.
   c. is more prevalent among those students who also use marijuana and alcohol.
   d. is most often in the form of smokeless tobacco.

3. Which of the following statements about smoking and race is true?
   a. Hispanic men are less likely to smoke than Hispanic women.
   b. Native Americans smoke less than African Americans and Asian Americans.

c. Smoking is culturally unacceptable among Southeast Asian men.

d. Caucasian college students smoke more than African-American and Asian-American students.

4. Women smokers

a. are more likely to die from breast cancer than lung cancer.

b. are less fertile than nonsmokers.

c. are less likely to develop osteoporosis.

d. bear children with fewer birth defects.

5. Which of the following statements about tobacco and its components is true?

a. Nicotine affects the central nervous system in eight seconds.

b. Tobacco stimulates the kidneys to form urine.

c. Carbon monoxide contained in tobacco smoke is an addictive substance.

d. The tar in burning tobacco impairs oxygen transport in the body.

6. Cigarette smokers

a. are more likely to die of lung cancer than heart disease.

b. usually develop lung problems after years of tobacco use.

c. have two to three times the risk of suffering a stroke than nonsmokers.

d. may completely reverse the damage to their blood vessels if they quit smoking.

7. Which of the following statements is *false?*

a. Using chewing tobacco can lead to lesions on the mucous membranes of the mouth.

b. Bidis come in several flavors.

c. The active ingredient in cloves lowers sensation in the throat, so clove-cigarette smokers inhale more deeply.

d. Smoking cigars is safe if you don't inhale.

8. Quitting smoking

a. usually results in minor withdrawal symptoms.

b. will do little to reverse the damage to the lungs and other parts of the body.

c. can be aided by using nicotine replacement products.

d. is best done by cutting down on the number of cigarettes you smoke over a period of months.

9. Ways to help yourself quit include all of the following *except*

a. join a support group.

b. make your home a smoke-free zone.

c. try acupuncture.

d. switch to bidis.

10. Secondhand tobacco smoke is

a. the smoke inhaled by a smoker.

b. more hazardous than outdoor pollution as a cancer-causing agent.

c. less hazardous than mainstream smoke.

d. less likely to cause serious health problems in children than in adults.

Answers to these questions can be found on page 587.

Critical Thinking

1. Has smoking become unpopular among your friends or family? What social activities continue to be associated with smoking? Can you think of any situation in which smoking might be frowned upon?

2. How would you motivate someone you care about to stop smoking? What reasons would you give for them to stop? Describe your strategy.

3. According to the chapter, environmental tobacco smoke is even more dangerous than mainstream smoke. If you're a nonsmoker, how would you react to someone who's smoking in the same room you occupy? Define the rights of smokers and nonsmokers.

Media Menu

Health Now™

Throughout the chapter, this icon introduces a list of resources on the Health-Now website at **http://healthnow.brookscole.com/ith** that will:

• Help you evaluate your knowledge of the material.

• Allow you to take an exam-prep quiz.

• Provide a Personalized Learning Plan targeting resources that address areas you should study.

• Coach you through identifying target goals for behavior change and creating and monitoring your personal change plan throughout the semester.

INTERNET CONNECTIONS

Tobacco Information and Prevention Source (TIPS)

www.cdc.gov/tobacco

This comprehensive feature on the Centers for Disease Control and Prevention (CDC) website provides educational information, research, a report from the U.S. Surgeon General, tips on how to quit, and much more.

Joe Chemo—an antismoking site

www.joechemo.org

Based on the character Joe Chemo, an antismoking parody of Joe Camel, this site is highly interactive and allows visitors to test their "Tobacco IQ," get a personalized "Smoke-o-Scope," and send free Joe Chemo e-cards. There is also extensive information for teachers, antismoking activists, health-care providers, journalists, and smokers who wish to quit.

Tobacco Facts

www.tobaccofacts.org

This excellent site provides access to many facts and resources regarding tobacco use.

Tobacco Control Resource Center and Tobacco Products Liability Project (TPLP)

www.tobacco.neu.edu

This site provides current information on tobacco-related litigation and legislation.

Self Survey ▪ Are You Addicted to Nicotine?

Answer the following questions as honestly as you can by placing a check mark in the appropriate column:

	Yes	No
1. Do you smoke every day?	___	___
2. Do you smoke because of shyness and to build up self-confidence?	___	___
3. Do you smoke to escape from boredom and worries or while under pressure?	___	___
4. Have you ever burned a hole in your clothes, carpet, furniture, or car with a cigarette?	___	___
5. Have you ever had to go to the store late at night or at another inconvenient time because you were out of cigarettes?	___	___
6. Do you feel defensive or angry when people tell you that your smoke is bothering them?	___	___
7. Has a doctor or dentist ever suggested that you stop smoking?	___	___
8. Have you ever promised someone that you would stop smoking, then broken your promise?	___	___
9. Have you ever felt physical or emotional discomfort when trying to quit?	___	___
10. Have you ever successfully stopped smoking for a period of time, only to start again?	___	___
11. Do you buy extra supplies of tobacco to make sure you won't run out?	___	___
12. Do you find it difficult to imagine life without smoking?	___	___
13. Do you choose only those activities and entertainments during which you can smoke?	___	___
14. Do you prefer, seek out, or feel more comfortable in the company of smokers?	___	___
15. Do you inwardly despise or feel ashamed of yourself because of your smoking?	___	___
16. Do you ever find yourself lighting up without having consciously decided to?	___	___
17. Has your smoking ever caused trouble at home or in a relationship?	___	___
18. Do you ever tell yourself that you can stop smoking whenever you want to?	___	___
19. Have you ever felt that your life would be better if you didn't smoke?	___	___
20. Do you continue to smoke even though you are aware of the health hazards posed by smoking?	___	___

If you answered Yes to one or two of these questions, there's a chance that you are addicted or are becoming addicted to nicotine. If you answered Yes to three or more of these questions, you are probably already addicted to nicotine.

Source: Nicotine Anonymous World Services, San Francisco.

InfoTrac College Edition Activities Log on, insert **tobacco use** into the Keyword search box, and limit your search to the past year. When you get the results, Mark articles to review, then Select one to read. Summarize three or four key points from the article.

You can find additional readings related to personal health with InfoTrac College Edition, an online library of more than 900 journals and publications. Follow the instructions for accessing InfoTrac College Edition that were packaged with your textbook; then search for articles using a keyword search.

For additional links, resources, and suggested readings on the InfoTrac College Edition, visit our Health and Wellness Resource Center at **http://health .wadsworth.com.**

Key Terms

The terms listed are used on the page indicated. Definitions of the terms are in the Glossary at the end of this book.

aversion therapy 379
bidis 377
bupropion 381
carbon monoxide 374
environmental tobacco smoke 382
mainstream smoke 382
nicotine 373
sidestream smoke 382
tar 373

YOUR ACTION PLAN FOR KICKING THE HABIT

Here's a six-point program to help you or someone you love quit smoking. (*Caution:* Don't undertake the quit-smoking program until you have a two- to four-week period of relatively unstressful work and study schedules or social commitments.)

1. *Identify your smoking habits.* Keep a daily diary (a piece of paper wrapped around your cigarette pack with a rubber band will do) and record the time you smoke, the activity associated with smoking (after breakfast, in the car), and your urge for a cigarette (desperate, pleasant, or automatic). For the first week or two, don't bother trying to cut down; just use the diary to learn the conditions under which you smoke.

2. *Get support.* It can be tough to go it alone. Phone your local chapter of the American Cancer Society or Nicotine Anonymous or otherwise get the names of some ex-smokers who can give you support.

3. *Begin by tapering off.* For a period of one to four weeks, aim at cutting down to, say, 12 or 15 cigarettes a day; or change to a lower-nicotine brand and concentrate on not increasing the number of cigarettes you smoke. As indicated by your diary, begin by cutting out those cigarettes you smoke automatically. In addition, restrict the times you allow yourself to smoke. Throughout this period, stay in touch, once a day or every few days, with your ex-smoker friend(s) to discuss your problems.

4. *Set a quit date.* At some point during the tapering-off period, announce to everyone—friends, family, and ex-smokers—when you're going to quit. Do it with flair. Announce it to coincide with a significant date, such as your birthday or anniversary.

5. *Stop.* A week before Q-day, smoke only five cigarettes a day. Begin late in the day, say after 4:00 P.M. Smoke the first two cigarettes in close succession. Then, in the evening, smoke the last three, also in close succession, about 15 minutes apart. Focus on the negative aspects of cigarettes, such as the rawness in your throat and lungs. After seven days, quit and give yourself a big reward on that day, such as a movie or a fantastic meal or new clothes.

6. *Follow up.* Stay in touch with your ex-smoker friend(s) during the following two weeks, particularly if anything stressful or tense occurs that might trigger a return to smoking. Think of the person you're becoming—the very person cigarette ads would have you believe smoking makes you. Now that you're quitting smoking, you're becoming healthier, sexier, more sophisticated, more mature, and better looking—and you've earned it!

Sources: American Cancer Society, National Cancer Institute.

CASE IN POINT

Student: Kylie, 21

Goal: To quit smoking

Action Plan:

▌ Get her roommate's agreement to declare their dorm room a smoke-free zone

▌ Put off her first cigarette by half an hour every other day

▌ Start swimming at the campus pool every day so she avoids putting on weight and keeps busy with an activity absolutely incompatible with smoking

▌ Cut down on the number of puffs per cigarette so she smokes less and less of each one

▌ Talk to a health counselor about nicotine replacement therapy

Health ☺ Now ™   If you want to write your own goals for tobacco use, go to the **Wellness Journal** at HealthNow http://healthnow.brookscole.com/ith

Protecting Your Health

© M. Möllenberg/zefa/CORBIS

Every day you make choices that affect both the quantity and the quality of your life. The right choices aren't always easy to make or to sustain. The chapters in this section can help by providing information you can use in making and implementing healthful decisions. By understanding the risks to your health, you can prepare to overcome them—and not simply live life, but celebrate it every day.

14 Defending Yourself Against Infectious Diseases

There's something I have to tell you." Anise knew, just by the sound of her boyfriend's voice, that the "something" wasn't good news.

"My herpes is back."

Stunned, Anise tried to absorb all the information packed into this short sentence: She'd had no idea that the man she'd been sleeping with for several months had a sexually transmitted infection (STI). How did he get it? What else hadn't he told her about his past? What did he mean that it was "back"? Could she have caught it? And, finally, she asked the all-too-human question: How could this have happened to me?

By their very nature, infectious diseases take people by surprise. Throughout history, they have claimed more lives than any military conflict or natural disaster. Although modern medicine has won many victories against the agents of infection, we remain vulnerable to a host of infectious illnesses. Drug-resistant strains of tuberculosis and *Staphylococcus* bacteria challenge current therapies. New infectious diseases, such as SARS and West Nile Virus, are emerging and traveling around the world. Agents of infection also can be used as weapons of bioterrorism.

Some of today's most common and dangerous infectious illnesses spread primarily through sexual contact, and their incidence has skyrocketed. The federal government estimates that 65 million Americans have a sexually transmitted infection.[1] These diseases cannot be prevented in the laboratory. Only you, by your behavior, can prevent and control them.

This chapter is a lesson in self-defense against all forms of infection. The information it provides can help you boost your defenses, recognize and avoid enemies, protect yourself from sexually transmitted infections, and realize when to seek help.

(FAQ) **Frequently Asked Questions**

- **How do you catch an infection?** *p. 393*
- **Who's at highest risk of infectious diseases?** *p. 399*
- **Are college students at higher risk of colds and flu?** *p. 402*
- **What is SARS?** *p. 408*
- **How common are STIs on campus?** *p. 410*

After studying the material in this chapter, you should be able to:

- **Explain** how the different agents of infection spread disease.

- **Describe** how your body protects itself from infectious disease.

- **List** and **describe** some common infectious diseases.

- **Identify** the sexually transmitted infections and the symptoms and treatment for each.

- **List** the methods of STI transmission.

- **Define** HIV infection and **describe** its symptoms.

- **Explain** some practical methods for preventing HIV infection and other sexually transmitted infections.

UNDERSTANDING INFECTION

We live in a sea of microbes. Most of them don't threaten our health or survival; some, such as the bacteria that inhabit our intestines, are actually beneficial. Yet in the course of history, disease-causing microorganisms have claimed millions of lives. The twentieth century brought the conquest of infectious killers such as cholera and scarlet fever. Although modern science has won many victories against the agents of infection, infectious illnesses remain a serious health threat.

Infection is a complex process, triggered by various **pathogens** (disease-causing organisms) and countered by the body's own defenders. Physicians explain infection in terms of a **host** (either a person or a population) that contacts one or more agents in an environment. A **vector**—a biological or physical vehicle that carries the agent to the host—provides the means of transmission.

AGENTS OF INFECTION

The types of microbes that can cause infection are viruses, bacteria, fungi, protozoa, and helminths (parasitic worms).

Viruses

The tiniest pathogens—**viruses**—are also the toughest; they consist of a bit of nucleic acid (DNA or RNA, but never both) within a protein coat. Unable to reproduce on its own, a virus takes over a body cell's reproductive machinery and instructs it to produce new viral particles, which are then released to enter other cells.

The most common viruses are these types:

- **Rhinoviruses and adenoviruses,** which get into the mucous membranes and cause upper-respiratory tract infections and colds.
- **Coronaviruses,** named for their corona, or halo-like appearance, are second only to rhinoviruses in causing the common cold and other respiratory infections. A coronavirus is the prime suspect in severe acute respiratory syndrome (SARS).
- **Influenza viruses,** which can change their outer protein coats so dramatically that individuals resistant to one strain cannot fight off a new one.
- **Herpes viruses,** which take up permanent residence in the cells and periodically flare up.
- **Papilloma viruses,** which cause few symptoms in women and almost none in men but may be responsible, at least in part, for a rise in the incidence of cervical cancer among younger women.
- **Hepatitis viruses,** which cause several forms of liver infection, ranging from mild to life-threatening.
- **Slow viruses,** which give no early indication of their presence but can produce fatal illnesses within a few years.

- **Retroviruses,** which are named for their backward (*retro*) sequence of genetic replication compared to other viruses. One retrovirus, human immunodeficiency virus (HIV), causes acquired immune deficiency syndrome (AIDS).
- **Filoviruses,** which resemble threads and are extremely lethal.

The problem in fighting viruses is that it's difficult to find drugs that harm the virus and not the cell it has commandeered. **Antibiotics** (drugs that inhibit or kill bacteria) have no effect on viruses. **Antiviral drugs** don't completely eradicate a viral infection, although they can decrease its severity and duration. Because viruses multiply very quickly, antiviral drugs are most effective when taken before an infection develops or in its early stages.

Bacteria

Simple one-celled organisms, **bacteria** are the most plentiful microorganisms as well as the most pathogenic. Most kinds of bacteria don't cause disease; some, like certain strains of *Escherichia coli* that aid in digestion, play important roles within our bodies. Even friendly bacteria, however, can get out of hand and cause acne, urinary tract infections, vaginal infections, and other problems.

Bacteria harm the body by releasing either enzymes that digest body cells or toxins that produce the specific effects of such diseases as diphtheria or toxic shock syndrome. In self-defense, the body produces specific proteins (called *antibodies*) that attack and inactivate the invaders. Tuberculosis, tetanus, gonorrhea, scarlet fever, and diphtheria are examples of bacterial diseases.

Because bacteria are sufficiently different from the cells that make up our bodies, antibiotics can kill them without harming our cells. Antibiotics work only against specific types of bacteria. If your doctor thinks you have a bacterial infection, tests of your blood, pus, sputum, urine, or stool can identify the particular bacterial strain.

Fungi

Single-celled or multicelled organisms, **fungi** consist of threadlike fibers and reproductive spores. Fungi lack chlorophyll and must obtain their food from organic material, which may include human tissue. Fungi release enzymes that digest cells and are most likely to attack hair-covered areas of the body, including the scalp, beard, groin, and external ear canals. They also cause athlete's foot. Treatment consists of antifungal drugs.

Protozoa

These single-celled, microscopic animals release enzymes and toxins that destroy cells or interfere with their function. Diseases caused by **protozoa** are not a major health problem in this country, primarily because of public health measures. Around the world, however, some 2.24 billion people (more than 40 percent of the world's population) are at risk

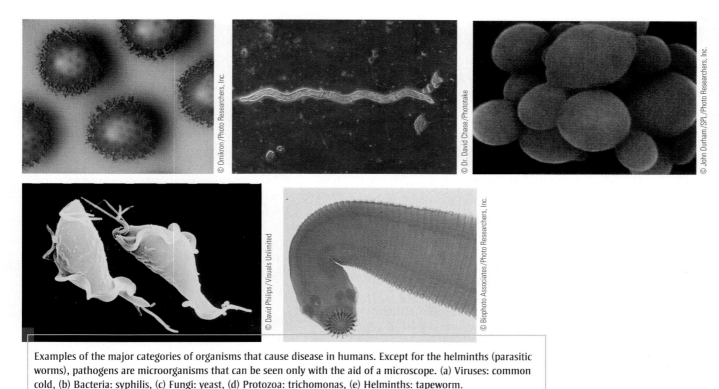

Examples of the major categories of organisms that cause disease in humans. Except for the helminths (parasitic worms), pathogens are microorganisms that can be seen only with the aid of a microscope. (a) Viruses: common cold, (b) Bacteria: syphilis, (c) Fungi: yeast, (d) Protozoa: trichomonas, (e) Helminths: tapeworm.

for acquiring malaria—a protozoan-caused disease. Up to 3 million die from this disease annually. Many more come down with amoebic dysentery. Treatment for protozoa-caused diseases consists of general medical care to relieve the symptoms, replacement of lost blood or fluids, and drugs that kill the specific protozoan.

The most common disease caused by protozoa in the United States is *giardiasis,* an intestinal infection caused by microorganisms in human and animal feces. It has become a threat at day-care centers, as well as among campers and hikers who drink contaminated water. Symptoms include nausea, lack of appetite, gas, diarrhea, fatigue, abdominal cramps, and bloating. Many people recover in a month or two without treatment. However, in some cases the microbe causes recurring attacks over many years. Giardiasis can be life-threatening in small children and the elderly, who are especially prone to severe dehydration from diarrhea. Treatment usually consists of antibiotics.

Helminths (Parasitic Worms)

Small parasitic worms that attack specific tissues or organs and compete with the host for nutrients are called **helminths.** One major worldwide health problem is *schistosomiasis,* a disease caused by a parasitic worm, the fluke, that burrows through the skin and enters the circulatory system. Infection with another helminth, the tapeworm, may be contracted from eating undercooked beef, pork, or fish containing larval forms of the tapeworm. Helminthic diseases are treated with appropriate medications.

(FAQ) HOW DO YOU CATCH AN INFECTION?

The major vectors, or means of transmission, for infectious disease are animals and insects, people, food, and water.

Animals and Insects

Disease can be transmitted by house pets, livestock, birds, and wild animals. Insects also spread a variety of diseases. The housefly may spread dysentery, diarrhea, typhoid fever, or trachoma (an eye disease rare in the United States but common in other parts of the world). Other insects, including mosquitoes, ticks, mites, fleas, and lice, can transmit such diseases as malaria, yellow fever, encephalitis, dengue fever (a growing threat in Mexico), and Lyme disease.

New threats in the United States include West Nile virus (WNV), which can be spread to humans by mosquitoes that bite infected birds, and monkeypox virus, carried by various animals, including prairie dogs. Concern is also growing about avian influenza, or bird flu. (These illnesses are discussed later in this chapter.)

People

The people you're closest to can transmit pathogens through the air, through touch, or through sexual contact. To avoid infection, stay out of range of anyone who's coughing, sniffling, or sneezing, and don't share food or dishes. Carefully wash your dishes, utensils, and hands, and abstain from sex or make self-protective decisions about sexual partners. (See "Your Life Coach: Safer, Smarter Sex" later in this chapter.)

Food

Every year foodborne illnesses strike millions of Americans, sometimes with fatal consequences. Bacteria account for two-thirds of foodborne infections, and thousands of suspected cases of infection with *Escherichia coli* bacteria in undercooked or inadequately washed food have been reported.

Every year as many as 4 million Americans have a bout with *Salmonella* bacteria, which have been found in about a third of all poultry sold in the United States. These infections can be serious enough to require hospitalization and can lead to arthritis, neurological problems, and even death. Consumers can greatly reduce the number of salmonella infections by proper handling, cooking, and refrigeration of poultry (see Chapter 6).

Water

Waterborne diseases, such as typhoid fever and cholera, are still widespread in less developed areas of the world. They have been rare in the United States, although outbreaks caused by inadequate water purification have occurred.

THE PROCESS OF INFECTION

If someone infected with the flu sits next to you on a bus and coughs or sneezes, tiny viral particles may travel into your nose and mouth. Immediately, the virus finds or creates an opening in the wall of a cell, and the process of infection begins. During the **incubation period,** the time between invasion and the first symptom, you're unaware of the pathogen multiplying inside you. In some diseases, incubation may go on for months, even years; for most, it lasts several days or weeks.

The early stage of the battle between your body and the invaders is called the *prodromal period.* As infected cells die, they release chemicals that help block the invasion. Other chemicals, such as *histamines,* cause blood vessels to dilate, thus allowing more blood to reach the battleground. During all of this, you feel mild, generalized symptoms, such as headache, irritability, and discomfort. You're also highly contagious. At the height of the battle—the typical illness period—you cough, sneeze, sniffle, ache, feel feverish, and lose your appetite.

Recovery begins when the body's forces gain the advantage. With time, the body destroys the last of the invaders and heals itself. However, the body is not able to develop long-lasting immunity to certain viruses, such as colds, flu, or HIV.

HOW YOUR BODY PROTECTS ITSELF

Various parts of your body safeguard you against infectious diseases by providing **immunity,** or protection, from these health threats. Your skin, when unbroken, keeps out most potential invaders. Your tears, sweat, skin oils, saliva, and mucus contain chemicals that can kill bacteria. Cilia, the tiny hairs lining your respiratory passages, move mucus, which traps inhaled bacteria, viruses, dust, and foreign matter, to the back of the throat, where it is swallowed; the digestive system then destroys the invaders.

When these protective mechanisms can't keep you infection-free, your body's immune system, which is on constant alert for foreign substances that might threaten the body, swings into action. The immune system includes structures of the lymphatic system—the spleen, thymus gland, lymph nodes, and lymph vessels—that help filter impurities from the body (Figure 14-1). More than a dozen different types of white blood cells (lymphocytes) are concentrated in the organs of the lymphatic system or patrol the entire body by way of the blood and lymph vessels.

Some of these white blood cells are generalists and some are specialists. The generalists include *macrophages,* which are large scavenger cells with insatiable appetites for foreign cells, diseased and run-down red blood cells, and other biological debris (see photo). The specialists are the *B cells* and *T cells,* which respond to specific invaders.

An *antigen* is any substance the white blood cells recognize as foreign. B cells create antibodies, which are proteins that bind to antigens and mark them for destruction by other white blood cells. Antigens are specific to the pathogen, and the antibody to a particular antigen binds only to that antigen (Figure 14-2). Once the human body produces antibodies against a specific antigen—the mumps virus, for instance—you're protected against that antigen for life. If you're again exposed to mumps, the antibodies previously produced prevent another episode of the disease. This protection is called **antibody-mediated immunity** (or humoral immunity). Antibody-mediated immunity is generally effective against bacterial or viral infections.

But you don't have to suffer through an illness to acquire immunity. Inoculation with a vaccine containing synthetic or weakened antigens can give you the same protection. The type of long-lasting immunity in which the body makes its own antibodies to a pathogen is called *active immunity.* Immunity produced by the injection of **gamma globulin,** the antibody-containing part of the blood from another person or animal that has developed antibodies to a disease, is called *passive immunity.*

The various types of T cells are responsible for **cell-mediated immunity.** T cells are white blood cells manufactured in the bone marrow and carried to the thymus for maturation. Cell-mediated immunity mainly protects against parasites, fungi, cancer cells, and foreign tissue. Thousands of different T cells work together to ward off disease.

IMMUNE RESPONSE

Attacked by pathogens, the body musters its forces and fights. Sometimes the invasion is handled like a minor border skirmish; other times a full-scale battle is waged throughout the body. Together, the immune cells work like an internal police force. When an antigen enters the body, the T cells aided by macrophages engage in combat with the invader. Certain T cells (cytotoxic T cells) can destroy infected body

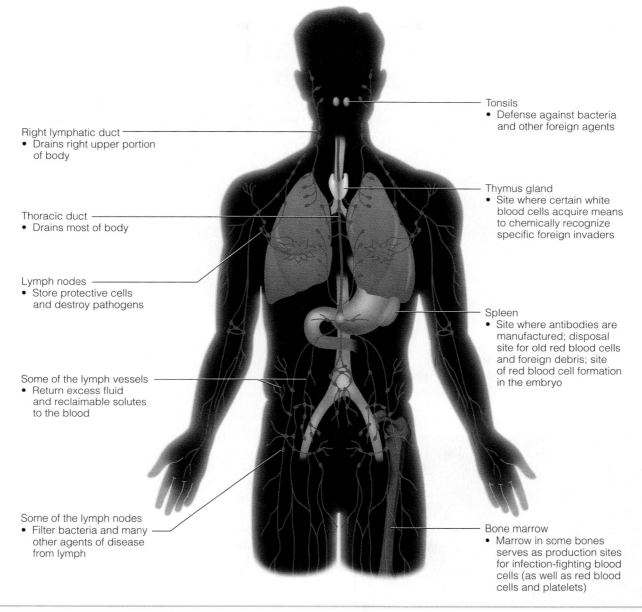

Tonsils
• Defense against bacteria
  and other foreign agents

Right lymphatic duct
• Drains right upper portion
  of body

Thymus gland
• Site where certain white
  blood cells acquire means
  to chemically recognize
  specific foreign invaders

Thoracic duct
• Drains most of body

Lymph nodes
• Store protective cells
  and destroy pathogens

Spleen
• Site where antibodies are
  manufactured; disposal
  site for old red blood cells
  and foreign debris; site
  of red blood cell formation
  in the embryo

Some of the lymph vessels
• Return excess fluid
  and reclaimable solutes
  to the blood

Some of the lymph nodes
• Filter bacteria and many
  other agents of disease
  from lymph

Bone marrow
• Marrow in some bones
  serves as production sites
  for infection-fighting blood
  cells (as well as red blood
  cells and platelets)

FIGURE 14-1   The Human Lymphatic System and Its Functions
The lymphatic system helps filter impurities from the body.

cells or tumor cells by "touch-killing." Meanwhile, the B cells churn out antibodies, which rush to the scene and join in the fray. Also busy at surveillance are natural killer cells that, like the elite forces of a SWAT team, seek out and destroy viruses and cancer cells (Figure 14-2).

The **lymph nodes,** or glands, are small tissue masses in which some protective cells are stored. If pathogens invade your body, many of them are carried to the lymph nodes to be destroyed. This is why your lymph nodes often feel swollen when you have a cold or the flu.

If the microbes establish a foothold, the blood supply to the area increases, bringing oxygen and nutrients to the fighting cells. Tissue fluids, as well as antibacterial and antitoxic proteins, accumulate. You may develop redness, swelling, local warmth, and pain—the signs of **inflammation.** As more tissue is destroyed, a cavity, or **abscess,** forms, and fills with fluid, battling cells, and dead white blood cells (pus). If the invaders aren't killed or inactivated, the pathogens are able to spread into the bloodstream and cause what is known as **systemic disease.**

Some people have an **immune deficiency**—either inborn or acquired. A very few children are born without an effective immune system; their lives can be endangered by any infection. Although still experimental, therapy to implant a missing or healthy gene may offer new hope for a normal life.

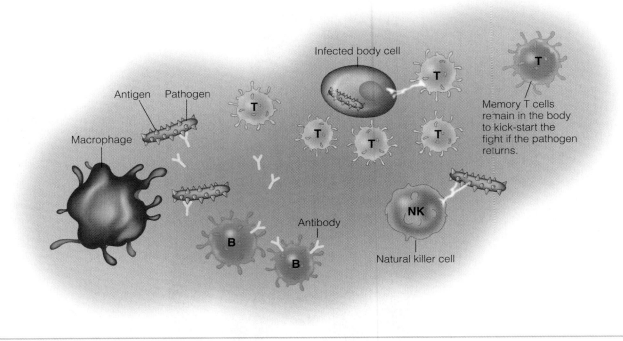

FIGURE 14-2   The Immune Response
Some T cells can touch-kill infected body cells. B cells churn out antibodies to tag pathogens for destruction by macrophages and other white blood cells.

© Boehringer Ingelheim International GmbH, photo by Lennart Nilsson

Bacterial cells ——   Cytoplasmic extension of macrophage

Electron micrograph of macrophage (red), with extensions that are making contact with bacterial cells (green). Bacteria are engulfed by this type of white blood cell.

IMMUNITY AND STRESS

Whenever we confront a crisis, large or small, our bodies produce powerful hormones that provide extra energy. However, this stress response dampens immunity, reducing the number of some key immune cells and the responsiveness of others.

Stress affects the body's immune system in different ways, depending on two factors: the controllability or uncontrollability of the stressor and the mental effort required

to cope with the stress. An uncontrollable stressor that lasts longer than 15 minutes may interfere with cytokine interleukin-6, which plays an essential role in activating the immune defenses. Uncontrollable stressors also produce high levels of the hormone cortisol, which suppresses immune system functioning. The mental efforts required to cope with high-level stressors produce only brief immune changes that appear to have little consequence for health. However, stress has been shown to slow pro-inflammatory cytokine production, which is essential for wound healing.

IMMUNE DISORDERS

Sometimes our immune system overreacts to certain substances, mistakes the body's own tissues for enemies, or doesn't react adequately. The result is an immune disorder such as allergies and autoimmune disorders.

Allergies

An **allergy** represents a hypersensitivity to a substance in our environment or diet. More than half of Americans between ages 6 and 59 are sensitive to one or more allergens.[2] Millions of them suffer unnecessarily because they don't know about effective treatment options, such as allergy shots (immunotherapy).

Allergy sufferers run annual tabs of up to $2 billion in doctor visits, diagnostic tests, prescriptions, and decreased productivity. Every year they account for more than

10 million workdays missed; every day they keep 10,000 children out of school.

Allergies are common on campus. In one study of 251 college seniors, more than half (58 percent) reported some allergy symptoms during the previous year. More than nine in ten took medications for relief—prescription drugs, over-the-counter agents, or a combination of both. Even though more than half of allergy sufferers described the effects of medications as comparable to three or four drinks of alcohol, about a third reported taking over-the-counter antihistamines, with or without prescription drugs prior to a test.[3]

Allergy symptoms are many and miserable: itching, nasal congestion, eye irritation, coughing, wheezing, hives, vomiting, and diarrhea (from food allergies), even sudden, life-threatening collapse (from anaphylaxis, the most extreme allergic reaction). While victims seldom die of allergies, they just as rarely recover. And when individuals try to outrun allergies by moving away from one region's irritants, they often end up acquiring new sensitivities on their new home ground.

A list of allergic triggers, or allergens, reads like an inventory of creation, including life's pleasures (such as foods and flowers), perils (insect stings and poison ivy), and inescapable realities (like mold and dust). The very air we breathe can be a danger. The symptoms of allergy and of its more sinister sister-disease, asthma, increase along with pollutants, such as diesel fumes, and the number of small particles in the environment.

Thanks to treatment breakthroughs, allergy sufferers no longer have to choose between feeling better or feeling alert. Treatment options include nonsedating oral medications, nasal sprays, and **immunotherapy,** which consists of a series of injections of small but increasing doses of an allergen.

Immunotherapy has proved to have long-term, perhaps permanent, benefits. In one study, traditional allergen immunotherapy with a grass-pollen extract, administered for three to four years, induced a clinical remission that persisted for at least three years after treatment. Immunotherapy in patients allergic to insect stings also induces long-lasting immunologic changes and reduces their risk of potentially fatal reactions. Immunotherapy has the greatest benefit, relative to the investment of time and cost, for

allergies that persist for more than one season or throughout the year.

Autoimmune Disorders

For unknown reasons, the immune system sometimes declares war on the cells, tissues, or organs it normally protects. This misfiring can cause more than 80 **autoimmune disorders,** including rheumatoid arthritis, myasthenia gravis, and systemic lupus erythematosus. Striking women three times as often as men, these illnesses afflict some 14 to 22 million Americans and rank among the top ten killers and top four disablers of women under age 65 (see Table 14-1, "Diseases That Discriminate").

Genetics accounts for about half of vulnerability to autoimmune disorders, which tend to cluster in families. Environmental factors—drugs, chemicals, bacteria and viruses—also may play a role. Recent research has led to new understanding of why the body sometimes turns on itself as well as breakthroughs in diagnosis and treatment, such as new biological agents that target specific proteins involved in inflammation.

 GENDER DIFFERENCES IN SUSCEPTIBILITY

When the flu hits a household, the last one left standing is likely to be Mom. The female immune system responds more vigorously to common infections, offering extra protection against viruses, bacteria, and parasites. But this enhanced immunity doesn't apply to sexually transmitted infections (STIs). A woman who has unprotected sex with an infected man is more likely to contract an STI than a man who has sex with an infected woman. Symptoms of STIs also tend to be more "silent" in women, so they often go undetected and untreated, leading to potentially serious complications.

The genders also differ in their vulnerability to allergies and autoimmune disorders. Although both men and women frequently develop allergies, allergic women are twice as likely to experience potentially fatal anaphylactic shock. A woman's robust immune system also is more likely to overreact and turn on her own organs and tissues. On average, three of four people with autoimmune disorders, such

---

Strategies for Prevention :: Fighting Hidden Allergens

- *Switch to feather pillows.* Researchers in the United Kingdom found significantly higher levels of house dust mite allergens in synthetic pillows.

- *Use bleach rather than detergent.* Very low concentrations of bleach are more effective in removing allergens from various surfaces around the house than other common cleaners.

- *Cover mattresses and pillows with tightly woven fabrics.* These materials, compared with nonwoven or semipermeable synthetic fabrics, effectively block cat and dust allergens even after repeated washings.

- *Store clothing in sealed containers with moth-killing products.* Products such as moth balls or crystals and lavandin oil

packets also kill house dust mites and their eggs.

- *Put comforters in the clothes dryer.* An hour of dry heat in a home dryer dramatically reduces the number of house dust mites in comforters and duvets filled with synthetic materials.

TABLE 14-1 DISEASES THAT DISCRIMINATE

Autoimmune Diseases	Characteristics	Prevalence in Women vs. Men	Common Symptoms
Systemic lupus erythematosus (lupus)	A chronic autoimmune disorder that can affect any tissue or organ system including the joints, kidneys, heart, lungs, brain, blood, or skin.	9:1	Achy joints; frequent fever of 100 °F or higher; anemia; fatigue; arthritis; skin rash; butterfly-shaped rash across cheek and nose; hair loss.
Graves' disease	A thyroid condition characterized by an overactive thyroid gland, which produces too much thyroid hormone.	7:1	Nervousness and irritability; weight loss; fast/irregular heart rate; heat intolerance/increased perspiration; increased appetite; sleep disturbances (such as insomnia); muscle weakness; trembling hands; irregular menstrual periods; exophthalmos (bulging eyes); appearance of a goiter (a swelling in the neck caused by enlargement of the thyroid gland).
Scleroderma	Proliferation of immune cells that produce scar tissue in the skin, some internal organs, and small blood vessels.	3:1	Reynaud's phenomenon, a condition characterized by decreased blood flow, usually to the fingers, and often brought on by cold temperatures; swelling and puffiness of the fingers or hands, followed by skin thickening a few months later; skin ulcers on the fingers; joint stiffness in the hands; sore throat; diarrhea.
Rheumatoid arthritis	Develops when the immune system attacks the synovium (the membranes that surround joints) causing inflammation, which gradually destroys cartilage, making movement of the joints painful and difficult. May also affect muscles, lungs, and liver.	2.5:1	Inflamed, swollen, and tender joints that may eventually become deformed; weakness or loss of function of joints; morning stiffness, fatigue, or general sense of malaise. Often affects joints in a symmetrical pattern: If one knee or hand is affected, usually the other one also is impaired.
Multiple sclerosis	Occurs when the immune system attacks the myelin sheath—the fatty insulation surrounding nerve cells in the brain and spinal cord. The myelin sheath enables high-speed transmission of messages between these centers and the rest of the body; gradually, as scar tissue develops in different areas of myelin, nerve messages are disrupted, affecting the body in a variety of ways.	2:1	Fatigue; short-term memory problems; temporary weakness, tingling, or paralysis in one or more limbs; loss of coordination or unsteady gait; balance problems; blurred vision; difficulty swallowing; any or all symptoms may appear and then subside, then appear again, weeks, months, or years later.

Sources: American Autoimmune Related Diseases Association, Inc.; American Diabetes Association; American Thyroid Association; Lupus Foundation of America; National Graves' Disease Foundation; National Institute of Diabetes and Digestive and Kidney Diseases; National Institute of Arthritis and Musculoskeletal and Skin Diseases; National Multiple Sclerosis Society.

as multiple sclerosis, Hashimoto's thyroiditis, and scleroderma, are women (Table 14-1).

Why are there such large gender differences in susceptibility? Scientists believe that the sex hormones have a great impact on immunity. Through a woman's childbearing years, estrogen, which protects heart, bone, brain, and blood vessels, also bolsters the immune system's response to certain infectious agents. Women produce greater numbers of antibodies when exposed to an antigen; after immunization, they show increased cell-mediated immunity.

In contrast, testosterone may dampen this response—possibly to prevent attacks on sperm cells, which might otherwise be mistaken as alien invaders. When the testes are removed from mice and guinea pigs, their immune systems become more active.

Pregnancy dampens a woman's immune response, probably to ensure that her natural protectors don't attack the fetus as a foreign invader. This impact is so great that pregnant women with transplanted kidneys may require lower doses of drugs to prevent organ rejection. Pregnant women with multiple sclerosis and rheumatoid arthritis typically experience decreased symptoms during the nine months of gestation, then return to their prepregnancy state after giving birth. Oral contraceptives also can diminish symptoms of multiple sclerosis and rheumatoid arthritis. Neither pregnancy nor birth control pills has such an impact on lupus.

IMMUNIZATIONS FOR COLLEGE STUDENTS

One of the great success stories of modern medicine has been the development of vaccines that provide protection against many infectious diseases. Immunization has reduced cases of measles, mumps, tetanus, whooping cough, and other life-threatening illnesses by more than 95 percent.

Although many people think that vaccines are only for children, they remain an important part of protection throughout life. The American College Health Association has provided recommendations for immunizations, consistent with current guidelines, for incoming students (see Table 14-2).

INFECTIOUS DISEASES

Although infections can be unavoidable at times, the more you know about their causes, the more you can do to protect yourself.

(FAQ) WHO IS AT HIGHEST RISK OF INFECTIOUS DISEASES?

Like human bullies, the viruses responsible for the most common infectious illnesses tend to pick on those least capable of fighting back. Among the most vulnerable are the following groups:

▪ **Children and their families.** Youngsters get up to a dozen colds annually; adults average two a year. When a flu epidemic hits a community, about 40 percent of school-age boys and girls get sick, compared with only 5 to 10 percent of adults. But parents get up to six times as many colds as other adults.

▪ **The elderly.** Statistically, fewer older men and women are likely to catch a cold or flu, yet when they do, they face greater danger than the rest of the population. People over 65 who get the flu have a one in ten chance of being hospitalized for pneumonia or other respiratory problems, and a one in fifty chance of dying from the disease.

▪ **The chronically ill.** Lifelong diseases, such as diabetes, kidney disease, or sickle-cell anemia, decrease an individual's ability to fend off infections. Individuals taking medications that suppress the immune system, such as steroids, are more vulnerable to infections, as are those with medical conditions that impair immunity, such as infection with HIV.

▪ **Smokers and those with respiratory problems.** Smokers are a high-risk group for respiratory infections and serious complications, such as pneumonia. Chronic breathing disorders, such as asthma and emphysema, also greatly increase the risk of respiratory infections.

▪ **Those who live or work in close contact with someone sick.** Health-care workers who treat high-risk patients, nursing home residents, and others living in close quarters—such as students in dormitories—face greater odds of catching others' colds and flus.

▪ **Residents or workers in poorly ventilated buildings.** Building technology has helped spread certain airborne illnesses, such as tuberculosis, via recirculated air. Indoor air quality can be closely linked with disease transmission in winter, when people spend a great deal of time in tightly sealed rooms.

COMMON COLD

There are more than 200 distinct cold viruses. Although in a single season you may develop a temporary immunity to one or two, you may then be hit by a third. Americans come down with 1 billion colds annually.

Every year, about 25 million cold sufferers in the United States visit their family doctors with uncomplicated upper respiratory infections. The common cold results in about 20 million days of absence from work and 22 million days of absence from school.

Colds can strike in any season, but different cold viruses are more common at different times of years. Rhinoviruses cause most spring, summer, and early fall colds and tend to cause more symptoms above the neck (stuffy nose, headache, runny eyes). Adenoviruses, parainfluenza viruses, coronaviruses, influenza viruses, and others that strike in the winter are more likely to get into the bronchi and trachea (the breathing passages) and cause more fever and bronchitis.

Cold viruses spread by coughs, sneezes, and touch. Cold sufferers who sneeze and then touch a doorknob or countertop leave a trail of highly contagious viruses behind them. The best preventive tactics are frequent hand-washing, replacing toothbrushes regularly, exercising regularly, and avoiding stress overload. High levels of stress increase the risk of becoming infected by respiratory viruses and developing cold symptoms. People who feel unable to deal with

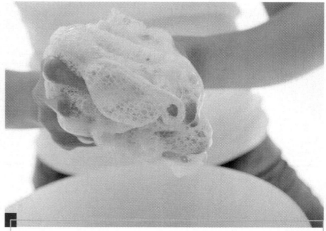

© CORBIS

Washing your hands frequently is one of your best defenses against cold viruses.

TABLE 14-2 RECOMMENDATIONS FOR ADULT IMMUNIZATION

Vaccine	Recommended for	Schedule
Influenza	All adults older than 50 Adults living or working with at-risk people Women who will be pregnant during flu season All health-care workers Persons who provide essential community services Students or other persons in institutional settings (such as dormitories) Travelers going to areas where flu activity exists Anyone wishing to reduce the likelihood of catching the flu	Given every year
Pneumococcal disease (includes bacterial pneumonia and ear infection)	All adults older than 65 Adults with chronic illness or other risk factors	One-time dose
Hepatitis B	All adolescents High-risk adults, including: • household contacts and sex partners of persons with hepatitis B • users of illicit injectable drugs • heterosexuals with more than one sex partner in 6 months • men who have sex with men • people with recently diagnosed STIs • patients receiving dialysis • health-care workers and public safety workers who are exposed to blood • clients and staff of institutions for the developmentally disabled • inmates of long-term correctional facilities • certain international travelers	Three doses over 6 months
Hepatitis A	People who travel outside the United States (except for Canada, western Europe, New Zealand, Australia, and Japan) People with chronic liver disease Illicit drug users Men who have sex with men People with clotting-factor disorders Some food handlers	Two doses over 6 months
Tetanus, diphtheria	All adolescents and adults	Booster dose every 10 years
Measles, mumps, rubella	Adults older than 18 who did not receive a dose after their first birthday Adults in high-risk groups, including: • health-care workers • students entering college and other post–high school educational institutions • international travelers All women of childbearing age	One or two doses over 4 weeks
Varicella (chickenpox)	All susceptible adults, including: • health-care workers and family contacts of people with compromised immune systems • teachers of young children, day-care employees • residents and staff in institutional settings such as colleges and correctional institutions • nonpregnant women of childbearing age	Two doses within 8 weeks
Polio	Not routinely recommended for adults	
Meningococcal disease	People with risk factors	

Source: CDC and the Immunization Action Coalition

everyday stresses have an exaggerated immune reaction that may intensify cold or flu symptoms once they've contracted a virus. Those with a positive emotional outlook are less vulnerable.[4]

Until scientists develop truly effective treatments, experts advise against taking aspirin and acetaminophen (Tylenol), which may suppress the antibodies the body produces to fight cold viruses and increase symptoms such as nasal stuffiness. A better alternative for achiness is ibuprofen (brand names include Motrin, Advil, and Nuprin), which doesn't seem to affect immune response. Children, teenagers, and young adults should never take aspirin for a cold or flu because of the danger of Reye's syndrome, a potentially deadly disorder that can cause convulsions, coma, swelling of the brain, and kidney damage.

The main drawback of antihistamines, the most widely used cold remedy, is drowsiness, which can impair a person's ability to safely drive or operate machinery. Another common ingredient, pseudoephedrine, opens and drains sinus passages without drowsiness but can speed up heart rate and cause complications for individuals with high blood pressure, diabetes, heart disease, or thyroid disorders. Nasal sprays clear a stuffy nose, but they invariably cause a rebound effect.

In general, doctors recommend treating specific symptoms—headache, cough, chest congestion, sore throat—rather than taking a multisymptom medication. For a cough, the ingredient to look for in any suppressant is dextromethorphan, which turns down the brain's cough reflex. In expectorants, the only medicine the FDA has deemed effective is guaifenesin, which helps liquefy secretions so you can bring up mucus from the chest. Unless you're coughing up green or foul yellow mucus (signs of a secondary bacterial infection), antibiotics won't help. They have no effect against viruses and may make your body more resistant to such medications when you develop a bacterial infection in the future.

 Many Americans try alternative remedies for colds. Vitamin C and extracts of the plant *Echinacea* are widely used to prevent the common cold, but there is no conclusive evidence that they help. In a recent, carefully controlled study of college students, echinacea tablets proved no more effective than placebos in reducing the duration or severity of a cold.[5] Zinc lozenges, another popular alternative treatment in recent years, have not proved to be clearly beneficial.

Although colds and sore throats—a frequent cold symptom—are caused by viruses, many people seek treatment with antibiotics, which are effective only against bacteria. An estimated 5 to 17 percent of sore throats in adults are caused by bacteria (*Group A streptococci*). In others, antibiotics have a modest effect, if any.

Excess prescribing for antibiotics accounts for more than half of all prescriptions and costs $726 million a year.[6] In addition to their costs, antibiotics may increase risks to users and their contacts. An increasing number of studies show that antibiotics foster the growth of one or more strains of antibiotic-resistant bacteria for at least two to six months inside the person taking the pills—who can pass on this drug-resistant bug to family, roommates, and others.

Your own immune system can do something modern science cannot: cure a cold. All it needs is time, rest, and plenty of fluids. Usually, cold symptoms last for one to two weeks, although chest colds (bronchitis) may last two or three weeks. Warmth is important because the aptly named "cold" viruses replicate at lower temperatures. Hot soups and drinks (particularly those with a touch of something pungent, like lemon or ginger) raise body temperature and help clear the nose. Tea may enhance the immune system. Even more important is getting off your feet. Taking it easy reduces demands on the body, which helps speed recovery.

INFLUENZA

Although similar to a cold, **influenza**—or the flu—causes more severe symptoms that last longer. Every year 10 to 20 percent of Americans develop influenza, more than 200,000 are hospitalized, and 36,000 die.[7]

Flu viruses, transmitted by coughs, sneezes, laughs, and even normal conversation, are extraordinarily contagious, particularly in the first three days of the disease. The usual incubation period is two days, but symptoms can hit hard and fast. Two varieties of viruses—influenza A and influenza B—cause most flus. In recent years, the deadliest flu epidemics have been caused by various forms of influenza A viruses.

The CDC has set priorities for individuals who should get a flu shot because they are at higher risk for flu complications, such as heart disease, diabetes, and asthma. They are:

- **Individuals aged 65 years and older,** with and without chronic health conditions.
- **Residents of long-term care facilities.**
- **Individuals aged 2 to 64 years** with chronic health conditions.
- **Children aged 6 to 23 months.**
- **Pregnant women.**
- **Health-care personnel** who provide direct patient care.
- **Household contacts and caregivers** of children under six months.

In older individuals, flu shots may offer significant protection against strokes and heart disease. The only individuals who should steer clear are those allergic to eggs, since the inactivated flu viruses are grown in chick embryos.

Vaccination with the live, nasal-spray flu vaccine (FluMist®) is an option for healthy people aged 5 to 49 years who are not pregnant. The aerosol vaccine significantly reduces flu severity, days lost from work, health-care visits, and the use of over-the-counter medication. The spray represents a particular advantage for children since more than 30 percent of youngsters get the flu, but most don't receive a flu shot.

For those who don't get vaccinated this year, antiviral drugs, such as Relenza (zanamivir) and Tamiflu (oseltamivir), are the next best line of defense. These agents act against both influenza A and influenza B viruses and cause few side effects. In research trials, they shortened the duration of flu by up to two days and decreased the likelihood of complications such as bronchitis, sinusitis, and ear infections. However, to be effective, treatment with either medication must begin within 36 to 48 hours of the first flu symptom. Although approved only for use as a treatment, antiviral drugs also can prevent flu from spreading through a family, workplace, or school.

(FAQ) ARE COLLEGE STUDENTS AT HIGHER RISK OF COLDS AND FLUS?

 College and university students are at increased risk for colds and influenza-like illnesses. In one study that followed more than 3,000 students from fall to spring, nine in ten had at least one cold or flu-like illness. These infections were responsible for 6,023 days in bed, 4,263 days of missed class, 3,175 days of missed work, and 45,219 days of illness. Flu caused more and more severe symptoms than colds (see Student Snapshot: "Colds and Flu on Campus"). About 20 percent of the sick students sought health care; 16 percent received antibiotics.[8]

Flu shots are now advised for almost everyone, but the majority of college health centers report vaccinating fewer than 20 percent of their students.[9]

Those living in dormitories are at higher risk of influenza than those in nondormitory settings.[10] Researchers have identified the specific aspects of dormitory life that increase the risk of flu symptoms, including the number of roommates

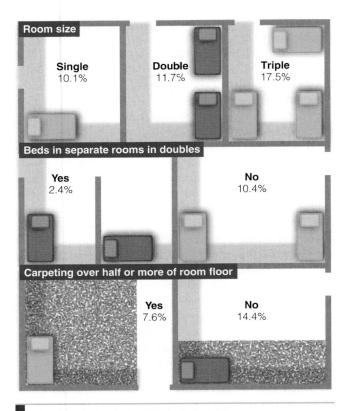

FIGURE 14-3 Rate of Flu in College Dorms

In a survey of 540 undergraduates, the rate of flu was highest for students living three to a room and lowest for those living alone. Students living in uncarpeted rooms had a higher flu rate than those living in carpeted rooms.

Source: Tsuang, Wayne, et al. "Influenza-like Symptoms in the College Dormitory Environment." *Journal of Environmental Health,* Vol. 66, No. 8, April 2004, p. 39.

and the presence/absence of carpeting. Students living in "triples," with three beds to a room; those sleeping in the same room with a roommate in a double; and those with uncarpeted floors have higher rates of flu symptoms, such as fever, sore throat, and fatigue (Figure 14-3).

MENINGITIS

Meningitis, or invasive meningococcal disease, attacks the membranes around the brain and spinal cord and can result in hearing loss, kidney failure, and permanent brain damage. An estimated 2,400 to 3,000 cases occur every year; approximately 10 percent are fatal. One of the most common types is caused by the bacterium *Neisseria meningitidis,* which is spread through coughing; kissing; sharing drinks, eating utensils, or cigarettes; or prolonged exposure to infected individuals. Viral meningitis is typically less severe.

 Most common in the first year of life, the incidence of bacterial meningitis rises in young people between ages 15 and 24. Adolescents and young adults account for nearly 30 percent of all cases of meningitis in the United States. Approximately 100 to 125 cases of

Student Snapshot

COLDS AND FLU ON CAMPUS

Symptom	Percentage of Students with Colds	Percentage of Students with Flu
Fever	12.7%	100.0%
Chills	22.9	75.4
Muscle aches	33.3	67.7
Cough	54.4	100.0
Headache	60.3	84.5
Sore throat	60.9	82.6
Runny nose	82.9	89.8

Symptoms reported by 362 students with influenzalike illnesses and 929 students with colds at the University of Minnesota.
Source: Nichol, Kristin, et al. "Colds and Influenza-like Illnesses in University Students: Impact on Health, Academic and Work Performance, and Health Care Use." *Clinical Infectious Diseases,* Vol. 40, No. 9, May 1, 2005, p. 1263(8).

Myrleen Ferguson Cate/PhotoEdit

meningococcal disease occur on college campuses each year, and 5 to 15 students will die as a result.

Campus lifestyle factors, such as crowded living situations, patronizing bars, active or passive smoking, irregular sleep patterns, and sharing personal items increase the risk for students, particularly those living in residence halls or dorms.

In an analysis of data from 50 state health departments and 231 college health centers, CDC researchers found that the risk of meningitis is three times greater for freshmen in dorms than for other college students.[11]

Symptoms may include fever, stiff neck, rash, nausea, and vomiting. The disease progresses very rapidly and can easily be misdiagnosed as the flu. Students should seek medical attention if any of these symptoms are present and unusually sudden or severe. If not treated early, meningitis can lead to death or permanent disabilities. One in five of those who survive will suffer from long-term side effects, such as brain damage, hearing loss, seizures, or limb amputation. Fatality rates are five times higher among 15- to 24-year-olds.

Protecting Yourself Against Meningitis

With the approval of a safer reformulated meningococcal vaccine that provides longer protection, the American College Health Association, as well as the CDC's Advisory Committee on Immunization Practices, has called for immunization of all incoming college freshmen living in

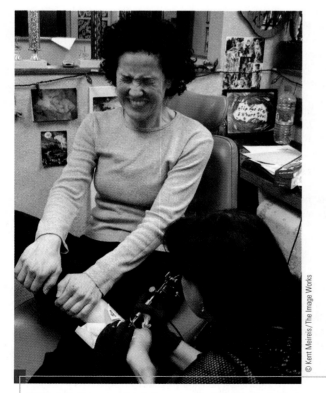

Getting a tattoo or a piercing can pose health risks, including bacterial infection and hepatitis.

dormitories or residence halls. Other college students under 25 years of age may choose to receive meningococcal vaccination to reduce their risk for the disease. Immunizing a large proportion of the student population is likely to protect even those who are not vaccinated.

 At most schools, the cost of vaccination ranges from $50 to $75. Research into the success of meningococcal vaccination programs on college campuses has shown that women are more likely than men to be vaccinated and that vaccination rates for all nonwhite ethnic groups are somewhat lower than rates for whites. Students majoring in science-oriented fields have higher vaccination rates than those majoring in the humanities. More younger students living on campus than older ones get vaccinations, possibly because of greater parental influence or because they see themselves as being at higher risk.

HEPATITIS

An estimated 500,000 Americans contract hepatitis each year. At least five different viruses, referred to as **hepatitis** A, B, C, Delta, and E, can cause this inflammation of the liver. Newly identified viruses also may be responsible for some cases of what is called "non-A, non-B" hepatitis.

All forms of hepatitis target the liver, the body's largest internal organ. Symptoms include headaches, fever, fatigue, stiff or aching joints, nausea, vomiting, and diarrhea. The liver becomes enlarged and tender to the touch; sometimes the yellowish tinge of jaundice develops. Treatment consists of rest, a high-protein diet, and the avoidance of alcohol and drugs that may stress the liver. Alpha interferon, a protein that boosts immunity and prevents viruses from replicating, may be used for some forms.

Most people begin to feel better after two or three weeks of rest, although fatigue and other symptoms can linger. As many as 10 percent of those infected with hepatitis B and up to two-thirds of those with hepatitis C become carriers of the virus for several years or even life. Some have persistent inflammation of the liver, which may cause mild or severe symptoms and increase the risk of liver cancer.

Hepatitis A

Hepatitis A, a less serious form, is generally transmitted by poor sanitation, primarily fecal contamination of food or water, and is less common in industrialized nations than in developing countries. As many as 30 percent of individuals in the United States show evidence of past infection with the virus.[12] Among those at highest risk in the United States are children and staff at day-care centers, residents of institutions for the mentally handicapped, sanitation workers, and workers who handle primates such as monkeys. Gamma globulin can provide short-term immunity; vaccines against hepatitis A have been approved by the FDA. The CDC recommends routine immunization against hepatitis A in states with high rates, as well as for travelers to countries where hepatitis A is common, men who have sex with men, and persons who use illegal drugs.

Hepatitis B

Hepatitis B, a potentially fatal disease transmitted through the blood and other bodily fluids, infects an estimated 350,000 people around the world each year. Once spread mainly by contaminated tattoo needles, needles shared by drug users, or transfusions of contaminated blood, hepatitis B is now transmitted mostly through sexual contact. It can cause chronic liver infection, cirrhosis, and liver cancer.

Hepatitis B is a particular threat to young people; 75 percent of new cases are diagnosed in those between ages 15 to 39. They usually contract hepatitis B through high-risk behaviors such as multiple sex partners and use of injected drugs. Individuals who have tattoos or body piercing may also be at risk if procedures are not done under regulated conditions. At highest risk are male homosexuals, heterosexuals with multiple sex partners, health-care workers with frequent contact with blood, injection drug users, and infants born to infected mothers. Vaccination can prevent hepatitis B and is recommended for all newborns.

Hepatitis C

Hepatitis C virus (HCV) is four times as widespread as HIV, infecting about 2 percent of Americans. A simple blood test can show if you are infected with HCV. However, few of the estimated 3 to 4 million carriers in the United States realize

---

Savvy Consumer :: Before You Get a Tattoo or Piercing

"Body art"—tattoos and piercings—may seem harmless, but health officials warn of hidden risks, including Hepatitis B and C infection and transmission of HIV. In a survey of undergraduates at a university in New York, 51 percent reported body piercings, and 23 percent had gotten tattoos. Almost one in five of those with piercings reported medical complications. Bacterial infection was the most common, followed by bleeding and injury or tearing at the site.

With no state or federal regulations of "body artists," unsafe tattooing and piercing practices can put consumers in danger. In one survey of "skin-penetration operators," only half said that they followed governmental guidelines for infection control. Many were not knowledgeable about standard infection-control principles and practices.

Epidemiologists have identified tattooing as a strong, independent risk factor for testing positive for hepatitis C virus (HCV) but not with development of acute hepatitis. In other words, individuals with tattoos may acquire HCV but may not develop symptoms themselves. This does not mean that they will never become symptomatic or that they cannot transmit HCV to others.

Even so-called temporary tattooing with henna is not without risk. Dermatologists have reported an increasing number of skin reactions. The culprit is an ingredient in many henna preparations called paraphenylenediamine (PPD). Allergic reactions to henna itself can occur, but are much rarer. Piercings of the tongue, lips, or cheeks present different dangers, including recessed gums; loose, chipped, or fractured teeth; pain; infection; inflammation; nerve damage; and tooth loss.

You may think you're safe if you go to a licensed tattoo or piercing salon. However, there are no formal schools, no certification requirements, and no diplomas for these practitioners. In many states it is possible to get a license without the benefit of any kind of training. Your best assurance of quality is making sure that basic safety principles are followed:

- **Ask to see certification that the autoclave, a high-temperature pressure cooker used for medical instruments, has been sterilized.** Ask to see the autoclave itself. Is it clean? More importantly, are the shop personnel happy to show it to you, or do they seem to have something to hide? Autoclaves need to be regularly tested to ensure that they are working properly. Ask to see the results of their latest spore test. Check the date. The results should be no more than two months old.

- **Make sure the artist is wearing standard medical latex gloves.** Check the fit. If the gloves are too big or too small, the artist runs the risk of either poking a hole in the gloves or tearing them. All it takes is a pinhole to run the risk of cross-contamination.

- **Find out if the artist is vaccinated for hepatitis B.** As this infection has spread, vaccination has become essential for a tattoo artist's own safety as well as that of clients. If artists claim to be vaccinated, never just take their word for it. Can they show you proof, such as a doctor's record, that they were vaccinated? If they tell you they don't remember if they've been vaccinated, they're probably lying.

Most people vividly remember the vaccinations.

- **Make sure the artist uses only new sterile needles.** The needles should not be removed from the autoclave bag, the sort of pouch you see in dentists' offices, until you are ready for your tattoo. Ask to see the sterile confirmation logo on the bag itself. Usually the name of the company that made the bag will be visible on the front of the bag only when the equipment has been properly autoclaved. To determine if the needles are new and not just sterilized after previous use, check the color. They should be bright silver, not stained with ink or brownish looking.

- **Ask how the artist disposes of used needles.** They should be placed in a sharps container, a plastic container, usually red, with a biohazard symbol on the outside, and removed in a timely manner.

- **Always ask to see photos of the artist's finished work.** Examine the designs up close to check precision and skill. If you have the time, watch the artist work on another client before you go ahead with your tattoo.

- **If you require prophylactic antibiotics for dental cleanings or other procedures, do not get a tattoo.** Consumers with rheumatic heart disease and other conditions that increase their risk of infections have died as a result of bacterial infection contracted from a tattoo.

they are infected. Of those infected with HCV, 80 percent have no symptoms.[13]

The risk factors for HCV infection are blood transfusion or organ transplant before 1992, exposure to infected blood, illegal drug use, tattoos, or body piercing. If you choose to have a body piercing, avoid piercing guns, and make certain that the piercing equipment has been sterilized[14] (see Savvy Consumer: "Before You Get a Tattoo or Piercing"). Hepatitis C virus is not spread by casual contact, such as hugging, kissing, or sharing food utensils. There is controversy over whether HCV also can be transmitted sexually.

About three-quarters of those infected with HCV develop chronic or long-term hepatitis. About one-quarter develop progressive, irreversible liver damage, with scar tissue (cirrhosis) gradually replacing healthy liver tissue.

The most common treatment for Hepatitis C is a combination of interferon, which stops the virus from making copies of itself; and ribavirin, an antiviral medication. If the liver no longer functions adequately, a patient may require liver transplantation.

MONONUCLEOSIS

You can get **mononucleosis** through kissing—or any other form of close contact. "Mono" is a viral disease that targets people 15 to 24 years old. Its symptoms include a sore throat, headache, fever, nausea, and prolonged weakness. The spleen is swollen and the lymph nodes are enlarged. You may also develop jaundice or a skin rash similar to rubella (German measles).

The major symptoms usually disappear within two to three weeks, but weakness, fatigue, and often depression may linger for at least two more weeks. The greatest danger is from physical activity that might rupture the spleen, resulting in internal bleeding. The liver may also become inflamed. A blood test can determine whether you have mono. However, there's no specific treatment other than rest.

CHRONIC FATIGUE SYNDROME (CFS)

As many as 500,000 Americans have the array of symptoms known as **chronic fatigue syndrome (CFS).** Diagnosis of CFS remains difficult, although numerous studies have found significant immune abnormalities, such as high levels of certain immune cells (B lymphocytes and cytokines) that act as if they were constantly battling a viral infection. Researchers are working to develop a blood test that will definitively diagnose CFS.

PNEUMONIA

An inflammation of the lungs, **pneumonia** fills the fine, spongy networks of the lungs' tiny air chambers with fluid. It can be caused by bacteria, viruses (including flu), or foreign material in the lungs (such as smoke). The symptoms of classic bacterial pneumonia are fever, shortness of breath, and general weakness. Along with influenza, pneumonia is the fifth leading killer of Americans and the most common infectious cause of death.

The typical signs of pneumonia include cough, a fever of more than 101°F, difficulty breathing, chills, and excessive yellow-green phlegm. Symptoms of pneumonia can develop either gradually or else so quickly that a person's life is in danger within hours. Antibiotics can control bacterial pneumonia, but they must be given before microbes erode local tissues and spread through the blood elsewhere in the body, causing a condition known as septicemia, or blood poisoning. Because of the dangers of pneumonia, you should see a doctor if there's any chance you have it. Severe cases may require hospitalization and high doses of antibiotics.

Vaccination against pneumonia is recommended for those who've had pneumonia in the past, those with impaired immune function, and those over age 65. The pneumonia vaccine greatly reduces the risk of this disease, especially for women and those with impaired immunity.

TUBERCULOSIS

A bacterial infection of the lungs that was once the nation's leading killer, **tuberculosis (TB)** still claims the lives of more people than any acute infectious disease other than pneumonia (Figure 14-4). About 30 percent of the world's population is infected with the TB organism, although not all develop active disease. In the United States, immigration from countries where TB is common, poverty, homelessness, alcoholism and drug abuse, the HIV/AIDS epidemic, and the emergence of resistant strains of TB account for most new cases of TB. Approximately 15 million Americans have the disease.[15]

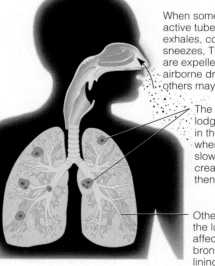

When someone with active tuberculosis exhales, coughs, or sneezes, TB bacteria are expelled in tiny airborne droplets that others may inhale.

The TB bacteria lodge mainly in the lungs, where they slowly multiply, creating patches, then cavities.

Other parts of the lung are affected, including bronchi and the lining of the lung.

FIGURE 14-4 How Tuberculosis Spreads
If untreated, TB can eventually spread to and damage the brain, bone, eyes, liver and kidneys, spine, and skin.

Although TB is most prevalent among high-risk groups, the overall danger increases as more people develop active disease because TB is highly contagious. TB outbreaks have occurred throughout the country in hospitals, nursing homes, prisons, and office buildings, where inadequate ventilation increases the risk of infection.

Symptoms vary, depending on the organs that are infected. They include fever and sweating (particularly at night), unexplained weight loss, loss of appetite, fatigue, persistent cough that may produce bloody sputum, and difficulty breathing or chest pain when breathing.

Most TB patients recover completely after six months of taking a combination of three different medicines. Drug-resistant forms of the tuberculosis microorganism strike mostly patients who start drug treatment but don't follow through with it. Because they don't take enough of the medication to kill all the TB bacteria in their system, those that survive become resistant. Even with full treatment, the risk of dying from drug-resistant tuberculosis is 50 percent. HIV infection greatly increases susceptibility to infection with TB and the risk of dying if infected with treatment-resistant forms.

If you think you may have been exposed to TB or if you develop suspicious symptoms (loss of appetite and weight, low-grade fever, fatigue, chills, night sweats, coughing), see your doctor for a TB test. This consists of an injection just under the skin. The area of the arm where the test was administered should be checked by a health-care professional to determine the presence of the TB bacteria; further tests confirm the diagnosis. If the skin test is positive, indicating that TB is present, you'll be monitored with yearly chest X rays. You may also require treatment which usually requires three to four antibiotics taken daily for at least 6 to 9 months.

GROUP A AND GROUP B STREP INFECTION

Sore throats are common winter complaints, but those caused by group A streptococcus bacteria—*strep throats*—are more than a trivial threat. If not treated promptly with antibiotics, strep bacteria can travel to the kidneys, the liver, or the heart, where they can cause rheumatic fever—an inflammation of the heart that can cause weakness, shortness of breath, joint pain, and an abnormal heartbeat. In recent years clusters of rheumatic fever have sprung up in several major cities. Pediatricians are urging parents to consult their doctors if a youngster complains of a sore throat or if strep is widespread in the community. Rapid new diagnostic tests can identify strep within minutes. If the test is positive, treatment with penicillin or a similar antibiotic is indicated. Brief treatment (five days) with Omnicef, a new antibiotic, has proved as effective as ten days of oral penicillin.

Toxic streptococcal shock syndrome, or toxic strep, is an invasive form of the disease in which strep gains access to the blood and causes a drop in blood pressure, a very high fever, and the production of exotoxins (substances that can attack various organs, such as the kidneys, heart, or in rare cases, flesh). Toxic strep is rather rare and usually doesn't occur with strep throats. Prompt treatment is critical.

Group B streptococcus (GBS), the leading cause of life-threatening perinatal infections in the United States, is primarily a threat to newborns. Because some 15 to 40 percent of pregnant women carry GBS but have no symptoms, the American Academy of Pediatrics has called for universal screening of expectant mothers. Each year 12,000 newborns are infected, most of them during childbirth; more than 1,600 die; and another 1,600 suffer permanent brain damage from meningitis. Women at high risk of infecting their newborns with GBS are those who have premature labor, early rupture of their amniotic membranes, fever, and a high group B strep count before or during pregnancy, or who have previously borne an infant infected with GBS. Also at risk are diabetics, poor women, and those under age 20.

TOXIC SHOCK SYNDROME

As discussed in Chapter 9, **toxic shock syndrome (TSS)** is a potentially deadly disease associated with the use of tampons, particularly high-absorbency types. It is caused by *Staphylococcus aureus* and group A *Streptococcus pyogenes* bacteria that release toxins (poisonous waste products) into the bloodstream. Symptoms include a high fever; a rash that leads to peeling of the skin on the fingers, toes, palms, and soles; dizziness; dangerously low blood pressure; and abnormalities in several organ systems (the digestive tract and the kidneys) and in the muscles and blood.

In addition to women who use high-absorbency tampons, or leave their tampons in too long, those who have given birth within the preceding six to eight weeks are at greater risk. Children (including newborns), men, and post-menopausal women also have developed TSS, which usually has been traced to bacteria in skin abscesses, boils, cuts, or postsurgical wounds.

Without prompt treatment, TSS can cause severe and permanent damage, including muscle weakness, partial paralysis, amnesia, disorientation, an inability to concentrate, and impaired lung and kidney function. Sometimes toxic shock weakens the blood vessels, increasing the risk of heart problems. Victims can enter the life-threatening crisis called shock, in which blood flow throughout the body is inadequate to sustain life. Treatment usually consists of immediate hospitalization, intravenous administration of fluids, medications to raise blood pressure, and powerful antibiotics; intravenous administration of immunoglobins that attack the toxins produced by these bacteria may also be beneficial.

INSECT- AND ANIMAL-BORNE INFECTIONS

Common insects and animals, including ticks and mosquitoes, can transmit dangerous infections. Lyme disease is the most widespread in the United States, while West Nile virus continues to spread. The first outbreak of animal-borne monkeypox virus occurred in 2003.

Lyme Disease

Lyme disease, a bacterial infection, is spread by ticks carrying a particular bacterium—the spirochete *Borrelia burgdorferi.* An infected person may have various symptoms, including joint inflammation, heart arrhythmias, blinding headaches, and memory lapses. The disease can also cause miscarriages and birth defects. Lyme disease is by far the most commonly reported vector-borne infectious disease in the United States. The vast majority of all reported cases have occurred in just ten states, including New York, New Jersey, Connecticut, Pennsylvania, and Wisconsin.

The FDA has licensed a vaccine to prevent Lyme disease in individuals 15 to 70 years old. LYMErix, like most vaccines, stimulates the immune system to produce antibodies, in this case against the bacterium that causes Lyme disease. But the vaccine, administered in three doses over a one-year period, is not 100 percent effective and should not be considered a substitute for protective clothing and tick repellent.

The primary culprit in most cases of Lyme disease is the deer tick, although other ticks, including the western black-legged tick, the dog tick, and the Lone Star tick, also may transmit the bacterium that causes Lyme disease.

Hunters and campers are more likely to test positive for Lyme disease. Pet owners are not at additional risk. The most important preventive step is to check yourself for ticks whenever you come in from the outdoors. However, detecting some types of ticks can be difficult. In their nymphal stage, when they're most likely to bite, ticks are about the size of a poppyseed. Even as adults, some ticks are no bigger than a sesame seed.

Regardless of whether or not they've spotted a tick, residents of infested areas should check regularly for signs of a bite. About two-thirds of those bitten develop some skin changes from two days to four weeks afterward. The classic skin lesion is a small, clear-centered red doughnut that expands, but most people simply have a red blotch or two blotches. However, the rash always expands, usually to about 2 inches in diameter. In some cases, it may cover a person's entire chest or thigh; others develop rashes far from the

Ticks are responsible for the spread of Lyme disease. If you spot a tick, remove it as soon as possible with tweezers or small forceps. Put it in a plastic bag or sealed bottle and save it. If you develop a rash or other symptoms, take it with you to the doctor.

© Scott Camazine/Photo Researchers, Inc.

bite, caused by spirochetes that travel through the bloodstream. More sensitive diagnostic tests allow detection of extremely low numbers of spirochetes and make earlier diagnosis possible.

West Nile Virus

West Nile virus (WNV) is transmitted by a mosquito that feeds on an infected bird and then bites a human. The first cases in the United States occurred in 1999. Experts now see WNV as a seasonal epidemic that flares up in the summer and continues into the fall. WNV also can be spread through blood transfusions, organ transplants, breast-feeding, and from mother to fetus during pregnancy.

WNV interferes with normal central nervous system functioning and causes inflammation of brain tissue. The risk of catching WNV is low. Relatively few mosquitoes carry WNV, and fewer than 1 percent of people who are bitten by mosquitoes experience any symptoms. Repellents that contain DEET, picaridin, and oil of lemon eucalyptus can protect against WNV.[16]

There is no specific treatment for WNV infection. People with more severe cases usually require hospitalization and supportive treatment, including intravenous fluids and help with breathing. An antiviral drug, interferon, which might lessen the symptoms and duration of the illness in infected patients, is undergoing testing.

Strategies for Prevention :: Protecting Yourself from Insect-Borne Diseases

- :: Apply insect repellent containing DEET (N,N-diethyl-meta-toluamide), which provides the longest-lasting protection against bites, when you're outdoors.

- :: When possible, wear long-sleeved clothes and long pants treated with repellents containing permethrin or DEET since insects may bite through thin clothing. Do not apply repellents

containing permethrin directly to exposed skin. If you spray your clothing, there is no need to spray repellent containing DEET on the skin under your clothing.

- :: Consider staying indoors at dawn, dusk, and in the early evening, which are peak mosquito-biting times.

- :: After spending time outdoors, examine yourself for ticks or bites every day.

Check less obvious places, such as the scalp and behind the ears.

- :: If you do spot a tick, remove it right away. Using tweezers or forceps, grasp the tick firmly as close to its head and as near to your skin as possible. Gently pull backward, without squeezing the tick's body, until its hold is released. Wash your hands thoroughly. Treat the wound with rubbing alcohol.

Monkeypox Virus

This rare viral disease occurs mainly in Africa, where it was first identified in monkeys. Researchers have since recovered monkeypox from other animals, including rats, mice, and rabbits, as well as humans.

The signs and symptoms of monkeypox are similar to those of smallpox but milder. People can catch monkeypox from an infected animal's bite, blood, or body fluids. It can spread from person to person during long periods of face-to-face contact or by touching the body fluids of a sick person or bedding or clothing contaminated with the virus. There is no specific treatment.

Avian Influenza

Avian influenza, or bird flu, is caused by viruses that occur naturally among wild birds. Domesticated birds, such as chickens and ducks, that become infected can become very sick and die.

Bird flu viruses do not usually infect humans, but more than 100 confirmed cases of human infection with bird flu viruses have occurred since 1997, mostly individuals who have close contact with birds or fowl. The spread of avian influenza viruses from one ill person to another is very rare. However, fear of a possible mutation in the virus that would increase human-to-human transmission has sparked global concern of a flu *pandemic,* a worldwide outbreak of disease. Medical and public health personnel are working to diagnose and prevent the spread of avian influenza.

The CDC advises travelers to countries with known outbreaks of avian influenza to avoid poultry farms, contact with animals in live food markets, and any surfaces that appear to be contaminated with feces from poultry or other animals.

NEW INFECTIOUS THREATS

The twenty-first century has ushered in new agents of infection and new apprehension about the potential use of infectious diseases as instruments of terror and mass destruction.

FAQ What Is SARS?

Severe acute respiratory syndrome (SARS) became a new global health threat in 2003, with major outbreaks in several Asian countries, including China and Hong Kong, and in Toronto.

Another outbreak occurred in China in 2004. SARS-associated coronavirus (SARS-CoV) spreads by close face-to-face contact, most often by droplets expelled into the air when an infected person coughs or sneezes. The virus is believed capable of living outside the body for at least 24 hours. A few persons may be especially infectious and are more likely to spread the SARS virus to others in the same airplane, household, school, workplace, or hospital. Doctors do not know how long a person remains contagious.

The average incubation period for SARS is six to ten days. Symptoms include high fever, coughing, headache, chills, muscle aches, and shortness of breath. Most of those infected develop pneumonia. There are no specific treatments

Although used by many in an outbreak, surgical masks do not offer complete protection against the SARS virus.

for SARS. Patients receive supportive care, such as fluids to prevent dehydration and ventilators to aid breathing. Scientists are developing possible vaccines and antiviral agents.

The best defenses against SARS are avoiding travel to regions with high numbers of cases and frequent, thorough handwashing with soap and water. Although many people in areas of SARS outbreaks wear surgical masks as protection, the CDC does not recommend their routine use, because they are not 100 percent effective in blocking the SARS virus.

Bioterror Threats

Americans have learned firsthand that certain infectious agents can be used as weapons of terrorism and war. Bioterror agents, such as anthrax and, potentially, smallpox or botulism, have been added to the ranks of emerging infectious diseases.

Anthrax Anthrax, which is found naturally in wild and farm animals, can also be produced in a laboratory. The disease is spread through exposure to anthrax spores, not through exposure to an infected person.

Smallpox Smallpox is a serious, contagious, and sometimes fatal infectious disease. Smallpox was eradicated decades ago after a successful worldwide vaccination program. The last case of smallpox in the United States was in 1949. The last naturally occurring case in the world was in Somalia in 1977. There is no treatment, and up to 30 percent of those infected with smallpox die.

Because of fear that terrorists might use smallpox as a biological weapon, the U.S. government has stockpiled enough vaccine to inoculate everyone in the event of an emergency. Most individuals vaccinated before 1972, when mandated smallpox immunization ended in the United States, retain some immunity for many years, some for up to 75 years. However, half of all Americans have never received the smallpox vaccine, and many scientists believe protection wanes over time for those who did. Those vaccinated in the past can safely be revaccinated for optimum protection. An Institute of Medicine committee has recommended against vaccinating the entire population at this time.

Botulism Botulism is a muscle-paralyzing disease caused by a toxin made by the bacterium *Clostridium botulinum*. Botulinum toxin is among the most lethal substances known, and it can kill within 24 hours. Botulism causes muscle weakness and eventual paralysis that starts at the top of your body and works its way down. The disease kills by paralyzing muscles you use to breathe. The CDC and some state health departments keep an antidote to botulinum toxin in storage. Treatment includes taking the antidote and possibly using a ventilator for breathing until the toxin works its way out of your system.

Tularemia Tularemia is an illness that normally infects wild animals, such as rabbits and squirrels. Humans can acquire the illness by coming in contact with the blood or body fluids of infected animals, from the bite of a fly or tick that carries blood from an infected animal, or from contaminated food or water. As a biological weapon, tularemia-causing bacteria could be dispersed through the air and inhaled. Signs and symptoms vary but include fever, headache, chills, weakness, enlarged and tender lymph nodes, and an ulcerated sore if bitten by an infected fly or tick. Intravenous (IV) antibiotics can be used to treat tularemia. Even without treatment, it's fatal in less than 2 percent of cases. Tularemia is not passed from person to person.

REPRODUCTIVE AND URINARY TRACT INFECTIONS

Reproductive and urinary tract infections are very common. Many are not spread exclusively by sexual contact, so they are not classified as sexually transmitted diseases.

Vaginal Infections

Vaginal complaints account for approximately 10 million medical office visits a year.[17] The most common are trichomoniasis, candidiasis, and bacterial vaginosis (Table 14-3).

Protozoa (*Trichomonas vaginalis*) that live in the vagina can multiply rapidly, causing itching, burning, and discharge—all symptoms of **trichomoniasis.** Male carriers usually have no symptoms, although some may develop urethritis or an inflammation of the prostate and seminal vesicles. Anyone with this infection should be screened for syphilis, gonorrhea, chlamydia, and HIV. Sexual partners must be treated with oral medication (metronidazole, trade name Flagyl), even if they have no symptoms, to prevent reinfection.

Populations of a yeast called *Candida albicans*—normal inhabitants of the mouth, digestive tract, and vagina—are usually held in check. Under certain conditions, however (such as poor nutrition, stress, or antibiotic use), the microbes multiply, causing burning, itching, and a whitish discharge, and producing what is commonly known as a yeast infection. Common sites for **candidiasis,** which is also called *moniliasis,* are the vagina, vulva, penis, and mouth. The women most likely to test positive for candidiasis have never been pregnant, use condoms for birth control, have sexual intercourse more than four times a month, and have taken antibiotics in the previous 15 to 30 days. Vaginal medications, such as GyneLotrimin and Monistat, are nonprescription drugs that provide effective treatment. Male sexual partners may be advised to wear condoms during outbreaks of candidiasis. Women should keep the genital area dry and wear cotton underwear.

Bacterial vaginosis is characterized by alterations in the microorganisms that live in the vagina, including depletion of certain bacteria and overgrowth of others. It typically causes a white or gray vaginal discharge with a distinctive fishy odor similar to that of trichomoniasis. Its underlying cause is unknown, although it occurs most frequently in women with multiple sex partners. Long-term dangers include pelvic inflammatory disease (PID, discussed later in this chapter) and pregnancy complications. Metronidazole,

---

TABLE 14-3 COMMON REPRODUCTIVE TRACT INFECTIONS

Infection	Transmission	Symptoms	Treatment
Bacterial vaginosis	Most common causative agent, *Gardnerella vaginalis* bacterium, sometimes transmitted through coitus	Women: Fishy- or musty-smelling, thin discharge, like flour paste in consistency and usually gray Men: Mostly asymptomatic	Metronidazole (Flagyl) by mouth or intravaginal applications of topical metronidazole gel or clindamycin cream
Candidiasis (yeast infection)	*Candida albicans* fungus may accelerate growth when the chemical balance of the vagina is disturbed; also transmitted through sexual interaction	Women: White, "cheesy" discharge; irritation of vaginal and vulval tissues	Vaginal suppositories or topical cream, such as clotrimazole (GyneLotrimin) and miconazole (Monistat), or oral fluconazole
Trichomoniasis	Protozoan parasite *Trichomonas vaginalis*, usually passed through genital sexual contact	Women: White or yellow vaginal discharge with an unpleasant odor; sore and irritated vulva Men: No symptoms	Metronidazole (Flagyl) for both women and men

either in the form of a pill or a vaginal gel, is the primary treatment. According to CDC guidelines, treatment for male sex partners appears to be of little benefit, but some health practitioners recommend treatment for both partners in cases of recurrent infections.

Urinary Tract Infections

A urinary tract infection (UTI) can be present in any of the three parts of the urinary tract: the urethra, the bladder, or the kidneys. An infection involving the urethra is known as **urethritis.** If the bladder is also infected, it's called **cystitis.** If it reaches the kidneys, it's called **pyelonephritis.**

An estimated 40 percent of women report having had a UTI at some point in their lives. Three times as many women as men develop UTIs, probably for anatomical reasons. A woman's urethra is only 1.5 inches long; a man's is 6 inches. Therefore, bacteria, the major cause of UTIs, have a shorter distance to travel to infect a woman's bladder and kidneys. About one-fourth to one-third of all women between ages 20 and 40 develop UTIs, and 80 percent of those who experience one infection develop recurrences.

Conditions that can set the stage for UTIs include irritation and swelling of the urethra or bladder as a result of pregnancy, bike riding, irritants (such as bubble bath, douches, or a diaphragm), urinary stones, enlargement of the prostate gland in men, vaginitis, and stress. Early diagnosis is critical because infection can spread to the kidneys and, if unchecked, result in kidney failure. Symptoms include frequent burning, painful urination, chills, fever, fatigue, and blood in the urine.

Recurrent UTIs, a frequent problem among young women, have been linked with a genetic predisposition, sexual intercourse, and the use of diaphragms. Postintercourse treatment with antibiotics can lower the risk.

SEXUALLY TRANSMITTED INFECTIONS

Venereal diseases (from the Latin *venus,* meaning *love* or *lust*) are called **sexually transmitted infections (STIs),** or sexually transmitted diseases (STDs). Around the world, some 50 million cases of curable STIs occur each year (not including HIV and herpes). Almost 700,000 people are infected every day with one of the over 20 STIs tracked by world health officials. STIs are much more widespread in developing nations because of lack of adequate health standards, prevention practices, and access to treatment.

More Americans are infected with STIs now than at any other time in history. According to the Institute of Medicine, the odds of acquiring an STI during a lifetime are one in four. STIs are among the top ten most frequently reported diseases in the United States. The major cause of preventable sterility in America, STIs have tripled the rate of ectopic (tubal) pregnancies, which can be fatal if not detected early. STI complications, including miscarriage, premature delivery, and uterine infections after delivery, annually affect more than

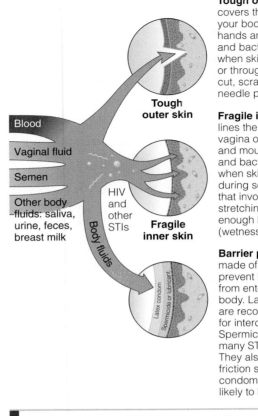

Tough outer skin
covers the outside of your body, including hands and lips. Viruses and bacteria enter when skin is chapped or through a hangnail, cut, scrape, sore, or needle puncture.

Fragile inner skin
lines the inside of your vagina or penis, anus, and mouth. Viruses and bacteria can enter when skin is torn during sexual contact that involves rubbing, stretching, or not enough lubrication (wetness).

Barrier protection
made of latex helps prevent body fluids from entering your body. Latex condoms are recommended for intercourse. Spermicides help kill many STI microbes. They also reduce friction so latex condoms are less likely to break.

FIGURE 14-5 How HIV Infection and Other STIs Are Spread
Most STIs are spread by viruses or bacteria carried in certain body fluids.

100,000 women. Moreover, infection with an STI greatly increases the risk of HIV transmission (discussed later in this chapter). The incidence of STIs is highest in 16- to 24-year-olds, particularly older teenagers, and homosexual men. Others affected by STIs include unborn and newborn children who can "catch" potentially life-threatening infections in the womb or during birth.

Although each STI is a distinct disease, all STI pathogens like dark, warm, moist body surfaces, particularly the mucous membranes that line the reproductive organs; they hate light, cold, and dryness (Figure 14-5). It is possible to catch or have more than one STI at a time. Curing one doesn't necessarily cure another, and treatments don't prevent another bout with the same STI (Table 14-4).

Many STIs, including early HIV infection and gonorrhea in women, may not cause any symptoms. As a result, infected individuals may continue their usual sexual activity without realizing that they're jeopardizing others' well-being.

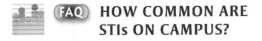 **(FAQ) HOW COMMON ARE STIs ON CAMPUS?**

Young people of college age account for about half of new cases of sexually transmitted infections (STIs). The college years are a prime time for contracting STIs. According to the

TABLE 14-4 COMMON SEXUALLY TRANSMITTED INFECTIONS (STIS): MODE OF TRANSMISSION, SYMPTOMS, AND TREATMENT

STI	Transmission	Signs and Symptoms	Treatment
Chlamydia (p. 414)	*Chlamydia trachomatis* bacterium transmitted primarily through sexual contact (can also be spread by fingers from one body site to another)	Men: Watery discharge; pain when urinating Women: Usually asymptomatic; sometimes a similar discharge to men's; leading cause of pelvic inflammatory disease (PID)	Antibiotics: doxycycline, azithromycin, ofloxacin, levofloxacin
Human papilloma virus (HPV) (genital warts) (p. 414)	Spread primarily through vaginal, anal, or oral-genital sexual interaction	Cauliflowerlike growths in genital and rectal areas	Removal of lesions by laser surgery or chemicals
Herpes simplex (p. 415)	Genital herpes virus (HSV-2) transmitted primarily by vaginal, anal, or oral-genital intercourse. Oral herpes virus (HSV-1) transmitted primarily by kissing	Small, painful red bumps (papules) in the genital region (genital herpes) or mouth (oral herpes). The papules become painful blisters that eventually rupture to form wet, open sores.	No known cure. Treatment may reduce symptoms; acyclovir, famcyclovir, or valacyclovir promote healing and suppress recurrent outbreaks
Gonorrhea ("clap") (p. 417)	*Neisseria gonorrhoeae* bacterium ("gonococcus") spread through genital, oral-genital, or genital-anal contact	Men: Pus discharge from urethra; burning during urination Women: Usually asymptomatic; can lead to PID and sterility in both men and women	Antibiotics: ceftriaxone, cefixime, or spectinomycin
Nongonococcal urethritis (NGU) (p. 417)	Bacteria, most commonly transmitted through sexual intercourse	Men: Discharge from the penis and irritation during urination Women: Mild discharge of pus from the vagina but often no symptoms	A single dose of azithromycin or doxycycline for seven days
Syphilis (p. 418)	*Treponema pallidum* bacterium ("spirochete") transmitted from open lesions during genital, oral-genital, or genital-anal contact	Primary: Chancre Secondary: Rash Latent: Asymptomatic Late: Irreversible damage to central nervous system, cardiovascular system	Penicillin or other antibiotic
Chancroid (p. 418)	*Haemophilus ducrevi* bacterium transmitted by sexual interaction	Men: Painful irregular chancre on penis Women: Chancre on labia	Tetracycline
Viral hepatitis (p. 403)	Hepatitis A primarily spread via the fecal-oral route, but oral-anal sexual contact a common mode. Hepatitis B virus transmitted by blood, semen, vaginal secretions, and saliva. Manual, oral, or penile stimulation of the anus strongly associated with the spread of this virus	Vary from nonexistent to mild, flulike symptoms to an incapacitating illness characterized by high fever, vomiting, and severe abdominal pain	Bed rest and adequate fluid intake; combination therapy with interferon and ribavarin possibly effective for hepatitis C infections
Pubic lice ("crabs") (p. 419)	*Phthirus pubis* spread easily through body contact or through shared clothing or bedding	Persistent itching; visible lice often located in pubic hair or other body hair	1% permethrin cream for body areas; 1% Lindane shampoo for hair
HIV/AIDS (p. 419)	HIV transmitted in blood and semen, primarily through sexual contact or needle sharing among injection drug users	Asymptomatic at first; opportunistic infections	Combination of three or more antiretroviral drugs (termed highly active antiretroviral therapies, or HAART) plus other specific treatment for opportunistic infections and tumors

American College Health Association, chlamydia and HPV have reached epidemic levels at many schools—although many of those infected aren't even aware of it.

In the National College Health Assessment, infection with human papilloma virus (HPV) was the most commonly reported STI on campus; 1.6 percent of students said they had HPV in the past school year. Chlamydia, reported by 1.4 percent, ranked second, while 0.8 percent of students had genital herpes and 0.6 had pelvic inflammatory disease.[18]

Rates of specific STIs vary by region. In California colleges, for instance, 3.8 percent of women and 3 percent of men had chlamydia.[19] (All of these infections are discussed in the following pages.) As noted in Table 14-5, about half of students used condoms the last time they had vaginal intercourse; less than a quarter used condoms for anal intercourse.[20]

Contracting STIs may increase the risk of being infected with HIV, and half of new HIV infections occur in

TABLE 14-5 CONDOM USE ON CAMPUS

Type of Sexual Activity	Students Using Condoms Last Time They Had Sex		
	Total	Women	Men
Oral intercourse	3.3%	2.9%	3.9%
Vaginal intercourse	48.6%	46.2%	53.9%
Anal intercourse	23%	17.3%	32.5%

Source: American College Health Association. "The American College Health Association's National College Health Assessment (ACHA-NCHA), Spring 2003 Reference Group Report." *Journal of American College Health,* Vol. 53, No. 5, March–April 2005, p. 199, www.acha.org.

people under age 25. Because college students have more opportunities to have different sexual partners and may use drugs and alcohol more often before sex, they are at greater risk. More than half of 13- to 24-year-old women with HIV are infected heterosexually.

Schools vary in the STI services, including screening, diagnosis, and treatment, that they offer. In a national survey, about half of colleges and universities made condoms available to students—some free in an open display, some free on request, and some for a fee or in vending machines. Larger schools, those with health centers, and those with on-campus housing are more likely to provide STI education and services.[21]

RISK FACTORS AND RISK CONTINUUMS

Various factors put young people at risk of STIs, including:

- **Feelings of invulnerability,** which lead to risk-taking behavior. Even when they are well informed of the risks, adolescents and young adults may remain unconvinced that anything bad can or will happen to them.
- **Multiple partners.** Figure 14-6 illustrates how STI risks increase as relationships become less

familiar and exclusive. In surveys of students, a significant minority report having had four or more sexual partners during their lifetime.

- **Failure to use condoms.** Among those who reported having had sexual intercourse in the previous three months, fewer than half reported condom use. Figure 14-7 shows the risk continuum for protected and nonprotected sexual behaviors. STI risks increase as sexual activities become unprotected and receptive. Students who'd had four or more sexual partners were significantly less likely to use condoms than those who'd had fewer partners.
- **Substance abuse.** Individuals who drink or use drugs are more likely to engage in sexually risky behaviors, including sex with partners whose health status and history they do not know, and unprotected intercourse.

Rate your own sexual health risk by taking the Self Survey on page 424.

Your Life Coach

Safer, Smarter Sex

How can you tell if someone you're dating or hope to date has been exposed to an STI? The bad news is you can't. But the good news is it doesn't matter—as long as you avoid sexual activity that could put you at risk of infection. Ideally, before engaging in any such behavior, both of you should talk about your prior sexual history (including number of partners and sexually transmitted infections) and other high-risk behavior, such as the use of injection drugs. If you know someone well enough to consider having sex with that person, you should be able to talk about STIs. If the person is unwilling to talk, you shouldn't have sex.

Keep in mind that no "protection" is 100 percent "safe." For instance, nonoxynol-9, the most widely used spermicide in the world, does not protect women from

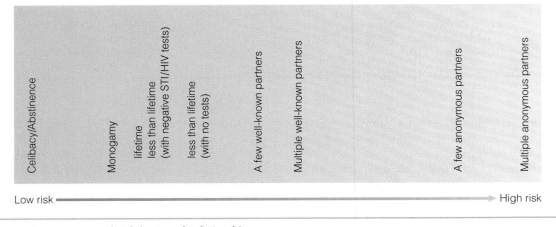

FIGURE 14-6 **Continuum of Risk for Sexual Relationships**
STI risks increase as relationships become less familiar and exclusive.

Noninsertive	Insertive and protected (condoms, other barriers)	Insertive and not protected (withdrawal)	Insertive, not protected, including ejaculation

Low risk ━━━━━━━━━━━━━━━━━━━━━━━━━━━━━━━━━▶ High risk

i = insertive partner
r = receptive partner

FIGURE 14-7   A Continuum of Risk for Sexual Behaviors
STI risks increase as sexual activities become unprotected and receptive.

gonorrhea or chlamydia. Here are some specific steps to lower your risk of STIs:

■ **Abstain.** Abstinence from vaginal and anal intercourse is free, available to everyone, extremely effective at preventing both pregnancy and sexually transmitted infections, and has no medical or hormonal side effects. Even without vaginal or anal penetration, other sexual activity such as oral sex can expose you to STIs.

■ **Practice monogamy.** For men and women who are sexually active, a mutually faithful sexual relationship with just one healthy partner is the safest option.

■ **If you are sexually active and are not in a mutually monogamous relationship, protect yourself:**

   ■ **Use a new condom** each and every time you engage in any form of intercourse.

   ■ **Do not use spermicide containing nonoxynol-9.** Contrary to past advice, experts now advise against choosing safer sex products with nonoxynol-9. According to recent research, nonoxynol-9 without condoms is ineffective against HIV transmission. Even with condoms, it does not protect women from the bacteria that cause gonorrhea and chlamydia.

   ■ **If a condom fails** during vaginal or anal intercourse, remove it carefully. If you continue sexual activity, replace it with a new condom.

   ■ **Make sure the package says that the condoms are meant to prevent disease.** If not, the condoms may not provide adequate protection, even though they may be the most expensive ones you can buy.

■ Because bacteria can be transmitted by hand, **wash your hands with hot water** and antibacterial soap after sex.

■ **If You Are A Women:**

   ■ Keep in mind that your risk of getting an infection is greater than a man's because a woman's vagina and rectum are more easily infected than a man's penis.

   ■ Don't think you don't have to worry just because you have no symptoms. Because many sexual infections are "silent" in women, you are less likely to know if you are infected and may have pelvic inflammatory disease, which puts you at risk of infertility and ectopic pregnancy.

   ■ At your check-up talk to your doctor about whether you should be tested for sexually transmitted infections. You need to ask for these tests, or else they won't be done.

■ **If You Are A Man:**

   ■ Use a new condom each and every time you engage in any form of intercourse. Try different brands to find the ones you like best.

   ■ After potential exposure to an STI, give yourself a little extra protection by urinating and washing your genitals with an antibacterial soap.

   ■ At your check-up talk to your doctor about whether you should be tested for sexually transmitted infections. You need to ask for these tests, or else they won't be done.

▪ **If you have oral sex,** make it safer by using effective barrier methods such as condoms or latex dental dams. In the absence of barrier methods, men should avoid ejaculating in their partners' mouths.

  ▪ **Be aware of sores and discharge or unpleasant odors** from your partner's genitals. These are signs to avoid oral sex.

  ▪ Don't floss or brush teeth before oral sex. It might tear the lining of the mouth, increasing exposure to viruses.

  ▪ **Avoid aggressive and deep thrusting in oral sex,** which can damage throat tissues and increase susceptibility for throat-based gonorrhea, herpes, and abrasions.

  ▪ **Remember that oral sex can transmit various STIs,** including herpes, gonorrhea, syphilis, and HIV.

About half of campuses in one national survey make condoms available to students—for free, on request, or in vending machines. Although condoms are one of the most effective forms of protection from sexually transmitted infections, some feel that providing condoms shows approval of casual sexual involvement. Should colleges encourage condom use by distributing them on campus? Or should condom use be a student's personal responsibility and choice? **You decide.**

CHLAMYDIA

The most widespread sexually transmitted bacterium in the United States is *Chlamydia trachomatis,* which causes an estimated 3 million cases of **chlamydia** each year.[22] One in 25 young Americans is infected with chlamydia, according to a recent nationwide study.

 Chlamydia is six times more prevalent in young black adults than in young white adults, with almost 14 percent of young black women and more than 11 percent of black men testing positive.[23] Chlamydial infections are more common in younger than in older women, and they also occur more often in both men and women with gonorrhea.

Those at greatest risk of chlamydial infection are individuals 25 years old or younger who engage in sex with more than one new partner within a two-month period and women who use birth control pills or other nonbarrier contraceptive methods. The U.S. Preventive Services Task Forces recommend regular screening for chlamydia for all sexually active women under age 25 and for older women with multiple sexual partners, a history of STIs, or inconsistent use of condoms.

As many as 75 percent of women and 50 percent of men with chlamydia have no symptoms or symptoms so mild that they don't seek medical attention. Without treatment, up to 40 percent of cases of chlamydia can lead to pelvic inflammatory disease, a serious infection of the woman's fallopian tubes that also can damage the ovaries and uterus. Also, women infected with chlamydia may have three to five times the risk of getting infected with HIV if exposed. Babies exposed to chlamydia in the birth canal during delivery can be born with pneumonia or with an eye infection called conjunctivitis, both of which can be dangerous unless treated early with antibiotics. Symptomless women who are screened and treated for chlamydial infection are almost 60 percent less likely than unscreened women to develop pelvic inflammatory disease. Chlamydia may also be linked to cervical cancer.[24]

The use of condoms with spermicide can reduce, but not eliminate, the risk of chlamydial infection. Sexual partners should be examined and treated if necessary. The CDC, in its most recent guidelines, recommends that all women with chlamydia be rescreened three to four months after treatment is completed. The reason is that re-infection, which often happens because a patient's sex partners were not treated, increases the risk of pelvic inflammatory disease and other complications. Immediately treating the partners of people infected with gonorrhea or chlamydia can reduce rates of recurrence of these infections.[25]

HUMAN PAPILLOMA VIRUS

Infection with **human papilloma virus (HPV),** a pathogen that can cause *genital warts,* is the most common viral STI. At least 15 percent of sexually active adults in the United States have genital HPV infection. The highest rates of HPV infection occur in young adults between ages 18 and 28. Young women who engage in sexual intercourse at an early age are more likely than those with later sexual debuts to become infected with HPV. Their risk also increases if they have multiple sexual partners or a history of a sexually transmitted disease, use drugs, or have partners with multiple sexual partners. An estimated 9.2 million young adults have been infected with HPV and could spread the virus.[26]

 College-age women are among those at greatest risk of acquiring HPV infection. In various studies conducted in college health centers, 10 to 46 percent of female students (mean age 20 to 22) had a cervical HPV infection—and increased risk of precancerous cell changes. Risk factors include smoking, use of oral contraceptives, multiple sex partners, anal as well as vaginal intercourse, alcohol consumption at the time of engaging in vaginal intercourse, and sex partners with a history of HPV.

HPV infections in young women tend to be of short

Human papilloma virus, which causes genital warts, is the most common viral STI.

(a) Herpes simplex virus (HSV-1) as a mouth sore; (b) Herpes simplex virus (HSV-2) as a genital sore.

duration. In a three-year study, 60 percent of 608 college women became infected with the virus; the average duration of infection was eight months. According to the researchers, many young women who get HPV may not require treatment, because the condition often regresses on its own.

HPV is transmitted primarily through vaginal, anal, and oral-genital sex. More than half of HPV-infected individuals do not develop any symptoms. After contact with an infected individual, genital warts may appear from three weeks to eighteen months, with an average period of about three months. The warts are treated by freezing, cauterization, chemicals, or surgical removal. Recurrences are common because the virus remains in the body.

HPV infection may invade the urethra and cause urinary obstruction and bleeding. It greatly increases a woman's risk of developing a precancerous condition called *cervical intraepithelial neoplasia,* which can lead to cervical cancer. There also is a strong association between HPV infections and cancer of the vagina, vulva, urethra, penis, and anus.

HPV may be the single most important risk factor in 95 percent of all cases of cervical cancer. Adolescent girls infected with HPV appear to be particularly vulnerable to developing cervical cancer. It is not known if HPV itself causes cancer or acts in conjunction with cofactors (such as other infections, smoking, or suppressed immunity).

Most HPV infections are asymptomatic in men, who may unwittingly increase their partners' risk. Men who test positive for HPV typically report significantly more sex partners than those who do not. A woman's risk of cervical cancer is strongly related to the number of her partner's current and lifetime female partners.[27] Women are five to eleven times as likely to get cervical cancer if their steady sexual partner has had 20 or more previous partners.

 Women who have had an HPV infection should examine their genitals regularly and get an annual Pap smear. However, this standard diag-

nostic test for cervical cancer doesn't identify HPV infection. A new laboratory test can detect the presence of HPV, including the high-risk types associated with the development of cervical cancer. The HPV DNA test does not test for cancer, but for the HPV viruses that can cause cell changes in the cervix. If left untreated, these changes can eventually lead to cancer in some women. Surgery or laser therapy can prevent further damage.

 HPV may also cause genital warts in men and increase the risk of cancer of the penis. HPV-infected men, who may not develop any symptoms, can spread the infection to their partners. People with visible genital warts also may have asymptomatic or subclinical HPV infections that are extremely difficult to treat.

No form of therapy has been shown to completely eradicate HPV, nor has any single treatment been uniformly effective in removing warts or preventing their recurrence. CDC guidelines suggest treatments that focus on the removal of visible warts—cryotherapy (freezing) and topical applications of podofilox, podophyllin, or trichloroacetic acid—and then eradication of the virus. At least 20 to 30 percent of treated individuals experience recurrence. In experimental studies, interferon, a biologic substance produced by virus-infected cells that inhibits viral replication, has proved helpful.

HERPES

Herpes (from the Greek word that means *to creep*) collectively describes some of the most common viral infections in humans. Characteristically, **herpes simplex** causes blisters on the skin or mucous membranes. Herpes simplex exists in several varieties. *Herpes simplex virus 1 (HSV-1)* generally causes cold sores and fever blisters around the mouth. *Herpes simplex virus 2 (HSV-2)* may cause blisters on the penis, inside the vagina, on the cervix, in the pubic area, on the buttocks, or on the thighs. With the increase of oral-genital sex, some doctors report finding type 2 herpes lesions in the mouth and throat.

Genital herpes has skyrocketed during the last three decades, yet only a minority of infections with HSV-2 are recognized by those infected. About 40 percent of new cases of genital herpes occur in young people ages 15 to 24. An estimated 4.2 million young adults in this age range—11 percent of the population—have been infected.[28]

Research has shown that individuals without any obvious symptoms shed the virus subclinically, whether or not they have lesions. Most people with herpes contract it from partners who were not aware of any symptoms or of their own contagiousness. Standard methods of diagnosing genital herpes in women, which rely primarily on physical examination and viral cultures, may miss as many as two-thirds of all cases. Newly developed blood tests are more effective in detecting unrecognized and subclinical infections with HSV-2.

In the past, patients and most doctors thought people with herpes could safely have unprotected sex when they had no symptoms. The herpes virus is present in genital secretions even when patients do not notice any signs of the disease, and people infected with genital herpes can spread it even between flare-ups when they have no symptoms. There is growing evidence that genital herpes promotes the spread of HIV.

HSV transmission occurs through close contact with mucous membranes or abraded skin. Condoms help prevent infection but aren't foolproof. When herpes sores are present, the infected person is highly contagious and should avoid bringing the lesions into contact with someone else's body through touching, sexual interaction, or kissing.

A newborn can be infected with genital herpes while passing through the birth canal, and the frequency of mother-to-infant transmission seems to be increasing. Most infected infants develop typical skin sores, which can be cultured to confirm a herpes diagnosis. Some physicians recommend treatment with acyclovir. Because of the risk of severe damage and possible death, caesarean delivery may be advised for a woman with active herpes lesions.

The virus that causes herpes never entirely goes away; it retreats to nerves near the lower spinal cord, where it remains for the life of the host. Herpes sores can return without warning weeks, months, or even years after their first occurrence, often during menstruation or times of stress, or with sudden changes in body temperature. Of those who experience HSV recurrence, 10 to 35 percent do so frequently—that is, about six or more times a year. In most people, attacks diminish in frequency and severity over time. Herpes, like other STIs, can trigger feelings of shame, guilt, and depression.

Antiviral drugs, such as acyclovir (Zovirax), have proven effective in treating and controlling herpes. Available as an ointment, in capsules, and in injection form,

acyclovir relieves the symptoms but doesn't kill the virus. Whereas the ointment works only for the initial bout with herpes, acyclovir in injectable and pill form dramatically reduces the length and severity of herpes outbreaks. Continuing daily oral acyclovir can reduce recurrences by about 80 percent. However, its safety in pregnant women has not been established. Infection with herpes viruses resistant to acyclovir is a growing problem, especially in individuals with immune-suppressing disorders.

Various treatments—compresses made with cold water, skim milk, or warm salt water; ice packs; or a mild anesthetic cream—can relieve discomfort. Herpes sufferers should avoid heat, hot baths, or nylon underwear. Some physicians have used laser therapy to vaporize the lesions. Clinical trials of an experimental vaccine to protect people from herpes infections are underway.

PELVIC INFLAMMATORY DISEASE

Infection of a woman's fallopian tubes or uterus, called **pelvic inflammatory disease (PID),** is not actually an STI, but rather a complication of STIs. About one in every seven women of reproductive age has PID; half of all adult women may have had it. Each year, about 1 million new cases are reported.

Ten to 20 percent of initial episodes of PID lead to scarring and obstruction of the fallopian tubes severe enough to cause infertility. Other long-term complications are ectopic pregnancy and chronic pelvic pain. The risk of these complications rises with subsequent PID episodes, bacterial vaginosis (discussed earlier in this chapter), and use of an IUD. Smoking also may increase the likelihood of PID. Two bacteria—gonococcus (the culprit in gonorrhea) and chlamydia—are responsible for one-half to one-third of all cases of PID. Other organisms are responsible for the remaining cases.

Most cases of PID occur among women under age 25 who are sexually active. Gonococcus-caused cases tend to affect poor women; those caused by chlamydia range across all income levels. One-half to one-third of all cases are transmitted sexually, and others have been traced to some IUDs that are no longer on the market. Several studies have shown that women with PID are more likely to have used douches than those without the disease. Consistent condom use may decrease PID risk.

PID is a silent disease that in half of all cases produces no noticeable symptoms as it progresses and causes scarring of the fallopian tubes. Experts are encouraging women with mild symptoms, such as abdominal pain or tenderness, to seek medical evaluation and are encouraging physicians to test these patients for infections. Urine testing is a cost-effective method of detecting gonorrhea and chlamydia in young women and can prevent development of PID. For women with symptoms, magnetic resonance imaging (MRI) is highly accurate in establishing a diagnosis of PID and detecting other diseases that may be responsible for the symptoms. Treatment may require hospitalization and intensive antibiotics therapy. PID causes an estimated 15 to 30 percent of all cases of infertility every year and about half of all cases of ectopic pregnancy.

GONORRHEA

Gonorrhea (sometimes called "the clap" in street language) is one of the most common STIs in the United States. After steady declines from the 1970s to the late 1990s, gonorrhea infections have increased, with about 60 percent of new cases occurring in young adults.[29] The incidence is highest among teenagers and young adults. Sexual contact, including oral-genital sex, is the primary means of transmission.

Most men who have gonorrhea know it. Thick, yellow-white pus oozes from the penis and urination causes a burning sensation. These symptoms usually develop two to nine days after the sexual contact that infected them. Men have a good reason to seek help: It hurts too much not to. Women also may experience discharge and burning on urination. However, as many as eight out of ten infected women have no symptoms.

Gonococcus, the bacterium that causes gonorrhea, can live in the vagina, cervix, and fallopian tubes for months, even years, and continue to infect the woman's sexual partners. Approximately 5 percent of sexually active American women have positive gonorrhea cultures but are unaware that they are silent carriers.

If left untreated in men or women, gonorrhea spreads through the urinary-genital tract. In women, the inflammation travels from the vagina and cervix, through the uterus, to the fallopian tubes and ovaries. The pain and fever are similar to those caused by stomach upset, so a woman may dismiss the symptoms. Eventually these symptoms diminish, even though the disease spreads to the entire pelvis. Pus may ooze from the fallopian tubes or ovaries into the peritoneum (the lining of the abdominal cavity), sometimes causing serious inflammation. However, this, too, can subside in a few weeks. Gonorrhea, the leading cause of sterility in women, can cause PID. In pregnant women, gonorrhea becomes a threat to the newborn. It can infect the infant's external genitals and cause a serious form of conjunctivitis, an inflammation of the eye that may lead to blindness. As a preventive step, newborns may have penicillin dropped into their eyes at birth.

In men, untreated gonorrhea can spread to the prostate gland, testicles, bladder, and kidneys. Among the serious complications are urinary obstruction and sterility caused by blockage of the vas deferens (the excretory duct of the testis). In both sexes, gonorrhea can develop into a serious, even fatal, bloodborne infection that can cause arthritis in the joints, attack the heart muscle and lining, cause meningitis, and attack the skin and other organs.

Although a blood test has been developed for detecting gonorrhea, the tried-and-true method of diagnosis is still a microscopic analysis of cultures from the male's urethra, the female's cervix, and the throat and anus of both sexes.

Because gonorrhea often occurs along with chlamydia, practitioners often prescribe an agent effective against both, such as ofloxacin. In some parts of the United States, gonorrhea has become so resistant to certain antibiotics such as fluoroguinolone that they are no longer advised for use in its treatment.[30] Antibiotics taken for other reasons may not affect or cure gonorrhea because of their dosage or type. And you can't develop immunity to gonorrhea; within days of recovering from one case, you can catch another.

NONGONOCOCCAL URETHRITIS

The term **nongonococcal urethritis (NGU)** refers to any inflammation of the urethra that is not caused by gonorrhea. NGU is the most common STI in men, accounting for 4 to 6 million visits to a physician every year. Three microorganisms—*Chlamydia trachomatis, Ureaplasma urealyticum,* and *Mycoplasma genitalium*—are the primary causes; the usual means of transmission is sexual intercourse. Other infectious agents, such as fungi or bacteria, allergic reactions to vaginal secretions, or irritation by soaps or contraceptive foams or gels also may lead to NGU.

In the United States, NGU is more common in men than gonococcal urethritis. The symptoms in men are similar to those of gonorrhea, including discharge from the penis (usually less than with gonorrhea) and mild burning during urination. Women frequently develop no symptoms or very mild itching, burning during urination, or discharge. Symptoms usually disappear after two or three weeks, but the infection may persist and cause cervicitis or PID in women and, in men, may spread to the prostate, epididymis, or both. Treatment usually consists

© Science VU/Visuals Unlimited

A cloudy discharge is symptomatic of gonorrhea.

of doxycycline or azithromycin and should be given to both sexual partners after testing.

SYPHILIS

A corkscrew-shaped, spiral bacterium called *Treponema pallidum* causes **syphilis.** This frail microbe dies in seconds if dried or chilled but grows quickly in the warm, moist tissues of the body, particularly in the mucous membranes of the genital tract. Entering the body through any tiny break in the skin, the germ burrows its way into the bloodstream. Sexual contact, including oral sex or intercourse, is a primary means of transmission. Genital ulcers caused by syphilis may increase the risk of HIV infection, while individuals with HIV may be more likely to develop syphilis.

Public education programs, expanded screening and surveillance, increased tracing of contacts, and condom promotion have helped control the spread of syphilis in some areas. Syphilis rates have fallen to the lowest ever reported in the United States. The decline has been particularly significant in African Americans and people living in the South.

Syphilis has clearly identifiable stages:

- **Primary syphilis.** The first sign of syphilis is a lesion, or *chancre* (pronounced "shanker"), an open lump or crater the size of a dime or smaller, teeming with bacteria. The incubation period before its appearance ranges from 10 to 90 days; three to four weeks is average. The chancre appears exactly where the bacteria entered the body: in the mouth, throat, vagina, rectum, or penis. Any contact with the chancre is likely to result in infection.

- **Secondary syphilis.** Anywhere from one to twelve months after the chancre's appearance, secondary-stage symptoms may appear. Some people have no symptoms. Others develop a skin rash or a small, flat rash in moist regions on the skin; whitish patches on the mucous membranes of the mouth or throat; temporary baldness; low-grade fever; headache; swollen glands; or large, moist sores around the mouth and genitals. These are loaded with bacteria; contact with them, through kissing or intercourse, may transmit the infection. Symptoms may last for several days or several months. Even without treatment, symptoms eventually disappear as the syphilis microbes go into hiding.

- **Latent syphilis.** Although there are no signs or symptoms, no sores or rashes at this stage, the bacteria are invading various organs inside the body, including the heart and brain. For two to four years, there may be recurring infectious and highly contagious lesions of the skin or mucous membranes. However, syphilis loses its infectiousness as it progresses: After the first two years, a person rarely transmits syphilis through intercourse.

  After four years, even congenital syphilis is rarely transmitted. Until this stage of the disease, however, a pregnant woman can pass syphilis to her unborn child. If the fetus is infected in its fourth month or earlier, it may be disfigured or even die. If infected late in pregnancy, the child may show no signs of infection for months or years after birth, but may then become disabled with the symptoms of tertiary syphilis.

- **Tertiary syphilis.** Ten to 20 years after the beginning of the latent stage, the most serious symptoms of syphilis emerge, generally in the organs in which the bacteria settled during latency. Syphilis that has progressed to this stage has become increasingly rare. Victims of tertiary syphilis may die of a ruptured aorta or of other heart damage, or may have progressive brain or spinal cord damage, eventually leading to blindness, insanity, or paralysis. About a third of those who are not treated during the first three stages of syphilis enter the tertiary stage later in life.

Health experts are urging screening for syphilis for everyone who seeks treatment for an STI, especially adolescents; for everyone using illegal drugs; and for the partners of these two groups. They also recommend that anyone diagnosed with syphilis be screened for other STIs and be counseled about voluntary testing for HIV.

Penicillin is the drug of choice for treating primary, secondary, and latent syphilis. The earlier treatment begins, the more effective it is. Those allergic to penicillin may be treated with doxycycline, ceftriaxone, or erythromycin. An added danger of not getting treatment for syphilis is an increased risk of HIV transmission.

CHANCROID

A **chancroid** is a soft, painful sore or localized infection caused by the bacterium *Haemophilus ducrevi* and usually acquired through sexual contact. Half of the cases heal by themselves. In other cases, the infection may spread to the lymph glands near the chancroid, where large amounts of pus can accumulate and destroy much of the local tissue. The incidence of this STI, widely prevalent in Africa and tropical and semitropical regions, is rapidly increasing in the United States, with outbreaks in several states, including Louisiana, Texas, and New York. Chancroids, which may increase susceptibility to HIV infection, are believed to be a major factor in the heterosexual spread of HIV. This infection is treated with antibiotics (ceftriaxone, azithromycin, or erythromycin)

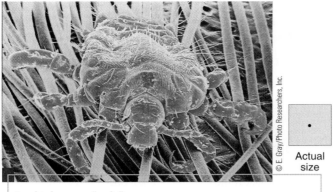

A pubic louse, or "crab."

and can be prevented by keeping the genitals clean and washing them with soap and water in case of possible exposure.

PUBIC LICE AND SCABIES

These infections are sometimes, but not always, transmitted sexually. *Pubic lice* (or "crabs") are usually found in the pubic hair, although they can migrate to any hairy areas of the body. Lice lay eggs called nits that attach to the base of the hair shaft. Irritation from the lice may produce intense itching. Scratching to relieve the itching can produce sores. *Scabies* is caused by a mite that burrows under the skin, where they lay eggs that hatch and undergo many changes in the course of their life cycle, producing great discomfort, including intense itching.

Lice and scabies are treated with applications of permethrin cream and Lindane shampoo to all the areas of the body where there are concentrations of body hair (genitals, armpits, scalp). You must repeat treatment in seven days to kill any newly developed adults. Wash or dry-clean clothing and bedding.

HIV AND AIDS

Thirty years ago, no one knew about **human immuno-deficiency virus (HIV).** No one had ever heard of **acquired immune deficiency syndrome (AIDS).** Once seen as an epidemic affecting primarily gay men and injection drug users, AIDS has taken on a very different form. Today, heterosexuals in developing countries have the highest rates of infection and mortality. And HIV infection continues to spread, doubling at an estimated rate of every ten years.

About 39.4 million people worldwide are infected with HIV; 15,000 more individuals are infected every day. AIDS now claims about 3 million lives—more than half children—around the world a year.[31] According to the CDC, 1,039,000 to 1,185,000 people are living with HIV or AIDS

in the United States, with about 40,000 new infections every year.[32]

Federal health officials fear that a new generation may not be using adequate safer sex precautions, because they have grown complacent about the dangers of HIV/AIDS. Efforts to prevent sexual transmission of HIV have taken a new focus: counseling those who already have HIV in an attempt to get them to stop spreading it.

Breakthrough drugs are indeed allowing HIV-infected people to live longer. However, new dangers have emerged. Up to 15 percent of new HIV cases in the country may stem from drug-resistant strains of the virus. "Superinfection" with more than one strain of HIV seems more common than previously thought. As a result, HIV-infected people who initially were doing well without drugs may become ill after contracting a second strain of the AIDS virus.

Efforts to prevent nonsexual forms of HIV transmission have been very effective. Screening the blood supply has reduced the rate of transfusion-associated HIV transmission by 99.9 percent. Treatment with antiretroviral drugs during pregnancy and birth has reduced transmission by about 90 percent in optimal conditions. Among drug users in some settings, programs that combine addiction treatment and needle exchange reduced the incidence of HIV infection by 30 percent.

Men who have sex with men now account for 57 percent of AIDS diagnoses among men. Homosexual and bisexual men, particularly those who are young or of color and living in metropolitan areas, are at particularly high risk. The percentage of individuals who acquired HIV through heterosexual contact has increased to 31 percent. However, many heterosexual adults are not aware of their partners' HIV status and may not see themselves as being at risk of HIV infection. According to the CDC, about a third of the HIV-infected individuals in the United States have not been diagnosed.

 African Americans and Latinos account for a disproportionate share of new AIDS diagnoses (Figure 14-8). Almost half of all living with HIV/AIDS in the United States are African American. The AIDS case rate per 100,000 people is 9.5 times that of whites. African Americans are less likely to survive after a diagnosis of AIDS than other ethnic or racial groups. HIV/AIDS is the third leading cause of death among African Americans between ages 25 and 34 and the sixth leading cause of death for whites and Latinos in this age group.

Although HIV/AIDS is often seen as a threat to men, more than a quarter of new HIV infections in the United States occur among women. About a quarter of Americans living with HIV/AIDS are women. Women of color, particularly African Americans, have been hardest hit. While African-American women make up just 13 percent of the female population of the United States, they account for 67 percent of newly diagnosed cases. HIV/AIDS is most prevalent among women in their childbearing years.[33]

 Epidemiologists have identified outbreaks of HIV in men on campuses in several southern states, with most occurring in North Carolina. All but two of the

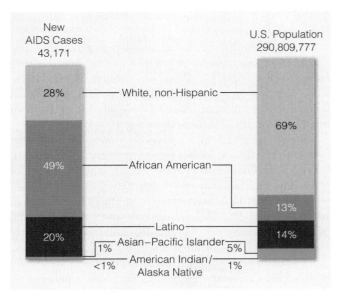

FIGURE 14-8 **The Impact of AIDS by Race**

Racial and ethnic minorities have been disproportionately affected by HIV/AIDS since the beginning of the epidemic, and minority Americans now represent the majority of new AIDS cases and of those living with AIDS.

Source: "The HIV/AIDS Epidemic in the United States." *Kaiser Family Foundation HIV/AIDS Policy Fact Sheet,* September 2005. This information is reprinted with permission from the Henry J. Kaiser Family Foundation. The Kaiser Family Foundation, based in Menlo Park, California, is a nonprofit, independent health care philanthropy and is not associated with Kaiser Permanente or Kaiser Industries.

men had sex at least once with another man, but they typically did not consider themselves gay or bisexual. The majority were black, met sexual partners on the Internet, used ecstasy or club drugs, and were 34 times more likely than noncollege men to have sex with other college students.[34] Following these outbreaks, HIV/AIDS infection among young heterosexual black women in North Carolina rose to a rate 14 times higher than that for whites in the same age range.[35]

REDUCING THE RISK OF HIV TRANSMISSION

HIV/AIDS can be so frightening that some people have exaggerated its dangers, whereas others understate them. The fact is that although no one is immune to HIV, you can reduce the risk if you abstain from sexual activity, remain in a monogamous relationship with an uninfected partner, and do not inject drugs.

If you're not in a long-term monogamous relationship with a partner you're sure is safe, and you're not willing to abstain from sex, there are things you can do to lower your risk of HIV infection. Remember that the risk of HIV transmission depends on sexual behavior, not sexual orientation. Among young men, the prevalence and frequency of sexual risk behaviors are similar regardless of sexual orientation, ethnicity, or age. Homosexual, heterosexual, and bisexual

individuals all need to know about the kinds of sexual activity that increase their risk.

Here's what you should know about HIV transmission:

- Casual contact does *not* spread HIV infection. You cannot get HIV infection from drinking from a water fountain, contact with a toilet seat, or touching an infected person.
- Compared to other viruses, HIV is extremely difficult to get.
- HIV can live in blood, semen, vaginal fluids, and breast milk.
- Many chemicals, including household bleach, alcohol, and hydrogen peroxide, can inactivate HIV.
- In studies of family members sharing dishes, food, clothing, and frequent hugs with people with HIV infection or AIDS, those who have contracted the virus have shared razor blades, toothbrushes, or had other means of blood contact.
- You cannot tell visually whether a potential sexual partner has HIV. A blood test is needed to detect the antibodies that the body produces to fight HIV, thus indicating infection.
- HIV can be spread in semen and vaginal fluids during a single instance of anal, vaginal, or oral sexual contact between heterosexuals, bisexuals, or homosexuals. The risk increases with the number of sexual encounters with an infected partner.
- Teenage girls may be particularly vulnerable to HIV infection because the immature cervix is easily infected.
- Anal intercourse is an extremely high-risk behavior because HIV can enter the bloodstream through tiny breaks in the lining of the rectum. HIV transmission is much more likely to occur during unprotected anal intercourse than vaginal intercourse.
- Other behaviors that increase the risk of HIV infection include having multiple sexual partners, engaging in sex without condoms or virus-killing spermicides, sexual contact with persons known to be at high risk (for example, prostitutes or injection drug users), and sharing injection equipment for drugs.
- Individuals are at greater risk if they have an active sexual infection. Sexually transmitted infections, such as herpes, gonorrhea, and syphilis, facilitate transmission of HIV during vaginal or rectal intercourse.
- No cases of HIV transmission by deep kissing have been reported, but it could happen. Studies have found blood in the saliva of healthy people after kissing; other lab studies have found HIV in saliva. Social (dry) kissing is safe.
- Oral sex can lead to HIV transmission. The virus in any semen that enters the mouth could make its way into the bloodstream through tiny nicks or

sores in the mouth. A man's risk in performing oral sex on a woman is smaller because an infected woman's genital fluids have much lower concentrations of HIV than does semen.

▮ HIV infection is not widespread among lesbians, although there have been documented cases of possible female-to-female HIV transmission. In each instance, one partner had had sex with a bisexual man or male injection drug user or had injected drugs herself.

HIV INFECTION

HIV infection refers to a spectrum of health problems that results from immunologic abnormalities caused by the virus when it enters the bloodstream. In theory, the body may be able to resist infection by HIV. In reality, in almost all cases, HIV destroys the cell-mediated immune system, particularly the CD4+ T-lymphocytes (also called *T4 helper cells*). The result is greatly increased susceptibility to various cancers and opportunistic infections (infections that take hold because of the reduced effectiveness of the immune system).

Researchers now know that HIV triggers a state of all-out war within the immune system. Almost immediately following infection with HIV, the immune system responds aggressively by manufacturing enormous numbers of CD4+ cells. It eventually is overwhelmed, however, as the viral particles continue to replicate, or multiply. The intense war between HIV and the immune system indicates that the virus itself, not a breakdown in the immune system, is responsible for disease progression.

Shortly after becoming infected with HIV, individuals may experience a few days of flulike symptoms, which most ignore or attribute to other viruses. Some people develop a more severe mononucleosis-type syndrome. After this stage, individuals may not develop any signs or symptoms of disease for a period ranging from weeks to more than 12 years.

HIV symptoms, which tend to increase in severity and number the longer the virus is in the body, may include any of the following:

▮ Swollen lymph nodes.

▮ Fever, chills, and night sweats.

▮ Diarrhea.

▮ Weight loss.

▮ Coughing and shortness of breath.

▮ Persistent tiredness.

▮ Skin sores.

▮ Blurred vision and headaches.

▮ Development of other infections, such as certain kinds of pneumonia.

HIV infection is associated with a variety of HIV-related diseases, including different cancers and dangerous infections, including tuberculosis. HIV-infected individuals may develop persistent generalized lymphadenopathy, enlargement of the lymph nodes at two or more different sites in the body.

Electron micrograph of a white blood cell being attacked by HIV (*light blue particles*), the virus that causes AIDS.

This condition typically persists for more than three months without any other illness to explain its occurrence. Diminished mental function may appear before other symptoms. Tests conducted on infected but apparently healthy men have revealed impaired coordination, problems in thinking, or abnormal brain scans.

HIV TESTING

Nearly half of American adults over age 18 have been tested for HIV. In general, minorities are more likely to have sought testing than whites.[36] In one study of 246 sexually active heterosexual college students, 21 percent had been tested for HIV, and most had disclosed the results to their intimate partners. Five percent admitted to telling a potential partner that they were HIV-negative, even though they had not been tested.[37] About 11,600 facilities provide publicly funded HIV testing and counseling in the United States; approximately 2 million tests are performed annually at these sites.

All HIV tests measure antibodies, cells produced by the body to fight HIV infection. A negative test indicates no exposure to HIV. It can take three to six months for the body to produce the telltale antibodies, however, so a negative result may not be accurate, depending on the timing of the test.

HIV testing can be either confidential or anonymous. In confidential testing, a person's name is recorded along with the test results, which are made available to medical personnel and, in 32 states, the state health department. In anonymous testing, no name is associated with the test results. Anonymous testing is available in 39 states.

 Different groups of individuals at risk prefer different tests. Asian–Pacific Islander and white men who have sex with men are most likely to choose anonymous testing; African-American men who have sex with men are much more likely to choose confidential test-

Lennart Nilsson © Boehringer Ingelheim International GmbH

ing. Consumers must be wary of bogus HIV tests offered via the Internet.

The following HIV tests are currently available in the United States:

- **EIA** (enzyme immune assay) or **ELISA** (enzyme-linked immunosorbent assay). These standard blood tests are the most commonly used HIV screens. A health-care provider draws a blood sample, which is analyzed for antibodies produced to fight against HIV particles. Results are available within a few days to two weeks.

- **Oral HIV tests.** These tests have become available in some doctors' offices and health clinics. A health-care worker swabs a tissue sample from the inside of the mouth. The only oral test approved by the Food and Drug Administration (FDA) is the OraSure.

- **Rapid tests.** Different types, such as the OraQuick Rapid HIV-1/2 Antibody Test, can detect HIV antibodies in blood or oral fluid. The advantage is fast results—usually in 20 or 30 minutes.

- **Western blot.** This more accurate and expensive test is used to confirm the results of a positive HIV test.

- **HomeAccess.** This test—the only home HIV test approved by the FDA—is available in drug stores or online for $40 to $50. An individual draws a blood sample by pricking a finger and sends it to a laboratory along with a personal identification number. Results are given over the phone by a trained counselor, usually within several days.

- **Urine test.** This alternative to a blood test must be ordered by a health-care provider. A urine sample is screened by a laboratory. Results are generally available in a few days to two weeks.

Newly developed blood tests can determine how recently a person was infected with HIV and distinguish between long-standing infections and those contracted within the previous four to six months.

DIAGNOSING AIDS

A diagnosis of AIDS applies to anyone with HIV whose immune system is severely impaired, as indicated by a CD4 count of less than 200 cells per cubic millimeter of blood, compared to normal CD4 cell counts in healthy people not infected with HIV of 800 to 1,200 per cubic millimeter of blood. In addition, AIDS is diagnosed in persons with HIV infection who experience recurrent pneumonia, invasive cervical cancer, or pulmonary tuberculosis.

People with AIDS also may experience persistent fever, diarrhea that persists for more than one month, or involuntary weight loss of more than 10 percent of normal body weight. Neurological disease—including dementia (confusion and impaired thinking) and other problems with thinking, speaking, movement, or sensation—may occur. Secondary infectious diseases that may develop in people with AIDS include *Pneumocystis carinii* pneumonia, tuberculosis, or oral candidiasis (thrush). Secondary cancers associated with HIV infection include Kaposi's sarcoma and cancer of the cervix.

TREATING HIV/AIDS

New forms of therapy have been remarkably effective in boosting levels of protective T cells and reducing *viral load*—the amount of HIV in the bloodstream. People with high viral loads are more likely to progress rapidly to AIDS than people with low levels of the virus.

The current "gold-standard" approach to combating HIV is known as HAART (highly active antiretroviral therapies), which dramatically reduces viral load even though it does not eradicate the virus. This complex regimen uses one of 250 different combinations of three or more antiretroviral drugs. Since the development of HAART, the number of deaths among persons with AIDS in the United States has declined by 70 percent, and the number of those living with AIDS has risen.

Because HAART can drastically lower viral load, there is some evidence that it also may reduce the risk of infectiousness of HIV-positive individuals. Fearing that this could lead to unsafe sex, researchers did a meta-analysis of

Strategies for Prevention :: Should I Be Tested for HIV?

Health officials recommend HIV testing for the following individuals:

- Men who have had sex with other men, regardless of whether they consider themselves homosexual.
- Anyone who uses injection drugs or has shared needles.
- Anyone who has had sex with someone who uses injection drugs or has shared needles.

- Women who have had sex with bisexual men.
- Anyone who has had sex with someone from an area with a high incidence of HIV infection.
- Individuals who have had sex with people they do not know well.

- Individuals diagnosed with an STI such as chlamydia or gonorrhea.
- Anyone who received blood transfusions or blood products between 1978 and 1985, their sexual partners, and, if they are new mothers, their infants.

HAART recipients and found no increased sexual risk behavior. Even when HIV levels are undetectable, they note, this does not mean the infected person is "cured," nor does it eliminate the possibility of transmitting HIV.

In the last two years, several new drugs have become available, and many of these antiretroviral agents can be taken just once or twice a day, rather than more. New antiretroviral agents and new types of drugs are currently in clinical trials. Work is also continuing toward an AIDS vaccine. As more effective therapies have emerged, there has been a major shift in attitude: Physicians are more optimistic about long-term treatments, and hope is replacing despair as more individuals are living productive lives with HIV.

Learn It / Live It

The Best Defense

Some day medical science may develop vaccines or other means of providing total protection against infectious diseases. Until then your best defense is to take commonsense steps to promote well-being and reduce the risks of infection. Here are some basic principles of self-defense:

- **Eat a balanced diet** to be sure you get essential vitamins and minerals. Severe deficiencies in vitamins B_6, B_{12}, and folic acid impair immunity. Keep up your iron and zinc intake. Iron influences the number and vigor of certain immune cells, whereas zinc is crucial for cell repair. Too little vitamin C also may increase susceptibility to infectious diseases.
- **Avoid fatty foods.** A low-fat diet can increase the activity of immune cells that hunt down and knock out cells infected with viruses.
- **Get enough sleep.** Without adequate rest, your immune system cannot maintain and renew itself.
- **Exercise regularly.** Aerobic exercise stimulates the production of an immune-system booster called interleukin-2.
- **Don't smoke.** Smoking decreases the levels of some immune cells and increases susceptibility to respiratory infections.
- **Control your alcohol intake.** Heavy drinking interferes with normal immune responses and lowers the number of defender cells.
- **Wash your hands frequently** with hot water and soap. In a public restroom, use a paper towel to turn off the faucet after you wash your hands, and avoid touching the doorknob. Wash objects used by someone with a cold.
- **Don't share food, drinks, silverware, glasses,** and other objects that may carry infectious microbes.
- **Spend as little time as possible in crowds** during cold and flu season, especially closed

places, such as elevators and airplanes. When out, keep your distance from sneezers and coughers.

- **Don't touch your eyes, mouth, and nose** after being with someone who has cold symptoms.
- **Use tissues** rather than cloth handkerchiefs, which may harbor viruses for hours or days.
- **Avoid irritating air pollutants** whenever possible.
- **Always use safer sex practices.**
- **Get tested immediately** if you have any reason to suspect that you may have been exposed to an STI.

Making This Chapter Work for You

Review Questions

1. Which of the following statements about disease-causing microbes is *false?*
   a. Helminths cause malaria, one of the major worldwide diseases.
   b. AIDS is caused by a retrovirus.
   c. In the United States, the most common protozoan disease is giardiasis.
   d. Salmonella is a foodborne illness caused by bacteria.

2. Which of the following statements about the immune system is *false?*
   a. The immune system has two types of white blood cells: B cells, which produce antibodies that fight bacteria and viruses, and T-cells, which protect against parasites, fungi, and cancer cells.
   b. Immune system structures include the spleen, tonsils, thymus gland, and lymph nodes located throughout the body.
   c. Inoculation with a vaccine confers active immunity.
   d. The effect of stress on the human immune system depends on whether you can control the stressor and on the mental effort required to cope.

3. College students should have all of the following immunizations *except*
   a. hepatitis A.
   b. hepatitis B.
   c. measles.
   d. tetanus.

4. Which of the following statements about the common cold and influenza is true?
   a. Influenza is just a more severe form of the common cold.
   b. Aspirin should be avoided by children and young adults who have a cold or influenza.

(continued on p. 426)

Self Survey ▪ Assessing Your STI Risk

This Self Survey looks at your risk of acquiring or transmitting any sexually transmitted infection (STI).

STI Quiz

1. **True** or **False:** A person can have an STI and not know it.
2. **True** or **False:** It is normal for women to have some vaginal discharge.
3. **True** or **False:** Once you have had an STI and have been cured, you can't get it again.
4. **True** or **False:** HIV is mainly present in semen, blood, vaginal secretions, and breast milk.
5. **True** or **False:** Chlamydia and gonorrhea can cause pelvic inflammatory disease.
6. **True** or **False:** A pregnant woman who has an STI can pass the disease on to her baby.
7. **True** or **False:** Most STIs go away without treatment, if people wait long enough.
8. **True** or **False:** STIs that aren't cured early can cause sterility.
9. **True** or **False:** Birth control pills offer excellent protection from STIs.
10. **True** or **False:** Condoms can help prevent the spread of STIs.
11. **True** or **False:** If you know your partner, you can't get an STI.
12. **True** or **False:** Chlamydia is the most common bacterial STI.
13. **True** or **False:** A sexually active woman should get an annual pap test from her doctor.

Answers

1. **True** Some of the most common symptoms of an STI infection include: Abnormal discharge, painful urination, burning, itching or tingling in the genital area, but it is important to remember that many women and men who have an STI often do not experience any symptoms at all. Chlamydia, for example, often has no symptoms.

2. **True** Normal vaginal discharge has several purposes: cleaning and moistening the vagina and helping to prevent and fight infections. Although it's normal for the color, texture, and amount of vaginal fluids to vary throughout a woman's menstrual cycle, some changes in discharge may indicate a problem.

   If you think you may have a problem, you should see a doctor as soon as possible. First, though, it helps to learn some of the differences between what is normal and abnormal vaginal discharge for you.

3. **False** Having an STI and being cured from it does not mean that your body now has a built in immunity to the bacteria that causes the infection. You must protect yourself from becoming infected again by using a condom. Remember, it is your body!

4. **True** Although small traces of HIV can be found in tears, saliva, urine and perspiration, extensive studies have shown that there is not enough of the virus or the virus is not strong enough to be transmitted. Only blood, semen, vaginal secretions, and breast milk have been proven to transmit the HIV virus and Hepatitis B. HIV cannot be passed on by casual contact.

5. **True** Many different organisms can cause PID, but most cases are associated with gonorrhea and genital chlamydial infections, two very common STIs. Scientists have found that bacteria normally present in small numbers in the vagina and cervix also may play a role.

6. **True** STIs can be passed from a pregnant woman to the baby before, during, or after the baby's birth. Some STIs (like syphilis) cross the placenta and infect the baby while it is in the uterus (womb). Other STIs (like gonorrhea, chlamydia, hepatitis B, and genital herpes) can be transmitted from the mother to the baby during delivery as the baby passes through the birth canal. HIV can cross the placenta during pregnancy, infect the baby during the birth process, and unlike most other STIs, can infect the baby through breastfeeding.

7. **False** Even if symptoms appear to go away, the infected person will still have the infection and is able to pass the infection on to others until he/she gets treatment. STIs that aren't cured early can cause sterility.

8. **True** If the fallopian tubes are blocked at one or both ends, the egg can't travel through the tubes into the uterus. Blocked tubes may result from pelvic inflammatory disease, which is often caused by untreated STIs.

9. **False** The birth control pill does not protect against sexually transmitted infections. For those having sex, condoms must always be used along with birth control pills to protect against STIs. Abstinence (the decision to not have sex) is the only method that always prevents pregnancy and sexually transmitted infections.

10. **True** Most condoms are made of latex. Those made of lambskin may offer less protection against some sexually transmitted infections, including HIV, so use of latex condoms is recommended. For people who may have an allergic skin reaction to latex, both male and female condoms made of polyurethane are available.

   When properly used, latex and plastic condoms are effective against most STIs. Condoms do not protect against infections spread from sores on the skin not covered by a condom (such as the base of the penis or scrotum).

11. **False** As stated in question number 1, a person can have an STI and not know it. If they can't tell, how can you?

12. **True** The U.S. Centers for Disease Control and Prevention estimates that more than 4 million new cases of chlamydia occur each year. The highest rates of chlamydial infection are in 15- to 19-year-old adolescents regardless of demographics or location.

13. **True** The Pap test is a way to find cell changes on the cervix. Abnormal cells may lead to cancer, so having a Pap test can find and treat them early, before they have time to progress to cancer.

   Although Pap tests do not test for STIs, some STIs such as HPV (human papillomavirus infection) can cause abnormal Pap test results. Certain types of HPV are linked to cancer in both women and men.

Copyright 2002 by SmarterSex.org.

YOUR ACTION PLAN FOR COPING WITH STIS

What to Do If You Have an STI

▪ If you suspect that you have an STI, don't feel too embarrassed to get help through a physician's office or a clinic. Treatment relieves discomfort, prevents complications, and halts the spread of the disease.

▪ Following diagnosis, take oral medication (which may be given instead of or in addition to shots) exactly as prescribed.

▪ Try to figure out from whom you got the STI. Be sure to inform that person, who may not be aware of the problem.

▪ If you have an STI, never deceive a prospective partner about it. Tell the truth—simply and clearly. Be sure your partner understands exactly what you have and what the risks are.

Telling a Partner You Have an STI

Even though the conversation can be awkward and embarrassing, you need to talk honestly about any STI that you may have been exposed to or contracted. What you don't say can be hazardous to your partner's health. Here are some guidelines:

▪ **Talk before you become intimate.** A good way to start is simply by saying, *"There is something we need to talk over first."*

▪ **Be honest.** Don't downplay any potential risks.

▪ **Don't blame.** Even if you suspect that your partner was the source of your infection, focus on the need for medical attention.

▪ **Be sensitive to your partner's feelings.** Anger and resentment are common reactions when someone feels at risk. Try to listen without becoming defensive.

▪ **Seek medical attention.** Do not engage in sexual intimacies until you obtain a doctor's assurance that you are no longer contagious.

Source: Bacchus and Gamma Peer Education Network, www.smartersex.org.

CASE IN POINT

Student: Brady, 26

Goal: Tell a potential partner that he has a history of human papillomavirus (HPV) infection

Action Plan:

▪ Become thoroughly infomed about HPV and its risks to both himself and female partners

▪ Get regular testing for asymptomatic HPV

▪ Seek prompt treatment in case of a recurrence of visible warts

▪ Talk to his physician about preventing transmission

▪ Bring up the subject before the couple becomes intimate

Health(🕭)Now™ If you want to write your own goals for preventing infectious diseases, go to the **Wellness Journal HealthNow** at http://healthnow.brookscole.com/ith

  c. The flu vaccine is also effective against most of the viruses that cause the common cold.

  d. Antibiotics are appropriate treatments for colds but not for influenza.

5. Which of the following statements about specific infectious diseases is *false?*

  a. Yeast infections can be treated with nonprescription drugs.

  b. Symptoms of UTIs include burning urination, chills, fever, and blood in the urine.

  c. Hepatitis A is usually transmitted through contaminated needles, transfusions, and sexual contact.

  d. College freshmen are at higher risk for contracting meningitis than the general population of young people between the ages of 18 and 23.

6. Sexually transmitted infections

  a. are the major cause of preventable sterility in the United States.

  b. can result in a severe kidney disease called pylonephritis.

  c. have declined in incidence in developing nations due to improving health standards.

  d. do not increase the risk of being infected with HIV.

7. Viral agents cause all of the following STIs *except* for

  a. herpes.

  b. genital warts.

  c. hepatitis B.

  d. candidiasis.

8. Jake is sexually active but doesn't want to use a condom. His other choices to protect himself against STIs include all of these *except*

  a. abstinence.

  b. a sexual relationship with a longtime friend.

  c. a sexual relationship with one STI-free partner.

  d. masturbation only.

9. Which of the following statements about HIV transmission is true?

  a. Individuals are not at risk for HIV if they are being treated for chlamydia or gonorrhea.

  b. HIV can be transmitted between lesbians.

  c. Heterosexual men who do not practice safe sex are at less risk for contracting HIV than homosexual men who do practice safe sex.

  d. HIV cannot be spread in a single instance of sexual intercourse.

10. A person with AIDS

  a. has a low viral load and a high number of T4 helper cells.

  b. can no longer pass HIV to a sexual partner.

  c. may suffer from secondary infectious diseases and cancers.

  d. will not respond to treatment.

Answers to these questions can be found on page 587.

Critical Thinking

1. Prior to reading this chapter, describe what you did to avoid contracting infectious disease. Now that you have read the chapter, will you be making any changes in your practices? Briefly explain the convenience, advantages, and disadvantages of each practice that you have and/or will be using to prevent infection.

2. The U.S. military and some employers routinely screen personnel for HIV. Some hospitals test patients and note their HIV status on their charts. Some insurance companies test for HIV before selling a policy. Do you believe that an individual has the right to refuse to be tested for HIV? Should a physician be able to order an HIV test without a patient's consent? Can a surgeon refuse to operate on an HIV-infected patient or one who refuses HIV testing? Do patients have the right to know if their doctors, dentists, or nurses are HIV-positive?

3. A man who developed herpes sued his former girlfriend. A woman who became sterile as a result of pelvic inflammatory disease (PID) took her ex-husband to court. A woman who contracted HIV infection from her dentist, who had died of AIDS, filed suit against his estate. Do you think that anyone who knowingly transmits a sexually transmitted disease should be held legally responsible? Do you think such an act should be a criminal offense?

Media Menu

Health�Now™

Throughout the chapter, this icon introduces a list of resources on the Health-Now website at **http://healthnow.brookscole.com/ith** that will:

- Help you evaluate your knowledge of the material.
- Allow you to take an exam-prep quiz.
- Provide a Personalized Learning Plan targeting resources that address areas you should study.
- Coach you through identifying target goals for behavior change and creating and monitoring your personal change plan throughout the semester.

INTERNET CONNECTIONS

Immunization Action Coalition
www.immunize.org
This site features comprehensive vaccination information for children, adolescents, and adults.

National Institute of Allergy and Infectious Diseases
www3.niaid.nih.gov
This institute is part of the National Institutes for Health. Its website provides information about current research, and includes fact sheets about all manner of topics related to allergies and infectious diseases.

National Center for HIV, STD, and TB Prevention
www.cdc.gov/hiv/dhap.htm
This site, sponsored by the Centers for Disease Control and Prevention (CDC) features current information, fact

sheets, conferences, media campaigns, publications, the 20-year history of HIV/AIDS, information on prevention and treatment, FAQ section, as well as the most current HIV/AIDS statistics.

HIV InSite: Gateway to AIDS Knowledge
http://hivinsite.ucsf.edu
This site, sponsored by the University of California San Francisco School of Medicine, provides statistics, education, prevention, and new developments related to HIV/AIDS.

InfoTrac College Edition Activities Log on, insert **infectious diseases** into the Keyword search box, and limit your search to the past year. When you get the results, Mark articles to review, then Select one to read. Summarize three or four key points from the article.

You can find additional readings related to personal health with InfoTrac College Edition, an online library of more than 900 journals and publications. Follow the instructions for accessing InfoTrac College Edition that were packaged with your textbook; then search for articles using a keyword search.

For additional links, resources, and suggested readings on the InfoTrac College Edition, visit our Health and Wellness Resource Center at **http://health .wadsworth.com.**

Key Terms

The terms listed are used on the page indicated. Definitions of the terms are in the Glossary at the end of his book.

abscess 395
acquired immune deficiency syndrome (AIDS) 419
allergy 396
antibiotics 392
antibody-mediated immunity 394
antiviral drug 392
autoimmune disorder 397
bacteria 392
bacterial vaginosis 409
candidiasis 409
cell-mediated immunity 394
chanchroid 418
chlamydia 414
chronic fatigue syndrome (CFS) 405
cystitis 410
fungi 392
gamma globulin 394
gonorrhea 417
helminth 393
hepatitis 403
herpes simplex 415
host 392
human immunodeficiency virus (HIV) 419
human papilloma virus (HPV) 414
immune deficiency 395
immunity 394
immunotherapy 397
incubation period 394
inflammation 395
influenza 401
Lyme disease 407
lymph nodes 395
meningitis 402
mononucleosis 405
nongonococcal urethritis (NGU) 417
pathogen 392
pelvic inflammatory disease (PID) 416
pneumonia 405
protozoa 392
pyelonephritis 410
sexually transmitted infections (STIs) 410
syphilis 418
systemic disease 395
toxic shock syndrome (TSS) 406
trichomoniasis 409
tuberculosis (TB) 405
urethritis 410
vector 392
virus 392

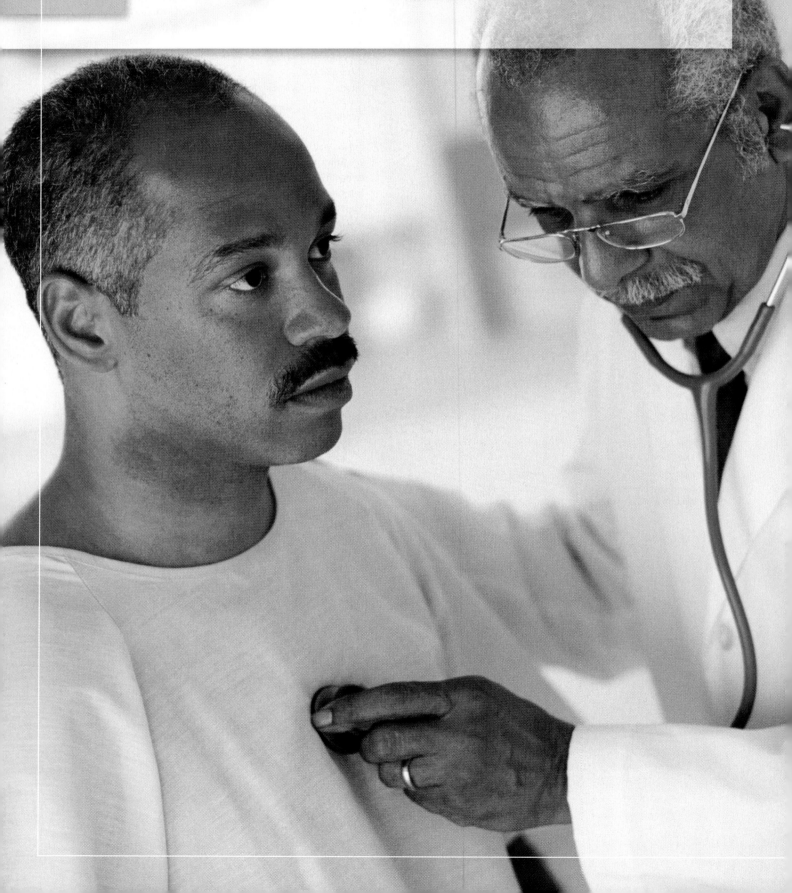

Keeping Your Heart Healthy

Jamal never forgot the terror he felt when his Dad had his first heart attack. Only ten, he couldn't understand why this towering giant of a man had fallen to the ground, his face twisted in pain, his fist pressed against his chest. His father seemed different when he came home from the hospital, as if something had gone out of him. But his face would still light up with an impish grin, especially when he'd sneak a cigarette and wink at Jamal so he wouldn't tell his mother. The second heart attack came four years later. This time Jamal's Dad didn't come home.

Jamal promised his mother that he'd take better care of his heart. He wouldn't smoke; he'd watch his blood pressure and weight; he'd keep tabs on his diet; he'd exercise regularly. Jamal didn't forget these promises as time passed. But like many college students, he felt invincible. He was shocked when a sports physical revealed that his blood pressure was high and his levels of the most dangerous type of cholesterol were elevated. But he also felt lucky: "I got my wake-up call," he explains. "And I'm not going to ignore it."

As Jamal realizes, it's never too soon, or too late, to start being heart smart. The World Health Organization reports that an estimated 16.7 million—or 29 percent of total global deaths—result from various forms of cardiovascular disease. In the United States, death rates have dropped by 60 percent since 1950, one of the major U.S. health achievements of the twentieth century. The medical advances described in this chapter have contributed to this decline, but much of the credit goes to lifestyle changes, such as quitting smoking and making dietary changes that lower blood pressure and cholesterol levels.

Yet we still have a long way to go to keep the hearts of all Americans healthy. Nearly 2,600 Americans die of heart disease every day—that's one every 34 seconds. More than 64 million Americans have heart disease.[1] Each year an estimated one million Americans suffer a heart attack; nearly half of them die.

This chapter provides the information you need about risk factors, silent dangers such as high blood pressure and cholesterol, and medical advances that can improve your chances to have a healthier heart and a longer life.

FAQ Frequently Asked Questions

- Why should I worry about heart disease? *p. 431*
- What is a healthy blood pressure? *p. 441*
- What is a healthy cholesterol reading? *p. 442*
- Should I take a statin to prevent heart disease? *p. 444*
- How do I know it's a heart attack? *p. 447*
- What causes a stroke? *p. 451*

After studying the material in this chapter, you should be able to:

- **Name** three changes you can make to keep your heart healthy.
- **Identify** the risk factors for cardiovascular disease that you can control and those that you cannot control.
- **Define** hypertension, and **discuss** why it is dangerous and ways to prevent it.
- **Describe** the types of cholesterol that compose your lipoprotein profile and the effects of each on heart health.
- **Identify** three strategies for lowering LDL cholesterol and C-reactive protein.
- **Explain** what happens during a myocardial infarction (MI) and what can be done to prevent and treat such attacks.
- **Define** stroke and transient ischemic attacks (TIAs), and **list** five risk factors for them.

HOW THE HEART WORKS

The heart is a hollow, muscular organ with four chambers that serve as two pumps (see Figure 15-1). It is about the size of a clenched fist. Each pump consists of a pair of chambers formed of muscles. The upper two—each called an **atrium**—receive blood, which then flows through valves into the lower two chambers, the **ventricles,** which contract to pump blood out into the arteries through a second set of valves. A thick wall divides the right side of the heart from the left side; even though the two sides are separated, they contract at almost the same time. Contraction of the ventricles is called **systole;** the period of relaxation between contractions is called **diastole.** The heart valves, located at the entrance and exit of the ventricular chambers, have flaps that open and close to allow blood to flow through the chambers of the heart.

The *myocardium* (heart muscle) consists of branching fibers that enable the heart to contract or beat between 60 and 80 times per minute, or about 100,000 times a day. With each beat, the heart pumps about 2 ounces of blood. This may not sound like much, but it adds up to nearly 5 quarts of blood pumped by the heart in one minute, or about 75 gallons per hour.

The heart is surrounded by the *pericardium,* which consists of two layers of a tough membrane. The space between the two contains a lubricating fluid that allows the heart muscle to move freely. The *endocardium* is a smooth membrane lining the inside of the heart and its valves.

Blood circulates through the body by means of the pumping action of the heart, as shown in Figure 15-2. The right ventricle (on your own right side) pumps blood, via the *pulmonary arteries,* to the lungs, where it picks up oxygen (a gas essential to the body's cells) and gives off carbon dioxide (a waste product of metabolism). The blood returns from the lungs via the *pulmonary veins* to the left side of the heart, which pumps it, via the **aorta,** to the arteries in the rest of the body.

The arteries divide into smaller and smaller branches and finally into **capillaries,** the smallest blood vessels of all (only slightly larger in diameter than a single red blood cell). The blood within the capillaries supplies oxygen and nutrients to the cells of the tissues and takes up various waste products. Blood

returns to the heart via the veins: The blood from the upper body (except the lungs) drains into the heart through the *superior vena cava,* while blood from the lower body returns via the *inferior vena cava.*

The workings of this remarkable pump affect your entire body. If the flow of blood to or through the heart or to the rest of the body is reduced, or if a disturbance occurs in the small bundle of highly specialized cells in the heart that generate electrical impulses to control heartbeats, the result may at first be too subtle to notice. However, without diagnosis and treatment, these changes could develop into a life-threatening problem.

FIGURE 15-1   The Healthy Heart

(a) The heart muscle is nourished by blood from the coronary arteries, which arise from the aorta. (b) The cross section shows the four chambers and the myocardium, the muscle that does the heart's work. The pericardium is the outer covering of the heart.

(a)

(b)

FIGURE 15-2   The Path of Blood Flow

Blood is pumped from the right ventricle into the pulmonary arteries, which lead to the lungs, where gas exchange (oxygen for carbon dioxide) occurs. Oxygenated blood returning from the lungs drains into the left atrium and is then pumped into the left ventricle, which sends the blood into the aorta and its branches. The oxygenated blood flows through the arteries, which extend to all parts of the body. Again, gas exchange occurs in the body tissues; this time oxygen is "dropped off" and carbon dioxide "picked up."

From E. S. Ford, et al., "Prevalence of the metabolic syndrome among U.S. adults: Findings from the third national health and nutrition examination survey," *JAMA,* 2002: 287–358.

Perhaps the biggest breakthrough in the field of cardiology has been not a test or a treatment but a realization: Heart disease is not inevitable. We can keep our hearts healthy for as long as we live, but the process of doing so must start early and continue throughout life.

PREVENTING HEART PROBLEMS

For the first time ever, the number of deaths from heart disease for Americans under age 85 has dropped lower than those caused by cancer.[2] This decline reflects the success of new treatments that can save damaged hearts, but it is also testimony to the power of prevention.

As years of research have confirmed, heart disease does not have to happen. However, avoiding or delaying it must start early. Some of the risk factors for heart disease discussed in this chapter begin in childhood with too much time in front of the television, too many fatty foods, and too many extra pounds. Other behaviors that endanger a heart's health begin in adolescence and young adulthood, including tobacco use, high-fat diets, sedentary lifestyles, and high stress. The choices that you make in your college years can affect your heart's health for decades to come.

As research shows, young women with a low-risk profile for heart disease—that is, who don't smoke, who exercise 30 minutes or more a day, who have BMIs under 25, who consume alcohol only moderately (one drink a day for women), and who eat healthfully—have a much lower risk of heart disease and fatal heart attacks throughout life. In the Nurses Health Study, only 3 percent of the more than 84,000 female participants were low risk, but their odds of having heart problems were 83 percent lower than the other women. These women also were less likely to die of any cause over a 31-year period.[3]

Simplying holding the line on weight can make a difference. In a 15-year study that followed over 5,000 men and women initially aged 18 to 30, those who maintained their starting weight showed no significant change in risk factors for heart disease as they reached middle age. However, only about one in five of the study participants managed to avoid gaining weight with the passing years.[4]

(FAQ) WHY SHOULD I WORRY ABOUT HEART DISEASE?

Many people, including college students and other young adults, are unaware of habits and conditions that put their hearts at risk. In a survey of almost 1,500 undergraduates, the majority viewed heart disease as mainly a problem for white men and underestimated the risks for women and ethnic groups (see Student Snapshot: "How Heart-Smart Are College Students?"). Students rated their own knowledge of heart disease as lower than that of sexually transmitted infections and psychological disorders. Most—88 percent—said a doctor had never discussed heart disease with them.[5] Yet heart disease is the third leading cause of death among adults aged 25 to 44.

In another study of undergraduates enrolled in physical activity classes at a large university, 68 percent rated their risk of heart disease as lower or much lower than that of their peers, reflecting what researchers called "a clear optimistic bias." The undergraduates who exercised regularly rated their risk as lower than those who did not. Men and women did not realize that diabetes, family history, and other risk factors increase their likelihood of heart disease.[6]

Student Snapshot

HOW HEART-SMART ARE COLLEGE STUDENTS?

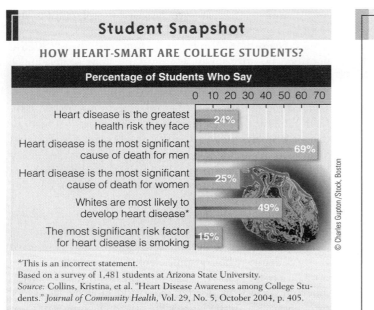

Percentage of Students Who Say

Heart disease is the greatest health risk they face	24%
Heart disease is the most significant cause of death for men	69%
Heart disease is the most significant cause of death for women	25%
Whites are most likely to develop heart disease*	49%
The most significant risk factor for heart disease is smoking	15%

© Charles Gupton/Stock, Boston

*This is an incorrect statement.
Based on a survey of 1,481 students at Arizona State University.
Source: Collins, Kristina, et al. "Heart Disease Awareness among College Students." *Journal of Community Health,* Vol. 29, No. 5, October 2004, p. 405.

Even college students who indicate that they're aware of cardiovascular risks often behave in ways that do not reflect their knowledge. In one study of 226 students at a New Jersey college, half or more ate a high-fat diet or reported moderate to severe stress. Many did not exercise frequently; some already had high cholesterol or high blood pressure.[7]

Young athletes face special risks. Each year seemingly healthy teens or young adults die suddenly on playing fields and courts. The culprit in one of every three cases of sudden cardiac death in young athletes is a silent condition called hypertrophic cardiomyopathy (HCM), an excessive thickness of the heart muscle. Because of HCM, the heart is more prone to dangerous heart irregularities (see "You Decide").

Every year some seemingly healthy young athletes die suddenly on playing fields or courts, often because of heart abnormalities. Some health officials argue that colleges should screen competitive athletes before allowing them to join a team. Others argue that screening should be an individual choice. Should college athletes be required to undergo testing for potentially lethal health risks? Or should they have the right to choose whether or not to be tested and whether to take the risks of playing their sport? **You decide.**

Your Life Coach

Making Heart Healthy Changes

Chances are that you don't have any noticeable symptoms of heart disease: no pain, no swelling, no breathlessness when you walk or climb stairs. But that doesn't mean that you're home safe. Depending on your age, family history, blood pressure, cholesterol levels, and other risk factors, your heart's health may be in jeopardy.

Yes, advances in treatment can help if you eventually develop heart disease. But changes in lifestyle can do even more: They can prevent or reverse heart-related symptoms. In one recent study, a 12-week program of therapeutic life changes, sometimes called TLC, helped lower blood pressure, cholesterol, blood sugar, and weight without medications.[8]

If you don't feel any need to make changes, you are in the precontemplation stage of behavioral change (see Chapter 2 for a complete discussion). Read this entire chapter with an open mind, and think of family members or friends who have heart disease or who are clearly at risk because they smoke or are overweight. What effect have their habits had on their health? Make a list of the benefits heart-healthy habits might have for you.

If you do want to make some heart-healthy changes, select some of the behavioral modifications that follow:

CHANGES YOU CAN MAKE TODAY

- Eat a good breakfast: whole-grain cereal, juice, yogurt, and so forth.
- Take a walk after lunch.
- Skip dessert at dinner.
- Eat one more serving of vegetables.
- Eat one more piece of fruit.
- Drink one more glass of water.
- Take the stairs for one or two flights rather than riding the elevator in your dorm or classroom building.
- Get seven to eight hours of sleep tonight.

CHANGES YOU CAN MAKE THIS WEEK

- **Block out time for exercise on your calendar.** Try for at least 30 minutes of physical activity most days.
- **If you haven't had your lipoproteins checked** within the last year, schedule a test.
- **If you don't know your blood pressure,** find out what it is. If you know it, compare your reading with those in Table 15-1 (page 442) to determine if it is too high.

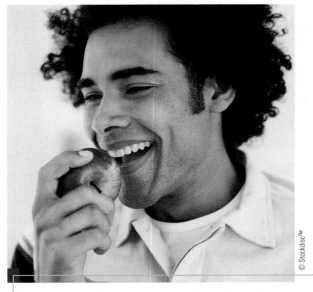

You can do something today to prevent heart disease in your future: Eat some fruit.

Regular physical activity can lower your risk of heart disease.

- **Make a list of stress-reducing activities,** such as meditation or listening to music. Select two or three to do this week.
- **Get in touch with an old friend,** and enjoy catching up on each other's lives.

CHANGES YOU CAN MAKE THIS TERM

- **Look for new ways to meet your goals.** For example, try new and different healthy foods each week, or join a volleyball team.
- **Be patient.** Don't get discouraged if change seems harder and slower than you thought it would be.
- **If you slip up and smoke again or blow your diet, don't give up.** Analyze what triggered your relapse. Was it the smell of smoke at the party Saturday night? Did you try to console yourself for a poor grade with a carton of chocolate ice cream? Think of how you might handle similar situations differently in the future, such as staying away from smokers at parties or taking a walk to lift your mood rather than turning to food.
- **Develop and use a support system of friends and family members.** Identify individuals you can talk to, work out with, or call.

GETTING PHYSICAL

Physical activity prevents or reduces many of the risk factors for heart disease discussed later in this chapter by:

- **Reducing body weight.**
- **Reducing blood pressure.**
- **Reducing harmful low-density-lipoprotein** (LDL) and total cholesterol.
- **Increasing beneficial high-density lipoprotein** (HDL) cholesterol.
- **Increasing insulin sensitivity** (and lowering the risk of diabetes).[9]
- **Lowering C-reactive protein,** a marker of inflammation.

Sometimes exercise alone can lower an individual's risk of heart problems; in other cases exercise enhances the benefits of other treatments, such as cholesterol-lowering medications.

To maintain cardiovascular fitness, many medical groups, including the American Heart Association, American College of Sports Medicine, and the CDC, recommend 30 to 60 minutes or more of moderate-intensity physical activity such as brisk walking on most, if not all, days of the week. Simply meeting this recommendation for activity would reduce heart disease by 30 to 40 percent. The greatest cardiovascular gains occur in people who go from being sedentary to engaging in low-intensity to moderate activities, such as gardening, walking, and housecleaning. Their blood pressure falls; they lose weight; their hearts function more efficiently.

The greater the exercise "dose," the more benefits it yields. In studies that compared individuals of different fitness levels, the least fit were at much greater risk of dying. In men, more rigorous exercise, such as jogging, produces greater protection against heart disease and boosts longevity. (See Chapter 5 on fitness.)

In women, exercise capacity, adjusted for a woman's age, is a key predictor of cardiac health. Women who score less than 85 percent of the usual exercise capacity for women their age are more than twice as likely to die of heart disease or any other cause.[10]

CHOOSING HEART-HEALTHY FOODS

A balanced, low-fat diet is the best recipe for a healthy heart. Fruits and vegetables, in particular, are associated with a reduced risk of cardiovascular disease, including lower blood pressure.

The American Heart Association (AHA) also recommends including cholesterol-lowering foods, such as oats, barley, soy protein, and nuts, in your daily diet. A diet rich in bran, one of the major components of whole grains, lowers the risk of heart disease. In a study of 43,000 men, those who ate the most oatmeal, brown rice, and other whole grain products had the lowest rates of heart disease.[11]

Another dietary heart helper is fish. Eating fish two times a week, as the AHA recommends, can reduce blood pressure, decrease levels of the blood fats known as triglycerides, and increase HDL ("good") cholesterol levels. The more fish you eat, the slower your heart beats. This may protect against the fast irregular heart beats that can lead to sudden death.[12] Even five ounces of fish a week reduces the risk of "acute" coronary events, such as chest pain and heart attack.[13]

Clinical trials generally have found no cardiovascular benefits from antioxidant supplements, such as vitamins C and E, and some evidence suggests that they may have harmful effects, such as interfering with cholesterol-lowering drugs.[14]

RISK FACTORS FOR CARDIOVASCULAR DISEASE

Heart disease, contrary to a common misperception, generally does not strike "out of the blue." According to research, 80 to 90 percent of those who develop heart disease and 95 percent of those who suffer a fatal heart attack have at least one major risk factor. Recognition of the risk factors for heart disease has helped prevent many heart-related problems and saved countless lives.

Approximately 25 percent of adults have multiple risk factors, some form of heart disease, or type 2 diabetes. These high-risk men and women should work with their physicians on specific strategies to protect their hearts. Roughly 40 percent of adults with one or more elevated risk factors are at intermediate risk. They should undergo regular testing by a physician.[15]

RISK FACTORS YOU CAN CONTROL

The choices you make and the habits you follow can have a significant impact on whether or not your heart remains healthy. You can choose to avoid the following potential risks for the sake of your heart's health.

Physical Inactivity

As discussed in Chapter 5, about one-quarter of U.S. adults are sedentary and another third are not active enough to reach a healthy level of fitness. (See the Self Survey to assess your own level of activity.) The risk for heart disease is 1.5 to 2.4 times higher for people who are inactive compared with those who engage in regular physical activity.[16]

Women who report higher levels of physical fitness have less risk of cardiovascular disease, regardless of their body mass index (BMI), waist circumference, or waist-hip ratio (see Chapter 7). This suggests that fitness may be more important than overweight or obesity per se for women's cardiovascular risk.[17] A minimum of 30 minutes a day of moderate activity at least five days a week, can lift a woman from the "low-fitness category" and lessen her risk of heart disease.[18]

In men, more rigorous exercise produced greater protection against heart disease.[19] Those who ran for an hour or more per week reduced their risk of heart disease by 42 percent, compared with an 18 percent reduction for those who walked briskly for a half-hour per day or more. With walking, pace, not duration, was linked with lower danger of heart disease.

Tobacco

Smoking may be the single most significant risk factor for cardiovascular disease—and quitting may do more to reduce the risk of mortality among heart disease patients who smoke than any other intervention or treatment. Each year smoking causes more than 250,000 deaths from cardiovascular disease—far more than it causes from cancer and lung disease. Smokers who have heart attacks are more likely to die from them than are nonsmokers. Smoking is the major risk factor for *peripheral vascular disease*, in which the vessels that carry blood to the leg and arm muscles become hardened and clogged.

Cigar smoking causes a moderate but significant increase in an individual's risk for coronary artery disease, as well as for cancers of the upper digestive tract and chronic obstructive pulmonary disease.

Both active and passive smoking accelerate the process by which arteries become clogged and increase the risk of heart attacks and strokes.[20] Overall, nonsmokers exposed to

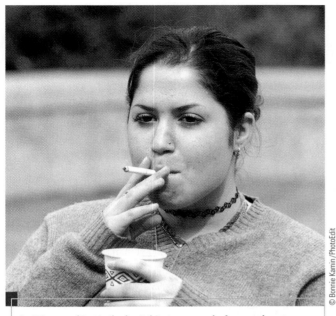

Quitting smoking is the best thing you can do for your heart—no matter what age you are.

environmental tobacco smoke are at a 25 percent higher relative risk of developing coronary heart disease than non-smokers not exposed to environmental tobacco smoke.

In various studies, quitting has reduced the risk of heart disease and subsequent death among patients with heart disease by as much as 50 percent. After 18 years without cigarettes, the risk of dying of heart disease among ex-smokers is no greater than that of never-smokers.[21]

Obesity

Obesity has emerged as an increasingly common and dangerous risk factor for cardiovascular disease, increasing the risk for hypertension, diabetes, coronary artery disease, and congestive heart failure in both men and women. BMI and measurement of waist circumference, discussed in Chapter 7, are good indicators of increased risk.

According to the National Heart, Lung and Blood Institute (NHLBI), losing weight at any age can help reduce the risk of heart problems. For women, obesity is as great a cause of death and disability from heart disease as smoking and heavy drinking. Even mild-to-moderately obese women are more likely to suffer chest pain or a heart attack than thinner women. Weight loss significantly reduces high blood pressure, another risk factor for heart disease. (See Chapter 7 for a discussion of obesity.)

High Blood Pressure (Hypertension)

Blood pressure is a result of the contractions of the heart muscle, which pumps blood through your body, and the resistance of the walls of the vessels through which the blood flows. Each time your heart beats, your blood pressure goes up and down within a certain range. It's highest when the heart contracts; this is called **systolic blood pressure.** It's lowest between contractions; this is called **diastolic blood pressure.** A blood pressure reading consists of the systolic measurement "over" the diastolic measurement, recorded in millimeters of mercury (mm Hg) by a sphygmomanometer (see Figure 15-3).

High blood pressure, or **hypertension,** occurs when the artery walls become constricted so that the force exerted as the blood flows through them is greater than it should be. Physicians see blood pressure as a continuum: The higher the reading, the greater the risk of stroke and heart disease. New guidelines have lowered the levels considered dangerous and identified *prehypertension* as a potential threat to the heart's health. (See the discussion of high blood pressure later in this chapter.)

As a result of the increased work in pumping blood, the heart muscle of a person with hypertension can become stronger and also stiffer. This stiffness increases resistance to filling up with blood between beats, which can cause shortness of breath with exertion. Hypertension can also act on the kidney arteries, which can lead to kidney failure in some cases. In addition, hypertension accelerates the development of plaque buildup within the arteries. Especially when combined with obesity, smoking, high cholesterol levels, or diabetes, hypertension increases the risks of cardiovascular problems several times. However, you can control high blood pressure through diet, exercise, and if necessary, medication.

Blood Fats (Lipids)

Cholesterol is a fatty substance found in certain foods and also manufactured by the body. The measurement of cholesterol in the blood is one of the most reliable indicators of the formation of plaque, the sludgelike substance that builds up on the inner walls of arteries. You can lower blood cholesterol levels by cutting back on high-fat foods and exercising more, thereby reducing the risk of a heart attack. According to the NHLBI, for every 1 percent drop in blood cholesterol, studies show a 2 percent decrease in the likelihood of a heart attack.

Lipoproteins are compounds in the blood that are made up of proteins and fat. The different types are classified by their size or density. The heaviest are *high-density lipoproteins,* or HDLs, which have the highest proportion of protein. These "good guys," as some cardiologists refer to them, pick up excess cholesterol in the blood and carry it back to the liver for removal from the body. An HDL level of 40 mg/dL or lower substantially increases the risk of heart disease. (Cholesterol levels are measured in milligrams of cholesterol per deciliter of blood—mg/dL.) The average HDL for men is about 45 mg/dL; for women, it is about 55 mg/dL.

Low-density lipoproteins, or (LDLs), and very low-density lipoproteins (VLDLs) carry more cholesterol than HDLs and deposit it on the walls of arteries—they're the "bad guys." The higher your LDL cholesterol, the greater

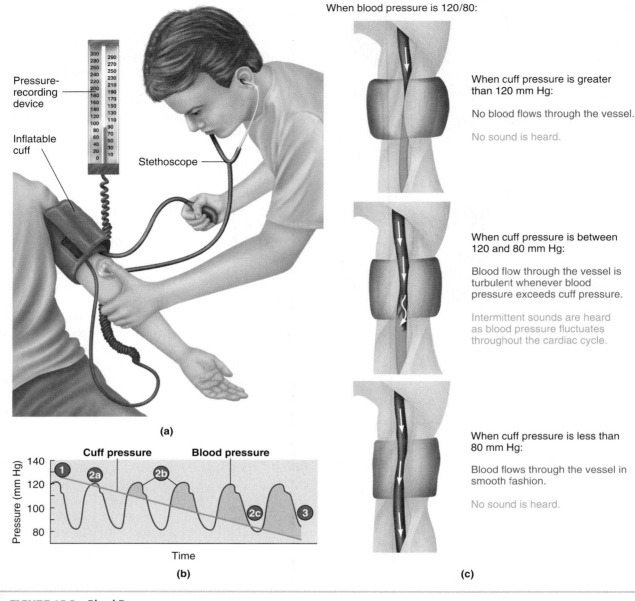

When blood pressure is 120/80:

When cuff pressure is greater than 120 mm Hg:

No blood flows through the vessel.

No sound is heard.

When cuff pressure is between 120 and 80 mm Hg:

Blood flow through the vessel is turbulent whenever blood pressure exceeds cuff pressure.

Intermittent sounds are heard as blood pressure fluctuates throughout the cardiac cycle.

When cuff pressure is less than 80 mm Hg:

Blood flows through the vessel in smooth fashion.

No sound is heard.

FIGURE 15-3   Blood Pressure

Three steps in measuring blood pressure: (1) Increasing cuff pressure until no blood flows through (① in graph). (2) Releasing the cuff slowly so blood starts to flow through (②a, ②b, ②c)—your systolic pressure is at ②a. (3) As release of the cuff pressure continues, your diastolic pressure is the point when no sound is heard (③ on graph).

your risk for heart disease. If you are at high risk of heart disease, any level of LDL higher than 100 mg/dL may increase your danger. (See "Your Lipoprotein Profile" later in this chapter.)

Triglycerides are fats that flow through the blood after meals and have been linked to increased risk of coronary artery disease, especially in women. Triglyceride levels tend to be highest in those whose diets are high in calories, sugar, alcohol, and refined starches. High levels of these fats may increase the risk of obesity, and cutting back on these foods can reduce high triglyceride levels.

Metabolic Syndrome

Metabolic syndrome, once called Syndrome X or insulin-resistant syndrome, is emerging as a major risk factor for heart disease.[22] This condition is not a disease but a cluster of disorders of your body's metabolism—including high blood pressure, high insulin levels, abdominal obesity, and abnormal cholesterol levels—that make you more likely to develop diabetes, heart disease, or stroke. Each of these conditions is by itself a risk factor for other diseases. In combination, they dramatically boost your chances of potentially life-threatening illnesses.

FIGURE 15-4 Prevalence of the Metabolic Syndrome

Source: Darwin, Deen. "Metabolic Syndrome: What Is It and What Can I Do about It?" *American Family Physician,* Vol. 69, No. 12, June 15, 2004, p. 2887.

 This dangerous syndrome has become so widespread that health officials describe it as an epidemic that affects one in three Americans. As Figure 15-4 shows, it is especially common in Hispanic men and women. College-age men and women who maintain their weight as they get older are much less likely to develop metabolic syndrome.[23] However, about one in four undergraduates already has one risk factor for metabolic syndrome.[24] Young adults with metabolic syndrome are more likely than others their age to have thicker neck arteries, an indicator of atherosclerosis, the buildup of fatty plaques in arteries (discussed on page 445).[25]

According to the National Institutes of Health, three or more of the following characteristics indicate metabolic syndrome:[26]

- **Waist measurement of 40 inches or more** in men and 35 inches or more in women (for Asians and individuals with a genetic pre disposition to diabetes, 37 to 39 inches in men and 31 to 35 inches in women).
- **Triglyceride level of 150 mg/dL** or more.

- **High-density lipoprotein (HDL)**—"good" cholesterol—level of less than 40 mg/dL in men or 50 mg/dL in women.
- **Blood pressure of 130 mmHg** systole over 85 mmHg diastole (130/85), or higher.
- **Fasting blood sugar of 100 mg/dL** or higher.

Men with three factors of metabolic syndrome are nearly twice as likely to have a heart attack or stroke and more than three times more likely to develop heart disease than those with none. Men with four or five characteristics of the syndrome have nearly four times the risk of heart attack or stroke and more than 24 times the risk of diabetes.

In a study of more than 3,000 people with metabolic syndrome, lifestyle changes—including moderate exercise and weight loss—and a common glucose-lowering drug both had an impact on metabolic syndrome. However, changing health habits had greater benefits, with 41 percent of those who made lifestyle changes no longer having metabolic syndrome at the end of the study, compared with 17 percent of those taking medication.[27]

Diabetes Mellitus

Diabetes mellitus, a disorder of the endocrine system discussed in depth in Chapter 16, increases the likelihood of hypertension and atherosclerosis, thereby increasing the risk of heart attack and stroke. A physician can detect diabetes and prescribe a diet, exercise program, and if necessary, medication to keep it in check. Even before developing diabetes, individuals at high risk for this disease—those who are overweight, have a family history of the disease, have mildly elevated blood pressure and blood sugar levels, and above-ideal levels of harmful blood fats—may already be at increased risk of heart disease. Up to one-half of diabetics also have hypertension, another risk factor.

Individuals with diabetes who have never had a heart attack are as likely to experience what physicians call a "cardiac event" as nondiabetics who have had heart attacks. Diabetics who develop heart disease are more likely to die if they suffer a heart attack or develop heart failure. Two-thirds of people with diabetes die from cardiovascular disease.

Strategies for Prevention :: Overcoming Metabolic Syndrome

The following steps have proved effective in reversing metabolic syndrome and reducing the risks associated with it:

:: Eat a low-fat, low-calorie diet.

:: Engage in a minimum of 150 calories a week of moderate exercise, such as walking.

:: Reduce your body weight by 5 to 7 percent.

:: If these strategies don't work for you, talk to your doctor about taking a glucose-lowering medication.

Type 2 diabetes, a strong risk factor for coronary heart disease in all women, is especially common in black women. If combined with other risk factors, it puts them at very high risk of cardiovascular disease.

Psychosocial Factors

How you respond to everyday sources of stress can affect your heart as well as your overall health. While you may not be able to control the sources of stress, you can change how you habitually respond to it.

Researchers classify psychological risk factors for heart disease into three categories: chronic, episodic, and acute. Chronic factors, such as job strain or lack of social support, play an important role in the buildup of artery-clogging plaque.[28] Episodic factors, such as depression, can last from several weeks to two years and may lead to the creation of "unstable" plaque (discussed later in this chapter), which is more likely to break off and block a blood vessel within the heart. Short-term or acute psychological risk factors, such as an angry outburst, can directly trigger a heart attack in people with underlying heart disease.

These factors may act alone or combine and exert different effects at different ages and stages of life. They may influence behaviors such as smoking, diet, alcohol consumption, and physical activity, as well as directly cause changes in physiology.

Depression and heart disease often occur together. People with heart disease are more likely to be depressed, and some seemingly healthy people with depression are at greater risk of heart problems. Depressed women younger than age 60 are twice as likely to suffer a heart attack than those who do not suffer from depression. After a heart attack, depression is common in both men and women, but physicians are less likely to recognize and treat depression in African-American patients.[29]

Patients who suffer heart attacks and develop clinical depression have higher rates of complications and an increased risk of dying from another heart attack or other heart problems. People who are physically healthy with no risk factors for heart disease but who are prone to anger, hostility, and mild depression have higher levels of C-reactive protein, a substance linked to increased risk of heart disease.

In addition to stress and depression, other psychological traits can increase the risk of heart disease. Based on more than a decade of research, Dutch scientists have identified a "Type D" (for distressed) personality type. Type D people tend to be anxious, self-conscious, irritable, insecure, negative, and go to great lengths not to say or do anything that others might not like.[30] In the Dutch study, almost four times as many Type D individuals as others in cardiac rehabilitation programs died within an eight-year period. Other studies have linked Type D personality to other heart-related problems, such as chronic heart failure.[31]

In the past, other personality types have been linked to disease, for example, hard-charging, hostile Type As to heart disease and conflict-avoiding, emotion-suppressing Type Cs to cancer. However, these traits have not proved to be sig-

nificant risk factors for these illnesses. Much more research is needed to evaluate the importance of Type D traits. Until we know more, regular aerobic exercise and relaxation techniques such as meditation may ease distress as well as keep the heart healthy.[32]

Drug Use

Illegal Drugs Illegal drugs pose many dangers—one of the most serious is their potentially deadly impact on the cardiovascular system. Ecstasy, amphetamines, and cocaine can cause a sudden rise in blood pressure, heart rate, and contractions of the left ventricle (the pumping chamber) of the heart, which can increase the risk of a heart attack.

The hallucinogens lysergic acid diethylamide (LSD) and psilocybin (psychoactive mushrooms) also have the potential for triggering irregular heartbeats and heart attacks, although less serious cardiac complications, such as a temporary rise in blood pressure, are more common. Morphine and heroin, which account for almost half of drug-related deaths, can lower blood pressure and affect the heart rate. Inhalants can produce fatal heartbeat irregularities. Marijuana, the most widely used illegal drug among young adults, can affect blood pressure and heart rate, but it is not known whether it can trigger a heart attack.

Prescription Painkillers Legal prescription drugs also can endanger the heart. Vioxx, a popular painkiller, was removed from the market in 2004 because of increased risks of heart attacks and strokes in patients taking it for more than 18 months. The Food and Drug Administration (FDA) estimates that Vioxx may have contributed to as many as 80,000 to 140,000 cases of serious heart disease, many of them fatal.[33] Similar drugs in the category known as COX-2 inhibitors, used primarily to relieve arthritis pain, may also increase the risk of heart problems[34] (see Chapter 11).

RISK FACTORS YOU CAN'T CONTROL

Heredity

Anyone whose parents, siblings, or other close relatives suffered heart attacks before age 50 is at increased risk of developing heart disease. Certain risk factors, such as abnormally high blood levels of lipids, can be passed down from generation to generation. Although you can't rewrite your family history, individuals with an inherited vulnerability to cardiovascular disease can lower the danger by changing the risk factors within their control. Your heart's health depends to a great extent on your behavior, including the decisions you make about the foods you eat or the decision not to smoke. As an added preventive step, cardiologists may prescribe a small daily dose of aspirin to individuals with a history of coronary artery disease who are at risk of forming clots that could block blood supplies to the heart, brain, and other organs. (Note: Daily aspirin is not advised for individuals who are not at risk because of their age or health history.)

Know your family history. If a close relative had a heart attack before age 50, your risk of heart disease is higher.

 ### Race and Ethnicity

Heart disease and its risk factors occur at higher rates among ethnic minority populations such as African Americans, Hispanic Americans, and Native Americans. Nearly four in every ten black adults have cardiovascular disease. Among Hispanic Americans, nearly three in ten have cardiovascular disease.[35]

African Americans are twice as likely to develop high blood pressure as whites. African Americans also suffer strokes at an earlier age and of greater severity. Poverty may be an unrecognized risk factor for members of this minority group, who are less likely to receive medical treatments or undergo corrective surgery. Family history, lifestyle, diet, and stress may also play a role, starting early in life. However, researchers have found no single explanation for why African-American youngsters, like their parents, tend to have higher blood pressure than white children.

 Black women are twice as likely as white women to suffer heart attacks and to die from heart disease. Common risk factors—high blood pressure, diabetes, and high cholesterol—account for this increased jeopardy. In addition, black women are less likely to receive common medications, such as aspirin and cholesterol-lowering drugs, to lower their risk.

Age

Almost four out of five people who die of a heart attack are over age 65. Heart disease accounts for more than 40 percent of deaths among people between 65 and 74 and almost 60 percent at age 85 and above. However, the risk factors that are likely to cause heart disease later in life, including high blood pressure and high levels of "bad" cholesterol, may begin to develop in childhood. Nevertheless, although cardiovascular function declines with age, heart disease is not an inevitable consequence of aging. Many 80- and 90-year-olds have strong, healthy hearts.

 ### Gender

Many people still think of heart disease as a "guy problem." Men have a higher incidence of cardiovascular problems than women before age 45. The onset of heart disease in women lags behind that in men by 10 to 15 years. However, for the U.S. population as a whole, as many women as men eventually die of heart disease. Although the same risk factors jeopardize the hearts of men and women, each gender also faces some unique heart-related issues, including male pattern baldness and menopause.

 Male pattern baldness (the loss of hair at the vertex, or top, of the head) is associated with increased risk of heart attack in men under age 55. The speed at which men lose their hair also may be an indicator of risk. Men with male pattern baldness who lose their hair quickly may metabolize male sex hormones differently than others, thereby increasing the likelihood of heart disease. Although it's premature to say that baldness is definitely bad news for the heart, health experts advise bald men to follow basic guidelines, such as not smoking and controlling their cholesterol levels, to lower any possible risk.

Heart disease is the fourth leading cause of death among women aged 30 to 34, third among women aged 35 to 39, second among women aged 40 to 64, and first among women over age 65. A woman's risk increases sharply after menopause (discussed in Chapter 18).

Researchers long believed that postmenopausal hormone therapy (HT) protected women from heart disease. However, this has been proved wrong. Based on large-scale studies that showed little, if any, benefit and some potential harm to the hearts of postmenopausal women, combined hormone therapy is no longer recommended for the prevention of heart disease and stroke.

Bacterial Infection

Certain bacteria may indeed put the heart at risk. *Streptococcus sanguis,* the bacterium found in dental plaque, has been implicated in the buildup of atherosclerotic plaque. Individuals with periodontal disease are at increased risk of heart disease and stroke. Regular brushing, flossing, and dental visits can reduce this danger.

Another common bacterium, *Chlamydia pneumoniae,* long linked to respiratory infections, also may threaten the heart. Individuals with high levels of antibodies to this bacteria are more likely to suffer a heart-related problem. Researchers have reported that antibiotics, taken to treat common infections, may protect against first-time heart attacks. A national clinical trial to determine whether antibiotics can reduce the risk of heart attack and stroke is under way.

HIGH BLOOD PRESSURE (HYPERTENSION)

Blood pressure refers to the force of blood against the walls of arteries. When blood pressure remains elevated over time—a condition called hypertension—it forces the heart

Eye damage
Prolonged high blood pressure can damage delicate blood vessels on the retina, the layer of cells at the back of the eye. If the damage, known as retinopathy, remains untreated, it can lead to blindness.

Stroke
High blood pressure can damage vessels that supply blood to the brain, eventually causing them to rupture or clog. The interruption in the blood flow to the brain is known as a stroke.

Damage to artery walls
Artery walls are normally smooth, allowing blood pressure to flow easily. Over time, high blood pressure can wear rough spots in artery walls. Fatty deposits can collect in the rough spots, clogging arteries and raising the risk of a heart attack or stroke.

Heart attack
High blood pressure makes the heart work harder to pump sufficient blood through narrowed aterioles (small blood vessels). This extra effort can enlarge and weaken the heart, leading to heart failure. High blood pressure also damages the coronary arteries that supply blood to the heart, sometimes leading to blockages that can cause a heart attack.

Rough artery walls   Clogged artery

Kidney failure
Prolonged high blood pressure can damage blood vessels in the kidney, where wastes are filtered from the bloodstream. In severe cases, this damage can lead to kidney failure and even death.

FIGURE 15-5 Consequences of High Blood Pressure
If left untreated, elevated blood pressure can damage blood vessels in several areas of the body and lead to serious health problems.

to pump harder than is healthy. Because the heart must force blood into arteries that are offering increased resistance to blood flow, the left side of the heart becomes enlarged. If untreated, high blood pressure can cause a variety of cardiovascular complications, including heart attack and stroke—two of the three leading causes of death among U.S. adults—as well as kidney failure and blindness (Figure 15-5).

The World Health Organization estimates that hypertension causes one in every eight deaths globally, making it the third leading killer in the world. In the United States, high blood pressure is responsible for about a third of cardiovascular problems like heart attack or stroke and a quarter of all premature deaths.

About a third of adults age 18 and older in the United States—some 65 million men and women—have high blood pressure.[36] In the last decade, hypertension grew by about 8 percent, with a 30 percent jump in the total number of adults with high blood pressure. Blood pressure has also increased among children and adolescents over the last decade, with the highest rates among black and Mexican-American children. The primary culprit is the increase in obesity in the young. No one knows why African Americans are more vulnerable, although some speculate that overweight or dietary factors may contribute.

 Family history also plays a role. "If you study healthy college students with normal blood pressures, those who have one parent with hypertension will have blood pressure that's a little higher than average," notes Rose Marie Robertson, M.D., of the American Heart Association. "If two parents have high blood pressure, their levels will be a little higher, and they're destined to go higher still. If your parents have high blood pressure, have yours checked regularly."[37]

Men and women are equally likely to develop hypertension, but in women, blood pressure tends to rise around the time of menopause. Half of all women over age 45 have hypertension. For individuals who smoke, are overweight, don't exercise, or have high cholesterol levels, hypertension multiplies the risk of heart disease and stroke. Overweight people with high blood pressure have twice the risk of dying of a heart attack or stroke as those with normal blood pressure.[38] At ultrahigh risk are people with diabetes or kidney disease.

In its most recent report, the Joint National Committee on Prevention, Detection, Evaluation, and Treatment of High Blood Pressure identified the following key messages:[39]

■ Beginning at 115/75 mmHG, cardiovascular disease risk doubles for each increment of 20/10 mmHg.

■ In those older than age 50, a systolic blood pressure greater than 140 mmHg is a more important risk factor for cardiovascular disease than diastolic blood pressure.

■ Men and women with normal blood pressure at age 55 have a 90 percent lifetime risk of developing hypertension.

In a young person even mild hypertension can cause organs such as the heart, brain, and kidneys to start to deteriorate. By age 50 or 60, the damage may be irreversible.

 Different races suffer different consequences of high blood pressure. An African American with the same elevated blood pressure reading as a Caucasian faces a greater risk of stroke, heart disease, and kidney problems.

PREVENTING HYPERTENSION

Prevention pays off when it comes to high blood pressure. The most effective preventive measures involve lifestyle changes. Losing weight is the best approach for individuals with high normal values. Exercise may be effective in lowering mildly elevated blood pressure. High intake of folate, a B vitamin discussed in Chapter 6, can significantly reduce the risk of hypertension. In a study of women under age 35, those who consumed the most folate had one-third the risk of developing high blood pressure as those consuming very little.[40] Among the approaches that have not proved effective are dietary supplements, such as calcium, magnesium, potassium, and fish oil.

The National Heart, Lung and Blood Institute has developed what is known as the DASH diet. Following DASH, which stands for Dietary Approaches to Stop Hypertension, has proved as effective as drug therapy in lowering blood pressure. An additional benefit: The DASH diet also lowers harmful blood fats, including cholesterol and low-density lipoprotein, and the amino acid homocysteine (one of the new suspects in heart disease risk).

Restriction of sodium intake also helps. Most Americans consume more salt than they need. The 2005 *Dietary Guidelines for Americans* recommend limiting sodium to 2,300 milligrams a day—about a teaspoonful—including

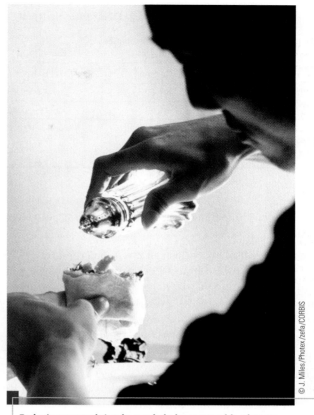

Reducing your salt intake can help lower your blood pressure.

© J. Miles/Photex/zefa/CORBIS

salt used at the table and in cooking. Diets of less than 1,500 milligrams of sodium produce greater benefits and help blood pressure medicines work better.

The lower the amount of sodium in the diet, the lower the blood pressure for both those with and those without hypertension and for both genders and all racial and ethnic groups. However, reducing dietary sodium has an even greater effect on blood pressure in blacks than whites, in women than men, and in individuals with hypertension.

(FAQ) WHAT IS A HEALTHY BLOOD PRESSURE?

Current guidelines (Table 15-1) categorize a reading of 120/80 as **prehypertension,** a condition that is likely to worsen in time. A healthy reading is 115/75 mmHg. Once blood pressure rises above this threshold, the risk of cardiovascular disease may increase.

In healthy adults, blood pressure screening should begin at age 21, with repeat evaluations at least every two years, or more often depending on your current health, medical history, and risk factors for cardiovascular disease.

To get an accurate blood pressure reading, you should visit the doctor's office at least twice and have your blood pressure taken two or more times while you're seated. The average of those measurements determines how your blood pressure is classified.

TABLE 15-1 WHAT YOUR BLOOD PRESSURE MEANS

Top Number (systolic)		Bottom Number (diastolic)	Your Group	What to Do
Below 120	and	Below 80	Normal blood pressure	Maintain a healthy lifestyle
120–139	or	80–89	Prehypertension	Adopt a healthy lifestyle
140–159	or	90–99	Stage 1 hypertension	Adopt a healthy lifestyle; take medication
160 or more	or	100 or more	Stage 2 hypertension	Adopt a healthy lifestyle; take more than one medication

Numbers are expressed in millimeters of mercury (mm Hg).

The new guidelines classify hypertension into two categories:

■ **Stage 1.** This consists of a systolic pressure ranging from 140 to 159 or a diastolic pressure ranging from 90 to 99.

■ **Stage 2.** The most severe form of hypertension occurs with a systolic pressure of 160 or higher or a diastolic reading of 100 or higher.

Only one of the numbers—the top or bottom—needs to be high to meet these criteria. In people over age 50, systolic pressure is more important than diastolic. If it rises to 140 mmHg or higher, doctors advise treatment regardless of the diastolic pressure.

CONTROLLING HIGH BLOOD PRESSURE

Lifestyle changes are a first-line weapon in the fight against high blood pressure. Rather than making a single change, a combination of behavioral changes, including losing weight, eating heart-healthy foods, reducing sodium, and exercising more, yields the best results. For uncomplicated hypertension, the recommended treatment is a thiazide diuretic, either alone or combined with other antihypertensive medications.

Making healthy lifestyle modifications can help reduce Stage 1 hypertension, but most people also require a medication. Those with Stage 2 hypertension typically need at least two types of high blood pressure medications (antihypertensives) to reduce blood pressure to a safer level. The goal for most people with hypertension is to reduce blood pressure to below 140/90 mmHg.

 According to research, a beta blocker called nebivolol is significantly better than placebo in reducing systolic and diastolic blood pressure among African-American hypertensive patients.

Only about one-third of people with hypertension have it effectively controlled—below 140/90 mmHg. Reducing systolic blood pressure 12 mmHg for 10 years can prevent one death in every 11 people treated for hypertension. In those with existing cardiovascular disease or organ damage, such as kidney disease, that reduction has an even bigger benefit, preventing one death in every nine people treated.

YOUR LIPOPROTEIN PROFILE

Medical science has changed the way it views and targets the blood fats that endanger the healthy heart. In the past, the focus was primarily on total cholesterol in the blood. The higher this number was, the greater the risk of heart disease. The NHLBI's National Cholesterol Education Program has recommended more comprehensive testing, called a *lipoprotein profile,* for all individuals age 20 or older (see Savvy Consumer: "What You Need to Know About Your Lipoprotein Profile").

This blood test, which should be performed after a 9- to 12-hour fast and repeated at least once every five years, provides readings of:

■ **Total cholesterol.**

■ **LDL (bad) cholesterol,** the main culprit in the buildup of plaque within the arteries.

■ **HDL (good or *H*ealthy) cholesterol,** which helps prevent cholesterol buildup.

■ **Triglycerides,** the blood fats released into the bloodstream after a meal.

FAQ WHAT IS A HEALTHY CHOLESTEROL READING?

Total cholesterol is the sum of all the cholesterol in your blood. The higher your total cholesterol, the greater your risk for heart disease. The National Heart, Lung and Blood Institute uses the following levels to assess overall risk of heart disease:

Total Cholesterol

Less than 200 mg/dL	"Desirable" level that puts you at lower risk for heart disease
200 to 239 mg/dL	"Borderline-high"
240 mg/dL and above	"High" blood cholesterol. A person with this level has more than twice the risk of heart disease compared to someone whose cholesterol is below 200 mg/dL.

Total cholesterol is not the only crucial number you should know. Because LDL increases your risk for heart disease, you always should find out your LDL level. Even if your total cholesterol is higher than 200, you may not be at high risk for a heart attack. Some people—such as women before menopause and young, active men who have no other risk factors—may have high HDL cholesterol and desirable LDL levels. Ask your doctor to interpret your results so you both know your numbers and understand what they mean.

The updated guidelines of the National Cholesterol Education Program (NCEP) focus on the greatest threat to your heart's health: LDL cholesterol. However, the degree of danger of a higher reading depends not just on the number itself but on whether or not you have other risk factors for heart disease. These include age (over 45 in men, over 55 in women), smoking, high blood pressure, high blood sugar, diabetes, abdominal obesity ("belly" fat), and a family history of heart disease. The new guidelines set lower target goals for LDL cholesterol, particularly for those at greatest risk of a heart attack or death from cardiovascular disease (Table 15-2).

HDL, good cholesterol, also is important, particularly in women. Federal guidelines define an HDL reading of less than 40 mg/dL as a major risk factor for developing heart disease. HDL levels of 60 mg/dL or more are protective and lower the risk of heart disease.

Triglycerides, the free-floating molecules that transport fats in the bloodstream, ideally should be below 150 mg/dL. Individuals with readings of 150 to 199 mg/dL, considered borderline, as well as those with higher readings, may benefit from weight control, physical activity, and if necessary, medication.

 Whether you are male, female, white, or black, if you have high blood pressure and high cholesterol, you are at greater risk of heart disease and stroke than those without these combined conditions. According

TABLE 15-2 NEW TARGETS FOR LOWERING LDL

Risk Category	LDL Goal
Low Risk (1 or 0 risk factors for heart disease)	Less than 160 mg/dL
Moderate Risk (2 or more risk factors that create a 10 percent or lower risk of a heart attack in the next 10 years)	Less than 130 mg/dL
Moderately High Risk (2 or more risk factors that create a 10 to 20 percent chance of a heart attack in next 10 years)	Less than 130 mg/dL
High Risk (heart disease or diabetes, diseased blood vessels, 2 or more risk factors)	Less than 100 mg/dL
Very High Risk (heart disease and multiple, severe, or poorly controlled risk factors, especially smoking, or a history of heart attack or angina)	Less than 70 mg/dL

Source: Based on the National Cholesterol Education Program Adult Treatment Panel III Guidelines, www.circulationaha.org.

to epidemiological research, black men and women have the highest combined rates of systolic blood pressure and total cholesterol.[41]

LOWERING CHOLESTEROL

According to federal guidelines, about one in five Americans may require treatment to lower their cholesterol level and the risk of dying from heart disease. The National Cholesterol Education Program (NCEP) estimates that some 36 million

Savvy Consumer :: What You Need to Know About Your Lipoprotein Profile

- Go to your primary health-care provider to get a lipoprotein profile. Although cholesterol tests at shopping malls or health fairs can help identify people at risk, the analyzers are often not certified technicians, and the readings may be inaccurate. In addition, without a health expert to counsel them, some people may be unnecessarily frightened by a high reading—or falsely reassured by a low one.

- Ask about accuracy. Even at first-rate laboratories, cholesterol readings are often inaccurate. Find out if the lab is using the National Institutes of Health standards, and ask about the lab's margin for error (which should be less than 5 percent).

- Fast beforehand. Cholesterol tests are most accurate after a 9- to 14-hour fast. Schedule the test before breakfast if you can. Women may not want to get tested at the end of their menstrual cycles, when minor elevations in cholesterol levels occur because of lower estrogen levels. Cholesterol levels can also rise 5 to 10 percent during periods of stress. Reschedule the test if you come down with an intestinal flu because the viral infection could interfere with the absorption of food and thus with cholesterol levels. Let your doctor know if you're taking any drugs. Common medications, including birth control pills and hypertension drugs, can affect cholesterol levels.

- Sit down before allowing blood to be drawn or your finger to be pricked; fluids pool differently in the body when you're standing than when you're sitting. Don't let a technician squeeze blood from your finger, which forces fluid from cells, diluting the blood sample and possibly leading to a falsely low reading.

- Get real numbers. Don't settle for "normal" or "high," because laboratories can inaccurately label results. Find out exactly what your reading is: your LDL, HDL, and triglyceride levels.

Americans should be watching their diet and exercising more. Another 65 million should be taking cholesterol-lowering drugs. Depending on your lipoprotein profile and an assessment of other risk factors, your physician may recommend that you take steps to lower your LDL cholesterol.

Lifestyle Changes

Some individuals with elevated cholesterol can improve their lipoprotein profile with lifestyle changes:

- **Dietary changes.** In the past, dietary changes reduced cholesterol by only 4 to 13 percent, relatively modest improvements compared to the effects of medications, which can cut cholesterol by as much as 35 percent. However, a diet consisting of cholesterol-lowering foods, including nuts, soy, oats, and plant sterols (in margarine and green leafy vegetables), reduced LDL cholesterol by about 30 percent. An added benefit: a reduction in C-reactive protein, discussed below. Researchers are recommending this diet as an effective first treatment for individuals with high cholesterol levels, particularly when coupled with exercise and weight loss.

- **Weight management.** For individuals who are overweight, losing weight can help lower LDL. This is especially true for those with high triglyceride levels and/or low HDL levels and those who have a large waist measurement (more than 40 inches for a man and more than 35 inches for a woman).

- **Physical activity.** The recommended amount is 30 minutes on most, if not, all days. Regular activity can help lower LDL, lower blood pressure, reduce triglycerides, and, particularly importantly, raise HDL. Again, these benefits are especially important for those with high triglyceride levels or large waist measurements.

Lifestyle changes can lower harmful LDL levels by 5 to 10 percent. However, a greater reduction of 30 to 40 percent requires either the kind of intensive lifestyle changes promoted by Dr. Dean Ornish, including an extremely low-fat diet (described on page 446), or the addition of cholesterol-lowering medication.

Medications

The last decade has seen a revolution in treatment for high cholesterol, thanks to a new class of drugs called statins—better known by brand names such as Lipitor, Mevacor, Pravachol, and Zocor. These medications can cut the risk of dying of a heart attack by as much as 40 percent. Initially tested in men, statins have proved equally beneficial for women, including those whose cholesterol levels rise after menopause. Statins are currently used by an estimated 11 million Americans. Because LDL targets are now lower, the number of people on statins could rise to about 50 million.

Statins work in the liver to block production of cholesterol. When the liver can't make cholesterol, it draws LDL cholesterol from the blood to use as raw material. This means that less LDL is available to trigger or promote the artery-clogging process known as atherosclerosis. Statins also appear to stabilize cholesterol-filled deposits in artery walls and to cool down inflammation. All of these actions can help prevent a heart attack or other forms of cardiovascular trouble. Long-term therapy with statins reduces the risk for death, heart attack, and stroke among people with heart disease, even when LDL levels are not elevated. The lower the LDL, the lower the risk.

All medications, including the ones used to lower LDL, cost money and sometimes cause side effects. However, if you are at high risk of having a heart attack, their benefits far outweigh the costs and risks.

Raising HDL—which can be done with lifestyle changes, vitamins such as niacin, or a combination of both—can both stop and reverse the progression of cardiovascular plaque. Other medications, called fibrates, can help lower triglycerides, the main fat-carrying particle in the blood.

(FAQ) SHOULD I TAKE A STATIN TO PREVENT HEART DISEASE?

With so many ads touting the benefits of cholesterol-lowering statin drugs, many people who don't have heart disease wonder if they have anything to gain and nothing to lose by taking one of these medications. However, medical experts caution that taking a statin or any cholesterol-lowering drug could do more harm than good. Statins can cause liver and muscle damage, and they require close monitoring. A far safer option would be to make lifestyle changes, such as not smoking, controlling your weight, eating a heart-healthy diet, and getting regular exercise.

For those who already have heart disease or are at high risk for it because of a condition such as diabetes, taking a statin in addition to lifestyle measures to lower LDL ("bad") cholesterol is probably a good idea. Women with heart disease may benefit even more than men.

In addition to their cholesterol-lowering benefits for those at risk, statins have other positive effects in the body. They seem to ease inflammation, which (as discussed on page 445) is a major player in the development of atherosclerosis. Their use has been linked with improved blood vessel growth, stronger bones, prevention of heart rhythm abnormalities, and even a lower risk of depression. When given within 24 hours of a heart attack, they reduce complications and the risk of dying.

▌OTHER RISK INDICATORS

C-REACTIVE PROTEIN (CRP)

C-reactive protein (CRP), produced in the liver, rises whenever the body responds to inflammation. As scientists recognized the role of inflammation in heart disease (see the discussion of atherosclerosis on page 445), they developed

---

Strategies for Change ❖ Lowering LDL and C-Reactive Protein

- Stop smoking.
- Eat a diet rich in fruit and vegetables.
- Increase your daily servings of whole grains and bran-containing foods.
- Cut back on high-fat foods.

- Exercise regularly for at least 30 minutes each day.
- Aim for a healthy weight by thinking long-term and making gradual changes.

- Know your numbers, including blood pressure and lipoprotein levels, and follow your doctor's advice on whether you would benefit from medication.

---

the high-sensitivity CRP test (hsCRP), which detects coronary artery inflammation by measuring small changes in CRP. Several investigations have shown that CRP can predict heart disease before any other risk factors become evident, particularly in women. Individuals with the highest CRP levels (Table 15-3) are two to seven times more likely to develop heart disease than those with the lowest levels.[43] High concentrations of CRP also may predict greater risk of sudden death.[44] The test seems most useful in combination with a lipoprotein profile and assessments of other blood components.[45]

Does lowering CRP reduce the dangers of inflammation or prevent damage to the arteries? Medical researchers don't know for sure. However, individuals with lower CRP levels have less risk of developing or dying from heart disease. Various strategies can reduce CRP. These include lifestyle changes (healthy diet, exercise, weight control, and not smoking) and medications (aspirin and, as needed, drugs to lower cholesterol and blood pressure).

Exercise may be particularly effective. In studies that compared people who got little or no exercise, those who exercised at moderate levels were somewhat less likely to have elevated CRP levels, while those who exercised vigorously had a significantly lower risk than couch potatoes. In people who've had heart attacks or been diagnosed with heart disease, exercise lowers CRP, regardless of whether they also lose weight and take cholesterol-lowering statins.

While CRP testing is not yet a standard screening tool, doctors are using it for those at intermediate or high risk of developing coronary artery disease in the next ten years. The results can help them decide on the need for further evaluations and more aggressive therapy.

HOMOCYSTEINE

Homocysteine is an amino acid in the blood. Higher levels have been linked to a greater risk of heart disease and stroke. Homocysteine may have an effect on atherosclerosis by damaging the inner lining of arteries and promoting blood clots. Several clinical trials are under way to test whether lowering homocysteine will reduce the risk of heart disease.

Folic acid and vitamins B_6 and B_{12} break down homocysteine in the body and lower blood levels. The widespread consumption of folate-fortified foods has reduced the average level of homocysteine in the U.S. population. Green leafy vegetables also are a good source of folic acid.

TABLE 15-3 C-REACTIVE PROTEIN (CRP) LEVELS AND CARDIOVASCULAR RISK

CRP (milligrams per liter)	Level of Cardiovascular Risk
Less than 0.5 mg/L	Lowest
Less than 1 mg/L	Low
1–3 mg/L	Moderate
Greater than 3 mg/L	High (risk doubles)

Measuring homocysteine levels can help in assessing an individual's cardiovascular risks. This may be particularly true in patients with a personal or family history of heart disease who do not have the usual well-established risk factors, such as elevated cholesterol or high blood pressure.

CRISES OF THE HEART

CORONARY ARTERY DISEASE

The general term for any impairment of blood flow through the blood vessels, often referred to as "hardening of the arteries," is **arteriosclerosis.** The most common form is **atherosclerosis,** a disease of the lining of the arteries in which **plaque**—deposits of fat, fibrin (a clotting material), cholesterol, other cell parts, and calcium—narrows the artery channels. However, twenty-first century research has revealed that inflammation also plays a crucial role.

Atherosclerosis

This process begins when LDL cholesterol penetrates the wall of an artery. Ideally, HDL cholesterol carries the cholesterol out of the artery wall to the liver for disposal. However, if LDL accumulates, the artery responds by releasing chemical messengers called cytokines, which trigger active inflammation in the artery wall. T-lymphocytes and macrophages, specialized white blood cells that are part of the body's defensive immune system, move from the bloodstream into the artery and engulf the LDL. As they ingest the LDL, the macrophages enlarge and become foam cells, which rupture, releasing cholesterol into the artery wall, where the cycle of damage begins again. In response, the

Red blood cell

LDL

Macrophage

Hard fibrous cap

Plaque

Foam cells

FIGURE 15-6   How Atherosclerosis Happens

LDL cholesterol penetrates an artery wall, and the accumulation of LDL cholesterol triggers an inflammation. Macrophages engulf the LDL and become foam cells. The artery wall creates a fibrous cap over this plaque, and the artery is narrowed. If the plaque ruptures, blood clots can block blood flow to the heart or to the brain.

smooth muscle cells in the artery wall create a fibrous cap over the inflamed area (Figure 15-6).[46]

These hard-capped plaques are dangerous: They narrow arteries, reduce the flow of blood, and produce angina (chest pain). However, the usual culprits in heart attacks are smaller, softer plaques that can rupture. As the body responds with clotting factors, platelets, and blood cells, a blood clot, or thrombus, forms on the disrupted plaque's surface. The clot ultimately blocks the artery and kills heart muscle cells. Similar clots can block blood flow to the brain and lead to other complications, including kidney failure and circulation problems in the legs and feet.

An early sign that this insidious process is underway is a rise in C-reactive protein. Although CRP levels can help determine if individuals are at high risk and might benefit from aggressive preventive measures, including both lifestyle changes and medications, doctors are still learning when to measure CRP levels and how to use the readings to guide therapy.[47] However, they advise commonsense steps such as regular exercise and a heart-healthy diet to lower both CRP and harmful LDL cholesterol and reduce the dangers of atherosclerosis.

Unclogging the Arteries

Reversing the buildup of plaque inside the arteries is possible with cholesterol-lowering drugs and a low-fat diet. A strict program of dietary and lifestyle change without any medication, developed by Dean Ornish, M.D., of the University of California, San Francisco, also has proved effective in reversing coronary artery disease. The following are the key elements of this approach:

▪ **A very low-fat, vegetarian diet,** including non-fat dairy products and egg whites, keeping fat intake to below 8 percent of total calories consumed. Ornish's recommended diet allows no meat, poultry, fish, butter, cheese, ice cream, or any form of oil.

▪ **Moderate exercise,** consisting of an hour of aerobic activity three times a week. Walking is recommended because more rigorous exercise might be dangerous for heart patients, who may develop increased risk of blood clots, irregular heartbeats, or coronary artery spasms during exertion.

▪ **Stress counseling.** Ornish's patients learn how the body's stress response can cause a rapid heartbeat and narrowing of the arteries, and how stress reduction can reduce cholesterol levels.

▪ **An hour a day of yoga, meditation, breathing, and progressive relaxation.** Some patients use visualization, for instance, imagining their arteries being cleared by a tunneling machine.

ANGINA PECTORIS

A temporary drop in the supply of oxygen to the heart tissue causes feelings of pain or discomfort in the chest known as **angina pectoris.** Some people suffer angina only when the demands on their hearts increase, such as during exercise or when under stress. Many people have angina for years and yet never suffer a heart attack; in some, the angina even disappears. However, angina should be considered a warning of danger if it becomes more severe or more frequent, occurs with less activity or exertion, begins to waken a person from a sound sleep at night, persists for more than ten to fifteen minutes, or causes unusual perspiration.

CORONARY ARTERY SPASMS

Sometimes the arteries tighten suddenly or go into a spasm, cutting off or reducing blood flow. Spasms can produce heart attacks, as well as angina, and can be fatal. Several factors may trigger spasms in the heart, including the following:

▪ **Clumping of platelets.** When *platelets* (a type of blood cell) clump together, they produce a substance called thromboxane A-2, which causes the narrowing of a blood vessel.

- **Smoking.** When some angina victims stop smoking, their chest pain declines or disappears.

- **Stress.** No one knows exactly how stress may lead to spasms, but many heart specialists believe that it's a culprit.

- **Increased calcium flow.** Calcium regularly flows into smooth muscle cells; too much calcium, however, may lead to a spasm. (This calcium flow is not regulated by the amount of calcium in your diet.)

HEART ATTACK (MYOCARDIAL INFARCTION)

Each year, about 1.1 million Americans suffer a heart attack. About 460,000 are fatal. Half of the deaths occur within an hour of the start of symptoms and before the person reaches the hospital. The medical name for a heart attack, or coronary, is **myocardial infarction (MI).** The *myocardium* is the cardiac muscle layer of the wall of the heart. It receives its blood supply, and thus its oxygen and other nutrients, from the coronary arteries. If an artery is blocked by a clot or plaque, or by a spasm, the myocardial cells do not get sufficient oxygen, and the portion of the myocardium deprived of its blood supply begins to die. Although such an attack may seem sudden, usually it has been building up for years, particularly if the person has ignored risk factors and early warning signs.

FAQ **How Do I Know It's a Heart Attack?**

If they experience the following symptoms, individuals should seek immediate medical care and take an aspirin (325 milligrams) to keep the blood clot in a coronary artery from getting any bigger:

- A tight ache, heavy, squeezing pain, or discomfort in the center of the chest, which may last for 30 minutes or more and is not relieved by rest.

- Chest pain that radiates to the shoulder, arm, neck, back, or jaw.

- Anxiety.

- Sweating or cold, clammy skin.

- Nausea and vomiting.

- Shortness of breath.

- Dizziness, fainting, or loss of consciousness.

 Women often experience heart attacks differently than men. In the month before an attack, many report unusual fatigue and disturbed sleep. Far fewer women than men experience chest pain. More common symptoms are shortness of breath, weakness and fatigue, a clammy sweat, dizziness, and nausea.

If you're with someone who's exhibiting the classic signs of heart attack, and if they last for two minutes or more, act at once. Expect the person to deny the possibility of anything as serious as a heart attack, but insist on taking prompt action.

Time is of the essence when a heart attack occurs. If you develop symptoms or if you're with someone who does, call the emergency system (911 in most places) immediately. The sooner emergency personnel get to a heart attack and administer cardiac life support, the greater the odds of survival. Yet according to the American Heart Association, most patients wait three hours after the initial symptoms begin before seeking help. By that time, half of the affected heart muscle may already be lost.

Saving Hearts

State-of-the-art treatments for heart attacks include clot-dissolving drugs, early administration of medications to thin the blood, intravenous nitroglycerin, and, in some cases, a beta-blocker (which blocks many of the effects of adrenaline in the body, particularly its stimulating impact on the heart).

Clot-dissolving drugs called thrombolytic agents are the treatment of choice for acute myocardial infarction in most clinical settings. Administered through a *catheter* (flexible tube) threaded through the arteries to the site of the blockage (the more effective method of delivery) or injected intravenously (the faster, cheaper method of delivery), these agents can save lives and dissolve clots, but don't remove the underlying atherosclerotic plaque.

Two clot-thinning drugs may be better than one for treating heart attacks. One drug, called a thrombolytic, dissolves blood clots. The second drug, a platelet receptor blocker, keeps platelets from clumping and forming the blood clots that can obstruct blood flow and thereby trigger a heart attack or stroke.

Emergency balloon **angioplasty** has shown greater effectiveness than clot-dissolving medication in restoring blood flow in arteries immediately after an attack. With this approach, arteries are less likely to close down again and patients have shorter hospital stays and fewer hospital readmissions. Angioplasty patients also are less likely to die of the heart attack or to experience repeat attacks.

 Women who have heart attacks are less likely than men to survive over both the short and the long term. A woman's risk of dying within a month of a heart attack is up to 75 percent higher than a man's, in part because women typically take an hour longer to get to the hospital than men. Women also have more complications than men during hospitalization and a higher death rate. Men are more likely to receive therapy with aspirin, beta-blockers, or angiotensin-converting enzyme inhibitors and to undergo angioplasty or bypass surgery.

Cardiopulmonary Resuscitation (CPR) and Defibrillation

Cardiac arrest occurs when the heart stops beating. If circulation isn't restored within four or five minutes, the brain shuts down completely, and the person dies. **Cardiopulmonary resuscitation (CPR),** a combination of mouth-

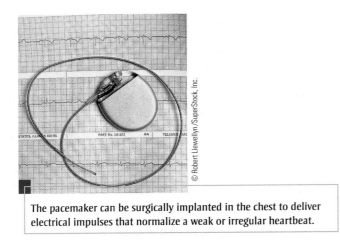

The pacemaker can be surgically implanted in the chest to deliver electrical impulses that normalize a weak or irregular heartbeat.

to-mouth breathing and chest compressions, can keep individuals with cardiac arrest alive until they can be treated in a hospital.

Only about one in twenty people who have a cardiac arrest outside a hospital survive, even if they receive CPR.[48] The reason may be that even trained health professionals do not perform CPR correctly.[49] CPR is most effective when started within minutes of a cardiac arrest by trained medical personnel who arrive within 8 to 12 hours. If performed incorrectly, CPR may be ineffective or harmful.

Automated external defibrillators (AEDs), portable computerized devices, can actually restart a heart with a lethal rhythm (ventricular fibrillation) or that is not beating at all. The machines, widely available on airplanes and in public places like stadiums and terminals, also can be purchased for about $1,500. Written and voice instructions allow lay people as well as trained professionals to use them in case of emergency. A combination of CPR and defibrillation boosts the survival rate much higher than from CPR alone.[50]

OTHER HEART DISORDERS

Arrhythmias (Heart Rate Abnormalities)

The heart has its own electrical system, which produces an evenly timed, regular beat. When relaxed, most adults have a heart rate of between 60 and 80 beats per minute—slower if they're in good physical condition. During strenuous activity or stress, the heart beats faster. Sometimes the heart seems to skip a beat or experience premature (or early) heartbeats. In many cases, these irregularities, or **arrythmias,** are no cause for alarm; but they can be dangerous in an MI victim. Caffeine, long suspected of triggering irregular heartbeats, doesn't seem to be a culprit.

A very fast heart rate (over 100 beats per minute) is known as **tachycardia;** a very slow one (under 60 beats per minute) is **bradycardia.** Resting heart rates of under 60 beats per minute aren't necessarily signs of illness, even though they meet the definition of bradycardia; in fact, they may reflect excellent physical condition.

Treatment options include medications, an artificial pacemaker about the size of a small beeper (to ensure that the heart keeps beating regularly), and radio frequency ablation, a nonsurgical procedure that has revolutionized arrhythmia therapy. In this treatment, cardiologists thread a catheter with an electrode at its tip into the blood vessels of the heart. Using drugs to trigger an irregular heartbeat, they pinpoint its source and administer pulses of radio frequency energy (similar to microwave heat) that destroy the cells sending errant signals. The risks are low, and more than 90 percent of patients report a complete cure.

As both sexes age, other arrhythmias, often linked with coronary artery disease, increase—and become increasingly perilous. Half of all deaths associated with coronary artery disease are due to arrhythmias.

More than 680 Americans die each day because their hearts suddenly stop beating. Cardiac arrest, which results from the extremely rapid, chaotic quivering of the heart's lower chambers (a condition called ventricular fibrillation), often is reversible—if treated within a few minutes with an electric shock to the heart from a defibrillator, a device that can allow a normal rhythm to resume.

Mitral-Valve Prolapse

Mitral-valve prolapse (MVP) is a condition in which a valve in the heart is abnormally long and floppy. Normally, after blood rushes from the left atrium to the left ventricle, the valve between the two chambers slaps shut. But in some people, the closed valve bulges or prolapses back into the atrium. This often occurs because the valve doesn't close completely and blood leaks back into the atrium. This leakage, also called regurgitation, is what doctors may hear as a murmur when listening to your heart.

In the past doctors calculated that up to 30 percent of otherwise healthy young people had MVP. However, this problem is substantially less common and less serious than previously believed. According to recent estimates, MVP affects about 2 percent of the population rather than the 5 to 35 percent of the population previously believed. MVP, once thought to be more common in women, affects men and women equally.

In addition to being thought to have a high prevalence rate, MVP was seen as a disease with frequent and serious complications, including stroke and heart failure. New data show that these complications do not occur at higher rates among patients with mitral-valve prolapse compared to those patients without prolapse.

Congestive Heart Failure

When the heart's pumping power is well below normal capacity, fluid begins to collect in the lungs, hands, and feet. The heart is then said to be in failure. As blood fluids accumulate in the lungs, pulmonary congestion occurs, causing shortness of breath. In other parts of the body, fluid seeps through the thin capillary walls and causes swelling (edema), especially in the ankles and legs. **Congestive heart failure** usually results from myocardial infarction but can also be the result of rheumatic fever, birth defects, hypertension, or atherosclerosis. As many as 4.7 million Americans develop congestive heart failure, which causes 250,000 deaths a year. It is treated by reducing the workload on the heart, modifying salt intake, administering drugs that rid the body of excess fluid, and using medications (such as digitalis) to improve the heart's pumping efficiency. Adding the medication spironolactone, a standard diuretic, can reduce heart failure deaths by 30 percent.

Rheumatic Fever

Rheumatic fever, which strikes most often between the ages of 5 and 15, is a disease that causes painful, swollen joints; skin rashes; and heart damage in half its victims. It is always preceded by a streptococcal infection (see Chapter 14 on infectious diseases). A new strain of streptococcal bacteria has caused a resurfacing of rheumatic fever, which had been considered a disease of the past. The first step to prevention is early identification of the streptococcal infection; the second is treatment with antibiotics to avoid permanent scarring of the heart valves.

Congenital Defects

Approximately 8 out of every 1,000 children born in the United States have congenital heart disease. The most common defects are holes in the ventricular septum, the wall dividing the lower chambers of the heart. Holes may also occur in the atrial septum, the wall between the upper chambers. Sometimes the arteries delivering blood to the body and lungs are transposed and thus attached to the wrong ventricles. Such babies have a bluish color because their blood isn't carrying sufficient oxygen.

HEART SAVERS

A generation ago physicians had no way of detecting problems before the symptoms of heart disease began and could offer little more than bed rest as a therapy after they struck.

Tremendous progress has been made in the diagnosis and treatment of heart problems. Today men and women with heart problems can learn of possible dangers much earlier than in the past and undergo treatments that may add years to their lives.

DIAGNOSTIC TESTS

The **electrocardiogram (ECG, EKG),** a recording of the electrical activity of the heart, is the traditional method of evaluating the heart's health (Figure 15-7). An exercise ECG—or *stress test*—is one method of finding out whether an area of the heart begins to run out of blood during the stress of an athletic workout. The subject walks or jogs on a treadmill while the ECG monitors the heart's response. This test is less accurate in women because of a high rate of false positives.

Thallium scintigraphy uses radioactive isotopes that are injected into the bloodstream. A special imaging device called a *scintillation,* or gamma camera, picks up the rays emitted by the isotopes; a computer translates these signals into images of the heart as it pumps. The test can be performed while the patient is either resting or exercising on a treadmill or bicycle. Adding a thallium scan to an exercise ECG increases the probability of detecting existing heart disease by 70 to 90 percent. A stress echocardiogram uses ultrasound to study the heart.

In **coronary angiography,** the most complete and accurate diagnostic test for heart problems, a thin tube is threaded through the blood vessels of the heart, a radiopaque dye is injected, and X rays are taken to detect any blockage of the arteries. Angiography is extremely precise, but it's also costly and risky: About one of every 1,500 patients dies as a result of the test.

A wave of advances in cardiac imaging may change the way doctors diagnose and treat heart disease. They include

(a)

(b)

© Bruce Ayres/Stone/Getty Images

FIGURE 15-7   ECG Readings
(a) A recording of normal electrical activity in the heart. (b) Grossly irregular activity seen in an acute heart attack.

CT scans show a healthy heart (left) and one with a stent in place.

improvements in CT (computed tomography) scanning, which uses highly specialized X-ray machines to take multiple, finely layered pictures of the heart and surrounding blood vessels (see photos). Sophisticated computer programs generate intricately detailed, three-dimensional images. Advances in other techniques like MRI (magnetic resonance imaging) also provide clear images of the inner workings of the heart. However, the tests are so new that cardiologists are still sorting out which scan is best for which patient and insurance companies may not reimburse for all.

TREATMENTS

Most people with heart disease can be treated successfully with medications. Other alternatives are bypass surgery, balloon angioplasty, heart transplants, and external and implanted mechanical devices. Patients who respond positively, remain optimistic, and are conscientious in taking prescribed medications significantly reduce their risk of death, a subsequent heart attack, or another coronary event.

Aspirin and the Heart

Daily aspirin has been recommended as a preventive step for people at high risk of cardiovascular disease because it reduces the stickiness of platelets (cells that cause blood clotting). This lowers the risk of blood clots, which can block a blood vessel and trigger a heart attack or stroke. Several research studies, such as the Hypertension Optimal Treatment study, have demonstrated an association between aspirin use and reductions in heart attacks in men.

 Low-dose aspirin has not proved equally beneficial for women. In the landmark Women's Health Study, women under age 65 who took aspirin every other day did not lower their chances of having a first heart attack. However, aspirin did lower their risk of a first-ever stroke. And in women over age 65, aspirin reduced both strokes and heart attacks.[51] This is not true for men. While aspirin lowers the likelihood of heart attack, it may slightly increase stroke risk.

Who should consider aspirin therapy? Patients and their doctors should always make the decision, but in general those who might benefit include:

▪ Men over age 40 with several risk factors for having a heart attack.

▪ Men in their 50s, even if they don't have any risk factors.

▪ Women age 65 or older.

▪ Men and women with diabetes and at least one other risk factor.

▪ Anyone who has cardiovascular disease.

Aspirin can produce side effects, including gastrointestinal bleeding, allergic reactions, and peptic ulcers. However, the very low doses recommended for heart disease prevention generally do not cause serious problems. They are not advised for people taking anticlotting medication, who have stomach ulcers, or who have kidney or liver disease. Some individuals are aspirin-resistant and do not benefit from its protective effects.

Medications

The main types of drugs used to treat high blood pressure and heart disease include diuretics; beta-blockers; calcium channel blockers; and angiotensin-converting enzyme (ACE) inhibitors, which block the hormone angiotensin

A catheter with a tiny balloon is used in balloon angioplasty to widen a clogged artery.

that strongly influences blood pressure. Side effects range from lethargy and fatigue to an increased risk of chest pain and heart attack if certain drugs are discontinued abruptly. Calcium channel blockers and ACE inhibitors have become more popular, even though they have not proved more effective than older medications such as diuretics and beta-blockers. Unlike the older drugs, the new ones are less likely to cause side effects such as impotence, insomnia, lethargy, and depression. The newer drugs can be taken in lower doses with negligible side effects.

Surgical Procedures and Mechanical Aids

A **coronary bypass** is a procedure in which an artery from the patient's leg or chest wall is grafted onto a coronary artery to detour blood around the blocked area. Each year hundreds of thousands of coronary bypasses are performed in the United States; about 1 to 5 percent of these patients die as a result of surgical complications. Surgery or angioplasty to improve blood flow in patients with moderate to severe levels of blood flow restriction to the heart reduces the risk of cardiac death more than drugs alone.

Coronary bypasses do not extend life for individuals with mild to moderate angina unless the left main coronary artery was the one that was blocked. If drugs fail to control angina, a coronary bypass can eliminate pain. But surgery is not a cure for the atherosclerotic process that caused the blockage.

A **stent**—a metal mesh tube that may be coated with medication—helps maintain blood flow and prevent a new blockage. Stents that release medication reduce the risk of a renarrowing of an artery.[52]

Percutaneous transluminal coronary angioplasty (PTCA), also called balloon angioplasty, is the most often performed heart operation. Less costly and less risky than bypass surgery, PTCA opens blood vessels in the heart that are narrowed but not completely blocked. PTCA involves a precise, time-consuming technique called *cardiac catheterization*—the threading of a narrow tube or catheter through

an artery to the heart. An X ray taken with a special dye injected into the arteries reveals the location and extent of a blockage. By inflating a tiny balloon at the tip of the catheter, physicians can break up the clog and widen the narrowed artery. When they deflate the balloon, circulation is restored. Stents can help prevent balloon-opened arteries from clogging again.

For a variety of heart disorders in which the heart muscle has become so damaged that it can no longer effectively pump blood throughout the body, the only hope is a heart transplant. In recent years the survival rates for transplant recipients have improved dramatically. *Left-ventricular-assist devices (LVADs)* enhance the pumping action of the heart. Until a donor heart becomes available, fully implantable models may someday serve as permanent blood-pumping devices.

STROKE

When the blood supply to a portion of the brain is blocked, a cerebrovascular accident, or **stroke,** occurs. Someone in the United States suffers a stroke every 53 seconds; more than a quarter are under age 65. An estimated 20 percent of stroke victims die within three months; 50 to 60 percent are disabled. About half of those who have a stroke are partially paralyzed on one side of their body; between a quarter and a half are partially or completely dependent on others for daily living; a third become depressed; a fifth cannot walk.

Strokes rank third, after heart disease and cancer, as a cause of death in this country. Worldwide, stroke is second only to heart disease as a cause of death. After decades of steady decline, the number of strokes per year has begun to rise. The main reasons seem to be that more people in the United States are living longer, advanced medical care is allowing more people to survive heart disease, and doctors are better able to diagnose and detect strokes. Yet 80 percent of strokes are preventable, and key risk factors can be modified through either lifestyle changes or drugs. The most important steps are treating hypertension, not smoking, managing diabetes, lowering cholesterol, and taking aspirin.

Strokes continue to occur 40 percent more often in the Southeast (the so-called Stroke Belt) than in other regions of the United States. However, stroke rates have fallen in Mississippi and Alabama, while they've increased in Oregon, Washington, and Arkansas.

(FAQ) WHAT CAUSES A STROKE?

There are two types of stroke: *ischemic stroke,* which is the result of a blockage that disrupts blood flow to the brain, and *hemorrhagic stroke,* which occurs when blood vessels rupture. One of the most common causes of ischemic stroke is the blockage of a brain artery by a thrombus, or blood clot—a *cerebral thrombosis.* Clots generally form around deposits sticking out from the arterial wall. Sometimes a wandering

---

Strategies for Prevention ⬛ How to Recognize a Stroke

Prompt treatment can stop a stroke in its track—but only with prompt treatment. Researchers have found that the following steps can identify facial weakness, arm weakness, and speech problems, all signs of a stroke:

■ Ask the individual to smile.

■ Ask him or her to raise both arms.

■ Ask the person to speak a simple sentence, such as "It is sunny out today."

If he or she has trouble with any of these tasks, call 9-1-1 immediately and describe the symptoms to the dispatcher.

---

blood clot (embolus), carried in the bloodstream, becomes wedged in one of the cerebral arteries. This is called a *cerebral embolism,* and it can completely plug up a cerebral artery.

In hemorrhagic stroke, a diseased artery in the brain floods the surrounding tissue with blood. The cells nourished by the artery are deprived of blood and can't function, and the blood from the artery forms a clot that may interfere with brain function. This is most likely to occur if the patient suffers from a combination of hypertension and atherosclerosis. Hemorrhage (bleeding) may also be caused by a head injury or by the bursting of an aneurysm, a blood-filled pouch that balloons out from a weak spot in the wall of an artery.

Brain tissue, like heart muscle, begins to die if deprived of oxygen, which may then cause difficulty speaking and walking, and loss of memory. These effects may be slight or severe, temporary or permanent, depending on how widespread the damage and whether other areas of the brain can take over the function of the damaged area. About 30 percent of stroke survivors develop dementia, a disorder that robs a person of memory and other intellectual abilities.

TRANSIENT ISCHEMIC ATTACKS (TIAs)

Sometimes a person will suffer **transient ischemic attacks (TIAs),** "little strokes" that cause minimal damage but serve as warning signs of a potentially more severe stroke. One of three people who suffer TIAs will have a stroke during the following five years if they don't get treatment. The two major types of TIAs are:

■ **Transient monocular blindness.** Blurring, a blackout or whiteout of vision, a sense of a shade coming down, or another visual disturbance in one eye.

■ **Transient hemispheral attack.** Diminished blood flow to one side of the brain, causing numbness or weakness of one arm, leg, or side of the face, or problems speaking or thinking.

Many TIAs are caused by a narrowing of blood vessels in the neck (carotid arteries) because of a buildup of plaque. Specialists can diagnose this problem by feeling and listening to the arteries, by ultrasound, by measuring the pressure or circulation rate from the carotid arteries to the eyes, or by arterial angiography (injection of a dye into the arteries as X rays are taken), a procedure that can be dangerous, even deadly, or lifesaving.

Surgery to widen the carotid arteries may be recommended for individuals under age 60 with significant narrowing (50 to 80 percent or more). For other patients, aspirin and other drugs that make platelets less sticky and interfere with clotting may be effective.

RISK FACTORS FOR STROKES

Other risk factors, like those for heart disease, include some that can't be changed (such as gender and race) and some that can be controlled:

■ **Gender.** Men have a greater risk of stroke than women. However, women are at increased risk at times of marked hormonal changes, particularly pregnancy and childbirth. Past studies have shown an association between oral contraceptive use and stroke, particularly in women over age 35 who smoke. The newer low-dose oral contraceptives have not shown an increased stroke risk among women ages 18 to 44. A woman's stroke risk may increase markedly at menopause.

■ **Race.** The incidence of strokes is two to three times greater in blacks than whites in the same communities. Hispanics also are more likely to develop hemorrhagic strokes than whites.

■ **Age.** A person's risk of stroke more than doubles every decade after age 55.

■ **Hypertension.** Detection and treatment of high blood pressure are the best means of stroke prevention.

■ **High red blood cell count.** A moderate to marked increase in the number of a person's red blood cells increases the risk of stroke.

■ **Heart disease.** Heart problems can interfere with the flow of blood to the brain; clots that form in the heart can travel to the brain, where they may clog an artery.

■ **Blood fats.** Although the standard advice from cardiologists is to lower harmful LDL levels, what may be more important to lower stroke risk is a drop in the levels of protective HDL.

▪ **Diabetes mellitus.** Diabetics have a higher incidence of stroke than nondiabetics.

▪ **Estrogen therapy.** In 2004, the Women's Health Initiative—a series of clinical trials of hormone therapy for post-menopausal women—halted its study of estrogen-only therapy because of an increase in the risk of stroke. Women on estrogen experienced 12 more strokes per 10,000 persons, compared to women not taking hormones.[53]

▪ **A diet high in fat and sodium.** Individuals consuming the largest amounts of fatty foods and sodium are at much greater risk then those eating low-fat, low-salt diets.[54]

TREATMENTS FOR STROKES

A small ("baby") aspirin a day cuts in half the risk of strokes caused by abnormal heartbeats, which strike 75,000 Americans each year. Extremely rapid beating of the heart's upper chambers causes blood clots to form; they may enter the bloodstream and travel to the brain, where they can get stuck and choke off the blood supply. In the past, the only way to prevent such strokes was regular use of a medication called warfarin, which inhibits blood clotting and therefore increases the risk of severe bleeding. However, aspirin proved as effective as warfarin—without that dangerous side effect.[55]

Increasingly, surgeons are operating on carotid arteries that may have been narrowed by a buildup of atherosclerotic plaque—a condition that contributes to 20 to 30 percent of strokes, some in individuals with no symptoms—by cleaning them out in a procedure called *carotid endartectomy*. This procedure has been shown to be effective in preventing stroke in patients with and without early symptoms of stroke. An alternative is brain angioplasty, in which surgeons thread a catheter tipped with a tiny inflatable balloon into an artery and gently inflate it to restore blood flow.

It now seems possible to save brain cells during a brief period immediately after a thrombotic stroke occurs. Thrombolytic drugs such as tissue-type plasminogen activator (tPa), can restore brain blood flow after a thrombotic stroke; other medications called heparinoids can reduce the blood's tendency to clot. For thrombolytic drugs to be effective, they must be administered within three hours after the stroke; heparinoids must be given within 24 hours. However, the average person does not seek help for 22 hours or longer.

Physicians also are experimenting with ways to tie off tiny, bleeding, cranial arteries with tiny "clothespins" or to suction off blood that is exerting pressure on the brain. Using stereotactic radio imagery, which relies on a three-dimensional imaging system, surgeons can focus an X-ray beam on a clot or hemorrhage and destroy it.

Learn It / Live It

Protecting Your Heart

Heart disease is not inevitable. We can keep our hearts healthy for as long as we live, but the process of doing so must start early and continue throughout life.

▪ **Don't smoke.** There's no bigger favor you can do your heart—and lungs!

▪ **Watch your weight.** Even relatively modest gains can have a big effect on your risk of heart disease.

▪ **Cut down on saturated fats and cholesterol.** This can help prevent high blood cholesterol levels, obesity, and heart disease.

▪ **Get moving.** Engage in regular physical activity. A little is better than none; more is even better.

▪ **Lower your stress levels.** If too much stress is a problem in your life, try the relaxation techniques described in Chapter 4.

▪ **Know your family history.** Inheriting a predisposition to high blood pressure or heart disease means that your heart needs extra preventive care.

▪ **Get your blood pressure checked regularly.** Knowing your numbers can alert you to a potential problem long before you develop any symptoms.

▪ **Tame your temper.** Hostility can be hazardous to the heart. Look for other ways of releasing anger and frustration.

▪ **Get a lipoprotein profile.** You can't know if your heart is in danger unless you know your cholesterol and lipoprotein levels. Get a blood test at your next physical, and discuss the results with your physician.

▪ **Take appropriate medications.** Those with high cholesterol or high blood pressure should seek their physicians' advice.

Making This Chapter Work for You

Review Questions

1. The heart
   a. has four chambers, which are responsible for pumping blood into the veins for circulation through the body.
   b. pumps blood first to the lungs where it picks up oxygen and discards carbon dioxide.
   c. beats about 10,000 times and pumps about 75 gallons of blood per day.
   d. has specialized cells that generate electrical signals to control the amount of blood that circulates through the body.

Self Survey ▦ What Is Your Physical Activity and Heart Disease IQ?

Mark each statement true or false.

T   F   1. Regular physical activity can reduce your chances of getting heart disease.
T   F   2. Most people get enough physical activity from their normal daily routine.
T   F   3. You don't have to train like a marathon runner to become more physically fit.
T   F   4. Exercise programs do not require a lot of time to be very effective.
T   F   5. People who need to lose some weight are the only ones who will benefit from regular physical activity.
T   F   6. All exercises give you the same benefits.
T   F   7. The older you are, the less active you need to be.
T   F   8. It doesn't take a lot of money or expensive equipment to become physically fit.
T   F   9. There are many risks and injuries that can occur with exercise.
T   F   10. You should consult a doctor before starting a physical activity program.
T   F   11. People who have had a heart attack should not start any physical activity program.
T   F   12. To help stay physically active, include a variety of activities.

Check your answers:

1 **True** Heart disease is almost twice as likely to develop in inactive people. Being physically inactive is a risk factor for heart disease along with cigarette smoking, high blood pressure, high blood cholesterol, and being overweight. The more risk factors you have, the greater your chance for heart disease. Regular physical activity (even mild to moderate exercise) can reduce this risk.

2 **False** Most Americans are very busy but not very active. Every American adult should make a habit of getting 30 minutes of low to moderate levels of physical activity daily. This includes walking, gardening, and walking up stairs. If you are inactive now, begin by doing a few minutes of activity each day. If you only do some activity every once in a while, try to work something into your routine everyday.

3 **True** Low- to moderate-intensity activities, such as pleasure walking, stair climbing, yardwork, housework, dancing, and home exercises can have both short- and long-term benefits. If you are inactive, the key is to get started. One great way is to take a walk for 10 to 15 minutes during your lunch break, or take your dog for a walk every day. At least 30 minutes of physical activity everyday can help improve your heart health.

4 **True** It takes only a few minutes a day to become more physically active. If you don't have 30 minutes in your schedule for an exercise break, try to find two 15-minute periods or even three 10-minute periods. These exercise breaks will soon become a habit you can't live without.

5 **False** People who are physically active experience many positive benefits. Regular physical activity gives you more energy, reduces stress, and helps you to sleep better. It helps to lower high blood pressure and improves blood cholesterol levels. Physical activity helps to tone your muscles, burns off calories to help you lose extra pounds or stay at your desirable weight, and helps control your appetite. It can also increase muscle strength, help your heart and lungs work more efficiently, and let you enjoy your life more fully.

6 **False** Low-intensity activities—if performed daily—can have some long-term health benefits and can lower your risk of heart disease. Regular, brisk, and sustained exercise for at least 30 minutes, three to four times a week, such as brisk walking, jogging, or swimming, is necessary to improve the efficiency of your heart and lungs and burn off extra calories. Other activities, depending on the type, may give you other benefits such as increased flexibility or muscle strength.

7 **False** Although we tend to become less active with age, physical activity is still important. In fact, regular physical activity in older persons increases their capacity to do everyday activities. In general, middle-aged and older people benefit from regular physical activity just as young people do. What is important, at any age, is tailoring the activity program to your own fitness level.

8 **True** Many activities require little or no equipment. For example, brisk walking requires only a comfortable pair of walking shoes. Many communities offer free or inexpensive recreation facilities and physical activity classes. Check your shopping malls, as many of them are open early and late for people who do not wish to walk alone, in the dark, or in bad weather.

9 **False** The most common risk in exercising is injury to the muscles and joints. Such injuries are usually caused by exercising too hard for too long, particularly if a person has been inactive. To avoid injuries, try to build up your level of activity gradually, listen to your body for warning pains, be aware of possible signs of heart problems (such as pain or pressure in the left or mid-chest area, left neck, shoulder, or arm during or just after exercising, or sudden light-headedness, cold sweat, pallor, or fainting), and be prepared for special weather conditions.

10 **True** You should ask your doctor before you start (or greatly increase) your physical activity if you have a medical condition such as high blood pressure, have pains or pressure in the chest and shoulder, feel dizzy or faint, get breathless after mild exertion, are middle-aged or older and have not been physically active, or plan a vigorous activity program. If none of these apply, start slow and get moving.

11 **False** Regular, physical activity can help reduce your risk of having another heart attack. People who include regular physical activity in their lives after a heart attack improve their chances of survival and can improve how they feel and look. If you have had a heart attack, consult your doctor to be sure you are following a safe and effective exercise program that will help prevent heart pain and further damage from overexertion.

12 **True** Pick several different activities that you like doing. You will be more likely to stay with it. Plan short-term and long-term goals. Keep a record of your progress, and check it regularly to see the progress you have made. Get your family and friends to join in. They can help keep you going.

Source: National Heart, Lung, and Blood Institute; National Institutes of Health

YOUR ACTION PLAN FOR LOWERING HEART DISEASE RISK

1. **Maintain a healthy weight.**
   - Check with your health-care provider to see if you need to lose weight.
   - If you do, lose weight slowly using a healthy eating plan and engaging in physical activity.

2. **Be physically active.**
   - Engage in physical activity for a minimum of 30 minutes on most days of the week.
   - Combine everyday chores with moderate-level sporting activities, such as walking, to achieve your physical activity goals.

3. **Follow a healthy eating plan.**
   - Set up a healthy eating plan with foods low in saturated fat, total fat, and cholesterol, and high in fruits, vegetables, and low fat dairy foods.
   - Write down everything that you eat and drink in a food diary. Note areas that are successful or need improvement.
   - If you are trying to lose weight, choose an eating plan that is lower in calories.

4. **Reduce sodium in your diet.**
   - Choose foods that are low in salt and other forms of sodium.
   - Use spices, garlic, and onions to add flavor to your meals without adding more sodium.

5. **Drink alcohol only in moderation.**
   - In addition to raising blood pressure, too much alcohol can add unneeded calories to your diet.
   - If you drink alcoholic beverages, have only a moderate amount—one drink a day for women, two drinks a day for men.

6. **Take prescribed drugs as directed.**
   - If you need drugs to help lower your blood pressure or cholesterol, you still must follow the lifestyle changes mentioned here.
   - Use notes and other reminders to help you remember to take your drugs.

CASE IN POINT

Student: April, 22

Goal: Get her blood pressure under control

Action Plan:

- Find out specifics of her family's history of high blood pressure
- Talk to her doctor about how being African American may affect her blood pressure
- Reduce the salt in her diet by cutting back on processed and fast foods
- Increase her exercise by walking to classes instead of taking a shuttle bus
- Use the guidelines in Chapter 7 to get her weight under control

Health Now™   If you want to write your own goals for avoiding heart problems, go to the **Wellness Journal HealthNow** at http://healthnow.brookscole.com/ith

2. You can help maintain a healthy heart by doing all the following *except*
   a. getting regular moderate levels of exercise every day.
   b. stopping smoking and avoiding regular exposure to secondhand smoke.
   c. taking vitamin E supplements daily.
   d. controlling your blood pressure.

3. Which of the following statements about blood pressure is true?
   a. Blood pressure increases when the heart relaxes.
   b. Systolic blood pressure is the pressure of the blood entering the atrium of the heart.
   c. High blood pressure is usually the cause of sudden cardiac death in young athletes.
   d. Blood pressure decreases during diastole.

4. You can control all of these risk factors for heart disease *except*
   a. male pattern baldness.
   b. diabetes mellitus.
   c. sedentary lifestyle.
   d. blood fat cells.

5. Hypertension
   a. is diagnosed when blood pressure is consistently lower than 130/85 mm Hg.
   b. may be treated with dietary changes, which include eating low-fat foods and avoiding sodium.
   c. can cause fatty deposits to collect on the artery walls.
   d. usually does not respond to medication, especially in severe cases.

6. In your lipoprotein profile, having a high level of this blood element is a good thing:
   a. LDL cholesterol
   b. HDL cholesterol
   c. C-reactive protein
   d. triglyceride

7. Which of the following statements about coronary artery disease is *false*?
   a. In atherosclerosis, arteries are narrowed by deposits of plaques on the arterial walls.
   b. One successful approach to treatment combines a very low-fat diet, moderate exercise, and stress reduction.
   c. Once plaque appears in the arteries, it is impossible to reverse the effects of coronary artery disease.
   d. A coronary thrombosis may occur if a coronary artery is blocked by a blood clot.

8. A heart attack
   a. occurs when the myocardium receives an excessive amount of blood from the coronary arteries.
   b. is typically suffered by individuals who have irregular episodes of atherosclerosis.
   c. can be treated successfully up to four hours after the event.
   d. occurs when the myocardial cells are deprived of oxygen-carrying blood, causing them to die.

9. Treatments for heart disease include all the following *except*
   a. diuretics and beta-blockers.
   b. coronary bypass surgery to detour blood around a blocked artery.
   c. electrocardiogram to normalize the electrical activity of the heart.
   d. balloon angioplasty to open narrowed blood vessels.

10. Which of the following statements about stroke is true?
    a. A stroke occurs when the blood supply to the aorta is blocked.
    b. Ischemic stroke is usually caused by a blood clot in the brain.
    c. Little strokes, also called transient ischemic attacks, can cause permanent blindness and paralysis of one side of the body.
    d. Risk factors for stroke include gender and occupation.

Answers to these questions can be found on page 587.

Critical Thinking

1. Have you had your blood pressure checked lately? If your reading was high, what steps are you now taking to help reduce your blood pressure?

2. Have you had a lipoprotein profile lately? Do you think it's necessary for you to obtain one? If your reading was/is borderline or high, what lifestyle changes can you make to help control your cholesterol level?

3. The costs for a heart transplant are over $100,000. The annual price tag for a year's worth of cyclosporine, the drug that prevents rejection and must be taken for the rest of a transplant recipient's life, is about $5,000. The total medical bill can come to hundreds of thousands of dollars—enough to fund programs to improve the nutrition of poor pregnant women, to treat alcoholism, or to provide regular preventive care. Does treatment of any single individual justify such huge costs? Should our society try to balance the costs versus the benefits of such heroic measures as heart transplants? How would you go about making such decisions?

Media Menu

Health ⊗ Now™

Throughout the chapter, this icon introduces a list of resources on the Health-Now website at **http://healthnow.brookscole.com/ith** that will:
- Help you evaluate your knowledge of the material
- Allow you to take an exam-prep quiz
- Provide a Personalized Learning Plan targeting resources that address areas you should study
- Coach you through identifying target goals for behavior change and creating and monitoring your personal change plan throughout the semester.

INTERNET CONNECTIONS

National Cholesterol Education Program

http://www.nhlbi.nih.gov/chd/

This comprehensive site features interactive sessions on planning a low-cholesterol diet and lots more. It provides you with information to prevent heart disease as well as information for people who already have heart disease. You can also hear radio messages from the Heart Beat Radio Network. This site is highly recommended.

American Heart Association

http://www.americanheart.org/

This comprehensive site features a searchable database of all major cardiovascular diseases, plus information on healthy lifestyles, current research, CPR, cardiac warning signs, risk awareness, low-cholesterol diets, and family health. The interactive Heart Profilers® provides personalized information about treatment options for common cardiovascular conditions such as hypertension, heart failure, and cholesterol.

HeartSite.com

http://www.heartsite.com/

This site, developed by two prominent cardiologists at the Medical College of Georgia, features many color diagrams to illustrate cardiac disease, including diagnostic tests, procedures, and treatment. The site also features a multi-media lecture on heart disease and heart failure with slides and accompanying audio lecture.

The Heart: An Online Exploration

http://www.fi.edu/biosci/heart.html

This interesting site, developed by the Franklin Institute of Science, provides an interactive multimedia tour of the heart, as well as statistics, resources, links, and information on how to monitor your heart's health by becoming aware of your vital signs.

InfoTrac College Edition Activities Log on, insert **cardiovascular disease** into the Keyword search box, and limit your search to the past year. When you get the results, Mark articles to review, then Select one to read. Summarize three or four key points from the article.

You can find additional readings related to personal health with InfoTrac College Edition, an online library of more than 900 journals and publications. Follow the instructions for accesssing InfoTrac College Edition that were packaged with your textbook; then search for articles using a keyword search.

For additional links, resources, and suggested readings on the InfoTrac College Edition, visit our Health and Wellness Resource Center at **http://health .wadsworth.com.**

Key Terms

The terms listed are used on the page indicated. Definitions of the terms are in the Glossary at the end of this book.

angina pectoris 446

angioplasty 447

aorta 430

arrhythmia 448

arteriosclerosis 445

atherosclerosis 445

atrium 430

bradycardia 448

capillary 430

cardiopulmonary resuscitation (CPR) 447

cholesterol 435

congestive heart failure 448

coronary angiography 449

coronary bypass 451

diabetes mellitus 437

diastole 430

diastolic blood pressure 435

electrocardiogram (ECG, EKG) 449

homocysteine 445

hypertension 435

lipoprotein 435

male pattern baldness 439

metabolic syndrome 436

mitral-valve prolapse 448

myocardial infarction (MI) 447

percutaneous transluminal coronary angioplasty (PTCA) 451

plaque 445

prehypertension 441

stent 451

stroke 451

systole 430

systolic blood pressure 435

tachycardia 448

thallium scintigraphy 449

transient ischemic attack (TIA) 452

triglyceride 436

ventricle 430

Celine knows that she inherited her mother's brown eyes and buoyant sense of humor. She wonders whether she's also inherited "the bad gene"—the cancer-causing one that killed her grandmother and great-grandmother. Celine's mother was 42 years old when she learned that she, too, had cancer. She died two years later, leaving behind eight sisters. Within the next decade, six had developed breast or ovarian cancer.

Unlike most college students, Celine never thinks of cancer as something that affects only people much older than she. Three of her five sisters have tested positive for what is called "the breast cancer gene." Celine is struggling to decide whether she too will undergo testing.

An estimated 10 percent of cancers are hereditary, but no one is immune from the threat of cancer or other serious diseases.

Cancer has overtaken heart disease as the number-one killer of Americans under age 85. Yet many of the almost 500,000 deaths caused by cancer each year could be prevented. A third of cancers are related to smoking; another third, to obesity, poor diet, and lack of exercise.[1] Many of the other serious illnesses discussed in this chapter, including diabetes mellitus, epilepsy, asthma, and digestive disorders, also can be prevented or improved by lifestyle changes and appropriate immunizations.

This chapter is a lesson in self-defense against the illnesses that can threaten your well-being and your survival. The information that it provides can help you boost your defenses, recognize and avoid health threats, protect yourself, and realize when to seek medical help.

© Roger Charity/Stone/Getty Images

(FAQ) Frequently Asked Questions

- Who is at risk for developing cancer? *p. 460*
- Are you addicted to tanning? *p. 467*
- Who is at risk for developing diabetes? *p. 474*
- What should I do in case of an asthma attack? *p. 478*

After studying the material in this chapter, you should be able to:

- **Explain** how cancer develops.
- **List** the risk factors for cancer, and **describe** ways you can reduce your risk of cancer.
- **Discuss** the most common types of cancer, and **describe** the treatments for each.
- **Explain** the disease process of diabetes mellitus, and **describe** the early symptoms and treatment for this disease.
- **Describe** common major respiratory, liver, kidney, digestive, skeletal-muscular, and skin diseases.

UNDERSTANDING CANCER

The uncontrolled growth and spread of abnormal cells causes cancer. Normal cells follow the code of instructions embedded in DNA (the body's genetic material); cancer cells do not. Think of the DNA within the nucleus of a cell as a computer program that controls the cell's functioning, including its ability to grow and reproduce itself. If this program or its operation is altered, the cell goes out of control. The nucleus no longer regulates growth. The abnormal cell divides to create other abnormal cells, which again divide, eventually forming **neoplasms** (new formations), or tumors.

HOW CANCER SPREADS

Tumors can be either *benign* (slightly abnormal, not considered life-threatening) or *malignant* (cancerous). The only way to determine whether a tumor is benign is by microscopic examination of its cells. Cancer cells have larger nuclei than the cells in benign tumors; they vary more in shape and size; and they divide more often.

At one time cancer was thought to be a single disease that attacked different parts of the body. Now scientists believe that cancer comes in countless forms, each with a genetically determined molecular "fingerprint" that indicates how deadly it is. With this understanding, doctors can identify how aggressively a tumor should be treated.

Without treatment, cancer cells continue to grow, crowding out and replacing healthy cells. This process is called **infiltration,** or invasion. Cancer cells may also **metastasize,** or spread to other parts of the body via the bloodstream or lymphatic system (Figure 16-1). For many cancers, as many as 60 percent of patients may have metastases (which may be too small to be felt or seen without a microscope) at the time of diagnosis.

WHO IS AT RISK FOR DEVELOPING CANCER?

According to the American Cancer Society, 1.37 million individuals are diagnosed with cancer each year; about 570,280 die of it. Cancer death rates have decreased in men by about 1 percent per year since 1992. The five-year survival rate for all cancer is 64 percent, up from 50 percent three decades ago.[2]

Since the occurrence of cancer increases over time, most cases affect adults who are middle-aged or older (Table 16-1). In the United States, men have a one in two lifetime risk of developing cancer; for women, the risk is one in three (Figure 16-2).

The term **relative risk** compares the risk of developing cancer in people with a certain exposure or trait to the risk in those who do not have this exposure or trait. Smokers, for instance, have a ten-times-greater relative risk of developing lung cancer than nonsmokers. Most relative risks are smaller. For example, women who have a first-degree (mother, sister,

TABLE 16-1   AGE AND THE RISK OF CANCER (ALL SITES)

	Men	Women
Birth to age 39	1 in 64	1 in 51
Ages 40 to 59	1 in 12	1 in 11
Ages 60 to 79	1 in 3	1 in 4
Birth to death	1 in 2	1 in 3

Source: Cancer Facts & Figures 2005. Atlanta, GA: American Cancer Society, 2005.

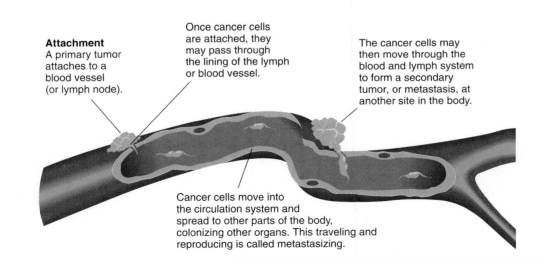

Attachment A primary tumor attaches to a blood vessel (or lymph node).

Once cancer cells are attached, they may pass through the lining of the lymph or blood vessel.

The cancer cells may then move through the blood and lymph system to form a secondary tumor, or metastasis, at another site in the body.

Cancer cells move into the circulation system and spread to other parts of the body, colonizing other organs. This traveling and reproducing is called metastasizing.

FIGURE 16-1   Metastasis, or Spread of Cancer

Cancer cells can travel through the blood vessels to spread to other organs, or through the lymphatic system to form secondary tumors.

Strategies for Prevention :: Seven Warning Signs of Cancer

If you note any of the following seven warning signs, immediately schedule an appointment with your doctor:

:: Change in bowel or bladder habits.

:: A sore that doesn't heal.

:: Unusual bleeding or discharge.

:: Thickening or lump in the breast, testis, or elsewhere.

:: Indigestion or difficulty swallowing.

:: Obvious change in a wart or mole.

:: Nagging cough or hoarseness.

Estimated New Cases*		Estimated Deaths	
Male	**Female**	**Male**	**Female**
Prostate 232,090 (33%)	Breast 211,240 (32%)	Lung and bronchus 90,490 (31%)	Lung and bronchus 73,020 (27%)
Lung and bronchus 93,010 (13%)	Lung and bronchus 79,560 (12%)	Prostate 30,350 (10%)	Breast 40,410 (15%)
Colon and rectum 71,820 (10%)	Colon and rectum 73,470 (11%)	Colon and rectum 28,540 (10%)	Colon and rectum 27,750 (10%)
Urinary bladder 47,010 (7%)	Uterine corpus 40,880 (6%)	Pancreas 15,820 (5%)	Ovary 16,210 (6%)
Melanoma of the skin 33,580 (5%)	Non-Hodgkin's lymphoma 27,320 (4%)	Leukemia 12,540 (4%)	Pancreas 15,980 (6%)
Non-Hodgkin's lymphoma 29,070 (4%)	Melanoma of the skin 26,000 (4%)	Esophagus 10,530 (4%)	Leukemia 10,030 (4%)
Kidney and renal pelvis 22,490 (3%)	Ovary 22,220 (3%)	Liver 10,330 (3%)	Non-Hodgkin's lymphoma 9,020 (3%)
Leukemia 19,640 (3%)	Thyroid 19,190 (3%)	Non-Hodgkin's lymphoma 10,150 (3%)	Uterine corpus 7,310 (3%)
Oral cavity 19,100 (3%)	Urinary bladder 16,200 (2%)	Urinary bladder 8,970 (3%)	Multiple myeloma 5,640 (2%)
Pancreas 16,100 (2%)	Pancreas 16,080 (2%)	Kidney and renal pelvis 8,020 (3%)	Brain and nervous system 5,480 (2%)
All sites 710,040 (100%)	All sites 662,870 (100%)	All sites 295,280 (100%)	All sites 275,000 (100%)
All sites 699,560	All sites 668,470	All sites 290,890	All sites 272,810

FIGURE 16-2 Sex Differences in Cancer Rates and Deaths

Source: ©2005, American Cancer Society, Inc., Surveillance Research.

or daughter) family history of breast cancer have about a twofold increased risk of developing breast cancer compared with women who do not have a family history of the disease. This means that they are about twice as likely to develop breast cancer.

HEREDITY

An estimated 13 to 14 million Americans may be at risk of a hereditary cancer. In hereditary cancers, such as retinoblastoma (an eye cancer that strikes young children) or certain colon cancers, a specific cancer-causing gene is passed down from generation to generation. The odds of any child with one affected parent inheriting this gene and developing the cancer are fifty/fifty.

Other people are born with genes that make them susceptible to having certain cells grow and divide uncontrollably, which may contribute to cancer development. The most well-known are mutations of the BRCA gene, linked with increased risk of breast, colon, and ovarian cancer.

© Michael Doolittle / The Image Works

By age 39, 1 in 64 men and 1 in 51 women will develop cancer. Consider your risk factors and lifestyle: What do you think are your odds of getting cancer?

Researchers recently recognized an even more common inherited cancer susceptibility gene, known as TGFRB1*6A, carried by nearly one in eight people, that increases cancer risk by 26 percent.[3]

Genetic tests can identify some individuals who are born with an increased susceptibility to cancer. By spotting a mutated gene in an individual, doctors can sometimes detect cancer years earlier through increased cancer screening. The most likely sites for inherited cancers to develop are the breast, brain, blood, muscles, bones, and adrenal glands. The telltale signs of inherited cancers include:

▪ **Early development.** Genetic forms of certain diseases strike earlier than noninherited cancers. For example, the average age of women diagnosed with breast cancer is 62. But if breast cancer is inherited, the average age at diagnosis is 44, an 18-year difference.

▪ **Family history.** Anyone with a close relative (mother, father, sibling, child) with cancer has about three times the usual chance of getting the same type of cancer.

▪ **Multiple targets.** The same type of hereditary cancer often strikes more than once—in both breasts or both kidneys, for instance, or in two separate parts of the same organ.

▪ **Unusual gender pattern.** Genes may be responsible for cancers that generally don't strike a certain gender—for example, breast cancer in a man.

▪ **Cancer family syndrome.** Some families, with unusually large numbers of relatives affected by cancer, seem clearly cancer-prone. For instance, in Lynch syndrome (a form of colon cancer), more than 20 percent of the family members in at least two generations develop cancer of both the colon and the endometrium.

RACIAL AND ETHNIC GROUPS

More cases of cancer occur in black Americans than in any other racial or ethnic group.[4] Blacks are 30 percent more likely to die of cancer than whites. African-American women have the highest incidence of colorectal and lung cancers of any ethnic group, while black men have the highest rates of prostate, colorectal, and lung cancer. African Americans also have higher rates of incidence and deaths from other cancers, including those of the mouth, throat, esophagus, stomach, pancreas, and larynx.

Cancer rates also vary in other racial and ethnic groups. Hispanics have six times lower risk of developing melanoma than Caucasians, yet tend to have a worse prognosis than Caucasians when they do develop this skin cancer. The incidence of female breast cancer is highest among white women and lowest among Native American women. Cervical cancer is most common in Hispanic women.

OBESITY

Long recognized as threats to cardiovascular health, overweight and obesity may play a role in an estimated 90,000 cancer deaths each year. According to American Cancer Society researchers who examined the relationship between body mass index (BMI) and risk of dying from cancer, 14 percent of cancer deaths in men and 20 percent of cancer deaths in women may stem from excess weight.

The higher an individual's BMI, the greater the likelihood of dying of cancer. A woman with a BMI of 25 to 30 faces a 30 percent higher risk of breast cancer, while the risk is 63 percent higher for women with BMIs in the 30 to 35 range and 70 percent higher for those with a BMI between 35 and 40. The heaviest men had a 52 percent higher death rate from all cancers, while the heaviest women had a 62 percent higher death rate.[5]

An unhealthy body weight increases the risk of many types of cancer, including breast (in postmenopausal women), colon and rectum, kidney, cervix, ovary, uterus, esophagus, gallbladder, stomach (in men), liver, pancreas, prostate, non-Hodgkin's lymphoma, and multiple myeloma.

The degree to which extra pounds affect cancer risk varies by site. Obesity elevates the risk of esophageal cancer fivefold; increases the risk of breast or uterine cancer by two to four times; and boosts the risk for colon cancer by 35 percent to twofold.[6]

INFECTIOUS AGENTS

Worldwide, an estimated 17 percent of cancers can be attributed to infection. In economically developing countries, infections cause or contribute to 26 percent of cancers. In developed countries, they play a role in 7 percent of new cases of cancer.[7]

Among the cancers that have been linked with infectious agents are human papilloma virus (HPV) with cervical cancer and *Helicobacter pylori* with stomach cancer. Viruses have been implicated in certain leukemias (cancers of the blood system) and lymphomas (cancers of the lymphatic system), cancers of the nose and pharynx, liver cancer, and cervical cancer. Human immune deficiency virus (HIV) can lead to certain lymphomas and leukemias and to a type of cancer called Kaposi's sarcoma.

Generally, the presence of a bacterium or a virus per se is not enough to cause cancer. A predisposing environment and other cofactors—most still unknown—are needed for cancer development and growth.

Your Life Coach

Lowering Your Cancer Risk

Environmental factors may cause between 80 and 90 percent of cancers. At least in theory, these cancers can be prevented by avoiding cancer-causing substances (such as tobacco and sunlight) or using substances that protect against cancer-causing factors (such as antioxidants and vitamin D). How do you start protecting yourself? Simple changes in lifestyle—smart eating, losing excess weight, not smoking, protecting yourself from the sun, exercising regularly—are essential. Despite their initial promise, neither aspirin[8] nor vitamin E[9] has proven effective in preventing specific cancers or cancer in general.

STAY SMOKE-FREE

Cigarette smoking is the single most devastating and preventable cause of cancer deaths in the United States. If you don't smoke, don't start and limit the time you spend around smokers. If you smoke, read Chapter 13 for advice on quitting. Your life could depend on it.

People who smoke two or more packs of cigarettes a day are 15 to 25 times more likely to die of cancer than nonsmokers. Cigarettes cause most cases of lung cancer and increase the risk of cancer of the mouth, pharynx, larynx, esophagus, pancreas, and bladder. Pipes, cigars, and smokeless tobacco also increase the danger of cancers of the mouth and throat.

Environmental tobacco smoke can increase the risk of cancer even among those who've never smoked. For example, exposure to others' tobacco smoke for as little as three hours a day can increase the risk of developing cancer. (See the discussion of environmental tobacco smoke in Chapter 13.)

EAT SMART

The links between diet and cancer are complex, and medical advice is constantly evolving. According to recent studies, cutting down on high-fat foods, particularly in middle age, does little to reduce the risk of breast and colon cancer.[10] In large epidemiological studies, increasing fruits and vegetables did not significantly lower rates of breast cancer.[11] However, there is evidence linking red meat consumption and colon cancer.[12]

The best approach is to follow the guidelines designed for overall well-being. The same foods that keep your heart healthy, your blood pressure low, your bones strong, and your weight under control are most likely to help you reduce your risk of cancer and other major illnesses.

Pay attention to food processing and preparation. Whenever possible, select foods close to their natural state, grown locally and without pesticides. Avoid cured, pickled, or smoked meats. When cooking, try not to fry or barbecue often; these cooking methods can produce mutagens that have induced cancer in animal testing. The process of smoking or charcoal-grilling releases carcinogenic tar that may increase the risk of cancer of the stomach and esophagus.

MAINTAIN A HEALTHY WEIGHT

Obesity, as discussed earlier, causes one in six cancer deaths. Excess weight may account for 14 to 20 percent of all cancers.

 Women who gain more than 20 pounds from age 18 to midlife double their risk of breast cancer compared to those whose weight remains stable. Too much body fat increases cancer risk in several ways: It raises the amount of estrogen in a woman's blood, which may contribute to cancers of the female reproductive system. It also raises levels of insulin, which prompts the body to create a hormone that causes cells to multiply. Obesity also makes various types of cancer harder to diagnose and treat.

LIMIT EXPOSURE TO ENVIRONMENTAL RISKS

Although it may not be possible to avoid all possible **carcinogens** (cancer-causing chemicals), you can take steps to minimize your danger. Many chemicals used in industry, including nickel, chromate, asbestos, and vinyl

Follow workplace safety precautions to avoid unnecessary exposure to carcinogens.

© David Hoffman Photo Library/Alamy

chloride, are carcinogens; employees as well as people living near a factory that creates smoke, dust, or gases are at risk. If your job involves their use, follow safety precautions at work. If you are concerned about possible hazards in your community, check with local environmental protection officials.

Very dark shades of permanent coloring have been linked with several types of cancer, but more recent research did not find strong evidence of a marked increase in cancer risk among personal hair dye users. A ban on potential carcinogens in hair dyes may be the reason for the decline.[13]

Chapter 20 discusses pesticides and other environmental threats.

BE VIGILANT

Proven methods of cancer prevention and early detection could save more than 60,000 lives a year. Screening examinations, conducted regularly by a health-care professional, can lead to early diagnosis of cancers of the breast, colon, rectum, cervix, prostate, testicles, and oral cavity, and can improve the odds of successful treatment. Self-examinations for cancers of the breast, testicles, and skin may also result in detection of tumors at earlier stages. The five-year relative survival rate for all these cancers is about 81 percent. If all Americans participated in regular cancer screenings, this rate could increase to more than 95 percent. (See Your Action Plan for the latest guidelines on cancer screenings.)

COMMON TYPES OF CANCER

Cancer refers to a group of more than a hundred diseases characterized by abnormal cell growth. Although all cancers have similar characteristics, each is distinct. Some cancers are relatively simple to cure, whereas others are more threatening and mysterious. The earlier any cancer is found, the easier it is to treat and the better the patient's chances of survival.

Cancers are classified according to the type of cell and the organ in which they originate, such as the following:

- **Carcinoma,** the most common kind, which starts in the epithelium, the layers of cells that cover the body's surface or line internal organs and glands.
- **Sarcoma,** which forms in the supporting, or connective, tissues of the body: bones, muscles, blood vessels.
- **Leukemia,** which begins in the blood-forming tissues: bone marrow, lymph nodes, and the spleen.
- **Lymphoma,** which arises in the cells of the lymph system, the network that filters out impurities.

SKIN CANCER

Skin cancer is diagnosed in more than 1.5 million Americans every year.[14] One of every five Americans can expect to develop skin cancer in their lifetimes. Once scientists thought exposure to the B range of ultraviolet light (UVB), the wavelength of light responsible for sunburn, posed the greatest danger. However, longer-wavelength UVA, which penetrates deeper into the skin, also plays a major role in skin cancers. An estimated 80 percent of total lifetime sun exposure occurs during childhood, so sun protection is especially important in youngsters. Tanning salons and sunlamps also increase the risk of skin cancer because they produce ultraviolet radiation. A half-hour dose of radiation from a sunlamp can be equivalent to the amount you'd get from an entire day in the sun.

 Young adults spend the most time in the sun and also frequent tanning salons. Even when they perceive the seriousness of skin cancer, college students—particularly women—describe suntanned skin as attractive, healthy, and athletic-looking and view the benefits of getting a suntan as outweighing the risks of skin cancer or premature aging.

A third of college students do not use sunscreen on their faces; about half don't apply sunscreen to their bodies while sunbathing. Even fewer use sunscreen on a routine basis[15] (see Student Snapshot: "Under the Campus Sun"). College athletes who spend a great deal of time in the sun practicing and competing are even less likely to protect their skin. In a study conducted during August and September of soccer and cross-country teams from four colleges, only 6 percent used sunscreens during the previous three days; 15 percent did so in the past week. There were no significant differences between students' genders, ages, school years, or schools. Fair-skinned athletes did report using sunscreen more often than those with darker skin. None reapplied sunscreen during practice.[16]

	Percent of Time
Use sunscreen while sunbathing	
On face	67%
On body	51%
Use sunscreen during incidental sun exposure	
On face	42%
On body	22%
Family history of skin cancer	42%

Based on a study of 146 college students.
Source: Mahler, Heike, et al. "Effects of UV Photographs, Photoaging Information, and Use of Sunless Tanning Lotion on Sun Protection." *Archives of Dermatology,* Vol. 141, March 2005, p. 373, www.archdermatol.com.

The most common skin cancers are *basal-cell* (involving the base of the epidermis, the top level of the skin) and *squamous-cell* (involving cells in the epidermis). Figure 16-3 shows the skin layers and the cells where these cancers originate. Their incidence is increasing among men and women under the age of 40.[17] Long-term exposure to the sun is the biggest risk factor for these cancers.

Every year more than 5 million Americans develop skin lesions known as actinic keratoses (AKs), rough red or brown scaly patches that develop in the upper layer of the skin, usually on the face, lower lip, bald scalp, neck, and back of the hands and forearms. Forty percent of squamous cell carcinomas, the second leading cause of skin cancer deaths, begin as AKs. Treatments include surgical removal, cryosurgery (freezing the skin), electrodesiccation (heat generated by an electric current), topical chemotherapy, and removal with lasers, chemical peels, or dermabrasion.

Smoking and exposure to certain hydrocarbons in asphalt, coal tar, and pitch may increase the risk of squamous-cell skin cancer. Other risk factors include occupational exposure to carcinogens and inherited skin disorders, such as xeroderma pigmentosum and familial atypical multiple-mole melanoma.

Malignant *melanoma,* the deadliest type of skin cancer, causes 1 to 2 percent of all cancer deaths. During the 1930s, the lifetime risk of melanoma was about 1 in 1,500.

Squamous-cell cancer

Melanoma

Basal-cell cancer

Courtesy of the Skin Cancer Foundation (all)

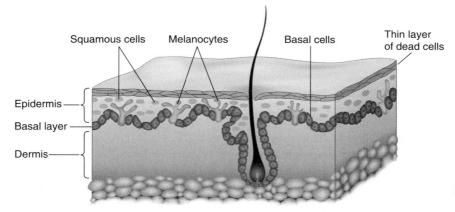

FIGURE 16-3   Three Types of Skin Cancer
Squamous-cell cancer arises from the squamous cells in the epidermis. Malignant melanoma, the deadliest form of skin cancer, arises from melanocyte cells. Basal-cell cancer arises from the basal cells.

Strategies for Prevention ▓ Scanning and Saving Your Skin

▓ Once a month, stand in front of a full-length mirror to examine your front and back, and your left and right sides with your arms raised. Check the backs of your legs, the tops and soles of your feet, and the surfaces between your toes. Use a hand mirror to check the back of your neck, behind your ears, and your scalp.

▓ Watch for changes in the size, color, number, and thickness of moles. Suspicious moles are likely to be asymmetrical (one half doesn't match the other), with ragged, notched, or blurred edges. Also look for any signs of darkly pigmented growth, oozing, scaliness, bleeding, or a change in sensation, itchiness, tenderness, or pain.

▓ Don't put too much faith in sunscreens. Wearing sunscreen (with a sun protection factor, or SPF, of at least 15) is good, but protective clothing is better—and staying in the shade is best. Check your shadow. One simple guideline for reducing the risk of skin cancer is avoiding the sun anytime your shadow is shorter than you are. According to the National Cancer Institute (NCI), this shadow method—based on the principle that the closer the sun comes to being directly overhead, the stronger its ultraviolet rays—works for any location and at any time of year.

▓ Check for photosensitivity. If you are taking any drugs, ask your doctor or pharmacist to see if the medication could make you more sensitive to sun damage. Be especially cautious about sun exposure if you have been using a synthetic preparation derived from vitamin A (Retin A) as an acne or anti-wrinkle treatment; it can increase your susceptibility.

▓ Use extra caution near water, snow, and sand since they reflect the damaging rays of the sun and increase the risk of sunburn. Wear protective clothing, such as a wide-brimmed cap or hat, whenever possible.

Today it is 1 in 75. This increase in risk is due mostly to overexposure to UV radiation. The use of a tanning bed ten times or more a year doubles the risk for individuals over age 30.

Both the amount and the intensity of lifetime sun exposure play key roles in determining risk for melanoma. People living in areas where the sun's ultraviolet rays reach the earth with extra intensity, such as tropical or high-altitude regions, are at increased risk. Although melanoma occurs more often among people over 40, it is increasing in younger people, particularly those who had severe sunburns in childhood. The rate of increase in melanoma also has risen more in men (4.6 percent a year) than for women (3.2 percent). Men are more likely than women to be diagnosed with melanoma after age 40.

Individuals with any of the following characteristics are at increased risk:

▌ **Fair skin,** light eyes, or fair hair.

▌ **A tendency to develop freckles** and to burn instead of tan.

▌ **A history of childhood sunburn** or intermittent, intense sun exposure.

▌ **A personal or family history** of melanoma.

▌ **A large number of nevi,** or moles (200 or more, or 50 or more if under age 20), or dysplastic (atypical) moles.

Detection

The most common predictor for melanoma is a change in an existing mole or development of a new and changing pigmented mole. The most important early indicators are change in color, an increase in diameter, and changes in the borders of a mole (Figure 16-4). An increase in height signals a corresponding growth in depth under the skin. Itching in a new or long-standing mole also should not be ignored.

Asymmetry: One half doesn't match the other half

Border irregularity: The edges are ragged, notched, or blurred

Color: Rather than uniform pigmentation, there are shades of tan, brown, and black, with possible dashes of red, white, and blue.

Diameter: The mole is larger than 6 mm (about the size of a pencil eraser). (The melanoma shown here is magnified about 20 times its actual size.)

Courtesy of the Skin Cancer Foundation

FIGURE 16-4   ABCD: The Warning Signs of Melanoma

An estimated 95 percent of cases of melanoma arise from an existing mole. A normal mole is usually round or oval, less than 6 millimeters (about 1/4 inch) in diameter, and everly colored (black, brown, or tan). Seek prompt evaluation of any moles that change in ways shown in the photo.

Source: American Academy of Dermatology. All rights reserved.

Treatment

If caught early, melanoma is highly curable, usually with surgery alone. Once it has spread, chemotherapy with a single drug or a combination can temporarily shrink tumors in some people. However, the five-year survival rate for metastatic melanoma is 14 percent.

 ARE YOU ADDICTED TO TANNING?

You know that exposure to ultraviolet rays increases your risk of developing skin cancer, but maybe you still can't stay out of the sun or a tanning booth. Why? Researchers theorize that repetitive tanning behavior may be the result of a kind of addiction.[18]

Texas beachgoers, asked questions about their tanning habits, gave replies similar to those who gamble or drink compulsively. About a quarter of those interviewed were classified as "ultraviolet light (UVL) dependent" because of their answers to the CAGE screening test (see Chapter 11), which asks the following questions:

- **C**ut: Ever felt you ought to cut down on your behavior?
- **A**nnoyed: Have people annoyed you by criticizing your behavior?
- **G**uilt: Ever felt bad or guilty about your behavior?
- **E**ye Opener: Ever engaged in your behavior to steady your nerves in the morning?

Answering yes to two of the CAGE questions is a strong indication for an addictive behavior; answering yes to three confirms it.

 BREAST CANCER

Every 3 minutes a woman in the United States learns that she has breast cancer. Every 12 minutes a woman dies of breast cancer. Many women misjudge their own likelihood of developing breast cancer, either overestimating or underestimating their susceptibility. In a national poll, one in every ten surveyed considered herself at no risk at all. This is never the case. Every woman is at risk for breast cancer simply because she's female.

However, not all women's risks are equal. The National Cancer Institute (NCI) has developed a computerized Breast Cancer Risk Assessment Tool, based on data from more than 280,000 women, that allows a woman to sit down with her doctor and discuss her own odds of developing breast cancer within the next five years and over her entire lifetime.

The most common risk factors include the following:

- **Age.** As shown in Figure 16-5, at 25, a woman's chance of developing breast cancer is 1 in 19,608; by age 45, it has increased to 1 in 93; by 65, it is 1 in 17. The mean age at which women are diagnosed is 63.

By age 25	1 in 19,608
By age 30	1 in 2,525
By age 35	1 in 622
By age 40	1 in 217
By age 45	1 in 93
By age 50	1 in 50
By age 55	1 in 33
By age 60	1 in 24
By age 65	1 in 17
By age 70	1 in 14
By age 75	1 in 11
By age 80	1 in 10
By age 85	1 in 9
Ever	1 in 8

 FIGURE 16-5 A Woman's Risk of Developing Breast Cancer

Source: Surveillance Program, National Cancer Institute.

- **Family history.** The overwhelming majority of breast cancers—90 to 95 percent—are not due to strong genetic factors. However, having a first-degree relative—mother, sister, or daughter—with breast cancer does increase risk, and if the relative developed breast cancer before menopause, the cancer is more likely to be hereditary. Genetic testing, controversial but sometimes recommended for women in cancer-prone families, can identify these defects. However, it's not yet clear how many women with a defective gene actually will develop breast cancer; estimates range from 50 to 80 percent, or higher in families with many affected members.

- **Long menstrual history.** Women who had their first period before age 12 are at greater risk than women who began menstruating later. The reason is that the more menstrual cycles a woman has, the longer her exposure to estrogen, a hormone known to increase breast cancer danger. For similar reasons, childless women, who menstruate continuously for several decades, are also at greater risk.

- **Age at birth of first child.** An early pregnancy—in a woman's teens or twenties—changes the actual maturation of breast cells and decreases risk. But if a woman has her first child in her forties, precancerous cells may actually flourish with the high hormone levels of the pregnancy.

- **Breast biopsies.** Even if laboratory analysis finds no precancerous abnormalities, women who require such tests are more likely to develop breast cancer. Fibrocystic breast disease, a term often used for "lumpy" breasts, is not a risk factor.

- **Race.** Breast cancer rates are lower in Hispanic and Asian populations than in whites and in African-American women.

Caucasian women over 40 have the highest incidence rate for breast cancer in this country, but African-American women at every age have a greater likelihood of dying from breast cancer. Researchers don't know if the reason is unequal access to care, a lack of optimal care, or greater aggressiveness of the disease itself in black women.

■ **Occupation.** Based on two decades of following more than a million women, Swedish researchers have developed a list of jobs linked with a high risk of breast cancer. These include pharmacists, certain types of teachers, schoolmasters, systems analysts and programmers, telephone operators, telegraph and radio operators, metal platers and coaters, and beauticians.

■ **Alcohol.** Women's risk of breast cancer increases with the amount of alcohol they drink. Those who take two or more drinks per day are 40 percent more likely to develop breast cancer than women who don't drink at all. For a nondrinking woman, the lifetime risk of breast cancer by age 80 is 1 in 11. For heavy drinkers it's about 1 in 7, regardless of race, education, family history, use of hormone therapy, or other risk factors.[19]

■ **Hormone therapy.** After years of debate over postmenopausal hormone therapy (HT), several studies confirmed an increased risk with a combination of estrogen and progestin, particularly in women who use combination HT for five years or longer.[20] Women taking combination HT are more likely to have abnormal mammograms requiring further testing and to be diagnosed at a more advanced stage of breast cancer. Researchers theorize that estrogen and progestin may stimulate breast cancer growth and hinder cancer diagnosis by increasing breast density. Women using only estrogen did not have an elevated rate of breast cancer.

■ **Obesity.** Excess weight, particularly after menopause, increases the risk of getting breast cancer. Overweight women, both pre- and postmenopausal, with breast cancer are more likely to die of their disease.

■ **Sedentary lifestyle.** According to the World Health Organization, regular physical activity may cut the risk of developing breast cancer by 20 to 40 percent, regardless of a woman's menopausal status or the type or intensity of the activity. The reason may be that exercise lowers levels of circulating ovarian hormones. Exercise may also boost survival in women who've been diagnosed with breast cancer. In one recent study, women who performed the equivalent of walking three to five hours a week at a moderate pace survived longer than those who did not exercise. Among the activities the women engaged in were walking, bicycling, and aerobics classes.[21]

Detection

Doctors long advised women to perform monthly breast self-exams (BSE) after their periods (Figure 16-6). In its newest guidelines, the American Cancer Society now describes BSE as "an option" for women starting in their twenties and

Feeling

1. Lie flat on your back. Place a pillow or towel under one shoulder, and raise that arm over your head. With the opposite hand, you'll feel with the pads, not the fingertips, of the three middle fingers, for lumps or any change in the texture of the breast or skin.

2. The area you'll examine is from your collarbone to your bra line and from your breastbone to the center of your armpit. Imagine the area divided into vertical strips. Using small circular motions (the size of a dime), move your fingers up and down the strips. Apply light, medium, and deep pressure to examine each spot. Repeat this same process for your other breast.

3. Gently squeeze the nipple of each breast between your thumb and index finger. Any discharge, clear or bloody, should be reported to your doctor immediately.

FIGURE 16-6   Breast Self-Exam
The best time to examine your breasts is after your menstrual period every month.

urges all women to report any breast changes promptly. It recommends a breast exam by a trained practitioner every three years for women in their twenties and thirties and every year for women 40 and over and a yearly mammogram for all women, starting at age 40.[22]

The best tool for early detection is the diagnostic X-ray exam called **mammography.** Women whose breast cancer is detected by screening mammography have a significantly better prognosis than those whose cancer is found another way—even if the cancer has already spread to their lymph nodes. A likely reason is that mammography can detect tumors that are both slower growing and less biologically lethal than others.[23] In the future, digital mammography, which allows doctors to break down images of breast cancer into slices, may reveal cancerous tissue even sooner.[24] Mammograms can detect a tumor two to three years before it can be detected by manual exam.

Treatment

Breast cancer can be treated with surgery, radiation, and drugs (chemotherapy and hormonal therapy). Doctors may use one of these options or a combination, depending on the type and location of the cancer and whether the disease has spread.

Most women undergo some type of surgery. **Lumpectomy,** or breast-conserving surgery, removes only the cancerous tissue and a surrounding margin of normal tissue. A modified radical **mastectomy** includes the entire breast and some of the underarm lymph nodes. Radical mastectomy, in which the breast, lymph nodes, and chest wall muscles under the breast are removed, is rarely performed today, because modified radical mastectomy has proved just as effective. Removing underarm lymph nodes is important to determine if the cancer has spread, but a technique called sentinel node biopsy allows physicians to pinpoint the first lymph node into which a tumor drains (the sentinel node) and remove only the nodes most likely to contain cancer cells.

Radiation therapy is treatment with high-energy rays or particles to destroy cancer. In almost all cases, lumpectomy is followed by six to seven weeks of radiation. Chemotherapy is used to reach cancer cells that may have spread beyond the breast—in many cases even if no cancer is detected in the lymph nodes after surgery.

The use of drugs such as **tamoxifen** and aromatase inhibitors, in addition to standard chemotherapy, can significantly lower the risk of recurrence. Biological therapies—monoclonal antibodies that zero in on cancer cells like miniature guided missiles—have shown promise against some aggressive breast tumors. The drug Herceptin, for instance, targets a defective growth-promoting gene (HER-2/neu) found in about 30 percent of women with breast cancer. The combination of monoclonal antibodies and standard chemotherapy has significantly improved survival rates in women with both early-stage and metastatic cancers.[25]

CERVICAL CANCER

An estimated 16,370 cases of invasive cervical cancer are diagnosed in the United States every year, with about 3,710 annual deaths from this disease. The highest incidence rate occurs among Vietnamese women; Alaskan Native, Korean, and Hispanic women also have higher rates than the national average. The mortality rate for African-American women is more than twice that of whites, largely because of a high number of deaths among older black women.

The primary risk factor for cervical cancer is infection with certain types of the human papilloma virus (HPV), discussed in Chapter 14. HPV occurs in more than 99.7 percent of cervical cancer cases. However, not every HPV infection becomes cervical cancer, and while HPV infection is very common, cervical cancer is not. Other risk factors for cervical cancer include early age of first intercourse, multiple sex partners, genital herpes, and smoking or significant exposure to passive smoke.

The standard screening test for cervical cancer is the Pap smear. New, more precise forms of Pap testing and new screening tests for HPV may help detect cases of cervical cancer at earlier stages. Warning signs for cervical cancer include irregular bleeding or unusual vaginal discharge. In precancerous stages, cervical cells can be destroyed by laser surgery or freezing during a visit to a doctor's office.

The National Cancer Institute (NCI) recommends a combination of chemotherapy and radiation rather than the standard use of radiation alone for invasive tumors. For women whose cervical cancer is detected early, cryotherapy (use of extreme cold), electrocoagulation (intense heat), or surgery are standard treatments.

OVARIAN CANCER

Ovarian cancer is the leading cause of death from gynecological cancers. Risk factors include a family history of ovarian cancer; personal history of breast cancer; obesity; infertility (because the abnormality that interferes with conception may also play a role in cancer development); and low levels of transferase, an enzyme involved in the metabolism of dairy foods. Often women develop no obvious symptoms until the advanced stages, although they may experience painless swelling of the abdomen, irregular bleeding, lower abdominal pain, digestive and urinary abnormalities, fatigue, backache, bloating, and weight gain.

The lifetime risk of ovarian cancer in a woman with no affected relatives is 1 in 70. The risk for a woman with one first-degree relative with ovarian cancer is 1 in 20, and the risk increases with additional affected relatives. For women who may have a hereditary ovarian cancer syndrome and have mutations in genes BRCA-1 or BRCA-2, the lifetime risk may be as high as 1 in 2. Routine screening is not recommended for women who are not at known risk. For those at increased risk, a National Institutes of

Health (NIH) consensus panel has recommended annual pelvic and rectal exams, as well as ultrasound imaging of the pelvic region and a blood test for a substance called CA125 every six months. In cases of very high risk, some oncologists (cancer specialists) recommend prophylactic removal of the ovaries when childbearing is completed or by no later than age 35. Treatment involves surgery, radiation therapy, and chemotherapy. The five-year survival rate is 53 percent.

TESTICULAR CANCER

In the last 20 years the incidence of testicular cancer has risen 51 percent in the United States—from 3.61 to 5.44 per 100,000. It is not clear why testicular cancer is on the rise, although researchers speculate that changing environmental or socioeconomic risk factors could have a role. Testicular cancer occurs mostly among young men between the ages of 18 and 35, who are not normally at risk of cancer. At highest risk are men with an undescended testicle (a condition that is almost always corrected in childhood to prevent this danger). To detect possibly cancerous growths, men should perform monthly testicular self-exams, as shown in Figure 16-7.

Although college-age men are among those at highest risk of testicular cancer, three in four do not know how to perform a testicular self-examination.

Often the first sign of this cancer is a slight enlargement of one testicle. There also may be a change in the way it feels when touched. Sometimes men with testicular cancer report a dull ache in the lower abdomen or groin, along with a sense of heaviness or sluggishness. Lumps on the testicles also may indicate cancer.

A man who notices any abnormality should consult a physician. If a lump is indeed present, a surgical biopsy is necessary to find out if it is cancerous. If the biopsy is positive, a series of tests generally is needed to determine whether the disease has spread.

Treatment for testicular cancer generally involves surgical removal of the diseased testis, sometimes along with radiation therapy, chemotherapy, and the removal of nearby lymph nodes. The remaining testicle is capable of maintaining a man's sexual potency and fertility. Only in rare cases is removal of both testicles necessary. Testosterone injections following such surgery can maintain potency. The chance for a cure is very high if testicular cancer is spotted early.

COLON AND RECTAL CANCER

Colon and rectal, or colorectal, cancer is the third most common cancer and accounts for 10 percent of cancer deaths. Most cases occur after age 50. Both age and gender influence the risk of colon cancer. Older individuals and men are more likely to develop polyps (nonmalignant growths that may turn cancerous at some point) and tumors in the colon than young people and women.

Risk factors include age (over 50), personal or family history of colon and rectal cancer, polyps in the colon or rectum, ulcerative colitis, smoking, alcohol consumption, prolonged high consumption of red and processed meat,[26] high-fat or low-fiber diet, and inadequate intake of fruits and vegetables. Nonsteroidal anti-inflammatory drugs, such as aspirin and ibuprofen, and regular exercise may reduce the risk.[27] Vitamin B_6, whether from food or supplements, may help prevent colorectal cancer in women.[28]

The simplest test for colon cancer, the fecal occult blood test, detects blood in a person's stool. It involves placing a small sample of feces on a card and then adding a chemical solution. If the result indicates blood, further testing is needed to detect its source. While simple and easy, it does not detect all colon cancers.

New guidelines recommend screening for colon cancer beginning at age 50, earlier for those at higher risk based on personal, family, or medical history. The initial screening is crucial because it detects the largest, most dangerous polyps, which can then be removed.

Flexible sigmoidoscopy places a lighted tube into the lowest part of the colon after enemas to cleanse the lower part of the bowel. Even a single sigmoidoscopy reduces mortality from cancers in the areas examined by two-thirds. Its primary limitation is inability to screen about half of the bowel, so half of potentially cancerous polyps might not be detected. An estimated 1 to 3 percent of adults have cancerous growths that would not be detected by sigmoidoscopy alone.[29] Current recommendations call for repeat sigmoidoscopies every five years, but some researchers recommend a shorter time interval of every three years.

FIGURE 16-7 Testicular Self-Exam

The best time to examine your testicles is after a hot bath or shower, when the scrotum is most relaxed. Place your index and middle fingers under each testicle and the thumb on top, and roll the testicle between the thumb and fingers. If you feel a small, hard, usually painless lump or swelling, or anything unusual, consult a urologist.

In a colonoscopy, a physician inserts a lighted tube with a camera at its end through the rectum after laxative solutions have cleared feces from the bowel. The colonoscope can be used to sample suspicious areas in the colon and to remove polyps (small growths) that may be precancerous. Colonoscopy is more sensitive and specific than sigmoidoscopy or fecal blood testing, but it also is more expensive and entails greater risks. This screening test should be repeated every ten years.

A large-scale study has detected a crucial difference between the sexes when it comes to detecting and preventing colon cancer: only colonoscopy can detect advanced precancerous polyps in women. In previous studies of men, fecal occult blood testing (which identifies microscopic amounts of blood in stool) and flexible sigmoidoscopy (which examines the lower 25 percent of the colon) were able to identify more than 70 percent of men with advanced pre-cancerous polyps. However, these tools are not as effective in women. The reason: Men and women do not develop polyps in the same area of the colon. Advanced precancerous polyps in men tend to grow in the lower portion of the colon, whereas women's polyps tend to grow deeper in the colon, beyond a flexible sigmoidoscopy's reach.[30]

Early signs of colorectal cancer are bleeding from the rectum, blood in the stool, or a change in bowel habits. Treatment may involve surgery, radiation therapy, and/or chemotherapy.

LEUKEMIA

Risk factors for this cancer of the blood include Down's syndrome and other inherited abnormalities and excessive exposure to radiation or certain chemicals, such as benzene. Leukemia can be difficult to detect early because its symptoms are often similar to those of less serious conditions, such as influenza. Diagnosis is based on blood tests and a bone marrow biopsy. Treatment may involve chemotherapy, drugs, blood transfusions, and bone marrow transplants.

LUNG CANCER

Cigarettes cause most cases of lung cancer, which is the leading cause of cancer deaths in women and in men. Risk factors include cigarette smoking; exposure to certain industrial substances, particularly asbestos; radiation or radon exposure; and environmental tobacco smoke. Family members of individuals with lung cancer are at greater risk themselves, particularly if they are black and smoke.[31] A smoker's risk of developing lung cancer drops almost to that of a nonsmoker within ten years after his or her last cigarette, although the lungs may still be damaged.

 Nonsmoking women are more likely than nonsmoking men to develop lung cancer. The small amount of research available suggests that, when exposed to an environmental carcinogen, nonsmoking women are more susceptible to DNA damage than nonsmoking men.

Warning signs include a persistent cough, sputum streaked with blood, chest pain, recurring bronchitis, or pneumonia. Diagnosis is based on a chest X ray, sputum cytology (cell) testing, and fiber-optic bronchoscopy (direct examination of the lungs by means of a specially lighted tube). The use of CT scans, which can detect tiny tumors, and molecular markers in sputum can lead to earlier diagnosis and might improve survival rates. Treatment generally involves surgery, chemotherapy, and/or radiation. The five-year survival rate for all stages combined is just 15 percent.

ORAL CANCER

Heavy smoking of cigarettes, cigars, or pipes; excessive drinking; and the use of chewing tobacco increase the risk of oral cancer. Those who drink as well as smoke are particularly vulnerable. More young Americans are being diagnosed with oral and tongue cancer.

Early signs include a mouth sore that bleeds easily and doesn't heal; a lump or thickening; a reddish or whitish patch; and difficulty chewing, swallowing, or moving the tongue or jaws. Regular exams by your dentist or primary care physician can detect oral cancers. Surgery and radiation are the standard treatments.

PROSTATE CANCER

After skin cancer, prostate cancer is the most common form of cancer in American men. The risk of prostate cancer is 1 in 6; the risk of death due to metastatic prostate cancer is 1 in 30. More than a quarter of men diagnosed with cancer have prostate cancer. The disease strikes African-American men more often than white; Asian and American Indian men are affected less often.

The risk of prostate cancer increases with age, family history, exposure to the heavy metal cadmium, high number of sexual partners, and history of frequent sexually transmitted diseases. An inherited predisposition may account for 5 to 10 percent of cases. A purported link between vasectomy and prostate cancer has been disproved.

The development of a simple annual screening test that measures levels of a protein called prostate-specific antigen (PSA) in the blood has revolutionized the diagnosis of prostate cancer. PSA testing is recommended for men at high risk (African Americans and men with close relatives with prostate cancer) starting at age 45 and for all men at age 50. It remains controversial, however. Some claim that PSA testing saves lives; others, that it leads to unnecessary and potentially harmful treatments.

Treatment may include hormones, chemotherapy, and radiation. About 60,000 men undergo radical prostate surgery in the United States every year.[32] The five-year survival rate has increased from 67 percent to 99 percent over the past 20 years.[33]

NEW HOPE AGAINST CANCER

Every year for more than a decade the death rate from cancer has fallen by 1 percent. In part, this is due to preventive steps such as not smoking. But advances in treatment also are having a dramatic effect.

As scientists have unraveled the processes by which cancer grows and spreads, they have identified more ways in which they can intervene. Rather than traditional chemotherapy, which kills both cancerous and healthy tissues, new treatments hone in and destroy only the malignant cells. Because targeted drugs are so precise, side effects are relatively minimal. One such drug, Gleevec, has turned the prognosis around for two deadly cancers: chronic myeloid leukemia and a form of advanced stomach cancer called gastrointestinal stomach cancer.

Another frontier is the study of *angiogenesis,* the process by which tumors create new blood vessels. A new therapy called antiangiogenesis cuts off the blood supply needed for tumor growth. When added to conventional chemotherapy, it has extended survival times for patients with some forms of lung cancer, colorectal cancer, and metastatic breast cancer. Researchers are developing personalized vaccines that capture a particular cancer's "fingerprint" and use it to trigger the body's immune system and attack a specific cancer.

CANCER SURVIVORSHIP

Nearly 10 million cancer survivors are living active, productive lives years after diagnosis and treatment.[34] Many have had no evidence of cancer for years; others are in remission, a state in which the spread of cancerous cells is presumed to be temporarily stopped.

But for millions of men, women, and children who "win" their battle against cancer, survival—even when they live past the milestone five-year mark—does not mark the end of their cancer experience. Many cancer survivors encounter difficulties that persist for years after initial diagnosis and treatment. These include physical problems, such as pain and fatigue, that can stem from the cancer itself or from cancer treatments. Sexual problems are a common consequence, affecting many women surviving breast and gynecologic cancers and many men surviving prostate cancer. Coping with cancer also causes psychological and emotional difficulties that can lead to depression, posttraumatic stress disorder, and profound fear of recurrence. Another source of anxiety is the cost of medical treatments, which, along with the loss of wages or a job, can be financially devastating.

Cancer survivors also are at risk of another bout with cancer. Patients surviving one cancer have almost twice the risk of developing a second cancer as the general population has of developing an initial cancer. Children under age 15 who have survived cancer have eight times the risk. Young women treated with radiation for Hodgkin's disease remain at exceptionally high risk of breast cancer for 25 or more years and require lifetime surveillance.

> *In the not distant future genomic scans might be able to identify any disease-causing genes. Such tests could reveal an individual's odds of developing serious, potentially life-threatening illnesses long before symptoms occur. Would you opt for such testing, even if there were nothing you could do to avoid the disease? Or would you rather not live under a shadow of apprehension about your health?* **You decide.**

Savvy Consumer :: Alternative Cancer Treatments

About one-third of cancer patients use alternative medicine, such as meditation, reflexology, herbal medicine, food supplements, or homeopathy. None of these can cure cancer, but some may help ease patient suffering when used to complement mainstream treatments. Nonetheless, alternative therapies that are overused or used in lieu of mainstream treatments can be dangerous to a patient's health. Keep these points in mind when evaluating unconventional treatments for cancer:

:: Special diets, especially those rich in high-antioxidant foods, may help prevent cancer. No diet can cure cancer.

:: Vitamins, even in very high doses, cannot cure cancer. Excessive amounts of vitamins and minerals can be harmful and may even speed tumor growth.

:: Over-the-counter herbal remedies for cancer can be contaminated or diluted with useless leaves.

:: Detoxification regimens, such as high colonic irrigation to remove toxins thought to cause cancer, can be dangerous and have resulted in infection and death.

:: Among the alternative therapies that can decrease pain and improve the quality of a cancer patient's life are relaxation techniques, massage, and aromatherapy.

:: Patients should never put their trust in an alternative practitioner who encourages them to avoid or stop conventional cancer therapy.

:: Many websites offering cancer information, particularly about unproven or alternative therapies, are unreliable. Always check that the website creators are clearly identified, that their credentials are reputable, and that the posting date is recent.

DIABETES MELLITUS

About 100 million people around the world, including more than 18 million in the United States, have **diabetes mellitus,** a disease in which the body doesn't produce or respond properly to insulin, a hormone essential for daily life. In those with diabetes, the pancreas, which produces insulin (the hormone that regulates carbohydrate and fat metabolism) doesn't function as it should. When the pancreas either stops producing insulin or doesn't produce sufficient insulin to meet the body's needs, almost every body system can be damaged.

The prevalence of diabetes has nearly doubled since 1990, and health experts describe it as a global epidemic. About 6.3 percent of Americans have diabetes; a third are not aware that they have it because certain types develop insidiously with no visible symptoms.

The risk of premature death among people with diabetes is about twice that of people without the disease. According to the American Diabetes Association, the total economic cost of diabetes totals more than $132 billion a year. Diabetes accounts for $1 of every $10 spent on health care in the United States.[35]

UNDERSTANDING DIABETES

Glucose is the primary form of sugar that the body cells use for energy. When a person without diabetes eats a meal, the level of glucose in the blood rises, triggering the production and release of insulin by special cell clusters in the pancreas.

Insulin enhances the movement of glucose into various body cells, bringing down the level of glucose in the blood. In those who have diabetes, however, insulin secretion is either nonexistent or deficient. Without sufficient insulin, the glucose in the blood is unable to enter most body cells, so the cells' energy needs aren't met. The levels of glucose in the blood rise higher and higher after each meal. This unused glucose eventually passes through the kidneys, which are unable to process the excessive glucose, and out of the body in urine (Figure 16-8).

Deprived of the fuel it needs, the body begins to break down stored fat as a source of energy. This process produces weak acids, called ketones. A buildup of ketones leads to ketoacidosis, an upheaval in the body's chemical balance that brings on nausea, vomiting, abdominal pain, lethargy, and drowsiness. Severe ketoacidosis can lead to coma and eventual death.

Before the development of insulin injections, diabetes was a fatal illness. Today diabetics can have normal lifespans. However, diabetes still can lead to devastating complications. Uncontrolled glucose levels slowly damage blood vessels throughout the body; thus, individuals who become diabetic early in life may face devastating complications even before they reach middle age. Diabetes is the number one cause of blindness, nontraumatic amputations, and kidney failure, and diabetes increases by two or three times the risk of heart attack or stroke.

Diabetic women who become pregnant face higher risks of miscarriage and babies with serious birth defects; however, precise control of blood sugar levels before conception and in early pregnancy can lower the likelihood of these problems.

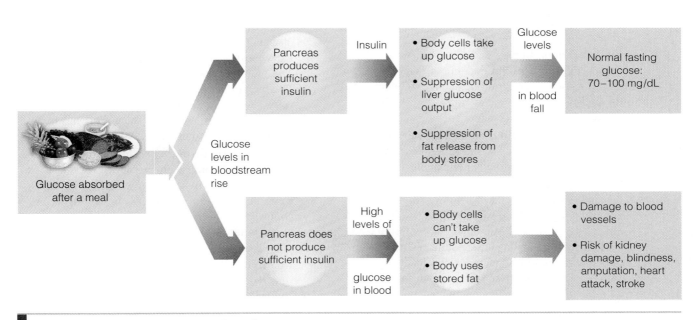

FIGURE 16-8   How Diabetes Affects the Body
Diabetes affects almost every organ system of the body in complex and often subtle ways.

TYPES OF DIABETES

Diabetes includes several conditions in which the body has difficulty controlling levels of glucose in the bloodstream. After an overnight fast, most people have blood glucose levels between 70 and 100 milligrams of glucose per deciliter of blood (mg/dL). This is considered normal. Abnormal readings can indicate the following:

▪ **Prediabetes.** In this condition, blood glucose levels are higher than normal but are not high enough for a diagnosis of diabetes. If your fasting blood glucose is consistently 126 mg/dL or higher, you have diabetes. However, if your fasting blood glucose level is between 101 and 125 mg/dL, you have prediabetes, which also is called hyperglycemia or glucose intolerance.

   People with prediabetes are at increased risk for developing type 2 diabetes and for heart disease and stroke. An estimated 41 million children and adults in the United States have prediabetes. Recent research has shown that some long-term damage to the body, especially the heart and circulatory system, already may be occurring during prediabetes. If people with prediabetes take action to manage their blood glucose, they can delay or prevent type 2 diabetes from developing.

▪ **Type 1 diabetes.** In this form of diabetes (once called juvenile-onset or insulin-dependent diabetes), the body's immune system attacks the insulin-producing beta cells in the pancreas and destroys them. The pancreas then produces little or no insulin and therefore blood glucose cannot enter the cells to be used for energy. Type 1 diabetes develops most often in young people but can appear in adults. Individuals with type 1 diabetes require insulin therapy because their own bodies no longer supply this vital hormone.

▪ **Type 2 diabetes.** In type 2 diabetes (once called adult-onset or non–insulin-dependent diabetes), either the pancreas does not make enough insulin or the body is unable to use insulin correctly. Its two characteristic problems are:

   ▪ **Insufficient insulin** produced by the pancreas. Over time the body produces less and less insulin and eventually none at all.

   ▪ **Insulin resistance.** When muscles and body tissue become resistant to insulin, glucose accumulates in the bloodstream. This results in high blood glucose levels (hyperglycemia). Exactly why the cells become insulin resistant is uncertain, although excess weight, inactivity, and fatty tissue seem to be important factors.

   Type 2 diabetes, which accounts for 90 percent of cases of diabetes, develops most often in middle-aged and older adults, but increasingly is appearing in young people, including adolescents and children. Diet, weight loss, exercise, and medications are the first line of treatment for type 2 diabetes, but insulin also may be required.

▪ **Gestational diabetes.** Women who get diabetes while they are pregnant are more likely to have a family history of diabetes, especially on their mothers' side; they are at greater risk of developing diabetes later in life.

(FAQ) WHO IS AT RISK FOR DEVELOPING DIABETES?

Although type 1 and type 2 diabetes have different causes, two factors are important in both: an inherited predisposition to the disease and something in the environment that triggers diabetes. Genes alone are not enough. In most cases of type 1 diabetes, people need to inherit risk factors from both parents and to experience some environmental trigger, which might involve prenatal nutrition, a virus, or an unknown agent.[36]

In type 2 diabetes, family history is one of the strongest risk factors for getting the disease, but only in Westernized countries. African Americans, Mexican Americans, and Native Americans have the highest rates, but people who live in less developed nations tend not to get type 2 diabetes, no matter how high their genetic risk.

Other risk factors for type 2 diabetes include:

▪ **Weight.** Excess weight is most risky for young people and for people who have been obese for a long time. However, you can improve your glucose levels simply by losing weight. Even a small loss can be beneficial.

▪ **Waist circumference.** As discussed in Chapter 7, apple-shaped people who carry most of their excess weight around their waists are at greater risk of diabetes than are pear-shaped individuals who carry most of their excess weight below their waist. The more visceral fat that you have, the more resistant your body's cells become to the effects of your own insulin. A measurement of more than 40 inches in men and more than 35 inches in women indicates increased health risks.

▪ **Metabolic syndrome.** As discussed in Chapter 15, this condition is a cluster of disorders of your body's metabolism—including high blood pressure, high insulin levels, excess body weight, and abnormal cholesterol levels—that make you more likely to develop diabetes as well as heart disease or stroke.

▪ **Inactivity.** The less active you are, the greater your risk of diabetes. Physical activity helps you control your weight, uses up glucose, makes your cells more sensitive to insulin, increases blood flow, and improves circulation in even the smallest blood vessels. Exercise also helps build muscle mass, which is important because most of the glucose in your blood is absorbed into your muscles. When you have less muscle tissue, more glucose stays in your blood.

- **Age.** Your risk of type 2 diabetes increases as you get older, especially past the age of 45. This may be because people tend to exercise less, lose muscle mass, and gain weight as they age. More often than not, weight gain involves a diet high in carbohydrates and fat. However, diabetes is also increasing dramatically among younger people.

- **Race.** For reasons that aren't entirely clear, people of some races are more likely to develop diabetes. Blacks and Hispanics have double the rate for whites. The incidence is even higher among American Indians. Among the Pima Indians of Arizona, half of all adults have type 2 diabetes, one of the highest rates of diabetes in the world.

- **Depression.** If you're a younger adult who has received a diagnosis of depression, you may be at higher risk of developing type 2 diabetes than may someone without depression. Researchers speculate that this is because people with depression often gain weight and are inactive.

DIABETES SIGNS AND SYMPTOMS

About a third of individuals with type 2 diabetes do not realize they have the illness. If you have risk factors for the disease, watch for the following warning signs:

- **Increased thirst and frequent urination.** Excess glucose circulating in your body draws water from your tissues, making you feel dehydrated. Drinking water and other beverages to quench thirst leads to more frequent urination.

- **Flu-like symptoms.** Type 2 diabetes can sometimes feel like a viral illness, with such symptoms as extreme fatigue and weakness. When glucose, your body's main fuel, doesn't reach cells, you may feel tired and weak.

- **Weight loss or weight gain.** Because your body is trying to compensate for lost fluids and glucose, you may eat more than usual and gain weight, or the opposite may occur. Although eating more than normal, you may lose weight because your muscle tissues don't get enough glucose to generate growth and energy.

- **Blurred vision.** High levels of blood glucose pull fluid from body tissues, including the lenses of the eyes, which affects ability to focus. Vision should improve with treatment of diabetes.

- **Slow-healing sores or frequent infections.** Diabetes affects the body's ability to heal and fight infection. Bladder and vaginal infections can be a particular problem for women.

- **Nerve damage (neuropathy).** Excess blood glucose can damage the small blood vessels to your nerves, leading to symptoms such as tingling and loss of sensation in hands and feet.

- **Red, swollen, tender gums.** Diabetes increases the risk of infection in your gums and in the bones that hold your teeth in place.

DETECTING DIABETES

To identify individuals with this disease as early as possible, the American Diabetes Association now recommends screening every three years for all men and women beginning at age 45. The American College of Endocrinology recommends screening at age 30 for individuals at risk, including those who are overweight, sedentary, have a family history of diabetes, or have high blood pressure or heart disease.[37]

Tests that can detect diabetes include:[38]

- **Random blood sugar test.** Because you don't necessarily fast for this test, your blood glucose may be high because you've just eaten. Even so, it shouldn't be higher than 200 mg/dL.

- **Fasting blood glucose test.** In general, glucose is lowest after an overnight fast. That's why the preferred way to test your blood sugar is after you've fasted overnight or for at least eight hours.

Strategies for Prevention :: How to Lower Your Risk of Prediabetes and Type 2 Diabetes

The Diabetes Prevention Program (DPP), a landmark study sponsored by the National Institutes of Health, found that people at increased risk for type 2 diabetes can prevent or delay the onset of the disease by taking the following steps:

- Exercise 30 minutes on at least five days of the week.

- If you're overweight or obese, lose weight. Aim for 5 to 7 percent of your initial weight.

- Eat a diet rich in complex carbohydrates (bread and other starches) and high-fiber foods, and low in sodium and fat.

- Eat fruits and vegetables that are rich in antioxidants, substances that prevent oxygen damage to cells.

- If your doctor advises, take medications, such as metformin (Glucophage), to help lower your blood sugar.

▪ **Glucose challenge test.** Often used to screen pregnant women for gestational diabetes, this test measures glucose before drinking 8 ounces of an extremely sweet liquid after fasting for six hours, then every hour for a three-hour period. If your blood sugar rises more than expected and doesn't return to normal by the third hour, you likely have diabetes.

DIABETES MANAGEMENT

Unlike many other medical conditions, patients must take charge of their diabetes and monitor their blood glucose regularly to prevent or delay the serious complications of the disease. Diabetes educators teach patients a new set of ABCs: Manage your **A**1c (blood glucose or sugar), **B**lood pressure, and **C**holesterol:

▪ **A** is for the **A1c test.** This test measures the amount of glucose attached to hemoglobin molecules, the iron-rich molecules in red blood cells that deliver oxygen to the body. The higher your blood glucose levels, the more hemoglobin molecules you will have with glucose attached—and the greater the risk of damage to eyes, kidneys, and feet. In general, the life cycle of a red blood cell is 75 to 90 days, which is why the A1c test shows average blood glucose levels for the past two to three months. The American Diabetes Association recommends a goal for A1c of less than 7 percent. The American College of Endocrinology recommends a goal of 6.5 percent. (Normal A1c levels are below 6.) Individuals with diabetes should have their A1c levels checked at least twice a year.

▪ **B** is for **blood pressure.** As discussed in Chapter 15, the goal for most people is 120/80. High blood pressure can cause heart attack, stroke, and kidney disease.

▪ **C** is for **cholesterol.** The LDL goal for most people is less than 100. Bad cholesterol, or LDL, can build up and clog your blood vessels.[39]

Treatment

The goal for diabetics is to keep blood sugar levels as stable as possible to prevent complications, such as kidney damage. Home glucose monitoring including new continuous glucose monitors, allow diabetics to check their blood sugar levels as many times a day as necessary and to adjust their diet or insulin doses as appropriate.

Types of insulin differ in how long it takes to start working after injection (onset), when it works hardest (peak), and how long it lasts in the body (duration). Individuals with diabetes may use different types in various combinations, depending on time of day and timing of meals. New insulin inhalers offer an alternative to injections for those with type 2 diabetes.

An insulin pump delivers insulin to the body 24 hours a day through a thin plastic tube inserted just under the skin, usually on the abdomen.

© BSIP/Phototake

Those with type 1 diabetes require daily doses of insulin via injections, an insulin infusion pump, or oral medication. Those with type 2 diabetes can control their disease through a well-balanced diet, exercise, and weight management. However, insulin therapy may be needed to keep blood glucose levels near normal or normal, thereby reducing the risk of damage to the eyes, nerves, and kidneys. New medications help control weight and lower blood pressure and cholesterol.

Medical advances hold out bright hopes for diabetics. Laser surgery, for instance, is saving eyesight. Bypass operations are helping restore blood flow to the heart and feet. Dialysis machines and kidney and pancreas transplants save many lives. Researchers are exploring various approaches to prevention, including antibody therapies that delay the onset of type 1 diabetes.[40] Transplanting insulin-producing cells from healthy pancreases has helped a small number of patients, but many problems remain.

OTHER MAJOR ILLNESSES

Other noninfectious diseases besides cancer and diabetes have a debilitating effect on many people. But most of the diseases discussed in this section can be controlled, if not cured.

EPILEPSY AND SEIZURE DISORDERS

About 10 percent of all Americans will have at least one seizure at some time. Between 0.5 and 1 percent of all Americans have recurrent seizures. Derived from the Greek word for seizure, **epilepsy** is the term used to refer to a variety of neurological disorders characterized by sudden attacks (seizures) of violent muscle contractions and unconsciousness. Epilepsy is rarely fatal; the primary danger to life is to suffer an attack while driving or swimming.

Seizures can be major, referred to as *grand mal;* minor, referred to as *petit mal;* or psychomotor. In a grand-mal seizure, the person loses consciousness, falls to the ground, and experiences convulsive body movements. Petit-mal seizures are brief, characterized by a loss of consciousness for 10 to 30 seconds, by eye or muscle flutterings, and occasionally by a loss of muscle tone. About 90 percent of all epileptics have grand-mal seizures; 40 percent suffer both petit-mal and grand-mal seizures. The frequency of attacks defines the severity of the epilepsy. Diagnosis is based on a history of recurring attacks and a study of the brain's electrical activity, called an electroencephalogram (EEG).

About half of all cases of epilepsy have no known cause and are therefore classified as *idiopathic*. All others stem from conditions that affect the brain, such as trauma, tumors, congenital malformations, or inflammation of the membranes covering the brain. Idiopathic epilepsy usually begins between the ages of 2 and 14. Seizures before age 2 are usually related to developmental defects, birth injuries, or a metabolic disease affecting the brain. (Fever-induced convulsions are not related to epilepsy.) Seizures after age 14 are generally symptoms of brain disease or injury.

Seizure disorders don't reflect or affect intellectual or psychological soundness; people who suffer from them have normal intelligence. Therapy with anticonvulsant drugs can control seizures in most people, and once seizures are under control, epileptics can live full, normal lives by continuing to take their medications. However, many of the 2.3 million Americans with epilepsy "are undertreated because of old-fashioned ideas about the disease," says neurologist William Theodore, M.D., chief of the clinical epilepsy section at the National Institute of Neurological Disease and Stroke. "Recent advances in neuroimaging and basic science have revolutionized our understanding of epilepsy, but physicians who aren't experts are still telling patients that they have to live with seizures."[41]

Such advice can be more harmful than doctors once thought. A growing body of scientific evidence shows that seizures damage the brain, kill brain cells, lead to bodily injury, and increase the risk of dying. Seizures interfere with learning and memory, so they affect every aspect of a child's development or an adult's functioning.

People with uncontrolled epilepsy have lower levels of marriage, education, and employment and higher rates of depression and disability. "The longer that patients have seizures, especially if they begin in childhood and continue into adolescence and early adulthood, the more likely they are to suffer irreversible psychological and social consequences," says Jerome Engel, Jr., M.D., director of UCLA's epilepsy center. "Early, aggressive treatment—with medication or, if that fails, surgery—is critical to rescue people from a lifetime of disability."[42]

About two-thirds of patients with drug-resistant temporal lobe epilepsy (the most common form) who undergo epilepsy surgery become seizure free; the others still require medication. Yet of the more than 100,000 people with uncontrollable seizures who might benefit, fewer than 3,000 opt for the operation every year, usually as a last resort. In various studies, the average time from first seizure to surgery is about 20 years. For patients with uncontrolled epilepsy who cannot undergo surgery because of the number or location of their seizure centers, the best hope may come from pioneering new brain implants currently in clinical trials.[43]

If you're with a person who suffers a grand-mal seizure, make sure he or she isn't injured during the attack. Don't try to restrain the person or interfere with his or her movements, and don't try to force anything into the person's mouth.

RESPIRATORY DISEASES

See Chapter 14 for the major infectious respiratory diseases and Chapter 13 for smoking-induced problems. In addition to the diseases discussed below, chronic bronchitis and emphysema can also be causes of disability and death.

Asthma

Asthma is a disease characterized by constriction of the breathing passages. As with allergy, asthma rates have skyrocketed in the last two decades. Approximately 20 million Americans have asthma. Asthma-related problems account for more than half a million hospital stays each year and 14 deaths each day in the United States, according to the Asthma and Allergy Foundation of America.

 Asthma is more common among inner-city residents and blacks. The disease disproportionately affects African Americans. A black man in New York City is 11 times more likely to die from asthma than other men in the city.

While asthma is not always linked to allergy, the two are related. Among people with asthma, 90 percent of the children, 70 percent of young adults, and 50 percent of older adults also have allergies. According to epidemiologic research, 23 percent of youngsters diagnosed with allergies by age 1 develop asthma by age 6. Of those diagnosed after age 1, 13 percent eventually become asthmatic. Symptoms include wheezing, coughing, shortness of breath, and chest tightness. If the symptoms are untreated or undertreated, they can worsen and damage the lungs.

 The number of people with asthma continues to increase into adulthood. However, as shown by a study that followed college students for 23 years, most report that their symptoms improve or disappear.

The two main approaches to asthma treatment are control of the underlying inflammation by means of anti-inflammatory drugs, such as corticosteroids, cromolyn sodium, and nedocromil, and short-term relief of symptoms with bronchodilators, such as albuterol, which expand the breathing passages. In its most recent official guidelines, the National Heart, Lung and Blood Institute encouraged more frequent use of inhaled steroids and less reliance on bronchodilators, which have little effect on the underlying inflammation.

Although medications can help relieve asthma symptoms in the short term, prolonged use of the most popular drugs, the short-acting beta-agonists, actually can produce the opposite effect by closing air passages. Many people with severe asthma use more medication as their symptoms worsen—but the drugs actually exacerbate their condition. The reason, researchers theorize, may be that continuous use of asthma medications changes how the airway contracts in ways that intensify the constriction and make breathing more difficult.

(FAQ) What Should I Do in Case of an Asthma Attack?

If you have asthma, here are some steps you should take:

▪ **Get away from the asthma trigger** (cigarette smoke, cat, pollen, etc.).

▪ **Assess the severity of the attack.** The most precise way to do so is with a peak flow meter. If your peak flow is less than half your best value, the attack is severe.

▪ **Use a quick reliever.** The fastest way to relieve an asthma attack is to use a quick-acting bronchodilator such as albuterol.

▪ **Suppress inflammation.** Quick-relief bronchodilators treat only the constricted muscles surrounding the bronchial tubes. Treating the overproduction of mucus requires an anti-inflammatory medication, typically a corticosteroid, such as prednisone.

▪ **Know when to call for help.** Severe asthma attacks can be dangerous. If you don't feel improvement, get help immediately from your doctor or an urgent care or emergency health care center, or call 911.

Chronic Obstructive Lung Disease (COLD)

Chronic obstructive lung disease (COLD), also called chronic obstructive pulmonary disease (COPD), is characterized by progressively more limited flow of air into and out of the lungs. COLD consists of two separate but closely related conditions: chronic bronchitis and emphysema. Most COLD patients develop both forms. The major cause is cigarette smoking, although air pollution may also play a role.

In chronic bronchitis, the bronchial passageways are constantly inflamed, and individuals develop a persistent, sputum-producing cough; shortness of breath; and wheezing. They must stop smoking, lose excess weight, exercise, and avoid or reduce contact with air pollutants.

Chronic bronchitis can lead to emphysema, a deterioration of the lungs that may begin in adolescence. Eventually, the alveoli, tiny air sacs in the lungs, tear, reducing the lungs' ability to exhale. This condition can lead to heart failure.

ANEMIAS

The **anemias** are diseases affecting the oxygen-carrying capacity of the blood. Usually there's a reduced number of red blood cells or a reduced amount of hemoglobin, the

Sickle-cell anemia. (a) Normal mature red blood cells are disk-shaped and concave. (b) In sickle-cell anemia, the red blood cells are crescent-shaped and jagged, causing them to pile up and obstruct small blood vessels. Areas of the body are thus deprived of oxygen and nutrients.

oxygen-carrying component of red blood cells. Anemia can be caused by nutritional inadequacies; loss of blood, including heavy menstrual bleeding; deficiencies in red-cell production; or genetic disorders. Iron-deficiency anemia is a form of anemia caused by a lack of dietary iron, an essential component of the hemoglobin molecule that carries oxygen. It's the most common form of anemia and often goes undiagnosed in women.

▪ **Sickle-cell anemia** is a genetic blood disorder that occurs when the hemoglobin contained in the red blood cells is abnormal. The red blood cells become crescent or sickle-shaped and unable to supply oxygen to body tissues (see photos). This disease causes crippling, severe pain, and premature death. About 8 to 10 percent of African Americans carry the gene for sickle-cell anemia.

▪ **Pernicious anemia** results from a lack of vitamin B_{12} (cobalamine), which causes a deficiency in the formation of red blood cells. Although B_{12} is usually present in the diet, some people lack a substance needed to absorb it into their blood. Injections of B_{12} can control this condition.

▪ **Aplastic anemia,** most common in young adults and adolescents, interferes with the bone marrow's ability to form blood. Usually it results from ingesting a toxic agent, often a medication; symptoms include multiple internal hemorrhages. Whole-blood transfusions are the primary therapy, but the condition is usually fatal.

LIVER DISORDERS

Cirrhosis is characterized by significant loss of liver cells and the formation of scar tissue that can interfere with circulation in the liver. The major cause of one of the most common forms of cirrhosis, Laennec's cirrhosis, is chronic alcoholism. Each year, about 30,000 Americans die of alcohol-related liver disorders (see Chapter 12).

Early signs of liver damage include an enlarged liver (which your doctor can feel during a physical exam) and tiny, spiderlike blood vessels on the surface of the skin. Blood tests may show abnormal levels of certain enzymes or enlarged red blood cells. Even people with advanced liver disease feel better and live longer once they've stopped drinking alcohol. Cirrhosis symptoms, which occur only in the advanced stages of the disease, include yellow discoloration of the skin and eyes (jaundice), accumulation of fluid in the abdomen, and mental confusion.

Liver transplants are the only hope for those with advanced liver disease. With improvements in surgical techniques and the use of antirejection drugs (including cyclosporin, a combination of cyclosporin and an antifungal medication, and a drug called FK-506), 70 percent or more of liver-transplant recipients—including some in their sixties and seventies—now live for at least a year. Some liver transplant recipients have lived longer than 20 years.

KIDNEY DISEASES

A wide range of diseases can affect the kidneys and their ability to process fluids and waste. Some are acute, temporary problems; others are chronic, progressive illnesses that permanently impair kidney function.

Nephrosis refers to a cluster of symptoms indicating chronic damage to the kidneys, including chronic proteinuria (the loss of more than 1 gram of protein a day in the urine), hypercholesteremia (high levels of fats in the blood), and edema (fluid retention). The kidney damage can be the result of diabetes, heavy metal poisoning, allergic reactions to insect stings, or other disorders.

Kidney stones can form either from calcium salts or from minerals (the causes are unknown). Most stones eventually pass out of the body in urine, which can be extremely painful. They don't usually obstruct the flow of urine or interfere with kidney function. However, infection can develop behind a stone. Larger stones can be surgically removed or painlessly shattered into harmless fragments by high-frequency sound waves.

The various chronic and inflammatory diseases of the kidney can all lead to kidney failure. A mechanical process of clearing waste fluids from the body, called *dialysis,* can do the kidneys' job temporarily. Another alternative is a kidney transplant, either from a living, related donor or from a cadaver whose kidney has been carefully tissue matched to the recipient to minimize the risk of rejection. On average, a transplanted kidney continues to function for only nine years. Kidneys that came from cadaver donors are especially likely to deteriorate slowly but steadily. The antirejection drugs that transplant recipients must take may themselves cause side effects and impair the functioning of the new kidney over time. High blood pressure and high glucose and cholesterol levels also can be harmful. A lack of organ donors remains a critical obstacle to performing more of these lifesaving operations.

DIGESTIVE DISEASES

Most disorders of the digestive tract affect only one section: either the esophagus, the stomach and duodenum, the small intestine, the large intestine, the liver, the pancreas, the gallbladder, or the rectum. The most dangerous are Crohn's disease and ulcerative colitis. According to the National Digestive Diseases Advisory Board, almost half of the U.S. population will suffer a digestive problem at some time in their lives.

Ulcers

Open sores, often more than an inch wide, that develop in the lining of the stomach or the duodenum (the first part of the small intestine) are called **ulcers.** They are caused by excessive acidic digestive juices. The major symptom is a burning pain felt throughout the upper abdomen. The pain may come and go, lasting up to three hours. It may begin either right after eating or several hours later.

One in five men and one in ten women get ulcers of the stomach or duodenum, but the number of ulcers is declining. Risk factors include heavy use of cigarettes, alcohol, or caffeine; the ingestion of large amounts of painkillers that contain aspirin or ibuprofen; and advanced age. Bleeding is not common but may be dangerous, even life-threatening. An untreated stomach ulcer can lead to serious weight loss and anemia.

Researchers have identified a bacterium, *Helicobacter pylori,* that may infect the digestive system and set the stage for ulcers. According to various studies, most ulcer patients carry this organism. One theory is that infection leads to an inflammation of the stomach lining called gastritis, which increases vulnerability to other stressors, such as smoking, alcohol, or anxiety.

H. pylori can be detected in several ways. A blood test can reveal the presence of infection by detecting antibodies against *H. pylori.* However, a blood test can be positive even if someone has long been free of the bacteria. The most definitive test requires endoscopy, a procedure in which a physician examines the lining of the stomach or duodenum by passing a thin flexible tube (an endoscope) down the patient's throat and snips a small bit of tissue for laboratory analysis to detect bacteria. Researchers are experimenting with a simpler diagnostic breath test in which patients drink a special liquid that triggers a response by *H. pylori* bacteria

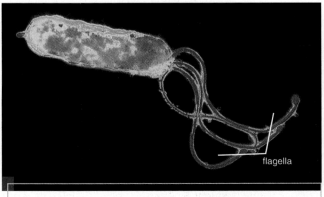

The bacterium *Helicobacter pylori* has flagella that enable it to tunnel beneath the protective layer coating the stomach lining.

in the stomach. Treatment with antibiotics leads to improvement in most patients.

Conventional therapy for ulcers includes self-help measures, such as avoiding aspirin; eating small, frequent meals; taking antacids; and not smoking or drinking alcohol or caffeine. Drugs such as cimetidine, ranitidine, and sucralfate can reduce the amount of acid produced by the stomach and relieve ulcer symptoms. If a stomach ulcer doesn't heal after six to eight weeks of drug treatment, physicians may recommend surgery to remove the ulcer.

Inflammatory Bowel Disease (IBD)

As many as 2 million Americans—many in the prime of life—suffer from one of the two forms of **inflammatory bowel disease (IBD):** *Crohn's disease,* which causes inflammation anywhere in the digestive tract, and *ulcerative colitis,* which creates severe ulcers in the inner lining of the colon and rectum. Both illnesses can trigger frequent and intense diarrhea, abdominal pain, gas, fever, and rectal bleeding.

The specific causes of IBD remain unknown, but scientists speculate that some irritating substance—perhaps a bacterium, virus, or chemical or environmental agent—somehow leaks through the intestine's thin lining into the bowel's deep inner wall. Inflammation develops, setting into motion a chain of harmful reactions by the body's protective immune system and causing swelling, pain, and damage to the intestinal wall. Ulcers (small perforations or holes) may form, exposing cells and tissues to destructive intestinal bacteria and enzymes. Blood and fluid from body tissues may leak into the intestines, showing up as diarrhea or blood in the stool. Twenty percent of cases involve a genetic or familial predisposition.

Treatment for IBD consists primarily of drugs, including powerful steroids, antibiotics, and medications that fight inflammation. Dietary changes can also help. Crohn's patients who don't improve on medication or who develop life-threatening complications, such as a severe intestinal blockage, may undergo surgery to remove or bypass the diseased part of the intestine and reconnect two healthy segments. However, the disease very often recurs in another part of the intestinal tract. For those with ulcerative colitis, removal of the entire colon brings an end to troubling symptoms—and to the increased risk of colon cancer that these individuals face. Most gastroenterologists advise patients with ulcerative colitis to undergo annual colonoscopies to detect precancerous changes in cells.

Irritable Bowel Syndrome

Irritable bowel syndrome (also called irritable colon or spastic colon) is a common problem caused by intestinal spasms. The muscular contractions that move waste material through the intestines become irregular and uncoordinated, causing frequent feelings of a need to defecate, nausea, cramping, pain, gas, and a sensation that the rectum is never emptied.

Diagnostic tests, including X rays, stool samples, and sigmoidoscopy, can rule out colon cancer and other problems. Travel, stress, changes in diet, and smoking often worsen these symptoms. Many people respond well to a high-fiber diet; others prefer a bland diet. There's no standard medical treatment for irritable bowel syndrome; some physicians prescribe stool softeners, laxatives, or drugs to reduce intestinal spasms.

Gallstones

An estimated 25 million Americans—about 10 percent of the population—have **gallstones:** clumps of solid material, usually cholesterol, that form in bile stored in the gallbladder. One-third to one-half of all gallstones produce no symptoms. However, some gallstones, carried out of the liver with bile, get stuck in the bile duct and cause intense pain that lasts for several hours. Ultrasound and special X rays called cholecystograms can detect gallstones.

During an attack of gallstone pain, a physician may recommend a painkiller. Some gallstones can be dissolved by long-term drug treatment. Another alternative to traditional gallbladder surgery is laparoscopic surgery, in which gallstones are removed without having to cut through the major abdominal muscles.

DISORDERS OF THE MUSCLES, JOINTS, AND BONES

Because they're constantly being used, muscles, joints, and bones are more susceptible to damage from injury than are most other parts of the body.

Arthritis

More than 22 million people suffer from some form of **arthritis,** an inflammatory disease of the joints that takes over a hundred forms. Rheumatoid arthritis is an autoimmune disease in which the body attacks its own connective tissue; it's fairly common among younger people. Degenerative arthritis, or osteoarthritis, characterized by changes in bone tissue and cartilage, primarily at the joints, seems to be the result of normal wear and tear.

Women are generally affected by arthritis three times more often than are men, until the seventh or eighth decade of life. Race and occupation don't seem to be factors; climate affects symptoms but not causes.

Aggressive treatment of arthritis pays off, but to be successful, early diagnosis before cartilage destruction occurs is critical. The most effective therapies include anti-inflammatory agents, which prevent or delay joint destruction, and new drugs called COX-2 inhibitors. An educational arthritis self-help course can reduce physician visits by 40 percent and pain perception by about 20 percent. Relaxation training and cognitive-behavioral techniques also have proved highly effective in controlling arthritis pain.

The goal of all treatments for arthritis is to maintain the patient's ability to function. Drugs can relieve pain and reduce inflammation; surgical treatments, including total joint replacement, and physical therapy are also used to maintain motion and strength, and to correct deformities.

Hernias

A **hernia** is a bulge of soft tissue that forces its way through or between strained or weakened muscles. Hernias can occur in many parts of the body, but they're most common in the abdominal wall. A surgeon can push the protruding tissue back into place and tighten or sew together the loose muscles.

Backaches

The average person has an 80 percent chance of experiencing low back pain in the course of a lifetime.[44] Back pain strikes slightly more women than men and is most common between the ages of 20 and 55. You are at greater risk if you smoke or if you're overstressed, overweight, or out of shape. Back pain, which accounts for 40 percent of sickness absences, causes more lost workdays and costs the country more than any other chronic condition.

Anyone from a college athlete to a retired grandparent can suffer a back injury, but the risks increase with time as the deeper muscles and tendons surrounding the spine become less resilient. Yet age itself is rarely the only factor in a disabling back attack; almost always tense, injured, or weak muscles are to blame. Other risk factors include extra pounds, particularly if stuffed into a pot belly; lack of exercise; poor posture; and bending from the waist to hoist a heavy load.

Strain from use or abuse accounts for 80 percent of back ailments. Most vulnerable is the lower, or lumbar, part of the spine, which bears the greatest pressure when bending and lifting. Five to 10 percent of back problems involve the discs between the vertebrae. Most common is the protrusion (or herniation) of the soft center of a disc through the casing so that it presses on spinal nerves. Another 10 percent of back problems involve structural defects, which may be the result of injuries, tumors, arthritis, congenital malformations, osteoporosis (the weakening of the bones), or scoliosis (side-to-side curving of the spine). Sometimes a sore back is a symptom of diseases of other organs, such as the kidneys, gallbladder, or stomach. A physical exam and various tests, including electrodiagnostic studies, X rays, CT scans, and MRIs (magnetic resonance imaging), may be necessary to pinpoint the problem.

Most severe back pain lasts only a few days, although less severe symptoms may persist for many months, and most patients will have intermittent recurrences of back pain.

Once bedrest was the primary treatment for back pain, but now doctors urge patients to avoid it. Even two to seven days of bedrest may provide little, if any, benefit. Acetaminophen (Tylenol), is the first-line therapy for pain relief. If that doesn't work, doctors recommend nonsteroidal anti-inflammatory drugs, such as ibuprofen (Motrin or Advil). Muscle relaxants seem to be effective for a spasm in the lower back. The sooner that patients return to normal activity, the

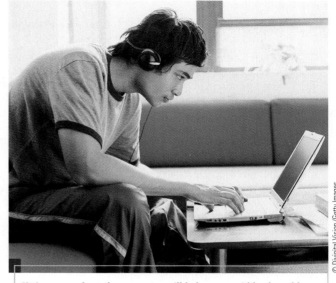

Sitting properly at the computer will help you avoid back problems.

less pain medication they require and the less long-term disability they suffer.[45]

So many people have been disappointed with the treatment provided by their doctors that an entire industry of alternative therapies has sprung up. Many swear by chiropractic manipulation (discussed in Chapter 17), but studies have not shown that it works better than other approaches.[46] Popular treatments involving ice, heat, and ultrasound are probably harmless but have never been shown to be effective in scientific studies. Biofeedback, shoe insoles and shoe lifts, or special corsets and supports have not proved to make any difference in easing back pain. There also is no clear evidence that spinal surgery is more effective than an adequate rehabilitation program for chronic low-back pain.[47] Fewer than 1 percent of patients with chronic low-back pain benefit from surgery.

SKIN DISORDERS

Your skin is the largest organ of your body. Because of its visibility, none of its problems may seem trivial. Two serious skin diseases are discussed next.

Eczema and Dermatitis

Dermatitis is any inflammation of the skin. *Eczema,* a specific type of dermatitis usually caused by allergies, is a skin inflammation that results from internal processes. Symptoms of eczema include redness, flaking, blistering, and thickening of the skin. Self-help treatments include avoiding irritants, such as dishwater, and using steroid creams containing 0.5 percent hydrocortisone.

Psoriasis

In **psoriasis,** the rate of skin cell production is speeded up. As skin cells pile up faster than they can be shed, they produce scaly, deep pink, raised patches on the skin. Triggers of

Strategies for Prevention   Preventing Back Problems

- When standing, shift your weight from one foot to the other. If possible, place one foot on a stool, step, or railing 4 to 6 inches off the ground. Hold in your stomach, tilt your pelvis toward your back, and tuck in your buttocks to provide crucial support for the lower back.

- Because sitting places more stress on the lower back than standing, try to get up from your seat at least once an hour to stretch or walk around. Whenever possible, sit in a straight chair with a

firm back. Avoid slouching in over-stuffed chairs or dangling your legs in midair. When driving, keep the seat forward so that your knees are raised to hip level; your right leg should not be fully extended. A small pillow or towel can help support your lower back.

- Sleep on a flat, firm mattress. The best sleep position is on your side, with one or both knees bent at right angles to your torso. The pillow should keep your head in line with your body so

that your neck isn't bent forward or to the side.

- When lifting, bend at the knees, not from the waist. Get close to the load. Tighten your stomach muscles, but don't hold your breath. Let your leg muscles do the work.

- Don't smoke. Smoking may interfere with circulation to the lower back; and a chronic smoker's cough can be so irritating that it provokes a back spasm.

---

psoriasis are stress, skin damage, and illness. Self-help measures include sunbathing or using ultraviolet light to clear up the psoriasis. Physicians usually prescribe ointments, creams, or pastes, including some steroid preparations, or ultraviolet treatment.

SPECIAL NEEDS FOR DIFFERENT ABILITIES

Physical or mental impairments include blindness, deafness, disorders of the muscles or nerves, paralysis, loss of limbs, or mental retardation, that substantially limit one or more major life activities. Most are the result of illnesses, such as strokes, arthritis, or heart disease, and affect the ability to walk, speak, or live independently. Some congenital disorders, such as cerebral palsy, cause speech problems, muscular weakness, and mental retardation. Accidents are responsible for other disabilities, including paralysis.

Individuals with special needs and abilities can live full, happy, and productive lives. Famous people who've made major contributions to the world despite disabilities include the composer Ludwig van Beethoven, who wrote some of his most famous music after becoming deaf; the inventor Thomas A. Edison, who was deaf throughout much of his life; and President Franklin D. Roosevelt, who became paralyzed in both legs at the age of 39.

Few such problems can be cured, but a great deal can be done to overcome them. **Rehabilitation medicine,** the specialty dedicated to improving the condition of the disabled, can provide treatments such as surgery for certain types of blindness or deafness, medications to ease the crippling pain of arthritis, and physical therapy, including special exercises to build up endurance and muscle strength. Mechanical devices, such as electric wheelchairs, artificial limbs, and hearing aids, can open up wider worlds to people with disabilities. Occupational therapy teaches skills to help them gain confidence, and vocational training prepares them to find employment.

Individuals with special needs face special challenges in their daily lives. Some are primarily physical, such as difficulty bathing, lifting groceries, opening cans and bottles, or going someplace. They also face many social and economic challenges. Because some people feel uncomfortable about disabilities, they may not treat individuals with special needs with the same acceptance and respect that they show to others. This can lead to discrimination from employers.

The Americans with Disabilities Act protects people with disabilities from discrimination by private employers, requires wheelchair access to public buildings and mass transportation, and orders telephone companies to provide telephone relay services that allow people with impaired speech or hearing to make and receive calls. Many states require insurers to provide coverage for high-risk individuals such as cancer survivors. The names of many of the organizations that help the disabled, such as the National Coalition for Cancer Survivorship and the National Library Service for the Blind and Physically Handicapped, are in "Your Health Almanac" at the back of the book.

Learn It / Live It

Preventing Serious Illness

You may not be able to control every risk factor in your life or environment, but you can protect yourself from the obvious ones.

- **Don't smoke.** There's no bigger favor you can do for yourself and those who live and work near you. Smoking decreases the levels of some immune cells and increases susceptibility to respiratory infections.

- **Eat a balanced diet** to be sure you get essential vitamins and minerals. Severe deficiencies in vitamins B_6, B_{12}, and folic acid impair immunity. Keep up your iron and zinc intake. Iron influences the number and vigor of certain immune cells, whereas zinc is crucial for cell repair. Too little vitamin C may also increase susceptibility to infectious diseases.

■ **Avoid fatty foods.** A low-fat diet can increase the activity of immune cells that hunt down and knock out cells infected with viruses.

■ **Watch your weight.** Overweight and obesity are associated with increased risk for cancers at several sites: breast (among postmenopausal women), colon, endometrium, esophagus (adenocarcinoma), and kidney.

■ **Get enough sleep.** Without adequate rest, your immune system cannot maintain and renew itself.

■ **Exercise regularly.** Aerobic exercise stimulates the production of an immune-system booster called interleukin-2.

■ **Avoid excessive exposure to ultraviolet light.** If you spend a lot of time outside, you can protect your skin by using sunscreen and wearing long-sleeve shirts and a hat. Also, wear sunglasses to protect your eyes. Don't purposely put yourself at risk by binge-sunbathing or by using sunlamps.

■ **Avoid obvious cancer risks.** Besides ultraviolet light, other environmental factors that have been linked with cancer include tobacco, asbestos, and radiation.

■ **Control your alcohol intake.** Heavy drinking interferes with normal immune responses and lowers the number of defender cells. The risk of cancers of the mouth, pharynx, larynx, esophagus, liver, and breast increases substantially with intake of more than 2 drinks per day for men or one drink for women.

■ **Be alert to changes in your body.** You know your body's rhythms and appearance better than anyone else, and only you will know if certain things aren't right. Changes in bowel habits, skin changes, unusual lumps or discharges—anything out of the ordinary—may be clues that require further medical investigation.

Making This Chapter Work for You

Review Questions

1. Which of the following statements about cancer is true?
   a. When cancer cells spread to another part of the body, the process is called infiltration.
   b. Cancer occurs when abnormal cells grow and spread uncontrollably until they form an ectoplasm.
   c. Those cancers that have been shown to be triggered by viruses are contagious.

   d. Every cancer has a genetically determined "fingerprint" that indicates how deadly it is.

2. Signs that a cancer might be inherited include all of the following *except*
   a. family history.
   b. late development of the disease.
   c. a diagnosis of retinoblastoma.
   d. an unusual gender pattern in the incidence of the disease.

3. You can protect yourself from certain types of cancer by
   a. eating a diet rich in antioxidants.
   b. avoiding people who have had cancer.
   c. wearing sunscreen with an SPF of less than 15.
   d. using condoms during sexual intercourse.

4. Which of the following statements about skin cancer is true?
   a. Individuals with a large number of moles are at decreased risk for melanoma.
   b. The most serious type of skin cancer is squamous-cell carcinoma.
   c. The safest way to get a tan and avoid skin cancer is to use tanning salons and sunlamps instead of sunbathing in direct sunlight.
   d. Individuals with a history of childhood sunburn are at increased risk for melanoma.

5. A woman's risk of developing breast cancer increases if
   a. she is Caucasian over the age of 40.
   b. she had her first child when in her teens or twenties.
   c. her husband's mother had breast cancer.
   d. she began menstruating when she was 15 or 16.

6. Prostate cancer
   a. occurs mostly among men between the ages of 18 and 35.
   b. is usually more aggressive in white men.
   c. has a low survival rate.
   d. can be detected through a screening test that measures the levels of prostate-specific antigen in the blood.

7. Which of the following statements about diabetes mellitus is *false?*
   a. Individuals with type 2 diabetes can often control the disease without taking insulin.
   b. The incidence of diabetes has decreased in the last decade, especially among African Americans, Native Americans, and Latinos.
   c. Individuals with diabetes must measure the levels of glucose in their blood to ensure that it does not rise to unsafe levels.
   d. Untreated or uncontrolled diabetes can lead to coma and eventual death.

8. With asthma,
   a. the most common symptom is a persistent, sputum-producing cough.

(continued on p. 486)

Self Survey ‖ Are You at Risk of Cancer?

Answer the following questions:

1. Do you protect your skin from overexposure to the sun? _____
2. Do you abstain from smoking or using tobacco in any form? _____
3. If you're over 40 or if family members have had colon cancer, do you get routine digital rectal exams? _____
4. Do you eat a balanced diet that includes the recommended Daily Value for vitamins A, B, and C? _____
5. If you're a woman, do you have regular Pap tests and pelvic exams? _____
6. If you're a man over 40, do you get regular prostate exams? _____
7. If you have burn scars or a history of chronic skin infections, do you get regular checkups? _____
8. Do you avoid smoked, salted, pickled, and high-nitrite foods? _____
9. If your job exposes you to asbestos, radiation, cadmium, or other environmental hazards, do you get regular checkups? _____
10. Do you limit your consumption of alcohol? _____
11. Do you avoid using tanning salons or home sunlamps? _____
12. If you're a woman, do you examine your breasts every month for lumps? _____
13. Do you eat plenty of vegetables and other sources of fiber? _____
14. If you're a man, do you perform regular testicular self-exams? _____
15. Do you wear protective sunglasses in sunlight? _____
16. Do you follow a low-fat diet? _____
17. Do you know the cancer warning signs? _____

Scoring:

If you answered no to any of the questions, your risk for developing various kinds of cancer may be increased.

YOUR ACTION PLAN FOR EARLY DETECTION OF CANCER

Site	Recommendation
Breast	▪ Yearly mammograms are recommended starting at age 40. The age at which screening should be stopped should be individualized by considering the potential risks and benefits of screening in the context of overall health status and longevity.
	▪ Clinical breast exam should be part of a periodic health exam, about every 3 years for women in their twenties and thirties, and every year for women 40 and older.
	▪ Women should know how their breasts normally feel and report any breast change promptly to their health care providers. Breast self-exam is an option for women starting in their twenties.
	▪ Women at increased risk (e.g., family history, genetic tendency, past breast cancer) should talk with their doctors about the benefits and limitations of starting mammography screening earlier, having additional tests (i.e., breast ultrasound and MRI), or having more frequent exams.
Colon and Rectum	Beginning at age 50, men and women should begin screening with one of the examination schedules that follow: ▪ A fecal occult blood test (FOBT) or fecal immunochemical test (FIT) every year ▪ A flexible sigmoidoscopy (FSIG) every 5 years ▪ Annual FOBT or FIT and flexible sigmoidoscopy every 5 years* ▪ A double-contrast barium enema every 5 years ▪ A colonoscopy every 10 years

*Combined testing is preferred over either annual FOBT or FIT, or FSIG every 5 years, alone. People who are at moderate or high risk for colorectal cancer should talk with a doctor about a different testing schedule.

Site	Recommendation
Prostate	The PSA test and the digital rectal examination should be offered annually, beginning at age 50, to men who have a life expectancy of at least 10 years. Men at high risk (African-American men and men with a strong family history of one or more first-degree relatives diagnosed with prostate cancer at an early age) should begin testing at age 45. For both men at average risk and high risk, information should be provided about what is known and what is uncertain about the benefits and limitations of early detection and treatment of prostate cancer so that they can make an informed decision about testing.
Uterus	**Cervix:** Screening should begin approximately 3 years after a woman begins having vaginal intercourse, but no later than 21 years of age. Screening should be done every year with regular Pap tests or every 2 years using liquid-based tests. At or after age 30, women who have had three normal test results in a row may get screened every 2 to 3 years. Alternatively, cervical cancer screening with human papilloma virus (HPV) DNA testing and conventional or liquid-based cytology could be performed every 3 years. However, doctors may suggest that a woman get screened more often if she has certain risk factors, such as HIV infection or a weak immune system. Women 70 years and older who have had three or more consecutive normal Pap tests in the last 10 years may choose to stop cervical cancer screening. Screening after total hysterectomy (with removal of the cervix) is not necessary unless the surgery was done as a treatment for cervical cancer. **Endometrium:** The American Cancer Society recommends that at the time of menopause all women should be informed about the risks and symptoms of endometrial cancer, and strongly encouraged to report any unexpected bleeding or spotting to their physicians. Annual screening for endometrial cancer with endometrial biopsy beginning at age 35 should be offered to women with or at risk for hereditary nonpolyposis colon cancer (HNPCC).
Cancer-Related Checkup	For individuals undergoing periodic health examinations, a cancer-related checkup should include health counseling, and, depending on a person's age and gender, might include examinations for cancers of the thyroid, oral cavity, skin, lymph nodes, testes, and ovaries, as well as for some nonmalignant diseases.

Source: American Cancer Society, Cancer Facts and Figures-2005. © 2005 American Cancer Society, Inc. *www.cancer.org.* Reprinted with permission.

CASE IN POINT: SAVING YOUR SKIN

Student: Cory, 23

Goal: Prevent skin cancer

Action Plan:

▮ Apply sunscreen to face every day

▮ Use high-protection sunscreen for body whenever spending time outdoors

▮ Reapply sunscreen regularly during each day at the beach and when lifeguarding during the summer

▮ Check skin for changes regularly throughout the year

▮ Have a full-body dermatologic examination every year

Health🜨Now™   If you want to write your own goals for lowering your cancer risk, go to the **Wellness Journal in HealthNow at http://healthnow .brookscole.com/ith** *b.* the recommended treatments include antibiotics to eliminate the underlying infection and bronchodilators to expand the breathing passages.

c. an individual experiences wheezing and shortness of breath because of constricted breathing passages.

d. if the disease is untreated, it may lead to emphysema.

9. Major disorders of the digestive system include all of the following *except*

a. irritable bowel disease.

b. Crohn's disease.

c. gallstones.

d. abdominal hernia.

10. Which of the following statements is *false?*

a. Psoriasis is the most severe form of dermatitis.

b. In rheumatoid arthritis, the body attacks its own connective tissue.

c. Sickle-cell anemia is a fatal genetic blood disorder of African Americans.

d. Cirrhosis of the liver is commonly caused by chronic alcoholism.

Answers to these questions can be found on page 587.

Critical Thinking

1. Do you have family members who have had cancer? Were these individuals at risk for cancer because of specific environmental factors, such as long-term exposure to tobacco smoke? If no particular cause was identified, what other factors could have triggered their diseases? Are you concerned that you might have inherited a genetic predisposition to any particular type of cancer because of your family history?

2. A friend of yours, Karen, discovered a small lump in her breast during a routine self-examination. When she mentions it, you ask if she has seen a doctor. She tells you that she hasn't had time to schedule an appointment; besides, she says she's not sure it's really the kind of lump one has to worry about. It's clear to you that Karen is in denial and procrastinating about seeing a doctor. What advice would you give her?

3. Because of advances in antirejection treatment, organ transplants have proved highly successful in helping many people who otherwise might have died. Even elderly patients have clearly benefited from donated kidneys and livers. However, because the demand for organs to transplant greatly exceeds the supply, health experts have debated setting priorities. Should a 30-year-old be placed higher on the waiting list for a particular organ than a 70-year-old? Should a nurse who needs a liver because she contracted hepatitis on the job get priority over an alcoholic whose liver has been destroyed by cirrhosis? Who, if anyone, should make such decisions? Would a lottery be a fair way to determine who receives an available organ?

Media Menu

Health ⊛ Now™

Throughout the chapter, this icon introduces a list of resources on the Health-Now website at **http://healthnow.brookscole.com/ith** that will:

- Help you evaluate your knowledge of the material.
- Allow you to take an exam-prep quiz.
- Provide a Personalized Learning Plan targeting resources that address areas you should study.
- Coach you through identifying target goals for behavior change and creating and monitoring your personal change plan throughout the semester.

INTERNET CONNECTIONS

Cancer Prevention

www.cancer.org/docroot/PED/ped_0.asp

This site from the American Cancer Society features information on prevention, emphasizing nutrition and environmental toxins.

American Diabetes Association

www.diabetes.org

Here you will find the latest information on both type 1 and type 2 diabetes mellitus, including suggestions regarding diet and exercise. The online bookstore features meal planning guides, cookbooks, and self-care guides. Type in your zip code to find community resources.

Cancer Prevention and Control

www.cdc.gov/cancer/index.htm

This site, sponsored by the Centers of Disease Control and Prevention (CDC), features current information on cancer of the breast, cervix, prostate, skin, and colon. The site also provides monthly spotlights on specific cancers, as well as links to the National Comprehensive Cancer Control Program and the National Program of Cancer Registries.

Women's Cancer Network

www.wcn.org

Sponsored by Health Net, this site features a detailed personal breast cancer risk analysis; screening information about self-exams, clinical exams, and mammograms; and teaching aids and resources.

InfoTrac College Edition Activities Log on, insert **skin cancer** into the Keyword search box, and limit your search to the past year. When you get the results, Mark articles to review, then Select one to read. Summarize three or four key points from the article.

You can find additional readings related to personal health with InfoTrac College Edition, an online library of more than 900 journals and publications. Follow the instructions for accessing InfoTrac College Edition that were packaged with your textbook; then search for articles using a keyword search.

For additional links, resources, and suggested readings on the InfoTrac College Edition, visit our Health and Wellness Resource Center at **http://health .wadsworth.com.**

Key Terms

The terms listed are used on the page indicated. Definitions of the terms are in the Glossary at the end of this book.

anemia 478

arthritis 480

asthma 477

carcinogen 463

chronic obstructive lung disease (COLD) 478

cirrhosis 478

dermatitis 481

diabetes mellitus 473

epilepsy 476

gallstones 480

hernia 481

infiltration 460

inflammatory bowel disease (IBD) 480

irritable bowel syndrome 480

kidney stones 479

lumpectomy 469

mammography 469

mastectomy 469

metastasize 460

neoplasm 460

nephrosis 479

psoriasis 481

rehabilitation medicine 482

relative risk 460

tamoxifen 469

ulcer 479

17 Health-Care Consumerism and Complementary/Alternative Medicine

Long after she immigrated to the United States from India, Tapu's grandmother refused to go to Western doctors. She preferred practitioners who used the herbs and techniques she had relied on in her homeland. Tapu's father, an American-trained physician, would argue with his mother-in-law about what he considered her old-fashioned views. As a doctor's son, Tapu grew up believing in the superiority of Western medicine.

In his sophomore year at college, Tapu found out that he needed oral surgery. To his surprise, the oral surgeon suggested an alternative method of controlling postoperative pain: acupuncture. "My dad's never going to approve," he said. "And he's the one who's still paying my medical bills." The doctor referred Tapu—and his father—to recent studies conducted by National Institute of Health researchers on acupuncture's efficacy in relieving postsurgical pain. After doing more research online, Tapu agreed to try acupuncture following his operation.

Like Tapu, millions of Americans are turning to complementary and alternative medicine (CAM), a term that includes a broad range of healing philosophies, approaches, and therapies not traditionally taught in medical schools or provided in hospitals. But consumers are learning that they have to be just as savvy—and skeptical—about these therapies and practitioners as they are with any other form of health care.

Because there are so many health-care choices, you face a greater responsibility for your personal well-being. Whether you are monitoring your blood pressure, taking medication, or deciding whether to try an alternative therapy, you need to gather information, ask questions, weigh advantages and disadvantages, and take charge of your health. The reason: No one cares more about your health than you do, and no one will do more to promote your well-being than you.

(FAQ) Frequently Asked Questions

After studying the material in this chapter, you should be able to:

■ **List** ways of becoming an informed health-care consumer.

■ **Discuss** strategies for self-care, as well as how to get the best possible health care.

■ **Describe** common medical exam procedures and medical tests.

■ **Identify** strategies for maintaining good oral health.

■ **List** your rights as a medical consumer.

■ **Describe** the different types of complementary and alternative therapies and explain what research has shown about their effectiveness.

■ **Compare** and **contrast** the different types of health-care practitioners and health-care facilities.

■ **Explain** what managed care is.

SAFEGUARDING YOUR HEALTH

It's up to you. By learning how to maintain your health, evaluate medical information, and spot early signs of a problem, you're more likely to get the best possible care—and to keep down your medical bills. Self-care means head-to-toe maintenance, including good oral care, appropriate screening tests, knowing your medical rights, and understanding the health-care system.

Chances are that you've tried—or will try—alternative therapies. Many use a "whole-person" approach that addresses all the dimensions of health. You need to be just as savvy a consumer when considering a complementary or alternative treatment as you would with a more mainstream one. You also need to continue your best healthy practices throughout your life so you can function at your best for as long as possible. But your future begins with the healthy choices you make today and every day.

HEALTH CARE AND THE COLLEGE STUDENT

All of the more than 14 million men and women enrolled in institutions of higher learning need some health-care services, regardless of their age or general health. The Preventive Services Task Force of the U.S. Public Health Service recommends that all adolescents and young adults have periodic screenings for high blood pressure, obesity, and problem alcohol consumption and that they receive regular counseling concerning the use of drugs, tobacco, and alcohol; sexually transmitted infections; effective contraception; a healthy diet; exercise; oral health; and prevention of motor vehicle injuries and other accidents.

In addition to the medical services available at student health centers, colleges provide health information. According to a CDC survey of approximately 4,600 undergraduates at 136 colleges and universities, about three-quarters of undergraduates have received some form of health information. About half of all students surveyed had been given some information on prevention of alcohol and drug use and HIV infection and AIDS.

 Black students were more likely than white students to say they'd been taught about AIDS and HIV in college classes. African-American, Hispanic, or students of other racial and ethnic groups also were more likely than whites to report receiving information on any health topic. More traditional full-time students between ages 18 and 24 who had never been married and were not working full-time had received health information, compared to part-time, older, nontraditional students.

 Because undergraduates are remarkably diverse, they also vary in their health beliefs and practices, particularly when born outside the United States in countries with different medical traditions. A study that compared the health beliefs of undergraduates born in the United States, China, and India found unexpected similarities and differences. Regardless of their origins, students identified the same four factors as very important for keeping healthy: enough rest and sleep, physical exercise, proper weight, and eating proper foods. The students also agreed on the need for rest and sleep in recovering from an illness. Only 20 percent of American-born students—compared with 40 percent of those born in China and 48 percent of those born in India—said seeing a nurse or doctor promptly was very important for recovering from illness. More of the India-born students placed great importance on eating proper foods, taking vitamins, and religious faith for recovery. The largest proportion of each group placed their greatest faith in doctors and in their families to help them when sick.[1]

Your Life Coach

Making Smart Health-Care Decisions

Although you may not realize it, you make crucial decisions that affect your health every day. You choose what you eat, whether you exercise, if you smoke or drink, when to fasten your seat belt. You decide when to see health professionals, what to tell them, and whether to follow their advice.

The responsibility for making smart choices about your health lies with you. Never before has so much information about health been available in so many forms and formats. However, not all of it is accurate, objective, or helpful. In order to base your decisions on a solid scientific basis, you have to develop and apply your critical-thinking skills.

The following sections can help.

(FAQ) HOW CAN I FIND GOOD ADVICE ONLINE?

An estimated 85 million Americans—three in four Internet users—are "e-health" consumers who seek information or support, communicate with health-care providers, or buy medical products online.[2] "They use the Internet as an adjunct to physicians, who remain their primary source of health advice," says Mark Bard, president of Manhattan Research, a health-care marketing firm.[3] As noted in Student Snapshot: "Going Online for Health Information," about 3 in 4 college students have used the Internet to get health information.[4]

According to Manhattan Research, 57 percent of doctors suggest specific sites to patients. The American College of Physicians Foundation has launched an "Information Rx" campaign that refers patients to a website (www.medlineplus.gov) operated by the National Library of Medicine. Table 17-1 lists some doctor-endorsed websites.

About one in four doctors uses e-mail with patients. That number is expected to grow as more physicians realize that e-mail is an efficient, effective way of

TABLE 17-1 DOCTOR-RECOMMENDED WEBSITES

National Library of Medicine: MedlinePlus   **www.medlineplus.gov**

MedlinePlus contains links to information on hundreds of health conditions and issues. The site also includes a medical dictionary, an encyclopedia with pictures and diagrams, and links to physician directories.

FDA Center for Drug Evaluation and Research   **www.fda.gov**

Click on Drugs@FDA for information on approved prescription drugs and some over-the-counter medications.

WebMD   **www.webmd.com**

WebMD is full of information to help you manage your health. The site's quizzes and calculators are a fun way to test your medical knowledge. Get diet tips, information on drugs and herbs, and check out special sections on men's and women's health.

MayoClinic   **www.mayoclinic.com**

The renowned Mayo Clinic offers a one-stop health resource website. Use the site's Health Decision Guides to make decisions about prevention and treatment. Learn more about complementary and alternative medicine, sports medicine, and senior health in the Healthy Living Centers.

Centers for Disease Control   **www.cdc.gov**

Stay up to date on the latest public health news and get the CDC's recommendations on travelers' health, vaccines and immunizations, and protecting your health in case of a disaster.

Medscape   **www.medscape.com**

Medscape delivers news and research specifically tailored to your medical interests. The site requires (free) registration.

Student Snapshot

GOING ONLINE FOR HEALTH INFORMATION

	Percentage
Students who have used the Internet to get health information for themselves	74%
Did so in the past day or week	15%
Did so in the last month	32%
Said that online information improved the way they took care of their health	37%
Searched for information on fitness/exercise	50%
Searched for information on diet/nutrition	47%

Based on a survey of 743 undergraduates at two southeastern universities. *Source:* Escoffery, Cam, et al. "Internet Use for Health Information among College Students." *Journal of American College Health*, Vol. 53, No. 4, January–February 2005, p. 183.

© 2000 Photo Disc, Inc.

---

communicating with patients. Contrary to assumptions, e-health consumers aren't likely to seek more health care than others. In a Stanford University study, more than 90 percent of respondents said their use of e-mail and the Internet had no effect on how often they called or visited a doctor.[5] However, the new digital age is changing the way patients use health services, with increasing numbers going online to make appointments, refill prescriptions, or view electronic medical records.[6]

If you go to other websites for medical information, here are some guidelines for evaluating them:

■ **Check the creator.** Websites are produced by health agencies, health support groups, school health programs, health-product advertisers, health educators, and health-education organizations. Read site headers and footers carefully to distinguish biased commercial advertisements from unbiased sites created by scientists and health agencies.

■ **If you are looking for the most recent research,** check the date the page was created and last updated as well as the links. Several nonworking links signal that the site isn't carefully maintained or updated.

■ **Check the references.** As with other health-education materials, web documents should provide the reader with references. Unreferenced suggestions may be scientifically unsound and possibly unsafe.

■ **Consider the author.** Is he or she recognized in the field of health education or otherwise qualified to publish a health-information web document? Does the author list his or her occupation, experience, and education?

■ **Look for possible bias.** Websites may be attempting to provide healthful information to consumers, but they also may be attempting to sell a product. Many sites are merely disguised advertisements.

EVALUATING HEALTH NEWS

Cure! Breakthrough! Medical miracle! These words make headlines. Remember that although medical breakthroughs and cures do occur, most scientific progress is made one small step at a time. Rather than putting your faith in the most recent report or the hottest

Reprinted with special permission of King Features Syndicate.

trend, try to gather as much background information and as many opinions as you can. Weigh them carefully—ideally with a trusted physician—and make the decision that seems best for you.

When reading a newspaper or magazine story or listening to a radio or television report about a medical advance, look for answers to the following questions:

- **Who are the scientists involved?** Are they recognized, legitimate health professionals? What are their credentials? Are they affiliated with respected medical or scientific institutions? Be wary of individuals whose degrees or affiliations are from institutions you've never heard of, and be sure that the person's educational background is in a discipline related to the area of research reported.

- **Where did the scientists report their findings?** The best research is published in peer-reviewed professional journals, such as the *New England Journal of Medicine*. Research developments also may be reported at meetings of professional societies.

- **Is the information based on personal observations?** Does the report include testimonials from cured patients or satisfied customers? If the answer to either question is yes, be wary.

- **Does the article, report, or advertisement include words like *amazing, secret, or quick?*** Does it claim to be something the public has never seen or been offered before?

Such sensationalized language is often a tip-off to a dubious treatment.

- **Is someone trying to sell you something?** Manufacturers who cite studies to sell a product have been known to embellish the truth.

- **Does the information defy all common sense?** Be skeptical. If something sounds too good to be true, it probably is.

MAKING SENSE OF MEDICAL RESEARCH

Medical research is the only way that anyone, physician or consumer, can assess the quality of diagnostic methods, medications, or surgical treatments. The principal rule of science is that nothing works until it's been proved.

Researchers rely on a variety of studies to determine whether a new approach to prevention, diagnosis, or treatment works. These include:

- **Epidemiological studies,** in which scientists assess the health status of a large, defined group of people, such as the population of a country or region. They may look at various health habits, such as alcohol consumption, to determine whether those who practice these habits have a higher likelihood of developing certain diseases.

- **Animal studies, or preclinical trials,** in which scientists administer a drug or try a procedure on various laboratory animals to assess its safety and determine its effects.

■ **Clinical trials,** in which volunteers agree to act as test subjects—"human guinea pigs," as it were. Patients must give written permission in order to participate. Clinical trials generate data for the purpose of evaluating one or more diagnostic or therapeutic approaches in a population. Well-designed clinical trials, which must have strict eligibility criteria, a standardized intervention, follow-up, and measures of outcome, set the "gold standard" for new diagnostic tests or medical or surgical treatments.

In *controlled studies,* the group receiving an experimental drug or treatment is compared with a group receiving no treatment or standard therapy. In *single-blind studies,* the subjects don't know whether they're receiving the experimental drug or treatment, or an inactive substance. In *double-blind studies,* neither the subjects nor the researchers have this information. In *prospective studies,* patients are selected, assessed, participate in the trial, and are then followed for a preset period. In *retrospective studies,* investigators look back at their past experiences with a certain group of patients.

The results of even the most careful studies aren't considered conclusive in and of themselves. The FDA reviews every new drug, as well as the research methods used to test it, before it's allowed on the market. And a new therapy is widely accepted (or rejected) only after publication of study results in a *peer-reviewed* journal (one in which scientists in the same field critique the research methods before accepting the paper) and after *replication* (the repetition of the same investigation by other researchers with similar results). In recent years, a technique called **meta-analysis,** which summarizes and reviews research in a particular area, has been used to evaluate the results of several large trials in a uniform manner.

One reason why study results must be confirmed is that, no matter what treatment patients receive, one-third to one-half of all patients improve temporarily. This well-documented but little-understood phenomenon is called the *placebo effect.* Scientific trials of a new treatment must show that the patients receiving the experimental medication or therapy improve *more* than those receiving a sugar pill or mock procedure (the placebo).

EVIDENCE-BASED MEDICINE

One of the ways in which physicians are working to improve the quality of care is by basing diagnostic testing and treatments on solid evidence produced by rigorous research studies (usually randomized controlled trials).[7] Evidence-based medicine is not an entirely new concept of medical care but a methodical approach that establishes a solid and conscientious scientific basis for decision making about health care. Evidence-based medicine pays particular attention to **outcomes,** that is, the impact that a specific medication or treatment has on a patient's condition, overall health, and quality of life.

Outcomes research is designed to answer questions such as: Is treatment better or worse than no treatment? Is one treatment better than another? If a treatment is effective, is a little just as good as a lot? Does quality of life change because of treatment? Are the benefits of treatment worth the cost or the risks to the patient?

Studies of outcomes look at how patients fared with or without a specific treatment, the costs involved, and the impact of undergoing or not undergoing treatment in terms of the patients' quality of life. Outcomes research can help determine which of several therapies or approaches provides the best results at the most reasonable costs.

When you are diagnosed with a health problem, ask your doctor if your treatment is based on the latest evidence and clinical guidelines. The National Guideline Clearinghouse provides a comprehensive database of evidence-based clinical practice guidelines for many common health problems, available at www.guideline.gov.

SELF-CARE

Most people do treat themselves. You probably prescribe aspirin for a headache, chicken soup or orange juice for a cold, or a weekend trip to unwind from stress. At the very least, you should know what your **vital signs** are and how they compare against normal readings (Table 17-2).

TABLE 17-2 TAKE YOUR OWN VITAL SIGNS

Vital Sign	Normal Values
Temperature	98.9° F in the morning or 99.9° F later in the day is upper limit of the normal oral temperature for people 40 years old or younger. • Women's temperatures are slightly higher than men's. • African-Americans' temperatures are slightly higher than white Americans. Measure your temperature with a mercury or digital thermometer.
Blood pressure	Below 120 (systolic) and below 80 (diastolic). You can measure your own blood pressure if you want to invest in blood pressure equipment. Check your local drugstore to purchase a blood pressure cuff or digital blood pressure monitor.
Pulse	72 beats per minute. Take your pulse rate at your wrist or at the carotid artery in your neck.
Respiration rate	15–20 breaths per minute.

Once a thermometer was the only self-testing equipment found in most American homes. Now hundreds of home tests are available to help consumers monitor everything from fertility to blood pressure to cholesterol levels (Table 17-3). More convenient and less expensive than a visit to a clinic or doctor's office, the new tests are generally as accurate as those administered by a professional.

TABLE 17-3 HOME HEALTH TESTS: A CONSUMER'S GUIDE

Type of Test	What It Does
Pregnancy	Determines if a woman is pregnant by detecting the presence of human chorionic gonadotropin in urine. Considered 99 percent accurate.
Fertility	Measures levels of luteinizing hormone (LH), which rise 24 to 36 hours before a woman conceives. Can help women increase their odds of conceiving.
Blood pressure	Measures blood pressure by means of an automatically inflating armband or a cuff for the finger or wrist; helps people taking hypertension medication or suffering from high blood pressure monitor their condition.
Cholesterol	Checks cholesterol in blood from a finger prick; good for anyone concerned about cholesterol.
Colon cancer	Screening test to detect hidden blood in stool; recommended for anyone over 40 or concerned about colorectal disease.
Urinary tract infection	Diagnoses infection by screening for certain white blood cells in urine; advised for women who get frequent UTIs and whose doctors will prescribe antibiotics without a visit.
HIV infection	Detects antibodies to HIV in a blood sample sent anonymously to a lab. Controversial because no face-to-face counseling is available for those who test positive.

Self-care also can mean getting involved in the self-help movement, which has grown into a major national trend. An estimated 20 million people participate in self-help support groups. Many others join virtual support communities online.

ORAL HEALTH

Oral health involves more than healthy teeth—it refers to the entire mouth, including all the structures that allow us to talk, bite, chew, taste, swallow, smile, scream, or scowl. Oral health is a critical part of overall health. Research has revealed links between chronic oral infection and heart and lung diseases, stroke, low birthweight, premature births, and diabetes.

Thanks to fluoridated water and toothpaste and improved dental care, Americans' oral health is better than in the past. However, without good self-care, you probably will lose some teeth to decay and gum disease. The best way to prevent such problems is through proper and regular brushing and flossing.

Gum, or periodontal, **disease** is an inflammation that attacks the gum and bone that hold your teeth in place. The culprit is **plaque,** the sticky film of bacteria that forms on teeth. More than 300 species of bacteria live under the gum line, and about half a dozen have been linked to serious gum problems. The early stage of gum disease is called **gingivitis.** If untreated, it develops into a more serious form known as **periodontitis,** in which plaque moves down the tooth to the roots, which then become infected. In advanced periodontitis, the infection destroys the bone and fibers that hold teeth in place.

Symptoms of gum disease include bleeding during brushing or flossing, redness and puffiness of gums, tenderness or pain, persistent bad breath or a bad taste in the

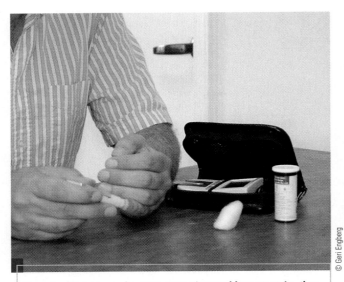

Home health tests can be more convenient and less expensive than a trip to a clinic or doctor's office.

Flossing every day helps prevent gum disease and other health problems. Using a gentle sawing motion, work the floss down to your gum line. Move the floss up and down to scrape the sides of each tooth. Clean between all your teeth, using a fresh section of floss for each tooth.

Strategies for Prevention ▪▪ Taking Care of Your Mouth

▪▪ Brush your teeth every morning and every night. Oral bacteria reach their highest count during sleep because fluids in the mouth accumulate. Nighttime cleaning reduces the bacterial population; morning cleaning lets you reduce the buildup.

▪▪ Use a toothpaste that has the American Dental Association (ADA) seal of acceptance and a toothbrush with soft, rounded bristles. Replace your toothbrush every three months.

▪▪ Hold the brush at a 45-degree angle from your gums. Pay particular attention to the space between your teeth and gums, especially on the inside,

toward your tongue. Brush for two to five minutes. Don't brush too vigorously. If you scrub as hard as you can, you may damage your teeth and gums. Abrasion—a problem for more than half of American adults—erodes tooth surfaces, weakens teeth, and increases sensitivity to hot and cold foods. There is some evidence that powered toothbrushes are better at removing plaque and reducing the risk of gum disease than are ordinary manual toothbrushes.

▪▪ Because brushing can't reach plaque and food trapped between teeth, daily flossing is essential. Using waxed or

unwaxed floss, start behind the upper and lower molars at one side of your mouth and work toward the other side.

▪▪ See your dentist twice a year for routine cleaning and examination. Your dentist should take a complete medical history from you and update it every six months, examine your mouth for signs of cancer, and thoroughly outline all treatment options.

▪▪ Make sure that everyone who works on the inside of your mouth wears a mask and rubber gloves to reduce the risk of disease transmission (that is, bacterial and viral infections, such as hepatitis, herpes, and HIV).

mouth, receding gums, shifted or loosened teeth, and changes in the way your teeth fit together when you bite. New treatments, which offer an alternative to traditional gum surgery, include a single antibiotic injection or the implant of a small antibiotic chip in the periodontal pockets to promote healing.

Taking care of your mouth isn't important only for dental health: It may affect how long you live. Gingivitis and periodontitis trigger an inflammatory response that causes the arteries to swell, which leads to a constriction of blood flow that can increase the incidence of cardiovascular disease. Periodontal disease also leads to a higher white blood cell count, an indicator that the immune system is under increased stress. The good news: You can prevent these problems by flossing daily and brushing your teeth and your tongue (to get rid of bacteria that can cause gum disease and bad breath).

GETTING THE BEST HEALTH CARE

Once patients simply put their faith in physicians and assumed that they knew best and would make the correct medical decisions. Today health care has become far more complex and impersonal. Increasingly, doctors as well as consumer advocates insist that patients need to take responsibility for their own care. Rather than assuming that healthcare providers will do whatever is necessary and appropriate, you must take the initiative to ensure that you get quality care.

THE DOCTOR-PATIENT PARTNERSHIP

Once the family doctor was indeed part of the family. The family doctor brought babies into the world, shepherded them through childhood, comforted and counseled them,

stood by their bedside in their darkest hours. Patients entrusted the doctor with their cares, their confidences, their very lives. Dramatic breakthroughs in diagnosing and treating illness shifted the focus in medicine from the family physician to the specialist, from basic caring to high-tech medical care. Patients today are more likely to be cured of a vast array of illnesses than were patients a century ago. However, they often complain of insensitive, uncaring physicians who focus on their diseases rather than on them as individuals.

As more physicians have joined managed-care organizations (discussed later in this chapter), which emphasize efficiency, they sometimes feel pressure to see more patients a day, to spend less time with each, and to discourage expensive tests and treatments.

In a recent survey, nearly one in three doctors reported sometimes not informing patients about "useful" medical services not covered by their health insurance companies. Physicians whose salaries are closely tied to controlling costs are more likely than other doctors to withhold information.[8] Because physicians have less time and less autonomy, patients today must do more. Your first step should be learning more about your body, any medical conditions or problems you develop, and your options for treatment. You can find a great deal of information via computer online services, patient advocacy and support organizations (see the Hales Health Almanac at the end of this book for listings), and libraries.

This information can help you know what questions to ask and how to evaluate what your doctor says. But you have to be willing to speak up. Busy doctors give patients less than a minute on average during a routine visit to say what's bothering them before they interrupt. This doesn't mean your doctor isn't interested, but it does mean that you have to develop good communication skills so you can tell physicians what they need to know to help you.

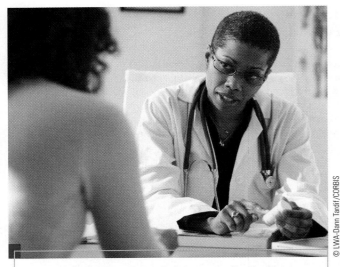

Take charge of your health by educating yourself and asking your doctor questions about your health and treatments.

(FAQ) HOW SHOULD I CHOOSE MY PRIMARY CARE PHYSICIAN?

Why does a healthy young adult need a doctor? To stay healthy as long as possible. At some point in early adulthood, you should establish a relationship with a physician who will do basic screening tests (Table 17-4), record your family history, and help you prevent problems down the road. The primary care physicians who are playing increasingly important roles in American health care include family practitioners, general internists, and pediatricians.

 Obstetrician-gynecologists serve as the primary providers of health care for more than half of all women. If you're a woman and your gynecologist is the only physician you see, make sure that he or she performs other tests, such as measuring your blood pressure, in addition to a pelvic and breast exam. If you develop other symptoms or health concerns, ask for an appropriate referral.

At college health centers, clinics, and some health-care organizations, consumers may be assigned to a primary physician or restricted to certain doctors. Even if your choices are limited, don't suspend your critical judgment. If your assigned physician does not listen to your concerns or is not providing adequate care, you can—and should—request another physician. Your rapport with your primary physician and the feelings of mutual trust and respect that develop between you can have as much of an impact on your well-being as your doctor's technical expertise.

One key to making the health-care system work for you lies in choosing a good physician. After seeing your primary care physician, ask yourself the following questions to evaluate the quality of care you are getting.

- Did your physician take a comprehensive history? Was the physical examination thorough?
- Did your physician explain what he or she was doing during the exam?

TABLE 17-4 SCREENING TESTS AND RECOMMENDATIONS

Anemia

Beginning in adolescence, all nonpregnant women should be screened every five to ten years until menopause.

Clinical Breast Exam/Mammography

Women ages 20 to 39 should receive a clinical breast exam every three years. Women age 40 and older should receive an annual clinical breast exam and mammography.

Cervical Cancer Screening (Pap Smear)

Three years after first sexual intercourse or by age 21, whichever comes first, until age 30, women should receive an annual Pap smear. After age 30, the screening rate may decrease. See "Your Action Plan for Early Detection of Cancer" in Chapter 16.

Cholesterol and Lipids

Adults over age 20 should have a lipoprotein panel test every five years.

Colorectal Cancer Screening

Adults age 50 and older should receive an annual fecal occult blood test and sigmoidoscopy every five years or colonoscopy every ten years.

Type 2 Diabetes

Beginning at age 45, adults should have a fasting plasma glucose test every three years.

Hypertension Screening

Adults age 18 and older should have an annual blood pressure (BP) check. If the BP is less than 130/85, it should be checked every two years. If the blood pressure is between 130–139/85–89, it should be checked annually. After age 60, blood pressure should be checked annually.

Osteoporosis

Women age 65 and older should have a baseline bone mineral density test. To reduce the risk of fractures, women should increase dietary calcium and vitamin D, perform weight-bearing exercise, stop smoking, and moderate alcohol intake.

Prostate Cancer Screening

Men age 50 and older should discuss potential benefits and known harms of screening with PSA and digital rectal exam.

Skin Cancer Screening

Between the ages of 20 to 39, adults should receive a skin exam every three years. After age 40, adults should receive an annual skin exam.

Visual Exam

Adults age 18 to 40 should have a complete visual examination every two to three years; ages 41 to 60, every 2 years; and ages 61 and older, every year.

- Did he or she spend enough time with you?
- Did you feel free to ask questions? Did your physician give you straight answers? Did he or she reassure you when you were worried?
- Does your physician seem willing to admit that he or she doesn't know the answers to some questions?
- Does your physician hesitate to refer you to a specialist even when you have a complex problem that warrants such care?

Strategies for Change ❚❚ How to Talk with Your Doctor

❚❚ Prepare in advance. Write down your questions, organize them in a logical fashion, and select the top ten queries you want answered. Make a copy of all your questions to review and leave with your doctor.

❚❚ Ask about a "question hour." Many health-care practitioners set aside a specific time of day for patients with call-in questions. Find out if your college health center offers this service. Does a nurse field all calls? Can you get specific advice?

❚❚ Go online. Many doctors' offices answer queries by e-mail. Ask your doctor if you can e-mail follow-up questions or progress reports on how you're feeling.

❚❚ Interrupt the interrupter. If you're having difficulty explaining what's wrong, say so. If your doctor tries to put words in your mouth, say, "Please just listen so I can tell you the whole story without getting sidetracked."

Look back at your answers. If they make you feel uneasy, have a talk with your physician. Or find a physician or a health plan that provides better service.

YOUR MEDICAL EXAM

Although analysts have not found evidence that an annual screening physical is warranted for healthy adults, primary care physicians feel differently. In a recent survey about two-thirds agreed that an annual physical examination is necessary. The benefits, as doctors see them, include time to counsel patients about preventive health services, detection of underlying illnesses before symptoms develop, and improved patient-physician relationships.[9]

Your physician will want a past **medical history,** including major illnesses, surgery, and treatments. Report any allergies you have, particularly to drugs, and the medications you take, including aspirin, antacids, sleeping pills, oral contraceptives, and recreational drugs, even if illegal. Your physician may also want to know about topics you consider private, such as sexually transmitted infections. Remember that he or she needs all this information to provide you with comprehensive treatment. Note, too, that a physician must report certain information—for example, certain sexually transmitted diseases—to health authorities.

After the physician has asked you questions about your complaints, medical history, and lifestyle, he or she will probably perform the standard tests described next (Figure 17-1). During the examination, point out any pains, lumps, or skin growths you've noticed. If you feel pain when the physician palpates (feels) any part of your body, say so.

❚ **Head.** Using a flashlightlike instrument called an *ophthalmoscope,* the physician will look at the lens, retina, and blood vessels of your eyes. For patients over 40, he or she may test for a treatable eye disease called *glaucoma* (a disorder characterized by increased pressure within the eye), which can cause blindness if not detected early. The physician presses against the surface of each eye a soft instrument that measures the pressure within the eye and checks to see if the reading is normal. He or she also will examine your ears, mouth, tongue, teeth, and gums.

❚ **Neck.** Feeling around your neck, the physician will check for enlarged lymph glands (a sign of infection), for lumps in the thyroid gland, and for warning signs of stroke in the neck arteries.

❚ **Chest.** With a *stethoscope,* the physician will listen to the sounds made by your heart, to detect heart murmurs and irregular contractions, and by your lungs, to detect asthma or emphysema. By tapping on your chest and back with his or her fingers, the physician can tell the size and shape of your heart, which may reveal some forms of heart disease, and whether any fluid has collected in your lungs. The physician will also check for abnormal lumps in a woman's breasts.

❚ **Abdomen.** Here the physician uses his or her fingers to probe for tender spots and malformations of the liver and other organs, which may reveal signs of alcoholism, hepatitis, or hernias.

❚ **Rectum and genitals.** With a gloved hand, the physician can feel in the rectum for growths and hemorrhoids. A rectal examination can also reveal enlargement of the male's prostate gland. The physician will check male testicles and spermatic cords for abnormalities.

❚ **Pelvic examination.** During a pelvic examination, a woman lies on her back, with her heels in stirrups at the end of the examining table and her legs spread out to the sides. The physician inspects the labia, clitoris, and vaginal opening. Using two gloved, lubricated fingers, the physician will check for abnormalities in the vagina, uterus, fallopian tubes, and ovaries. Many physicians will also perform a rectal or rectovaginal (one finger in the rectum and one in the vagina) examination. A nurse or other health-care worker should be present throughout the exam.

The *speculum* is a medical instrument that spreads the walls of the vagina so that the inside can be seen. The physician will gently scrape cells

Looking into the eyes. With an ophthalmoscope, your doctor will look for changes in eye's blood vessels or the optic nerve. These can signal severe diabetes, high blood pressure, or a tumor in the brain.

Examining the throat. Your doctor will look for signs of infection and other abnormalities.

Listening to the heart, lungs, and abdomen. Your doctor will use a stethoscope to listen to the heart sounds to detect heart murmurs and other abnormalities. He or she will listen for wheezing or crackling sounds in your lungs, which could indicate asthma, bronchitis, or pneumonia. Your abdomen should make gurgling sounds. If it doesn't, the bowel may not be working properly.

Probing the abdomen. A swelling on the right side may indicate a liver problem. A swelling on the left may mean that the spleen is enlarged, which could be a sign of infection or another condition.

FIGURE 17-1 Standard Tests Performed During a Medical Checkup

from the cervix for a **Pap smear,** a procedure that identifies abnormal cells that may indicate an infection or, more seriously, cervical cancer, a slow-growing cancer that's usually curable if detected early (see Chapter 16). All women should start having regular Pap smears once they begin having intercourse, or at age 18. While there has been debate about how often women should have Pap smears, many health-care providers recommend Pap smears every year for women who are sexually active or have other risk factors, such as infection with the human papilloma virus (see Chapter 14).

■ **Extremities.** The physician may check your knees and other joints for reflexes, which can indicate nerve disorders, and look for tremors in outstretched hands or in the face. The color, elasticity, and wetness or dryness of your skin can alert him or her to nutritional problems, or can indicate diabetes or skin cancer. Hair and nails can give indications of internal health, such as blood disorders. Swelling of the ankles can be an indication of heart, kidney, or liver disease.

■ **Pulse and blood pressure.** Your physician may check your pulse in various places, looking for signs of poor circulation. The rhythm and speed of the heart may also signal diseases of the heart or thyroid gland. High blood pressure can be an early warning sign of possible heart attack, stroke, or kidney damage.

MEDICAL TESTS

Besides the diagnostic tests just listed, the physician may order some laboratory and other tests, including the following:

■ **Chest X ray.** A chest X ray can reveal abnormalities of the heart and lungs; if you're a smoker, the physician may insist on one.

■ **Electrocardiogram.** The *electrocardiogram,* performed while you're at rest, records the electrical activity of your heart. It can show irregularities in heart rhythm or muscle damage, as well as hardening of the arteries.

- **Urinalysis.** Your urine may be analyzed by a medical laboratory. If sugar (glucose) is found in your urine, your physician may order a separate blood test to check for diabetes. The presence of blood cells may indicate infection of the bladder or kidneys. Abnormal amounts of albumin (protein) in the urine may also suggest kidney disease.

- **Blood tests.** The physician or laboratory technician may draw blood to do a blood cell count. An excess of white blood cells may indicate an infection or, occasionally, leukemia. A deficiency of red blood cells may indicate anemia. Your blood also may be analyzed to measure the levels of its various components. High levels of glucose can indicate diabetes, and high levels of uric acid may mean gout or kidney stones. Your lipoprotein profile may indicate cardiac risk (see Chapter 15).

See the Hales Health Almanac at the back of this book for a comprehensive guide to medical tests.

MEN AND WOMEN AS HEALTH-CARE CONSUMERS

The genders differ significantly in the way they use health-care services in the United States. Women see more doctors than men, take more prescription drugs, are hospitalized more, and control the spending of three of every four health-care dollars. In a national telephone poll, 76 percent of American women—but only 60 percent of men—said they had had a health exam in the last 12 months.

Many experts believe that the need for birth control and reproductive health services gets women into the habit of making regular visits to health-care professionals, primarily gynecologists. There are no comparable specialists for men, who tend to visit urologists, specialists in male reproductive organs, only when they develop problems. Men also are conditioned to take a stoic, tough-it-out attitude to early symptoms of a disease.

Men feel they are not allowed to manifest illness unless it's overt, says family practitioner Martin Miner, M.D., who has conducted research on men and health care. One reason men die earlier than women is because of the length of time they wait to go for treatment.

The genders also differ in the symptoms and syndromes they develop. For instance, men are more prone to back problems, muscle sprains and strains, allergies, insomnia, and digestive problems. Men develop heart disease about a decade earlier in life than women. More men develop ulcers and hernias; women are more likely to get gallbladder disease and irritable bowel syndrome. An estimated 3 to 6 percent of men suffer from migraines, compared with 15 to 17 percent of women. Yet women and men spend similar proportions of their lifetimes—about 81 percent—free of disability. For men, whose lifespans are shorter, this translates into an average of 58.8 years; for women, 63.9 years.

The genders also differ in access to health services.

Women are more likely than men to lack health insurance, and the lower a woman's income and education, the less her likelihood of getting important preventive services, such as an annual Pap smear or prenatal care. Women and men are about equally likely to use complementary and alternative medicine—but different types. Men outnumber women in use of chiropractic services and acupuncture, while women are more likely to try herbal medicine, mind-body remedies, folk remedies, movement and exercise techniques, and prayer or spiritual practices. Both genders turn to alternative treatments for the same reason: a desire for greater control over their health.

ELECTIVE TREATMENTS

As medical technology has developed new options, millions of Americans are trying elective procedures and products that are not medically necessary but that promise to enhance health or appearance. Some are new alternatives for correcting common problems, such as poor vision, while others offer the promise of looking younger or more attractive.

VISION SURGERY

Millions of people in the United States have undergone laser surgery to correct their vision. In LASIK (laser-assisted in situ keratomileusis), the most common technique, a surgeon uses a razorlike instrument to lift a flap of the cornea—the clear stiff outer layer over the colored iris—and then reshapes the exposed area using a laser. The surgery alters the way the eye focuses light, correcting nearsightedness, farsightedness, and some astigmatism. Laser surgery cannot make an aging eye's lens flexible again to improve close-up vision in middle-aged adults. Numbing eye drops make the treatment painless, although burning and scratchiness are normal for a couple of hours. An estimated 10 to 30 percent of patients require additional surgery, or "enhancements," to sharpen their vision. Other complications include glare, sensitivity to bright lights, and poor night vision.

Prices have fallen, but ophthalmologists have warned consumers that some laser surgery centers have cut corners to cut prices, such as hiring inexperienced surgeons or using optometrists or technicians rather than MDs for pre- and postoperative checkups. A qualified eye surgeon should have a record of 100 or more LASIK procedures and at least 25 enhancements—but no more than 20 percent of his or her patients should require enhancements. Ideally, the surgeon should also be the one doing your pre- and post-procedure checks.

COSMETIC SURGERY

Approximately 9.2 million cosmetic treatments are performed every year. About a quarter of those undergoing plastic surgery are between the ages of 18 and 29.[10] The number of teenagers opting for cosmetic procedures—primarily

---

Strategy for Prevention: :: When Is LASIK Not for Me?

You are probably NOT a good candidate for refractive surgery if:

:: **You are not a risk taker.** Certain complications are unavoidable in a percentage of patients, and there are no long-term data available for current procedures.

:: **Cost is an issue.** Most medical insurance will not pay for refractive surgery. Although the cost is coming down, it is still significant.

:: **You required a change in your contact lens or glasses prescription in the past year.** This is called refractive instability. Patients who are in their early twenties or younger, whose hormones are fluctuating due to disease such as diabetes, who are pregnant or breastfeeding, or who are taking medications that may cause fluctuations in vision are more likely to have refractive instability and should discuss the possible additional risks with their doctor.

:: **You have a disease or are on medications that may affect wound healing.** Certain conditions, such as autoimmune diseases and diabetes, and some medications may prevent proper healing after a refractive procedure.

:: **You actively participate in contact sports.** If you participate in boxing, wrestling, martial arts, or other activities in which blows to the face and eyes are a normal occurrence, LASIK is probably not right for you.

:: **You are under 18.** Currently, no lasers are approved for LASIK on persons under the age of 18.

:: **It will jeopardize your career.** Some jobs, including certain military assignments, prohibit refractive procedures.

Source: Food and Drug Administration, www.fda .gov/cdrh/LASIK/when.htm.

---

liposuction, nose reshaping, and breast augmentation—is increasing. Nonsurgical cosmetic procedures such as injections of synthetic collagen and botulinum toxin (Botox®) also have become more popular. Health insurance rarely covers cosmetic procedures, which range from $300 to upwards of $10,000.

The most common cosmetic operation is liposuction, the removal of fatty tissue by means of a vacuum device. It can be performed on many areas of the body, from sagging jowls to midsection "love handles." The doctor first flushes the target area with a solution of lidocaine (a local anesthetic with a numbing effect), saline, and epinephrine (a drug that reduces bleeding by constricting blood vessels). Inserting a hollow wandlike cannula under the skin, the doctor breaks up fatty deposits and suctions them, along with other body fluids, with a vacuum device.

Risks and complications include infection, numbness, bleeding, discoloration, lumpiness, and, if too much tissue is removed without proper cautions, potentially fatal complications. The American Society of Plastic and Reconstructive Surgeons estimates the mortality rate is one in 5,000 liposuction patients. Several states are considering legislation to tighten restrictions on training and credentialing doctors who perform liposuction.

Breast augmentation is the second most common cosmetic procedure, and surgeons report a 300 percent increase in demand in the last six years. The Institute of Medicine, after reviewing all available evidence, has reported that there appears to be no link between breast implants and autoimmune disease, connective tissue disorders, or cancer. However, today's surgeons use implants filled with a saltwater solution. Patients still face possible complications, including rupture, scarring, infection, and leaking or hardening of their implants.

YOUR MEDICAL RIGHTS

As a consumer, you have basic rights that help ensure that you know about any potential dangers, receive competent diagnosis and treatment, and retain control and dignity in your interactions with health-care professionals. Many hospitals publish a patient's bill of rights, including your rights to know whether a procedure is experimental; to refuse to undergo a specific treatment; to designate someone else to make decisions about your care if and when you cannot; and to leave the hospital, even against your physician's advice.

You have the right to be treated with respect and dignity, including being called "Mr." or "Ms." or whatever you wish, rather than by your first name. Make clear your preferences. If you feel that health-care professionals are being condescending or inconsiderate, say so—in the same tone and manner that you would like others to use with you. If you're hospitalized, find out if there's a patient advocate or representative at your hospital. These individuals can help you communicate with physicians, make any special arrangements, and get answers to questions or complaints.

You have the right to give consent to donate an organ while alive, or have your organs removed in the event of an accident, injury, or illness that leaves you brain-dead. However, you cannot agree to donate a body part for money or other compensation. Congress has prohibited the marketing of organs; any attempt to do so is a felony punishable by up to five years in jail and a $50,000 fine.

YOUR RIGHT TO INFORMATION

By law, a patient must give consent for hospitalization, surgery, and other major treatments. **Informed consent** is a right, not a privilege. Use this right to its fullest. Ask questions. Seek other opinions. Make sure that your expectations are realistic and that you understand the potential risks, as well as the possible benefits, of a prospective treatment.

YOUR RIGHT TO PRIVACY AND ACCESS TO MEDICAL RECORDS

Your medical records are your property. You have the right to see them whenever you choose and to limit who else can see them. Federal standards protecting the privacy of patients' medical information guarantee patients access to their medical records, give them more control over how personal health information is disclosed, and limit the ways that health plans, pharmacies, and hospitals can use personal medical information.

Key provisions include:

■ **Access to medical records.** As a patient, you should be able to see and obtain copies of your medical records and request corrections if there are errors. Health-care providers must provide these within 30 days; they may charge for the cost of copying and mailing records.

■ **Notice of privacy practices.** Your providers must inform you of how they use personal medical information. Doctors, nurses, and other providers may not disclose information for purposes not related to your health care.

■ **Prohibition on marketing.** Pharmacies, health plans, and others must obtain specific authorization before disclosing patient information for marketing.

■ **Confidentiality.** Patients can request that doctors take reasonable steps to ensure confidential communications, such as calling a cell phone rather than home or office.[11]

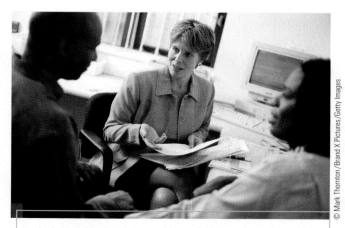

In the hospital, you can discuss the hospital's patient's bill of rights as well as individual concerns with a patient advocate.

YOUR RIGHT TO GOOD, SAFE, CARE

According to recent court rulings, patients have the right to sue health insurers that refuse to authorize medically necessary treatment. This enables patients to hold health plans accountable for their role in medical decision making.

Preventing Medical Errors

Medical errors, which can occur whenever something goes wrong with a test or treatment, are a leading cause of injury and death. An average of 195,000 people in the United States die due to potentially preventable, hospital medical errors each year, according to a recent study of 37 million patient records.[12]

The risks associated with hospitalization include what health workers call the "terrible I's": infection; inactivity; incorrect actions; and the inherent risks of drugs, X rays, and false lab tests. The simplest method for preventing hospital-acquired infection—handwashing—is often ignored by health-care providers.

Errors, which may involve diagnosis, equipment, lab reports, medications, or surgery, are more likely to occur when doctors and their patients have problems communicating. The single most important thing you can do to prevent errors is take part in every decision about your health care. Make sure you understand what may be wrong with you, as well as which medications you are taking and why:

■ **When your doctor writes you a prescription** make sure you can read it and know why and how you are to take the medication.

■ **Ask for information about your medicines** in terms you can understand, including explanations of possible interactions with other drugs or dietary supplements and potential side effects.

■ **If you must undergo surgery** and you can choose a hospital, select one at which many patients have had the procedure or surgery you need.

■ **Consider asking all health-care workers** in direct contact with you whether they have washed their hands. This simple step prevents the spread of infections.

■ **Speak up if you have questions or concerns.** Ask a family member or friend to be your advocate and speak up for you if you can't.

Malpractice

The essence of a **malpractice** suit is the claim that the physician failed to meet the standard of care required of a reasonably skilled and careful medical doctor. Although physicians don't have to guarantee good results to their patients and aren't held liable for unavoidable errors, they are required to use the same care and judgment in treatment that other physicians in the same specialty would use under similar circumstances. To protect themselves financially,

---

Strategies for Prevention ⋮⋮ Protecting Yourself Against Quackery

⋮⋮ Arm yourself with up-to-date information about your condition or disease from appropriate organizations, such as the American Cancer Society or the Arthritis Foundation, which keep track of unproven and ineffective methods of treatment.

⋮⋮ Ask for a written explanation of what a treatment does and why it works, evidence supporting all claims (not just testimonials), and published reports of the studies, including specifics on numbers treated, doses, and side effects. Be skeptical of self-styled "holistic practitioners," treatments supported by crusading groups, and endorsements from self-proclaimed experts or authorities.

⋮⋮ Don't part with your money quickly. Be especially careful because insurance companies won't reimburse for unproven therapies.

⋮⋮ Don't discontinue your current treatment without your physician's approval. Many physicians encourage supportive therapies—such as relaxation exercises, meditation, or visualization—as a supplement to standard treatments.

---

physicians, particularly those in surgical specialties who are most likely to be sued, pay tens of thousands of dollars a year in malpractice insurance premiums. Some of this cost is passed on to patients.

Because of fear of malpractice, many physicians practice "defensive" medicine and order more tests, refer more patients, prescribe more medications, and suggest biopsies more often than necessary for legal rather than medical reasons. In some states the cost of malpractice insurance has soared, forcing some physicians to change specialties or relocate. Health policy experts have suggested replacing the current system of handling malpractice claims with special medical courts staffed by medical experts.[13]

Most lawsuits are based on negligence and assert that a physician failed to render diagnosis and treatment with appropriate professional knowledge and skill. Other cases are brought for failure to provide information, obtain consent, or respect a patient's confidentiality. However, analysis of malpractice cases has shown that, in 70 to 80 percent, a doctor's attitude and inability to communicate effectively—by devaluing patients' views, delivering information poorly, failing to understand patients' perspectives, or displaying an air of superiority—also played a role.

The Public Citizen Health Research Group has compiled a national directory of "questionable physicians," which lists physicians disciplined by state medical boards or the federal government for offenses ranging from overprescribing drugs to sexual misconduct to negligent or substandard care. Some of these physicians committed minor misdeeds, such as failing to complete continuing medical education requirements. Consumer advocates urge patients to find out why a particular name appears on the list by calling the state licensing board. At the federal level, the agencies most involved in ensuring quality health care are the Food and Drug Administration (FDA), which approves the production and labeling of drugs, and the Federal Trade Commission (FTC), which oversees advertising and prohibits deceptive or false claims.

Quackery

Every year millions of Americans go searching for medical miracles that never happen. In all, they spend more than $10 billion on medical **quackery,** unproven health products and services. Those who lose only money are the lucky ones. Many also waste precious time, during which their conditions worsen. Some suffer needless pain, along with crushed expectations. Far too many risk their lives on a false hope—and lose (see Savvy Consumer: "Spotting Health Hoaxes").

Savvy Consumer ⋮⋮ Spotting Health Hoaxes

Promoters of fraudulent health products often use similar claims and practices to trick consumers into buying their products. Be suspicious when you see:

⋮⋮ Claims that a product is a "scientific breakthrough," "miraculous cure," "secret ingredient," or "ancient remedy."

⋮⋮ Claims that the product is an effective cure for a wide range of ailments. No product can cure multiple conditions or diseases.

⋮⋮ Claims that use impressive-sounding medical terms. They're often covering up a lack of good science.

⋮⋮ Undocumented case histories of people who've had amazing results. It's too easy to make them up. And even if true, they can't be generalized to the entire population. Anecdotes are not a substitute for valid science.

⋮⋮ Claims that the product is available from only one source and payment is required in advance.

⋮⋮ Claims of a "money-back" guarantee.

⋮⋮ Websites that fail to list the company's name, physical address, phone number, or other contact information.

To file a complaint with the Federal Trade Commission (FTC) or to get free information on consumer topics, call 1-877-FTC-HELP (1-877-382-4357), or use the complaint form at www.ftc.gov.

Source: Federal Trade Commission, www.ftc .gov/bcp/conline/features/healthclaims.htm.

COMPLEMENTARY AND ALTERNATIVE MEDICINE

The medical research community uses the term **complementary and alternative medicine (CAM)** to apply to all health-care approaches, practices, and treatments not widely taught in medical schools and not generally used in hospitals.[14] CAM includes many healing philosophies, approaches, and therapies, including preventive techniques designed to delay or prevent serious health problems before they start and **holistic** methods that focus on the whole person and the physical, mental, emotional, and spiritual aspects of well-being. Some approaches are based on the same physiological principles as traditional Western methods; others, such as acupuncture, are based on different healing systems.

According to a recent nationwide government survey of more than 31,000 adults aged 18 and over, 50 percent have used CAM at some time and 46 percent have tried some form of complementary and alternative medicine in the last year. When CAM includes megavitamins and prayer specifically for health, the number reporting they ever used some form of CAM rises to 75 percent; 62 percent did so in the past year.[15]

 CAM use varies among different groups. Those most likely to use CAM include women, people with higher education, those hospitalized within the past year, and former smokers (compared to current smokers or those who never smoked). African-American adults are more likely than white or Asian adults to use CAM practices, including megavitamin therapy and prayer (Figure 17-2).

Some states have mandated health insurance coverage for CAM therapies, which also are becoming more common in Canada and Europe. Many medical schools now include training in CAM in their curricula. **Integrative medicine,** which combines selected elements of both conventional and alternative medicine in a comprehensive approach to diagnosis and treatment, has gained greater acceptance within the medical community.

WHY PEOPLE USE CAM THERAPIES

Rather than turning to CAM as an alternative to conventional treatments, consumers combine the two approaches. About half (55 percent of those surveyed) use CAM because they believe that it could help them when combined with conventional medical care; 50 percent thought CAM would be interesting to try. Almost one in three (28 percent) used CAM because they believed conventional medical treatments would not help their health problem. About a quarter used CAM because a conventional medical professional suggested it; 13 percent turned to CAM because they felt that conventional medicine was too expensive.

Consumers turn to CAM most often for chronic or recurring pain—of the back, neck, or joints—and for colds,

FIGURE 17-2 **CAM Use by U.S. Adults and by Race/Ethnicity**

Source: NCCAM, http://nccam.nih.gov.

anxiety, or depression. Most use CAM as a form of self-care; only about 12 percent seek care from a licensed CAM practitioner, suggesting that most people who use CAM do so without consulting a practitioner. According to the survey, the ten most commonly used CAM therapies are:

- **Prayer** for own health (used by 43 percent)
- **Prayer by others** for the respondent's health (24 percent)
- **Natural products,** such as herbs, other botanicals, and enzymes (19 percent)
- **Deep-breathing** exercises (12 percent)
- **Participation in prayer** group for own health (10 percent)
- **Meditation** (8 percent)
- **Chiropractic care** (8 percent)
- **Yoga** (5 percent)
- **Massage** (5 percent)
- **Diet-based therapies** (such as Atkins, Pritikin, Ornish, and Zone diets) (4 percent)

Individuals with a psychiatric disorder are significantly more likely to use a CAM therapy than the general population. Those with severe depression or anxiety disorders use CAM most often. Most patients who use CAM for mental health problems also use conventional therapies. The most popular CAM therapies in mental health care are relaxation techniques and "spiritual healing." The efficacy and safety of most CAM therapies used to self-treat or treat mental health problems are not yet established.

An estimated 10 to 50 percent of cancer patients try alternative treatments, many without their physicians' knowledge. These include dietary changes, antioxidant vitamins, soy, herbs, and other natural products, acupuncture, massage, exercise, and psychological and mind-body interventions. Based on the best evidence available, cancer specialists have ranked these approaches on a continuum ranging from "recommend" to "discourage."

A reduction in dietary fat was deemed acceptable, but the use of antioxidant vitamins A, C, and E may cause more harm than benefit because of the risks of cancer progression and effects on blood clotting. Doctors discourage the use of soy supplements in women with breast cancer but accept their use by men with prostate cancer. The efficacy of shark cartilage remains unclear. Acupuncture was deemed acceptable to help control chemotherapy-related nausea and vomiting among cancer patients. Massage has not demonstrated any positive effect on cancer progression or pain relief. Psychologic and mind-body therapies such as individual and group therapy, relaxation, imagery, hypnosis, and meditation can relieve distress and pain as well as some of the physical symptoms of disease and side effects of conventional therapy.

(FAQ) WHAT SHOULD I KNOW BEFORE I TRY CAM?

You should never decide on any treatment—traditional or CAM—without fully evaluating it. Here are some key questions to ask:

- **Is it safe?** Be particularly wary of unregulated products.
- **Is it effective?** Check the website of the National Center for CAM: http://nccam.nih.gov.
- **Will it interact with other medicines or conventional treatments?** Many widely used alternative remedies can interact with prescription medications in dangerous ways.
- **Is the practitioner qualified?** Find out if your state licenses practitioners who provide acupuncture, chiropractic services, naturopathy, herbal medicine, homeopathy, and other treatments.
- **What has been the experience of others?** Talk to people who have used CAM for a similar problem, both recently and in the past.
- **Can you talk openly and easily with the practitioner?** You should feel comfortable asking questions and confident in the answers you receive. And the practitioner's office should put you at ease.

- **What are the costs?** Many CAM services are not covered by HMOs or health insurers.

EVIDENCE-BASED CAM

Many have criticized health-care providers for giving alternative therapies "a free ride" by not demanding the same proof and regulation required of traditional treatments.[16] While many CAM treatments have been in use for a long time (sometimes for centuries), they do not have the same sort of scientific basis gained from studies of conventional medicine. Individuals who use them may be at risk for serious side effects, for example, from taking the wrong dose or using a treatment in the wrong way. Scientists are working to apply the same standards of evidence-based medicine used for conventional treatment to CAM. Recent studies that have applied rigorously scientific standards to popular alternative therapies have revealed unexpected risks, confirmed benefits from some forms of CAM, and disproved the alleged positive effects of others.[17]

TYPES OF CAM

The National Center for Complementary and Alternative Medicine (NCCAM) has classified CAM therapies into five categories (Figure 17.3).

- **Alternative medical systems**
- **Mind-body medicine**
- **Biologically based therapies**
- **Manipulative and body-based methods**
- **Energy therapies**

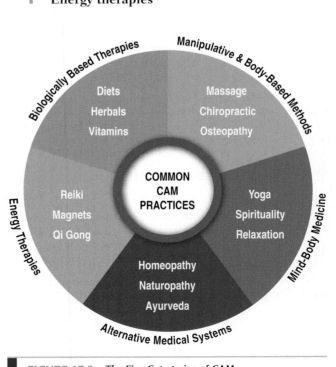

FIGURE 17-3 The Five Categories of CAM

Source: NCCAM, http://nccam.nih.gov.

Alternative Medical Systems

Systems of theory and practice other than traditional Western medicine are included in this group. They include acupuncture, Eastern medicine, t'ai chi, external and internal qi, Ayurvedic medicine, naturopathy, and unconventional Western systems, such as homeopathy and orthomolecular medicine.

Acupuncture is an ancient Chinese form of medicine, based on the philosophy that a cycle of energy circulating through the body controls health. Pain and disease are the result of a disturbance in the energy flow, which can be corrected by inserting long, thin needles at specific points along longitudinal lines, or *meridians,* throughout the body. Each point controls a different corresponding part of the body. Once inserted, the needles are rotated gently back and forth or charged with a small electric current for a short time. Western scientists aren't sure exactly how acupuncture works, but some believe that the needles alter the functioning of the nervous system.

A National Institute of Health (NIH) consensus development panel that evaluated current research into acupuncture concluded that there is "clear evidence" that acupuncture can control nausea and vomiting in patients after surgery or while undergoing chemotherapy and relieve postoperative dental pain. The panel said that acupuncture is "probably" also effective in the control of nausea in early pregnancy and that there were "reasonable" studies showing satisfactory treatment of addiction to illicit drugs and alcohol (but not to tobacco), stroke rehabilitation, headache, menstrual cramps, tennis elbow, general muscle pain, low back pain, carpal tunnel syndrome, and asthma. Ongoing studies are evaluating its efficacy for chronic headaches and migraines.

Considered alternative in this country, **Ayurveda** is a traditional form of medical treatment in India, where it has evolved over thousands of years. Its basic premise is that illness stems from incorrect mental attitudes, diet, and posture. Practitioners use a discipline of exercise, meditation, herbal medication, and proper nutrition to cope with such stress-induced conditions as hypertension, the desire to smoke, and obesity.

Homeopathy is based on three fundamental principles: like cures like; treatment must always be individualized; and less is more—the idea that increasing dilution (and lowering the dosage) can increase efficacy. By administering doses of animal, vegetable, or mineral substances to a large number of healthy people to see if they all develop the same symptoms, homeopaths determine which substances may be given, in small quantities, to alleviate the symptoms. Some of these substances are the same as those used in conventional medicine: nitroglycerin for certain heart conditions, for example, although the dose is minuscule.

Naturopathy emphasizes natural remedies, such as sun, water, heat, and air, as the best treatments for disease. Therapies might include dietary changes (such as more vegetables and no salt or stimulants), steam baths, and exercise. Some naturopathic physicians (who are not MDs) work closely with medical doctors in helping patients.

Mind-Body Medicine

Mind-body medicine uses techniques designed to enhance the mind's capacity to affect bodily function and symptoms. Some techniques that were considered alternative in the past have become mainstream (for example, patient support groups and cognitive-behavioral therapy). Other mind-body approaches are still considered CAM, including meditation, prayer (see Chapter 3), yoga, t'ai chi, visual imagery, mental healing, and therapies that use creative outlets such as art, music, or dance. About 30 percent of Americans report using relaxation techniques and imagery, biofeedback, and hypnosis; 50 percent use prayer.

The physical and emotional risks of using mind-body interventions are minimal. Although we need much more research on how these approaches work and when to apply them most effectively, there is considerable evidence that mind-body interventions have positive effects on psychological functioning and quality of life and may be particularly helpful for patients coping with chronic illnesses.

Mind-body medicine is ancient, dating back more than 2,000 years to the healing approaches of traditional Chinese and Ayurvedic medicine. In the West, Hippocrates, the great Greek healer, recognized the moral and spiritual aspects of treating illnesses. However, by the sixteenth and seventeenth centuries, Western science separated spiritual and emotional dimensions from the physical body. Fixing or curing an illness became a matter of science and technology and took precedence over healing the soul.

During World War II, the importance of belief regained credibility. When morphine for wounded soldiers ran out, doctors discovered that they could often control pain by saline injections. Research into this "placebo effect" showed that up to 35 percent of a therapeutic response to any medical treatment could be the result of belief in it. Since the 1960s, researchers have demonstrated more benefits of

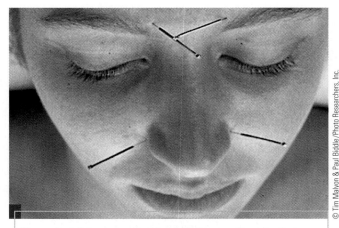

The ancient Chinese practice of acupuncture produces healing through the insertion and manipulation of needles at specific points throughout the body.

© Tim Malyon & Paul Biddle/Photo Researchers, Inc.

mind-body interventions, such as biofeedback and hypnosis. We know much less about the use of other popular CAM approaches like meditation and yoga.

Mind-body approaches definitely have won some acceptance in modern medical care. Scientists now recognize that psychological factors can play a significant role in the development and progression of coronary artery disease. Along with standard medical treatments, they help reduce death rates and heart attacks in people with heart disease. Mind-body interventions also are effective in treating arthritis; they reduce pain and the number of physician visits. Multiple studies with various types of cancer patients suggest that mind-body treatments improve mood, quality of life, and coping, as well as relieve disease- and treatment-related symptoms, such as nausea, vomiting, and pain. Techniques such as hypnosis have proved helpful in reducing discomfort and complications during and after various surgical procedures. An array of mind-body therapies (e.g., imagery, hypnosis, relaxation), when used presurgically, can improve recovery time and reduce pain following surgical procedures.[18]

Biofeedback uses machines that measure temperature or skin responses and then relays this information to the subject. In this way, people can learn to control usually involuntary functions, such as circulation to the hands and feet, tension in the jaws, and heartbeat rates. Biofeedback has been used to treat dozens of ailments, including asthma, epilepsy, pain, and Reynaud's disease (a condition in which the fingers become painful and white when exposed to cold). Many health insurers now cover biofeedback treatments.

Creative **visualization,** or imaging, helps patients, including some diagnosed as terminally ill with cancer, heal. On the premise that positive and negative beliefs and attitudes have a great deal to do with whether people get well or die of disease, patients imagine themselves getting well—they "see," for instance, immune-system cells marching to conquer cancer cells. Other patients use visualization in different ways—for example, to create a clear idea of what they want to achieve, whether the goal is weight loss or relaxation.

Biologically Based Therapies

Biologically based CAM therapies use substances such as herbs, foods, and vitamins. They include botanical medicine or phytotherapy, the use of individual herbs or combinations; special diet therapies, such as macrobiotics, Ornish, McDougall, and high fiber; Mediterranean orthomolecular medicine (use of nutritional and food supplements for preventive or therapeutic purposes); and use of other products (such as shark cartilage) and procedures applied in an unconventional manner.

Herbal medicine has become an estimated $4 billion-a-year industry, yet questions about the safety and effectiveness of herbal supplements persist. Although more than 1,500 different preparations are on the U.S. market, just a few single-herb preparations account for about half the

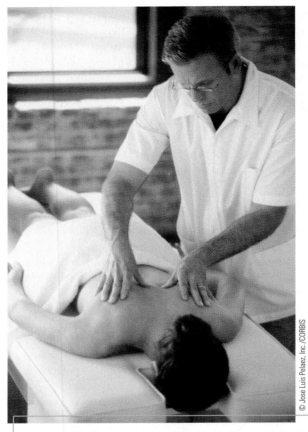

Massage and body work are among the popular "manipulative" forms of complementary and alternative medicine.

sales in the United States: echinacea, garlic, ginkgo, ginseng, kava, St. John's wort, and valerian. Unlike medications, herbal products are exempt from the FDA's regulatory scrutiny. The ingredients and the potency of active ingredients can vary from batch to batch.

Rigorous research studies are producing the first scientific evidence on the safety and efficacy of herbal supplements.[19] Their benefits, if any, have proved modest (Table 17-5). Ginkgo biloba, for instance, temporarily boosts memory, but no more so than eating a candy bar.[20] Other agents, such as saw palmetto or garlic, produce slight benefits but far less than available medications.

Most of the herbs tested have proved generally safe, although side effects such as headache and nausea can occur. However, some herbs can cause serious, even fatal dangers. Echinacea, widely used as a cold remedy, may cause liver damage if taken in combination with anabolic steroids.

Several widely used herbs, including ginger, garlic, and ginkgo, are dangerous if taken prior to surgery—yet it's been estimated that more than 70 percent of patients fail to disclose their use of herbal medicine before an operation. Herbs such as ginseng and goldenseal can cause unexpected rises in blood pressure and heart rate during an operation, while St. John's wort and kava may interact with and

TABLE 17-5 EVIDENCE-BASED EVALUATIONS OF HERBAL SUPPLEMENTS

Herb	Evidence
Saw Palmetto	Reduces an enlarged prostate, but the effect is small compared with prescription medication
Ginseng	No demonstrated benefits or proven effect on energy
Echinacea	No proven benefits as a cold remedy; can trigger an allergic reaction
Kava	May reduce anxiety, but can cause liver damage
Gingko biloba	No improvement in memory or thinking in the healthy elderly, but a small benefit for patients with dementia
Garlic	Lowers cholesterol when taken in higher doses than you would get with food; much less effective than cholesterol-lowering medications
Black Cohosh	Currently under study as a treatment for hot flashes; long-term effects unknown

© David Young-Wolff/PhotoEdit, Inc.

prolong anesthesia medications. All herbal supplements should be discontinued for periods of several days or longer prior to surgery.

The most dangerous herbal products, sold as ephedra, ma huang, sinica, and sida cordifolia, contain ephedrine, which stimulates the heart to beat faster and increases blood pressure. The FDA prohibited the sale of dietary supplements containing ephedra, which was linked with dozens of deaths and more than 1,000 adverse reactions.[21] It has issued warnings on other potentially dangerous herbs, including chaparral, comfrey, yohimbe, lobelia, germander, willow bark, jin bu huan, and products containing magnolia or stephania.[22]

Manipulative and Body-Based Methods

CAM therapies based on manipulation and/or movement of the body are divided into three subcategories:

- **Chiropractic medicine**
- **Massage therapy and body work** (including osteopathic manipulation, Swedish massage, Alexander technique, reflexology, Pilates, acupressure, and rolfing)
- **Unconventional physical therapies** (including colonics, hydrotherapy, and light and color therapies)

Chiropractic is a treatment method based on the theory that many human diseases are caused by misalignment of the bones (subluxation). Chiropractors are licensed in all 50 states, but chiropractic is considered a mainstream therapy by some and a form of CAM by others. Significant research in the last ten years has demonstrated its efficacy for acute lower-back pain. NIH is funding research on other potential benefits, including headaches, asthma, middle ear inflammation, menstrual cramps, and arthritis.

Chiropractors, who emphasize wellness and healing without drugs or surgery, may use X rays and magnetic resonance imaging (MRI) as well as orthopedic, neurological, and manual examinations in making diagnoses. However, chiropractic treatment consists solely of the manipulation of misaligned bones that may be putting pressure on nerve tissue and affecting other parts of the body. Many HMOs offer chiropractic services, which are the most widely used alternative treatment among managed care patients.

Energy Therapies

Various approaches focus on energy fields believed to exist in and around the body. Some use external energy sources, such as electromagnetic fields. Magnets are marketed to relieve pain but there is little scientific evidence of their efficacy. Others, such as therapeutic touch, use a therapist's healing energy to repair imbalances in an individual's biofield.

© Design Pics Inc./Alamy

Many people seek chiropractic services after suffering a painful injury.

THE HEALTH-CARE SYSTEM

In the past, getting health care was fairly simple. When people were sick, they went to their family physician and paid in cash. If they didn't have enough money, the physician would still provide care. Today health care involves many more people, places, and processes.

As a college student, you can turn to the student health service if you get sick. There, a nurse, nurse practitioner, physician's assistant, or medical doctor may evaluate your symptoms and provide basic care. However, you may rely on a primary care physician in your hometown to perform regular checkups or manage a chronic condition like asthma. If you're injured in an accident, you probably will be treated at the nearest emergency room. If you become seriously ill and require highly specialized care, you may have to go to a university-affiliated medical center to receive state-of-the-art treatment.

Most students can continue their health-care coverage under their parents' policy until the age of 23. However, if a parent belongs to an HMO with a local network of providers, the student may not be covered for anything outside the plan's service area except emergency care. A more open plan, like a preferred provider organization, may allow students to see doctors near school, but the costs may be high.

Most colleges offer some type of health insurance plan, with the student health center acting as the primary care provider. Many schools require enrollment if the student is not covered under any other plan. Check the plan carefully. Physicals, gynecological visits, and other preventive care may not be covered. College plans also may not cover pre-existing conditions, such as asthma.

HEALTH-CARE PRACTITIONERS

Fewer than 10 percent of health-care practitioners are physicians; other types of health professionals are assuming more important roles in delivering primary, or basic, health services. As a consumer, you should be aware of the range and special skills of the most common types of health-care providers.

Physicians

A medical doctor (MD) trained in American medical schools usually takes at least three years of premedical college courses (with an emphasis on biology, chemistry, and physics) and then completes four (but sometimes three or five) years of medical school. The first two years of medical school are devoted to the study of human anatomy, embryology, pharmacology, and similar basic subjects. During the last two years, students work directly with physicians in hospitals. Medical students who pass a series of national board examinations then enter a one-year internship in a hospital, followed by another two to five years of residency (depending on their specialty), which leads to certification in a particular field, or specialty.

About 500,000 of the nation's 700,000 physicians are specialists or subspecialists, who focus on a specific part of the body, organ system, type of disease, or type of treatment. Traditionally, they have had greater status and earned much larger incomes than primary care physicians—family practitioners, pediatricians, and internists—who provide preventive care, regular checkups, and routine treatments of uncomplicated medical conditions. However, changes in health policy (such as increases in Medicare payments to primary care physicians) and in the delivery of services have given a more prominent role to primary care physicians. They now often function as "gatekeepers" who decide whether a patient needs to see a medical specialist.

Nurses

A registered nurse (RN) graduates from a school of nursing approved by a state board and passes a state board examination. RNs may have a bachelor's or an associate degree and may specialize in certain areas, such as intensive care or nurse-midwifery. Nurse practitioners, RNs with advanced training and experience, may run community clinics or provide screening and preventive care at group medical practices. Some have independent practices.

Licensed practical nurses (LPNs), also called licensed vocational nurses, are licensed by the state. After graduating from state-approved schools of practical nursing, they must take a board exam. They work under the supervision of RNs or physicians. Nursing aides and orderlies assist registered and practical nurses in providing services directly related to the comfort and well-being of hospitalized patients.

Specialized and Allied-Health Practitioners

More than 60 types of health practitioners work with physicians and nurses in providing medical services. Some, such as *occupational therapists,* have at least a bachelor's degree. Allied-health professionals may specialize in a variety of fields. *Clinical psychologists* have graduate degrees and provide a wide range of mental health services but don't prescribe medications—as do *psychiatrists. Optometrists,* trained in special schools of optometry, diagnose visual abnormalities and prescribe lenses or visual aids; however, they don't prescribe drugs, diagnose or treat eye diseases, or perform surgery—functions performed by *ophthalmologists. Podiatrists* are specially trained, licensed health-care professionals who specialize in problems of the feet.

Dentists

Most dental students earn a bachelor's degree and then complete two more years of training in the basic sciences and two years of clinical work before graduating with a degree of D.D.S. or D.M.D. (Doctor of Dental Surgery or

Doctor of Medical Dentistry). To qualify for a license, graduates must pass both a written and a clinical examination. Dentists may work in general practice or choose a specialty, such as *orthodontics* (straightening teeth).

Chiropractors

Chiropractors hold the degree of Doctor of Chiropractic (D.C.), which signifies that they have had two years of college-level training, plus four years in a health-care school specializing in chiropractic, described earlier in this chapter.

HEALTH-CARE FACILITIES

As a prospective patient, you can choose from various options: a physician's office, a clinic, an emergency room, or a hospital. Most **primary care**—also referred to as ambulatory or outpatient care—is provided by a physician in an office, emergency room, or clinic. *Secondary care* usually is provided by specialists or subspecialists in either an outpatient or inpatient (hospital) setting. *Tertiary care,* available at university-affiliated hospitals and regional referral centers, includes special procedures such as kidney dialysis, open-heart surgery, and organ transplants.

College Health Centers

The American College Health Association estimates that 1,500 institutions of higher learning provide direct health services. Student health centers, initially developed by departments of physical education and hygiene, range in size from small dispensaries staffed by nurses to large-scale, multispecialty clinics that provide both inpatient and outpatient care and are fully accredited by the Joint Commission on Accreditation of Healthcare Organizations. Some serve only students; others provide services for faculty, staff, and family members.

On some campuses, health educators work with the student health centers to provide counseling on such topics as nutrition; tobacco, drug, and alcohol abuse; exercise and fitness; sexuality; and contraception. Some college health centers provide psychological counseling, as well as dental, pharmacy, and optometric services. Some campuses also provide sports-medicine services for student athletes. Services are paid for by various combinations of prepaid health fees, general university funds, fee-for-service charges, and health-insurance reimbursements.

Outpatient Treatment Centers

Increasingly, procedures that once required hospitalization, such as simple surgery, are being performed at outpatient centers, which may be freestanding or affiliated with a medical center. Patients have any necessary tests performed beforehand, undergo surgery or receive treatment, and return home after a few hours to recuperate. Outpatient centers can handle many common surgical procedures, including cataract removal, tonsillectomy, breast biopsy, dilation and curettage (D and C), vasectomy, and face-lifts.

Without the high overhead costs of a hospital, outpatient surgery costs run only about 30 to 50 percent of standard hospital fees. Today, 70 percent of hospitals do outpatient, or "in-and-out," surgery. To cut health-care costs, insurance companies are encouraging, or in some cases requiring, their policyholders to choose outpatient surgery. However, operations requiring prolonged general anesthesia or extensive postoperative care still must be performed on an inpatient basis.

Freestanding emergency or urgent-care centers (those not part of a hospital) claim that they deliver high-quality medical treatment with maximum convenience in minimal time. Rather than going to crowded hospital emergency rooms when they slice a finger in the kitchen, patients can go to a freestanding emergency center and receive prompt attention.

Hospitals and Medical Centers

Different types of hospitals offer different types of care. The most common type of hospital is the *private,* or community, *hospital,* which may be run on a profit or a nonprofit basis, generally contains 50 to 400 beds and provides more personalized care than public hospitals do. The quality of care individual patients receive depends mostly on the physicians themselves. Public *hospitals* include city, county, public health service, military, and Veterans Administration hospitals. The quality of patient care depends on the overall quality of the institution.

Of the more than 6,500 hospitals nationwide, about 300 are major *academic medical centers* or teaching hospitals. Affiliated with medical schools, they generally provide the most up-to-date and experienced care, because staff physicians must stay current in order to teach their students. These centers, with the best equipment, researchers, and resources, offer high-technology care—at a price. The cost

Is there a student health center on your campus? Have you used its services?

© AP Photo

of treatment at all teaching hospitals averages approximately 20 percent higher than at nonteaching hospitals. At major teaching hospitals with large graduate training programs for physicians and other health providers, the costs are as much as 45 percent higher than those at nonteaching hospitals.

The Joint Commission on the Accreditation of Health-care Organizations (JCAH) reviews all hospitals every three years. Eighty percent of hospitals qualify for JCAH accreditation. If you have to enter a hospital and your health insurance or plan allows a choice, try to find out as much as you can about the alternatives available to you:

■ Talk to your physician about a hospital and why he or she recommends it.

■ As a cost-cutting strategy, many hospitals have cut back on the use of registered nurses. Check with the local nursing association about the ratio of patients to nurses, and the ratio of RNs to LPNs.

■ Find out room rates and charges for ancillary services, including tests, lab work, X rays, and medications. Check with your health plan to see whether you need preapproval for any of these costs and ask what you will be expected to pay.

■ Ask how many times in the past year the hospital has performed the procedure recommended for you, and what the success and complication rates have been. Ask about the hospital's nosocomial (hospital-caused) infection rate and accident rate. You also have the right to information on the number and types of malpractice claims filed against a hospital.

■ If possible, go on a tour of the hospital. Does the setting seem comfortable? Is the staff courteous? Does the hospital seem clean and efficiently run?

Emergency Services Hospital emergency rooms should be used only in a true emergency. Most are overwhelmed, understaffed, and underfinanced—particularly in big cities. Patients usually see a different physician each time; he or she deals with the main complaints but doesn't have time for a full examination. Extensive tests and procedures are difficult to arrange in an emergency room, and patients who don't have truly urgent problems may have to wait for a long time. Emergency-room fees are higher than those for standard office visits and are not always covered by medical insurance.

Inpatient Care Inpatient hospital care remains the most expensive form of health care. Health-insurance companies and health-care plans (described on pages 511–512) often demand a second opinion or make their own evaluation before approving coverage of an elective, or nonemergency, hospital admission. As another means of controlling costs, health insurers (including Medicare) may limit hospital stays or pay for hospital care on the basis of **diagnostic-related groups,** or **DRGs.** Under this system, hospitals are paid according to a patient's diagnosis—for example, a set number of dollars for every appendectomy. If the hospital

can treat and discharge patients more quickly than the national average for that DRG, it makes money. On the other hand, if a patient develops unexpected complications or is slow to recover, the hospital loses money.

Because hospital stays are shorter than in the past, patients often leave "quicker and sicker"—after a shorter stay and not as far along in their recovery. Nevertheless, the benefits of shorter hospital stays, including reduced risk of infection and more rapid resumption of normal life activities, may outweigh the slightly increased risks associated with early discharge.

Home Health Care

With hospitals discharging patients sooner, **home health care**—the provision of equipment and services to patients in the home to restore or maintain comfort, function, and health—has become a major industry. Advances in technology have made it possible for treatments once administered only in hospitals—such as kidney dialysis, chemotherapy, and traction—to be performed at home at 10 to 40 percent of the cost. The physician's house call, once considered an anachronism, has also come back in fashion. According to various surveys, the majority of primary care physicians see patients in their homes.

Hospital discharge planners usually arrange home health care for patients who've been hospitalized. Families can also contact health aides, nurses, and other needed professionals on their own. According to the Health Insurance Association of America, most private insurance policies offer some coverage for these home health-care costs.

PAYING FOR HEALTH CARE

Health insurance did not become common as a standard benefit until World War II, when the government imposed wage controls and businesses offered free health-insurance policies to lure prospective employees. For the next 50 years, patients went to the physicians of their choice, with insurance companies usually paying part or all of their fees.

As technological breakthroughs, such as new imaging techniques and bone-marrow transplants, transformed modern medicine, subspecialists multiplied, and medical costs spiraled upward. Finally, in the 1990s, health care policymakers and the employers that had footed the bills agreed that health costs, which had grown to almost 14 percent of the gross domestic product, had to be controlled. This led to the emergence of **managed care,** a new way of delivering and paying for health-care services. Managed-care organizations provide health care or health-care insurance at lower costs to employers. The tradeoff for such savings is that a third party makes the final decision on when or if a medical visit or treatment is necessary. This differs from traditional *fee-for-service* medicine, in which patients decide when to seek care and choose which physician to see.

Both fee-for-service and managed-care systems have drawbacks. Fee-for-service medicine errs on the side of doing too much and providing unneeded tests and therapies. Managed-care organizations are more likely to do too little so they can keep costs low.

Traditional Health Insurance

In the past, most working Americans relied on conventional **indemnity** insurance policies to pay major medical expenses. Policyholders paid a percentage (generally 20 percent) of hospitalization costs and a deductible (a minimum paid out each year before the insurance company pays anything). While indemnity insurance gave patients freedom to choose physicians and hospitals, it often failed to cover routine physical exams and screening tests. Individuals with "preexisting" conditions often could not qualify for coverage or were not reimbursed for treatments related to these conditions. In the last decade, as health-care costs skyrocketed, insurers increasingly refused to pay claims, canceled groups with high medical bills, or denied coverage to people in high-risk occupations.

Managed Care

Managed care has become the predominant from of health care in the United States. Managed-care organizations, which take various forms, deliver care through a network of physicians, hospitals, and other health-care professionals who agree to provide their services at fixed or discounted rates. Nine in ten physicians in the United States have contracted with managed care companies.

Consumers in a managed-care group must follow certain procedures in advance of seeking care (for example, getting prior approval for a test or treatment) and must abide by a limit on reimbursement for certain services. Some procedures may be deemed unnecessary and not be covered at all. Patients who choose to see a physician who is not a participating member of the medical-insurance coverage group may have to pay the entire fee themselves.

Managed-care plans have been criticized for pressuring providers to "undertreat" patients—for example, sending them home from the hospital too soon or denying them costly tests or treatments. Members have complained of long waits, the need to switch primary physicians if their doctor leaves the plan, difficulty getting approval for needed services, and a sense that providers pay more attention to the bottom line than to the health needs of their patients.

As dissatisfaction with managed care has grown, consumers have demanded more choice of physicians, direct access to specialists, and the ability to go "out of network." In response to patients' complaints, many states have approved "patient protection acts" or "comprehensive consumer bills of rights."

According to the National Committee for Quality Assurance, managed-care plans have shown improvement in the delivery of care, but health-care costs continue to rise. As a result, employers are cutting back coverage and asking employees to shoulder more of the burden of their health care in the belief that consumers will seek more efficient care when they are required to pay more out of pocket.

Health Maintenance Organizations (HMOs)

Health maintenance organizations, or **HMOs,** are managed-care plans that emphasize routine care and prevention by providing complete medical services in exchange for a predetermined monthly payment. In a *group-model* HMO, physicians provide care in offices at a clinic run by the HMO. In an *individual practice association (IPA),* or network HMO, independent physicians provide services in their own offices. HMOs generally pay a fixed amount per patient to a physician or hospital, regardless of the type and number of services actually provided. This is called *capitation.*

Members of HMOs pay a regular, preset fee that usually includes diagnostic tests, routine physical exams, and vaccinations as well as treatment of illnesses. HMOs usually do not require a deductible, and copayments for medications or services are small. The primary drawback of standard HMOs is that the consumer is limited to a particular health-care facility and staff.

(FAQ) How Do I Choose an HMO?

When deciding on an HMO or PPO, use these questions as a guide:

- How many doctors can I choose from?
- Is the network made up of private or group practice physicians?
- Which doctors are accepting new patients?
- Can I change my primary care physician?
- What is the procedure for referrals to specialists?
- How easy is it to get an appointment?
- How far in advance must routine visits be scheduled?
- What arrangements are there for handling emergency care?
- What health-care services are offered?
- Are there limits on medical tests, surgery, or other services?
- What if I want or need a special service that is not covered?
- Which hospitals do you admit patients to?
- What happens if I'm out of town and need medical attention?
- What is the yearly total for monthly premiums?
- Are there any copayments? For which services and how much?

Preferred Provider Organizations (PPOs)

In a **preferred provider organization (PPO),** a third party—a union, an insurance company, or a self-insured business—contracts with a group of physicians and hospitals to treat members at a discount. PPO members may choose any physician within the network, and usually pay a 10 percent copayment for care within the system and a higher percentage (20 to 30 percent) for care elsewhere. PPOs generally require prior approval for expensive tests or major procedures.

A *point-of-service (POS)* plan is a PPO that permits patients to use physicians outside the network. Consumers pay the difference between the preferred provider's discounted fee and the outside physician's fee. A *gatekeeper* plan requires members to choose a primary physician, as in an HMO, who must approve all referrals to specialists.

Government-Financed Insurance Plans

The government, through programs like Medicare and Medicaid, funds 45 percent of total U.S. health spending.[23] Under Medicare, the federal government pays 80 percent of most medical bills, after a deductible fee, for people over age 65. Medicare also offers options for coverage of prescription medications.

Medicaid, a federal and state insurance plan that protects people with very low or no incomes, is the chief source of coverage for the unemployed. However, many unemployed Americans don't qualify because their family incomes are above the poverty line. Publicly insured patients are more likely than those with private insurance to receive inadequate care and to experience adverse health outcomes.

THE UNINSURED

The United States is the only industrialized nation that does not have national health insurance.[24] More Americans lack health insurance coverage than a decade ago—a total of more than 43 million. Many more experience temporary lapses in coverage or are underinsured, meaning that they don't have adequate coverage and are less likely to receive preventive care or routine checkups.[25]

The primary reason people are uninsured is that they can't afford health insurance, even if they have jobs. Eight in ten come from working families.[26] Most are not offered health benefits by an employer and have few, if any, affordable insurance options.

 Racial and ethnic minorities are much more likely to be uninsured than white Americans. More than a third of the Hispanic population and over a quarter of Native Americans are uninsured, compared to 12 percent of whites. The uninsured rates among African Americans and Asian Americans are also much higher than among whites. Nearly one-third of the uninsured are Latino, despite the fact that Latinos make up just 13 percent of the population. This disparity results from several factors, including citizenship issues and language barriers.[27]

Young adults, 18 to 24 years of age, are more likely than any other age group to be uninsured. Of Americans between the ages of 18 and 24 years, almost a third are without medical insurance. Many commercial policies no longer cover young people under their parents' policies, particularly if the young people are not enrolled full-time in college or other advanced training. Nationally, some 90 percent of private colleges in the United States with more than 1,000 students

require them to have health insurance. A quarter of public universities with more than 10,000 students have insurance requirements.[28]

According to the Institute of Medicine (IOM), the U.S. economy loses as much as $130 billion every year when people without health insurance get sick and die early, compared to the estimated $34 to $69 billion it would cost to provide universal health insurance.[29]

Public opinion surveys over time show that the majority of Americans believe decreasing the number of uninsured is an important policy priority. Part of the reason for this level of support may lie in a growing awareness that being in the workforce is no guarantee that job-based health coverage will always be available.[30]

A committee of the IOM, after years of exhaustive study, has urged federal leaders to provide health insurance for everyone living in the United States. The consequences of being uninsured, the IOM concluded, include "worse health and earlier death," including 18,000 deaths every year. It proposed that coverage be universal (for all residents, not just citizens), continuous, affordable, sustainable, and provided in such a way as to promote access to high-quality care.[31]

> *About 17 percent of Americans, including many families, have no health insurance. The Institute of Medicine has urged the government to provide coverage to all Americans. Critics charge that the costs would be too great. Do you think society has a responsibility for making sure all of its members get health-care services regardless of their ability to pay? Or should health insurance be a personal responsibility?* **You decide.**

Learn It / Live It
Becoming a Savvy Health-Care Consumer

You can do more to safeguard and enhance your well-being than any health-care provider. Here are some recommendations to keep in mind:

- **Trust your instincts.** You know your body better than anyone else. If something is bothering you, it deserves medical attention. Don't let your health-care provider—or your health plan administrator—dismiss it without a thorough evaluation.

- **Do your homework.** Go to the library or online and find authoritative articles that describe what you're experiencing. The more you know about possible causes of your symptoms, the more likely you are to be taken seriously.

- **Find a good primary care physician who listens carefully and responds to your concerns.** Look for a family doctor or general internist who takes a careful history, performs a thorough exam, and listens and responds to your concerns.

■ **See your doctor regularly.** If you're in your twenties or thirties, you may not need an annual exam, but it's important to get checkups at least every two or three years so you and your doctor can get to know each other and develop a trusting, mutually respectful relationship.

■ **Get a second opinion.** If you are uncertain of whether to undergo treatment or which therapy is best, see another physician and listen carefully for any doubts or hesitation about what you're considering.

■ **Seek support.** Patient support and advocacy groups can offer emotional support, information on many common problems, and referral to knowledgeable physicians.

■ **If your doctor cannot or will not respond to your concerns, get another one.** Regardless of your health coverage, you have the right to replace a physician who is not meeting your health-care needs.

■ **Speak up.** If you don't understand, ask. If you feel that you're not being taken seriously or being treated with respect, say so. Sometimes the only difference between being a patient or becoming a victim is making sure your needs and rights are not forgotten or overlooked.

■ **Bring your own advocate.** If you become intimidated or anxious talking to physicians, ask a friend to accompany you, to ask questions on your behalf, and to take notes.

Making This Chapter Work for You

Review Questions

1. Which of the following statements about health information on the Internet is true?
   a. Chat rooms are the most reliable source of accurate medical information.
   b. Physicians who have websites must adhere to a strict set of standards set by the American Medical Association.
   c. Government-sponsored sites such as that of the Centers for Disease Control and Prevention are excellent sources of accurate health-care information.
   d. The Internet is a safe and cost-effective source of prescription drugs.

2. In a preclinical trial,
   a. researchers examine the cost-effectiveness of a specific treatment.
   b. animals are used to test new medical treatments.

   c. humans are used to test new medical treatments.
   d. the health status of a large group of people who exhibit certain health habits is reviewed.

3. Periodontal disease
   a. results from poor eating habits.
   b. can lead to cardiovascular problems.
   c. in its early stage can be prevented by brushing alone.
   d. is caused by a variety of bacteria and viruses.

4. During a medical exam, your doctor will
   a. check your cardiovascular system by listening to your heart and feeling your neck arteries.
   b. check your lungs by probing for tender spots and malformations.
   c. look into your eyes to see if you have vision problems that require glasses or contact lenses.
   d. evaluate your joints by tapping on the knees and elbows.

5. Informed consent means that
   a. the patient has informed the doctor of his or her symptoms and has consented to treatment.
   b. the physician has informed the patient about the treatment to be given and has consented to administer the treatment.
   c. the patient has informed the doctor of his or her symptoms, and the doctor has consented to administer treatment.
   d. the physician has informed the patient about the treatment to be given, and the patient has consented to the treatment.

6. Patients have all the rights below *except* which of the following?
   a. access to their medical records
   b. medical care that meets accepted standards of quality
   c. to donate a body part for compensation
   d. to leave the hospital against their physician's advice

7. People use complementary and alternative therapies
   a. to spend less money on health care.
   b. to take an active role in their own treatment.
   c. to show their disdain for the medical establishment.
   d. to take more prescription drugs.

8. Which statement is *false*?
   a. Acupuncture has been shown to control nausea in patients after surgery.
   b. Reflexologists massage points on the foot or hand to relieve stress or pain in corresponding parts of the body.
   c. People can learn to control involuntary functions through biofeedback.
   d. Naturopathy is based on the premise that like cures like.

9. Which of the following statements about the health-care system is true?
   a. Primary care is usually provided by specialists in a hospital.

Self Survey ⠿ Are You a Savvy Health-Care Consumer?

1. You want a second opinion, but your doctor dismisses your request for other physicians' names as unnecessary. Do you:
   a. Assume that he or she is right and you would merely be wasting time.
   b. Suspect that your physician has something to hide and immediately switch doctors.
   c. Contact your health plan and request a second opinion.

2. As soon as you enter your doctor's office, you get tongue-tied. When you try to find the words to describe what's wrong, your physician keeps interrupting. When giving advice, your doctor uses such technical language that you can't understand what it means. Do you:
   a. Prepare better for your next appointment.
   b. Pretend that you understand what your doctor is talking about.
   c. Decide you'd be better off with someone who specializes in complementary/alternative therapies and seems less intimidating.

3. You feel like you're running on empty, tired all the time, worn to the bone. A friend suggests some herbal supplements that promise to boost energy and restore vitality. Do you:
   a. Immediately start taking them.
   b. Say that you think herbs are for cooking.
   c. Find out as much as you can about the herbal compounds and ask your doctor if they're safe and effective.

4. Your hometown physician's office won't give you a copy of your medical records to take with you to college. Do you:
   a. Hope you won't need them and head off without your records.
   b. Threaten to sue.
   c. Politely ask the office administrator to tell you the particular law or statute that bars you from your records.

5. Your doctor has been treating you for an infection for three weeks, and you don't seem to be getting any better. Do you:
   a. Talk to your doctor, by phone or in person, and say, "This doesn't seem to be working. Is there anything else we can try?"
   b. Stop taking the antibiotic.
   c. Try an herbal remedy that your roommate recommends.

6. Your doctor suggests a cutting-edge treatment for your condition, but your health plan or HMO refuses to pay for it. Do you:
   a. Try to get a loan to cover the costs.
   b. Settle for whatever treatment options are covered.
   c. Challenge your health plan.

7. You call for an appointment with your doctor and are told nothing is available for four months. Do you:
   a. Take whatever time you can get whenever you can get it.
   b. Explain your condition to the nurse or receptionist, detailing any symptoms and pain you're experiencing.
   c. Give up and decide you don't need to see a doctor at all.

8. Even though you've been doing sit-ups faithfully, your waist still looks flabby. When you see an ad for waist-whittling liposuction, do you:
   a. Call for an appointment.
   b. Talk to a health-care professional about a total fitness program that may help you lose excess pounds.
   c. Carefully research the risks and costs of the procedure.

9. You have a condition that you do not want anyone to know about, including your health insurer and any potential employer. Do you:
   a. Use a false name.
   b. Give your physician a written request for confidentiality about this condition.
   c. Seek help outside the health-care system.

---

b. Nurses can perform some surgical procedures once they are board certified.
c. Most hospitals in the United States are teaching hospitals and affiliated with medical schools.
d. The length of hospital stays may be determined by a patient's diagnosis rather than the person's pace of recovery.

10. Managed care features all of the following *except*
   a. health maintenance organizations.
   b. a fee-for-service system of insurance.
   c. preferred provider organizations.
   d. limitations on reimbursement for certain health services.

Answers to these questions can be found on page 587.

Critical Thinking

1. Think about an experience you've had with a traditional medical practitioner. How did you feel during the physical examination? Did you trust the practi-

10. Your doctor suggests a biopsy of a funny-looking mole that's sprouted on your nose. Rather than using a laboratory that specializes in skin analysis, your HMO requires that all samples be sent to a general lab, where results may not be as precise. Do you:
    a. Ask your doctor to request that a specialty pathologist at the general lab perform the analysis.
    b. Hope that in your case, the general lab will do a good-enough job.
    c. Threaten to change HMOs.

Answers:

1: c; 2: a; 3: c; 4: c; 5: a; 6: c; 7: b; 8: b and c; 9: b; 10: a

YOUR ACTION PLAN FOR PROTECTING YOURSELF FROM MEDICAL MISTAKES AND MISDEEDS

Just as physicians practice "defensive" medicine to protect themselves from legal liability, today's patients should take preventive steps to defend themselves from potentially harmful health services.

The Whats, Whys, and Hows of Medical Testing

- Before undergoing any test, find out why you need it. Get a specific answer, not a "just in case" or "for your peace of mind." If you've had the test before could the earlier results be used? Would a follow-up exam be just as helpful?

- Get some practical information as well: Should you do specific things before the test (such as not eat for a specified period)? How long will the test take? What will the test feel like? Will you need help getting home afterward?

- Check out the risks. Any invasive test—one that penetrates the body with a needle, tube, or viewing instrument—involves some risk of infection, bleeding, or tissue damage. Tests involving radiation also present risks, and some people develop allergic reactions to the materials used in testing.

- Get information on the laboratory that will be evaluating the test. Ask how often **false positives** or **false negatives** occur. (False positives are abnormal results indicating that you have a particular condition when you really don't; false negatives indicate that you don't have a particular condition when you really do.) Find out about civil or criminal **negligence** suits filed against the laboratory on charges such as failing to diagnose cervical cancer because of incorrect reading of Pap smears.

- You'll also want to know what happens when the test indicates a problem: Will the test be repeated? Will a different test be performed? Will treatment begin immediately? Could any medications you're taking (including nonprescription drugs, like aspirin) affect the testing procedures or results?

- If you have a test don't assume that no news is good news. Check back to get the results.

CASE IN POINT: AVOIDING MEDICAL ERRORS

Student: Mason, 24

Goal: Reducing risks before undergoing knee surgery

Action Plan:

- Get second opinion
- Find out if procedure is covered by university's insurance policy
- Do online research on possible complications
- Get suggestions from a primary care provider on ways to get into shape before surgery
- Check out surgeon's credentials and ask to talk to other patients who've had same operation

Health ⊗ Now™   If you want to write your own goals for getting good medical care on using CAM, go to the **Wellness Journal at HealthNow, http://healthnow.brookscole.com/ith**

tioner? Were you comfortable with the level of communication? Evaluate your experience and give your opinion of the value of the checkup.

2. Have you used any complementary or alternative approaches to health care? If so, were you satisfied with the results? How did your experience with the CAM therapist compare with your most recent experience with a traditional medical practitioner? Do you feel confident that you know the difference between alternative care and quackery?

3. If you're young and healthy, you'll have little problem getting health insurance. However, if you develop a chronic illness, sustain serious injuries in an accident, or simply get older, you may find insurance harder to get and more expensive to keep. What is your insurance coverage? Do you believe insurance companies have the right to turn down applicants with preexisting conditions, such as high blood pressure? Do they have the right to require screening for potentially serious health problems, such as HIV infection, or to can-

cel the policies of individuals who have run up high medical bills in the past?

4. Jocelyn has been experiencing a great deal of fatigue and frequent headaches for the past couple of months. She doesn't have health insurance and doesn't want to spend money on a doctor visit. So she did some research on the Internet about ways to relieve her symptoms and was considering taking a couple of herbal supplements that were touted as potential treatments. If she asked you for your advice, what would you tell her? Do you think that self-care is appropriate in this situation?

Media Menu

Health ⊗ Now™

Throughout the chapter, this icon introduces a list of resources on the Health-Now website at **http://healthnow.brookscole.com/ith** that will:

- Help you evaluate your knowledge of the material.
- Allow you to take an exam-prep quiz.
- Provide a Personalized Learning Plan targeting resources that address areas you should study.
- Coach you through identifying target goals for behavior change and creating and monitoring your personal change plan throughout the semester.

INTERNET CONNECTIONS

National Health Information Center

www.health.gov/nhic/

This excellent site, sponsored by the National Health Information Center (NHIC) of the U.S. Office of Disease Prevention and Health Promotion, is a health information referral service providing health professionals and consumers with a database of various health organizations. The site provides a searchable database, publications, and a list of toll-free numbers for health information.

National Center for Complementary and Alternative Medicine

http://nccam.nih.gov

This National Institutes of Health site features a variety of fact sheets on alternative therapies and dietary supplements, research, current news, and databases for the public as well as for practitioners.

MedicineNet

www.medicinenet.com

This comprehensive site is written for the consumer by board-certified physicians and contains medical news, a directory of procedures, a medical dictionary, a pharmacy, and first aid information. You can use the information at MedicineNet.com to prepare for a doctor visit,

learn about a diagnosis, or understand a prescribed treatment or procedure.

U.S. Food and Drug Administration

www.fda.gov

In addition to providing information on regulation and legislation relating to food and drugs, the FDA website offers information on strategies for evaluating health products and services.

InfoTrac College Edition Activities Log on, insert **complementary alternative medicine** into the Keyword search box, and limit your search to the past year. When you get the results, Mark articles to review, then Select one to read. Summarize three or four key points from the article.

You can find additional readings related to personal health with InfoTrac College Edition, an online library of more than 900 journals and publications. Follow the instructions for accessing InfoTrac College Edition that were packaged with your textbook; then search for articles using a keyword search.

For additional links, resources, and suggested readings on the InfoTrac College Edition, visit our Health and Wellness Resource Center at **http://health .wadsworth.com.**

Key Terms

The terms listed are used on the page indicated. Definitions of the terms are in the Glossary at the end of this book.

acupuncture 505	informed consent 500
Ayurveda 505	integrative medicine 503
biofeedback 506	malpractice 501
chiropractic 507	managed care 510
complementary and alternative medicine (CAM) 503	massage therapy 507
	medical history 497
diagnostic-related groups (DRG) 510	meta-analysis 493
	naturopathy 505
false negatives 515	negligence 515
false positives 515	outcomes 493
gingivitis 494	Pap smear 498
gum disease 494	periodontitis 494
health insurance organizations (HMO) 511	plaque 494
	preferred provider organization (PPO) 511
herbal medicine 506	
holistic 503	primary care 509
home health care 510	quackery 502
homeopathy 505	visualization 506
indemnity 511	vital signs 493

Health in Context

Ryan McVay

Personal health involves more than a single individual. We are social beings, and we live our lives as part of a network of family, friends, acquaintances, colleagues, neighbors. Our actions affect others; others' behaviors have a significant impact on our well-being.

Aging and dying are as much a part of the real world as life itself. The quest to find fulfillment in living and meaning in dying is one of the challenges of living.

For college students, staying safe is an essential part of staying healthy. Injury claims more lives of young Americans than illness. Threats such as violence and terrorism are too serious and widespread to ignore.

All of us share something else: our planet. The problems of creating a healthy environment are many and complex. They too demand our attention and commitment.

Corita didn't feel old until she enrolled in a college personal health course. Formal at first, the other students—young enough to be her children—started calling her "Mom." When the professor announced that the next week's topic would be aging, Corita beamed, "I'll be the expert!"

More of us can expect to do the same. In the United States, the number of persons over age 65 is expected to increase to an estimated 71 million in 2030, more than the number of school-age children.

Although **aging**—the characteristic pattern of normal life changes that occurs as humans, plants, and animals grow older—remains inevitable, you can do a great deal to influence the impact that the passage of time has on you. Whether you're in your teens, twenties, thirties, or older, now is the time to start taking the steps that will add healthy, active, productive years to your life.

This chapter provides a preview of the changes age brings, the steps you can take to age healthfully, and the ways you can make the most of all the years of your life.

Invariably, though, no one gets out of this life alive. Death is the natural completion of things, as much a part of the real world as life itself. In time we all lose people we cherish: grandparents, aunts and uncles, parents, friends, neighbors, coworkers, siblings. With each loss, part of us may seem to die, yet each loss also reaffirms how precious life is.

This chapter explores the meaning of death, describes the process of dying, provides information on end-of-life issues, and offers advice on comforting the dying and helping their survivors.

Masterfile (RM)/George Shelley

FAQ Frequently Asked Questions

▌ How long can I expect to live? *p. 520*

▌ What are advance directives? *p. 530*

▌ What do we know about near-death experiences? *p. 537*

▌ How can you help survivors of a loss? *p. 540*

After studying the material in this chapter, you should be able to:

▌ **List** the benefits that older Americans can gain from physical activity.

▌ **Name** three memory skills that diminish with age.

▌ **Discuss** hormone therapy for menopause symptoms.

▌ **Identify** some of the challenges of aging and **discuss** their risk factors and possible ways of preventing them.

▌ **Explain** the purposes of advanced directives, a living will, and a holographic will.

▌ **Define** death and **explain** the stages of emotional reaction experienced in facing death.

▌ **Name** some of grief's effects on health, and **explain** factors affecting the length and intensity of grief.

LIVING IN AN AGING SOCIETY

America is turning gray. People age 65 and older make up 13 percent of the U.S. population. By the year 2014, this group will grow to 15 percent. By the midpoint of the twenty-first century, 80 million Americans—one in five—will be seniors (65 or older).[1]

Throughout your life, you will confront a variety of issues related not just to your age, but also to that of the aging American population. These include:

▪ **Retirement costs.** Unless changes are made to decrease the demand on the Social Security system, Social Security taxes on workers may be increased.

▪ **Health costs.** Health-care costs for those over 65 years are three to five times greater than for younger men and women.[2]

▪ **Gray-power politics.** Senior citizens go to the polls in larger numbers than younger voters. With such voting power, programs for the elderly may make up a larger share of future federal budgets.

▪ **Anti-aging gimmicks.** As the population ages, health hucksters push an ever-growing number of unproven anti-aging treatments, such as melatonin or the hormone DHEA. Because some preparations have the potential to harm, consumers must be wary of all claims to turn back or slow down the biological clock.

FAQ HOW LONG CAN I EXPECT TO LIVE?

The answer depends on you. Statistically, you're likely to live longer than your parents or grandparents. Life expectancy has been increasing steadily over the last century, reaching an all-time high in the United States of 77.4 years. (The United States is not in the top five countries—see Table 18-1.) A child born in the United States in 2020 should expect to live 79.25 years; one born in 2050, 82.91 years.

Contrary to common belief, heredity doesn't determine how long you'll live or how well you'll age. Genes, as studies of identical twins have revealed, influence only about 30 percent of the rate and ways in which we age.[3]

When does a person become old? That answer may depend on your gender. In a survey of 441 undergraduates at a large southeastern university, men said that a person becomes "old" at age 58. Women viewed a person becoming "old" at age 62. But "old," like beauty, may be in the eye of the beholder. In other studies individuals between the ages of 65 and 74 identified 70 as the age at which a person becomes "old."[4]

One reason why men view individuals reaching old age faster may be the gender gap in life expectancy, discussed in the next section. White males born in 2005 are expected to die, on average, about six years sooner than white females (at age 74.5 years vs. 81.1 years). For African-American males and females, the average is close to seven years (69.9

TABLE 18-1 LIFE EXPECTANCIES AROUND THE WORLD (IN YEARS)

Top 5		Bottom 5	
Japan	81.6	Zambia	32.4
Sweden	80.1	Botswana	39.7
Hong Kong	79.9	Afghanistan	43.1
Iceland	79.8	Ethiopia	45.5
Canada	79.3	Laos	54.5

© David Young Wolf/PhotoEdit

Why do you think this student would probably say "old" is about 60, while the older person would likely say 70?

years vs. 76.8 years). Because women live longer, they may see themselves as becoming old "later."

THE LONGEVITY GENDER GAP

Women's lifespans average 5 to 10 percent longer than men's. No one knows exactly why. But the gender gap in longevity narrows over time. At birth a baby boy has a life expectancy about five years shorter than a girl's. By age 65, a man can expect to live an additional 15.1 years, just 3.8 years less than a woman. By age 85, the difference in projected life expectancies is down to 1.2 years.

The longevity gender gap also has been shrinking since 1990. According to the National Center for Health Statistics, life expectancy for American women now stands at 79.8 years; for men, it is a record high of 74.4 years. Women in other developed nations—Australia, Canada, France, Greece, Italy, Japan, the Netherlands, Norway, Spain, Sweden, Switzerland—live up to two years longer than those in the United States and about seven years longer than men. In the former Soviet Union, life expectancy for females is 13 years longer than for males.

The gender difference in mortality rates emerges from the moment of conception. Baby girls are less likely to die in the womb or after delivery than baby boys. Once past age 30, women consistently outnumber and outlive men. By age 85, there are three women for every man.

Why do men die sooner? The female edge may begin at conception with the extra X chromosome, which provides a backup for defects on the X gene and a double dose of the genetic factors that regulate the immune system. In addition, the female hormone estrogen bolsters immunity and protects heart, bone, brain, and blood vessels.

In some cancers, estrogen may somehow protect against distant metastases. In contrast, testosterone may dampen the immune response in males—possibly to prevent attacks on sperm cells that might otherwise be mistaken as alien invaders. When the testes are removed from mice and guinea pigs, their immune systems become more active. In men, lessened immunity may lower resistance to cancer as well as infectious disease. Half of all men—compared with a third of women—develop cancer. Smoking, which for a long time was much more prevalent among men, accounts for some of this difference. However, this is changing; 23 percent of American women smoke, and lung cancer rates in women have doubled since the early 1970s.

Testosterone also has been implicated in men's risk of heart disease and stroke. Originally designed to equip men with an instantaneous burst of power—essential for survival in Stone Age times—this potent male hormone may surge so intensely that it wreaks havoc throughout the cardiovascular system.

Males also die more often as a result of intentional and nonintentional injury. Overall, men are three times more likely than women to die in accidents, mainly in cars and on the job. Men also are four times more likely to die violently. Nine in ten murderers and eight in ten murder victims are men.

Your Life Coach

Staying Healthy Longer

If you want to feel young when you're older, the time to start taking care of yourself is now—whether you're 25, 45, or 65. The healthier you become now, the longer you're likely to stay healthy in the future.

Genes, as studies of identical twins have revealed, influence only about 30 percent of the rate and ways in which we age. "The rest is up to us," says Michael Roizen, M.D., coauthor of *You: The Owner's Manual*, who notes that it's possible to turn back the biological clock. "With relatively simple changes, someone whose chronological age is 69 can have a physiological age of 45. And the most amazing thing is that it's never too late to live younger—until one foot is six feet under."[5]

KEEP YOUR ARTERIES YOUNG

"You are as young—or as old—as your arteries," says Roizen. Problems like high blood pressure, high cholesterol, and buildup of atherosclerotic plaque increase the likelihood of stroke, heart disease, kidney problems, even memory impairment. If your arteries are healthy, you're much more likely to have a healthy heart and a healthy brain. People with "young" arteries tend to retain a higher level of cognitive functioning.

Premature aging of the arteries is largely self-inflicted; common culprits are a high-fat diet, lack of exercise, obesity, and a high-stress lifestyle. At any age, the unexercised body—though free of the symptoms of illness—will rust out long before it could ever wear out. Inactivity can make anyone old before his or her time. Just as inactivity accelerates aging, activity slows it down. The effects of ongoing activity are so profound that gerontologists sometimes refer to exercise as "the closest thing to an antiaging pill." Exercise slows many changes associated with advancing age, such as loss of lean muscle tissue, increase in body fat, and decreased work capacity. The bottom line: What you *don't* do may matter more than what you do do.

AVOID ILLNESS

In studies of centenarians, most have had no serious chronic illnesses. Among the most important strategies: not smoking, avoiding weight gain in middle age, and recognizing and treating conditions like elevated cholesterol and high blood pressure.

Also important is keeping up with immunizations against diseases, such as influenza and pneumococcal pneumonia, that take a greater toll on the elderly. For women at risk of osteoporosis, new options, including "designer estrogens" like raloxifene, can preserve their bones' health. A healthy diet, chockful of fruits and vegetables, also can contribute to a healthy old age, in part because they contain antioxidants that may ward off many age-related problems.

MAINTAIN YOUR ZEST FOR LIVING

Age may indeed be a matter of attitude. The healthiest seniors are "engaged" in life, resilient, optimistic, productive, and socially involved. While they are not immune to life's slings and arrows, successful agers bounce back after a setback and have a "can-do" attitude about the challenges they face. They also tend to be lifelong learners who may take up entirely new hobbies late in life—pursuits that stimulate production of more connections between neurons and may slow aging within the brain. Social interactions, such as entertaining friends and getting involved with religious activities, lead to greater life satisfaction as people get older.

Just as with muscles, the best advice to keep your brain healthy as you age is "use it or lose it." Some

Age is mainly a matter of attitude.

© Photo Network/PictureQuest

memory losses among healthy older people are normal—but reversible with training in simple methods, such as word associations, that improve recall.

STAY STRONG

For years, experts assumed that older meant weaker. Landmark research with frail nursing home residents in their eighties and nineties showed this isn't so. After just eight to ten weeks of strength training, even the oldest seniors increased muscle and bone, speeded up their metabolic rate, improved sleep and mobility, boosted their spirits, and gained in self-confidence. Other studies have found that exercise programs can increase lung capacity, double leg strength, and decrease the risk of disability and premature death.

❚ SUCCESSFUL AGING

Although the proportion of people who live beyond 100 years is still very small, the worldwide number is rapidly growing. The United Nations estimates that in 2050, there will be 3.2 million centenarians, an increase of about eighteen

times. The number of Americans living long enough to blow out 100 birthday candles has increased 35 percent from a decade ago.

Americans are living better as well as longer. Disability decreased steadily through the 1980s and 1990s, and the rate of improvement is accelerating. Nursing home use has fallen. Senior citizens are healthier and more independent. All in all, the mortality rates of senior citizens are declining by about 1 percent a year, and their disability rates are falling by about 2 percent a year.[6] Among the factors contributing to a longer healthspan are improved medical care, diet, exercise, and public health advances.

 When surveyed, about half of Americans aged 65 to 69 say, "These are the best years of my life." Many people in their seventies and eighties agree. Sixty percent of older black and 57 percent of older Hispanic respondents say these are their best years. When asked about the keys to a meaningful and vital life, older adults rate having family and friends and taking care of their health as most important, followed by spiritual life.[7]

PHYSICAL ACTIVITY: IT'S NEVER TOO LATE

No one is ever too old to get in shape. The American College of Sports Medicine encourages seniors to engage in the full range of physical activities, including aerobic conditioning. As much as 50 percent of the physiological declines commonly attributed to aging are due to sedentary living and can be dramatically reversed. With regular conditioning, 60-year-olds can regain the fitness they had at age 40 to 45.

Adults over the age of 72 who exercise more and smoke less than their peers are most likely to enjoy long, healthy, and happy lives, according to a study that followed 1,000 seniors for nine years. Proactive health-promoting behaviors, such as exercising and not smoking, contributed to high quality throughout life regardless of when they began.

 Older women who start exercising after the age of 65 live longer. Newly active women had a 36 percent lower risk of heart disease and a 51 percent lower risk of cancer than those who didn't exercise.[8]

Exercise can reverse many of the changes that occur with age, including increases in body fat and decreases in muscle strength. It lowers the risk of heart disease and stroke in the elderly—and greatly improves general health. Male and female runners over age 50 have much lower rates of disability and much lower health-care expenses than less active seniors. Even less intense activities, such as gardening, dancing, and brisk walking, can delay chronic physical disability and cognitive decline.

According to the U.S. surgeon general, physical activity offers older Americans additional benefits, including the following:

❚ **Greater ability to live independently.**
❚ **Reduced risk of falling and fracturing bones.**

- **Lower risk of dying from coronary heart disease** and of developing high blood pressure, colon cancer, and diabetes.
- **Reduced blood pressure** in some people with hypertension.
- **Fewer symptoms of anxiety** and depression.
- **Improvements in mood** and feelings of well-being.

Despite these potential benefits, many seniors are not active. By age 75, about one in three men and one in two women engage in no physical activity. Yet even sedentary individuals in their eighties and nineties can participate in an exercise program—and gain significant benefits.

Federal health officials recommend a moderate amount of physical activity, either in longer sessions of moderately intense activities (such as walking) or in shorter sessions of more vigorous activities (such as race-walking or stair-climbing). Seniors can gain additional health benefits by increasing the duration, intensity, or frequency of their workouts, but should avoid overdoing their training because of the risk of injury. Older adults should always consult with a physician before beginning a new physical activity program.

NUTRITION AND OBESITY

The most common nutritional disorder in older persons is obesity. Among Americans between 65 to 74 years old, approximately 34 percent of women and 44 percent of men are overweight; an additional 27 percent of women and 24 percent of men are obese.[9] They face higher risk of diabetes, heart disease, stroke, and other health problems, including arthritis.[10]

As many as 40 percent of elderly people who live independently do not get adequate amounts of one or more essential nutrients. The reasons are many: limited income, difficulty getting to stores, chronic illness, medications that interfere with the metabolism of nutrients, problems chewing or digesting, poor appetite, inactivity, illness, depression. Nutritionists urge the elderly, like other Americans, to concentrate on eating healthful foods; many also recommend daily nutritional supplements, which may provide the added benefit of improving cognitive function in healthy people over 65.

THE AGING BRAIN

Scientists used to think that the aging brain, once worn out, could never be fixed. Now they know that the brain can and does repair itself. When neurons (brain cells) die, the surrounding cells develop "fingers" to fill the gaps and establish new connections, or synapses, between surviving neurons. Although self-repair occurs more quickly in young brains, the process continues in older brains. Even victims of Alzheimer's disease, the most devastating form of senility, have enough healthy cells in the diseased brain to regrow

synapses. Scientists hope to develop drugs that someday may help the brain repair itself.

Mental ability does not decline along with physical vigor. Researchers have been able to reverse the supposedly normal intellectual declines of 60- to 80-year-olds by tutoring them in problem solving. Reaction time, intellectual speed and efficiency, nonverbal intelligence, and maximum work rate for short periods may diminish by age 75. However, understanding, vocabulary, ability to remember key information, and verbal intelligence remain about the same.

Memory

Between the ages of 30 and 90, the brain loses about 10 percent of its volume. Forgetfulness isn't an automatic result, however. Crossword puzzles, practicing the piano, and playing chess exercise the brain and can counteract natural changes in memory. Exercise also helps cognitive function.

Some memory skills, particularly the ability to retrieve names and quickly process information, inevitably diminish over time. What normal changes should you expect? Here is a preview:

- **Recalling information takes longer.** As individuals reach their mid- to late sixties, the brain slows down, but usually just by a matter of milliseconds. As long as they're not rushed, older adults eventually adapt and perform just as well as younger ones.
- **Distractions become more disruptive.** College students can study and listen to the stereo at the same time. Thirty-something moms can soothe the baby, field questions about homework, and prepare dinner all at once. But older individuals find it much more difficult to divide their attention or to remember details after having switched their attention to something else. Inability to ignore background information while focusing on a task may underlie the memory problems associated with aging.[11]
- **"Accessing" names gets harder.** The ability to remember names, especially those you don't use frequently, diminishes by as much as 50 percent between ages 25 and 65. Preventive strategies can help, such as repeating a person's name when introduced, writing down the name as soon as possible, and making obvious associations (the Golden Gate for a man named Bridges).
- **Learning new information is harder.** The quality of memory doesn't change, just the speed at which we receive, absorb, and react to information. That's why strategies like taking notes or outlining material become critical for older students, especially when learning new skills. However, adding to existing knowledge remains as easy as ever.
- **Wisdom matters.** In any memory test involving knowledge of the world, vocabulary, or judgment, older people outperform their younger counterparts.

PET Scan of a 20-year-old brain

PET Scan of an 80-year-old brain

In these PET scans, the red and yellow show greater neuron activity in the young adult. The brain of the older person shows less activity and more dark areas, indicating that the fluid-filled ventricles have grown larger.

WOMEN AT MIDLIFE

In the next two decades some 40 million American women will end their reproductive years. "The primary misconception is that this is a terrible time when all women suffer horrible symptoms," says Sherry Sherman, M.D., project officer for the National Institute of Aging's Study of Women Across the Nation, which has followed 3,300 women through midlife since 1996. Many earlier studies included only women seeking medical help for severe symptoms. "When you look at healthy women in the community in terms of what actually affects their lives, their periods stop. That's it."[12]

Perimenopause

While the average age of **menopause**—defined as the complete cessation of menstrual periods for 12 consecutive months—is 51.5, a woman's reproductive system begins changing more than a decade earlier. "Women think that because they're having a period, they're too young to think in terms of menopause," says psychiatrist Marsha Speller, M.D., author of *The Menopause Answer Book.* "But the change of life starts in our thirties with irregular menstrual cycles and then heats up in our forties with hot flashes and night sweats."[13]

For many women, **perimenopause**—the four-to-ten-year span before a woman's last period—is more baffling and bothersome than the years after.[14] During this time the egg cells, or oocytes, in a woman's ovaries start to *senesce* or die off at a faster rate. Eventually, the number of egg cells drops to a tiny fraction of the estimated 2 million packed into her ovaries at birth. Trying to coax some of the remaining oocytes to ripen, the pituitary gland churns out extra follicle-stimulating hormone (FSH). This surge is the earliest harbinger of menopause, occurring six to ten years before a woman's final periods. Eventually, the other menstrual messenger, luteinizing hormone (LH), also increases, but at a slower rate.

These hormonal shifts can trigger an array of symptoms. The most common are night sweats (a *subdromal hot flash,* in medical terms), which can be just intense enough to disrupt sleep. Women with lifelong history of depression are more likely to experience early perimenopause.

A woman's habits and health history also have an impact. Smokers experience more symptoms at an earlier age than nonsmokers. Heavier women—contrary to what medical experts long believed—also have more severe symptoms.

Menopause

About 10 to 15 percent of women breeze through this transition with only trivial symptoms. Another 10 to 15 percent are virtually disabled. The majority fall somewhere in between these extremes. Women who undergo surgical or medical menopause (the result of removal of their ovaries or chemotherapy) often experience abrupt symptoms, including flushing, sweating, sleeplessness, early morning awakenings, involuntary urination, changes in libido, mood swings, perception of memory loss, and changes in cognitive function.

Race and ethnicity profoundly affect women's experience. African-American women report more hot flashes and night sweats but have more positive attitudes toward menopause. Japanese and Chinese women experience more muscle stiffness and fewer hot flashes but view menopause more negatively. Hispanic women reach menopause a year or two earlier than Caucasian women; Asian women, a year or two later.[15]

Dwindling levels of estrogen subtly affect many aspects of a woman's health, from her mouth (where dryness, unusual tastes, burning, and gum problems can develop) to her skin (which may become drier, itchier, and overly sensitive to touch). The drop in estrogen levels also may cause hot flashes (bursts of perspiration that last from a few seconds to 15 minutes), which often happen at night, disturbing sleep and causing fatigue. With less estrogen to block them, a woman's androgens, or male hormones, may have a greater impact, causing acne, hair loss, and according to some anecdotal reports, surges in sexual appetite. (Other women, however, report a drop in sexual desire.)

At the same time, a woman's clitoris, vulva, and vaginal lining begin to shrivel, sometimes resulting in pain or bleeding during intercourse. Since the thinner genital tissues are less effective in keeping out bacteria and other pathogens, urinary tract infections may become more common. Some women develop breast or ovarian cysts, which usually go away on their own. Eventually, a woman's ovaries don't respond at all to her pituitary hormones. After the last ovulatory cycle, progesterone is no longer secreted, and estrogen levels decrease rapidly. A woman's testosterone level also falls.

In the United States, the average woman who reaches menopause has a life expectancy of about 30 more years. However, she faces risks of various diseases, including an increased risk of obesity, metabolic syndrome, heart disease, stroke, and breast cancer. Women can reduce these risks by exercise, good nutrition, and controlling weight both before and after menopause.[16]

"Exercise is the best thing a woman can do for herself at midlife," says JoAnn Pinkerton, M.D., of the National Women's Health Resource Center. "It improves your heart function so you have less chance of heart disease. It improves your cognition so you think better. It decreases your risk of breast cancer. It helps your mood. It lessens the likelihood of depression. It increases energy and protects your bones."[17]

Hormone Therapy

Many people, including physicians, long believed that **hormone therapy (HT)** would prevent heart disease and strokes and help women live longer.[18] But medical thinking on HT, particularly a combination of estrogen and progestin, has changed completely in recent years. Contrary to what once was standard practice, HT is no longer recommended for reasons other than short-term relief of symptoms such as hot flashes and night sweats.[19]

The Women's Health Initiative (WHI)—a series of clinical trials begun in 1991 on postmenopausal women—halted its study of combination estrogen/progestin therapy in July 2002 and its study of estrogen-only therapy in 2004 because of safety concerns. Combination therapy slightly increased the risk of breast cancer, heart disease, blood clots, and stroke. Estrogen-only therapy increased the risk of stroke, decreased the risk of hip fracture, and did not affect the incidence of heart disease in postmenopausal women ages 50 to 70.[20]

The Food and Drug Administration recommends hormone therapy for women with *acute* menopausal symptoms—but in the lowest possible dose and for the shortest possible time. For alternatives to HT, see Savvy Consumer: "What Are Some Alternatives to Relieve Menopausal Symptoms?"

In a follow-up study of women who discontinued hormone therapy following recommendations to do so, women most commonly reported hot flashes or night sweats, pain and stiffness, and fatigue and difficulty sleeping. However, 37 percent of women reported neither moderate nor severe symptoms. Among those reporting symptoms, lifestyle changes such as drinking more fluids, starting or increasing exercise, practicing yoga, meditation, or breathing exercises, and using fans or air conditioners often helped.[21] Researchers now think that many symptoms that had been linked with menopause, such as joint pain and stiffness, low backaches, and tiredness, are in fact related to aging or other conditions.[22]

MEN AT MIDLIFE

Although men don't experience the dramatic hormonal upheaval that women do, they do experience a decline by as much as 30 to 40 percent in their primary sex hor-

---

Savvy Consumer ■■ What Are Some Alternatives to Relieve Menopausal Symptoms?

For Hot flashes

■ **Lifestyle changes.** These include dressing and eating to avoid being too warm, sleeping in a cool room, and reducing stress. Avoid spicy foods and caffeine. Try deep breathing and stress reduction techniques, including meditation and other relaxation methods.

■ **Phytoestrogens.** Soybeans and some soy-based foods contain phytoestrogens, which are estrogen-like compounds. Plant sources of phytoestrogens include botanicals such as black cohosh, wild yam, dong quai, and red clover. However, there is no solid evidence that the phytoestrogens in soybeans, soy-based foods, other plant sources, or dietary supplements really do relieve hot flashes. The risks of taking the more concentrated forms of soy phytoestrogens, such as pills and powders, are not known. Dietary supplements with phytoestrogens do not have to meet the same quality standards as do drugs, and little is known about the safety or efficacy of these products.

■ **Antidepressants**, such as Effexor, Paxil, and Prozac. These medications have been proved moderately effective in clinical trials.

For Vaginal Dryness

■ **Vaginal lubricants** and moisturizers (available over the counter).

■ **Products that release estrogen** locally (such as vaginal creams, a vaginal suppository, called Vagifem, and a plastic ring, called an Estring)—these are used for more severe dryness. The ring, which must be changed every 3 months, contains a low dose of estrogen and may not protect against osteoporosis.

For Mood Swings

■ **Lifestyle behaviors**, including getting enough sleep and being physically active

■ **Relaxation exercises**

■ **Antidepressant** or anti-anxiety drugs

For Insomnia

■ **Over-the-counter sleep aids**

■ **Milk products**, such as a glass of milk or cup of yogurt—choose low-fat or fat-free varieties—consumed at bedtime

■ **Do physical activity** in the morning or early afternoon—exercising later in the day may increase wakefulness

■ **Hot shower or bath** immediately before going to bed

For Memory Problems

■ **Mental exercises**

■ **Lifestyle behaviors**, especially getting enough sleep and being physically active[23]

What life after 60 looks like.

mone, testosterone, between the ages of 48 and 70. This change, sometimes called *andropause,* may cause a range of symptoms, including decreased muscle mass, greater body fat, loss of bone density, flagging energy, lowered fertility, and impaired virility. Some researchers are experimenting with testosterone supplements, which in tests with young men, have been shown to increase lean body mass and decrease body fat—at least temporarily. However, other researchers warn that, particularly in older men, excess testosterone might raise the risk of prostate cancer and heart disease.

After age 40, the prostate gland, which surrounds the urethra at the base of the bladder, enlarges. This condition, called *benign prostatic hypertrophy,* occurs in every man. By age 50, half of all men have some enlargement of the gland; after 70, three-quarters do. As it expands, the prostate tends to pinch the urethra, decreasing urinary flow and creating a sense of urinary urgency, particularly at night. Other warning signs of prostate problems include difficult urination, blood in the urine, painful ejaculation, or constant lower-back pain.

The drug Proscar (generic name, finasteride), which shrinks an enlarged prostate, has provided an alternative to corrective surgery for many men. Other drugs are being tried experimentally. The older a man gets, the more likely he is to develop prostate cancer.

SEXUALITY AND AGING

Health and sexuality interact in various ways as we age. When they are healthy and have a willing partner, a substantial number of older men remain sexually active. The fittest men and women report more frequent sexual activity. Other research has found a relationship between sex and longevity. A Swedish study found that men, but not women, who had discontinued intercourse had higher death rates. A study of the entire male

For older couples, sexual desire and pleasure can be enhanced by years of intimacy and affection.

population of a small Welsh town found that the sexually active men had half the mortality of the inactive group. In a Duke University study, longevity in women correlated with enjoyment of sexual intercourse, rather than with its frequency.

Aging does cause some changes in sexual response: Women produce less vaginal lubrication. An older man needs more time to achieve an erection or orgasm and to attain another erection after ejaculating. Both men and women experience fewer contractions during orgasm. However, none of these changes reduces sexual pleasure or desire.

In a poll of more than 4,000 people between the ages of 40 and 80 in the United States, Canada, Australia, and New Zealand, around 30 percent of men aged 70 to 80 reported having sex five times in the past month, although only 8 percent of women reported doing so. Most women said the lack of sex was due to the absence of a partner. Some 40 percent of men reported problems such as erectile dysfunction.

THE CHALLENGES OF AGE

No matter how well we eat, exercise, and take care of ourselves, some physical changes are inevitable as we age. Figure 18-1 shows some of these changes, but most of them are not debilitating, and people can remain active and vital into extreme old age. Aging brains and bodies do become vulnerable to diseases like Alzheimer's and osteoporosis. Other common life problems, such as depression, substance misuse, and safe driving, become more challenging as we age.

ALZHEIMER'S DISEASE

About 15 percent of older Americans lose previous mental capabilities, a brain disorder called **dementia.** Sixty percent of these—a total of 4.5 million men and women over age 65—suffer from the type of dementia called **Alzheimer's disease,** a progressive deterioration of brain cells and mental capacity.

The percentage of people with Alzheimer's doubles for every five-year age group beyond 65. By age 85, nearly half of men and women have Alzheimer's. A person with the disease typically lives eight years after the onset of symptoms, but some live as long as 20 years. Some 13.2 million older Americans will develop Alzheimer's disease by 2050. The greatest increase will be among people age 85 and older.

Women are more likely to develop Alzheimer's than men, and women with Alzheimer's perform significantly worse than men in various visual, spatial, and memory tests. Initiating hormone therapy after age 60

Hair and nails Hair often turns gray and thins out. Men may go bald. Fingernails can thicken.

Brain The brain shrinks, but it is not known if that affects mental functions.

The senses The sensitivity of hearing, sight, taste, and smell can all decline with age.

Skin Wrinkles occur as the skin thins and the underlying fat shrinks, and age spots often develop.

Glands and hormones Levels of many hormones drop, or the body becomes less responsive to them.

Muscles Strength usually peaks in the twenties, then declines.

Immune system The body becomes less able to resist some pathogens.

Heart and blood vessels Cardiovascular problems become more common. The heart grows less efficient; buildup within arteries decreases oxygen and nutrients to cells.

Breasts Tissue degenerates after menopause, and breasts sag.

Lungs Lung capacity drops; risk of bronchitis and pneumonia grows.

Kidneys and urinary tract The kidneys become less efficient. The bladder can't hold as much, so urination is more frequent.

Digestive system Digestion slows down as the secretion of digestive enzymes decreases.

Reproductive system Women go through menopause, and testosterone levels drop for men.

Bones and joints Wear and tear can lead to arthritic joints, and osteoporosis is common, especially in women.

FIGURE 18-1   The Effects of Aging on the Body

increases the risk of Alzheimer's disease, but earlier use may reduce a woman's risk of this devastating illness.[24]

 African Americans have higher rates of Alzheimer's disease than Africans living in Africa, according to the first study to find differences in the incidence of this illness in an industrial and a nonindustrial country.

The early signs of dementia—insomnia, irritability, increased sensitivity to alcohol and other drugs, and decreased energy and tolerance of frustration—are usually subtle and insidious. Diagnosis requires a comprehensive assessment of an individual's medical history, physical health, and mental status, often involving brain scans and a variety of other tests.

Even though medical science cannot restore a brain that is in the process of being destroyed by an organic brain disease like Alzheimer's, medications can control difficult behavioral symptoms and enhance or partially restore cognitive ability. Often physicians find other medical or psychiatric problems, such as depression, in these patients; recognizing and treating these conditions can have a dramatic impact.

The FDA has approved several prescription drugs for people with mild to moderate Alzheimer's, including Cognex, Aricept, Exelon, and Reminyl. They all increase the level of the brain chemical acetylcholine. Researchers are studying other medications that might delay Alzheimer's or stop its progression.

OSTEOPOROSIS

Another age-related disease is **osteoporosis,** a condition in which losses in bone density become so severe that a bone will break after even slight trauma or injury (see photos). A chronic disease, osteoporosis is silent for years or decades before a fracture occurs.

 Women, who have smaller skeletons, are more vulnerable than men; in extreme cases, their spines may become so fragile that just bending causes severe pain. But although commonly seen as an illness of women, osteoporosis occurs frequently in men. One in every two women and one in four men over 50 will have an osteoporosis-related fracture in their lifetime (Figure 18-2).[25] An estimated 44 million men and women aged 50 and older currently have osteoporosis or low bone mass.[26]

Risk Factors

Osteoporosis doesn't begin in old age. The bone weakness that increases the risk of osteoporosis may actually begin before birth. Infants undernourished in the womb are small when born, remain smaller than their age peers at age 1, have low bone mass at 25, and an increased risk of fractures in late adulthood.[27] Other risk factors include:

- **Age**—risk increases as you grow older.
- **Being female**—Women have less bone tissue than do men and tend to experience a rapid loss of bone in the first few years after menopause.

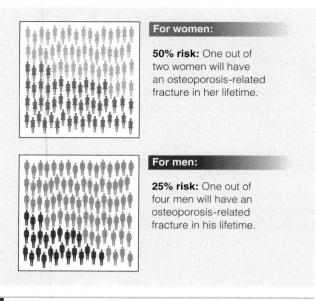

For women:

50% risk: One out of two women will have an osteoporosis-related fracture in her lifetime.

For men:

25% risk: One out of four men will have an osteoporosis-related fracture in his lifetime.

FIGURE 18-2 Osteoporosis risk in women and men

The Effect of Osteoporosis on Bone Density (a) Normal bone tissue. (b) After the onset of osteoporosis, bones lose density and become hollow and brittle.

Source: © Dr. P. Motta, Department of Anatomy, University "La Sapienza," Rome/Science Photo Library/Photo Researchers, Inc.

- **Body size**—small, thin-boned women are at greatest risk.
- **Ethnicity**—White and Asian women are at highest risk.
- **Having parents with a history of osteoporosis** as well as fractures in adulthood can place someone at increased risk for osteoporosis.
- **Sex hormones**—abnormal absence of menstrual periods (amenorrhea) or menopause.
- **Anorexia.**
- **Lifetime diet low in calcium and vitamin D.**

Strategies for Prevention :: Lowering Your Risk of Osteoporosis

Regardless of your age and gender, you can prevent future bone problems by taking some protective steps now. The most important guidelines are as follows:

:: Get adequate calcium. Increased calcium intake, particularly during childhood and the growth spurt of adolescence, can produce a heavier, denser skeleton and reduce the risk of the complications of bone loss later in life. College-age women also can strengthen their bones and reduce their risk of osteoporosis by increasing their

calcium intake and physical activity. Adequate dietary calcium and vitamin D in adulthood helps maintain bone density for years (Table 18-2).

:: If you do not get enough calcium in your diet, take daily supplements.

:: Drink alcohol only moderately. More than two or three alcoholic beverages a day impairs intestinal calcium absorption.

:: Don't smoke. Smokers tend to be thin and enter menopause earlier, thus

extending the period of jeopardy from estrogen loss.

:: Let the sunshine in (but don't forget your sunscreen). Vitamin D, a vitamin produced in the skin in reaction to sunlight, boosts calcium absorption.

:: Exercise regularly. Both aerobic exercise and weight training can help preserve bone density.

TABLE 18-2 DAILY CALCIUM REQUIREMENTS FOR EVERY STAGE OF LIFE

Age	Daily Calcium Requirements
1–3 years	500 mg
4–8 years	800 mg
9–18 years	1,300 mg
Adult women	1,000 mg
Pregnancy and lactation	1,000–1,200 mg
Postmenopause using hormones	1,200 mg
Postmenopause without hormones	1,500 mg
Adult men	
19–50 years	1,000 mg
51+ years	1,200 mg

▮ **Certain medications,** such as glucocorticoids (prescribed for various diseases, including arthritis, asthma, and lupus) and some anticonvulsants.

▮ **Physical inactivity** or extended bed rest.

▮ **Cigarette smoking.**

▮ **Excessive use of alcoholic beverages.**[28]

Treating Osteoporosis

Lifestyle changes, such as weight-bearing exercise, and medication can treat osteoporosis. Hormone therapy is used only if its potential benefits outweigh its risks. Other options include:

▮ **Raloxifene** is a selective estrogen receptor modulator (SERM), which preserves bone density and prevents fractures (although not hip fractures). Possible side effects include hot flashes and blood clots.

▮ **Alendronate** (brand name Fosamax) and risedronate (brand name Actonel) are bisphosphonates, drugs that slow the breakdown of bone, prevent fractures, and may reverse bone loss. Side effects may include nausea, heartburn, and pain in the stomach.

▮ **Calcitonin** is a naturally occurring nonsex hormone that increases bone mass in the spine, and it may prevent some fractures. It is used to treat women who are at least 5 years beyond menopause. The drug is taken by injection or nasal spray.

▮ **Teraparatide** (parathyroid hormone) may reverse bone loss.[29]

SUBSTANCE MISUSE AND ABUSE

Misuse and abuse of prescription and over-the-counter medications occur frequently among the elderly. In part this is because people over age 65 consume one-quarter of all drugs prescribed in the United States. Moreover, many older people have multiple health problems, requiring several medications at the same time. The drugs may interact and cause a confusing array of symptoms and reactions.

The most commonly misused drugs are sleeping pills, tranquilizers, pain medications, and laxatives. Sometimes a person innocently uses more than the prescribed dose or simultaneously takes several prescriptions of the same drug. Some older people are aware of their overreliance on drugs but don't like how they feel when they don't take the pills.

Problems remembering, concentrating, and thinking are the most common psychological side effects of drugs in the elderly. As people age, their bodies take longer to metabolize drugs, so medications like sleeping pills build up in the body. Almost any amount of alcohol can make mental confusion and memory problems worse. Whenever older people become confused, forgetful, or paranoid, family members should find out which medications they've been taking.

PREPARING FOR MEDICAL CRISES AND THE END OF LIFE

Throughout this book, we have stressed the ways in which you can determine how well and how long you live. You can also make decisions about the end of your life.

THE FIVE WISHES

An innovative document called "Five Wishes" helps the aged, the seriously ill, their loved ones, and caregivers prepare for medical crises. Written with the help of the American Bar Association's Commission on the Legal Problems of the Elderly, it enables individuals to specify:

- ▪ Which person they want to make health-care decisions for them when they are no longer able to do so.
- ▪ Which kinds of medical treatments they do or don't want.
- ▪ How comfortable they want to be made.
- ▪ How they want people to treat them.
- ▪ What they want loved ones to know.

The Five Wishes document (at www.agingwithdignity.org) is legally valid in 37 states. Churches, synagogues, hospices, hospitals, physicians, social service agencies, and employers also are distributing the document to help people plan for their own care or that of aging parents.

You also can assure that your wishes are heeded by advance directives, such as a health-care proxy, living will, or holographic will.

(FAQ) WHAT ARE ADVANCE DIRECTIVES?

Every state and the District of Columbia have laws authorizing the use of **advance directives** to specify the kind of medical treatment individuals want in case of a medical crisis. These documents are important because, without clear indications of a person's preferences, hospitals and other institutions often make decisions on an individual's behalf, particularly if family members are not available or disagree. Advance directives also help physicians, who often do not feel comfortable making these kinds of decisions about life-extending treatments for their terminally ill patients.[30]

According to the Patient Self-Determination Act, health-care facilities that receive Medicare or Medicaid reimbursements must advise patients of their right to sign advance directives for health-care decisions, including whether they want to be kept alive by artificial means. These statements allow medical professionals to know and follow an individual's wishes, or the wishes of a person to whom the patient has given authority to make decisions on his or her behalf. Figure 18-3 shows what you can include in an advance directive and the possible limitations on it because of differing state laws.

A *health-care proxy* is an advance directive that gives someone else the power to make decisions on your behalf. (Figure 18-4 on page 532 shows the Medical Power of Attorney form for Texas.) People typically name a relative or close friend as their agent. Let family and friends know that you have completed an advance directive. Tell your primary physician, but you should not designate your doctor as your agent. Many states prohibit this. Even when allowed, it is not a good idea because your doctor's primary responsibility is to administer care.

You can also sign an advance directive specifying that you want to be allowed to die naturally—you do not want to be resuscitated in case your heart stops beating. **Do-not-resuscitate (DNR)** orders apply mainly to hospitalized, terminally ill patients. However, in some states, it is possible to complete a *nonhospital DNR* form that specifies an individual's wish not to be resuscitated at home. Patients in the final stages of advanced cancer or AIDS may choose to use such forms to protect their rights in case paramedics are called to their home.

> *Even healthy young people may suffer injuries or illnesses that leave them capable of surviving only with artificial assistance. Some individuals would rather not face the possibility of making end-of-life decisions. Others argue that the surviving family should do what they feel is right. Is it better to make your preferences clear in an advance directive? Or can such difficult decisions be left until old age?* **You decide.**

LIVING WILLS

A **living will** isn't just for people who don't want to be kept alive by artificial means. Individuals can also use these advance directives to indicate that they want all possible medical treatments and technology used to prolong their lives. Living wills are most effective when they focus on priorities and goals, not so much on how to achieve them.[31]

Most states recognize living wills as legally binding, and a growing number of health-care professionals and facilities offer patients help in drafting living wills. You can obtain state-specific forms for living wills and health-care proxies free from Partnership for Caring (www.partnershipforcaring.org, 1-800-989-WILL). Computer software for preparing such documents is also available.

Once the forms are completed, make copies of your living will and other advance directives, and give them to anyone who might have input in decisions on your behalf. Also give copies to your physician or health-care organization, and ask that they be made part of your medical record.

Except in California, where they must be renewed every five years, directives are effective until they're revoked. Still, it's considered a good idea to initial and date your directive every few years to show that it still expresses your wishes.

"Imminent" is used on many directives to express the inevitability and timing of death, but it's open to varying interpretations. A recent Virginia court decision found that it doesn't necessarily mean "immediately, at once, within a few days," and that a comatose person who's within a few months of death falls within the definition.

Except in California, Idaho, and Oregon, directives will have a space to specify treatment you do or don't want. Ask your physician what to include here. You can:

- Ask for or prohibit use of artificial feeding tubes, cardiopulmonary resuscitation, antibiotics, dialysis, and respirators.
- Ask for pain medication to keep you comfortable.
- State whether you would prefer to die in the hospital or at home.
- Designate a proxy—someone to make decisions about your treatment when you're unable.
- Donate organs or other body parts.

DIRECTIVE TO PHYSICIANS

Directive made this _____ day of _____ (month, year). I, _____, being of sound mind, willfully and voluntarily make known my desire that my life shall not be artificially prolonged under the circumstances set forth below, and do hereby declare:

If at any time I should have an incurable condition caused by injury, disease, or illness certified to be a terminal condition by two physicians, and where the application of life-sustaining procedures would serve only to artificially prolong the moment of death and where my attending physician determines that my death is imminent whether or not life-sustaining procedures are utilized, I direct that such procedures be withheld or withdrawn, and that I be permitted to die naturally.

In the absence of my ability to give directions regarding the use of such life-sustaining procedures, it is my intention that this directive shall be honored by my family and physicians as the final expression of my legal right to refuse medical or surgical treatment and accept the consequences from such refusal.

If I have been diagnosed as pregnant and that diagnosis is known to my physician, this directive shall have no force or effect during the course of my pregnancy.

Other directions:
This directive shall be in effect until it is revoked. I understand the full import of this directive, and I am emotionally and mentally competent to make this directive. I understand that I may revoke this directive at any time.

Signed _____

City, County, and State of Residence _____

The declarant has been personally known to me and I believe him/her to be of sound mind. I am not related to the declarant by blood or marriage, nor would I be entitled to any portion of the declarant's estate on his/her decease, nor am I the attending physician of the declarant or an employee of the attending physician or a health facility in which the declarant is a patient, or a patient in the health care facility in which the declarant is a patient, or any person who has a claim against any portion of the estate of the declarant upon his/her decease.

Witness _____ Witness _____

"Life-sustaining procedures" are those that only prolong the process of dying. Most states include feeding and hydration tubes in this definition.

In some states a physician who will not carry out a patient's wishes must make a "good faith effort" to locate a doctor who will; other states require the physician to actually find someone and specify penalties—in some cases, jail terms—for failure to do so.

In some states the directive is valid for pregnant women. Others exclude women during all or part of their pregnancy, although that has been challenged on the grounds that a woman's right to privacy doesn't end when she becomes pregnant.

You can revoke or amend your directive at any time simply by making a statement to a physician, nurse, or other health-care worker.

Several states provide for the appointment of a proxy. In others decisions may be delegated through a document called a Durable Power of Attorney.

In some states your signature must be notarized. Elsewhere, the signature of the witnesses is adequate, although if you're in a hospital or nursing home, in some states you may need as an additional witness the chief of staff or medical director.

FIGURE 18-3 Preparing a Physician's Directive

Source: "A Guide to the Living Will." *Hippocrates*, May–June, 1988.

INSTRUCTIONS

TEXAS MEDICAL POWER OF ATTORNEY

PRINT YOUR NAME

DESIGNATION OF HEALTH CARE AGENT.

I, _____, appoint:

(name)

PRINT THE NAME, ADDRESS AND HOME AND WORK TELEPHONE NUMBERS OF YOUR AGENT

_____

(name of agent)

_____

(address)

_____   _____

(work telephone number)   *(home telephone number)*

as my agent to make any and all health care decisions for me, except to the extent I state otherwise in this document. This medical power of attorney takes effect if I become unable to make my own health care decisions and this fact is certified in writing by my physician.

STATE LIMITATIONS ON YOUR AGENT'S POWER (IF ANY)

LIMITATIONS ON THE DECISION MAKING AUTHORITY OF MY AGENT ARE AS FOLLOWS.

PRINT THE NAME, ADDRESS AND HOME AND WORK TELEPHONE NUMBERS OF YOUR FIRST AND SECOND ALTERNATE AGENTS

DESIGNATION OF ALTERNATE AGENT.

(You are not required to designate an alternate agent but you may do so. An alternate agent may make the same health care decisions as the designated agent if the designated agent is unable or unwilling to act as your agent. If the agent designated is your spouse, the designation is automatically revoked by law if your marriage is dissolved.)

If the person designated as my agent is unable or unwilling to make health care decisions for me, I designate the following persons to serve as my agent to make health care decisions for me as authorized by this document, who serve in the following order:

FIRST ALTERNATE

A. First Alternate Agent

_____

(name of first alternate agent)

_____

(home address)

_____   _____

(work telephone number)   *(home telephone number)*

SECOND ALTERNATE

B. Second Alternate Agent

_____

(name of second alternate agent)

_____

(home address)

_____   _____

(work telephone number)   *(home telephone number)*

LOCATION OF ORIGINAL

The original of this document is kept at: _____

LOCATION OF COPIES

The following individuals or institutions have signed copies:

Name: _____

Address: _____

Name: _____

Address: _____

DURATION.

I understand that this power of attorney exists indefinitely from the date I execute this document unless I establish a shorter time or revoke the power of attorney. If I am unable to make health care decisions for myself when this power of attorney expires, the authority I have granted my agent continues to exist until the time I become able to make health care decisions for myself.

EXPIRATION DATE (IF ANY)

(IF APPLICABLE) This power of attorney ends on the following date: _____

PRIOR DESIGNATIONS REVOKED.

I revoke any prior medical power of attorney.

ACKNOWLEDGMENT OF DISCLOSURE STATEMENT.

I have been provided with a disclosure statement explaining the effect of this document. I have read and understood that information contained in the disclosure statement.

(YOU MUST DATE AND SIGN THIS POWER OF ATTORNEY)

PRINT THE DATE

I sign my name to this medical power of attorney on _____

(date)

PRINT YOUR LOCATION

day of _____, at _____.

(month)   *(year)*   *(city and state)*

SIGN THE DOCUMENT

_____

(signature)

PRINT YOUR NAME

_____

(print name)

© 2000
PARTNERSHIP FOR CARING, INC.

...ESSING ...EDURE

... TWO ...ESSES ...IGN AND ...YOUR ...MENT ...OW

MUST PRINT NAMES ...ND ...ESSES

...SS #1

...SS #2

STATEMENT OF FIRST WITNESS.

I am not the person appointed as agent by this document. I am not related to the principal by blood or marriage. I would not be entitled to any portion of the principal's estate on the principal's death. I am not the attending physician of the principal or an employee of the attending physician. I have no claim against any portion of the principal's estate on the principal's death. Furthermore, if I am an employee of a health care facility in which the principal is a patient, I am not involved in providing direct patient care to the principal and am not an officer, director, partner or business office employee of the health care facility or any parent organization of the health care facility.

Signature: _____

Print Name: _____   Date: _____

Address: _____

SIGNATURE OF SECOND WITNESS

Witness Signature: _____

Print Name: _____   Date: _____

Address: _____

© 2000
PARTNERSHIP FOR CARING, INC.

Courtesy of Partnership for Caring, Inc.   9/99
1620 Eye Street, NW, Suite 202, Washington, DC 20006 800-989-9455

FIGURE 18-4   Health-Care Proxy

A medical power of attorney is another advance directive. This example is from the state of Texas.

Source: Reprinted by permission of Partnership for Caring Inc., Washington, DC 20006. 800-889-9455.

HOLOGRAPHIC WILLS

Perhaps you think that only wealthy or older people need to write wills. However, if you're married, have children, or own property, you should either hire a lawyer to draw up a will or at least write a **holographic will** yourself, specifying who you wish to raise your children and who should have your property. If you die *intestate* (without a will), the state will make these decisions for you. Even a modest estate can be tied up in court for a long period of time, depriving family members of money when they need it most.

A holographic will is a handwritten (not typed) statement that some states will recognize. You can:

- **Name a family member** or friend as the executor, the person who sees that your wishes are carried out.
- **List the things you own** and to whom you want them to go; include addresses and telephone numbers, if possible.
- **Select a guardian for your children** (if any), presumably someone whose ideas about raising children are similar to your own. Be sure that any named guardians are willing and able to accept this responsibility before writing them into your will.
- **Specify any funeral arrangements.**

Be sure to keep the will in a safe place, where your executor, family members, or closest beneficiary can find it quickly and easily; tell them where it is.

ETHICAL DILEMMAS

Modern medicine can do more to delay or defy death than was once thought possible. However, the ability to sustain life in patients with no hope of recovery has created wrenching medical and moral dilemmas. Increasingly, lawyers, ethicists, and consumer advocates are arguing that health-care providers must recognize a fundamental right of patients: the right to die.[32]

Health economists, noting that more than half of U.S. health-care dollars are spent in the last year of life, have questioned "heroic" measures to prolong the life of chronically ill elderly patients or those with fatal diseases. Policies on such aggressive measures vary from hospital to hospital and state to state; often medical staff are not aware of patients' wishes.

Some health-care facilities require that staff members try to resuscitate any patient whose heart stops unless a do-not-resuscitate (DNR) order has been written, usually with the family's permission.

Families may demand aggressive medical care near the end of life on the basis of religious grounds, such as a conviction that every moment of life is a gift from God worth preserving at any cost. However, doctors are not obliged to provide a treatment they consider medically inappropriate or inhumane simply because of the family's religious beliefs. Ideally, doctors and family members, perhaps with the aid of a chaplain, work together to reach a consensus on the appropriate limits to life-sustaining treatment.

Another major ethical concern is the fate of an estimated 5,000 to 10,000 unconscious Americans who are being kept alive by artificial means. Some are in a **coma,** a state of total unconsciousness. They may have no sense of where they are, no memory, and no experience of pain. Others are in a **persistent vegetative state,** in which they're awake and yet unaware. They open their eyes; their brain waves show the characteristic patterns of waking and sleep. They can usually breathe on their own after a few weeks on artificial respiration; they can cough; the pupils of their eyes respond to light; but they do not respond to pain.

About 20 percent of deaths in the United States occur in intensive care units. The majority involve either withholding or withdrawing life-sustaining treatments. The questions of when to use and when to discontinue artificial means of life support remain among the most challenging ethical dilemmas facing health-care workers and the families of critically ill patients.

THE GIFT OF LIFE

If you're at least 18 years old, you can fill out a donor card (Figure 18-5), agreeing to designate, in the event of your death, any organs or tissues needed for transplantation. Corneas may help a blind person see, for example. Kidneys, or even a heart, may be transplanted. The donation takes effect upon your death and is a generous way of giving others the possibilities for life that you have had yourself. The card should be filled out and signed; some must be signed in the presence of two witnesses. Attach the donor card to the back of your driver's license or I.D. card. (Whole-body donations may require other arrangements.)

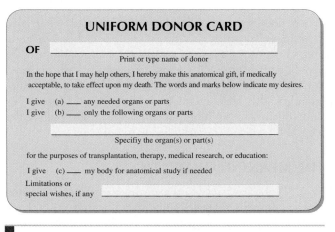

UNIFORM DONOR CARD

OF _____
Print or type name of donor

In the hope that I may help others, I hereby make this anatomical gift, if medically acceptable, to take effect upon my death. The words and marks below indicate my desires.

I give   (a) ____ any needed organs or parts
I give   (b) ____ only the following organs or parts

_____
Specifiy the organ(s) or part(s)

for the purposes of transplantation, therapy, medical research, or education:

I give   (c) ____ my body for anatomical study if needed
Limitations or
special wishes, if any _____

FIGURE 18-5 **Example of a Uniform Donor Card**

DEATH AND DYING

Some 2.4 million people die in the United States each year. Although most are older, death occurs in all age groups. The causes of death vary with both age and gender. Among those under age 35, intentional and nonintentional injury are the primary causes of death. Among older Americans, cancer and heart disease are the top killers. Men typically die at a younger age than women.

DEFINING DEATH

In our society, death isn't a part of everyday life, as it once was. Because machines can now keep alive people who, in the past, would have died, the definition of death has become more complex. Death has been broken down into the following categories:

- **Functional death.** The end of all vital functions, such as heartbeat and respiration.
- **Cellular death.** The gradual death of body cells after the heart stops beating. If placed in a tissue culture or, as is the case with various organs, transplanted to another body, some cells can remain alive indefinitely.
- **Death.** The moment when the heart stops beating.
- **Brain death.** The end of all brain activity, indicated by an absence of electrical activity (confirmed by an electroencephalogram, or EEG) and a lack of reflexes. The notion of brain death is bound up with what we consider to be the actual person, or self. The destruction of a person's brain means that his or her personality no longer exists; the lower brain centers controlling respiration and circulation no longer function.
- **Spiritual death.** The moment when the soul, as defined by many religions, leaves the body.

When does a person actually die? The traditional legal definition of death is failure of the lungs or heart to function. However, because respiration and circulation can be maintained by artificial means, most states have declared that an individual is considered dead only when the brain, including the brain stem, completely stops functioning. Brain-death laws prohibit a medical staff from "pulling the plug" if there is any hope of sustaining life.

THE MEANING OF DEATH

Death is not a mystery to those who have died. The living are the ones who struggle to find meaning in it. As far back as 60,000 years ago, prehistoric people observed special ceremonies when burying their dead. Many early cultures believed that people continued to exist after death and had the same needs that they did in life; hence they buried their loved ones with food, dishes, weapons, and jewels. Some religions, such as Christianity, believe that the dead will rise again; to them, the burial of the body is symbolic, like the planting of a seed in the earth to await rebirth. Many Eastern religions share the belief that death marks the end only of physical existence and of the limited view of reality that human beings can grasp.

Death itself is a remote experience in most lives today, something that takes place off-stage in a hospital or nursing home. In earlier times, dying was a much more visible part of daily living. Families, friends, and other loved ones in a community would share in caring for those at the end of life. Most deaths occurred at home, often following a brief illness and unaffected by the limited medical care available. Today, the process of dying has become invisible.

Our attitudes toward dying also have changed with the development of medical technology and the extension of the human lifespan. Some people will do anything to delay aging or defeat death itself through medical science or other means. Others see death as part of a natural biological process and work toward the goal of dying well, with dignity and without undue suffering.

DENYING DEATH

Most of us don't quite believe that we're going to die. A reasonable amount of denial helps us focus on the day-to-day realities of living. However, excessive denial can be life-threatening. Some drivers, for instance, refuse to buckle their seat belts because they refuse to acknowledge that a drunk driver might collide with them. Similarly, cigarette smokers deny that lung cancer will ever strike them, and people who eat high-fat meals deny that they'll ever suffer a heart attack.

One important factor in denial is the nature of the threat. It's easy to believe that death is at hand when someone's pointing a gun at you; it's much harder to think that cigarette smoking might cause your death 20 or 30 years down the road. The late Elisabeth Kübler-Ross, a psychiatrist who extensively studied the process of dying, described the downside of denying death in *Death: The Final Stage of Growth*.

> It is the denial of death that is partially responsible for people living empty, purposeless lives; for when you live as if you'll live forever, it becomes too easy to postpone the things you know that you must do. You live your life in preparation for tomorrow or in the remembrance of yesterday—and meanwhile, each today is lost. In contrast, when you fully understand that each day you awaken could be the last you have, you take the time that day to grow, to become more of who you really are, to reach out to other human beings.[33]

EMOTIONAL RESPONSES TO DYING

Kübler-Ross identified five typical stages of reaction that a person goes through when facing death (Figure 18-6).

FIGURE 18-6 Kübler-Ross's Five Stages of Adjustment to Facing Death

1. **Denial ("No, not me").** At first knowledge that death is coming, a terminally ill patient rejects the news. The denial overcomes the initial shock and allows the person to begin to gather together his or her resources. Denial, at this point, is a healthy defense mechanism. It can become distressful, however, if it's reinforced by the relatives and friends of the dying patient.

2. **Anger ("Why me?").** In the second stage, the dying person begins to feel resentment and rage regarding imminent death. The anger may be directed at God or at the patient's family and caregivers, who can do little but try to endure any expressions of anger, provide comfort, and help the patient on to the next stage.

3. **Bargaining ("Yes, me, but . . .").** In this stage, a patient may try to bargain, usually with God, for a way to reverse or at least postpone dying. The patient may promise, in exchange for recovery, to do good works or to see family members more often. Alternatively, the patient may say, "Let me live long enough to see my grandchild born" or "to see the spring again."

4. **Depression ("Yes, it's me").** In the fourth stage, the patient gradually realizes the full consequences of his or her condition. This may begin as grieving for health that has been lost and then become anticipatory grieving for the loss that is to come of friends, loved ones, and life itself. This stage is perhaps the most difficult: The dying person should not be left alone during this period. Neither should loved ones try to cheer up the patient, who must be allowed to grieve.

5. **Acceptance ("Yes, me; and I'm ready").** In this last stage, the person has accepted the reality of death: The moment looms as neither frightening nor painful, neither sad nor happy—only inevitable. The person who waits for the end of life may ask to see fewer visitors, to separate from other people, or perhaps to turn to just one person for support.

Several stages may occur at the same time and some may happen out of sequence. Each stage may take days or only hours or minutes. Throughout, denial may come back to assert itself unexpectedly, and hope for a medical breakthrough or a miraculous recovery is forever present.

Some experts dispute Kübler-Ross's basic five-stage theory as too simplistic and argue that not all people go through such well-defined stages in the dying process. The way a person faces death is often a mirror of the way he or she has faced other major stresses in life: Those who have had the most trouble adjusting to other crises will have the most trouble adjusting to the news of their impending death.

An individual's will to live can postpone death for a while. In a study of elderly Chinese women, researchers found that their death rate decreased before and during a holiday during which the senior women in a household play a central role; it increased after the celebration. A similar temporary drop occurs among Jews at the time of Passover. However, different events may have different effects. The prospect of an upcoming birthday postpones death in women but hastens it in men. The will to live typically fluctuates in terminal patients, varying along with depression, anxiety, shortness of breath, and a sense of well-being.

The family of a dying person experiences a spectrum of often wrenching emotions. Family members, too, may deny the verdict of death, rage at the doctors and nurses who can't do more to save their loved one, bargain with God to give up their own health if necessary, sink into helplessness and depression, and finally accept the reality of their anticipated loss.

HOW WE DIE

Life can end in very different ways. Sudden death, by accident or murder, for instance, brings an abrupt end to life in individuals who may have been in optimal health. A terminal illness, such as an aggressive and fatal cancer, can lead to a steep drop in functioning prior to death. When organs such as the kidneys fail, a patient's well-being tends to plummet and then recover but in a downward pattern. The frailty of old age leads to a gradual decline to ever lower levels of functioning and eventual death.

The death rate from all causes has dropped by almost a third since 1970, with the largest decreases for heart disease and stroke. However, diabetes and chronic obstructive pulmonary disease are claiming more lives.[34] College-age individuals are most likely to die as a result of accidents or assaults. (See Student Snapshot: "Dying Young" and Chapter 19.)

Most people who have a fatal or **terminal illness** prefer to know the truth about their health and chances for recovery. Even when they're not officially informed by a doctor or relative, most fatally ill people know or strongly suspect that they're dying. Dying people usually make it clear whether they want to talk about death and to what extent. The most frequent concern is how much time is left.

Student Snapshot

DYING YOUNG

The Five Leading Causes of Death for College-Age Americans:

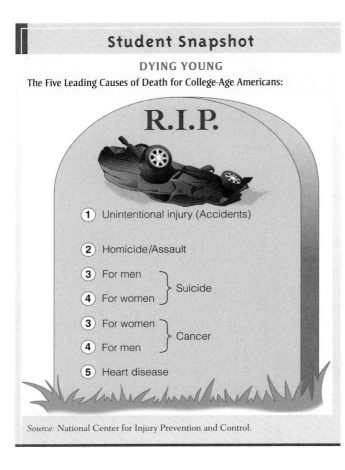

R.I.P.

① Unintentional injury (Accidents)

② Homicide/Assault

③ For men ⎤
④ For women ⎦ Suicide

③ For women ⎤
④ For men ⎦ Cancer

⑤ Heart disease

Source: National Center for Injury Prevention and Control.

Usually physicians can give only a rough estimate, such as "several weeks or months."

Once death was a taboo topic even between doctors and patients. Filled with a zeal to heal, physicians viewed death as the enemy; it caused a sense of medical impotence and failure that often led them to pull away from dying patients. However, surveys of physicians show changes in the last decades. Today's doctors are much more open to communicating with dying patients and their families on issues concerning death. They, too, benefit from open, honest conversations with their patients.

Most Americans die in institutions, such as nursing homes and hospitals. In one study of about 1,500 individuals, many families reported that their loved ones' needs for relief of pain, their breathing difficulties, physician communication, emotional support, and respect had not been met. Those whose loved ones died at home with hospice services reported greater satisfaction with both emotional and physical care.[35]

A "GOOD" DEATH

As life expectancy has increased and high-technology interventions have multiplied, many health-care professionals as well as citizens and social organizations have begun to demand a better way of caring for those who are dying. The Center to Improve Care of the Dying, in Washington, DC,

has set goals for reintegrating dying within living, thus enhancing the prospect for growth at the end of life. These experts talk of "dying well," "living while dying," and "physician-assisted living." They aim to change our way of thinking about dying so that we view the end of life as a time of love and reconciliation, and transcendence of suffering.

Physicians who care for the dying are being urged to do all that they can to eliminate pain. They are encouraged not to withhold opioid drugs, such as morphine, simply out of fear of addiction. More efforts are being made for patients to be taken care of at home, with appropriate support and well-informed guidance.

Various psychological factors can affect those at risk of dying. Elderly people who lack hope in the future are much more likely to die within the next few years. Researchers speculate that hopelessness may lead to biochemical and nervous system abnormalities or that hopeless individuals may not eat well, take medications as prescribed, or follow a doctor's recommendations.

Some terminally ill patients choose to stop eating and drinking because they are ready to die, see continued existence as pointless, and consider their quality of life poor. In a recent survey, hospice nurses reported that 85 percent of such patients die within 15 days after stopping food and fluids. On a scale from 0 (a very bad death) to 9 (a very good death), the median score for the quality of these deaths, as rated by the nurses, was 8.[36] The Oregon study found that patients choose to end their own lives by refusing food twice as often as they opt for physician-assisted suicide, which is legal only in that state.[37]

Spirituality also plays a major role. In various surveys, 41 to 94 percent of patients say they want their doctors and nurses to address their spiritual concerns. In one survey, even 45 percent of nonreligious patients thought physicians should inquire politely about patients' spiritual needs. However, some worry that such queries may be inappropriate or detract from a doctor's primary mission.

There are few data on the impact of spiritual approaches on the dying. In a survey of relatives of deceased patients, 63 percent thought that their loved one's faith was of help at the time of death. In a study of nursing home residents, traditional religious beliefs and values affected acceptance, endurance, coping, and security in the face of impending death.

CAREGIVING

When someone becomes terminally ill, a woman—usually the patient's wife, daughter, or sister—is most likely to provide day-to-day care, often for periods longer than a year. Caregiving takes a different toll on men and women. In one study of adult daughters and husbands caring for terminally ill breast cancer patients, the daughters experienced more symptoms of anxiety and depression and greater family strain.

The impact of caregiving continues even after the death of an ill spouse. In one study, the health of older caregivers who had experienced strain prior to a spouse's death did not deteriorate. They showed no increase in depressive symptoms or use of antidepressant drugs and did not lose weight. Those who had not been caregivers were more likely to experience depression and weight loss.

HOSPICE: CARING WHEN CURING ISN'T POSSIBLE

A **hospice** is a homelike health-care facility or program that helps dying men and women who can afford such care to live their final days to the fullest, as free as possible from disabling pain and mental anguish. Hospice workers generally work in teams, usually consisting of a nurse, physician, social worker, chaplain, and trained volunteers. Other professionals, such as a physical therapist, may join the team when needed. These workers provide the comfort, support, and care dying patients need until they do die.

Hospice programs offer a combination of medical and emotional care that involves not only the patient but also the family members or others concerned with caring for the patient. Most hospice patients have life expectancies of six months or less and are no longer receiving treatments aimed at curing their diseases. When someone is available to provide care, patients remain in their own homes. Hospice nurses regularly visit all home patients and are available around the clock.

For patients requiring care that the family cannot provide, round-the-clock care is available at the hospice facility. Unlike a traditional hospital, where the focus is on diagnosis, cure, and treatment, a hospice works to make what is left of life pain-free and comfortable. Visiting hours for relatives and friends are flexible, with no restrictions on visits by children and grandchildren. Hospice services are covered, in full or in part, by most major insurance companies.

(FAQ) WHAT DO WE KNOW ABOUT NEAR-DEATH EXPERIENCES?

Reports of **near-death experiences** have grown, thanks largely to advances in emergency medical care. Most are remarkably similar, whether they occur in children or adults, whether they're the result of accidents or illnesses, even whether the individuals actually are near death or only think they are. Some individuals who have survived a close brush with death report **autoscopy** (watching, from several feet in the air, resuscitation attempts on their own bodies) or **transcendence** (the sense of passing into a foreign region or dimension). Some see light, often at the end of a tunnel. Their vision seems clearer; their hearing, sharper. Some recall scenes from their lives or feel the presence of loved ones who have died. Many report profound feelings of joy, calm, and peace. Fewer than 1 percent of those who've reported near-death experiences described them as frightening or distressing, although a larger number recall transitory feelings of fear or confusion.

Humanitarian caregiving for both critically ill patients and their loved ones can take some of the fear out of death.

© David Young-Wolff/PhotoEdit

Many near-death experiences occur in individuals who've been sedated or given other medications; however, many others do not. Several studies have shown that individuals who received medication or anesthesia were actually less likely to remember near-death experiences than those who hadn't had any drugs. Some scientists have speculated that lack of oxygen, changes in blood gases, altered brain functioning, or the release of neurotransmitters (messenger chemicals in the brain) may play a role in near-death experiences. However, there's little solid evidence that physiological events are responsible. There's also no proof that wishful thinking, cultural conditioning, posttraumatic stress, or other psychological mechanisms may be at work. For now, the most that scientists can say for sure about this medical mystery is that it needs further study.

SUICIDE

Suicide increases with age and is most common in persons aged 65 years and older. This age group accounts for 18 percent of all suicides in the United States.[38] For every completed suicide, there are 10 to 40 unsuccessful attempts. (Chapter 3 presents a detailed discussion of the risk factors and warning signs of suicide.)

One of the main factors leading to suicide is illness, especially terminal illness. A great deal of debate centers on quality of life, yet there is no reliable or consistent way to measure this. Patients who are dying may feel some quality of life, even when others do not recognize it, or their evaluations of the quality of their lives may fluctuate. Dying patients who say their lives are not worth living may be suffering from depression; hopelessness is one of its characteristic symptoms.

"RATIONAL" SUICIDE

An elderly widow suffering from advanced cancer takes a lethal overdose of sleeping pills. A young man with several AIDS-related illnesses shoots himself. A woman in her fifties, diagnosed as having Alzheimer's disease, asks a doctor to help her end her life. Are these suicides "rational" because these individuals used logical reasoning in deciding to end their lives?

The question is intensely controversial. Advocates of the right to "self-deliverance" argue that individuals in great pain or faced with the prospect of a debilitating, hopeless battle against an incurable disease can and should be able to decide to end their lives. As legislatures and the legal system tackle the thorny questions of an individual's right to die, mental health professionals worry that, even in those with fatal diseases, suicidal wishes often stem from undiagnosed depression.

In one classic study of 44 terminally ill individuals, 34 had never been suicidal or wished for death. The remaining ten (seven who did desire early death and three who specifically considered suicide) all had severe depression. Their despair and preoccupation with dying may well have contributed to their willingness to consider suicide. Numerous studies have indicated that most patients with painful, progressive, or terminal illnesses do not want to kill themselves. The percentage of those who report thinking about suicide ranges from 5 to 20 percent; most of these have major depressions. Many mental health professionals argue that what makes patients with severe illnesses suicidal is depression, not their physical condition. Cognitive therapy (discussed in Chapter 3) has proved effective in reducing the risk of suicide in even extremely suicidal patients, many of whom were already taking drugs for depression.[39]

Because depression may indeed warp the ability to make a rational decision about suicide, mental health professionals urge physicians and family members to make sure individuals with chronic or fatal illnesses are evaluated for depression and given medication, psychotherapy, or both. It is also important for everyone to allow enough time—an average of three to eight weeks—to see if treatment for depression will make a difference in their desire to keep living.

PHYSICIAN-ASSISTED SUICIDE

 According to U.S. surveys, there is greater support for physician-assisted suicide and euthanasia among patients and the general public than among physicians.[40] More Caucasians support these practices than members of ethnic minority groups.[41]

If patients have a right to die, should doctors help them end their lives? Physicians could stop any extraordinary efforts to sustain life (for example, by withholding oxygen or ending intravenous feedings); such actions are referred to as passive **euthanasia,** or **dyathanasia.** Euthanasia, the active form of so-called mercy killing, has generally been viewed as illegal and unethical. Euthanasia is tolerated and legally pardoned in the Netherlands but remains illegal in all European countries. The demand for physician-assisted death in the Netherlands has not risen; and patients and physicians have become more reluctant to ask for or offer this option over the past few years.[42]

Oregon has passed the "Death with Dignity" act and is the first state to legalize physician-assisted suicide for terminally ill patients. Legal challenges to it continue. This law bars suicide assistance for anyone whose judgment may be impaired by a mental disorder.

In the 1990s, Jack Kevorkian, M.D., a Michigan pathologist, stirred public debate by using a "suicide machine" to help end the life (at their request) of dozens of people suffering from chronic, but not necessarily fatal, illnesses. He is serving a prison sentence for murder. Some medical groups, such as the American Medical Association, oppose as unethical any physician's involvement in euthanasia. Others argue that individuals have the right to end their own lives and that physicians who provide prescriptions for lethal doses of certain drugs are acting out of compassion and respect for patients' wishes.

THE PRACTICALITIES OF DEATH

At a time of great emotional pain, grieving family members must cope with medical, legal, and practical concerns, including obtaining a medical certificate of the cause of death, registering the death, and making funeral arrangements. They also may want to arrange for organ donations and, in some circumstances, an autopsy.

FUNERAL ARRANGEMENTS

A body can be either buried or cremated. Burial requires the purchase of a cemetery plot, which many families do decades before death. A burial is typically the third most expensive purchase of a lifetime, behind the cost of a house and car. The average national costs range as high as $6,000, although they vary considerably. Memorial societies are voluntary groups that help people plan in advance for death. They obtain services at moderate cost, keep the arrangements simple and dignified, and—most important, perhaps—ease the emotional and financial burden on the rest of the family when death finally does come.

If the body is to be cremated, you must comply with some additional formalities, with which the funeral director can help you. After a *cremation* (incineration of the remains), you can either collect the ashes to keep, bury, or scatter yourself, or ask the crematorium to dispose of them.

Funerals and memorial services help those in mourning to honor the deceased and to come to terms with their loss.

The tradition of a funeral may help survivors come to terms with the death, enabling them to mourn their loss and to celebrate the dead person's life. Funerals are usually held two to four days after the death. Many have two parts: a religious ceremony at a church or funeral home, and a burial ceremony at the grave site.

Alternatively, the body may be disposed of immediately, through burial, cremation, or bequeathal to a medical school, and a memorial service held later. In a memorial service, the body is not present, which may change the focus of the service from the person's death to his or her life.

AUTOPSIES

An autopsy is a detailed examination of a body after death, also called a postmortem exam. There are two types:

- **Medicolegal.** This type of autopsy is performed to establish the cause of death and to gather information about the death for use as evidence in any legal proceedings. It is done to detect any crimes and to help identify the proper person for prosecution, to investigate possible industrial hazards or contagious diseases that may endanger the public health, or to establish the cause of death for insurance purposes.

- **Medical/educational.** This type of autopsy is performed, usually in the hospital where the person died, to increase medical knowledge and to determine a more exact cause of death. It may be requested by the attending physician or the family, but it cannot be performed without the family's permission.

Autopsies can be extremely valuable in establishing an accurate cause of death, revealing a different diagnosis that might have led to a change in therapy and prolonged survival in about 10 percent of cases. Thirty years ago about 50 percent of patients who died in hospitals were autopsied. However, the autopsy rate in the United States has been steadily declining, and today about 10 to 20 percent of deaths in teaching hospitals are autopsied.

Physicians are arguing for an increase in autopsies as the best method for establishing the cause of death, helping to spot infectious diseases, aiding medical education, and helping assure the high quality of medical practice. Between 8 and 24 percent of autopsies pick up a condition that a patient's doctor missed and that may have been the actual cause of death. Between 4 and 7 percent may detect the most serious type of medical error—meaning that, if the doctor had properly diagnosed the condition, the patient might have lived.[43]

GRIEF

An estimated 8 million Americans lose a member of their immediate family each year. Each death leaves an average of five people bereaved.[44] Such loss may be the single most upsetting and feared event in a person's life. It produces a wide range of reactions, including anxiety, guilt, anger, and financial concern. Many may see the death of an old person as less tragic than the death of a child or young person. A sudden death is more of a shock than one following a long illness. A suicide can be particularly devastating, because family members may wonder whether they could have done anything to prevent it. The cause of death also can affect the reactions of friends and acquaintances. Some people express less sympathy and support when individuals are murdered or take their own lives.

Encountering death can make us feel alone and vulnerable. The most common and one of the most painful experiences is the death of a parent. When both parents die, individuals may feel like orphaned children. They mourn not just for the father and mother who are gone, but also for their lost role of being someone's child.

The death of a child can be even more devastating. Eventually parents may be able to resolve their grief and accept the death as "God's will" or as "something that happens." Time erases their pain and they feel a desire to get on with their lives, consciously putting the loss behind them. Others deal with their grief by keeping busy or by substituting other problems or situations to take their minds off their loss. Yet many parents who lose a child continue to grieve for many years. Although the pain of their loss diminishes with time, they view it as part of themselves and describe an emptiness inside—even though most have rich, meaningful, and happy daily lives.

The loss of a mate can also have a profound impact, although men's and women's responses to the death—and their subsequent health risks—may depend on how their spouses died. Men whose wives die suddenly face a much greater risk of dying themselves than those whose wives die after a long illness. On the other hand, women whose husbands die after a long illness face greater risk of dying than other widows. The reason may be that men whose wives were chronically ill learned how to cope with the loss of their nurturers, while women who spend a long time caring for an ill husband may be at greater risk because of the combined burdens of caregiving and loss of financial support.

 Bereavement is not a rare occurrence on college campuses, but it is largely an ignored problem. Counselors have called upon universities to help students who have lost a loved one through initiatives such as training nonbereaved students to provide peer support and raising consciousness about bereavement.

GRIEF'S EFFECTS ON HEALTH

Men and women who lose partners, parents, or children endure so much stress that they're at increased risk of serious physical and mental illness, and even of premature death.[45] Studies of the health effects of grief have found the following:

▪ Grief produces changes in the respiratory, hormonal, and central nervous systems, and may affect functions of the heart, blood, and immune systems.

▪ Grieving adults may experience mood swings between sadness and anger, guilt and anxiety.

▪ They may feel physically sick, lose their appetite, sleep poorly, or fear that they're going crazy because they "see" the deceased person in different places.

▪ Friendships and remarriage offer the greatest protection against health problems.

▪ Some widows may have increased rates of depression, suicide, and death from cirrhosis of the liver. The greatest risk factors are poor previous mental and physical health and a lack of social support.

▪ Grieving parents, partners, and adult children are at increased risk of serious physical and mental illness, suicide, and premature death.

Sometimes grief progresses from an emotionally painful but normal experience to a more persistent problem, called *complicated grief*.[46] Individuals who experience very long-lasting or severe symptoms, including inability to accept a loved one's death, persistent thoughts about the death, and preoccupation with the lost loved one, can benefit from a type of treatment called *interpersonal psychotherapy*.[47] (See Chapter 3.)

METHODS OF MOURNING

Grief is a psychological necessity, not self-indulgence. Psychotherapists refer to grief as work, and it is—slow, tedious, and painful. Yet only by working through grief—dealing with feelings of anger and despair, and adjusting emotionally and intellectually to the loss—can bereaved individuals make their way back to the living world of hope and love.

Some widows and widowers move through the grieving process without experiencing extreme distress. Others stop somewhere in the midst of normal grieving and continue to pine for the deceased, become overly reliant on others, or show signs of denial, avoidance, or anxiety. Individuals who lose children or spouses in car accidents are particularly likely to remain depressed and anxious years later. One of the most devastating losses is the death of a child killed by a drunk driver. Many years afterward parents often cannot find any meaning in what happened.

(FAQ) HOW CAN YOU HELP SURVIVORS OF A LOSS?

Although we grieve for the dead, the living are the ones who need our help. Bereavement is such an intense state that survivors may be too numb or too stunned to ask for help. Family and friends must take the initiative and spend time with those who are mourning the loss of a loved one, even if that means sitting together silently. Offer empathy and support, and let the grieving person know with verbal and nonverbal expressions that you care and wish to help. Simply being there is enough to let your friend know you care.

You may also wish to write a simple note expressing your sympathy. "I want to let you know I'm thinking of you and praying for you" can mean a great deal. A small gift, such as a book or plant, is also thoughtful. Or you can invite your friend to do something with you. Choose something you know your friend might enjoy—a walk in the country or a concert. And don't just give your help over the first few days

Strategies for Change :: Coping with Grief

:: **Accept your feelings**—sorrow, fear, emptiness, whatever—as normal. Don't try to deny emotions such as anger, guilt, despair, or relief.

:: **Let others help you**—by bringing you food, by taking care of daily necessities; by providing companionship and comfort. (It will make them feel better, too.)

:: **Face each day as it comes.** Let yourself live in the here-and-now until you're ready to face the future. Give yourself time—perhaps more than you ever imagined—for the pain to ebb, the scars to heal, and your life to move on.

:: **Don't think there's a right or wrong way to grieve.** Mourning takes many forms, and there's no set timetable for

working through the various stages of grief.

:: **Seek professional counseling** if you remain intensely distressed for more than six months or your grief does not ease over time. Therapy can help prevent potentially serious physical and psychological problems.

or weeks and then withdraw. Grieving people continue to need support for many months. The first anniversary of a death or the first holiday spent alone can be particularly difficult.

Most bereaved people don't need professional psychological counseling. In most instances, sharing their feelings with friends is all that's needed. However, you should urge a friend or relative to seek help if he or she shows no sign of grieving, or exhibits as much distress a year after the loss as during the first months. The family members of a suicide victim are those most likely to need, and benefit from, professional help in sorting out their feelings of failure, anger, and sorrow. Therapy and medication can be enormously helpful—and potentially life-saving.

Learn It / Live It

Living Long and Well

"Every man desires to live long," wrote Jonathan Swift, "but no man would be old." We all wish for long lives, yet we want to avoid the disease and disability that can tarnish our golden years. Here are the best ways to do so.

- **Exercise regularly.** By improving blood flow, staving off depression, warding off heart disease, and enhancing well-being, regular workouts help keep mind and body in top form.
- **Don't smoke.** Every cigarette you puff can snuff out seven minutes of your life, according to the Centers for Disease Control and Prevention.
- **Watch your weight and blood pressure.** Increases in these vital statistics can increase your risk of hypertension, cardiovascular disease, and other health problems.
- **Eat more fruits and vegetables.** These foods, rich in vitamins and protective antioxidants, can reduce your risk of cancer and damage from destructive free radicals.
- **Cut down on fat.** Fatty foods can clog the arteries and contribute to various cancers.

- **Limit drinking.** Alcohol can undermine physical health and sabotage mental acuity.
- **Cultivate stimulating interests.** Elderly individuals with complex and interesting lifestyles are most likely to retain sharp minds and memories beyond age 70.
- **Don't worry; be happy.** At any age, emotional turmoil can undermine well-being. Relaxation techniques, such as meditation, help by reducing stress.
- **Reach out.** Try to keep in contact with other people of all ages and experiences. Make the effort to invite them to your home or go out with them. On a regular basis, do something to help another person.
- **Make the most of your time.** Greet each day with a specific goal—to take a walk, write letters, visit a friend.

Making This Chapter Work for You

Review Questions

1. Factors that contribute to staying healthy longer include all of the following *except*
   a. avoiding illness.
   b. moderate smoking.
   c. regular exercise.
   d. lifelong learning.

2. Physically fit people over age 60
   a. have lower risk of dying from chronic heart disease.
   b. can regain the fitness level of a 25-year-old.
   c. show no difference in levels of anxiety and depression.
   d. have higher health-care expenses.

3. Which statement about the aging brain is *false?*
   a. When brain cells die, surrounding cells can fill the gaps to maintain cognitive function.
   b. Remembering names and recalling information may take longer.

(continued on p. 544)

Self Survey ▪▪ What is Your Aging I.Q.?

Answer true or false

T F 1. Everyone becomes "senile" sooner or later, if he or she lives long enough.

T F 2. American families have by and large abandoned their older members.

T F 3. Depression is a serious problem for older people.

T F 4. The numbers of older people are growing.

T F 5 The vast majority of older people are self-sufficient.

T F 6. Mental confusion is an inevitable, incurable consequence of old age.

T F 7. Intelligence declines with age.

T F 8. Sexual urges and activity normally cease around age 55–60.

T F 9. If a person has been smoking for 30 or 40 years, it does no good to quit.

T F 10. Older people should stop exercising and rest.

T F 11. As you grow older, you need more vitamins and minerals to stay healthy.

T F 12. Only children need to be concerned about calcium for strong bones and teeth.

T F 13. Extremes of heat and cold can be particularly dangerous to old people.

T F 14. Many older people are hurt in accidents that could have been prevented.

T F 15. More men than women survive to old age.

T F 16. Death from stroke and heart disease are declining.

T F 17. Older people on the average take more medications than younger people.

T F 18. Snake oil salesmen are as common today as they were on the frontier.

T F 19. Personality changes with age, just like hair color and skin texture.

T F 20. Sight declines with age.

Scoring

1. False. Even among those who live to be 80 or older, only 20–25 percent develop Alzheimer's disease or some other incurable form of brain disease. "Senility" is a meaningless term that should be discarded.

2. False. The American family is still the number one caretaker of older Americans. Most older people live close to their children and see them often; many live with their spouses. In all, 8 out of 10 men and 6 out of 10 women live in family settings.

3. True. Depression, loss of self-esteem, loneliness, and anxiety can become more common as older people face retirement, the deaths of relatives and friends, and other such crises—often at the same time. Fortunately, depression is treatable.

4. True. Today, 12 percent of the U.S. population are 65 or older. By the year 2030, one in five people will be over 65 years of age.

5. True. Only 5 percent of the older population live in nursing homes; the rest are basically healthy and self-sufficient.

6. False. Mental confusion and serious forgetfulness in old age can be caused by Alzheimer's disease or other conditions that cause incurable damage to the brain, but some 100 other problems can cause the same symptoms. A minor head injury, a high fever, poor nutrition, adverse drug reactions, and depression can all be treated and the confusion will be cured.

7. False. Intelligence per se does not decline without reason. Most people maintain their intellect or improve as they grow older.

8. False. Most older people can lead an active, satisfying sex life.

9. False. Stopping smoking at any age not only reduces the risk of cancer and heart disease, it also leads to healthier lungs.

10. False. Many older people enjoy—and benefit from—exercises such as walking, swimming, and bicycle riding. Exercise at any age can help strengthen the heart and lungs, and lower blood pressure. See your physician before beginning a new exercise program.

11. False. Although certain requirements, such as that for "sunshine" vitamin D, may increase slightly with age, older people need the same amounts of most vitamins and minerals as younger people. Older people in particular should eat nutritious food and cut down on sweets, salty snack foods, high-calorie drinks, and alcohol.

12. False. Older people require fewer calories, but adequate intake of calcium for strong bones can become more important as you grow older. This is particularly true for women, whose risk of osteoporosis increases after menopause. Milk and cheese are rich in calcium as are cooked dried beans, collards, and broccoli. Some people need calcium supplements as well.

13. True. The body's thermostat tends to function less efficiently with age and the older person's body may be less able to adapt to heat or cold.

14. True. Falls are the most common cause of injuries among the elderly. Good safety habits, including proper lighting, nonskid carpets, and keeping living areas free of obstacles, can help prevent serious accidents.

15. False. Women tend to outlive men by an average of 8 years. There are 150 women for every 100 men over age 65, and nearly 250 women for every 100 men over 85.

16. True. Fewer men and women are dying of stroke or heart disease.

17. True. The elderly consume 25 percent of all medications and, as a result, have many more problems with adverse drug reactions.
18. True. Medical quackery is a $10 billion business in the United States. People of all ages are commonly duped into "quick cures" for aging, arthritis, and cancer.
19. False. Personality doesn't change with age. Therefore, all old people can't be described as rigid and cantankerous. You are what you are for as long as you live. But you can change what you do to help yourself to good health.
20. False. Although changes in vision become more common with age, any change in vision, regardless of age, is related to a specific disease. If you are having problems with your vision, see your doctor.

Source: National Institute on Aging, www.counselingnotes.com/seniors/age/age_iq.htm.

YOUR ACTION PLAN FOR PREPARING FOR A MEDICAL CRISIS IN AN AGING RELATIVE

"Medical crises are more common and more likely to lead to serious complications after age 60," says Kenneth Brummel-Smith, M.D., former president of the American Geriatrics Society. As your parents, grandparents, and other relatives get older, here is what you can do in advance:

▪ **Watch for warning signals.** If your relative begins stumbling or having near-misses on the highway, make sure he or she sees a doctor before a serious fall or accident occurs. There may be a cure or, if not a cure, a way to improve functioning.

▪ **Suggest a surrogate.** Even if a couple has been married for 40 years, neither has the legal right to make medical decisions for a spouse. The same is true for children and other relatives. The only way to get that right is to fill out a form, usually called an advance directive or legal power of attorney (discussed on page 530).

▪ **Talk to loved ones.** "Waiting for something bad to happen doesn't make it any easier to talk about," says Dr. Brummel-Smith, who suggests sitting down for a formal discussion at some point after a relative reaches age 65 "but definitely before age 75."

▪ **Focus on values.** "You don't have to discuss every possible drug or surgery or intervention," says Dr. Brummel-Smith. "What's important is that you understand the older person's values. What are fates worse than death? Independence may be more important than living a longer life." Many families use the "Five Wishes" form (available online at www.aging withdignity.org and described on page 530) to discuss preferences for medical, personal, emotional, and spiritual care.

▪ **Involve the person's primary physician.** Often it's not a question of what doctors can do medically in a crisis, but of what they should do, which is the patient's decision. Encourage loved ones to discuss "what ifs" with their doctors and make their desires clear. For instance, a primary physician should know which treatments patients want (such as resuscitation during surgery) as well as those they don't want (such as remaining on a ventilator if unable to breathe on their own).

▪ **Investigate alternative living options.** Aging parents should visit retirement communities or nursing homes while they're still healthy, not with the idea of moving into them, but of knowing what's available. They also should find out if their health plan or HMO provides services for seniors after a medical crisis.

▪ **Make sure you know where to find key documents.** An easily accessible folder with copies of the latest lab reports, consultations, and advance directives helps to avoid unnecessary tests and get faster treatment when a crisis does occur.

CASE IN POINT

Student: Shayla, 20
Goal: To stay in touch with her aging grandparents
Health Action Plan:

▪ Send short notes or postcards every week or two
▪ Make a mix CD of music from her grandparents' youth
▪ Bring photo albums to reminisce about with them
▪ Do an oral history of her family
▪ Make a date to visit by phone at least once a month

Health ☾ Now ™   If you want to write your own goals for aging well, go to the **Wellness Journal** at **HealthNow**, http://healthnow.brookscole.com/ith

    c. "Use it or lose it."

    d. Mental ability and physical ability both decline with age.

4. Which statement about aging is *false?*

    a. The most common nutritional disorder in the elderly is obesity.

    b. In men, sexual activity and longevity are linked.

    c. Hormone therapy reduces the risk of heart disease in menopausal women.

    d. Seniors who take up new hobbies late in life may slow aging within the brain.

5. Which statement about age-related problems is correct?

    a. Osteoporosis affects only women.

    b. Alzheimer's disease is a form of dementia.

    c. Osteoporosis treatment includes surgery.

    d. Drug interactions do not occur in the elderly.

6. When should concern change to intervention?

    a. Uncle Charlie is 85 and continues to drive himself to the grocery store and to the Senior Center during the daytime.

    b. Nana takes pills at breakfast, lunch, and dinner but sometimes mixes them up.

    c. Mom's hot flashes have become a family joke.

    d. Your older brother can never remember where he put his car keys.

7. According to Elisabeth Kübler-Ross, an individual facing death goes through all of the following emotional stages *except*

    a. bargaining.

    b. acceptance.

    c. denial.

    d. repression.

8. The gender gap related to longevity

    a. is due to deficiencies in the Y chromosome.

    b. results from the presence of a mutant gene.

    c. may be due to the X chromosome and its hormonal influences on the immune system.

    d. is about 13 years in the United States.

9. An advance directive

    a. indicates who should have your property in the event you die.

    b. may authorize which individuals may not participate in your health care if you are unable to care for yourself.

    c. can specify your desires related to the use of medical treatments and technology to prolong your life.

    d. should specify which physician you designate to be your health-care proxy.

10. You can best help a friend who is bereaved by

    a. encouraging him to have a few drinks to forget his pain.

    b. simply spending time with her.

    c. avoiding talking about his loss because it is awkward.

    d. reminding her about all she still has in her life.

Answers to these questions can be found on page 587.

Critical Thinking

1. How are your parents or other mentors staying fit and alert as they age? Do you think you might use similar strategies?

2. Do you think that coming to terms with mortality allows an individual to live each day to its fullest, rather than putting off what he or she would like to do until tomorrow? How does this concept affect your own life? Explain. Do you believe in a next life? How does this affect your view of life and death?

3. Have your living parents and grandparents written advanced directives or a living will? Have you discussed with them their preferences regarding treatment in the event of a medical crisis? If you haven't had this discussion with your family, how can you begin the process of helping your parents or grandparents communicate their wishes?

4. As many as 10,000 people in this country are chronically unconscious, kept alive by artificial respirators and feeding tubes. If you were in an accident that left you in a vegetative state, would you want doctors to do everything possible to fight for your life? Would you want to spend months or even years totally unaware of your surroundings? Should health-care professionals have the right to declare that anyone is too old, too ill, or too frail to try to save? Should they have the right to insist that someone live on even if that person isn't experiencing much of a life?

Media Menu

Health�&Now™

Throughout the chapter, this icon introduces a list of resources on the Health-Now website at **http://healthnow.brookscole.com/ith** that will:

- Help you evaluate your knowledge of the material.
- Allow you to take an exam-prep quiz.
- Provide a Personalized Learning Plan targeting resources that address areas you should study.
- Coach you through identifying target goals for behavior change and creating and monitoring your personal change plan throughout the semester.

INTERNET CONNECTIONS

National Institute on Aging
www.nia.nih.gov

This government site features a comprehensive array of resources on aging, including publications on a variety of geriatric health topics, current news events, and a resource directory for older people.

RealAge

www.realage.com

This site features diet and exercise assessment tools—such as a BMI calculator, exercise estimator, and RealAge assessment quizzes on a variety of health topics—to help you determine your risk of disease and what you can do to reduce this risk. The main feature is an interactive online personal lifestyle assessment that also gives you options for "growing younger."

U.S. Administration on Aging

http://aoa.gov

This site, part of the Department of Health and Human Services, has information for seniors and their families on promoting healthy lifestyles and general aging topics.

The End of Life: Exploring Death in America

www.npr.org/programs/death/

This site, sponsored by National Public Radio, contains transcripts and resources from an *All Things Considered* series focusing on how Americans deal with death and dying. Features include personal stories, a place where you can tell your own story, and a comprehensive list of organizations that can help families who are coping with death, dying, and the diseases of old age.

InfoTrac College Edition Activities Log on, insert **advance directives** into the Keyword search box, and limit your search to the past year. When you get the results, Mark articles to review, then Select one to read. Summarize three or four key points from the article.

You can find additional readings related to personal health with InfoTrac College Edition, an online library of more than 900 journals and publications. Follow the instructions for accessing InfoTrac College Edition that were packaged with your textbook; then search for articles using a keyword search.

For additional links, resources, and suggested readings on the InfoTrac College Edition, visit our Health and Wellness Resource Center at **http://health .wadsworth.com.**

Key Terms

The terms listed are used on the page indicated. Definitions of the terms are in the Glossary at the end of this book.

advance directives 530	hormone therapy (HRT) 525
aging 519	hospice 537
Alzheimer's disease 527	living will 530
autoscopy 537	menopause 524
coma 533	near death experience 537
dementia 527	osteoporosis 528
do-not-resuscitate (DNR) 530	perimenopause 524
dyathanasia 538	persistent vegetative state 533
euthanasia 538	terminal illness 535
holographic will 533	transcendence 537

"This can't be happening to me!" This was the phrase that first ran through Parker's mind when the car swerved out of control. He kept repeating it to himself as he heard the sickening sound of metal hitting metal and felt a terrible crushing pain shoot up through his legs. Later at the hospital, when he woke up after surgery, it was his first thought. And all through the long months of rehabilitation, on the days when he thought life would never go back to normal, he'd try to tell himself that this too couldn't be happening to him.

Most young people think the same way. Accidents, injuries, assaults, crimes—all seem like things that happen only to other people, only in other places. But no one, regardless of how young, healthy, or strong, is immune from danger. The risks to college students include alcohol-associated injuries and illnesses, traffic accidents, and physical and sexual assaults.

Recognizing the threat of intentional and unintentional injury is the first step to ensuring your personal safety. You may think that the risk of something bad happening is simply a matter of chance, of being in the wrong place at the wrong time. That's not the case. Certain behaviors, such as using alcohol or drugs or not buckling your seat belt, greatly increase the risk of harm. Ultimately, you have more control over your safety than anyone or anything else in your life.

This chapter is a primer in self-protection that could help safeguard—perhaps even save—your life. Included are recommendations for common sense safety on the road, at home, and at work. This chapter also explores other serious threats to personal safety in our society: violence and sexual victimization.

After studying the material in this chapter, you should be able to:

▌ **List** and **explain** factors that increase the likelihood of an accident.

▌ **Describe** procedures for safety on the road, at work, and at home.

▌ **Define** hate crimes.

▌ **Define** sexual victimization, sexual harassment, stalking, and sexual coercion.

▌ **List** the different types of rape, and describe recommended actions for preventing rape.

▌ **Explain** the consequences of sexual violence.

PERSONAL SAFETY

The major threat to the lives of college students isn't illness but injury. Almost 75 percent of deaths among Americans 15 to 24 years old are caused by "unintentional injuries" (a term public health officials prefer), suicides, and homicides. The odds of dying from an injury in any given year are about 1 in 765; over a lifetime they rise to 1 in 23.[1] In all, injuries—intentional and unintentional—claim almost 150,000 lives a year. Accidents, especially motor vehicle crashes, kill more college-age men and women than all other causes combined; the greatest number of lives lost to accidents is among those 25 years of age.

UNINTENTIONAL INJURY: WHY ACCIDENTS HAPPEN

Some of the many factors that influence an individual's risk of accident or injury are these:

- **Age.** Injury is the leading cause of death during the first four decades of life in the United States. Most victims of fatal accidents are males, often in their teens and twenties. Feeling full of life and energy, they may take dangerous risks because they think they're invulnerable.

- **Alcohol.** An estimated 40 percent of Americans are involved in an alcohol-related accident sometime during their lives. Alcohol plays a role in about a quarter of fatal motor vehicle accidents and half of fatal motorcycle crashes.[2]

- **Stress.** When we're tense and anxious, we all pay less attention to what we're doing. One common result is an increase in accidents. If you find yourself having a series of small mishaps or near-misses, do something to lower your stress level, rather than wait for something more harmful to happen (see Chapter 4).

- **Situational Factors.** Some situations—such as driving on a curvy, wet road in a car with worn tires—are so inherently dangerous that they greatly increase the odds of an accident. But even when there's greater risk, you can lower the danger: For instance, you can make sure your tires and brakes are in good condition.

- **Thrill Seeking.** To some people, activities that others might find terrifying—such as skydiving or parachute jumping—are stimulating. These thrill seekers may have lower than normal levels of the brain chemicals that regulate excitement. Because the stress of potentially hazardous sports may increase the levels of these chemicals, they feel pleasantly aroused rather than scared.

(FAQ) WHAT SHOULD I DO IN AN EMERGENCY?

Life-threatening situations rarely happen more than once or twice in any person's life. When they do, you must think and act quickly to prevent disastrous consequences.

- **Stop, look, and listen.**
- Your immediate response to an emergency may be overwhelming fear and anxiety. Take several deep breaths. Start by assessing the circumstances. Look for any possible dangers to you or the victim, such as a live electrical wire or a fire. Listen for sounds, such as a cry for help or a siren. Don't attempt rescue techniques, such as cardiopulmonary resuscitation (CPR), unless you're trained.

- **Don't wait for symptoms to go away or get worse.** If you suspect that someone is having a heart attack or stroke, or has ingested something poisonous, *phone for help immediately.* A delay could jeopardize the person's life. Stay on the line long enough to give your name, address, and a brief description of the emergency.

- **Don't move a victim.** The person may have a broken neck or back, and attempting to move him or her could cause extensive damage or even death.

- **Don't drive.** Even if the hospital is just ten minutes away, you're better off waiting for a well-equipped ambulance with trained paramedics who can deliver emergency care on the spot. People rushing to emergency rooms are more likely to get into accidents themselves.

- **Don't do too much.** Often well-intentioned Good Samaritans make injuries worse by trying to tie tourniquets, wash cuts, or splint broken limbs. Also, don't give an injured person anything to eat or drink. (See "Emergency!" in the Hales Health Almanac at the back of this book for more on first-aid and emergency care.)

- **At home, keep a supply of basic first-aid items in a convenient place.** Beyond the emergency number 911, make sure that telephone numbers for your doctor and neighbors are handy.

BECOMING A SAFER DRIVER

With more drivers and more vehicles on the roads than ever before, the fatality rate per 100 million vehicle miles of travel has fallen to an all-time low.[3] However, despite the progress that has been made, our streets and highways remain dangerous. Eight nations now have lower fatality rates than the United States.

An average of 120 people die in motor vehicle crashes every day in the United States. Alcohol use is a factor in about 50 of these crashes; speeding, in about 40. Rollovers caused by drivers who lose control of their vehicles kill about 25 people daily. Crashes involving teen drivers result in about 25 fatalities each day.[4]

Motor vehicle accidents in the United States annually claim about 42,800 lives and injure almost three million people, more than any other form of unintentional injury. They are the leading cause of all deaths for people ages 2 to 33; only cancer and heart attacks claim more American lives. Driving accidents have killed more Canadians in the last 50 years than both World Wars.[5]

 College students aren't necessarily safer drivers than others their age. According to national data, full-time college students drink and drive more often than part-time students and other young adults, but they also are more likely to wear seat belts while driving and riding in cars.[6] How can you increase your odds of staying safe on the road? Some key factors are staying sober and alert, using your seat belt, making sure your vehicle has working air bags, and controlling road rage.

STAY SOBER AND ALERT

The number of fatalities caused by drunk driving, particularly among young people, has dropped. The NHTSA attributes this decline to increases in the drinking age, to educational programs aimed at reducing nighttime driving by teens, to the formation of Students Against Destructive Decisions (SADD; originally called Students Against Drunk Driving), and similar groups, and to changes in state laws that lowered the legal blood-alcohol concentration level for drivers under age 21 (some states have zero tolerance blood alcohol level (BAC) for drivers under 21).

Falling asleep at the wheel is second only to alcohol as a cause of serious motor-vehicle accidents. About half of drivers in the United States drive while drowsy. Nearly 14 million have fallen asleep at the wheel in the past year, according to the National Sleep Foundation. Men and young adults between the ages of 18 and 29 are at the highest risk for driving while drowsy or falling asleep at the wheel.

BUCKLE UP

Seat belt use has reached an all-time high, with three in four Americans buckling up. States with seat belt laws have even higher rates of use: 80 percent. However, young people are less likely to use seat belts. Men between ages 19 and 29 are least likely to wear seat belts while driving or riding in a car.[7] By official estimates, two-thirds of 15- to 20-year-olds killed in motor vehicle accidents were not wearing seat belts.[8]

Seat belts save an estimated 9,500 lives in the United States each year. When lap-shoulder belts are used properly, they reduce the risk of fatal injury to front-seat passengers by 45 percent and the risk of moderate to critical injury by 50 percent. Because an unrestrained passenger can

Buckling up is one of the simplest and most effective ways of protecting yourself from injury.

© Nick Clements

injure others during a crash, the risk of death is lowest when all occupants wear seat belts, according to federal analysts.[9] Seat belt use by everyone in a car may prevent about one in six deaths that might otherwise occur in a crash.[10]

CHECK FOR AIR BAGS

An air bag, either with or without a seat belt, has proved the most effective means of preventing adult death, somewhat more so for women than for men. However, they do not lower the risk of serious injury. A study of 15 million people involved in crashes found that seat belts provided the most protection. Air bags used in conjunction with seat belts did not significantly reduce the risk of injury; without seat belts, they increased the risk of injury, particularly to the head and legs.[11]

Because there is controversy over the potential hazard they pose to children, the American Academy of Pediatrics recommends that children be placed in the backseat, whether or not the car is equipped with a passenger air bag.

REIN IN ROAD RAGE

The emotional outbursts known as road rage are a factor in as many as two-thirds of all fatal car crashes and one-third of nonfatal accidents, according to the NHTSA. Psychologist

Arnold Nerenberg of Whittier, California, a specialist in motorway mayhem, estimates 1.78 billion episodes of road rage a year, resulting in more than 28,000 deaths and 1 million injuries.[12]

Some strategies for reducing road rage include the following:

- **Lower the stress in your life.** Take a few moments to breathe deeply and relax your shoulders before putting the key in the ignition.

- **Consciously decide not to let other drivers get to you.** Decide that whatever happens, it's not going to make your blood pressure go up.

- **Slow down.** If you're going five or ten miles over the speed limit, you won't have the time you need to react to anything that happens.

- **Modify bad driving habits one at a time.** If you tend to tailgate slow drivers, spend a week driving at twice your usual following distance. If you're a habitual horn honker, silence yourself.

- **Be courteous—even if other drivers aren't.** Don't dawdle in the passing lane. Never tailgate or switch lanes without signaling. Don't use your horn or high beams unless absolutely necessary.

- **Never retaliate.** Whatever another driver does, keep your cool. Count to ten. Take a deep breath. If you yell or gesture at someone who's upset with you, the conflict may well escalate.

- **If you do something stupid, show that you're sorry.** On its website, the AAA Foundation for Traffic Safety solicited suggestions for automotive apologies. The most popular: slapping yourself on your forehead or the top of your head to indicate that you know you goofed. Such gestures can soothe a miffed motorist—and make the roads a slightly safer place for all of us.

(FAQ) IS IT SAFE TO TALK ON THE PHONE WHILE DRIVING?

According to the National Highway Traffic Safety Administration, driver distraction from various causes plays a role in 20 to 30 percent of all motor vehicle crashes. People who use mobile phones while driving are four times more likely to have a serious crash.[13]

 Most college students with cell phones use them when driving. A third of these have been involved in a serious car accident.[14] In some states, it is now illegal to talk on a cell phone while driving.

Although many believe that hands-free car phones are less hazardous, researchers have shown this is not the case. Talking on a wireless phone while driving a car is just as dangerous with a hands-free or a handheld phone. The reason is that talking while driving distracts the brain as well as the eyes—much more so than talking to another person in the vehicle. Conversation on any type of phone disrupts a driver's attention to the visual environment, leading to what researchers call "inattention blindness," the inability to recognize objects encountered in the driver's visual field. This form of cognitive impairment may distract drivers for up to two minutes after the phone conversation has ended.[15]

On the other hand, mobile phones are helpful in alerting authorities to road hazards, congestion, or problem drivers and in summoning help in case of a breakdown or other emergency.

Car Phone Safety Tips

- Find out if cell phone use while driving is legal in your state.
- Do not dial new calls until you're stopped or in a safe low-traffic environment.
- Keep calls short, less than 1 or 2 minutes.

❚ Strategies for Prevention ❚❚ How to Drive Safely

- ❚❚ Don't drive while under the influence of alcohol or other drugs, including medications that may impair your reflexes, cause drowsiness, or affect your judgment. Never get into a car if you suspect the driver may be intoxicated or affected by a drug.

- ❚❚ Remain calm when dealing with drivers who are reckless or rude. Be alert and anticipate possible hazards. Don't let yourself be distracted by conversations, children's questions, arguments, food or drink, or scenic views.

- ❚❚ Don't get too comfortable. Alertness matters. Use the rearview mirror often.

- ❚❚ Don't let passengers or packages obstruct your view. Use turn signals when changing lanes or making a turn. If someone cuts you off, back off to a safe distance.

- ❚❚ Watch out for warning signs of fatigue, such as difficulty focusing, frequent blinking or heavy eyelids, trouble keeping one's head up; repeated yawning; trouble remembering the last few miles driven; and drifting from the lane or hitting the shoulder rumble strip.

- ❚❚ Drive more slowly if weather conditions are bad. Avoid driving at all during heavy rain, snow, or other conditions that affect visibility and road conditions. If you must drive in hazardous conditions, make sure that your car has the proper equipment, such as chains or snow tires, and that you know how to respond in case of a skid.

- ❚❚ Maintain your car properly, replacing windshield wipers, tires, and brakes when necessary. Keep flares and a fire extinguisher in your car for use in emergencies.

Any form of distraction, including talking on a cell phone, can put you and others at risk.

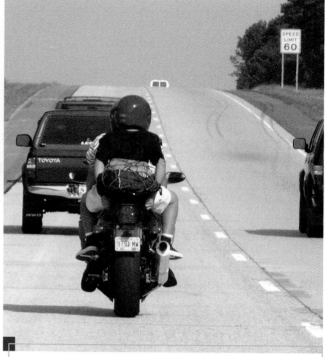

In states with motorcycle helmet laws, motorcyclist deaths and injuries have decreased significantly.

■ When you're on the phone, avoid difficult maneuvers, such as changing lanes, that require a lot of attention.

■ Have a passenger send or receive calls.

■ Invest in a hands-free model, especially if you use your phone regularly. While the cognitive distraction is the same, it helps to avoid the mechanical distraction.

SAFE CYCLING

Mile for mile, motorcycling is far more risky than automobile driving. The most common motorcycle injury is head trauma, which can lead to physical disability, including paralysis and general weakness, as well as problems reading and thinking. It can also cause personality changes and psychiatric problems, such as depression, anxiety, uncontrollable mood swings, and anger. Complete recovery from head trauma can take four to six years, and the costs can be staggering. Head injury can also result in permanent disability, coma, and death. To prevent head trauma, motorcycle helmets are required in most states.

Approximately 80.6 million people ride bicycles. Each year, bicycle crashes kill about 750 to 1,500 of these individuals and send 450,000 to 587,000 to emergency rooms. Men are more likely to suffer cycling injuries. Head injury is the cause of 70 to 85 percent of bicycle crash deaths.[16]

According to a national survey, 50 percent of all bicycle riders in the United States regularly wear bike helmets—43 percent every time they ride and 7 percent more than half the time. Wearing a helmet can reduce head injuries and deaths by an estimated 29 to 90 percent, depending on the type of helmet[17] (see Savvy Consumer: "Buying a Bicycle Helmet").

Savvy Consumer ■ Buying a Bicycle Helmet

What should you look for when buying a helmet? Here are some basic guidelines:

▪ A government regulation requires all helmets produced after 1999 to meet the Consumer Product Safety Commission standard; look for a CPSC sticker inside the helmet. The ASTM (American Society for Testing and Materials) standard is comparable to CPSC. The Snell Memorial Foundation's B-90 standard is even better.

▪ Check the fit. The helmet should sit level on your head, touching all around, comfortably snug but not tight. The helmet should not move more than about an inch in any direction, regardless of how hard you tug at it.

▪ Pick a bright color for visibility. Avoid dark colors, thin straps, or a rigid visor that could snag in a fall.

▪ Look for a smooth plastic outer shell, not one with alternating strips of plastic and foam.

▪ Watch out for excessive vents, which put less protective foam in contact with your head in a crash.

▪ Mirrors should have a breakaway mount; the wire type mounted on eyeglasses can gouge an eye in a fall.

SAFETY AT WORK

The workplace is second only to the home as the most frequent site of accidents. More than 5,500 injury deaths occur on the job every year.[18] The industries with the highest fatality rates are mining; transportation, communication, and public utilities; construction; and agriculture, forestry, and fishing. Whatever your job, find out about potential hazards and learn the proper safety regulations. (Chapter 19 discusses some potential environmental hazards at work, including noise and toxic substances.)

According to a report by the National Research Council and Institute of Medicine, annually about one million workers suffer musculoskeletal disorders of the lower back and upper extremities as a result of their "particular jobs and working conditions—including heavy lifting, repetitive and forceful motions, and stressful working conditions." Many can be prevented.[19]

(FAQ) CAN MY COMPUTER BE A HEALTH HAZARD?

As computers have become part of daily life for everyone from preschoolers to seniors, health professionals have learned a great deal about potential health problems, including repetitive motion injuries and vision-related difficulties.

REPETITIVE MOTION INJURIES

Repetitive motion injuries (RMI) have surpassed back and neck injuries as the number one claim for workers compensation injuries. Repeated motions—such as the hand and arm movements made while using a computer keyboard—all day, every day, can result in muscle and tendon strain and inflammation. About 20 percent of people with pain, tingling, or numbness in the hands may have carpal tunnel syndrome, an overuse injury caused by repetitive motions in the hands and wrists. Symptoms include pain, swelling, and numbness and weakness in the hands or the arms. If these problems are identified early, permanent damage can generally be avoided by altering the work environment and allowing for more breaks during the day.

The slope and height of a computer keyboard can affect the likelihood of repetitive motion injuries. If you work at a computer, good posture and correct positioning of the computer screen and keyboard can help prevent repetitive motion injuries, eyestrain, and back strain (Figure 19-1). Here are some additional tips:

- Place the keyboard so that your elbows are bent at a 90° angle and you don't have to bend your wrists to type.
- Use a chair that provides ample back support. Keep your thighs parallel to the floor and your feet on the floor. If your feet don't reach the floor, use a footrest.

The screen should be at eye level (22–26 inches higher than your seat).

Position the keyboard so that your elbows are bent at a 90° angle and your hands and wrists are straight.

Sit straight in your chair; for extra back support, place a rolled-up towel behind you.

Keep your hands and wrists relaxed.

FIGURE 19-1 Safe Computing

By paying attention to your posture and your computer's position, you can help protect yourself from repetitive motion injury, back strain, and eyestrain.

- If you experience neck strain, place a document holder next to your screen so that you can view the materials more easily.
- Every 15 minutes take a 30-second break, stretch your arms, and walk around the office. Take a 15-minute break at least once every two hours.

VISION PROBLEMS

Computer vision syndrome is a condition marked by tired and sore eyes, blurred vision, headaches, and neck, shoulder, and back pain. The American Optometric Association estimates that it afflicts nearly 90 percent of workers who use computers and also is common among children and students of all ages. The symptoms result from repeatedly stressing some aspect of the visual system, but they often disappear as soon as the person stops working at the computer.

The eye focuses on a computer image differently from the way it focuses on a printed one. The pixels that appear on a computer screen, unlike printed characters, are bright in the center and gradually fade away into the background color. This makes it difficult for the eye to sustain focus. Optometrists have developed a specific method, called a PRIO examination, that simulates how the eye responds to pixels on a computer screen. It can determine the need and proper prescription for computer-only eyeglasses.

SAFETY AT HOME

Every year home accidents cause nearly 25 million injuries. Poison poses the greatest threat, causing more than 17,000 deaths every year. Half a million children swallow poisonous materials each year; 90 percent are under age 5. Adults may also be poisoned by mistakenly taking someone else's prescription drugs or taking medicines in the dark and swallowing the wrong one. In most cities, you can call a poison control center for advice.

FALLS

Falls of all kinds are the second leading cause of death from unintentional injury in the United States. High heels or worn footgear, poor lighting, slippery or uneven walkways, broken stairs and handrails, loose or worn rugs, and objects left where people walk all increase the likelihood of a slip.

FIRES

You can prevent fires by making sure that the three ingredients of fire—fuel, a heat source, and oxygen—don't get a chance to mix. Almost anything can act as fuel for fire, including paper, wood, and flammable liquids such as oils, gasoline, and some paints. A heat source can be a spark from a lighted match, a pilot light, or an electrical wire. Oxygen is necessary for the chemical reaction between the fuel and heat source that causes combustion.

If a fire starts and it's small, you may be able to put it out with a portable fire extinguisher before it spreads. However, if the fire does get out of control, you might have only two to five minutes to get out of the house or building alive. A fire-escape plan can save time and lives. Sketch a plan of your house, apartment building, dormitory, or fraternity or sorority house. Identify two ways out of each room or apartment. Make sure everyone is familiar with these escape routes. Designate an area outside where all family members or dorm residents should meet after escaping from a fire. In a national survey, 67 percent of colleges had at least one dorm without a sprinkler system.[20] If a fire breaks out in your dorm room, get out as quickly as possible, but don't run. Before opening a room door, place your hand on it. If it's hot, don't open it. If the door feels cool, open it slightly to check for smoke; if there's none, leave by your planned escape route. If you're on an upper floor and your escape routes are blocked, open a window (top and bottom, if possible) and wait or signal from the window for help. Never try to use an elevator in a fire.

SAFETY AT PLAY

According to a study by the Johns Hopkins School of Public Health, every year 750,000 Americans are injured during recreational activities such as horseback riding, skiing, sledding, skating, and playground activities; 82,000 suffer head injuries requiring emergency room or hospital treatment.

■ **Drowning.** Over the last few decades, deaths from drowning have declined. Possible reasons include less use of alcohol by swimmers and boaters, and an increase in body fat, which makes floating easier. Toddlers under age 4 and teenage boys between 15 and 19 remain at greatest risk. Most drownings occur at unorganized facilities, such as ponds or pools with no lifeguard present. Among young children, 90 percent of drownings occur in residential swimming pools.

The causes of drowning, in order of frequency, are becoming exhausted, being swept into deep water, losing support, becoming trapped or entangled, having a cramp or other attack, and striking an underwater object. Many drowning victims were strong swimmers.

■ **Snowboarding.** Wrist fractures and arm/shoulder injuries are the most common injuries in snowboarding. Wrist fractures can be disabling and lead to early development of osteoarthritis, especially when the break goes through the joint line. Novice snowboarders are at greatest risk. Conventional wrist guards or an integrated glove/guard system can significantly reduce the danger.

■ **Cycling.** See p. 551.

■ See "Beyond the Gym" on p. 136 in Chapter 5.

(FAQ) ♀ WHICH GENDER IS AT GREATER RISK?

Just like illness, injury doesn't discriminate against either gender. Both men and women can find themselves in harm's way—but for different reasons. Here are some gender differences in vulnerability:

■ Men are ten times more likely to die of an occupational injury than women.

■ Males are most often the victims and the perpetrators of homicides in the United States. In about 68 percent of cases reported by the Bureau of Justice Statistics, both the offender and the victim were male.

■ Overall, men are 3.6 times more likely than women to be murdered and 9 times more likely to commit murder. Both men and women are more likely to kill or attempt to kill male victims than female victims.

■ Men are 1.5 times more likely than women to be assaulted as an adult. Each year 3.2 million men, compared with 1.9 million women, are physically attacked.

- Women are more often the targets of partner violence. Approximately 1.3 million women and 835,000 men are annually assaulted by an intimate partner. At some point in their lifetime, 22.1 percent of women—compared with 7.4 percent of men—report a physical attack by a spouse, partner, boyfriend or girlfriend, or date.

- Physical assaults are more likely to injure women than men. Of female assault victims, 39 percent—compared with 24.8 percent of male assault victims—reported being injured during their most recent attack.

- Thunderstorms kill twice as many men as women, according to the CDC. When lightning strikes, 85 percent of those killed are men. Men also are more likely to die from floods, tornados, and high winds.

INTENTIONAL INJURY: LIVING IN A DANGEROUS WORLD

Although the United States remains the most violent country in the Western world, the rate of violent crime is going down. The World Health Organization (WHO) defines violence as "the intentional use of physical force or power, threatened or actual, against oneself, another person, or a group or community, that either results in, or has a high likelihood of resulting in, injury, death, psychological harm, maldevelopment, or deprivation."[21]

Rates of violent crime in the United States have been dropping for more than a decade. Yet more than 300,000 people die each year as a result of violence, suicide or accidental injury. Interpersonal violence is the third leading cause of death among people 15 to 44 years old. Some studies show that a third of women age 16 to 49 have, at some point in their lives, been victims of sexual abuse.

VIOLENCE IN THE UNITED STATES

Gun-related injuries and deaths have declined, but guns remain the second leading cause of injury-related death in the United States after car accidents. About 260 Americans are injured by firearms every day; one-third die from their wounds.[22] Despite the decline in crime, gun violence annually takes the lives of nearly 30,000 Americans, including 10 children every day. The proportion of youth involved in crime has actually risen. Almost half the victims of violent crime are under 25 years of age.

Although men commit nine times more violent crimes than women, the rates are getting closer. Individuals with mental illness are somewhat more likely to become violent and to be the victims of violent crimes. There are ethnic and racial differences in patterns of violence. African Americans are at greater risk of victimization by violent crime than whites or persons of other racial groupings. Hispanics are at greater risk of violent

victimization than non-Hispanics. There is little difference between white women and nonwhite women in rape, physical assault, or stalking. Native American and Alaska Native women are significantly more likely than white women or African-American women to report being raped. Mixed-race women also have a significantly higher incidence of rape than white women. Native American and Alaska Native men report significantly more physical assaults than Asian and Pacific Islander men.

Alcohol availability increases the rates of total crime, violent crime, property crime, and homicides.

COPING WITH THE THREAT OF VIOLENCE AND TERRORISM

Uncertainty can be the most difficult aspect of living in a dangerous world. While you cannot eliminate risk, the following strategies can help you deal with it:

- **Focus on the here and now.** Make a daily to-do list. Check off each chore as you complete it. Break down large projects into a series of manageable steps.

- **Act despite fear.** Take that first step even if you are anxious, trusting that the second will be easier.

- **Adjust your attitude.** The way you appraise a situation—as a threat that endangers your life or as a challenge that can be overcome—has a tremendous impact on your psychological and physical responses.

- **Draw on your spiritual beliefs.** Faith and values provide a bridge over the unknown.

- **Dare to hope.** This may be the most life-affirming coping strategy of all.

HATE CRIMES

Recent years have seen the emergence of violent crimes motivated by hatred of a particular person's (or group of persons') race, ethnicity, religion, sexual orientation, or political values. These hate crimes have included the dragging death of a young African-American man, the beating death of a young gay man, the shooting of children and teachers at a Jewish community center, and the vandalizing of Muslim-owned businesses after the terrorist attacks of September 11, 2001. Politicians and government leaders have called for an expansion of hate-crime laws that would inflict especially severe sentences on those who commit violence on the basis of racism, sexism, homophobia, anti-Semitism, or other forms of prejudice.

More than half of hate crimes on campus are motivated by race; others by anti-Semitism and sexual orientation. These crimes can take the form of graffiti; verbal slurs; bombings, threatening notes, emails, or phone calls; and physical attacks. They often generate fear and intimidation in large groups of students, undermining health, academic work, and the basic security of a campus.[23]

INTIMATE PARTNER VIOLENCE

Violence doesn't stop at the front door of America's homes. According to the Federal Bureau of Investigation, the most common and least-reported violent crime is an attack in which the victim and the perpetrator knew each other at the time of or before the incident. One-third of all murders occur within families. Physical violence may occur in 20 to 30 percent of all American households. As with other forms of violent crime, there has been a decline in assaults and murders by intimates.

During her lifetime, at least one of every five women will be assaulted by a partner or ex-partner. Domestic violence is the single most common cause of injury to women—more common than car accidents, muggings, and rapes combined—and accounts for 42 percent of female murders.

Battered women (who outnumber battered men ten to one) are victims of severe, deliberate, and repeated physical assaults, often accompanied by psychological abuse and threats on their lives. A significant proportion of women who visit emergency departments seek help for symptoms related to ongoing abuse, yet only 5 percent are identified as victims of domestic violence by the physicians who treat them.

The primary factors contributing to physical abuse are the degree of frustration and stress a man is under, his use of alcohol (involved in up to 60 percent of battering cases), and whether he was raised in an abusive home. Only one in twenty men who beat their partners is violent outside the home. The risk of violence is highest in people with alcohol or drug misuse or dependence disorders.

Intimate partner violence often recurs. Two-thirds of both men and women physically assaulted by an intimate partner experience multiple incidents. Half of women raped by an intimate partner report being victimized by the same person several times. A high proportion of perpetrators of intimate partner violence report more depression, lower self-esteem, and greater aggression than others. They also may be more likely to have personality disorders. Alcohol abuse often plays a role in violence between partners. As the consumption of alcohol increases, so does the risk of serious injuries.

CRIME AND VIOLENCE ON CAMPUS

According to the Bureau of Justice, college students are victims of almost half a million violent crimes a year, including assault, robbery, sexual assault, and rape (see Student Snapshot: "Crime on Campus"). While this number may seem high, the overall violent crime rate has dropped by 54 percent since 1995.[24]

College students ages 18 to 24 are less likely to be victims of violent crime, including robbery and assault, than nonstudents of the same age. More than half (58 percent) of crimes against students are committed by strangers. More than nine in ten occur off campus, most often in an open area or street, on public transportation, in a place of business, or at a private home. In about two-thirds of the crimes, no weapon is involved. Most off-campus crimes occur at night, while on-campus crimes are more frequent in the day.[25]

Male college students are twice as likely to be victims of overall violence than female students. White undergraduates have higher rates of violent victimization than students of other races. Simple assault accounts for two-thirds of violent crimes against students; sexual assault or rape account for around 6 percent.[26]

About three in four campus crimes are never reported to the police. While students report half of aggravated assaults, only 22 percent of rapes and 18 percent of sexual assaults are reported. The main reasons students give for not reporting crimes are that they are too minor or private or they are not certain that it was a crime. Individuals also may be too ashamed or emotionally overwhelmed to contact authorities.

The Jeanne Clery Disclosure of Campus Security Policy and Campus Crime Statistics Act, originally known as the Student Right-to-Know and Campus Security Act, requires colleges to publish annual crime statistics for their campuses. However, the act excludes certain offenses, such as theft, threats, harassment, and vandalism, so the picture it presents may not be complete. The most recent crime statistics for the nation's 6,269 colleges, universities, and career schools are posted on the Internet at http://ope.ed.gov/security. How safe is your school? Take the Self Survey on page 564.

Because of concerns about safety on campus, more schools are taking tougher stands on student behavior. Many have established codes of conduct barring the use of alcohol and drugs, fighting, and sexual harassment. Many also have

© Bob Krist/CORBIS

A peaceful scene like this doesn't mean that a campus is safe. Do you know the crime statistics for your college?

Student Snapshot

CRIME ON CAMPUS

Crime	Percentage of Students
Engaged in a physical fight	7
Were physically assaulted	4
Were injured as a result of violence	25
Have been raped (female students)	15–20
Acknowledged forced intercourse or rape (male students)	5–15
Experienced harassment within last year (lesbian, gay, bisexual, and transgender students)	36

Sources: Carr, Joetta. *Campus Violence White Paper.* Baltimore, MD: American College Health Association, February 5, 2005. Baum, Katrina, and Patsy Klaus. "Violent Victimization of College Students, 1995–2002." *Bureau of Justice Statistics Special Report,* January 2005.

instituted policies requiring suspension or expulsion for students who violate this code.

Some types of violence occur mainly on college campuses. One is hazing, which refers to any activity that humiliates, degrades, or poses a risk of emotional or physical harm for the sake of joining a group or to maintain full status in that group. This behavior may occur in fraternities and sororities, athletic teams, or other campus organizations. Its forms include verbal ridicule and abuse, forced consumption of alcohol or ingestion of vile substances, sexual violation, sleep deprivation, paddling, beating, burning, or branding.

SEXUAL VICTIMIZATION

Sexual victimization refers to any situation in which a person is deprived of free choice and forced to comply with sexual acts. This is not only a woman's issue; in fact, men also are victimized. In recent years, researchers have come to view acts of sexual victimization along a continuum, ranging from street hassling, stalking, and obscene telephone calls to rape, battering, and incest.

A national survey found that the most common forms of sexual victimization on campus involved sexual or sexist remarks, catcalls, and whistles. One in five women reported obscene phone calls or being asked intrusive questions about her sex or romantic life. One in ten had false rumors spread about her sex life. About 6 percent confronted pornographic pictures, while 5 percent encountered a man exposing his sexual organs.

SEXUAL HARASSMENT

All forms of sexual harassment or unwanted sexual attention—from the display of pornographic photos to the use of sexual obscenities to a demand for sex by anyone in a position of power or authority—are illegal.

One in every two or three female undergraduates and more than one in ten male undergraduates have experienced some form of sexual harassment. Professors or supervisors may pressure students into sexual involvement for the sake of a grade, recommendation, or special opportunity. If a student tries to end a sexual relationship, the professor or supervisor may threaten reprisals. Most harassment comes from male faculty members, but both men and women report having been harassed by either male or female faculty. In a University of Washington study, college men were almost as likely as women to report unwanted sexual contact and coercion.

Sexual harassment can undermine students' well-being and academic performance. Its effects include diminished ambition and self-confidence, reduced ability to concentrate, sleeplessness, depression, physical aches, and numerous other ailments. Some students avoid classes or other contact with certain faculty members because of the risk of sexual advances. However, few victims of sexual harassment file official grievances.

Because college administrations can be held legally responsible for allowing a **hostile or offensive sexual environment,** many schools have set up committees to handle student complaints and to take action against faculty members. Universities also are discouraging and, in some cases, restricting consensual relationships between teachers and students, especially any dating of students by their academic professors or advisers. Although such relationships may seem consensual, in reality they may not be, because of the power faculty members have to determine students' grades and futures. In some cases, students have sued their universities for failing to protect them from professors who pressured them into sexual liaisons.

If you encounter sexual harassment as a student, report it to the department chair or dean. If you don't receive an adequate response to your complaint, talk with the campus representatives who handle matters involving affirmative action or civil rights. Federal guidelines prevent any discrimination against you in terms of grades or the loss of a job or scholarship if you report harassment. Schools that do not take measures to remedy harassment could lose federal funds.

Sexual harassment is not always directed at students. Recent research has documented that students of both sexes admit to harassing faculty members. In one survey, a third of undergraduates reported harassing a professor with uninvited gender-based remarks and, more rarely, unwanted sexual attention. Over two-thirds of professors reported having been targets of sexual harassment during their careers.[27]

Researchers theorize that "contrapower" harassment on college campuses may stem from gender-stereotyped notions of male dominance. Although a female faculty member has more organizational power than a male student, others may perceive her as lacking power because of her gender. This may explain why male students are far more likely than female students to engage in behaviors that could be perceived as sexually harassing. Women, whether students or faculty, perceive sexually harassing behaviors as more threatening, inappropriate, and bothersome than men do.

Sexual harassment can take many forms, ranging from suggestive comments to physical touching, and can occur in classrooms as well as offices and other workplaces.

STALKING

The "willful, repeated, and malicious following, harassing, or threatening of another person," as stalking is defined, is common on college campuses—perhaps more so than in the general population. In one survey, 13 percent of college women had been stalked since the start of the school year. In other studies, as many as 25 to 30 percent of female students and 11 to 17 percent of male students reported having been stalked.[28]

College students may be targeted for several reasons. Simply because they are young and still learning how to manage complex social relationships, some individuals may not recognize their behavior as stalking or even as disturbing. In addition, college students tend to live close to each other and to have flexible schedules and large amounts of unsupervised time. In a national survey at two- and four-year colleges, four of every five female victims knew their stalkers, who were most often boyfriends, ex-boyfriends, classmates, acquaintance, friends or coworkers. Only a small percentage of stalkers were strangers.

Stalking is not a benign behavior and can result in emotional or psychological distress, physical harm, or sexual assault. By some estimates, 10 percent of stalking incidents result in forced or attempted sexual contact. The most common consequence is psychological, with victims reporting emotional or psychological distress.

Most stalking victims try to avoid the stalker. Fewer than one in five confront the stalker or report the problem to the police. Other responses include ignoring emails or messages, changing residence, seeking a restraining order, filing a grievance with university officials, getting caller ID, going places only with a companion, and getting a weapon. Stalking laws vary from state to state.[29]

DATING VIOLENCE

Actual or threatened physical or sexual violence or psychological and emotional abuse of a current or former dating partner is a form of violence. It can occur between heterosexual, homosexual, or bisexual partners.

 According to the National College Health Assessment survey, 15 percent of women and 10 percent of men have been in emotionally abusive relationships in the last year, while 2.2 percent of women and 1.7 percent of men have been in a physically abusive relationship during the last school year (Figure 19-2).[30]

Over the course of five years (the national average for a college career), including summers and vacations, one of every four or five female students is raped. In a single academic year, 2.7 percent of coeds are raped—35 rapes for every 1,000 women. According to the Department of Justice, a campus with 6,000 coeds averages one rape a day every day for the entire school year.[31]

In nine surveys of male university students, between 3 and 6 percent had been raped by other men; up to 25 percent had been sexually assaulted. Like female rape victims, male victims suffer long-term psychological problems, physical injuries, and are at risk of contracting a sexually transmitted infection.[32]

NONVOLITIONAL SEX AND SEXUAL COERCION

Nonvolitional sex is sexual behavior that violates a person's right to choose when and with whom to have sex and what sexual behaviors to engage in. The more extreme forms of this behavior include sexual coercion or forced sex, rape, childhood sexual abuse, and violence against people with

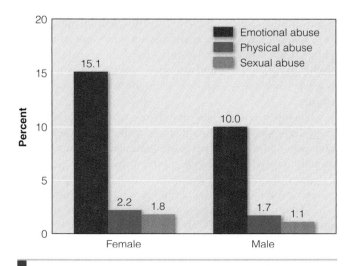

FIGURE 19-2   College Students in Abusive Relationships During Last School Year

Note: Spring 2003, Sample size *n* = 19,497

www.acha.org/projects_programs/ncha_sampledata_publix.cfm. © 2001 American College Health Association. Reprinted with permission.

nonconventional sexual identities. Other forms, such as engaging in sex to keep one's partner or to pass as heterosexual, are so common that many think of them as normal.

Sexual coercion can take many forms, including exerting peer pressure, taking advantage of one's desire for popularity, threatening an end to a relationship, getting someone intoxicated, stimulating a partner against his or her wishes, or insinuating an obligation based on the time or money one has expended. Men may feel that they need to live up to the sexual stereotype of taking advantage of every opportunity for sex. Women are far more likely than men to encounter physical force.

RAPE

Rape refers to sexual intercourse with an unconsenting partner under actual or threatened force. Sexual intercourse between a male over the age of 16 and a female under the age of consent (which ranges from 12 to 21 in different states) is called *statutory rape.* In *acquaintance rape,* or *date rape,* discussed in depth later in this chapter, the victim knows the rapist. In *stranger rape,* the rapist is an unknown assailant. Both stranger and acquaintance rapes are serious crimes that can have a devastating impact on their victims.

According to the National Violence Against Women survey, more than half of all women in the United States report an attempted or completed rape and/or physical assault. One in six women, compared with one in thirty-three men, has experienced an attempted or completed rape in the course of a lifetime.[33] In the previous 12 months, according to the survey, 0.3 percent of the women and 0.1 percent of the men had been raped. These findings indicate that some 302,091 women and 92,748 men are forcibly raped in the United States every year.

In the Harvard School of Public Health College Alcohol Study surveys of 119 schools, about 1 in 20 female students reported being raped. Nearly three quarters of the victims were raped while intoxicated. Women who were under 21, white, resided in sorority houses, used illicit drugs, drank heavily in high school, and attended colleges with high rates of heavy binge drinking were at higher risk of rape while intoxicated.[34]

The motives of rapists vary. Those who attack strangers often have problems establishing intimate relationships, have poor self-esteem, feel inadequate, and may have been sexually abused as children. Alcohol and drugs also play a major role. About 25 percent of both men and women report unwanted sexual experiences as a result of alcohol use. Many rapists drink prior to an assault, and alcohol may interfere with a victim's ability to avoid danger or resist attack.

For many years, the victims of rape were blamed for doing something to bring on the attack. However, researchers have shown that women are raped because they encounter sexually aggressive men, not because they look or act a certain way. Although no woman is immune to attack, many rape victims are children or adolescents. Women who were sexually abused or raped as children are at greater risk than others. Scientists are exploring the reasons for this greater vulnerability.

Women who successfully escape rape attempts do so by resisting verbally and physically, usually by yelling and fleeing. Women who use forceful verbal or physical resistance (screaming, hitting, kicking, biting, and running) are more likely to avoid rape than women who try pleading, crying, or offering no resistance.

Types of Rape

Although rape has long been viewed as an act of violence and domination, recent studies indicate that not all rapes fit into a single pattern. Within the broad category of rape are specific, but not mutually exclusive, subcategories of the crime, including anger rape, power rape, sadistic rape, gang rape, and sexual gratification rape.

Anger rape, usually on a total stranger, is motivated by hatred and a desire for revenge for the rejection the rapist feels he's suffered from women. Anger rapists often harbor long-standing hostility toward women, use far more physical violence than is needed for submission, and usually don't find the rape sexually gratifying.

Power rape is a generally premeditated attack motivated by a desire to dominate and control another person. Power rapists, unable to deal with stress and their sense of failure, may rape to regain a sense of power. They use only as much force as needed to make their victims submit and may find the rape sexually gratifying, even though that's not their primary motive.

Sadistic rape is a premeditated assault that often involves bondage, torture, or sexual abuse. Sadistic rapists find power and anger sexually arousing and may subject victims to rituals of humiliation or torture. They're often preoccupied with violent pornography; their motives are more complex and difficult to understand than those of other types of rapists.

Gang rape involves three or more rapists. Men in close groups that drink and party together—such as fraternities or athletic teams—are more likely to participate in such assaults. The reasons may go beyond aggression and sexual gratification to the excitement and camaraderie the men feel while sharing the experience.

Sexual gratification rape is usually an impulsive attack by someone willing to use physical coercion for the sake of sex. These rapists generally use no more force than needed to get a partner to submit and may stop the attack if it becomes clear they'll have to use extreme violence to overcome resistance. Many acquaintance rapes fit into this category.

Acquaintance, or Date, Rape

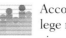 According to various studies, 25 to 60 percent of college men have engaged in some form of sexual coercion. Most often these men ignored a woman when she said no or protested. In addition, many college men reported engaging in sexual activity against their own wishes, most often because of male peer pressure or a desire to be popular.

The same factors that lead to other forms of sexual victimization can set the stage for date rape. Socialization into an aggressive role, acceptance of rape myths, and a view that force is justified in certain situations increase the likelihood of a man's committing date rape. Other factors can also play a role, including the following:

▪ **Personality and early sexual experiences.** Certain factors may predispose individuals to sexual aggression, including first sexual experience at a very young age, earlier and more frequent than usual childhood sexual experiences (both forced and voluntary), hostility toward women, irresponsibility, lack of social consciousness, and a need for dominance over sexual partners.

▪ **Situational variables (what happens during the date).** Men who initiate a date, pay all expenses, and provide transportation are more likely to be sexually aggressive, perhaps because they feel they can call all the shots.

▪ **Rape-tolerant attitudes.** As several studies have confirmed, college men hold more rape-tolerant attitudes than do college women. For example, college men are significantly more likely than college women to agree with statements such as, "Some women ask to be raped and may enjoy it" and "If a woman says 'no' to having sex, she means 'maybe' or even 'yes.'"[35]

In one study, 300 male and female college students read one of three vignettes, each using different language to describe a date rape situation. After reading the vignettes, each participant recommended one of five punishments for the perpetrator. Men recommended more lenient forms of punishment than women, including women who had read descriptions with language that diffused responsibility for the rape.[36]

Some social groups, such as fraternities and athletic teams, may encourage the use of alcohol; reinforce stereotypes about masculinity; and emphasize violence, force, and competition. The group's shared values, including an acceptance of sexual coercion, may keep individuals from questioning their behavior.

▪ **Drinking.** Alcohol use is one of the strongest predictors of acquaintance rape. Men who've been drinking may not react to subtle signals, may misinterpret a woman's behavior as a come-on, and may feel more sexually aroused. At the same time, drinking may impair a woman's ability to effectively communicate her wishes and to cope with a man's aggressiveness.

▪ **Date rape drugs.** Drugs such as Rohypnol (flunitrazepam) and GHB (gamma hydroxybutrate) have been implicated in cases of acquaintance, or date, rape. Since both drugs are odorless and tasteless,

Acquaintance rape and alcohol use are very closely linked. Both men and women may find their judgment impaired or their communications unclear as a result of drinking.

© 2000 PhotoDisc, Inc.

victims have no way of knowing whether their drink has been tampered with. The subsequent loss of memory leaves victims with no explanation for where they've been or what's happened.

Rohypnol—which can cause impaired motor skills and judgment, lack of inhibitions, dizziness, confusion, lethargy, very low blood pressure, coma, and death—has been outlawed in this country. Deaths also have been attributed to GHB overdoses.

▪ **Gender differences in interpreting sexual cues.** In research comparing college men and women, the men typically overestimated the woman's sexual availability and interest, seeing friendliness, revealing clothing, and attractiveness as deliberately seductive. In one study of date rape, the men reported feeling "led on," in part because their female partners seemed to be dressed more suggestively than usual.

Your Life Coach: Preventing Rape

Date Rape

According to data from the U.S. Bureau of Justice, nine in ten reported rapes and sexual assaults in the United States involve a single offender with whom the victim had a prior relationship.

Women

Beware of possible implied obligations for sex if a man appears interested in you and offers to buy you a drink.

At parties, mix your own drinks. At bars, watch when a bartender makes your drink. Use alcohol responsibly. Eighty to 90 percent of acquaintance rapes involve alcohol and/or drugs. You are more at risk.

Know that sex is not a male entitlement. **You can say "No" at any time.**

Beware of men who are hostile if you say no, who threaten, bully, or try to control you, try to make you feel guilty, accuse you of being uptight, put you down, or talk negatively about women.

If you feel pressured, afraid, or uncomfortable, leave, get help, or protest loudly.

Be clear about your desires, limits, and expectations. Ask and tell.

Don't listen to persuasion. You don't have to give reasons. Be assertive. State clearly what you want and do not want. Do not be afraid to set limits.

Consent to some sexual activity (kissing, touching, etc.) does NOT imply consent to all kinds of sexual activity.

Many women are in denial about what rape is. Get clear.

Threats, force, and coercion make it rape.

Getting drunk does not make rape OK. If you are too drunk to say no, it's rape, automatically.

Men

Be interested in women because you are truly interested, not as a means to getting sex.

Do not use alcohol as a means to increase the likelihood of sex. Make sure that nonalcoholic beverages are available. If you see a woman in trouble at a party, don't be afraid to intervene.

Know that sex is not a male entitlement. **It's safer and better to ask.**

Never force, pressure, or coerce anyone to have sex. Don't take silence as consent. Don't make or laugh at degrading jokes about women. Challenge abusive behavior when you witness it.

If you see a woman in trouble at a party, don't be afraid to intervene.

Be clear about your desires, limits, and expectations. Ask. Tell. No secret agenda. No LIES!

 Don't try to persuade or argue. Respect her "No" whether it is verbal or physical. Stop.

Consent to some sexual activity (kissing, touching, etc.) does NOT imply consent to all kinds of sexual activity.

Many men are in denial about what rape is. Get clear.

Threats, force, and coercion make it rape.

Don't have sex with someone who is too drunk to make responsible decisions, has passed out, or is asleep. Legally, it's rape.

Source: http://webits3. appstato.edu/apples/life/Rape/dating-guide.htm.

Both women and men report having been forced into sexual activity by someone they know. Many college students are in the age group most likely to face this threat: women aged 16 to 25 and men under 25. Women are most vulnerable and men are most likely to commit assaults during their senior year of high school and their first year of college.

Women who describe incidents of sexual coercion that meet the legal definition of rape often don't label it as such. They may have a preconceived notion that true rape consists of a blitzlike attack by a stranger. Or they may blame themselves for getting into a situation in which they couldn't escape. They may feel some genuine concern for others who would be devastated if they knew the truth (for example, if the rapist were the brother of a good friend or the son of a neighbor).

Here are some strategies that can lower your risk of being involved in a date rape:

 For men:

- Remember that it's okay not to "score" on a date.

- Don't assume that a sexy dress or casual flirting is an invitation to sex.

- Be aware of your partner's actions. If she pulls away or tries to get up, understand that she's sending you a message—one you should acknowledge and respect.

- Restrict drinking, drug use, or other behaviors (such as hanging out with a group known to be sexually aggressive in certain situations) that could affect your judgment and ability to act responsibly.

- Think of the way you'd want your sister or a close woman friend to be treated by her date. Behave in the same manner.

For women:

- If the man pays for all expenses, he may think he's justified in using force to get "what he paid for." If you cover some of the costs, he may be less aggressive.

- Back away from a man who pressures you into other activities you don't want to engage in on a date, such as chugging beer or drag racing with his friends.

- Avoid misleading messages and avoid behavior that may be interpreted as sexual teasing. Don't tell him to stop touching you, talk for a few minutes, and then resume petting.

- Despite your clearly stated intentions, if your date behaves in a sexually coercive manner, use a strategy of escalating forcefulness—direct refusal, vehement verbal refusal, and if necessary, physical force.

- Avoid using alcohol or other drugs when you definitely do not wish to be sexually intimate with your date.

The parallel guidelines on the facing page present the same information from the viewpoint of each gender. Read each point for the opposite gender first, then the corresponding one for your own gender. Any surprises?

STRANGER RAPE

Rape prevention consists primarily of making it as difficult as possible for a rapist to make you his victim:

- Don't advertise that you're a woman living alone. Use initials on your mailbox. Install and use secure locks on doors and windows, changing door locks after losing keys or moving into a new residence.

- Don't open your door to strangers. If a repairman or public official is at your door, ask him to identify himself and call his office to verify that he is a reputable person on legitimate business.

- Lock your car when it is parked, and drive with locked car doors. Should your car break down, attach a white cloth to the antenna and lock yourself in. If someone other than a uniformed officer stops to offer help, ask this person to call the police or a garage but do not open your locked car door.

- Avoid dark and deserted areas, and be aware of the surroundings where you're walking. Should a driver ask for directions when you're a pedestrian, avoid approaching his car. Instead, call out your reply from a safe distance.

- Have house or car keys in hand as you approach the door. Check the back seat before getting into your car.

- Carry a device for making a loud noise, like a whistle or, even better, a small pint-sized compressed air horn available in many sporting goods and boat supply stores. Sound the noise alarm at the first sign of danger.

- Take a self-defense class to learn techniques of physical resistance that can injure the attacker or distract him long enough for you to escape.

Date rape on campus is rarely reported to the police. However, even if a woman decides not to press criminal charges, she can turn to campus authorities. Should colleges establish a zero-tolerance policy and expel students for sexual coercion and assault? Or should colleges leave such matters to law enforcement? **You decide.**

MALE NONCONSENSUAL SEX AND RAPE

In a study of 247 young heterosexual men (mean age 18 years), one in four reported at least once incident of non-consensual sex (in this case, kissing/petting, sexual intercourse, or oral sex) with a woman or attempts by women to make them engage in nonconsensual sexual activity. In another study of 153 heterosexual men (mean age 22 years), 30 percent reported nonconsensual sexual interactions and 23.5 percent attempts at making them engage in non-consensual sex. In both samples, women exploited the man's inability to offer resistance. Kissing/petting was the most frequently reported unwanted sexual activity, followed by sexual intercourse and oral sex. Men were more likely to engage in nonconsensual sex with an ex-partner or friend than with an unknown woman. They described the experiences as moderately upsetting.

No one knows how common male rape is because men are less likely to report such assaults than women. In a recent survey in England, nearly 3 percent of men reported non-consensual sexual experiences as adults. Other researchers estimate that the victims in about 10 percent of acquaintance rape cases are men. These hidden victims often keep silent because of embarrassment, shame, or humiliation, as well as their own feelings and fears about homosexuality and conforming to conventional sex roles.

Although many people think men who rape other men are always homosexuals, most male rapists consider themselves to be heterosexual. Young boys aren't the only victims. The average age of male rape victims is 24. Rape is a serious problem in prison, where men may experience brutal assaults by men who usually resume sexual relations with women once they're released.

IMPACT OF RAPE

Rape-related injuries include unexplained vaginal discharge, bleeding, infections, multiple bruises, and fractured ribs. Victims of sexual violence often develop chronic symptoms, such as headaches, backaches, high blood pressure, sleep disorders, pelvic pain, and sexual fertility problems. But sexual violence has both a physical and a psychological impact. The psychological scars of a sexual assault take a long time to heal. Therapists have linked sexual victimization with hopelessness, low self-esteem, high levels of self-criticism, and self-defeating relationships. An estimated 30 to 50 percent of women develop posttraumatic stress disorder following a rape. Many do not seek counseling until a year or more after an attack, when their symptoms have become chronic or intensified.

Acquaintance rape may cause fewer physical injuries but greater psychological torment. Often too ashamed to tell anyone what happened, victims may suffer alone, without skilled therapists or sympathetic friends to reassure them. Women raped by acquaintances blame themselves more, see themselves less positively, question their judgment, have greater difficulty trusting others, and have higher levels of

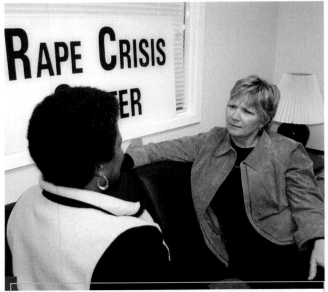

Counseling from a trained professional can help ease the trauma suffered by a rape victim.

psychological distress. Nightmares, anxiety, and flashbacks are common. The women may avoid others, become less capable of protecting themselves, and continue to be haunted by sexual violence for years. A therapist can help these victims begin the slow process of healing.

WHAT TO DO IN CASE OF RAPE

Women who are raped should call a friend or a rape crisis center. A rape victim should not bathe or change her clothes before calling. Semen, hair, and material under her fingernails or on her apparel all may be useful in identifying the man who raped her.

A rape victim who chooses to go to a doctor or hospital should remember that she may not necessarily have to talk to police. However, a doctor can collect the necessary evidence, which will then be available if she later decides to report the rape to police. All rape victims should talk with a doctor or health-care worker about testing and treatment for sexually transmitted infections and postintercourse conception.

Even an unsuccessful rape attempt should be reported because the information a woman may provide about the attack—the assaulter's physical characteristics, voice, clothes, car, even an unusual smell—may prevent another woman from being raped.

HALTING SEXUAL VIOLENCE

Sexual violence has its roots in social attitudes and beliefs that demean women and condone aggression. According to international research, much sexual violence takes place within families, marriage, and dating relationships. In many settings, rape is a culturally approved strategy to control and discipline women. In these places, laws and policies to improve women's status are critical to ending sexual coercion.

As colleges and universities have become more aware of the different forms of sexual danger, many have taken the lead in setting up primary prevention programs (including newspaper articles; seminars in dormitories, fraternities, and sororities; and lectures) to help students examine their attitudes and values, understand cultural influences, and develop skills for avoiding or escaping from dangerous situations. All men and women should recognize misleading rape myths and develop effective ways of communicating to avoid misinterpretation of sexual cues. Students should also know to whom they can turn to learn more about and seek help for sexual victimization: counselors, campus police, deans of student affairs, fraternity or sorority representatives, and campus ministers.

While most campuses provide self-defense seminars for potential female victims of rape and general campus safety measures, some have tried innovative approaches, such as Men Against Violence, a peer-education program that confronts male students' conceptions of manhood and appropriate gender roles to reduce their likelihood of sexual or physical violence. Such all-male, peer-guided approaches that challenge myths about rape and rape victims also have proven effective with college fraternity men.

In addition, practical institutional steps—such as providing adequate lighting, escort services, and clear policies against both violence and drug and alcohol abuse—can help. Self-defense classes teach women how to avoid becoming victims either by escaping or protecting themselves. Follow-up studies of college women have found that self-defense training increased their sense of control over their life, confidence, security, independence, and physical prowess.

Campuses are also providing secondary prevention by getting help to victims of sexual violence as soon as possible through rape-crisis teams and emergency mental-health services, and tertiary prevention by working with victims to ameliorate the long-term effects of their experience through psychotherapy, educational services, and medical care.

Learn It / Live It

Helping the Victims of Violence

As their numbers have grown and their anguish has been recognized, the victims of violence have received greater attention. Hundreds of shelters for battered wives and their children have been set up across the country. They offer physical and psychological treatment and a haven where women can begin to rebuild their shattered self-esteem, as well as their daily lives. Rape counseling and crisis centers on college campuses and in the community provide various forms of assistance to victims of rape. In many cities, the telephone directory lists hot lines and resources. More than 400 victims' advocacy groups have been set up across the country to advise those hurt by crime. Support organizations

help many survivors deal with the emotional aftermath of their experiences.

Sometimes well-intentioned friends and relatives add to the stress felt by the victims of violence. Here's how to offer comfort without implying criticism:

- **Don't try to deny that it happened.** Although it may be hard to talk about—or even listen to—what happened, the reality of the event must not be ignored. Denial makes victims doubt their own experience and question themselves at a time when they crave reassurance.

- **Don't pressure the victim to talk—or not to talk.** Some individuals need to go over every detail of what happened, again and again, until they work out their feelings of outrage and become ready to get on with their lives. Others find going into details too humiliating. Let the victim set the tone and limits for disclosure. Don't pry or prod.

- **Don't blame the victim.** Even when no one doubts that the victim is completely innocent, individuals may be plagued by regrets and self-accusation: Why didn't I lock the windows? Why did I park on that dark street? Any second-guessing or implied criticism adds to this burden of blame and shame.

- **Don't try to rush the victim to leave the past behind and get on with his or her life.** Recovery from any traumatic event takes time, and only the victim knows the appropriate pace. If, however, months pass without any lessening of symptoms or improvement in day-to-day functioning, family members and friends shouldn't hesitate to recommend that their loved one see a mental health professional.

Making This Chapter Work for You

Review Questions

1. When confronted with an emergency,
   a. move the victim to a safe place.
   b. move all electrical wires out of the way.
   c. wait to see whether someone else has taken matters in hand.
   d. assess the situation and call 911.

2. Which of the following factors affects an individual's risk of accident or injury?
   a. hunger level
   b. stress level
   c. amount of automobile insurance coverage
   d. knowledge of CPR

3. Safe-driving tips include all of the following *except*
   a. Avoid driving at night for the first year after getting a license.

(*continued on p. 566*)

Self Survey ▪ How Safe Is Your School?

Dormitory Security

YES	NO	**STUDENTS:**
____	____	Card swipe (like hotels)
____	____	Patented keys
____	____	Standard keys
____	____	Propped doors
____	____	Doors locked at night
____	____	Doors never locked
____	____	Doors always locked
____	____	Guards on duty (24 hrs.)

VISITORS:

____	____	Intercom at entrance
____	____	Show ID
____	____	Sign-in guests

DORM FEATURES:

____	____	Single sex dorms
____	____	Freshman dorms
____	____	Coed dorms
____	____	Senior dorms
____	____	Alcohol prohibited
____	____	Drugs prohibited
____	____	Substance-free
____	____	Propped door alarms
____	____	Fire sprinklers
____	____	Peep hole in room door
____	____	Dead bolt in room door
____	____	Safety chain on room door
____	____	Toilet in room
____	____	Shower in room
____	____	Bathrooms down hallway
____	____	Single sex bathrooms
____	____	Female hall bathrooms locked
____	____	Single sex floors locked
____	____	Secure windows (first and second floors)
____	____	Panic alarms in rooms

SECURITY PATROLS IN DORMS:

____	____	By police nightly
____	____	By security nightly
____	____	By students (unreliable)
____	____	By no one

ROOMMATES QUICKLY TRANSFERRED BY DEAN FOR:

____	____	Using illegal drugs
____	____	Having sex
____	____	Underage drinking
____	____	Vomiting after drinking
____	____	Noisy parties
____	____	Hate speech
____	____	Physical abuse
____	____	You have to move out instead!!

Campus Security

YES	NO	**CAMPUS SECURITY FORCE:**
____	____	Sworn police
____	____	Arrest power
____	____	Patrolling day
____	____	Patrolling night
____	____	Carry fire arms
____	____	Security guards
____	____	Bicycle patrols
____	____	Surveillance cameras
____	____	Emergency phones
____	____	Student amateurs
____	____	Escort services
____	____	Shuttle services

HEALTH SERVICES:

____	____	Rape crisis center
____	____	Alcohol-drug counselors
____	____	AA meetings on campus

Parental Involvement

		PARENTAL NOTIFICATION:
____	____	For underage drinkers
____	____	For alcohol poisoning
____	____	For illegal drug use
____	____	For acts of violence
____	____	For public drunkenness
____	____	For housing fire arms
____	____	For sexual assault
____	____	For hate crimes or speech
____	____	For academic probation
____	____	For disciplinary probation
____	____	For residence hall violations
____	____	For DUI convictions

CAMPUS JUDICIAL SYSTEM:

____	____	Open campus judicial hearings
____	____	Reveal names of campus sex offenders

Get campus crime statistics for the last three years from admissions office:

Criminal Offenses

Murder	
Forcible sex offenses	____
Nonforcible sex offenses	
Robbery	
Aggravated assault	____
Burglary	
Arson	
Motor vehicle theft	____
Hate crimes	
Total criminal offenses	____
Per student crime ratio	____

CAMPUS ARRESTS

Liquor law violations _____

Drug law violations _____

Weapons violations _____

TOTAL CAMPUS ARRESTS _____

Calculate campus crimes per thousand students and compare them with other schools. Also, attempt a balanced evaluation by combining your subjective impressions with any calculations.

Source: Security on Campus, Inc., www.securityoncampus.org.

YOUR ACTION PLAN FOR PERSONAL SAFETY ON CAMPUS

FUNDAMENTALS

▪ Freshmen should "respectfully decline" to have photo and personal information published for distribution to the campus community. Fraternities and upperclassmen have abused this type of publication to "target" naive freshmen.

▪ Study the campus and neighborhood with respect to routes between your residence and class/activities schedule. Know where emergency phones are located.

▪ Share your class/activities schedule with parents and a network of close friends, effectively creating a type of "buddy" system. Give network telephone numbers to your parents, advisors, and friends.

▪ Always travel in groups. Use a shuttle service after dark. Never walk alone at night. Avoid shortcuts.

▪ Survey the campus, academic buildings, residence halls, and other facilities while classes are in session and after dark to see that buildings, walkways, quadrangles, and parking lots are adequately secured, lit, and patrolled. Are emergency phones, escorts, and shuttle services adequate?

▪ To gauge the social scene, drive down fraternity row on weekend nights and stroll through the student hangouts. Are people behaving responsibly, or does the situation seem reckless and potentially dangerous? Remember, alcohol and/or drug abuse is involved in about 90 percent of campus crime. Carefully evaluate off-campus student apartment complexes and fraternity houses if you plan to live off-campus.

RESIDENCE

▪ Doors and windows to your residence hall should be equipped with quality locking mechanisms. Room doors should be equipped with peep holes and deadbolts. Always lock them when you are absent. Do not loan out your key. Rekey locks when a key is lost or stolen.

▪ Card access systems are far superior to standard metal key and lock systems. Card access enables immediate lock changes when keys are lost, stolen, or when housing arrangements change. Most hotels and hospitals have changed to card access systems for safety reasons. Higher education institutions need to adopt similar safety features.

▪ Always lock your doors and first and second floor windows at night. Never compromise your safety for a roommate who asks you to leave the door unlocked.

▪ Dormitories should have a central entrance/exit lobby where nighttime access is monitored, as well as an outside telephone which visitors must use to gain access.

▪ Dormitory residents should insist that residential assistants and security patrols routinely check for propped doors—day and night.

▪ Do not leave your identification, wallets, checkbooks, jewelry, cameras, and other valuables in open view.

▪ Program your phone's speed dial memory with emergency numbers that include family and friends.

▪ Know your neighbors and don't be reluctant to report illegal activities and suspicious loitering.

OFF-CAMPUS RESIDENTS

Off-campus residents should contact their student legal aid representative to draft leases that stipulate minimum standards of security and responsibility. Students and parents should also consult any "Neighborhood Watch" association active in the community or the municipal police regarding local crime rates.

Source: Reprinted with permission by Security on Campus, Inc., www.securityoncampus.org. Security on Campus assists victims of campus crime.

CASE IN POINT

Student: Kayla, 18

Goal: Staying safe on a new campus

Health Action Plan:

▪ Become familiar with the campus, including the routes to her dorm, classrooms, rec center, and so on, and find out if they are well lit and busy throughout the evening

▪ Be vigilant about locking her room door and making sure the dorm entrance doors lock behind her when she enters

▪ Take a course in self-defense

▪ Call for a campus escort when returning to her dorm late

▪ Avoid situations where people are drinking heavily, and be careful about what she drinks

Health ⊛ Now ™ If you want to write your own goals for staying safe, go to the **Wellness Journal at HealthNow,** http://healthnow.brookscole.com/ith

b. Make sure your car has snow tires or chains before driving in hazardous snowy conditions.

c. If riding with an intoxicated driver, keep talking to him so that he doesn't fall asleep at the wheel.

d. Don't let packages or people obstruct the rear or side windows.

4. Which of the following statements about home safety is true?

   a. Falls pose the greatest threat of injury in the home, followed by poison.

   b. The three ingredients of fire are fuel, a heat source, and oxygen.

   c. The risk of falls is lowest in the elderly.

   d. If you're on the top floor of the dorm when a fire breaks out, get to the elevator quickly.

5. You can avoid computer health hazards by

   a. positioning the monitor so that you are looking up at it.

   b. positioning the keyboard so that you don't have to bend your wrists to use it.

   c. sustaining focus on the screen with the PRIO method.

   d. taking a 15-minute break every 30 minutes.

6. Which of the following statements about violence in the United States is *false?*

   a. Almost half the victims of violent crime are under 25 years of age.

   b. More than half of hate crimes on campus are motivated by race.

   c. Gun-related deaths are the leading cause of death in the United States, followed by car accidents.

   d. Boys and men are most likely to be the perpetrators of homicide, domestic abuse, and hate-related crimes.

7. Which statement about violence on college campuses is *false?*

   a. Campus hazing often involves activities that would be called torture if perpetrated elsewhere.

   b. Most crimes against students occur on campus.

   c. Many campuses have codes of conduct on alcohol, drugs, and fighting.

   d. Crime statistics for colleges and universities are posted on the Internet.

8. Sexual victimization

   a. includes sexual harassment, sexual coercion, and rape.

   b. is gender-specific, affecting women who are violated emotionally or physically by men.

   c. is rare in academic environments such as college campuses.

   d. most commonly takes the form of physical assault and stalking.

9. Which of the following statements about rape is true?

   a. When a person is sexually attacked by a stranger, it is referred to as *rape.* When a person is sexually attacked by an acquaintance, it is referred to as *sexual coercion.*

   b. Statutory rape is defined as sexual intercourse initiated by a woman under the age of consent.

   c. Men who rape other men usually consider themselves heterosexuals.

   d. Women who flirt and dress provocatively are typically more willing to participate in aggressive sex than women who dress conservatively and do not flirt.

10. Ways to protect or prevent rape include:

    a. Use alcohol and drugs only in familiar surroundings.

    b. Take a self-defense class.

    c. To avoid angering a sexually aggressive person, become passive and quiet.

    d. Do not discuss your sexual limits on a first or second date because just talking about sex will encourage your date to think you are interested in a sexual relationship.

Answers to these questions can be found on page 587.

Critical Thinking

1. Can you name two risk factors in your daily life that might increase the likelihood of accidental injury? What actions have you taken to keep yourself safe? Are there other risk factors you could minimize or eliminate? What might you do about them?

2. A friend of yours, Eric, frequently makes crude or derogatory comments about women. When you finally call him on this, his response is, "I didn't say anything wrong. I like women." What might you say to him?

3. At one college, women raped by acquaintances on dates scrawled the names of their assailants on the walls of women's restrooms on campus. Several young men whose names appeared on the list objected, protesting that they were innocent and were being unfairly accused. How do you feel about this method of fighting back against date rape? Do you think it violates the rights of men? How do you feel about naming women who've been raped in news reports? Are there circumstances in which a woman's identity should be revealed? Would fewer women report a rape if not assured of privacy?

Media Menu
Health☉Now™

Throughout the chapter, this icon introduces a list of resources on the Health-Now website at **http://healthnow.brookscole.com/ith** that will:

- Help you evaluate your knowledge of the material.
- Allow you to take an exam-prep quiz.
- Provide a Personalized Learning Plan targeting resources that address areas you should study.
- Coach you through identifying target goals for behavior change and creating and monitoring your personal change plan throughout the semester.

INTERNET CONNECTIONS

RAINN-Rape Assault Incest National Network

www.rainn.org

This site provides great information from an organization fighting against rape, assault, and incest.

The Rape Crisis Center

www.rapecrisis.com

This private nonprofit organization provides support to victims of sexual violence and their families, including a 24/7 crisis hotline and several advocacy programs.

National Safety Council (NSC)

www.nsc.org

The mission of the NSC is to educate and influence society to adopt safety, health, and environmental policies, practices, and procedures that prevent human suffering and economic losses arising from preventable causes.

National Youth Violence Prevention Resource Center (NYVPRC)

www.safeyouth.org

This site is a gateway to resources for professionals, parents, youth, and individuals working to prevent and end violence committed by and against young people.

InfoTrac College Edition Activities Log on, insert **seat belts** into the Keyword search box, and limit your search to the past year. When you get the results, Mark articles to review, then Select one to read. Summarize three or four key points from the article.

You can find additional readings related to personal health with InfoTrac College Edition, an online library of more than 900 journals and publications. Follow the instructions for accessing InfoTrac College Edition that were packaged with your textbook; then search for articles using a keyword search.

For additional links, resources, and suggested readings on the InfoTrac College Edition, visit our Health and Wellness Resource Center at **http://health .wadsworth.com.**

Key Terms

The terms listed are on the page indicated. Definitions of the terms are in the Glossary at the end of this book.

computer vision syndrome 552

hostile or offensive sexual environment 556

nonvolitional sex 557

rape 558

repetitive motion injury (RMI) 552

sexual coercion 558

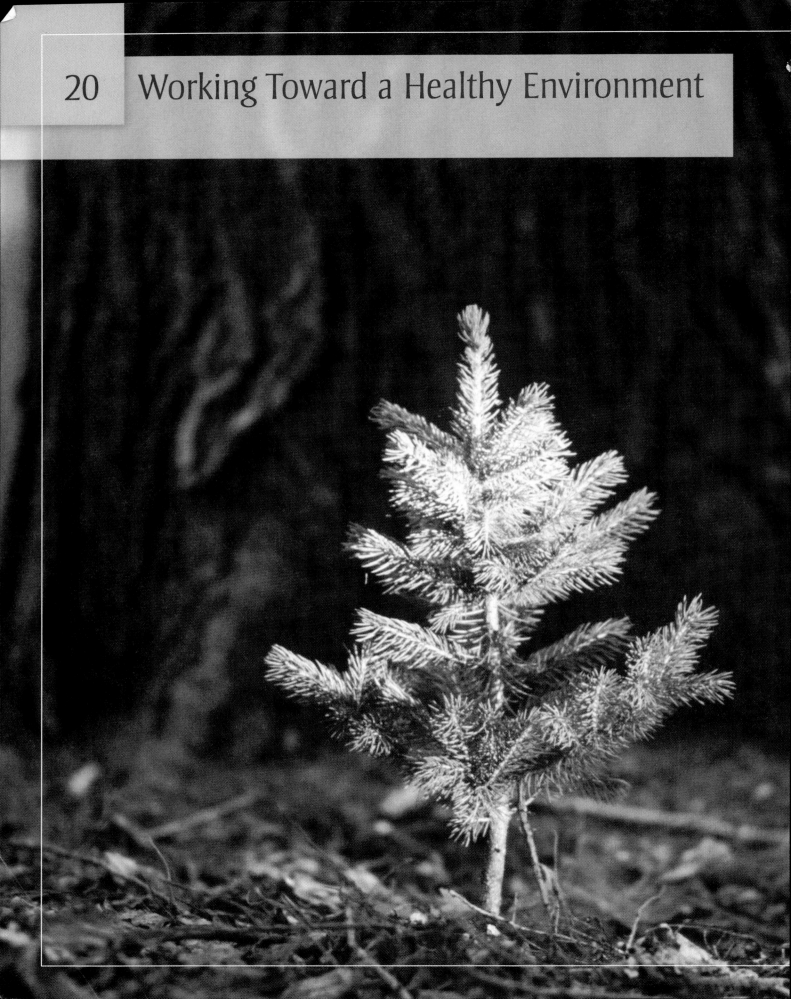

As a teenager, Ocean Robbins wanted to change the world. At age 16, he founded Youth for Environmental Sanity (YES!) to mobilize his generation to save the planet. Now in his thirties, Robbins has seen his California-based organization grow into what *Time* magazine describes as "a mini-movement that spans environmental consciousness raising, leadership training and community building." Since 1990, more than 620,000 students in seven countries have taken part in YES! events in schools, summer camps, and workshops. "Part of my mandate is to help my generation see the power we have," says Robbins.[1]

No one has more stake in the future of the planet than the young. Environmental concerns may seem so enormous that nothing any individual can do will have an effect. This is not the case. Some individuals, like Ocean Robbins, become international advocates. But all of us, as citizens of the world, can help find solutions to the challenges confronting our planet. The first step is realizing that you have a personal responsibility for safeguarding the health of your environment and, thereby, your own well-being.

This chapter explores the complex interrelationships between your world and your well-being. It discusses major threats to the environment—including atmospheric changes; air, water, and noise pollution; chemical risks; and radiation—and provides specific guidance on what you can do about them.

After studying the material in this chapter, you should be able to:

▮ **Discuss** the health effects of the major environmental hazards.

▮ **List** the major types of outdoor and indoor pollution.

▮ **List** and **describe** actions that individuals can take to protect the environment.

▮ **Describe** ways to protect your ears from noise-induced hearing loss.

▮ **Identify** the primary contaminants that affect water quality.

▮ **List** the key sources and health risks of electromagnetic fields.

THE ENVIRONMENT AND YOUR HEALTH

The planet Earth—once taken for granted as a ball of rock and water that existed for our use for all time—now is seen as a single, fragile **ecosystem** (a community of organisms that share a physical and chemical environment). Our environment is a closed ecosystem, powered by the sun. The materials needed for the survival of this planet must be recycled over and over again. Increasingly, we're realizing just how important the health of this ecosystem is to our own well-being and survival. However, as shown in Student Snapshot: "Do Students Care About the Environment?" the majority of undergraduates do not share this concern. Students at all-black colleges are more likely to express environmental concerns.[2]

Our environment affects our well-being both directly and indirectly. Changes in temperature and rainfall patterns disturb ecological processes in ways that can be hazardous to health. The environment may account for 25 to 40 percent of diseases worldwide. Children are the most vulnerable because of their greater sensitivity to toxic threats. In response to this trend, Congress has approved funding to create a nationwide system to track environmental links to chronic diseases.

No individual is immune to environmental health threats. Depletion of the ozone layer has already been implicated in the increase in skin cancers and cataracts. Global warming, according to some theorists, might lead to changes in one-third to one-half of the world's vegetation types and to the extinction of many plant and animal species. A warmer world is expected to produce more severe flooding in some places and more severe droughts in others, jeopardizing natural resources and the safety of our water supply. Warmer weather—a consequence of changes in atmospheric gases and climate—worsens urban-industrial air pollution and, if the air also is moist, increases concentrations of allergenic pollens and fungal spores. These are truly problems without borders.

For good or for ill, we cannot separate our individual health from that of the environment in which we live. The air we breathe, the water we drink, the chemicals we use all have an impact on the quality of our lives. At the same time, the lifestyle choices we make, the products we use, the efforts we undertake to clean up a beach or save wetlands affect the quality of our environment.

POLLUTION

Any change in the air, water, or soil that could reduce its ability to support life is a form of **pollution.** Natural events, such as smoke from fires triggered by lightning, can cause pollution. The effects of pollution depend on the concentration (amount per unit of air, water, or soil) of the **pollutant,** how long it remains in the environment, and its

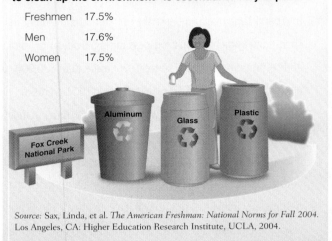
chemical nature. An *acute effect* is a severe immediate reaction, usually after a single, large exposure. For example, pesticide poisoning can cause nausea and dizziness, even death. A *chronic effect* may take years to develop or may be a recurrent or continuous reaction, usually after repeated exposures. The development of cancer after repeated exposure to a pollutant such as asbestos is an example of a chronic effect.

Environmental agents that trigger changes, or **mutations,** in the genetic material (the DNA) of living cells are called **mutagens.** The changes that result can lead to the development of cancer. A substance or agent that causes cancer is a *carcinogen:* All carcinogens are mutagens; most mutagens are carcinogens. Furthermore, when a mutagen affects an egg or a sperm cell, its effects can be passed on to future generations. Mutagens that can cross the placenta of a pregnant woman and cause a spontaneous abortion or birth defects in the fetus are called **teratogens.**

Pollution is a hazard to all who breathe. Deaths caused by air pollution exceed those from motor vehicle injuries. Those with respiratory illnesses are at greatest risk during days when smog or allergen counts are high. However, even healthy joggers are affected; carbon monoxide has been shown to impair their exercise performance. The effects of carbon monoxide are much worse in smokers, who already have higher levels of the gas in their blood.

Toxic substances in polluted air can enter the human body in three ways: through the skin, through the digestive system, and through the lungs. The combined interaction of two or more hazards can produce an effect greater than that of either one alone. Pollutants can affect an organ or organ system directly or indirectly.

Among the health problems that have been linked with pollution are the following:

- Headaches and dizziness.
- Eye irritation and impaired vision.
- Nasal discharge.
- Cough, shortness of breath, and sore throat.
- Constricted airways.
- Constriction of blood vessels and increased risk of heart disease.
- Chest pains and aggravation of the symptoms of colds, pneumonia, bronchial asthma, emphysema, chronic bronchitis, lung cancer, and other respiratory problems.
- Birth defects and reproductive problems.
- Nausea, vomiting, and stomach cancer.
- Allergy and asthma from diesel fumes in polluted air.[3]

 WHAT IS GLOBAL WARMING?

In the last century, Earth's average surface temperature has risen by an estimated 0.6 to 1.2 degrees Fahrenheit.[4] More of the warming has occurred over land than over water, more at night than during the day, and more in winter than in summer. No one can predict exactly the long-term impact of a continuing temperature rise, but experts believe that recent droughts and hurricanes and increases in carbon dioxide are early effects of global warming.

Why is our planet getting warmer? Figure 20-1 shows the normal greenhouse effect: Certain gases in Earth's atmosphere trap energy from the sun and retain heat somewhat like the glass panels of a greenhouse. These "greenhouse" gases include carbon dioxide, methane, and nitrous oxide. Human activities have increased the greenhouse gases in our atmosphere. We burn fossil fuels (oil, natural gas, coal) and wood products, which release carbon dioxide into the atmosphere. We produce coal, natural gas, and oil, which emit methane. Livestock and the decomposition of organic wastes also produce methane. Agricultural and industrial processes emit nitrous oxide. These emissions enhance the normal greenhouse effect, trapping more heat and raising the temperature of the atmosphere and Earth's surface. This is **global warming.**

Greenhouse gases have increased worldwide (Figure 20-2). The Intergovernmental Panel on Climate Change projects a global average warming of 2.5 to 10.4°F (1.4 to 5.8°C) by the year 2100, compared with the global average temperature in 1990.

For the last ten years, world leaders have been focusing on global warming and its potential consequences. Some 165 countries—not including the United States—have signed the first international treaty to fight global warming by implementing the rules known as the Kyoto Protocol. The treaty calls on about 40 industrialized nations to limit carbon emissions or reduce them to levels below those of 1990. The United States, which is responsible for 23 percent of greenhouse-gas emissions,[5] rejected the accord as harmful to the U.S. economy and unfair because it excused heavily polluting nations, such as India and China, from any obligation.

Global warming may have contributed to an increase in extremely powerful and dangerous hurricanes.

NOAA

CLEARING THE AIR

In most places in the United States, you can breathe easier today than you would have a quarter century ago. Smog has declined by about a third, although there are now 85 percent more vehicles being driven 105 percent more miles a year. Current model automobiles emit an average of 80 percent less pollution per mile than was emitted by new cars in 1970. However, tailpipe emissions from cars and trucks still account for almost a third of the air pollution in the United States.[6] Even a small shift of support away from fossil fuels toward clean renewable energy could save millions of lives and help avert global warming.[7]

According to the Harvard School of Public Health, living in a city with even moderately sooty air may shorten your lifespan by about a year. In fact, air pollution can be as harmful to breathing capacity as smoking. Residents of polluted cities are exposed to some of the same toxic gases, such as nitrogen oxide and carbon monoxide, found in cigarettes.

Air pollution of any sort can cause numerous ill effects. As pollutants destroy the hairlike cilia that remove irritants from the lungs, individuals may suffer chronic bronchitis,

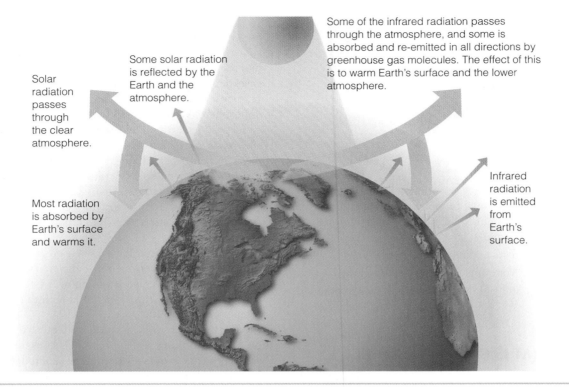

Some solar radiation is reflected by the Earth and the atmosphere.

Solar radiation passes through the clear atmosphere.

Some of the infrared radiation passes through the atmosphere, and some is absorbed and re-emitted in all directions by greenhouse gas molecules. The effect of this is to warm Earth's surface and the lower atmosphere.

Most radiation is absorbed by Earth's surface and warms it.

Infrared radiation is emitted from Earth's surface.

FIGURE 20-1   The Greenhouse Effect

The normal greenhouse effect warms the Earth to a hospitable temperature. An increase in greenhouse gases intensifies the greenhouse effect, trapping more heat and raising the Earth's temperature.

characterized by excessive mucus flow and continuous coughing. Emphysema may develop or worsen, as pollutants constrict the bronchial tubes and destroy the air sacs in the lungs, making breathing more difficult.

When air pollution levels are high, heart attacks, strokes, heart failure flare-ups, and lung troubles increase. Air contamination also has enduring effects on heart health and increases atherosclerosis and deaths due to heart disease, according to a long-term Harvard University study. Los Angeles residents living in areas with the highest average level of fine particulates in the air have thicker carotid arteries (a sign of more atherosclerosis) than those living in less polluted areas.[8]

For the elderly and people with asthma or heart disease, polluted air can be life-threatening. Even healthy individuals can be affected, particularly if they exercise outdoors during high-pollution periods.

SMOG

A combination of smoke and fog, **smog** is made up of chemical vapors from auto exhaust, industrial and commercial pollutants (volatile organic compounds, carbon monoxide, nitrogen oxides, sulfur oxides, particulates), and ozone. The

most obvious sources of these pollutants are motor vehicles, industrial factories, electric utility plants, and wood-burning stoves.

Gray-air, or *sulfur-dioxide,* smog, often seen in Europe and much of the eastern United States, is produced by burning oil of high sulfur content. Among the cities that must deal with gray-air smog are Chicago, Baltimore, Detroit, and Philadelphia. Like cigarette smoke, gray-air smog affects the cilia in the respiratory passages; the lungs are unable to expel particulates, such as soot, ash, and dust, which remain and irritate the tissues. This condition is hazardous to people with chronic respiratory problems.

Brown-air, or *photochemical,* smog is found in large traffic centers such as Los Angeles, Salt Lake City, Denver, Mexico City, and Tokyo. This type of smog results principally from nitric oxide in car exhaust reacting with oxygen in the air, forming nitrogen dioxide, which produces a brownish haze and, when exposed to sunlight, other pollutants.

One of these, *ozone,* the most widespread pollutant, can impair the body's immune system and cause long-term lung damage. (Ozone in the upper atmosphere protects us by repelling harmful ultraviolet radiation from the sun, but ozone in the lower atmosphere is a harmful component of air pollution.) Automobiles also produce carbon monoxide, a colorless and odorless gas that diminishes the ability of red blood

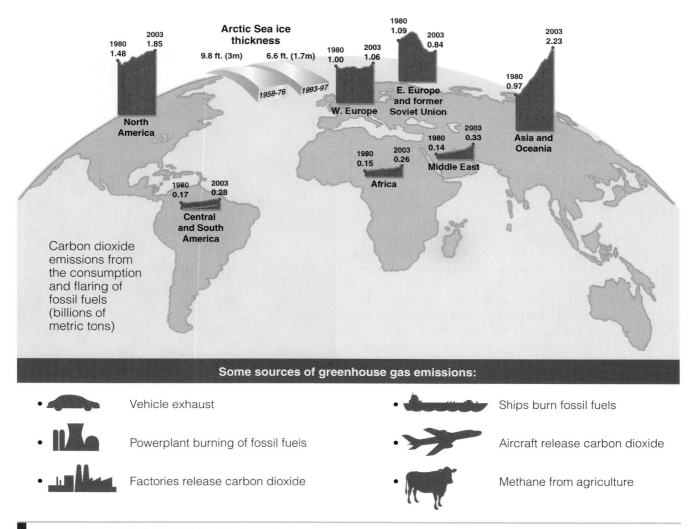

FIGURE 20-2   Why the World is Heating Up

The buildup of carbon dioxide and other greenhouse gases in the atmosphere could result in great climate change. A combination of factors, including the burning of fossil fuels and deforestation, is causing the atmosphere to retain heat. The graphs show the increase in carbon dioxide emissions from different areas of the world.

Source: Data from Energy Information Administration, Department of Energy, www.eia.doe.gov.

cells to carry oxygen. The resulting oxygen deficiency can affect breathing, hearing, and vision in humans and stunt the growth of plants and trees.[9]

> *Environmental issues, such as allowing drilling or logging in protected wildernesses or granting exemptions from clean air standards, often trigger fierce political debates. Should the needs or demands of today's businesses and consumers come first? Or should preserving and protecting open space and clean air take a higher priority?* **You decide.**

ACID RAIN

The burning of fossil fuels, such as oil and gas, and the smelting of certain ores, such as copper and nickel, can produce **acid rain**—rain, sleet, snow, mist, fog, and clouds containing sulfuric acid and nitric acid. These pollutants are carried through the atmosphere long distances from their sources and fall to Earth when it rains. Acid rain, which is believed to be declining in some regions, has damaged buildings, monuments, and other structures.

During the last 30 years, acid rain has contributed to the death of more than half of certain trees, including red spruce and sugar maples, in the Northeast. More than 15 years after the passage of the Clean Air Act in 1990, habitats in the northeastern states have not yet recovered from acid rain damage.

Your Life Coach

Going Green

By the choices you make and the actions you take, you can improve the state of the world. No one expects you to sacrifice every comfort or spend great amounts of money. However, for almost everyone, there's plenty of room for improvement. If enough people make small individual changes, they can have an enormous impact.

One basic environmental action is **precycling:** buying products packaged in recycled materials. According to Earthworks, a consumer group, packaging makes up a third of what people in the United States throw away. When you precycle, you consider how you're going to dispose of a product and the packaging materials before purchasing it. For example, you might choose eggs in recyclable cardboard packages, rather than in plastic cartons, and look for juice and milk in refillable bottles.

Recycling—collecting, reprocessing, marketing, and using materials once considered trash—has become a necessity for several reasons: We've run out of space for all the garbage we produce; waste sites are often health and safety hazards; recycling is cheaper than landfill storage or incineration (a major source of air pollution); and recycling helps save energy and natural resources. Different communities take different approaches to recycling. Many provide regular curbside pickup of recyclables, which is so convenient that a majority of those eligible for such services participate. Most programs pick up bottles, cans, and newspapers—either separated or mixed together. Other communities have drop-off centers where consumers can leave recyclables. Conveniently located and sponsored by community organizations (such as charities or schools), these centers accept beverage containers, newspapers, cardboard, metals, and other items.

Buyback centers, usually run by private companies, pay for recyclables. Many centers specialize in aluminum cans, which offer the most profit. Some operate in supermarket back rooms or parking lots; other centers have regular hours and staff members who carefully weigh and evaluate recyclables. In some places, reverse vending machines accept returned beverage containers and provide deposit refunds, in the form of either cash or vouchers.

Discarded computers, other electronic devices, and printer cartridges also should be recycled, by donating them to schools or charitable organizations. "Tech trash" buried in landfills is creating a new hazard because trace amounts of potentially hazardous agents, such as lead and mercury, can leak into the ground and water.

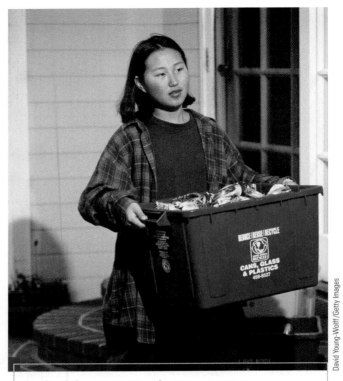

Recycling helps save energy and conserve resources.

David Young-Wolff/Getty Images

With *composting*—which some people describe as nature's way of recycling—the benefits can be seen as close as your backyard. Organic products, such as leftover food and vegetable peels, are mixed with straw or other dry material and kept damp. Bacteria eat the organic material and turn it into a rich soil. Some people keep a compost pile (which should be stirred every few days) in their backyard; others take their organic garbage (including mowed grass and dead leaves) to community gardens or municipal composting sites.

INDOOR POLLUTANTS

Because people in industrialized nations spend more than 90 percent of their time in buildings, the quality of the air they breathe inside can have an even greater impact on their well-being than outdoor pollution.

Indoor pollution accounts for 2.2 million deaths and costs the world between $150 billion and $750 billion per year—0.5 to 2.5 percent of the world's gross national product—mainly in lost production through sickness and death.[10]

TOXIC THREATS

The most hazardous form of indoor air pollution is cigarette smoke. Passive smoking—inhaling others' cigarette smoke—may rank behind active smoking and alcohol use as the third-leading preventable cause of death. Other threats include the following substances:

Formaldehyde

Unlike outdoor contaminants from exhaust pipes or smokestacks, indoor pollutants come from the very materials the buildings are made of and from the appliances inside them. For instance, formaldehyde, commonly used in building materials, carpet backing, furniture, foam insulation, plywood, and particle board, can cause nausea, dizziness, headaches, heart palpitations, stinging eyes, and burning lungs. Formaldehyde gas, which is colorless and odorless, has been shown to cause cancer in animals. Most manufacturers have voluntarily quit using it, but many homes already contain materials made with urea-formaldehyde, which can seep into the air. To avoid formaldehyde exposure, buy solid wood or nonwood products whenever possible, and ask about the formaldehyde content of building products, cabinets, and furniture before purchasing them.

Asbestos

Asbestos, a mineral widely used for building insulation, has been linked to lung and gastrointestinal cancer among asbestos workers and their families, although it may take 20 to 30 years for such cancers to develop. Fibers from asbestos home insulation or fireproofing that become airborne can cause progressive and deadly lung diseases, including cancer. More than 200,000 lawsuits have been filed for asbestos-related injuries, and as many as 300,000 American workers may have died from asbestos-linked diseases, including lung cancer. The danger may be greatest for those who smoke and are also exposed to asbestos.

If you're concerned about asbestos in your home, don't waste money searching for asbestos in the air. The results of such tests are meaningless. To check a building material for asbestos, put three small pieces in a film canister and send it to a laboratory approved by the U.S. Environmental Protection Agency (EPA). If you find asbestos in your house, sealing the source (for example, an old linoleum floor) may be safer than removing it. Contact your state or city health department for advice. If asbestos must be removed, have it done by professionals.

Lead

A danger both inside and outside our homes is lead, which lurks in some 57 million American homes, most built before 1960, with walls, windows, doors, and banisters coated with more than 3 million metric tons of lead-based paint. The percentage of children aged one to five with elevated levels of lead in their blood has dropped to 2.2 percent, half of what it was in the early 1990s.[11]

Fetuses and children under age 7 are particularly vulnerable to lead because their nervous systems are still developing and because their body mass is so small that they ingest and absorb more lead per pound than adults. Even 10 micrograms (millionths of a gram) of lead per deciliter of blood—the CDC standard for lead poisoning—can kill a child's brain cells and cause poor concentration, reduced short-term memory, slower reaction times, and learning disabilities.

Adults exposed to low levels of lead (which once were thought to be safe) may develop headaches, high blood pressure, irritability, tremors, and insomnia. Health effects increase with exposure to higher levels and include anemia, stomach pain, vomiting, diarrhea, and constipation. Long-term exposure can impair fertility and damage the kidneys. Workers exposed to lead may become sterile or suffer irreversible kidney disease, damage to their central nervous system, stillbirths, or miscarriages.

The CDC and the American Academy of Pediatrics recommend annual testing of blood levels of lead in all children from age 9 months to 6 years, regardless of where they live. High-risk youngsters—those who live or play in older housing (especially if a building is in poor condition or undergoing renovation), those who live with someone who uses lead for a job or hobby, and those who live near a lead smelter, a processing plant, or a heavily traveled road or highway—should be screened every two or three months until age 3 and every six months until age 6. High levels of ascorbic acid (vitamin C) have been associated with a lower rate of elevated blood lead levels.

Mercury

Some fish contain high levels of a form of mercury called methylmercury that can harm an unborn child's developing nervous system if eaten regularly. The FDA has advised that certain individuals—young children, women who are or might become pregnant, and nursing mothers—avoid eating shark, swordfish, king mackerel, and tilefish (all high in mercury); limit their consumption of fish and shellfish that are lower in mercury, such as shrimp, canned light tuna, salmon, pollock, and catfish, to 12 ounces (two average meals) a week; and keep consumption of canned albacore tuna (which is somewhat higher in mercury) to 6 ounces (one average meal) a week. They also should check local advisories about the safety of fish caught by family and friends in local lakes, rivers, and coastal areas. If no advice is available, the FDA advises eating a maximum of 6 ounces per week of local fish and no additional fish or shellfish.

While free of lead, some popular latex paints may contain potentially hazardous mercury, which manufacturers routinely added until a 1990 ban, to prevent the growth of mold and mildew. The threat of mercury poisoning is greatest during painting and immediately after.

Even mercury in medical devices, such as sphygmomanometers that measure blood pressure, can be a hazard. Symptoms of mercury poisoning include a racing heart-beat, sweating, aching limbs, kidney problems, hand tremors, peeling skin, and emotional problems. Levels of mercury in children and women of childbearing age have fallen in recent years.

Carbon Monoxide and Nitrogen Dioxide

Carbon monoxide (CO) gas, which is tasteless, odorless, colorless, and nonirritating, can be deadly. Produced by the incomplete combustion of fuel in space heaters, furnaces, water heaters, and engines, CO reduces the delivery of oxygen in the blood. Every year an estimated 10,000 Americans seek treatment for CO inhalation; at least 250 die because of this silent killer. Those most at risk are the chronically ill, the elderly, pregnant women, and infants. Typical symptoms of CO poisoning, which is most common in winter, are headache, nausea, vomiting, fatigue, and dizziness. More severe poisoning can damage the heart and cause respiratory distress, confusion, and coma. A blood test can measure CO levels; inhaling pure oxygen speeds removal of the gas from the body. Most people who don't lose consciousness as a result of CO poisoning recover completely.

Another dangerous gas, nitrogen dioxide, can reach very high levels if you use a natural gas or propane stove in a poorly ventilated kitchen. This gas may lead to respiratory illnesses. Pilot lights are a steady source of nitrogen dioxide; to reduce exposure, switch to spark ignition.

Radon

Radioactive radon—which diffuses from rock, brick, concrete building materials, and natural soil deposits under some homes—produces charged decay products that cling to dust particles. Once trapped inside a building, radon can reach levels that may increase the risk of lung cancer. The EPA estimates that the inhalation of indoor radon is responsible for approximately 14,000 lung cancer deaths per year. Radon levels tend to be highest in areas with granite and black shale topped with porous soil.

An estimated 10 million homes and over 30 million people are at risk from high levels of radon.[12] If you live in a high-radon area, don't panic. Your hypothetical risk of dying from radon-caused lung cancer is about equal to the known risk of dying in a home fire or fall. Check with the geology department at the nearest university or with your state health department to find out if they've performed radon tests in your area. If there may be danger, you can buy a radon detector. In most homes, the readings turn out to be low. If not, your state health department can provide guidelines for bringing them down.

FAQ IS MOLD DANGEROUS?

One of the oldest and most widespread substances on earth, mold—a type of fungus that decomposes organic matter and provides plants with nutrients—has emerged as a major health concern. Common molds include *Aspergillus, Penicillium,* and *Stachybotrys,* a slimy, dark green mold that has been blamed for infant deaths and various illnesses, from Alzheimer's disease to cancer, in adults that breathe in its spores. Faulty ventilation systems and airtight buildings have been implicated as contributing to the increased mold problem.

Experts agree that mold may trigger or worsen a number of health problems, including dizziness, breathing problems, nausea, and asthma attacks. However, mold usually is harmful only to allergic or sensitive individuals.[13] In the last decade, high-profile lawsuits have resulted in multimillion dollar judgments, despite a lack of scientific evidence linking mold exposure and cancer or brain damage.

Mold problems can range from small patches to large infestations of entire rooms or even a whole building. The first step to reduce mold exposure is moisture control, which may require new methods of keeping rainwater and ground water away from the interior and maintaining the heating ventilation and air conditioning systems appropriately. Bleach or soap and water can clean up small infestations. Larger ones may require appropriate protective respiratory equipment or professionally trained, licensed, and experienced contractors.

YOUR HEARING HEALTH

Hearing loss is the third most common chronic health problem, after high blood pressure and arthritis, among older Americans. Loud noises cause hearing loss in an estimated 10 million Americans every year. Only about one-fifth of the 28 million Americans suffering from hearing loss have sought professional help.[14]

Most hearing loss occurs on the job. The people at highest risk are firefighters, police, military personnel, construction and factory workers, musicians, farmers, and truck drivers. Other sources of danger include live or recorded

© Rune Hellestad/CORBIS

Besides listening to the music at your next concert, tune in to the noise level and how your ears are feeling.

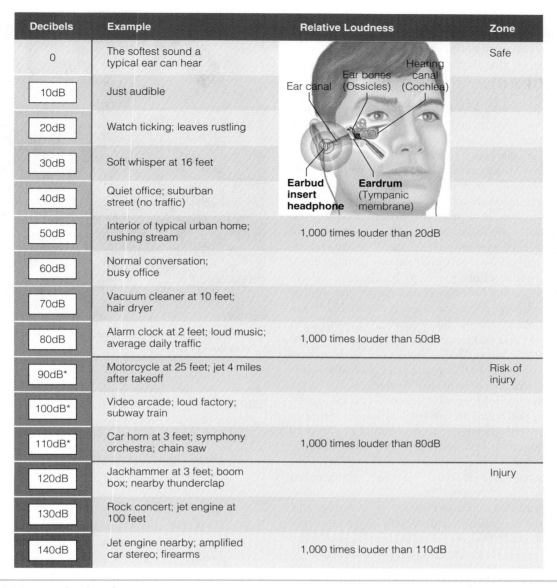

Decibels	Example	Relative Loudness	Zone
0	The softest sound a typical ear can hear		Safe
10dB	Just audible		
20dB	Watch ticking; leaves rustling		
30dB	Soft whisper at 16 feet		
40dB	Quiet office; suburban street (no traffic)		
50dB	Interior of typical urban home; rushing stream	1,000 times louder than 20dB	
60dB	Normal conversation; busy office		
70dB	Vacuum cleaner at 10 feet; hair dryer		
80dB	Alarm clock at 2 feet; loud music; average daily traffic	1,000 times louder than 50dB	
90dB*	Motorcycle at 25 feet; jet 4 miles after takeoff		Risk of injury
100dB*	Video arcade; loud factory; subway train		
110dB*	Car horn at 3 feet; symphony orchestra; chain saw	1,000 times louder than 80dB	
120dB	Jackhammer at 3 feet; boom box; nearby thunderclap		Injury
130dB	Rock concert; jet engine at 100 feet		
140dB	Jet engine nearby; amplified car stereo; firearms	1,000 times louder than 110dB	

FIGURE 20-3   Loud and Louder

The human ear perceives a 10-decibel increase as a doubling of loudness. Thus, the 100 decibels of a subway train sound much more than twice as loud as the 50 decibels of a rushing stream.

high-volume music, recreational vehicles, airplanes, lawn-care equipment, woodworking tools, some appliances, and chain saws.

HOW LOUD IS THAT NOISE?

Loudness, or the intensity of a sound, is measured in **decibels (dB).** A whisper is 20 decibels; a conversation in a living room is about 50 decibels. On this scale, 50 isn't two and a half times louder than 20, but 1,000 times louder: Each 10-dB rise in the scale represents a tenfold increase in the intensity of the sound. Very loud but short bursts of sounds (such as gunshots and fireworks) and quieter but

longer-lasting sounds (such as power tools) can induce hearing loss.

Sounds under 75 dB don't seem harmful. However, prolonged exposure to any sound over 85 dB (the equivalent of a power mower or food blender) or brief exposure to louder sounds can harm hearing. The noise level at rock concerts can reach 110 to 140 dB, about as loud as an air raid siren. Personal sound systems (boom boxes) can blast sounds of up to 115 dB. Cars with extremely loud music systems, known as boom cars, can produce an earsplitting 145 dB—louder than a jet engine or thunderclap (Figure 20-3).

Common "sound offenders" are nightclubs (with sustained levels of well over 100 decibels), restaurants (with levels of 80 to 96 decibels), and street traffic (80 decibels or more). However, even low-level office noise can undermine well-being and increase health risks.

EFFECTS OF NOISE

Noise-induced hearing loss is 100 percent preventable— and irreversible. Hearing aids are the only treatment, but they do not correct the problem; they just amplify sound to compensate for hearing loss.

The healthy human ear can hear sounds within a wide range of frequencies (measured in hertz), from the low-frequency rumble of thunder at 50 hertz to the high-frequency overtones of a piccolo at nearly 20,000 hertz. High-frequency noise damages the delicate hair cells that serve as sound receptors in the inner ear. Damage first begins as a diminished sensitivity to frequencies around 4,000 hertz, the highest notes of a piano.

Early symptoms of hearing loss include difficulty understanding speech and *tinnitus* (ringing in the ears). Brief, very loud sounds, such as an explosion or gunfire, can produce immediate, severe, and permanent hearing loss. Longer exposure to less intense but still hazardous sounds, such as those common at work or in public places, can gradually impair hearing, often without the individual's awareness.

Conductive hearing loss, often caused by ear infections, cuts down on perception of low-pitched sounds. Sensorineural loss involves damage or destruction of the sensory cells in the inner ear that convert sound waves to nerve signals.

Noise can harm more than our ears: High-volume sound has been linked to high blood pressure and other stress-related problems that can lead to heart disease, insomnia, anxiety, headaches, colitis, and ulcers. Noise frays the nerves; people tend to be more anxious, irritable, and angry when their ears are constantly barraged with sound.

(FAQ) IS LISTENING TO MUSIC THROUGH EARBUDS HAZARDOUS TO MY HEARING?

Although there is limited research, audiologists (who specialize in hearing problems) report seeing greater noise-induced hearing loss in young people. One probable culprit is extended use of earbuds, tiny earphones used with portable music players that deliver sound extremely close to the eardrum. Hearing loss can be temporary or permanent.[15]

The dangers to your hearing depend on how loud the music is and how long you listen. Because personal music players have long-lasting rechargeable batteries, people—especially young ones—both listen for long periods and turn up the volume. As long as the sound level is within safety levels (see Figure 20-3), you can listen as long as you'd like. If you listen to music so loud that someone else can hear two or three feet away, it's too loud.

For safe listening, limit listening to a portable music player with earphones at 60 percent of its potential volume

How loudly do you play your favorite music? How long do you listen through earbuds?

to one hour a day. At the very least, take a five-minute break after an hour of listening and keep the volume low.

Ask yourself the following questions to determine if you should have your hearing checked:

▪ Do you frequently have to ask people to repeat themselves?

▪ Do you have difficulty hearing when someone speaks in a whisper?

▪ Do people complain that you turn up the volume too much when watching television or listening to music?

▪ Do you have difficulty following conversation in a noisy environment?

▪ Do you avoid groups of people because of hearing difficulty?

▪ Have your friends or family suggested you might have hearing loss?

THE QUALITY OF YOUR DRINKING WATER

Worldwide 2.2 million people die annually as a result of contaminated water and poor sanitation.[16] Fears about the public water supply have led many Americans to turn off their taps. About two-thirds take steps to drink purer water, either by using filtration and distillation methods or by drinking bottled water. However, Consumer Union, a nonprofit advocacy group, maintains that the United States has the safest water supply in the world. The Environmental Protection Agency has set standards for some 80 contaminants. These include many toxic chemicals and heavy metals—including lead, mercury, cadmium, and chromium—that can cause kidney and nervous system damage and birth defects.

Each year the CDC reports an average of 7,400 cases of illness related to the water people drink. The most common culprits include parasites, bacteria, viruses, chemicals, and lead. Health officials suggest having your water tested if you live near a hazardous waste dump or industrial park, if the pipes in your house are made of lead or joined together with lead solder, if your water comes from a well, or if you purchase water from a private company. Check to see if your state health department or local water supplier will provide free testing. If not, use a state-certified laboratory that tests water in accordance with EPA standards.

IS BOTTLED WATER BETTER?

Is bottled water better? That's what consumers have often assumed. Bottled water sales have tripled in the past ten years. Women and college-age Americans make up the majority of bottled-water drinkers. Yet in the past, the Food and Drug Administration (FDA) simply defined bottled water as "sealed in bottles or other containers and intended for human consumption." Bottled water wasn't required to be "pure" or even to be tested for toxic chemicals. One survey found chemical contaminants associated with cancer in 22 of 100 brands tested.

The FDA has called for federal monitoring of the purity of bottled water. Some states, including California and New York, have their own bottled-water safety standards to ensure that bottled water is at least as safe as drinking water.

FLUORIDE

About two-thirds of Americans drink water containing fluoride, an additive to water and toothpaste that helps teeth resist decay. According to the American Dental Association, the incidence of tooth decay is a median of 29 percent lower among children and adolescents in areas with fluoridated water.[17] However, laboratory rats given fluoridated water

have shown a high rate of bone cancer. The more fluoride they drank in their water, the more likely they were to develop this cancer. But this type of cancer is extremely rare in humans, and the estimated lifetime risk to any individual from drinking fluoridated water is less than one in 5,000.

Federal health officials have found no evidence that fluoride causes cancer in humans and have concluded that its benefits far outweigh any risks. However, excessive fluoride can increase bone loss and fractures in pre- and postmenopausal women. Health professionals advise consumers to use only small amounts of fluoridated toothpaste, rinse thoroughly after brushing, and use fluoride supplements only when the home water supply is known to be deficient.

CHLORINE

Three-quarters of the population of the United States drinks water treated with chlorine to kill disease-causing bacteria. The Council on Environmental Quality has warned that people drinking chlorinated water have a 53 percent greater risk of getting colon and bladder cancer and a 13 to 93 percent greater risk of getting rectal cancer than those not drinking chlorinated water. There may even be a link between soft water and a higher rate of cardiovascular disease, perhaps because soft water in some areas tends to have more sodium in it.

LEAD

Long recognized as a hazard in paint and dust, lead can also leach into the drinking supply from pipes made of or soldered with lead. The highest risk exists in cities with older housing and with lead pipes or water lines.

CHEMICAL RISKS

Various chemicals, including benzene, asbestos, and arsenic, have been shown to cause cancer in humans. Probable carcinogens include DDT and PCB. Risks can be greatly increased with simultaneous exposures to more than one carcinogen, for example, tobacco smoke and asbestos.[18]

According to the CDC, the levels of potentially harmful chemicals, including pesticides and lead, in the country's blood supplies have declined.[19] Still, an estimated 50,000 to 70,000 U.S. workers die each year of chronic diseases related to past exposure to toxic substances, including lung cancer, bladder cancer, leukemia, lymphoma, chronic bronchitis, and disorders of the nervous system. **Endocrine disruptors,** chemicals that act as or interfere with human hormones, particularly estrogen, may pose a different threat. Scientists are investigating their impact on fertility, falling sperm counts, and cancers of the reproductive organs. Exposure to toxic chemicals causes about 3 percent of developmental defects.

(FAQ) WHAT HEALTH RISKS ARE CAUSED BY PESTICIDES?

High quantities of toxic chemical waste from unused or obsolete pesticides are posing a continuing and worsening threat to people and the environment in Eastern Europe, Africa, Asia, the Middle East, and Latin America.[20] In the United States, the FDA estimates that 33 to 39 percent of our food supply contains residues of pesticides that may pose a long-term danger to our health. Scientists have detected traces of pesticides in groundwater in both urban and rural areas.

No relationship has been found between fertility, as measured by time to pregnancy (that is, the time taken for a couple to conceive once they decide they want to), and male exposure to pesticides. Exposure to pesticides may, however, pose a risk to pregnant women and their unborn children. Men whose jobs routinely expose them to pesticide may be at increased risk of prostate cancer.[21] Parental exposure does not increase the likelihood of childhood brain cancer.[22]

© 2000 Paul Grebliunas/Stone/Getty Images

Pesticides protect crops from harmful insects, plants, and fungi but may endanger human health.

Chlorinated hydrocarbons include several high-risk substances—such as DDT, kepone, and chlordane—that have been restricted or banned because they may cause cancer, birth defects, neurological disorders, and damage to wildlife and the environment. They are extremely resistant to breakdown.

Organic phosphates, including chemicals such as malathion, break down more rapidly than the chlorinated hydrocarbons. Most are highly toxic, causing cramps, confusion, diarrhea, vomiting, headaches, and breathing difficulties. Higher levels in the blood can lead to convulsions, paralysis, coma, and death.

Farmworkers and those in the communities surrounding agricultural land are at greatest risk for pesticide exposure. However, even city dwellers aren't out of range. About half (52 percent) of the nation uses insect repellents, including some made with potent insecticides.

CHEMICAL WEAPONS

Terrorist threats include the possibility of the use of chemical weapons. Possible bioterror agents include poison gases, herbicides, and other types of chemical substances that can kill, maim, or temporarily incapacitate. Chemical agents can be dispersed as liquids, vapors, gases, and aerosols that attack nerves, blood, skin, or lungs. In contrast to biological weapons, chemical weapons can kill rapidly, often within hours or minutes, and sometimes with just a small drop. Possible protection against chemical weapons includes gas masks, shelters, and sealed suits and vehicles. Treatment and antidotes can sometimes help after exposure. If contaminated, you need to flush your eyes and skin immediately for at least five to ten minutes while awaiting emergency help.

Some common chemical agents include ricin, which when inhaled causes weakness, fever, chest tightness, cough, and severe respiratory problems, including potentially fatal fluid buildup in the lungs; sarin, a nerve gas that can cause death within minutes by paralyzing the muscles used for breathing; and VX, which kills within minutes by blocking the transmission of nerve impulses along the central nervous system, causing convulsions, respiratory paralysis, and death.

MULTIPLE CHEMICAL SENSITIVITY

The proliferation of chemicals in modern society has led to an entirely new disease, **multiple chemical sensitivity (MCS),** also called environmentally triggered illness, universal allergy, or chemical AIDS. MCS was first described almost a half century ago when a Chicago allergist treated a number of patients who reported becoming ill after being exposed to various petrochemicals. Since that time, many more cases of MCS have been reported, yet there is no agreed upon definition of the condition, no medical test that can diagnose it, and no proven treatment.

According to medical theory, people become chemically sensitive in a two-step process: First, they experience a major exposure to a chemical, such as a pesticide, a solvent, or a combustion product. The sensitized person then begins to react to low-level chemical exposures from ordinary substances, such as perfumes and tobacco smoke. In other words, these low-level exposures trigger a physiological response. Over time, chemically unrelated substances may induce symptoms such as chest pain, depression, difficulty remembering, dizziness, fatigue, headache, inability to concentrate, nausea, and aches and pains in muscles and joints.

INVISIBLE THREATS

Among the unseen threats to health are various forms of *radiation,* energy radiated in the form of waves or particles.

ELECTROMAGNETIC FIELDS

Any electrically charged conductor generates two kinds of invisible fields: electric and magnetic. Together they're called **electromagnetic fields (EMFs).** For years, these fields, produced by household appliances, home wiring, lighting fixtures, electric blankets, and overhead power lines, were considered harmless. However, epidemiological studies have revealed a link between exposure to high-voltage lines and cancer (especially leukemia, a blood cancer) in electrical workers and children.

Laboratory studies on animals have shown that alternating current, which changes strength and direction 60 times a second (and electrifies most of North America), emits EMFs that may interfere with the normal functioning of human cell membranes, which have their own electromagnetic fields. The result may be mood disorders, changes in circadian rhythms (our inner sense of time), miscarriage, developmental problems, or cancer. Researchers have documented increases in breast cancer deaths in women who worked as electrical engineers, electricians, or in other high-exposure jobs, and a link between EMF exposure and increased risk of leukemia and possibly brain cancer.

After six years of congressionally mandated research, the National Institute of Environmental Health Sciences concluded that the evidence of a risk of cancer and other human disease from the electric and magnetic fields around power lines is "weak." This finding applies to the extremely low frequency electric and magnetic fields surrounding both the big power lines that distribute power and the smaller but closer electric lines in homes and appliances. However, the researchers also noted that EMF exposure "cannot be recognized as entirely safe."

Expectant mothers who often use electric blankets or heated water beds during winter have a higher miscarriage rate than nonusers. Babies conceived in the winter by

© Tony Freeman/PhotoEdit

Although laboratory studies on animals indicate that EMFs affect human cell membranes, research on humans has found only a weak connection between EMFs and disease.

electric blanket-users grow more slowly in the womb and tend to have a lower birthweight than others. Federal officials urge "prudent avoidance" of electric blankets for women who are pregnant or hoping to conceive.

Cell phones emit low levels of electromagnetic energy (see Savvy Consumer: "Are Cell Phones Safe to Use?").

MICROWAVES

Microwaves (extremely high frequency electromagnetic waves) increase the rate at which molecules vibrate; this vibration generates heat. There's no evidence that existing levels of microwave radiation encountered in the environment pose a health risk to people, and all home microwave ovens must meet safety standards for leakage.

Another concern about the safety of microwave ovens stems from the chemicals in plastic wrapping and plastic containers used in microwave ovens. Chemicals may leak into food. In high concentrations, some of the chemicals (such as DEHA, which makes plastic more pliable) can cause cancer in mice. Consumers should be cautious about using clingy plastic wrap when reheating leftovers, and plastic-encased metal "heat susceptors" included in convenience foods such as popcorn and pizza. Although these materials seem safe when tested in conventional ovens at temperatures of 300° to 350° Fahrenheit, microwave ovens can boost temperatures to 500° Fahrenheit.

Savvy Consumer ▪ Are Cell Phones Safe to Use?

Since cellular phone service was introduced in the United States in 1984, mobile and handheld phones have become ubiquitous. More than 86 million people use cell phones, and concern has grown about their possible health risks. The federal government sets upper exposure limits to electromagnetic energy from cell phones known as the specific absorption rate, or SAR. A phone emits the most radiation during a call, but it also emits small amounts periodically whenever it's turned on.

Can exposure to low levels of electromagnetic energy that the body absorbs from a cell phone be harmful? More than

70 research papers on the potentially harmful effects of cell phone use have raised concerns about cancer, neurological disorders, sleep problems, or headaches; others have shown no association or were inconclusive. The Food and Drug Administration (FDA) and Federal Communications Commission (FCC) have stated that "the available scientific evidence does not show that any health problems are associated with using wireless phones. There is no proof, however, that wireless phones are absolutely safe." Additional studies are underway.

Swedish and Finnish researchers have found no "consistent evidence" of increased

risk of cancer from use for up to five years, but they did document protein changes in human cells exposed to cell phone radiation and an increased rate of benign brain tumors. Health experts in Britain, France, and Germany have discouraged children from using cell phones largely because of concerns that their developing nervous systems may be especially vulnerable.

A headset can keep the phone's antenna away from your head and body. Shields that claim to reduce exposure generally don't work as advertised, say the FDA and FCC.

IRRADIATED FOODS

The use of radiation on food, from either radioactive substances or devices that produce X rays, is known as **irradiation.** It doesn't make the food radioactive—its primary benefit is to prolong the food's useful life. Like the heat in canning, irradiation can kill all the microorganisms that might grow in food; the sterilized food can then be stored for years in sealed containers at room temperature without spoiling. In addition, low-dose irradiation can inhibit the sprouting of vegetables such as potatoes and onions, and delay the ripening of some fruits, such as bananas, mangoes, tomatoes, pears, and avocados—cost-saving benefits of great appeal to the food industry.

Irradiated foods are believed to be safe to eat, and the federal government has approved their distribution. Most research has focused on low-dose irradiation to delay ripening and destroy insects. Nutritional studies have shown no significant decreases in the quality of the foods, but high-dose treatments may cause vitamin losses similar to those that occur during canning. It's also possible that the ionizing effect of radiation creates new compounds in foods that may be mutagenic or carcinogenic. In meats, irradiation proved less effective than cooking in destroying bacteria.

IONIZING RADIATION

Radiation that possesses enough energy to separate electrons from their atoms, leaving charged ions, is called **ionizing radiation.** Its effects on health depend on many factors, including the amount, length of exposure, type, part of the body exposed, and the health and age of the individual.

We're surrounded by low-level ionizing radiation every day. Most comes from cosmic rays and radioactive minerals, which vary according to geography. (Denver has more than Atlanta, for instance, because of its altitude.) Man-made sources, including medical and dental X rays, account for

approximately 18 percent of the average person's lifetime exposure.

Radiation exposure in humans is measured in units called rads and rems. A *rad (radiation absorbed dose)* is a measure of the energy deposited by ionizing radiation when it's absorbed by an object. A *rem (roentgen equivalent man)* is a measure of the biological effect of ionizing radiation. Different types of radiation cause different amounts of damage. The rem measurement takes this into account. For X rays, rads and rems are equivalent. A quantity of 1 rad or 1 rem is a substantial dose of radiation. Smaller doses are measured in *millirads* (thousandths of a rad) or *millirems* (thousandths of a rem). The average annual radiation exposure for a person in the United States is about one-tenth of a rem.

Virtually any part of the body can be affected by ionizing radiation, although bone marrow and the thyroid are especially vulnerable. Radon exposures in homes can increase the risk of lung cancer. Although high levels of radiation are most dangerous, even low-level radiation can be harmful to health. According to the National Research Council, the risk of getting cancer from small amounts of radiation is four times more than had been previously estimated, and there's much greater danger of mental retardation among babies exposed to radiation in the womb from eight to fifteen weeks after conception.

DIAGNOSTIC X RAYS

The EPA estimates that 30 to 50 percent of the 700 million X rays taken every year in the United States are unnecessary. However, doctors sometimes prescribe X rays or newer imaging techniques involving radiation, such as CT scans, to protect themselves from malpractice suits, and hospitals benefit financially from the heavy use of X-ray equipment.

Dental X rays involve little radiation, but many people receive so many so often that they're second only to chest examinations in frequency. Dentists typically obtain radiographs of all the teeth at the beginning of a patient's care, and again every three to five years. However, you can cut down on total X rays by bringing previous films with you or having your dentist forward copies when you switch dentists.

Always ask why an X ray is being ordered. Don't give your consent unless there's a clear need. Keep a record of the date and location of every X-ray exam. Some of these X rays may someday provide information that would make more X rays unnecessary. Ask the radiologist to explain specifically how much radiation you'll be exposed to, and be sure to wear a protective leaded apron. There's no sense in refusing a needed medical X ray just because you're afraid of the radiation exposure. Under certain circumstances, the benefits far outweigh the risks.

Learn It / Live It:
Taking Care of Mother Earth

Environmental problems can seem so complex that you may think there's little you can do about them. That's not the case. This world can be made better instead of worse. The job isn't easy, and all of us have to do our part. Just as many diseases of the previous century have been eradicated, so in time we may be able to remove or reduce many environmental threats. Your future—and our planet's future—may depend on it.

- **Plant a tree.** Even a single tree helps absorb carbon dioxide and produces cooling that can reduce the need for air-conditioning.

- **Look for simply packaged items.** Whenever possible, choose items packed in recycled materials or something recyclable.

- **Bring your own bag.** Whenever possible, avoid using plastic or paper bags for items you could carry in a cloth or string carryall.

- **Hit the switch.** Turn off all electrical appliances (TVs, CD players, radios, lights) when you're not in the room or paying attention to them.

- **Avoid disposables.** Use a mug instead of a paper or Styrofoam cup, a sponge instead of a paper towel, a cloth napkin instead of a paper one.

- **Be water wise.** Turn off the tap while you shave or brush your teeth. Install water-efficient faucets, toilets, and shower heads. Wash clothes in cold water.

- **Cancel junk mail.** It consumes 100 million trees a year. To get off mailing lists, write: Direct Mail Association, Mail Preference Service, P.O. Box 9008, Farmingdale, NY 11735-9008

- **Spare the seas.** If you live near the coast or are picnicking or hiking near the ocean, don't use plastic bags (which are often blown into the water) or plastic six-pack holders (which can get caught around the necks of sea birds).

- **Don't buy products made of endangered substances.** Examples include coral, ivory, tortoise shell, or wood from endangered forests (teak, mahogany, ebony, rosewood).

- **Speak out.** E-mail your senators and congressional representatives, who vote on pollution controls, budgets for the enforcement of safety regulations, and the preservation of forests and wildlife. Identify the particular bill or issue you're addressing. Be as specific, brief, and to the point as possible. Go to www.senate.gov and click on "Senators" to find the e-mail addresses. To find your congressional representative, go to www.house.gov and click on "Write Your Representative."

Making This Chapter Work for You
Review Questions

1. Threats to the environment include
   a. an open ecosystem.
   b. depletion of the oxygen layer.
   c. ecological processes.
   d. global warming.

2. Mutagens
   a. are caused by birth defects.
   b. result in changes to the DNA of body cells.
   c. are agents that trigger changes in the DNA of body cells.
   d. are caused by repeated exposure to pollutants.

3. Which of the following statements about global warming is true?
   a. In 2001, the United States signed the first international treaty to fight global warming.
   b. Global warming may result in severe drought and a rise in ocean levels.
   c. Increasing tree cover and agricultural lands will contribute to global warming.
   d. Increasing carbon dioxide production will slow the progress of global warming.

4. One of the most important things you can do to help protect the environment is
   a. recycle paper, bottles, cans, and unwanted food.
   b. use as much water as possible to help lower the ocean water levels.
   c. avoid energy-depleting fluorescent bulbs.
   d. use plastic storage containers and plastic wrap to save trees from being cut down.

5. Which of the following statements about air pollution is *false*?
   a. Current model automobiles emit much less pollution per mile than new cars in 1970.
   b. The three types of smog include sulfur-dioxide smog, produced by burning oil; photochemical

Self Survey ▦ Are You Doing Your Part for the Planet?

You may think that there is little you can do, as an individual, to save Earth. But everyday acts can add up and make a difference in helping or harming the planet on which we live.

	Almost Never	Sometimes	Always
1. Do you walk, cycle, carpool, or use public transportation as much as possible to get around?	___	___	___
2. Do you recycle?	___	___	___
3. Do you reuse plastic and paper bags?	___	___	___
4. Do you try to conserve water by not running the tap as you shampoo or brush your teeth?	___	___	___
5. Do you use products made of recycled materials?	___	___	___
6. Do you drive a car that gets good fuel mileage and has up-to-date emission control equipment?	___	___	___
7. Do you turn off lights, televisions, and appliances when you're not using them?	___	___	___
8. Do you avoid buying products that are elaborately packaged?	___	___	___
9. Do you use glass jars and waxed paper rather than plastic wrap for storing food?	___	___	___
10. Do you take brief showers rather than baths?	___	___	___
11. Do you use cloth towels and napkins rather than paper products?	___	___	___
12. When listening to music, do you keep the volume low?	___	___	___
13. Do you try to avoid any potential carcinogens, such as asbestos, mercury, or benzene?	___	___	___
14. Are you careful to dispose of hazardous materials (such as automobile oil or antifreeze) at appropriate sites?	___	___	___
15. Do you follow environmental issues in your community and write your state or federal representatives to support "green" legislation?	___	___	___

Count the number of items you've checked in each column. If you've circled 10 or more in the "always" column, you're definitely helping to make a difference. If you've circled 10 or more in the "never" column, read this chapter carefully and "Your Action Plan for Protecting the Planet" to find out what you can do. If you've mainly circled "sometimes," you're moving in the right direction, but you need to be more consistent and more conscientious.

smog, resulting from car exhaust; and carbon-monoxide smog, caused by fossil fuels.

c. Ozone in the upper atmosphere protects us from harmful ultraviolet radiation from the sun, but in the lower atmosphere, it is a harmful air pollutant.

d. Air pollution can cause the same types of respiratory health problems as smoking.

6. Indoor pollutants include

a. lead, which is found in old paint and can result in nervous system damage in adults and impaired fertility and kidney damage in children.

b. radon, which is found in building materials and can cause heart disease.

c. asbestos, which may be found in building insulation and can cause lung diseases.

d. carbon monoxide, which can be produced by furnaces and engines and can result in chronic illnesses such as emphysema.

7. You can protect your hearing by

a. avoiding prolonged exposure to sounds under 75 decibels.

b. using foam earplugs when operating noisy tools or attending rock concerts.

c. limiting noise exposure to short bursts of loud sounds such as fireworks.

d. drinking alcohol in noisy environments to mute the sounds.

8. Drinking water safety

a. may be compromised if your water comes from a well.

b. is high in the United States because of the use of sodium chloride to kill disease-causing bacteria.

c. can be guaranteed by using bottled water, which is completely free of chemical contaminants.

d. has been significantly decreased in those communities that add fluoride to the water.

YOUR ACTION PLAN FOR PROTECTING THE PLANET

Simple steps can help save energy, lower carbon dioxide (CO_2) emissions, and cut down on energy costs. Here are some recommendations from the Environmental Defense and World Wildlife Fund:

▪ Wash laundry in warm or cold water, not hot. *Average annual CO_2 reduction: up to 500 pounds for two loads of laundry a week.*

▪ Buy products sold in the simplest possible packaging. Carry a tote bag or recycle shopping bags. *Average annual CO_2 reduction: 1,000 pounds because garbage is reduced 25 percent.*

▪ Switch from standard light bulbs to energy-efficient fluorescent ones. *Average annual CO_2 reduction: about 500 pounds per bulb.*

▪ Set room thermostats lower in winter and higher in summer. *Average annual CO_2 reduction: about 500 pounds for each two-degree reduction.*

▪ Run dishwashers only when full, and choose the energy-saving mode rather than the regular setting. *Average annual CO_2 reduction: 200 pounds.*

▪ Bike, carpool, or take mass transit whenever possible. *Average annual CO_2 reduction: 20 pounds for each gallon of gasoline saved.*

▪ Drive a car that gets high gas mileage and produces low emissions. Keep your speed at or below the speed limit.

▪ Keep your tires inflated and your engine tuned. Recycle old batteries and tires. (Most stores that sell new ones will take back old ones.)

▪ Turn off your engine if you're going to be stopped for more than a minute.

▪ Collect all fluids that you drain from your car (motor oil, antifreeze) and recycle or properly dispose of them.

CASE IN POINT

Student: Mike, 24

Goal: Become more environmentally responsible

Health Action Plan:

▪ Look for products made with recycled materials

▪ Check the energy efficiency of appliances and equipment he's planning to buy

▪ Set up recycling containers at his apartment complex

▪ Bike to class rather than drive

▪ Look into a high-mileage, hybrid vehicle the next time he buys a car

Health⊛Now™ If you want to write your own goals for working toward a healthy environment, go to the **Wellness Journal at HealthNow, http://healthnow .brookscole.com/ith**

---

9. Pesticide risks to health include:
   a. reduced male fertility.
   b. higher incidence of childhood brain cancer if parents have been exposed.
   c. higher incidence of cancer and birth defects from chlorinated hydrocarbons such as DDT.
   d. higher incidence of diabetes.

10. Which statement about radiation is *false?*
    a. Evidence indicates a weak link between electromagnetic fields around power lines and cancer and other diseases.
    b. Radio frequency signals from cell phones cause brain cancer.
    c. Irradiation can be used to kill microorganisms in food.
    d. Chemicals in plastic wrap may leak into foods heated in microwave ovens.

Answers to these questions can be found on page 587.

Critical Thinking

1. How do you contribute to environmental pollution? How might you change your habits to protect the environment?

2. An excerpt from a recent newspaper article stated, "Children living in a public housing project near a local refinery suffer from a high rate of asthma and allergies, and an environmental group says the plant may be to blame." The refinery has met all the local air quality standards, employs hundreds in the community, and pays substantial city taxes, which support police, fire, and social services. If you were a city council member, how would you balance health and environmental concerns with the need for industry in your community? What actions would you recommend in this particular situation?

3. In one Harris poll, 84 percent of Americans said that, given a choice between a high standard of living (but with hazardous air and water pollution and the depletion of natural resources) and a lower standard of living (but with clean air and drinking water), they would prefer clean air and drinking water and a lower standard of living. What about you? What exactly would you be willing to give up: air conditioning, convenience packaging and products, driving your own car rather than using public transportation? Do you think most people are willing to change their lifestyles to preserve the environment?

Media Menu

Health Now™

Throughout the chapter, this icon introduces a list of resources on the Health-Now website at **http://healthnow.brookscole.com/ith** that will:
- Help you evaluate your knowledge of the material.
- Allow you to take an exam-prep quiz.
- Provide a Personalized Learning Plan targeting resources that address areas you should study.
- Coach you through identifying target goals for behavior change and creating and monitoring your personal change plan throughout the semester.

INTERNET CONNECTIONS

Envirolink

www.envirolink.org

Envirolink is a nonprofit organization that brings together individuals and groups concerned about the environment and provides access to a wealth of online environmental resources.

Student Environmental Action Coalition

www.seac.org

Since 1988, the Student Environmental Action Coalition has been empowering students and youth to fight for environmental and social justice in our schools and communities.

Environmental Protection Agency

www.epa.gov

This comprehensive government site features environmental topics, including ecosystems, global warming, air and water pollution, compliance and enforcement, pesticides and toxins, accident prevention, and treatment.

National Center for Environmental Health (NCEH)

www.cdc.gov/nceh/

This site, sponsored by the U.S. Centers for Disease Control and Prevention, features a searchable database as well as fact sheets and brochures on a variety of environmental topics, from emergency preparedness and public health tracking to environmental hazards and lead poisoning prevention.

InfoTrac College Edition Activities Log on, insert **hearing** into the Keyword search box, and limit your search to the past year. When you get the results, Mark articles to review, then Select one to read. Summarize three or four key points from the article.

You can find additional readings related to personal health with InfoTrac College Edition, an online library of more than 900 journals and publications. Follow the instructions for accessing InfoTrac College Edition that were packaged with your textbook; then search for articles using a keyword search.

For additional links, resources, and suggested readings on the InfoTrac College Edition, visit our Health and Wellness Resource Center at **http://health .wadsworth.com.**

Key Terms

The terms listed are used on the page indicated. Definitions of the terms are in the Glossary at the end of this book.

acid rain 573	multiple chemical sensitivity (MCS) 580
chlorinated hydrocarbons 580	mutagen 570
decibel (dB) 577	mutation 570
ecosystem 570	organic phosphates 580
electromagnetic fields (EMFs) 581	pollutant 570
endocrine disruptors 580	pollution 570
global warming 571	precycling 574
ionizing radiation 582	recycling 574
irradiation 582	smog 572
microwaves 581	teratogen 570

Making This Chapter Work for You

ANSWERS TO MULTIPLE CHOICE QUESTIONS

CHAPTER 1

1. a; 2. d; 3. d; 4. c; 5. d; 6. b; 7. a; 8. c; 9. a; 10. c

CHAPTER 2

1. b; 2. c; 3. c; 4. c; 5. d; 6. a; 7. c; 8. d; 9. a; 10. c

CHAPTER 3

1. b; 2. d; 3. a; 4. c; 5. c; 6. a; 7. b; 8. a; 9. d; 10. b

CHAPTER 4

1. b; 2. d; 3. a; 4. a; 5. c; 6. c; 7. a; 8. b; 9. c; 10. d

CHAPTER 5

1. c; 2. b; 3. c; 4. b; 5. c; 6. d; 7. b; 8. b; 9. a; 10. d

CHAPTER 6

1. c; 2. a; 3. d; 4. a; 5. d; 6. c; 7. a; 8. a; 9. a; 10. b

CHAPTER 7

1. c; 2. b; 3. c; 4. c; 5. d; 6. c; 7. c; 8. c; 9. a; 10. c

CHAPTER 8

1. d; 2. c; 3. b; 4. a; 5. d; 6. b; 7. a; 8. d; 9. c; 10. c

CHAPTER 9

1. b; 2. d; 3. c; 4. d; 5. d; 6. b; 7. d; 8. c; 9. a; 10. a

CHAPTER 10

1. c; 2. d; 3. a; 4. c; 5. c; 6. b; 7. c; 8. a; 9. b; 10. d

CHAPTER 11

1. a; 2. c; 3. d; 4. b; 5. c; 6. c; 7. d; 8. a; 9. b; 10. d

CHAPTER 12

1. b; 2. c; 3. d; 4. a; 5. b; 6. b; 7. a; 8. d; 9. b; 10. d

CHAPTER 13

1. d; 2. c; 3. d; 4. b; 5. a; 6. c; 7. d; 8. c; 9. d; 10. b

CHAPTER 14

1. a; 2. c; 3. a; 4. b; 5. c; 6. a; 7. d; 8. b; 9. b; 10. c

CHAPTER 15

1. b; 2. c; 3. d; 4. a; 5. b; 6. b; 7. c; 8. d; 9. c; 10. b

CHAPTER 16

1. d; 2. b; 3. a; 4. d; 5. a; 6. d; 7. b; 8. c; 9. d; 10. a

CHAPTER 17

1. c; 2. b; 3. b; 4. a; 5. d; 6. c; 7. b; 8. d; 9. d; 10. b

CHAPTER 18

1. b; 2. a; 3. d; 4. c; 5. b; 6. b; 7. d; 8. c; 9. c; 10. b

CHAPTER 19

1. d; 2. b; 3. c; 4. b; 5. b; 6. c; 7. b; 8. a; 9. c; 10. b

CHAPTER 20

1. d; 2. c; 3. b; 4. a; 5. b; 6. c; 7. b; 8. a; 9. c; 10. b

Hales Health Almanac

HEALTH INFORMATION ON THE INTERNET

YOUR HEALTH DIRECTORY

EMERGENCY!

A CONSUMER'S GUIDE TO MEDICAL TESTS

USING THE INTERNET

What are the very latest statistics on the incidence of the flu? Are any new drugs in the works for the treatment of diabetes? How can I get in touch with others who suffer from asthma? Is it possible to make a low-fat chocolate cake? You can answer these kinds of questions with the help of the Internet. A gold mine of information for the student of health, the Internet can help you with research for your schoolwork and also with personal questions and concerns about your own health.

What are the practical uses of the Internet for the student of health and the health care consumer?

- **Research.** The Internet is a repository for many health journals, government statistics, archives, and other sources of scholarly information. Subscribing to a mailing list or posting to a newsgroup in an area of interest can yield new sources of information that would be hard to get elsewhere.
- **Self-help and support.** Dozens of newsgroups and mailing lists offer support and advice for people dealing with all kinds of health-related issues, from Alzheimer's caregivers to people with eating disorders to athletes comparing training programs.
- **Goods and services.** Online shopping for health-related products is easy.
- **Graduate school and career information.** If you are interested in a career in a health-related field, most graduate schools have websites that list their programs, entrance requirements, faculty profiles, and other information of interest to prospective students. And you can consult online listings of jobs available in many areas of health care.

SEARCHING THE WEB

One way to find websites of interest to you is to use a search engine. The large popular search engines are:

- **Google**   www.google.com
- **Yahoo!**   www.yahoo.com
- **AltaVista**   www.altavista.com

To use a search engine, go to the home page for the site, type one or more keywords or phrases into the "search" box. The engine will then search all the sites in its index and return a list to you, with hyperlinks and sometimes short descriptions, of those that contain your keywords.

No single search engine contains all the contents of the Internet. After connecting to a search engine for the first time, it is a good idea to read the tool's description, search options, and rules and restrictions. Each engine offers a different "view" of the Web and you'll want to tailor your query to make the best use of that system.

The key to an effective search is picking the right keywords. Try to find distinctive words or combinations of words. If you use several keywords, check your search engine's searching tips—in most cases you can use the plus sign, the minus sign, quotation marks and the word OR to make your search more precise. For example, the word "OR" broadens the search results. You may try searching "pregnancy teen OR adolescent," to find sites that refer to teen or adolescent pregnancy.

Your search may turn up hundreds or even thousands of results—or only a few. If you have more results than you can handle, try making the keywords in your search more precise or go to your search engine's advanced search section. If you have too few results, try another search engine, using synonyms or variations on your keywords, or be less specific in your query.

NEWS GROUPS/ DISCUSSION FORUMS

News groups and discussion forums are ways of discussing topics over the Internet with other people who share the same interests or concerns. They are a popular way to establish an online community, share information, and give and receive support. For example, a person suffering from a relatively rare

disorder may not know anyone else with the same problems and concerns on campus or in town, but he or she can frequent a news group specifically for people with that disorder to learn about other peoples' experiences, the latest treatments, and just to commiserate. Or a person who is trying to quit smoking can participate in a news group to share frustrations, tips, and successes. But, as always, be aware that not everything posted to a news group is necessarily true; you must be a critical thinker.

Many commercial online services offer members-only news groups to their subscribers, but many other news groups are available to anyone. To find a news group on a topic of interest to you, try going to http://groups.google.com.

News group addresses are grouped into several broad categories called hierarchies. Listed below are some of the standard hierarchies that relate to health.

- **alt**   groups generally alternative in nature (i.e., alt.sex)
- **bionet**   groups discussing biology and biological sciences (i.e., bionet.immunology)
- **misc**   groups that don't fit into other categories (i.e., misc.fitness)
- **rec**   groups discussing hobbies, sports, music, and art (i.e., rec.food)
- **sci**   groups discussing subjects related to the science and scientific research (i.e., sci.epidemiology)
- **soc**   groups discussing social issues including politics, social programs, etc. (i.e., soc.college)
- **talk**   public debating forums on controversial issues (i.e., talk.abortion)

Before you make a posting to a news group, you may want to "lurk" for awhile, that is, read the discussion without contributing your own posting. Lurking will give you a sense of the kinds of postings that are appropriate for that news group and what the news group culture is like. Read the news group's "FAQ," or list of answers to frequently asked questions before joining the discussion.

Postings to many news groups are updated frequently, so if an item is of interest to you, you should print it or save it to your computer since it may be gone the next day. After lurking for awhile, you can join in the discussion by posting a message to the news group. You may also want to reply only to the originator of a certain message. You may want to join in on the discussion of an already-existing topic, or start your own "thread."

Be cautious when providing your e-mail address to a site or news group. Spam is junk e-mail, and spammers scoop up e-mail addresses in news groups and chat rooms.

MAILING LISTS

You are probably already on a few mailing lists—they are used by retailers, organizations, politicians, educational institutions, and many other groups who e-mail large numbers of people. But mailing lists (or list serves) are also groups of people who "get together" via e-mail to discuss a specific topic. Mailing lists offer a way to participate in lively discussions, stay up on current research, or find out answers to burning questions. There are mailing lists on nearly every topic imaginable. Mailing lists are similar to news groups in that they are forums for discussion, but the messages are delivered to your e-mail account instead of to a public bulletin board. Here's how it works:

- First, find a mailing list dealing with a subject you are interested in discussing with others (i.e., attention deficit disorder).
- Then, you have to subscribe: send an e-mail to that mailing list's "subscribe" address with the word "subscribe" in the subject line and in the main body of the text.
- Usually, the mailing list will then subscribe you to the list and send you instructions on how to "post" to the group. "Posting" means that

you send out a comment to the entire mailing list that you have subscribed to.
- Every time any member posts to the list serve, all the subscribers get that posting as an e-mail message.
- Once you have subscribed you will begin to receive e-mail messages from the mailing list. Be careful though: Some discussion groups have a large following and you may find your mailbox filling up faster than you can read the messages.
- Again, evaluate carefully any information you get from a mailing list to make sure it is accurate.

THINKING CRITICALLY ABOUT HEALTH INFORMATION ON THE INTERNET

Unlike information in most books and journals, anyone can post information or advice on the Internet. Some of this information can be misleading or downright harmful, so it is important to use your best critical thinking skills to evaluate health information you find on the Internet. Ask yourself the following questions:

- **Who is the author or sponsor of the information?** The author of the site is usually listed at the top or bottom of a site's home page. Be very wary of any anonymous site. Sites that are maintained by established schools or universities, government agencies, professional organizations, or other established organizations like the American Cancer Society are probably trustworthy. Sites created by individuals or other groups may or may not contain valid information; see if you can verify their information in other places.

- **Is it current?** Many sites post the date of their last update. Look for sites where you can determine when the information was created or modified; many of the best sites are updated weekly or even daily.
- **What is the purpose of the site?** The hidden purpose of some health websites is to sell products or act as a vehicle for advertisements. Be wary of any site that tries to sell you things or get your money. Also beware of sites that seem to be trying to persuade you of things, promote "miracle cures" or anything that seems too good to be true. Some people also use news groups and other chat forums to sell or persuade. Be skeptical and use your common sense.
- **Who is the intended audience?** Some Internet information is intended for doctors and other health-care professionals; although the information may be accurate, it may be too difficult for a layperson to interpret. Other websites or Internet forums are targeted toward people with specific problems or disorders, students, or the general public.
- **Is the information verifiable?** To get a better perspective on information from the Internet, see if you can verify it with other sources. Before you follow any health advice you get from the Net, check it out with your physician.

HEALTH RESOURCES ON THE INTERNET

"Your Health Directory" (next pages) contains web addresses for many health-related organizations. And hundreds of health-related Internet addresses can be found at http://health.wadsworth.com.

In *An Invitation to Health,* I emphasize that you shoulder a great deal of responsibility for your health and the quality of your life. Given the complexity of our minds and bodies and the many social and environmental factors that affect us, this responsibility can be a very heavy burden. But your load can be made lighter if you know where to turn for health information, services, and support.

In this directory, you will find more than 100 health-related topics and about 250 resources, including addresses, phone numbers, and websites for government agencies, community organizations, professional associations, recovery groups, and Internet sources. Many of these organizations and groups have toll-free 800 or 888 phone numbers, and most have websites (one caution: as you may have experienced, website addresses—like street addresses and phone numbers—change on occasion). Much of the material available from these groups is free.

Also included in Your Health Directory are clearinghouses and information centers that are especially rich sources of health knowledge. Their main purpose is to collect, help manage, and disseminate information. Clearinghouses often perform other services as well, such as creating original publications and providing tailored responses to individual requests. These organizations also may provide referrals to other groups that can help you.

Many of the groups listed here have local offices or chapters. You can call, write, or visit the websites of these organizations to find out if there is a branch in your vicinity, or you can check your local telephone directory.

The purpose of this directory is to help you be in control of your health. If you know where to turn for answers to your questions and if you know what choices you have, you may find that you have more control over your life.

Resources by Topic

Abortion

National Abortion Federation
(provides information about abortion and referral for abortion services)
1755 Massachusetts Ave., N.W.
Suite #600
Washington, DC 20036
(202) 667-5881
(800) 772-9100
E-mail: naf@prochoice.org
www.prochoice.org

Accident Prevention

Centers for Disease Control and Prevention
1600 Clifton Rd. N.E.
Atlanta, GA 30333
(800) CDC-INFO
(404) 639-3534
(800) 311-3435
E-mail: cdcinfo@cdc.gov
www.cdc.gov

National Safety Council
1121 Spring Lake Dr.
Itasca, IL 60143-3201
(630) 285-1121
(800) 621-7619
E-mail: info@nsc.org
www.nsc.org

Adoption

AASK (Adopt a Special Kid)
(provides assistance to families who adopt older and handicapped children)
7700 Edgewater Drive, Suite 320,
Building B
Oakland, CA 94621
E-mail: info@aask.org
www.aask.org

Aging

Administration on Aging
U.S. Department of Health and Human Services
200 Independence Ave., S.W.
Washington, DC 20201
(800) 677-1116 (Eldercare Locator—to find services for an older person in his or her locality)

(202) 619-0724 (AoA's National Aging Information Center)
Fax: (202) 357-3555
E-mail: aoainfo@aoa.hhs.gov
www.aoa.gov

American Association of Retired Persons
601 E St., N.W.
Washington, DC 20049
(888) OUR-AARP
www.aarp.org

Gray Panthers
1612 K Street, N.W., Suite 300
Washington, DC 20006
(800) 280-5362
(202) 737-6637
E-mail: info@graypanthers.org
www.graypanthers.org

AIDS (Acquired Immunodeficiency Syndrome)

National Center for HIV, STD, and TB Prevention (NCHSTP)

Centers for Disease Control and Prevention
1600 Clifton Rd. N.E.
Atlanta, GA 30333
(800) HIV-0440
E-mail: contactus@aidsinfo.nih.gov
www.cdc.gov/hiv/dhap.htm

University of California at San Francisco HIV Insite
UCSF Center for HIV Information
4150 Clement St., Box 111V
San Francisco, CA 94121
Fax: (415) 379-5547
E-mail: info@hivinsite.ucsf.edu
www.hivinsite.ucsf.edu

Gay Men's Health Crisis
The Tisch Building
119 West 24th St.
New York, NY 10011
(212) 367-1000
(212) 807-6655 (hotline)
(800) AIDS-NYC
www.gmhc.org

National AIDS Hotline
(800) CDC-INFO (800-232-4636)
E-mail: cdcinfo@cdc.gov

San Francisco AIDS Foundation
995 Market St. #200
San Francisco, CA 94103
(415) 487-3000
(800) 367-AIDS (hotline)
E-mail: feedback@sfaf.org
www.sfaf.org

Alcohol Abuse and Alcoholism

Al-Anon and Alateen
(support groups for friends and
relatives of alcoholics)
1600 Corporate Landing Pkwy.
Virginia Beach, VA 23454
(757) 563-1600
Fax: (757) 563-1655
E-mail: wso@al-anon.org
www.al-anon-alateen.org
See also white pages of telephone
directory for listing of local chapter

Alcohol Hotline
(800) ALCOHOL

Alcoholics Anonymous
Street Address:
475 Riverside Dr., 11th Floor
New York, NY 10115
Mailing Address:
Alcoholics Anonymous
Grand Central Station
P.O. Box 459
New York, NY 10163
(212) 870-3400
www.alcoholics-anonymous.org
See also white pages or telephone
directory for listing of local chapter

**National Association of
Children of Alcoholics**
11426 Rockville Pike, Suite 100
Rockville, MD 20852
(888) 554-COAS (554-2627)
(301) 468-0985
E-mail: nacoa@nacoa.org
www.nacoa.org

**National Clearinghouse for
Alcohol and Drug Information**
P.O. Box 2345
Rockville, MD 20847-2345
(800) 729-6686
(301) 468-2600
www.health.org/

**National Institute on Alcohol
Abuse and Alcoholism**
5635 Fishers Lane
MSC 9304
Bethesda, MD 20892-9304
(301) 443-3860
www.niaaa.nih.gov
See also Drug Abuse; Drinking &
Driving Groups

Allopathic Medicine

American Medical Association
515 N. State St.
Chicago, IL 60610
(800) 621-8335
www.ama-assn.org

Alternative Medicine

**National Center for
Complementary and Alternative
Medicine (NCCAM)**
P.O. Box 7923
Gaithersburg, MD 20898
(888) 644-6226
International: (301) 519-3153
TTY: (866) 464-3615 (toll-free)
E-mail: info@nccam.nih.gov
www.nccam.nih.gov

Alzheimer's Disease

**Alzheimer's Association
National Office**
225 N. Michigan Ave., Fl. 17
Chicago, IL 60601-7663
(800) 272-3900
(312) 335-8700
Fax: (312) 335-1110
E-mail: info@alz.org
www.alz.org

Arthritis

Arthritis Foundation
P.O. Box 7669
Atlanta, GA 30357-0669
(800) 568-4045
(404) 872-7100
(404) 965-7888
www.arthritis.org

**National Institute of Arthritis
and Musculoskeletal and
Skin Diseases**
National Institutes of Health
1 Ams Circle
Bethesda, MD 20892-3675

(301) 495-4484
(877) 22-NIAMS (226-4267)
E-mail: NIAMSInfo@mail.nih.gov
www.nih.gov/niams

Asthma

**Asthma and Allergy Foundation
of America**
1233 20th St., N.W., Suite 402
Washington, DC 20036
(800) 7-ASTHMA (727-8462)
(202) 466-7643
Fax: (202) 466-8940
E-mail: Info@aafa.org
www.aafa.org

Lung Line
National Jewish Medical Research
Center
(information and referral service)
1400 Jackson St.
Denver, CO 80206
(800) 222-LUNG (5864)
(303) 388-4461
www.njc.org

Attention Deficit Disorder

**National Attention Deficit
Disorder Association
(National ADDA)**
P.O. Box 543
Pottstown, PA 19464
(484) 945-2101
Fax: (610) 970-7520
www.add.org

**Children and Adults with
Attention Deficit Disorder
(CHADD)**
8181 Professional Place, Suite 150
Landover, MD 20785
(800) 233-4050
(301) 306-7070
www.chadd.org/

Automobile Safety

**American Automobile
Association (AAA)**
1000 AAA Dr. #28
Heathrow, FL 32746-5080
(407) 444-4240
www.aaa.com
See also white or yellow pages of
telephone directory for listing of
local chapter

Insurance Institute for Highway Safety
1005 North Glebe Rd., Suite 800
Arlington, VA 22201
(703) 247-1500
www.highwaysafety.org/

National Highway Traffic Safety Administration
Office of Publications
400 7th St., S.W.
Washington, DC 20590
(888) 327-4236
(202) 366-0123
www.nhtsa.dot.gov

Auto Safety Hotline
(for consumer complaints about auto safety and child safety seats, and requests for information on recalls)
(800) 424-9393

Birth Control and Family Planning

Advocates for Youth
(develops programs and material to educate youth on sex and sexual responsibility)
2000 M Street N.W., Suite 750
Washington, DC 20036
(202) 419-3420
Fax: (202) 419-1448
E-mail: information@advocates foryouth.org
www.advocatesforyouth.org

American College of Obstetricians and Gynecologists
(provides literature and contraceptive information)
409 12th Street, S.W.
P.O. Box 96920
Washington, DC 20090-6920
(202) 638-5577
www.acog.com

Engender Health
(provides information and referrals to individuals considering tubal ligation or vasectomy)
440 Ninth Ave.
New York, NY 10001
(212) 561-8000
E-mail: info@engenderhealth.org
www.engenderhealth.org

Planned Parenthood Federation of America (PPFA)
434 West 33rd St.
New York, NY 10001
(212) 541-7800
www.plannedparenthood.org
See also white or yellow pages of telephone directory for listing of local chapter

Birth Defects

Cystic Fibrosis Foundation (CFF)
6931 Arlington Rd.
Bethesda, MD 20814
(800) FIGHT-CF (344-4823)
(301) 951-4422
Fax: (301) 951-6378
E-mail: info@cff.org
www.cff.org

March of Dimes Birth Defects Foundation
1275 Mamaroneck Ave.
White Plains, NY 10605
(888) 663-4637
(914) 428-7100
www.modimes.org

Blindness

American Foundation for the Blind
11 Penn Plaza, Suite 300
New York, NY 10001
(800) AFB-LINE (232-5463)
(212) 502-7600
E-mail: afbinfo@afb.net
www.afb.org

National Federation of the Blind
1800 Johnson St.
Baltimore, MD 21230
(800) 638-7518
(410) 659-9314
www.nfb.org

National Library Service for the Blind and Physically Handicapped
Library of Congress
1291 Taylor St., N.W.
Washington, DC 20011
(888) NLS-READ
(202) 707-5100
E-mail: nls@loc.gov
www.loc.gov/nls

Blood Banks

American Red Cross
2025 E Street, N.W.
Washington, DC 20006
(202) 303-4498
To make a donation: (800) HELP-NOW (800-435-7669)
www.redcross.org
See also white or yellow pages of telephone directory for listing of local chapter

Breast Cancer

Reach to Recovery
(support program for women who have undergone mastectomies as a result of breast cancer)
American Cancer Society
2200 Lake Blvd.
Atlanta, GA 30319
(800) 227-2345
(404) 816-7800
www.cancer.org

Cancer

American Cancer Society
American Cancer Society
2200 Lake Blvd.
Atlanta, GA 30319
(800) 227-2345
(404) 816-7800
www.cancer.org

Cancer Information Service
National Cancer Institute
Suite 3036A
6116 Executive Blvd.
Bethesda, MD 20892
(800) 4-CANCER (422-6237)
(301) 435-3848
www.cis.nci.nih.gov/

Leukemia & Lymphoma Society of America
1311 Mamaroneck Ave.
White Plains, NY 10605
(914) 949-5213
Fax: (914) 949-6691
www.leukemia.org

National Coalition for Cancer Survivorship
1010 Wayne Ave., Suite 770
Silver Spring, MD 20910-5600
(301) 650-9127
(877) NCCS-YES (622-7937)

Fax: (301) 565-9670
E-mail: info@canceradvocacy.org
www.canceradvocacy.org

**R. A. Bloch Cancer Foundation
(Cancer Connection)**
(support group that matches cancer
patients with volunteers who are
cured, in remission, or being treated
for same type of cancer)
4400 Main St.
Kansas City, MO 64111
(800) 433-0464
(816) 932-8453
www.blochcancer.org

Child Abuse

National Child Abuse Prevention
(provides services to children, adolescents, mentally retarded adults, and
elderly)
606 Delsea Drive
Sewell, NJ 08080
(908) 369-8972
E-mail: patstan1@patmedia.net
www.ncap.org

National Child Abuse Hotline
(800) 422-4453

**National Committee for the
Prevention of Child Abuse**
(provides literature on child abuse
prevention programs)
200 S. Michigan Ave., 17th Floor
Chicago, IL 60604-2404
(312) 663-3520
E-mail:
mailbox@preventchildabuse.org
www.preventchildabuse.org

Parents Anonymous
(self-help group for abusive parents)
675 W. Foothill Blvd., Suite 220
Claremont, CA 91711-3475
(909) 621-6184
Fax: (909) 625-6304
E-mail: Parentsanonymous@parents
anonymous.org
www.parentsanonymous.org

Childbirth

**American College of Nurse-
Midwives**
(R.N.s who provide services through
the maternity cycle)

8403 Colesville Rd, Suite 1550
Silver Spring, MD 20910
www.midwife.org

**American College of
Obstetricians and Gynecologists**
409 12th St., S.W.
P.O. Box 96920
Washington, DC 20090-6920
(202) 638-5577
www.acog.com

Lamaze International
2025 M St., Suite 800
Washington, DC 20036-3309
(800) 368-4404
(202) 367-1128
Fax: (202) 367-2128
E-mail: info@lamaze.org
www.lamaze.org

**International Childbirth
Education Association**
P.O. Box 20048
Minneapolis, MN 55420
(952) 854-8660
Fax: (952) 854-8772
E-mail: info@icea.org
www.icea.org

Child Health and Development

**National Center for Education
in Maternal and Child Health**
Georgetown University
Box 571272
Washington, DC 20007-2292
(202) 784-9770
Fax: (202) 784-9777
E-mail: mchlibrary@ncemch.org
www.ncemch.org

**National Institute of Child Health
& Human Development**
Bldg. 31, Rm. 2A32, MSC 2425
31 Center Dr.
Bethesda, MD 20892-2425
(800) 370-2943
E-mail: NICHDInformationResource
Center@mail.nih.gov
www.nichd.nih.gov

Chiropractic

**American Chiropractic
Association**
1701 Clarendon Blvd.
Arlington, VA 22209

(800) 986-4632
Fax: (703) 243-2593
E-mail: memberinfo@acatoday.org
www.amerchiro.org

Consumer Information

**Federal Consumer
Information Center**
(catalog of publications developed by
federal agencies for consumers)
Department WWW
Pueblo, CO 81009
(888) 878-3256
www.pueblo.gsa.gov

**U.S. Consumer Product
Safety Commission**
U.S. Consumer Product Safety
Commission
Washington, DC 20207-000
(800) 638-2772
(301) 504-7923
Fax: (301) 504-0124 and
(301) 504-0025
E-mail: info@cpsc.gov
www.cpsc.gov

**Consumers Union of
United States**
(tests quality and safety of consumer
products: publishes *Consumer Reports*
magazine)
101 Truman Ave.
Yonkers, NY 10703
(914) 378-2000
www.consumerreports.org

**Council of Better
Business Bureaus**
4200 Wilson Blvd., Suite 800
Arlington, VA 22203-1804
(703) 276-0100
Fax: (703) 525-8277
www.bbb.org
See also white or yellow pages of telephone directory for listing of local
chapter

**Food and Drug Administration
(FDA)**
Office of Consumer Affairs
Consumer Inquiries
5600 Fishers Lane
Rockville, MD 20857
(888) INFO-FDA (463-6332)
www.fda.gov

Crime Victims

Crisis Prevention Institute, Inc.
(offers programs on nonviolent physical crisis interventions)
3315-K North 124th St.
Brookfield, WI 53005
(800) 558-8976 (U.S. and Canada)
(262) 783-5787
E-mail: info@crisisprevention.com
www.crisisprevention.com

**National Center for
Victims of Crime**
2000 M Street, N.W., Suite 480
Washington, DC 20010
(202) 467-8700
Fax: (202) 467-8701
www.ncvc.org

Death and Grieving

Share
(support group for parents who have lost a newborn)
c/o St. Joseph's Health Center
300 First Capitol Dr.
St. Charles, MO 63301-2893
(800) 821-6819
(636) 947-6164
E-mail:
share@nationalshareoffice.com
www.nationalshareoffice.com

Dental Health

**American Dental Association
(ADA)**
211 E. Chicago Ave.
Chicago, IL 60611
(312) 440-2500
www.ada.org

**National Institute of Dental
and Craniofacial Research**
Public Information & Liaison Branch
45 Center Dr., MSC 6400
Bethesda, MD 20892-6400
(301) 402-7364
E-mail: nidcrinfo@mail.nih.gov
www.nidcr.nih.gov

Depressive Disorders

American Psychiatric Association
1000 Wilson Blvd., Suite 1825
Arlington, VA 22209-3901
(888) 357-7924
(703) 907-7300

E-mail: apa@psych.org
www.psych.org

**American Psychological
Association**
750 First St., N.E.
Washington, DC 20002-4242
(800) 374-2721
(202) 336-5510
TDD/TTY: (202) 336-6123
www.apa.org

**Depression & Bipolar
Support Alliance**
730 N. Franklin, Suite 501
Chicago, IL 60610-7204
(800) 826-3632
(312) 642-0049
Fax: (312) 642-7243
www.dbsalliance.org

DES (Diethylstibestrol)

DES Action, USA
(support group for persons exposed to DES)
158 S. Stanwood Rd
Columbus, OH 43209
(800) DES-9288
Fax: (510) 465-4815
E-mail: desaction@columbus.rr.com
www.desaction.org

Diabetes

American Diabetes Association
National Center
1701 North Beauregard St.
Alexandria, VA 22311
(800) DIABETES (342-2383)
(703) 549-1500
E-mail: AskADA@diabetes.org
www.diabetes.org

**Juvenile Diabetes Research
Foundation International
(JDRFI)**
120 Wall St.
New York, NY 10005-4001
(800) JDF-CURE (533-2873)
(212) 785-9500
Fax: (212) 785-9595
E-mail: info@jdrf.org
www.jdfcure.org

**National Diabetes Information
Clearinghouse**
1 Information Way
Bethesda, MD 20892-3560
(800) 860-8747

(301) 654-3327
E-mail: ndic@info.niddk.nih.gov
www.diabetes.niddk.nih.gov/

Digestive Diseases

**National Institute of Diabetes &
Digestive & Kidney Diseases
(NIDDK)**
Office of Communication & Public Liaison
NIDDK, NIH, Building 31
Room 9A04 Center Dr., MSC 2560
Bethesda, MD 20892-2560
(301) 654-3810
www.niddk.nih.gov

Disabled Services

**American Alliance for Health,
Physical Education, Recreation &
Dance (AAHPERD)**
(provides information about recreation and fitness opportunities for the disabled)
1900 Association Drive
Reston, VA 20191-1598
(800) 213-7193
Fax: (703) 476-9527
www.aahperd.org

**National Library Service
for the Blind and Physically
Handicapped**
Library of Congress
1291 Taylor St., N.W.
Washington, DC 20011
(888) 657-7323
(202) 707-5100
TDD: (202) 707-0744
Fax: (202) 707-0712
E-mail: nls@loc.gov
www.loc.gov/nls

**Special Olympics International
(SOI)**
1133 19th Street, N.W.
Washington, DC 20036
(202) 628-3630
Fax: (202) 824-0200
www.specialolympics.org

Domestic Violence

**National Coalition Against
Domestic Violence (NCADV)**
1120 Lincoln Street
Suite 1603
Denver, CO 80203

(303) 839-1852
Fax: (303) 831-9251
E-mail: mainoffice@ncadv.org
www.ncadv.org

**National Domestic
Violence Hotline**
(800) 799-SAFE (799-7233)

**National Network to
End Domestic Violence**
660 Pennsylvania, SE, Suite 303
Washington, DC 20003
(202) 543-5566
www.nnedv.org

Down Syndrome

National Down Syndrome Society
666 Broadway, 8th Floor
New York, NY 10012-2317
(800) 221-4602
(212) 460-9330
E-mail: info@ndss.org
www.ndss.org

**National Down
Syndrome Congress**
1370 Center Drive, Suite 102
Atlanta, GA 30338
(800) 232-6372
E-mail: NDSCcenter@aol.com
www.ndsccenter.org

Drinking and Driving Groups

Mothers Against Drunk Driving
511 E. John Carpenter Frwy.,
Suite 700
Irving, TX 75062
(800) GET-MADD (438-6233)
(214) 744-6233
www.madd.org
See also white or yellow pages of telephone directory for local chapter

**Students Against Destructive
Decisions (also Students Against
Driving Drunk (SADD))**
255 Main Street
Marlboro, MA 01752
(877) SADD-INC (723-3462)
(508) 481-3568
Fax: (508) 481-5759
E-mail: info@sadd.org
www.saddonline.com

Drug Abuse

**Cocaine Anonymous
World Services**
P.O. Box 2000
Los Angeles, CA 90049-8000 or
3740 Overland Ave., Ste. C
Los Angeles, CA 90034
(800) 347-8998
(310) 559-5833
E-mail: Cawso@ca.org
www.ca.org

Narcotics Anonymous (NA)
(support group for recovering
narcotics addicts)
P.O. Box 9999
Van Nuys, CA 91409
(818) 773-9999
Fax: (818) 700-0700
www.na.org
See also white or yellow pages of telephone directory for local chapter

National Cocaine Hotline
(800) COCAINE (262-2463)

National Institute on Drug Abuse
6001 Executive Blvd., Room 5213
Bethesda, MD 20892-9651
(301) 443-1124
Helpline: (800) 662-4357
E-mail: information@nida.nih.gov
www.nida.nih.gov

**Center for Substance Abuse
Prevention (CSAP)**
Substance Abuse and Mental Health
Administration
5600 Fishers Lane
Rockwall 2 Bldg.
Rockville, MD 20857
(301) 443-8956
www.prevention.samhsa.gov

Eating Disorders

**National Eating Disorders
Association (NEDA)**
(self-help groups that provide information and referrals to physicians and
therapists)
603 Stewart St., Suite 803
Seattle, WA 98101
(800) 931-2237
(206) 382-3587
E-mail: info@NationalEating
Disorders.org
www.nationaleatingdisorders.org

**Anorexia Nervosa and Related
Eating Disorders (ANRED)**
(provides information and referrals for
people with eating disorders)
P.O. Box 5102
Eugene, OR 97405
(541) 344-1144
www.anred.com

Environment

**U.S. Environmental
Protection Agency (EPA)**
Ariel Rios Bldg.
1200 Pennsylvania Ave., N.W.
Washington, DC 20460
(202) 272-0167
www.epa.gov

Greenpeace, USA
702 H St. N.W.
Washington, DC 20001
(800) 326-0959
(202) 462-1177
E-mail: info@wdc.greenpeace.org
www.greenpeace/usa.org

**Natural Resources
Defense Council**
40 West 20th St.
New York, NY 10011
(212) 727-2700
Fax: (212) 727-1773
E-mail: nrdcinfo@nrdc.org
www.nrdc.org

Sierra Club
85 2nd St., 2nd Floor
San Francisco, CA 94105-3441
(415) 977-5500
(415) 977-5799
E-mail: Information@sierraclub.org
www.sierraclub.org

World Wildlife Fund
1250 24th St., N.W.
P.O. Box 97180
Washington, DC 20090-7180
(800) CALL-WWF (225-5993)
(202) 293-4800
Fax: (202) 293-2911
www.wwfus.org

Epilepsy

Epilepsy Foundation of America
4351 Garden City Drive
Landover, MD 20785-7223

(800) EFA-1000 (332-1000)
(301) 459-3700
www.efa.org

Gay and Lesbian Organizations and Services

Human Rights Campaign
1640 Rhode Island Avenue, N.W.
Washington, DC 20036-3278
(202) 628-4160
(800) 777-4723
Fax: (202) 347-5323
E-mail: hrc@hrc.org
www.hrc.org

National Gay and Lesbian Task Force (NGLTF)
1325 Massachusetts Ave., N.W.,
Suite 600
Washington, DC, 20005
(202) 393-5177
Fax: (202) 393-2241
E-mail:
Thetaskforce@thetaskforce.org
www.ngltf.org

Parents, Families, and Friends of Lesbians and Gays (PFLAG)
1726 M St., N.W., Suite 400
Washington, DC 20036
(202) 467-8180
Fax: (202) 467-8194
E-mail: info@pflag.org
www.pflag.org

Genetics

American College of Medical Genetics
9650 Rockville Pike
Bethesda, MD 20814-3998
(301) 634-7127
Fax: (301) 571-0677
E-mail: acmg@faseb.org
www.acmg.net

The Human Genome Organization
HUGO Americas
Laboratory of Genetics
National Institute on Aging
NIH/NIA-IRP. GRC, Box 31
5600 Nathan Shock Dr.
Baltimore, MD 21224-6825
(410) 558-8337
Fax: (410) 558-8331
E-mail: schlessingerd@grc.nia.nih.gov

GeneTests—GeneClinics
(a database of information for patients and families with genetic disorders, providing access to support groups)
University of Washington School of Medicine
Seattle, WA
www.genetests.org

Hazardous Waste

Environmental Protection Agency (EPA)
Ariel Rios Bldg.
1200 Pennsylvania Ave., N.W.
Washington, DC 20460
(202) 260-2090
www.epa.gov

Hazardous Waste Hotline Information
(800) 424-9346

Health Care

Association for Applied and Therapeutic Humor (AATH)
(publishes a newsletter and sponsors seminars for people in the helping professions)
1951 W. Camelback Rd., Suite 445
Phoenix, AZ 85015
(602) 995-1454
FAX: (602) 995-1449
www.aath.org

American Medical Association
515 N. State St.
Chicago, IL 60610
(800) 621-8335
www.ama-assn.org

American Nurses Association
600 Maryland Ave., S.W.
Suite 100 West
Washington, DC 20024-2571
(800) 274-4ANA (274-4262)
(202) 651-7000
www.ana.org

Health Education

National Center for Chronic Disease Prevention and Health Promotion
Centers for Disease Control and Prevention
Mail Stop A34
1600 Clifton Rd., N.E.
Atlanta, GA 30333

(404) 639-3534
(800) 311-3435
E-mail: cdcinfo@cdc.gov
www.cdc.gov/nccdphp

Hearing Impairment

American Society for Deaf Children
(resource group for parents of hard of hearing and deaf children)
P.O. Box 3355
Gettysburg, PA 17325
(717) 334-7922
Fax: (717) 334-8808
(800) 942-ASDC (Parent Hotline)
www.deafchildren.org

Better Hearing Institute (BHI)
(provides educational and resource materials on deafness)
Better Hearing Institute
515 King St., Suite 420
Alexandria, VA 22314
(703) 684-3391
E-mail: mail@betterhearing.org
www.betterhearing.org

Heart Disease

American Heart Association (AHA)
7272 Greenville Ave.
Dallas, TX 75231
(800) 242-8721
(214) 373-6300
www.americanheart.org

National Heart, Lung, and Blood Institute
(provides information on cardio-vascular risk factors and disease)
Bldg. 31, Room 5A52
31 Center Dr., MSC 2486
Bethesda, MD 20892
(800) 575-9355
(301) 592-8573
E-mail: nhlbiinfo@nhlbi.nih.gov
www.nhlbi.nih.gov/index.htm

Helping Others

United Way of America
701 N. Fairfax St.
Alexandria, VA 22314-2045
(703) 836-7100
www.unitedway.org

Hospice

The National Hospice and Palliative Care Organization
1700 Diagonal Rd., Suite 625
Alexandria, VA 22314
(703) 837-1500
(800) 646-6460
E-mail: info@nhpco.org
www.nhpco.org

Immunization

National Immunization Program
Centers for Disease Control
Mail Stop E-05
1600 Clifton Rd., N.E.
Atlanta, GA 30333
(404) 639-3311
(800) 232-2522
www.cdc.gov/nip/diseases/adult-vpd
.htm

Immunization Action Coalition
(information for children, adolescents, and adults)
1573 Selby Ave., Suite 234
St. Paul, MN 55104
(651) 647-9009
Fax: (651) 647-9131
E-mail: admin@immunize.org
www.immunize.org

Infant Care

La Leche League International
(provides information and support to women interested in breast-feeding)
1400 N. Meacham Rd.
Schaumburg, IL 60168-4079
(800) LA-LECHE (525-3243)
(847) 519-7730
www.lalecheleague.org

Infectious Diseases

Centers for Disease Control and Prevention
1600 Clifton Rd., N.E.
Atlanta, GA 30333
(800) 311-3435
(404) 639-3534
E-mail: cdcinfo@cdc.gov
www.cdc.gov

Infertility

Resolve: The National Infertility Association
(offers counseling, information, and support to people with problems of infertility)
7910 Woodmont Avenue Suite 1350
Bethesda, MD 20814
(888) 623-0744
(301) 652-8585
E-mail: info@resolve.org
www.resolve.org

Kidney Disease

American Kidney Fund (AKF)
(provides information on financial aid to patients, organ transplants, and kidney-related diseases)
6110 Executive Blvd., Suite 1010
Rockville, MD 20852
(800) 638-8299
(301) 881-3052
E-mail: Helpline@kidneyfund.org
www.akfinc.org

American Association of Kidney Patients (AAKP)
3505 E. Frontage Rd., Suite 315
Tampa, FL 33607
(800) 749-2257
Fax: (813) 636-8122
E-mail: info@aakp.org
www.aakp.org

National Kidney Foundation (NKF)
30 East 33rd St., Suite 1100
New York, NY 10016
(800) 622-9010
(212) 889-2210
Fax: (212) 689-9261
www.kidney.org

Liver Disease

American Liver Foundation (ALF)
75 Maiden, Suite 603
New York, NY 10038
(800) 465-4837
(212) 668-1000
E-mail: info@liverfoundation.org
www.liverfoundation.org/

Lung Disease

American Lung Association
61 Broadway, 6th Floor
New York, NY 10006
(800) LUNG-USA
(800) 548-8252
(212) 315-8700
www.lungusa.org

National Heart, Lung, and Blood Institute
(provides information on cardio-vascular risk factors and disease)
Bldg. 31, Room 5A52
31 Center Dr., MSC 2486
Bethesda, MD 20892
(800) 575-9355
E-mail: nhlbiinfo@nhlbi.nih.gov
www.nhlbi.nih.gov/index.htm

Lupus Erythematosus

Lupus Foundation of America (LPA)
2000 L Street, N.W., Suite 710
Washington, DC 20036
(202) 349-1155
(800) 558-0121
Fax: (202) 349-1156
E-mail: info@lupus.org
www.lupus.org/

Marriage and Family

**Women Work!
The National Network for Women's Employment**
(national advocacy group for women over 35 who have lost their primary means of support through death, divorce, or disabling of spouse)
1625 K St. N.W., Suite 300
Washington, DC 20006
(202) 467-6346
E-mail: Info@womenwork.org
www.womenwork.org

Alliance for Children & Families
11700 West Lake Park Dr.
Milwaukee, WI 53224-3099
(414) 359-1040
Fax: (414) 359-1074
E-mail: info@alliance1.org
www.alliance1.org

Stepfamily Association of America

(provides information and publishes quarterly newsletter)
650 J St., Suite 205
Lincoln, NE 68508
(800) 735-0329
(402) 477-7837
Fax: (402) 477-8317
E-mail: stepfamfs@aol.com
www.saafamilies.org

Medications

(Prescriptions and Over-the-Counter)

Food and Drug Administration (FDA)

Office of Consumer Affairs Public Inquiries
5600 Fishers Lane (HFE-88)
Rockville, MD 20857-0001
(888) 463-6332 (INFO-FDA)
www.fda.gov

Mental Health

American Psychiatric Association

1000 Wilson Blvd., Suite 125
Arlington, VA 22209
(888) 357-7924
(703) 907-7300
E-mail: apa@psych.org
www.psych.org

American Psychological Association

750 First St., N.E.
Washington, DC 20002-4242
(800) 374-2721
(202) 336-5510
TDD/TTY: (202) 336-6123
www.apa.org

American Psychoanalytic Foundation

309 East 49th Street
New York, NY 10017
(212) 752-0450
E-mail: APF@cyberpsych.org
www.cyberpsych.org/apf

National Alliance for the Mentally Ill (NAMI)

(self-help advocacy organization for persons with schizophrenia and depressive disorders and their families)

Colonial Place Three
2107 Wilson Blvd., Suite 300
Arlington, VA 22201
(703) 524-7600
HelpLine: (800) 950-NAMI (950-6264)
www.nami.org/

National Institute of Mental Health

Information Resources and Inquiries Branch
6001 Executive Blvd., Room 8184
MSC 9663
Bethesda, MD 20892-9663
(301) 443-4513 (local)
(866) 615-6464
Fax: (301) 443-4279
TTY: (301) 443-8431
(866) 415-8051 (TTY toll-free)
E-mail: nimhinfo@nih.gov
www.nimh.nih.gov/

National Mental Health Association (NMHA)

2001 N. Beauregard St., 12 Floor
Alexandria, VA 22311
(800) 969-NMHA (969-6642)
(703) 684-7722
Fax: (703) 684-5968
www.nmha.org

Mental Retardation

Association for Retarded Citizens (ARC)

1010 Wayne Ave., Suite 650
Silver Spring, MD 20910
(301) 565-3842
E-mail: info@thearc.org
www.thearc.org

Missing and Runaway Children

Child Find of America

(800) I-AM-LOST (426-5678)
Runaway Hotline
(800) 621-4000
www.childfindofamerica.org

National Center for Missing and Exploited Children (NCMEC)

699 Prince St., Suite 550
Alexandria, VA 22314
(703) 274-3900
Fax: (703) 274-2200
24-hour Hotline:
(800) THE-LOST (843-5678)
www.missingkids.org

Neurological Disorders

National Institute of Neurological Disorders and Stroke

P.O. Box 5801
Bethesda, MD 20892
(800) 352-9424
(301) 496-5751
Fax: (301) 402-2186
E-mail: braininfo@ninds.nih.gov
www.ninds.nih.gov

Nutrition

American Dietetic Association

120 South Riverside Plaza, Suite 2000
Chicago, IL 60606-6995
(800) 877-1600
www.eatright.org

American Society for Nutritional Sciences

9650 Rockville Pike, Suite 4500
Bethesda, MD 20814-3990
(301) 530-7050
Fax: (301) 634-7892
E-mail: sec@nutrition.org
www.asnutrition.org

Food and Drug Administration (FDA)

Office of Consumer Affairs Public Inquiries
5600 Fishers Lane (HFE-88)
Rockville, MD 20857
(888) 463-6332 (INFO-FDA)
www.fda.gov

Food and Nutrition Information Center

U.S. Dept. of Agriculture
National Agricultural Library
10301 Baltimore Ave.
Beltsville, MD 20705-2351
(301) 504-5719
Fax: (301) 504-6409
TTY: (301) 504-6856
E-mail:fnic@nal.usda.gov
www.nal.usda.gov/fnic

Center for Nutrition in Sport and Human Performance

206A Chenoweth Lab
University of Massachusetts
Amherst, MA 01002
(413) 545-1076
Fax: (413) 545-1074
E-mail: volpe@nutrition.umass.edu
www.umass.edu/cnshp/

National Dairy Council
10255 W. Higgins Rd., Suite 900
Rosemont, IL 60018-5616
(800) 426-8271
E-mail: ndc@dairyinformation.com
www.nationaldairycouncil.org

Occupational Safety and Health

**Occupational Safety and
Health Administration (OSHA)**
U.S. Dept. of Labor
Office of Public Affairs, Room N3647
200 Constitution Ave.
Washington, DC 20210
(202) 693-1999
(800) 321-OSHA (6742)
TTY: (877) 889-5627
www.osha.gov

Organ Donations

The Living Bank (TLB)
(provides information and acts as registry and referral service for people
wanting to donate organs for research
or transplantation)
P.O. Box 6725
Houston, TX 77265
(800) 528-2971
E-mail: info@livingbank.org
www.livingbank.org

Osteopathic Medicine

**American Osteopathic
Association (AOA)**
142 East Ontario St.
Chicago, IL 60611
(800) 621-1773
(312) 202-8000
Fax: (312) 202-8200
E-mail: info@osteotech.org
www.osteopathic.org

Parent Support Groups

**National Organization of Mothers
of Twins Clubs (NOMOTC)**
P.O. Box 700860
Plymouth, MI 48170-0955
(877) 540-2200
(248) 231-4480
E-mail: Info@NOMOTC.ORG
www.nomotc.org

Parents Anonymous
(self-help group for abusive parents)
675 W. Foothill Blvd., Suite 220
Claremont, CA 91711-3475
(909) 621-6184
Fax: (909) 625-6304
E-mail: parentsanonymous@parents
anonymous.org
www.parentsanonymous.org

Parents Without Partners, Inc.
1650 South Dixie Highway, Suite 510
Boca Raton, FL 33432
(561) 391-8833
Fax: (561) 395-8557
E-mail: pwp@jti.net
www.parentswithoutpartners.org

Parenting

**National Parent
Information Network**
ERIC Clearinghouse on Elementary
and Early Childhood Education
University of Illinois at Urbana-
Champaign
Children's Research Center
51 Gerty Dr.
Champaign, IL 61820-7469
(800) 583-4135
(217) 333-1386
Fax: (217) 333-3767
www.npin.org

Phobias

**Anxiety Disorders Association
of America (ADAA)**
(provides information about phobias
and referrals to therapists and support
groups)
8730 Georgia Ave., Suite 600
Silver Spring, MD 20910
(240) 485-1001
Fax: (240) 485-1035
www.adaa.org

TERRAP Programs
(headquarters for national network of
treatment clinics for agoraphobia)
932 Evelyn St.
Menlo Park, CA 94025
(415) 327-1312
(800) 2-PHOBIA (274-6242)
www.terrap.com

Physical Fitness

See local yellow and white pages of
telephone directory for listing of local
health clubs and YMCAs, YWCAs,
and Jewish Community Centers

**Cooper Institutes for
Aerobics Research**
12330 Preston Rd.
Dallas, TX 75230
(972) 341-3200
Fax: (972) 341-3227
E-mail: courses@cooperinst.org
www.cooperinst.org

**President's Council on
Physical Fitness and Sports**
Dept. W 200 Independence Ave., S.W.
Room 738 H
Washington, DC 20201
(202) 690-9000
Fax: (202) 690-5211
www.fitness.gov

**American College of
Sports Medicine**
ACSM National Center
P.O. Box 1440
Indianapolis, IN 46206-1440
(317) 637-9200
www.acsm.org

**Center for Nutrition in Sport
and Human Performance**
206A Chenoweth Lab
University of Massachusetts
Amherst, MA 01002
(413) 545-1076
Fax: (413) 545-1074
E-mail: volpe@nutrition.umass.edu
www.umass.edu/cnshp/

Poisoning

See emergency numbers listed in the
front of your local phone directory

National Poison Hotline
(800) 222-1222

Pregnancy

**National Institute of Child Health
& Human Development**
Bldg. 31, Room 2A32, MSC 2425
31 Center Dr.
Bethesda, MD 20892-2425
(800) 370-2943

E-mail: NICHDInformationResource
Center@mail.nih.gov
www.nichd.nih.gov

Product Safety

**U.S. Consumer Product
Safety Commission**
Washington, DC 20207
(800) 638-CPSC (638-2772)
(301) 504-7923
www.cpsc.gov

Radiation Control and Safety

**Center for Devices and
Radiological Health**

**U.S. Food and
Drug Administration**
Office of Consumer Affairs
1350 Piccard Drive, HFZ-210
Rockville, MD 20850
(800) 638-2041
(301) 827-3990
www.fda.gov/cdrh/

**National Institute of
Environmental Health Sciences**

National Institutes of Health
P.O. Box 12233
Research Triangle Park, NC 27709
(919) 541-3345
www.niehs.nih.gov

Rape, Victimization

See white pages of telephone directory
for listing of local rape crisis and
counseling centers

**National Center for
Victims of Crime**
2000 M St., N.W., Suite 480
Washington, DC 20010
(202) 467-8700
Fax: (202) 467-8701
www.ncvc.org

**National Organization
for Victim Assistance (NOVA)**
NOVA
510 King Street, Suite 424
Alexandria, VA 22314
(800) TRY-NOVA (879-6682)
(703) 535-NOVA
Fax: (703) 535-5500
www.trynova.org

**National Sexual Violence
Resource Center**
123 North Enola Dr.
Enola, PA 17025
(877) 739-3895
(717) 909-0710
Fax: (717) 909-0714
TTY: (717) 909-0715
E-mail: resources@nsvrc.org
www.nsvrc.org

Reye's Syndrome

**National Reye's
Syndrome Foundation**
P.O. Box 829
Bryan, OH 43506-0829
(800) 233-7393 (U.S. only)
(419) 636-2679
Fax: (419) 636-9897
E-mail: nrsf@reyessyndrome.org
www.reyessyndrome.org

Self-Care/Self-Help

**National Self-Help
Clearinghouse (NSHC)**
(provides information about self-help
groups)
365 5th Ave., Suite 3300
New York, NY 10016
(212) 817-1822
http://selfhelpweb.org

Sex Education

**American Association of
Sex Educators, Counselors
and Therapists (AASECT)**
P.O. Box 1960
Ashland, VA 23005-1960
(804) 752-0026
Fax: (804) 752-0056
E-mail: aasect@aasect.org
www.aasect.org

Advocates for Youth
(develops programs and material to
educate youth on sex and sexual
responsibility)
2000 M Street N.W., Suite 750
Washington, DC 20005
(202) 419-3420
Fax: (202) 419-1448
E-mail: information@advocatesfor
youth.org
www.advocatesforyouth.org

**Planned Parenthood Federation
of America (PPFA)**
434 West 33rd St.
New York, NY 10001
(212) 541-7800
www.plannedparenthood.org

**Sexuality Information and
Education Council of the U.S.
(SIECUS)**
(maintains an information clearinghouse on all aspects of human
sexuality)
130 West 42nd St., Suite 350
New York, NY 10036-7802
(212) 819-9770
Fax: (212) 819-9776
E-mail: siecus@siecus.org
www.siecus.org

Sexual Abuse and Assault

**National Center for
Assault Prevention**
(provides services to children, adolescents, mentally retarded adults, and
elderly)
606 Delsea Dr.
Sewell, NJ 08080
(800) 258-3189
(908) 369-8972
www.ncap.org

Prevent Child Abuse America
200 S. Michigan Ave., Suite 1700
Chicago, IL 60604
(312) 663-3520
Fax: (312) 939-8962
E-mail:
mailbox@preventchildabuse.org
www.preventchildabuse.org

Sexually Transmitted Diseases

**Centers for Disease Control
and Prevention**
1600 Clifton Rd. N.E.
Atlanta, GA 30333
(800) CDC-INFO
(404) 639-3534
(800) 311-3435
E-mail: cdcinfo@cdc.gov
www.cdc.gov

**American Social
Health Association**
P.O. Box 13827
Research Triangle Park, NC 27709

(919) 361-8400
Fax: (919) 361-8425
E-mail: info@ashastd.org
www.ashastd.org

National Herpes Resource Center
American Social Health Association
P.O. Box 13827
Research Triangle Park, NC 27709-3827
(919) 361-8488
E-mail: hsvnet@ashastd.org
www.ashastd.org/hrc/index.html

National STD Hotline
(800) 227-8922

Sexuality Information and Education Council of the U.S. (SIECUS)
(maintains an information clearing-house on all aspects of human sexuality)
130 West 42nd St., Suite 350
New York, NY 10036-7802
(212) 819-9770
Fax: (212) 819-9776
E-mail: siecus@siecus.org
www.siecus.org

Sickle-Cell Disease

Sickle Cell Disease Association of America
231 East Baltimore St., Ste 800
Baltimore, MD 21202
(800) 421-8453
(410) 528-1555
E-mail: scdaa@sicklecelldisease.org
www.sicklecelldisease.org

The Sickle Cell Information Center
The Georgia Comprehensive Sickle Cell Center at Grady Health System
P.O. Box 109, Grady Memorial Hospital, 80 Jesse Hill Jr. Dr.
Atlanta, GA 30303
(404) 616-3572
Fax: (404) 616-5998
E-mail: aplatt@emory.edu
www.scinfo.org

Skin Diseases

American Academy of Dermatology
P.O. Box 4014
Schaumburg, IL 60168-4014

(888) 462-DERM (3376)
(847) 330-0230
Fax: (847) 330-0050
www.aad.org

University of Iowa Hospitals and Clinics

Department of Dermatology
200 Hawkins Drive BT 2045-1
Iowa City, IA 52242-1090
(319) 356-SKIN (7546)
(319) 384-6012
Fax: (319) 356-8317
www.tray.dermatology.uiowa.edu

National Psoriasis Foundation
6600 SW 92nd Ave., Suite 300
Portland, OR 97223-7195
(800) 723-9166
(503) 244-7404
Fax: (503) 245-0626
E-mail: getinfo@psoriasis.org
www.psoriasis.org

Sleep and Sleep Disorders

American Sleep Apnea Association
1424 K St., N.W., Suite 302
Washington, DC 20005
(202) 293-3650
Fax: (202) 293-3656
E-mail: asaa@sleepapnea.org
www.sleepapnea.org

American Academy of Sleep Medicine
One Westbrook Corporate Center, Suite 920
West Chester, IL 60154
(708) 492-0930
Fax: (708) 492-0943
www.aasmnet.org

Better Sleep Council
501 Wythe St.
Alexandria, VA 22314
(703) 683-8371
E-mail: spali@sleepproducts.org
www.bettersleep.org/

National Sleep Foundation
1522 K St., N.W., Suite 500
Washington, DC 20005
(202) 347-3471
Fax: (202) 347-3472
E-mail: nsf@sleepfoundation.org
www.sleepfoundation.org

Smoking and Tobacco

Action on Smoking and Health (ASH)
(provides information on nonsmokers' rights and related subjects)
2013 H St., N.W.
Washington, DC 20006
(202) 659-4310
http://ash.org

American Cancer Society
(provides information about quitting smoking and smoking cessation programs)
2200 Lake Blvd.
Atlanta, GA 30319
(800) 227-2345
(404) 816-7800
www.cancer.org

American Heart Association
(provides information about quitting smoking and smoking cessation programs)
7272 Greenville Ave.
Dallas, TX 75231
(800) 242-8721
(214) 373-6300
www.americanheart.org

American Lung Association
(provides information about quitting smoking and smoking cessation programs)
61 Broadway, 6th Floor
New York, NY 10006
(212) 315-8700
To reach your local American Lung Association: (800) LUNG-USA (586-4872)
www.lungusa.org

Americans for Nonsmokers' Rights
2530 San Pablo Ave., Suite J
Berkeley, CA 94702
(510) 841-3032
Fax: (510) 841-3071
E-mail: anr@no-smoke.org
www.no-smoke.org

Stress Reduction

American Institute of Stress
124 Park Ave.
Yonkers, NY 10703
(914) 963-1200
Fax: (914) 965-6267

E-mail: stress125@optonline.net
www.stress.org

American Psychological Association
750 First St., N.E.
Washington, DC 20002-4242
(800) 374-2721
(202) 336-5500
TDD/TTY: 202-336-6123
www.apa.org

Association for Applied Psychophysiology and Biofeedback
10200 W. 44th Ave., Suite 304
Wheat Ridge, CO 80033
(800) 477-8892
(303) 422-8436
E-mail: aapb@resourcenter.com
www.aapb.org

Stroke

Council on Stroke
American Stroke Association
National Center
7272 Greenville Ave.
Dallas, TX 75231
AHA: (800) AHA-USA-1
(800-242-8721)
ASA: (888) 4-STROKE
(888-478-7653)
www.strokeassociation.org

National Institute of Neurological Disorders and Stroke
National Institutes of Health
P.O. Box 5801
Bethesda, MD 20824
(800) 352-9424
(301) 496-5751
www.ninds.nih.gov/

Stuttering

National Center for Stuttering
200 East 33rd St.
New York, NY 10016
Hotline: (800) 221-2483
(212) 532-1460
www.stuttering.com

Sudden Infant Death Syndrome (SIDS)

First Candle/SIDS Alliance
(provides information and referrals to families who have lost an infant because of SIDS)
1314 Bedford Ave., Suite 210
Baltimore, MD 21208
(800) 221-7437
(410) 653-8226
Fax: (410) 653-8709
E-mail: info@firstcandle.org
www.sidsalliance.org

Suicide Prevention

American Association of Suicidology (AAS)
5221 Wisconsin Avenue, NW
Washington, DC 20015
(202) 237-2280; hotline
(800) 273-TALK (8255)
Fax: (202) 237-2282
E-mail: info@suicidology.org
www.suicidology.org

American Psychoanalytic Foundation
309 East 49th Street
New York, NY 10017
(212) 752-0450
www.cyberpsych.org/apf

Terminal Illness

Make-A-Wish Foundation of America (MAWFA)
(dedicated to granting the special wishes of terminally ill children)
3550 North Central Ave., Suite 300
Phoenix, AZ 85012-2127
(800) 722-WISH (722-9474)
(602) 279-WISH (279-9474)
Fax: (602) 279-0855
E-mail: mawfa@wish.org
www.wish.org

Make Today Count (MTC)
(self-help group for persons with terminal illness)
St. Johns Hospital
1235 E. Cherokee St.
Springfield, MO 65804
(800) 432-2273
(417) 885-3324
Fax: (417) 820-2587
E-mail: Info@stjohns.com
www.stjohns.com

Victimization

National Center for Victims of Crime
2000 M St., N.W., Suite 480
Washington, DC 20036
(202) 467-8700
Fax: (202) 467-8701
www.ncvc.org

National Coalition Against Domestic Violence
1120 Lincoln Street, Suite 1603
Denver, CO 80203
(303) 839-1852
Fax: (303) 831-9251
E-mail: mainoffice@ncadv.org
www.ncadv.org

National Coalition Against Sexual Assault
125 N. Enola Dr.
Enola, PA 17025
(717) 728-9764
Fax: (717) 728-9781
http://dreamingdesigns.com/other/indexncasa.html

National Organization for Victim Assistance (NOVA)
NOVA
510 King Street, Suite 424
Alexandria, VA 22314
(800) Try-NOVA (879-6682)
(703) 535-NOVA
Fax: (703) 535-5500
www.trynova.org

Weight Control

Overeaters Anonymous (OA)
P.O. Box 44020
Rio Rancho, NM 87174-4020
(505) 891-2664
Fax: (505) 891-4320
E-mail: info@overeatersanonymous.org
www.oa.org

Weight-Control Information Network (WIN)
National Institute of Diabetes and Digestive and Kidney Diseases
1 WIN Way
Bethesda, MD 20892-3665
(877) 946-4627
(202) 828-1025
Fax: (202) 828-1028
E-mail: win@info.niddk.nih.gov
www.win.niddk.nih.gov

Take Off Pounds Sensibly (TOPS)
P.O. Box 07360
4575 S. Fifth St.
Milwaukee, WI 53207-0360
(800) 932-8677
(414) 482-4620
www.tops.org

Weight Watchers International
175 Crossways Park West
Woodbury, NY 11797
(516) 390-1657
www.weight-watchers.com

Wellness

National Wellness Institute, Inc.
1300 College Court
P.O. Box 827
Stevens Point, WI 54481-0827
(800) 243-8694
(715) 342-2969
Fax: (715) 342-2979
E-mail: nwi@nationalwellness.org
www.nationalwellness.org

Wellness Associates of Chicago
(publishes *The Wellness Inventory*)
4250 Marine Dr., Suite 200
Chicago, IL 60613

(773) 935-6377
Fax: (773) 929-4446
E-mail: wellness-info@wellnessof
chicago.com
www.wellness-associates.com

Women's Health

**National Women's Health
Network (NWHN)**
514 10th St., N.W., Suite 400
Washington, DC 20004
(202) 347-1140
Health Info: (202) 628-7814
Fax: (202) 347-1168
E-mail: nwhn@nwhn.org
www.womenshealthnetwork.org

**National Women's Health
Information Center**

**U.S. Public Health Service on
Women's Health**
8270 Willow Oaks Corporate Drive
Fairfax, VA 22031
(800) 994-WOMAN (994-9662)
www.4women.gov

**GenneX Healthcare
Technologies, Inc.**

**Estronaut: A Forum
for Women's Health**
GenneX Healthcare Technologies,
Inc.
207 E. Ohio, 186
Chicago, IL 60611
(312) 335-0095
E-mail: ask@gennexhealth.com
www.estronaut.com

Planned Parenthood
434 West 33rd St.
New York, NY 10001
(212) 541-7800
Fax: (212) 245-1845
www.plannedparenthood.org
See also white or yellow pages of telephone directory for listing of local
chapter

By definition, an emergency is a situation in which you have to think and act fast. Start by assessing the circumstances. Shout for help if you're in a public place. Look for any possible dangers to you or the victim, such as a live electrical wire or a fire. Seek medical assistance as quickly as possible. Dial 911 or a local emergency phone number. Don't attempt rescue techniques, such as cardiopulmonary resuscitation (CPR), unless you are trained. If you have a car, be sure you know the shortest route from your home to the nearest 24-hour hospital emergency department.

SUPPLIES

Every home should have a kit of basic first aid supplies kept in a convenient location out of the reach of children. Stock it with the following:

- Bandages and sterile gauze pads
- Adhesive tape
- Scissors
- Cotton balls or absorbent cotton
- Cotton swabs
- Thermometer
- Antibiotic ointment
- Sharp needle
- Safety pins
- Calamine lotion

Keep a similar kit in your car or boat. You might want to add some extra items from your home, such as a flashlight, soap, blanket, paper cups, and any special equipment that a family member with a chronic illness may need.

BLEEDING

Blood loss is frightening and dangerous. Direct pressure stops external bleeding. Since internal bleeding can also be life-threatening, you must be aware of the warning signs.

FOR AN OPEN WOUND

1. Apply direct pressure over the site of the wound. Cover the entire wound.
2. Use sterile gauze, a sanitary napkin, a clean towel, sheet, or handkerchief or, if necessary, your washed bare hand. Ice or cold water in a pad will help stop bleeding and decrease swelling.
3. Apply firm, steady pressure for five to fifteen minutes. Most wounds stop bleeding within a few minutes.
4. If the wound is on a foot, hand, leg, or arm, use gravity to help slow the flow of blood. Elevate the limb so that it is higher than the victim's heart.
5. If the bleeding doesn't stop, press harder.
6. Seek medical attention if the bleeding was caused by a serious injury, if stitches will be needed to keep the wound closed, or if the victim has not had a tetanus booster within the last ten years.

FOR INTERNAL BLEEDING

1. Suspect internal bleeding if a person coughs up blood, vomits red or brown material that looks like coffee grounds, passes blood in urine or stool, or has black, tarlike bowel movements.
2. Do not let the victim take any medication or fluids by mouth until seen by a doctor, because surgery may be necessary.
3. Have the victim lie flat. Cover him or her lightly.
4. Seek immediate medical attention.

FOR A BLOODY NOSE

1. Have the victim sit down, leaning slightly forward so the blood does not run down his or her throat. The person should spit out any blood in his or her mouth.
2. Use the thumb and forefingers to pinch the nose. If the victim can do the pinching, apply a cold compress to the nose and surrounding area.
3. Apply pressure for ten minutes without interruption.
4. If pinching does not work, gently pack the nostril with gauze or a clean strip of cloth. Do not use absorbent cotton, which will stick. Let the ends hang out so you can remove the packing easily later. Pinch the nose, with the packing in place, for five minutes.
5. If a foreign object is in the nose, do not attempt to remove it. Ask the person to blow gently. If that does not work, seek medical attention.
6. The nose should not be blown or irritated for several hours after a nosebleed stops.

BREATHING PROBLEMS

If a person appears to be unconscious, approach carefully. The victim may be in contact with electrical current. If so, make sure the electricity is shut off before touching the victim. The first function you should check is respiration. Tap or shake the victim's shoulder gently, shouting, "Are you all right?" Look for any signs of breathing: Can you hear breath sounds? Can you feel breath on your cheek? If the person is breathing, do not perform mouth-to-mouth resuscitation.

If you aren't certain if the victim is breathing, or if there are no signs of breath, follow these steps:

1. Lay the person on his or her back on the floor or ground. Roll the victim over if necessary, being careful to turn the head with the remainder of the body as a unit to avoid possible neck injury. Loosen any tight clothing around the neck or chest.
2. Check for any foreign material in the mouth or throat and remove it quickly.

3. Open the airway by tilting the head back and lifting the chin up.
4. Pinch the nostrils shut with your thumb and index finger.
5. Take a deep breath, open your mouth wide and place it securely over the victim's, and give two slow breaths, each lasting 1 to 10 seconds. Remove your mouth, turn your head, and check to see if the victim's chest rises and falls. If you hear air escaping from the victim's mouth and see the chest fall, you know that you are getting air into the lungs.
6. Repeat once every five seconds (twelve breaths per minute) until professional help takes over, or the victim begins breathing on his or her own. It may take several hours to revive someone. If you stop, the victim may not be able to breathe on his or her own. Once the person does begin to breathe independently, always get professional help.
7. If air doesn't seem to be entering the chest, or the chest doesn't fall between breaths, tilt the head further back. If that doesn't work, follow the directions for choking emergencies later in this section.
8. If the victim is a child, do not pinch the nose shut. Cover both the mouth and nose with your mouth, and place your free hand very lightly on the child's chest. Use small puffs of air rather than big breaths. Feel the chest inflate as you blow, and listen for exhaled air. Repeat once every three seconds (twenty breaths per minute).

BROKEN BONES

If you suspect that a person has broken a leg, do not move him or her unless there is immediate danger.

1. Check for signs of breathing. If there is none or breathing is very weak, administer mouth-to-mouth resuscitation.
2. If the person is bleeding, apply direct pressure on the site of the wound.
3. Try to keep the victim warm and calm.
4. Do not try to push a broken bone back into place if it is sticking out of the skin. You can apply a moist dressing to prevent it from drying out.
5. Do not try to straighten out a fracture.
6. Do not allow the victim to walk.
7. Splint unstable fractures to prevent painful motion.

BURNS

1. If fire caused the burn, cool the affected area with water to stop the burning process.
2. Remove the victim's garments and jewelry and cover him or her with clean sheets or towels.
3. Call for help immediately.

4. If chemicals caused the burn, wash the affected area with cool water for at least 20 minutes. Chemical burns of the eye require immediate medical attention after flushing with water for 20 minutes.

CHOKING

A person with anything stuck in the throat and blocking the airway can stop breathing, lose consciousness, and die within four to six minutes. A universal signal of distress because of choking is clasping the throat with one or both hands. Other signs are an inability to talk and noisy, difficult breathing. You need to take immediate action, but NEVER slap the victim's back. This could make the obstruction worse.

If the victim can speak, cough, or breathe, do not interfere. Coughing alone may dislodge the foreign object. If the choking continues without lessening, call for medical help.

If the victim cannot speak, cough, or breathe but is conscious, use the Heimlich maneuver, as follows

1. Stand behind the victim (who may be seated or standing) and wrap your arms around his or her waist.
2. Make a fist with one hand and place the thumb side of your fist against the victim's abdomen, just above the navel. Grasp your fist with your other hand and press into his or her abdomen with a quick, upward thrust. Do not exert any pressure against the rib cage with your forearms.
3. Repeat this procedure until the victim is no longer choking or loses consciousness.
4. If the person is lying face down, roll the victim over. Facing the person, kneel with your legs astride his or her hips. Put the heel of one hand below the rib cage and place your other hand on top. Press into the abdomen with a quick, upward thrust. Repeat thrusts as needed.
5. If you start choking when you're by yourself, place your fist below your rib cage and above your navel. Grasp this fist with your other hand and press into your abdomen with a quick, upward thrust. You also can lean over a fixed, horizontal object, such as a table edge or chair back, and press your upper abdomen against it with a quick, upward thrust. Repeat as needed until you dislodge the object.

IF THE VICTIM IS UNCONSCIOUS

1. Place him or her on the ground and give mouth-to-mouth resuscitation as described earlier.
2. If the victim does not start breathing and air does not seem to be going into his or her lungs, roll the victim onto his or her back and give one or more manual thrusts: Place one of your hands on top of the other with the heel of the bottom hand in the middle of the abdomen, slightly above the navel and below the rib cage. Press into the abdomen with a quick, upward

thrust. Do not push to either side. Repeat six to ten times as needed.

3. Clear the airway. Hold the victim's mouth open with one hand and use your thumb to depress the tongue. Make a hook with the index finger of your other hand and, using a gentle, sweeping motion, reach into the victim's throat and feel for a swallowed foreign object in the airway.

4. Repeat the following steps in this sequence:
   ▪ Six to ten abdominal thrusts
   ▪ Probe in mouth
   ▪ Try to inflate lungs
   ▪ Repeat

5. If the victim suddenly seems okay, but no foreign material has been removed, take him or her directly to the hospital. A foreign object, such as a fish or chicken bone or other jagged object, could do internal damage as it passes through the victim's system.

IF THE VICTIM IS A CHILD

1. If the child is coughing, do nothing. The coughing alone may dislodge the object.

2. If the airway is blocked and the child is panicky and fighting for breath, do NOT probe the airway with your fingers to clear an unseen foreign object. You might push the material back into the airway, worsening the obstruction.

3. For an infant younger than a year, hang the child over your arm so that the head is lower than the trunk. Using the heel of your hand, administer four firm blows high on the back between the shoulder blades. For a bigger child, follow the same procedure, but invert the child over your knee rather than your arm.

4. After four back blows, perform four chest thrusts (the Heimlich maneuver as described above).

DROWNING

A person can die of drowning four to six minutes after breathing stops. Although prevention is the wisest course, follow these steps in case of a drowning emergency:

1. Get the victim out of the water fast. Be extremely cautious, because a drowning person may panic and grasp at a rescuer, endangering that individual as well. If possible, push a branch or pole within the victim's reach.

2. If the victim is unconscious, use a flotation device if at all possible. Carefully place the person on the device. Once out of the water, place the victim on his or her back.

3. If the victim is not breathing, start mouth-to-mouth resuscitation. Continue until the person can breathe unassisted or help arrives. (Note that it may take an hour or two for a drowning victim to resume indepen-

dent breathing.) Do not leave the victim alone for any reason.

4. Once the person is breathing without assistance, even if he or she is still coughing, you need only stay nearby until professional help arrives.

ELECTRICAL SHOCK

1. If you suspect that an electrical shock has knocked a person unconscious, approach very carefully. Do not touch the victim unless the electricity has been turned off.

2. Shut off the power at the plug, circuit breaker, or fuse box. Simply shutting off an appliance does not remove the shock hazard. Use a dry stick to move a wire or downed power line from the victim. Keep in mind that you also are in danger until the power is off.

3. If the person's breathing is weak or has stopped, follow the steps for mouth-to-mouth resuscitation.

4. Even if the victim returns to consciousness, call for medical help. While waiting, cover the victim with a blanket or coat to keep him or her warm. Place a blanket underneath the body if the surface is cold. Be sure the person lies flat if conscious, with legs raised. If the victim is unconscious, place him or her on one side, with a pillow supporting the head. Do not give the victim anything to eat or drink.

5. Electrical burns can extend deep into the tissue, even when they appear minor. Do not put butter, household remedies, or sprays on burns without a doctor's instruction. Do not use ice or cold water on an electrical burn that is more than 2 inches across.

HEART ATTACK

Chest pain can be caused by indigestion, strained muscles, or lung infections. The warning signs of a heart attack are:

▪ Intense pain that lasts for more than two minutes, produces a tight or crushing feeling, is centered in the chest, or spreads to the neck, jaw, shoulder, or arm
▪ Shortness of breath that is worse when the person lies flat and improves when the person sits
▪ Heavy sweating
▪ Nausea or vomiting
▪ Irregular pulse
▪ Pale or bluish skin or lips
▪ Weakness
▪ Severe anxiety, feeling of doom

If an individual develops these symptoms:

1. Call for emergency medical help immediately.

2. Have the person sit up or lie in a semi-reclining position. Loosen tight clothing. Keep him or her comfortably warm.

3. If the person loses consciousness, turn on his or her back and check for breathing and pulse. If vomiting occurs, turn the victim's head to one side and clean the mouth.

4. If the person has medicine for angina pectoris (chest pain) and is conscious, help him or her take it.

5. If the person is unconscious, and you are trained to perform cardiopulmonary resuscitation (CPR), check for a pulse at the wrist or neck. If there is none, begin CPR in conjunction with mouth-to-mouth resuscitation. Do not attempt CPR unless you are trained. It is not a technique you can learn from a book.

POISONING

Many common household substances, including glue, aspirin, bleaches, and paint, can be poisonous. If you think someone has been poisoned, call the National Poison Control Center: (800) 222-1222. Be prepared to provide the following information:

▪ The kind of substance swallowed and how much was swallowed
▪ If a child or adult swallowed the substance
▪ Symptoms
▪ Whether or not vomiting has occurred
▪ Whether you gave the person anything to drink
▪ How much time it will take to get to an emergency room

The Poison Control Center will tell you whether or not to induce vomiting or neutralize a swallowed poison. Here are some additional guidelines:

1. Always assume the worst if a small child has swallowed or might have swallowed something poisonous. Keep the suspected item or container with you to answer questions.

2. Do not give any medications unless a physician or the Poison Control Center instructs you to do so.

3. Do not follow the directions for neutralizing poisons on the container unless a doctor or the Poison Control Center confirms that they are appropriate measures to take.

4. If the child is conscious, give moderate doses of water to dilute the poison.

5. If a poisoning victim is unconscious, make sure he or she is breathing. If not, give mouth-to-mouth resuscitation. Do not give anything by mouth or attempt to stimulate the person. Call for emergency help immediately.

6. If the person is vomiting, make sure he or she is in a position in which he or she cannot choke on what is brought up.

7. While vomiting is the fastest way to expel swallowed poisons from the body, never try to induce vomiting if the person has swallowed any acid or alkaline substance, which can cause burns of the face, mouth, and throat (examples include ammonia, bleach, dishwasher detergent, drain and toilet cleaners, lye, oven cleaners, or rust removers), or petroleum-like products, which produce dangerous fumes that can be inhaled during vomiting (examples include floor polish, furniture wax, gasoline, kerosene, lighter fluid, turpentine, and paint thinner)

✔ What They Tell the Doctor

✔ How Often You Need Them

✔ What to Do About Abnormal Results

Do you wonder what the doctor sees when he looks into your eyes with that little light or what it means when your blood or urine test is normal? In this section we cover some of the most common tests your doctor does, what they tell, and how often they should be done.

GENERAL INFORMATION

▪ Always ask your doctor what tests are being done, why they are being ordered, what they involve, and what the results mean.

▪ No test is foolproof. If a result is unexpected, whether normal or abnormal, your doctor should repeat the test before making any decisions.

▪ Modern X-ray machines expose you to a minuscule amount of radiation. Nevertheless, be sure to tell the physician or X-ray technician if there is even a chance you may be pregnant.

▪ Often a doctor orders a test because that is the only way to prove you do not have a disease.

ALLERGY SKIN TESTING

▪ Skin testing is still the most reliable method.

▪ The physician either pricks your skin 20 to 40 or more times to introduce a tiny bit of potentially allergic material or injects a small amount.

▪ Children who are frightened by multiple needle sticks and are unlikely to sit still for as long as necessary may have blood (RAST) tests instead.

What the results mean. If you develop redness or a hivelike bump around an area, you are probably allergic to the injected substance. Sometimes you can avoid the offending material, but things like pollen and dust are everywhere. Your allergist may recommend desensitizing shots to reduce your reaction. The results of skin tests won't be reliable if you take antihistamines within 48 hours of the test.

How often to be tested. Skin tests are necessary only if you cannot get allergy relief from other measures such as over-the-counter medications, reducing mold and dust in the house, and staying away from animals.

BLOOD PRESSURE READING

▪ High blood pressure, a major cause of stroke and heart attacks, usually causes no symptoms.

▪ The upper number in a reading—the systolic—refers to peak amount of pressure generated when your heart pumps blood, the lower number—the diastolic—measures the least amount of pressure.

What the results mean. Most doctors today think the lower the pressure the better, which means a reading of 120/80 or less. Because the mere anxiety of having your blood pressure taken can cause a mild elevation, your doctor will want to repeat an abnormal test, ideally on a different day, before diagnosing high blood pressure.

How often to be tested. Everyone—no matter how healthy—should have a blood-pressure reading taken at least once a year, more often if you have high blood pressure.

BLOOD TESTS

▪ Blood may be taken from either a finger prick or, more commonly, a vein in your arm.

▪ See below for information on cholesterol testing, which is also done from a blood sample.

Complete Blood Count (CBC)

This is the most commonly performed of all blood tests.

What the results mean. A low red-cell count, called anemia, can be caused by something as simple as too little iron in your diet, as complex as an abnormality in your digestion, or as serious as a bone marrow problem or silent bleeding. Iron deficiency is the most frequent cause, with women who menstruate and limit their intake of red meat at the greatest risk. If your doctor diagnoses this problem, ask about making dietary changes as well as taking iron supplements.

A high white-cell count, a measure of the body's defenses against infection, usually indicates some kind of infection. Depending on the type of cell that predominates, your doctor may be able to identify whether you have a bacterial or viral infection.

Platelets, the first participants in blood clotting, may be decreased because of a viral infection, abnormal bleeding, or for no identifiable reason.

Chemistry Panels (Chem 12 or 18, SMA 12 or 24)

Kidney, bone, liver, pancreas, prostate, and some glandular functions are screened by these tests.

What the results mean. An abnormality may signal a problem that needs treatment. Because accuracy decreases when many tests are run together, any specific abnormal test should be repeated, especially if unexpected.

CAT (COMPUTERIZED AXIAL TOMOGRAPHY) SCAN

▪ A CAT scan is 100 times more sensitive than an X ray.

▪ You lie as motionless as possible in a large tube while an X-ray beam travels 360 degrees around you. The test takes about an hour.

What the results mean. The test can help diagnose such conditions as tumors, blood clots, cysts, and bleeding in the brain as well as in various other organs.

CHOLESTEROL TEST/LIPOPROTEIN PROFILE

- Anyone can have a high cholesterol level, but you are more apt to be at risk if there is a family history of early heart attacks, strokes, or high blood cholesterol.
- Your doctor will look at total blood cholesterol, high-density lipoprotein (HDL, the "good" cholesterol that prevents cholesterol from sticking to your blood vessels), low-density lipoprotein (LDL, the "bad" cholesterol that does the reverse), and triglycerides.

What the results mean. Experts today think optimum total cholesterol levels are below 200 mg/dL of blood. Persistently high cholesterol values will prompt your doctor to advise dietary and lifestyle changes—less fat intake, more exercise—and perhaps medication. Optimal LDL levels depend on your risk factors for heart disease, and optimal HDL levels are 60 mg/dL or higher.

How often to be tested. If your cholesterol level is under 200 and your LDL level is under 130, repeat the test every five years. If your test is borderline, repeat it annually. (Note that the test should be taken when you have not eaten for at least twelve hours.)

If you have a family history of cholesterol problems, have your children tested annually from age 2; if you don't, have them tested around age 10 and every few years thereafter. Children under 2 should not be given a low-cholesterol diet; they need extra fat to make brain tissue and hormones for growth.

FUNDOSCOPY

The doctor looks into your eye with a little light.

What the results mean. The beginnings of cataracts may be visible, as well as irregularities in the blood vessels that indicate damage from high cholesterol (fatty deposits in the blood vessels), high blood pressure (narrowing and notching), diabetes, or other diseases. If the optic nerve is swollen, there may be excess pressure inside your skull.

What your doctor *cannot* see are the early signs of glaucoma, which can lead to blindness if not treated. Over age 20, have a pressure check for glaucoma from an ophthalmologist or optometrist every three years—or every year if you have a family history of glaucoma.

HEART TESTS

- The following tests are listed from the simplest through the most complicated.
- Also see listings for blood pressure readings, cholesterol tests, and pulse.

Electrocardiogram (ECG, EKG)

A machine amplifies the electrical signals from your heart and records them on paper.

What the results mean. An EKG can detect such things as an enlarged heart, abnormal levels of potassium or calcium, disease of the small vessels of the heart, or the source of an abnormal heart rhythm. It is a nonspecific test, however, and more advanced studies should be done if serious disease is suspected.

Echocardiogram

In this painless test sound waves are used to produce a picture of the heart in action on a TV-type screen.

What the results mean. The test investigates the size of the heart chambers, the thickness of the walls, how the four heart valves are working, and the condition of the membrane surrounding the heart. Mitral valve prolapse, a common minor abnormality, often shows up on this test, as well as more serious problems.

Stress Test

Your heart rate, blood pressure, and EKG are constantly monitored as you exercise on a treadmill that goes faster and faster with a steeper and steeper incline. This test—also called an exercise tolerance test or treadmill test—should be performed in the presence of a cardiologist and in or near a hospital in case the strain causes heart problems that need emergency treatment. The test should be stopped immediately if you experience any light-headedness, chest pain, nausea, or palpitations.

What the results mean. The increasing strain on the heart causes changes that can tell your doctor if you are at risk of a heart attack. This is because a blockage in the coronary arteries—the blood vessels that feed your heart muscle—may show up only during exercise.

Angiography

A dye is injected into various arteries, and X rays are taken.

What the results mean. The doctor can detect blockages in the blood vessels that can lead to heart attack or stroke, as well as aneurysms (weakened spots in the blood-vessel walls). The test carries some risk of causing stroke.

KIDNEY TESTS

The two tests listed here involve taking X rays. Ultrasound (similar to an echocardiogram) can also be used to outline the kidneys.

Intravenous Pyelogram (IVP)

After an iodine-containing substance is injected into a vein, X rays are taken at five-minute intervals to show the outlines of the kidney, ureter, and bladder.

What the results mean.   Tumors, kidney stones, and swelling of the kidney tissue can be seen, as well as blockage to urine flow or a mass that may be pressing on the kidney. A kidney that is not functioning will not appear on the X ray, and one in an abnormal position can be found.

Voiding Cystourethrogram (VCUG)

A technician will fill your bladder with a dye injected through a catheter and take X rays while you urinate.

What the results mean.   If you have recurrent urinary-tract infections, the test will show if there is a significant backup of urine from the bladder into the ureter, in which case daily antibiotics may be needed to prevent infection. Investigating recurrent urinary tract infections is particularly important for children.

MAGNETIC RESONANCE IMAGING (MRI)

MRI uses no radiation but produces pictures of the brain that are much more detailed than those of a CAT scan.

What the results mean.   In addition to locating bleeding or tumors, as a CAT scan does, the test picks up subtle signs such as those of Parkinson's disease and multiple sclerosis in the brain or a herniated disc in the spinal column.

MAMMOGRAPHY

- Only a small amount of radiation is used to take the mammogram. You usually stand up and put your breast on a photographic plate where it is compressed with a plastic shield or balloonlike device. It shouldn't hurt. If your breasts are tender at certain times in your menstrual cycle, schedule your mammogram when they are least sensitive.
- Mammograms can detect breast abnormalities at easily treated stages before you can feel them, but they are not foolproof. Examine your breasts monthly.

What the results mean.   Mammograms can detect cysts, abscesses, and tumors. Whether a mass is benign or malignant is hard to tell in the early stages, so abnormalities usually need to be biopsied or removed totally to determine treatment.

How often to be tested.   Although there is controversy over the benefits of mammography for women under 50, many experts still recommend having a first mammogram between ages 35 and 40, followed by one every two years between 40 and 50, and yearly thereafter. If your mother or sister has had breast cancer, consult your doctor for an appropriate schedule. And if you have a lump, pain, or nipple discharge, have a mammogram right away, no matter what your age.

You also should have a breast examination by a doctor at least every three years between ages 20 and 40, and every year after 40.

PAP SMEAR

- A routine part of every gynecological examination.
- Your doctor takes a painless swab from the cervix and vaginal walls and sends it to a lab for analysis.

What the results mean.   Pap smears can detect not only cervical cancer but also inflammation and many infections, minor and more serious; they also provide important information about the state of your female hormones. A normal test is termed class I, and abnormal results are graded by degree into four classifications, with only the most severe—a class V test—signifying outright cancer. Treatment depends on the diagnosis and may range from doing nothing for a minor inflammation to, in rare cases, a hysterectomy for cancer. Because the error rate of Pap smears is high, the doctor should always repeat an abnormal test.

How often to be tested.   Women who are on birth control pills and are sexually active should have a Pap smear every six months; other women should be checked every year.

PHYSICAL EXAMINATION

The routine physical exam generally includes a pulse and blood-pressure reading, measure of height and weight, blood tests (including a lipoprotein profile), fundoscopy, and sometimes other tests as well, such as a fecal occult blood test.

What the results mean.   A physical exam serves as a general measure of health and sometimes picks up early signs of disease.

How often to have a physical exam.   Most doctors no longer recommend yearly physicals for everybody. A good schedule to follow instead is to have a complete checkup every four or five years under age 40, every three years between 40 and 50, every two years between 50 and 60, and every year after that. At any age, you should have more frequent examinations if you have chronic medical problems such as diabetes or high blood pressure, are obese, or smoke cigarettes.

PULSE

To take your own pulse, press two fingertips over the artery in your wrist, just below the base of the thumb. Count the beats in 20 seconds, then multiply by 3.

What the results mean.   The normal pulse rate—the speed at which your heart pumps blood—is 60–80 beats a minute; it should be regular, without skipped or extra beats. Abnormal rates can be due to thyroid problems (too high causes a fast rate, too low a slow one), heart problems, anxiety (even the stress of a physical exam), or weakness from an illness such as the flu or other problems.

The character of your pulse is also important. A discrepancy between the strength of the pulse on one side of the neck and the other may mean you are in danger of a stroke. A pulse that is abnormally strong and bounding can signal a problem with a heart valve. If the pulse is weak, you may have blockages in your blood vessels from diabetes, atherosclerosis (hardening of the arteries), or a variety of other disorders.

STOMACH AND INTESTINAL TESTS

Though most of these tests are uncomfortable, they generally are not painful.

Barium Enema

Barium, a radioactive material, is instilled in your large intestine through a tube inserted into your anus. Because barium is constipating, drink fluids afterward. Don't be alarmed if you have white stools for a day or two.

What the results mean. The doctor will be able to see tumors or polyps, any obstructions, and other abnormalities.

Colonoscopy and Sigmoidoscopy

In colonoscopy, for which you will be sedated, the doctor looks into the colon with a flexible tube inserted into your anus. The procedure is essentially the same for sigmoidoscopy, except that the doctor looks only into the lower third of the intestine.

What the results mean. Your doctor can see where bleeding comes from, remove a polyp, or biopsy a mass.

Upper GI Series

You will be asked to down a drink of barium so that X rays can be taken of the esophagus, stomach, duodenum, and sometimes the small intestine.

What the results mean. Your doctor can diagnose swallowing disorders, hiatus hernias, ulcers, tumors, and some inflammations of the stomach and small bowel.

Fecal Occult Blood Test (FOBT)

A small sample of stool that remains on the doctor's glove after a rectal exam or that is collected by you at home is tested for blood that is invisible to the eye.

What the results mean. This test is done routinely as part of a regular checkup to detect the earliest sign of cancer of the colon. It is also part of an investigation of anemia or abdominal pain. If your test is positive, tell your doctor if you recently ate radishes, turnips, or red meat, took large doses of vitamin C or iron pills, or had a nosebleed. All of these things can produce misleading results.

Urinalysis

Urine can tell about the health not only of the kidneys but also of other organ systems.

What the results mean. Specific gravity is the degree to which your urine is concentrated or diluted. If it is persistently too dilute, your doctor may ask for a first morning sample to see how well your kidneys concentrate your urine overnight. Urine that is too concentrated may indicate poor fluid intake, decreased kidney function, or dehydration from vomiting and diarrhea.

Acidity or alkalinity (pH) is useful information when there is a history or possibility of kidney stones, urinary tract infection, or kidney disease.

Glucose or sugar in the urine may mean you have diabetes. You will need a blood test to confirm the diagnosis, as some families filter sugar easily through their kidneys but do not have any disease. Inflammation of the pancreas and thyroid problems also may cause sugar in the urine.

Blood in the urine may mean infection, a stone, or an inflammation of the kidney. Excessive exertion such as running sometimes causes some blood to leak into the urine; this usually disappears after resting.

Protein molecules are large and under normal conditions should not filter into the urine. However, they may appear in small amounts in the urine after strenuous exercise or an illness, especially one with a fever. In large amounts, protein in the urine warrants a search for an underlying kidney problem.

Nitrites, substances produced when bacteria multiply, may be the earliest or only sign of an infection.

White blood cells may be present because of a urinary tract or vaginal infection.

X RAY

The simple X ray is a nonspecific test that is being replaced more and more by CAT scans, magnetic resonance imaging, and other tests.

What the results mean. An X ray can detect such things as an enlarged heart, a broken bone, a sinus infection, or pneumonia.

Glossary

abscess A localized accumulation of pus and disintegrating tissue.

absorption The passage of substances into or across membranes or tissues.

abstinence Voluntary refrainment from sexual intercourse.

acid rain Rain with a high concentration of acids produced by air pollutants emitted during the combustion of fossil fuels and the smelting of ores; damages plant and animal life and buildings.

acquired immune deficiency syndrome (AIDS) The final stages of HIV infection, characterized by a variety of severe illnesses and decreased levels of certain immune cells.

actin Thin myofilaments.

active stretching A technique that involves stretching a muscle by contracting the opposing muscle.

acupuncture A Chinese medical practice of puncturing the body with needles inserted at specific points to relieve pain or cure disease.

acute injuries Physical injuries, such as sprains, bruises, and pulled muscles, which result from sudden traumas, such as falls or collisions.

adaptive response The body's attempt to reestablish homeostasis or stability.

addiction A behavioral pattern characterized by compulsion, loss of control, and continued repetition of a behavior or activity in spite of adverse consequences.

additive Characterized by a combined effect that is equal to the sum of the individual effects.

additives Substances added to foods to enhance certain qualities, such as appearance, taste, or freshness.

adoption The legal process for becoming the parent to a child of other biological parents.

advance directives Documents that specify individual's preferences regarding treatment in a medical crisis.

aerobic circuit training Combining aerobic and strength exercises to build both cardiorespiratory fitness and muscular strength and endurance.

aerobic exercise Physical activity in which sufficient or excess oxygen is continually supplied to the body.

affirmation A single positive sentence used as a tool for behavior change.

aging The characteristic pattern of normal life changes that occur as humans grow older.

alcohol abuse Continued use of alcohol despite awareness of social, occupational, psychological, or physical problems related to its use, or use of alcohol in dangerous ways or situations, such as before driving.

alcohol dependence Development of a strong craving for alcohol due to the pleasurable feelings or relief of stress or anxiety produced by drinking.

alcoholism A chronic, progressive, potentially fatal disease characterized by impaired control of drinking, a preoccupation with alcohol, continued use of alcohol despite adverse consequences, and distorted thinking, most notably denial.

allergy A hypersensitivity to a particular substance in one's environment or diet.

allopathic medicine Conventional or orthodox Western medicine.

allostasis The body's ability to adapt to constantly changing environments.

altruism Acts of helping or giving to others without thought of self-benefit.

alveoli Tiny air sacs in the lungs where gas exchange takes place.

Alzheimer's disease A progressive deterioration of intellectual powers due to physiological changes within the brain; symptoms include diminishing ability to concentrate and reason, disorientation, depression, apathy, and paranoia.

amenorrhea The absence or suppression of menstruation.

amino acids Organic compounds containing nitrogen, carbon, hydrogen, and oxygen; the essential building blocks of proteins.

amnion The innermost membrane of the sac enclosing the embryo or fetus.

amphetamine Any of a class of stimulants that trigger the release of epinephrine, which stimulates the central nervous system; users experience a state of hyper-alertness and energy, followed by a crash as the drug wears off.

anabolic steroids Drugs derived from testosterone and approved for medical use, but often used by athletes to increase their musculature and weight.

anaerobic exercise Physical activity in which the body develops an oxygen deficit.

androgyny The expression of both masculine and feminine traits.

anemia A condition characterized by a marked reduction in the number of circulating red blood cells or in hemoglobin, the oxygen-carrying component of red blood cells.

angina pectoris A severe, suffocating chest pain caused by a brief lack of oxygen to the heart.

angioplasty Surgical repair of an obstructed artery by passing a balloon catheter through the blood vessel to the area of disease and then inflating the catheter to compress the plaque against the vessel wall.

anorexia nervosa A psychological disorder in which refusal to eat and/or an extreme loss of appetite leads to malnutrition, severe weight loss, and possibly death.

antagonistic Opposing or counteracting.

antibiotics Substances produced by microorganisms, or synthetic agents, that are toxic to other types of microorganisms; in dilute solutions, used to treat infectious diseases.

antidepressant A drug used primarily to treat symptoms of depression.

antioxidants Substances that prevent the damaging effects of oxidation in cells.

antiviral drug A substance that decreases the severity and duration of a viral infection if taken prior to or soon after onset of the infection.

anxiety A feeling of apprehension and dread, with or without a known cause; may range from mild to severe and may be accompanied by physical symptoms.

anxiety disorders A group of psychological disorders involving episodes of apprehension, tension, or uneasiness, stemming from the anticipation of danger and sometimes accompanied by physical symptoms, which cause significant distress and impairment to an individual.

aorta The main artery of the body, arising from the left ventricle of the heart.

appetite A desire for food, stimulated by anticipated hunger, physiological changes within the brain and body, the availability of food, and other environmental and psychological factors.

arrhythmia Any irregularity in the rhythm of the heartbeat.

arteriosclerosis Any of a number of chronic diseases characterized by degeneration of the arteries and hardening and thickening of arterial walls.

arthritis Inflammation of the joints.

artificial insemination The introduction of viable sperm into the vagina by artificial means for the purpose of inducing conception.

assertive Behaving in a confident manner to make your needs and desires clear to others in a nonhostile way.

asthma A disease or allergic response characterized by bronchial spasms and difficult breathing.

atherosclerosis A form of arteriosclerosis in which fatty substances (plaque) are deposited on the inner walls of arteries.

atrial fibrillation A condition characterized by an irregular, abnormally rapid heartbeat.

atrium (plural **atria**) Either of the two upper chambers of the heart, which receive blood from the veins.

atrophy A decrease in the size of muscles because of inactivity.

attention deficit/hyperactivity disorder (ADHD) A spectrum of difficulties in controlling motion and sustaining attention, including hyperactivity, impulsivity, and distractibility.

autoimmune disorder Resulting from the attack on body tissue by an immune system that fails to recognize the tissue as self.

autonomy The ability to draw on internal resources; independence from familial and societal influences.

autoscopy The sensation of one's self being outside its body, often experienced by individuals in near-death medical crises.

aversion therapy A treatment that attempts to help a person overcome a dependence or bad habit by making the person feel disgusted or repulsed by that habit.

axon The long fiber that conducts impulses from the neuron's nucleus to its dendrites.

axon terminal The ending of an axon, from which impulses are transmitted to a dendrite of another neuron.

ayurveda A traditional Indian medical treatment involving meditation, exercise, herbal medications, and nutrition.

bacteria (singular, **bacterium**) One-celled microscopic organisms; the most plentiful pathogens.

bacterial vaginosis A vaginal infection caused by overgrowth and depletion of various microorganisms living in the vagina, resulting in a malodorous white or gray vaginal discharge.

ballistic stretching Rapid bouncing movements.

barbiturates Antianxiety drugs that depress the central nervous system, reduce activity and induce relaxation, drowsiness, or sleep; often prescribed to relieve tension and treat epileptic seizures or as a general anesthetic.

barrier contraceptives Birth-control devices that block the meeting of egg and sperm, either by physical barriers, such as condoms, diaphragms, or cervical caps, or

by chemical barriers, such as spermicide, or both.

basal body temperature The body temperature upon waking, before any activity.

basal metabolic rate (BMR) The number of calories required to sustain the body at rest.

behavior therapy Psychotherapy that emphasizes application of the principles of learning to substitute desirable responses and behavior patterns for undesirable ones.

benign prostatic hypertrophy Enlargement of the prostate gland, resulting in a pinching of the urethra.

benzodiazepines Antianxiety drugs that depress the central nervous system, reduce activity and induce relaxation, drowsiness, or sleep; often prescribed to relieve tension, muscular strain, sleep problems, anxiety, and panic attacks; also used as an anesthetic and in the treatment of alcohol withdrawal.

bidis Skinny, sweet-flavored cigarettes.

binge drinking For a man, having five or more alcoholic drinks at a single sitting; for a woman, having four drinks or more at a single sitting.

binge eating The rapid consumption of an abnormally large amount of food in a relatively short time.

biofeedback A technique of becoming aware, with the aid of external monitoring devices, of internal physiological activities in order to develop the capability of altering them.

bipolar disorder Severe depression alternating with periods of manic activity and elation.

bisexual Sexually oriented toward both sexes.

blended family A family formed when one or both of the partners bring children from a previous union to the new marriage.

blood-alcohol concentration (BAC) The amount of alcohol in the blood, expressed as a percentage.

body composition The relative amounts of fat and lean tissue (bone, muscle, organs, water) in the body.

body mass index (BMI) A mathematical formula that correlates with body fat; the ratio of weight to height squared.

bone-marrow transplantation A cancer treatment involving high doses of radiation or chemotherapy during which the marrow is destroyed and then replaced with healthy bone marrow.

botulism Possibly fatal food poisoning, caused by a type of bacterium that grows and produces its toxin in the absence of air and is found in improperly canned food.

bradycardia An abnormally slow heart rate, under 60 beats per minute.

breech birth A birth in which the infant's buttocks or feet pass through the birth canal first.

bulimia nervosa Episodic binge eating, often followed by forced vomiting or laxative abuse, and accompanied by a persistent preoccupation with body shape and weight.

bupropion A drug, also known as Zyban, for treating nicotine addiction that is an alternative to the nicotine patch.

burnout A state of physical, emotional, and mental exhaustion resulting from constant or repeated emotional pressure.

caesarean delivery The surgical procedure in which an infant is delivered through an incision made in the abdominal wall and uterus.

calorie The amount of energy required to raise the temperature of 1 gram of water by 1 degree Celsius. In everyday usage related to the energy content of foods and the energy expended in activities, a calorie is actually the equivalent of a thousand such calories, or a kilocalorie.

candidiasis An infection of the yeast *Candida albicans*, commonly occurring in the vagina, vulva, penis, and mouth and causing burning, itching, and a whitish discharge.

capillary A minute blood vessel that connects an artery to a vein.

carbohydrates Organic compounds, such as starches, sugars, and glycogen, that are composed of carbon, hydrogen, and oxygen, and are sources of bodily energy.

carbon monoxide A colorless, odorless gas produced by the burning of gasoline or tobacco; displaces oxygen in the hemoglobin molecules of red blood cells.

carcinogen A substance that produces cancerous cells or enhances their development and growth.

cardiac muscle Heart muscle.

cardiopulmonary resuscitation (CPR) A method of artificial stimulation of the heart and lungs; a combination of mouth-to-mouth breathing and chest compression.

cardiorespiratory endurance Ability of the heart, lungs, and circulatory system to deliver oxygen to muscles working rhythmically over an extended period of time.

cardiorespiratory fitness The ability of the heart and blood vessels to circulate blood through the body efficiently.

cardiovascular system The heart and blood vessels; responsible for distributing nutrients and oxygen to the cells within the body and removing carbon dioxide and other waste materials from the body.

celibacy Abstention from sexual activity; can be partial or complete, permanent or temporary.

cell-mediated The portion of the immune response that protects against parasites, fungi, cancer cells, and foreign tissue, primarily by means of T cells, or lymphocytes.

certified social worker A person who has completed a two-year graduate program in counseling people with mental problems.

cervical cap A thimble-sized rubber or plastic cap that is inserted into the vagina to fit over the cervix and prevent the passage of sperm into the uterus during sexual intercourse; used with a spermicidal foam or jelly, it serves as both a chemical and a physical barrier to sperm.

cervix The narrow, lower end of the uterus that opens into the vagina.

chanchroid A soft, painful sore or localized infection usually acquired through sexual contact.

chemoprevention The use of natural or synthetic substances to reduce the risk of developing cancer.

chiropractic A method of treating disease, primarily through manipulating the bones and joints to restore normal nerve function.

chlamydial infections A sexually transmitted disease caused by the bacterium *Chlamydia trachomatis*, often asymptomatic in women, but sometimes characterized by urinary pain; if undetected and untreated, may result in pelvic inflammatory disease (PID).

chlorinated hydrocarbons Highly toxic pesticides, such as DDT and chlordane, that are extremely resistant to breakdown; may cause cancer, birth defects, neurological disorders, and damage to wildlife and the environment.

cholesterol An organic substance found in animal fats; linked to cardiovascular disease, particularly atherosclerosis.

chronic fatigue syndrome (CFS) A cluster of symptoms whose cause is not yet known; a primary symptom is debilitating fatigue.

chronic obstructive lung disease (COLD) Any one of several lung diseases characterized by obstruction of breathing, including emphysema and chronic bronchitis.

circumcision The surgical removal of the foreskin of the penis.

cirrhosis A chronic disease, especially of the liver, characterized by a degeneration of cells and excessive scarring.

clitoris A small erectile structure on the female, corresponding to the penis on the male.

club drugs Illegally manufactured psychoactive drugs that have dangerous physical and psychological effects.

cocaine A white crystalline powder extracted from the leaves of the coca plant which stimulates the central nervous system and produces a brief period of euphoria followed by a depression.

codependence An emotional and psychological behavioral pattern in which the spouses, partners, parents, children, and friends of individuals with addictive behaviors allow or enable their loved ones to continue their self-destructive habits.

cognitive therapy A technique used to identify an individual's beliefs and attitudes, recognize negative thought patterns, and educate in alternative ways of thinking.

cohabitation Two people living together as a couple, without official ties such as marriage.

coitus interruptus The removal of the penis from the vagina before ejaculation.

collagen White fibers that provide support and structure in the connective tissue.

colpotomy Surgical sterilization by cutting or blocking the fallopian tubes through an incision made in the wall of the vagina.

coma A state of total unconsciousness.

companion-oriented marriage A marital relationship in which the partners share interests, activities, and domestic responsibilities.

complementary and alternative medicine (CAM) A term used to apply to all health-care approaches, practices, and treatments not widely taught in medical schools, not generally used in hospitals, and not usually reimbursed by medical insurance companies.

complementary proteins Incomplete proteins that, when combined, provide all the amino acids essential for protein synthesis.

complete proteins Proteins that contain all the amino acids needed by the body for growth and maintenance.

complex carbohydrates Starches, including cereals, fruits, and vegetables.

computer vision syndrome A condition caused by computer use marked by tired and sore eyes, blurred vision, headaches, and neck, shoulder, and back pain.

conception The merging of a sperm and an ovum.

conditioning The gradual building up of the body to enhance one or more of the three main components of physical fitness: flexibility, cardiorespiratory or aerobic fitness, and muscular strength and endurance.

condom A latex sheath worn over the penis during sexual acts to prevent conception and/or the transmission of disease; some condoms contain a spermicidal lubricant.

congestive heart failure Inability of the heart to pump at normal capacity, resulting in decreased blood flow throughout the body, collection of blood fluids in the lungs, and pulmonary congestion.

constant-dose combination pill An oral contraceptive that releases synthetic estrogen and progestin at constant levels throughout the menstrual cycle.

contraception The prevention of conception; birth control.

coronary angiography A diagnostic test in which a thin tube is threaded through the blood vessels of the heart, a dye is injected, and X rays are taken to detect blockage of the arteries.

coronary bypass Surgical correction of a blockage in a coronary artery by grafting an artery from the patient's leg or chest wall onto the damaged artery to detour blood around the blockage.

corpus luteum A yellowish mass of tissue that is formed, immediately after ovulation, from the remaining cells of the follicle; it secretes estrogen and progesterone for the remainder of the menstrual cycle.

Cowper's glands Two small glands that discharge into the male urethra; also called bulbourethral glands.

crib death *See* sudden infant death syndrome (SIDS).

cross-training Alternating two or more different types of fitness activities.

crucifers Plants, including broccoli, cabbage, and cauliflower, that contain large amounts of fiber, proteins, and indoles.

culture The set of shared attitudes, values, goals, and practices of a group that are internalized by an individual within the group.

cunnilingus Sexual stimulation of a woman's genitals by means of oral manipulation.

cystitis Inflammation of the urinary bladder.

daily values (DV) Reference values developed by the FDA specifically for use on food labels.

decibel (dB) A unit for measuring the intensity of sounds.

defense mechanism A psychological process that alleviates anxiety and eliminates mental conflict; includes denial, displacement, projection, rationalization, reaction formation, and repression.

delerants Chemicals, such as solvents, aerosols, glue, cleaning fluids, petroleum products, and some anesthetics, that produce vapors with psychoactive effects when inhaled.

delirium tremens (DTs) The delusions, hallucinations, and agitated behavior following withdrawal from long-term chronic alcohol abuse.

dementia Deterioration of mental capability.

dendrites Branching fibers of a neuron that receive impulses from axon terminals of other neurons and conduct these impulses toward the nucleus.

dental dam A small sheet of latex used as a barrier between the vagina and the mouth during cunnilingus to prevent transmission of STIs.

depression In general, feelings of unhappiness and despair; as a mental illness, also characterized by an inability to function normally.

depressive disorders A group of psychological disorders involving pervasive and sustained depression.

dermatitis Any inflammation of the skin.

detoxification The supervised removal of a poisonous or harmful substance (such as a drug) from the body; a therapy for alcoholics in which they are denied alcohol in a controlled environment.

diabetes mellitus A disease in which the inadequate production of insulin leads to failure of the body tissues to break down carbohydrates at a normal rate.

diagnostic-related group (DRG) A category of conditions requiring hospitalization for which the cost of care has been determined prior to a client's hospitalization.

diaphragm A bowl-like rubber cup with a flexible rim that is inserted into the vagina to cover the cervix and prevent the passage of sperm into the uterus during sexual intercourse; used with a spermicidal foam or jelly, it serves as both a chemical and a physical barrier to sperm.

diastole The period between contractions in the cardiac cycle, during which the heart relaxes and dilates as it fills with blood.

diastolic blood pressure Lowest blood pressure between contractions of the heart.

dietary fiber The nondigestible form of carbohydrates found in plant foods, such as leaves, stems, skins, seeds, and hulls.

dilation and evacuation (D and E) A medical procedure in which the contents of the uterus are removed through the use of instruments.

distress A negative stress that may result in illness.

do-not-resuscitate (DNR) An advance directive expressing an individual's preference that resuscitation efforts not be made during a medical crisis.

drug Any substance, other than food, that affects bodily functions and structures when taken into the body.

drug abuse The excessive use of a drug in a manner inconsistent with accepted medical practice.

drug misuse The use of a drug for a purpose (or person) other than that for which it was medically intended.

dyathanasia The act of permitting death by the removal or ending of any extraordinary efforts to sustain life; passive euthanasia.

dynamic flexibility The ability to move a joint quickly and fluidly through its entire range of motion with little resistance.

dysfunctional Characterized by negative and destructive patterns of behavior between partners or between parents and children.

dysmenorrhea Painful menstruation.

dyspareunia A sexual difficulty in which a woman experiences pain during sexual intercourse.

dysthymia Frequent, prolonged mild depression.

eating disorders Bizarre, often dangerous patterns of food consumption, including anorexia nervosa and bulimia nervosa.

ecosystem A community of organisms sharing a physical and chemical environment and interacting with each other.

ecstasy (MDMA) A synthetic compound, also known as methylenedioxymethamphetamine, that is similar in structure to methamphetamine and has both stimulant and hallucinogenic effects.

ectopic pregnancy A pregnancy in which the fertilized egg has implanted itself outside the uterine cavity, usually in the fallopian tube.

edema An excessive accumulation of fluid in connective tissue, causing swelling and pain.

ejaculation The expulsion of semen from the penis.

ejaculatory duct The canal connecting the seminal vesicles and vas deferens.

elastin Yellow fibers that make the connective tissue elastic and flexible.

electrocardiogram (ECG, EKG) A graphic record of the electric current associated with heartbeats.

electromagnetic fields (EMFs) The invisible electric and magnetic fields generated by an electrically charged conductor.

embryo An organism in its early stage of development; in humans, the embryonic period lasts from the second to the eighth week of pregnancy.

emergency contraception Types of oral contraceptive pills usually taken within 72 hours after intercourse that can prevent pregnancy.

emotional health The ability to express and acknowledge one's feelings and moods.

emotional intelligence A term used by some psychologists to evaluate the capacity of people to understand themselves and relate well with others.

enabling To unwittingly contribute to a person's addictive or abusive behavior. Components of enabling include shielding or covering up for an abuser/addict; controlling them; taking over responsibilities; rationalizing addictive behavior; or cooperating with them.

enabling factors The skills, resources, physical and mental capabilities that shape our behavior.

endocrine disruptors Synthetic chemicals that interfere with the ways that hormones work in humans and wildlife.

endocrine system The group of ductless glands that produce hormones and secrete them directly into the blood for transport to target organs.

endometrium The mucous membrane lining the uterus.

endorphins Mood-elevating, pain-killing chemicals produced by the brain.

endothelium The specialized layer of tissue inside blood vessels.

endurance The ability to withstand the stress of continued physical exertion.

environmental tobacco smoke Secondhand cigarette smoke; the third leading preventable cause of death.

epididymis That portion of the male duct system in which sperm mature.

epidural block An injection of anesthesia into the membrane surrounding the spinal cord to numb the lower body during labor and childbirth.

epilepsy A variety of neurological disorders characterized by sudden attacks (seizures) of violent muscle contractions and unconsciousness.

erectile dysfunction The consistent inability to maintain a penile erection sufficient for adequate sexual relations.

ergogenic aids Dietary supplements that purport to boost strength and enhance athletic performance, such as androstenedione and creatine.

erogenous Sexually sensitive.

essential nutrients Nutrients that the body cannot manufacture for itself and must obtain from food.

estrogen The female sex hormone that stimulates female secondary sex characteristics.

ethyl alcohol The intoxicating agent in alcoholic beverages; also called ethanol.

eustress Positive stress, which stimulates a person to function properly.

euthanasia Any method of painlessly causing death for a terminally ill person.

failure rate The number of pregnancies that occur per year for every 100 women using a particular method of birth control.

fallopian tubes The pair of channels that transport ova from the ovaries to the uterus; the usual site of fertilization.

false negative A diagnostic test result that falsely indicates the absence of a particular condition.

false positive A diagnostic test result that falsely indicates the presence of a particular condition.

family A group of people united by marriage, blood, or adoption, residing in the same household, maintaining a common culture, and interacting with one another on the basis of their roles within the group.

fast-twitch fibers Muscle fibers that contract rapidly and forcefully but fatigue quickly.

fellatio Sexual stimulation of a man's genitals by means of oral manipulation.

fertilization The fusion of the sperm and egg nuclei.

fetal alcohol effects (FAE) Milder forms of FAS, including low birthweight, irritability as newborns, and permanent mental impairment as a result of the mother's alcohol consumption during pregnancy.

fetal alcohol syndrome (FAS) A cluster of physical and mental defects in the newborn, including low birthweight, smaller-than-normal head circumference, intrauterine growth retardation, and permanent mental impairment caused by the mother's alcohol consumption during pregnancy.

fetus The human organism developing in the uterus from the ninth week until birth.

fiber Indigestible materials in food that lower blood cholesterol or facilitate digestion and elimination.

FITT A formula that describes the frequency, intensity, type, and length of time for physical activity.

flexibility The range of motion allowed by one's joints; determined by the length of muscles, tendons, and ligaments attached to the joints.

folate Various chemical forms of a water-soluble B vitamin that can be obtained from a diet high in vegetables and citrus fruit.

folic acid A form of folate used in vitamin supplements and fortified foods.

food allergies Hypersensitivities to particular foods.

food toxicologists Specialists who detect toxins in food and treat the conditions toxins produce.

frostbite The freezing or partial freezing of skin and tissue just below the skin, or even muscle and bone; more severe than frostnip.

frostnip Sudden blanching or lightening of the skin on hands, feet, and face, resulting from exposure to high wind speeds and low temperatures.

functional fiber Isolated, nondigestible carbohydrates with beneficial effects in humans.

fungi (singular, **fungus**) Organisms that reproduce by means of spores.

gallstones Clumps of solid material, usually cholesterol, that form in bile stored in the gallbladder.

gamma globulin The antibody-containing portion of the blood fluid (plasma).

GBL gamma butyrolactone The main ingredient in gamma hydroxybutyrate (GHB), also known as the "date rape drug"; once ingested, GBL converts to GHB and can cause the ingestor to lose consciousness.

gender Maleness or femaleness, as determined by a combination of anatomical and physiological factors, psychological factors, and learned behaviors.

gene therapy A cancer treatment involving the insertion of genes into a patient.

general adaptation syndrome (GAS) The sequenced physiological response to a stressful situation; consists of three stages: alarm, resistance, and exhaustion.

generalized anxiety disorder (GAD) An anxiety disorder characterized as chronic distress.

generic Refers to products without trade names that are equivalent to other products protected by trademark registration.

GHB gamma hydroxybutyrate A brain messenger chemical that stimulates the release of human growth hormone; commonly abused for its high and its alleged ability to trim fat and build muscles. Also known as "blue nitro" or the "date rape drug."

gingivitis Inflammation of the gums.

glia Support cells for neurons in the brain and spinal cord that separate the brain from the bloodstream, assist in the growth of neurons, speed transmission of nerve impulses, and eliminate damaged neurons.

gonadotropins Gonad-stimulating hormones produced by the pituitary gland.

gonorrhea A sexually transmitted disease caused by the bacterium *Neisseria gonorrhoeae*; symptoms include discharge from the penis; women are generally asymptomatic.

guided imagery An approach to stress control, self-healing, or motivating life changes by means of visualizing oneself in the state of calmness, wellness, or change.

gum disease Inflammation of the gum and bones that hold teeth in place.

hallucinogen A drug that causes hallucinations.

hashish A concentrated form of a drug, derived from the cannabis plant, containing the psychoactive ingredient TCH, which causes a sense of euphoria when inhaled or eaten.

health A state of complete well-being, including physical, psychological, spiritual, social, intellectual, and environmental components.

health maintenance organization (HMO) An organization that provides health services on a fixed-contract basis.

health promotion An educational and informational process in which people are helped to change attitudes and behaviors in an effort to improve their health.

heart rate The number of heartbeats per minute.

heat cramps Painful muscle spasms caused by vigorous exercise accompanied by heavy sweating in the heat.

heat exhaustion Faintness, rapid heart beat, low blood pressure, an ashen appearance, cold and clammy skin, and nausea, resulting from prolonged sweating with inadequate fluid replacement.

heat stress Physical response to prolonged exposure to high temperature; occurs simultaneously with or after heat cramps.

heat stroke A medical emergency consisting of a fever of at least 105°F, hot dry skin, rapid heartbeat, rapid and shallow breathing, and elevated or lowered blood pressure, caused by the breakdown of the body's cooling mechanism.

helminth A parasitic roundworm or flatworm.

hemoglobin The oxygen-transporting component of red blood cells; composed of heme and globin.

hepatitis An inflammation and/or infection of the liver caused by a virus, often accompanied by jaundice.

herbal medicine An ancient form of medical treatment using substances derived from trees, flowers, ferns, seaweeds, and lichens to treat disease.

hernia The abnormal protrusion of an organ or body part through the tissues of the walls containing it.

herpes simplex A condition caused by one of the herpes viruses and characterized by lesions of the skin or mucous membranes; herpes virus type 2 is sexually transmitted and causes genital blisters or sores.

heterosexual Primary sexual orientation toward members of the other sex.

holistic An approach to medicine that takes into account body, mind, emotions, and spirit.

holographic will A will wholly in the handwriting of its author.

home health care Provision of medical services and equipment to patients in the home to restore or maintain comfort, function, and health.

homeopathy A system of medical practice that treats a disease by administering dosages of substances that would in healthy persons produce symptoms similar to those of the disease.

homeostasis The body's natural state of balance or stability.

homocysteine A naturally occurring amino acid that has recently been identified as a risk factor for heart disease.

homosexual Primary sexual orientation toward members of the same sex.

hormone Substance released in the blood that regulates specific bodily functions.

hormone replacement therapy (HRT) The use of supplemental hormones during and after menopause.

hospice A homelike health-care facility or program committed to supportive care for terminally ill people.

host A person or population that contracts one or more pathogenic agents in an environment.

hostile or offensive environment A workplace made hostile, abusive, or unbearable by persistent inappropriate behaviors of coworkers or supervisors.

human immunodeficiency virus (HIV) A type of virus that causes a spectrum of health problems, ranging from a symptomless infection to changes in the immune system, to the development of life-threatening diseases because of impaired immunity.

human papilloma virus (HPV) A pathogen that causes genital warts and increases the risk of cervical cancer.

humoral A portion of the immune response that provides lifelong protection against bacterial or viral infections, such as mumps, by means of antibodies whose production is triggered by the release of antigens upon first exposure to the infectious agent.

hunger The physiological drive to consume food.

hydrostatic weighing Weighing a person in water to distinguish buoyant fat from denser muscle.

hypertension High blood pressure occurring when the blood exerts excessive pressure against the arterial walls.

hypertrophy An increase in the size of muscles brought on by working the muscles harder than normal.

hypothermia An abnormally low body temperature; if not treated appropriately, coma or death could result.

hysterectomy The surgical removal of the uterus.

hysterotomy A procedure in which the uterus is surgically opened and the fetus inside it removed.

immune deficiency Partial or complete inability of the immune system to respond to pathogens.

immunity Protection from infectious diseases.

immunotherapy A series of injections of small but increasing doses of an allergen, used to treating allergies.

implantation The embedding of the fertilized ovum in the uterine lining.

impotence A sexual difficulty in which a man is unable to achieve or maintain an erection.

incomplete proteins Proteins that lack one or more of the amino acids essential for protein synthesis.

incubation period The time between a pathogen's entrance into the body and the first symptom.

indemnity A form of insurance that pays a major portion of medical expenses after a deductible amount is paid by the insured person.

indoles Naturally occurring chemicals found in foods such as winter squash, carrots, and crucifers; may help lower cancer risk.

infertility The inability to conceive a child.

infiltration A gradual penetration or invasion.

inflammation A localized response by the body to tissue injury, characterized by swelling and the dilation of the blood vessels.

inflammatory bowel disease (IBD) A digestive disease that causes frequent and intense diarrhea, abdominal pain, gas, fever, and rectal bleeding. Crohn's disease is an inflammation anywhere in the digestive tract, and ulcerative colitis causes severe ulcers in the inner lining of the colon and rectum.

influenza Any of a type of fairly common, highly contagious viral diseases.

informed consent Permission (to undergo or receive a medical procedure or treatment) given voluntarily, with full knowledge and understanding of the procedure or treatment and its possible consequences.

inhalants Substances that produce vapors having psychoactive effects when sniffed.

integrative medicine An approach that combines traditional medicine with alternative/complementary therapies.

intercourse Sexual stimulation by means of entry of the penis into the vagina; coitus.

interpersonal therapy (IPT) A technique used to develop communication skills and relationships.

intimacy A state of closeness between two people, characterized by the desire and ability to share one's innermost thoughts and feelings with each other either verbally or nonverbally.

intoxication Maladaptive behavioral, psychological, and physiologic changes that occur as a result of substance abuse.

intramuscular Into or within a muscle.

intrauterine device (IUD) A device inserted into the uterus through the cervix to prevent pregnancy by interfering with implantation.

intravenous Into a vein.

ionizing radiation A form of energy emitted from atoms as they undergo internal change.

irradiation Exposure to or treatment by some form of radiation.

irritable bowel syndrome A digestive disease caused by intestinal spasms, resulting in

frequent need to defecate, nausea, cramping, pain, gas, and a continual sensation of rectal fullness.

isokinetic Having the same force; exercise with specialized equipment that provides resistance equal to the force applied by the user throughout the entire range of motion.

isometric Of the same length; exercise in which muscles increase their tension without shortening in length, such as when pushing an immovable object.

isotonic Having the same tension or tone; exercise requiring the repetition of an action that creates tension, such as weight lifting or calisthenics.

joints The point or structure between two or more bones where movement occurs.

kidney stones Formations of calcium salts or minerals that form in the kidneys; may be passed out of the body in urine, surgically removed, or decomposed by high-frequency sound waves.

labia majora The fleshy outer folds that border the female genital area.

labia minora The fleshy inner folds that border the female genital area.

labor The process leading up to birth: effacement and dilation of the cervix; the movement of the baby into and through the birth canal, accompanied by strong contractions; and contraction of the uterus and expulsion of the placenta after the birth.

lactic acid A byproduct of the breakdown of glucose that causes muscle fatigue.

lacto-vegetarians People who eat dairy products as well as fruits and vegetables (but not meat, poultry, or fish).

Lamaze method A method of childbirth preparation taught to expectant parents to help the woman cope with the discomfort of labor; combines breathing and psychological techniques.

laparoscopy A surgical sterilization procedure in which the fallopian tubes are observed with a laparoscope inserted through a small incision, and then cut or blocked.

laparotomy A surgical sterilization procedure in which the fallopian tubes are cut or blocked through an incision made in the abdomen.

licensed clinical social worker (LCSW) *See* certified social worker.

lipoprotein A compound in blood that is made up of proteins and fat; a high-density lipoprotein (HDL) picks up excess cholesterol in the blood; a low-density lipoprotein (LDL) carries more cholesterol and deposits it on the walls of arteries.

listeria A bacterium commonly found in deli meats, hot dogs, and soft cheeses that can cause an infection called listeriosis.

living will A written statement providing instructions for the use of life-sustaining procedures in the event of terminal illness or injury.

lochia The vaginal discharge of blood, mucus, and uterine tissue that occurs after birth.

locus of control An individual's belief about the source of power and influence over his or her life.

lumpectomy The surgical removal of a breast tumor and its surrounding tissue.

Lyme disease A disease caused by a bacterium carried by a tick; it may cause heart arrhythmias, neurological problems, and arthritis symptoms.

lymph nodes Small tissue masses in which some immune cells are stored.

macronutrients Nutrients required by the human body in the greatest amounts, including water, carbohydrates, proteins, and fats.

mainstream smoke The smoke inhaled directly by smoking a cigarette.

major depression Sadness that does not end.

male pattern baldness The loss of hair at the vertex, or top, of the head.

malpractice The failure of a doctor or other health-care professional to provide appropriate and skillful medical or surgical treatment.

mammography A diagnostic X-ray exam used to detect breast cancer.

managed care Health-care services and reimbursement predetermined by third-party insurers.

marijuana The drug derived from the cannabis plant, containing the psychoactive ingredient THC, which causes a mild sense of euphoria when inhaled or eaten.

marriage and family therapist A psychiatrist, psychologist, or social worker who specializes in marriage and family counseling.

massage therapy A therapeutic method of using the hands to rub, stroke, or knead the body to produce positive effects on an individual's health and well-being.

mastectomy The surgical removal of an entire breast.

masturbation Manual (or nonmanual) self-stimulation of the genitals, often resulting in orgasm.

medical abortion Method of ending a pregnancy within 9 weeks of conception using hormonal medications that cause expulsion of the fertilized egg.

medical history The health-related information collected during the interview of a client by a health-care professional.

meditation A group of approaches that use quiet sitting, breathing techniques, and/or chanting to relax, improve concentration, and become attuned to one's inner self.

menarche The onset of menstruation at puberty.

meningitis An extremely serious, potentially fatal illness that attacks the membranes around the brain and spinal cord; caused by the bacterium *Neisseria meningitis*.

menopause The complete cessation of ovulation and menstruation for twelve consecutive months.

menstruation Discharge of blood from the vagina as a result of the shedding of the uterine lining at the end of the menstrual cycle.

mental disorder Behavioral or psychological syndrome associated with distress or disability or with a significantly increased risk of suffering death, pain, disability, or loss of freedom.

mental health The ability to perceive reality as it is, to respond to its challenges, and to develop rational strategies for living.

meta-analysis Summarization and review of research in a particular area to evaluate the results of several large clinical trials in a uniform manner.

metabolic syndrome A cluster of disorders of the body's metabolism that make diabetes, heart disease, or stroke more likely.

metastasize To spread to other parts of the body via the bloodstream or lymphatic system.

micronutrients Vitamins and minerals needed by the body in very small amounts.

microwaves Extremely high frequency electromagnetic waves that increase the rate at which molecules vibrate, thereby generating heat.

migraine headache Severe headache resulting from the constriction, then dilation of blood vessels within the brain; sometimes accompanied by vomiting and nausea.

mindfulness A method of stress reduction that involves experiencing the physical and mental sensations of the present moment.

minerals Naturally occurring inorganic substances, small amounts of some being essential in metabolism and nutrition.

minilaparotomy A surgical sterilization procedure in which the fallopian tubes are cut or sealed by electrical coagulation through a small incision just above the pubic hairline.

minipill An oral contraceptive containing a small amount of progestin and no estrogen, which prevents contraception by making the mucus in the cervix so thick that sperm cannot enter the uterus.

miscarriage A pregnancy that terminates before the twentieth week of gestation; also called spontaneous abortion.

mitral valve prolapse A condition in which a valve in the heart is abnormally long and floppy, which can cause heart murmurs.

mononucleosis An infectious viral disease characterized by an excess of white blood cells in the blood, fever, bodily dis-

comfort, a sore throat, and kidney and liver complications.

monophasic pill *See* constant-dose combination pill.

mons pubis The rounded, fleshy area over the junction of the female pubic bones.

mood A sustained emotional state that colors one's view of the world for hours or days.

multiphasic pill An oral contraceptive that releases different levels of estrogen and progestin to mimic the hormonal fluctuations of the natural menstrual cycle.

multiple chemical sensitivity (MCS) A sensitivity to low-level chemical exposures from ordinary substances, such as perfumes and tobacco smoke, that results in physiological responses such as chest pain, depression, dizziness, fatigue, and nausea. Also known as environmentally triggered illness.

muscular fitness The amount of strength and level of endurance in the body's muscles.

mutagen An agent that causes alterations in the genetic material of living cells.

mutation A change in the genetic material of a cell or cells that is brought about by radiation, chemicals, or natural causes.

myocardial infarction (MI) A condition characterized by the dying of tissue areas in the myocardium, caused by interruption of the blood supply to those areas; the medical name for a heart attack.

naturopathy An alternative system of treatment of disease that emphasizes the use of natural remedies such as sun, water, heat, and air. Therapies may include dietary changes, steam baths, and exercise.

near-death experiences *See* autoscopy *and* transcendence.

negligence The failure to act in a way that a reasonable person would act.

neoplasm Any tumor, whether benign or malignant.

nephrosis A cluster of symptoms indicating chronic damage to the kidneys.

neuron The basic working unit of the brain, which transmits information from the senses to the brain and from the brain to specific body parts; each nerve cell consists of an axon, an axon terminal, and dendrites.

neuropsychiatry The study of the brain and mind.

neurotransmitters Chemicals released by neurons that stimulate or inhibit the action of other neurons.

nicotine The addictive substance in tobacco; one of the most toxic of all poisons.

nocturnal emissions Ejaculations while dreaming; wet dreams.

nongonococcal urethritis (NGU) Inflammation of the urethra caused by organisms other than the gonococcus bacterium.

nonopioids Chemically synthesized drugs that have sleep-inducing and pain-relieving properties similar to those of opium and its derivatives.

norms The unwritten rules regarding behavior and conduct expected or accepted by a group.

nucleus The central part of a cell, contained in the cell body of a neuron.

nutrition The science devoted to the study of dietary needs for food and the effects of food on organisms.

obesity The excessive accumulation of fat in the body; a condition of having a BMI of 30 or above.

obsessive-compulsive disorder (OCD) An anxiety disorder characterized by obsessions and/or compulsions that impair one's ability to function and form relationships.

oncogene A gene that, when activated by radiation or a virus, may cause a normal cell to become cancerous.

opioids Drugs that have sleep-inducing and pain-relieving properties, including opium and its derivatives and nonopioid, synthetic drugs.

optimism The tendency to seek out, remember, and expect pleasurable experiences.

oral contraceptives Preparations of synthetic hormones that inhibit ovulation; also referred to as birth control pills or simply the pill.

organic Term designating food produced with, or production based on the use of, fertilizer originating from plants or animals, without the use of pesticides or chemically formulated fertilizers.

organic phosphates Toxic pesticides that may cause cancer, birth defects, neurological disorders, and damage to wildlife and the environment.

orgasm A series of contractions of the pelvic muscles occurring at the peak of sexual arousal.

osteopathy The manipulation of the spine and other structural parts of the body to treat disorders.

osteoporosis A condition common in older people in which the bones become increasingly soft and porous, making them susceptible to injury.

outcomes The ultimate impacts of particular treatments or absence of treatment.

ovary The female sex organ that produces egg cells, estrogen, and progesterone.

overload principle Providing a greater stress or demand on the body than it is normally accustomed to handling.

overloading Method of physical training involving increasing the number of repetitions or the amount of resistance gradually to work the muscle to temporary fatigue.

over-the-counter (OTC) drugs Medications that can be obtained legally without a prescription from a medical professional.

overtrain Working muscles too intensely or too frequently, resulting in persistent muscle soreness, injuries, unintended weight loss, nervousness, and an inability to relax.

overuse injuries Physical injuries to joints or muscles, such as strains, fractures, and tendinitis, which result from overdoing a repetitive activity.

overweight A condition of having a BMI between 25.0 and 29.9.

ovo-lacto-vegetarians People who eat eggs, dairy products, and fruits and vegetables (but not meat, poultry, or fish).

ovulation The release of a mature ovum from an ovary approximately 14 days prior to the onset of menstruation.

ovulation method A method of birth control based on the observation of changes in the consistency of the mucus in the vagina to predict ovulation.

ovum (plural, **ova**) The female gamete (egg cell).

oxytocin A hormone that has been linked to one's ability to bond with others; also plays a key role in inducing labor during childbirth.

panic attack A short episode characterized by physical sensations of light-headedness, dizziness, hyperventilation, and numbness of extremities, accompanied by an inexplicable terror, usually of a physical disaster such as death.

panic disorder An anxiety disorder in which the apprehension or experience of recurring panic attacks is so intense that normal functioning is impaired.

Pap smear A test in which cells removed from the cervix are examined under a microscope for signs of cancer; also called a Pap test.

passive stretching A stretching technique in which an external force or resistance (your body, a partner, gravity, or a weight) helps the joints move through their range of motion.

pathogen A microorganism that produces disease.

PCP (phencyclidine) A synthetic psychoactive substance that produces effects similar to other psychoactive drugs when swallowed, smoked, sniffed, or injected, but may also trigger unpredictable behavioral changes.

pelvic inflammatory disease (PID) An inflammation of the internal female genital tract, characterized by abdominal pain, fever, and tenderness of the cervix.

penis The male organ of sex and urination.

percutaneous transluminal coronary angioplasty (PTCA) A procedure for unclogging arteries; also called balloon angioplasty.

perimenopause The period from a woman's first irregular cycles to her last menstruation.

perinatology The medical specialty concerned with the diagnosis and treatment of pregnant women with high-risk conditions and their fetuses.

perineum The area between the anus and vagina in the female and between the anus and scrotum in the male.

periodontitis Severe gum disease in which the tooth root becomes infected.

persistent vegetative state A state of being awake and capable of reacting to physical stimuli, such as light, while being unaware of pain or other environmental stimuli.

phobia An anxiety disorder marked by an inordinate fear of an object, a class of objects, or a situation, resulting in extreme avoidance behaviors.

physical dependence The physiological attachment to, and need for, a drug.

physical fitness The ability to respond to routine physical demands, with enough reserve energy to cope with a sudden challenge.

phytochemicals Chemicals such as indoles, coumarins, and capsaicin, which exist naturally in plants and have disease-fighting properties.

placenta An organ that develops after implantation and to which the embryo attaches, via the umbilical cord, for nourishment and waste removal.

plaque The sludgelike substance that builds up on the inner walls of arteries; the sticky film of bacteria that forms on teeth.

pneumonia An inflammation of the lungs caused by infection or irritants.

pollutant A substance or agent in the environment, usually the by-product of human industry or activity, that is injurious to human, animal, or plant life.

pollution The presence of pollutants in the environment.

polyabuse The misuse or abuse of more than one drug.

postpartum depression The emotional downswing that occurs after having a baby due to hormonal changes, physical exhaustion, and psychological pressures.

posttraumatic stress disorder (PTSD) The repeated reliving of a trauma through nightmares or recollection.

potentiating Making more effective or powerful.

preconception care Health care to prepare for pregnancy.

precycling The use of products that are packaged in recycled or recyclable material.

predisposing factors The beliefs, values, attitudes, knowledge, and perceptions that influence our behavior.

preferred provider organization (PPO) A group of physicians contracted to provide health care to members at a discounted price.

prehypertension A condition of slightly elevated blood pressure, which is likely to worsen in time.

premature ejaculation A sexual difficulty in which a man ejaculates so rapidly that his partner's satisfaction is impaired.

premature labor Labor that occurs after the twentieth week but before the thirty-seventh week of pregnancy.

premenstrual dysphoric disorder (PMDD) A disorder that causes symptoms of psychological depression during the last week of the menstrual cycle.

premenstrual syndrome (PMS) A disorder that causes physical discomfort and psychological distress prior to a woman's menstrual period.

prevention Information and support offered to help healthy people identify their health risks, reduce stressors, prevent potential medical problems, and enhance their well-being.

primary care Ambulatory or outpatient care provided by a physician in an office, emergency room, or clinic.

progesterone The female sex hormone that stimulates the uterus, preparing it for the arrival of a fertilized egg.

progestin-only pill *See* minipill.

progressive overloading Gradually increasing physical challenges once the body adapts to the stress placed upon it to produce maximum benefits.

progressive relaxation A method of reducing muscle tension by contracting, then relaxing certain areas of the body.

proof The alcoholic strength of a distilled spirit, expressed as twice the percentage of alcohol present.

prostate gland A structure surrounding the male urethra that produces a secretion that helps liquefy the semen from the testes.

prostatitis Inflammation of the prostate gland.

protection Measures that an individual can take when participating in risky behavior to prevent injury or unwanted risks.

protein A substance that is basically a compound of amino acids; one of the essential nutrients.

protozoa Microscopic animals made up of one cell or a group of similar cells.

psoriasis A chronic skin disorder caused by stress, skin damage, or illness and resulting in scaly, deep-pink, raised patches on the skin.

psychiatric drugs Medications that regulate a person's mental, emotional, and physical functions to facilitate normal functioning.

psychiatric nurse A nurse with special training and experience in mental health care.

psychiatrist Licensed medical doctor with additional training in psychotherapy, psychopharmacology, and treatment of mental disorders.

psychoactive Mood-altering.

psychodynamic Interpreting behaviors in terms of early experiences and unconscious influences.

psychological dependence The emotional or mental attachment to the use of a drug.

psychologists Mental health-care professionals who have completed doctoral or graduate programs in psychology and are trained in a variety of psychotherapeutic techniques, but who are not medically trained and do not prescribe medications.

psychoneuroimmunology A scientific field that explores the relationships between and among the mind, the central nervous system, and the immune system.

psychoprophylaxis *See* Lamaze method.

psychotherapy Treatment designed to produce a response by psychological rather than physical means, such as suggestion, persuasion, reassurance, and support.

psychotropic Mind-affecting.

pyelonephritis Inflammation of the kidney.

quackery Medical fakery; unproven practices claiming to cure diseases or solve health problems.

quid pro quo A form of harassment in which a person in power or authority makes unwanted sexual advances as a condition for receiving a job, promotion, or favor.

range of motion The fullest extent of possible movement in a particular joint.

rape Sexual penetration of a female or a male by means of intimidation, force, or fraud.

rapid-eye-movement (REM) sleep Regularly occurring periods of sleep during which the most active dreaming takes place.

Rating of Perceived Exertion (RPE) A self-assessment scale that rates symptoms of breathlessness and fatigue.

receptors Molecules on the surface of neurons on which neurotransmitters bind after their release from other neurons.

recycling The processing or reuse of manufactured materials to reduce consumption of raw materials.

reflexology A treatment based on the theory that massaging certain points on the foot or hand relieves stress or pain in corresponding parts of the body.

refractory period The period of time following orgasm during which the male cannot experience another orgasm.

rehabilitation medicine The use of surgical procedures, medication, and physical therapy to improve the condition of patients with disabling conditions such as blindness, deafness, and arthritis.

reinforcement Reward or punishment for a behavior that will increase or decrease one's likelihood of repeating the behavior.

reinforcing factors Rewards, encouragement, and recognition that influence our behavior in the short run.

relapse prevention An alcohol recovery treatment method that focuses on social skills training to develop ways of preventing or minimizing a relapse.

relative risk The risk of developing cancer in persons with a certain exposure or trait compared to the risk in persons who do not have the same exposure or trait.

rep (or **repetition**) In weight training, a single performance of a movement or exercise.

repetitive motion injury (RMI) Inflammation of or damage to a part of the body due to repetition of the same movements.

rescue marriage A marital relationship in which one partner has had a traumatic childhood and views marriage as a way of healing the past.

resting heart rate The number of heartbeats per minute during inactivity.

reuptake Reabsorption by the originating cell of neurotransmitters that have not connected with receptors and have been left in synapses.

reversibility principle The physical benefits of exercise are lost through disuse or inactivity.

rhythm method A birth-control method in which sexual intercourse is avoided during those days of the menstrual cycle in which fertilization is most likely to occur.

romantic marriage A marital relationship in which sexual passion never fades.

rubella An infectious disease that may cause birth defects if contracted by a pregnant woman; also called German measles.

satiety A feeling of fullness after eating.

saturated fat A chemical term indicating that a fat molecule contains as many hydrogen atoms as its carbon skeleton can hold. These fats are normally solid at room temperature.

schizophrenia A general term for a group of mental disorders with characteristic psychotic symptoms, such as delusions, hallucinations, and disordered thought patterns during the active phase of the illness, and a duration of at least six months.

scrotum The external sac or pouch that holds the testes.

secondary sex characteristics Physical changes associated with maleness or femaleness, induced by the sex hormones.

self-actualization A state of wellness and fulfillment that can be achieved once certain human needs are satisfied; living to one's full potential.

self-disclosure Sharing personal information and experiences with another that he or she would not otherwise discover; self-disclosure involves risk and vulnerability.

self-efficacy Belief in one's ability to accomplish a goal or change a behavior.

self-esteem Confidence and satisfaction in oneself.

self-talk Repetition of positive messages about one's self-worth to learn more optimistic patterns of thought, feeling, and behavior.

semen The viscous whitish fluid that is the complete male ejaculate; a combination of sperm and secretions from the prostate gland, seminal vesicles, and other glands.

seminal vesicles Glands in the male reproductive system that produce the major portion of the fluid of semen.

set-point theory The proposition that every person has an unconscious control system for keeping body fat (and therefore weight) at a predetermined level, or set point.

sets In weight training, the number of repetitions of the same movement or exercise.

sex Maleness or femaleness, resulting from genetic, structural, and functional factors.

sexual addiction A preoccupation with sex so intense and chronic that an individual cannot have a normal sexual relationship with a spouse or lover; sexual compulsion.

sexual coercion Sexual activity forced upon a person by the exertion of psychological pressure by another person.

sexual compulsion *See* sexual addiction.

sexual dysfunction The inability to react emotionally and/or physically to sexual stimulation in a way expected of the average healthy person or according to one's own standards.

sexual health The integration of the physical, emotional, intellectual, and social aspects of sexual being in ways that are positively enriching and that enhance personality, communication, and love.

sexuality The behaviors, instincts, and attitudes associated with being sexual.

sexually transmitted infections (STIs) Any of a number of diseases that are acquired through sexual contact.

sidestream smoke The smoke emitted by a burning cigarette and breathed by everyone in a closed room, including the smoker; contains more tar and nicotine than mainstream smoke.

simple carbohydrates Sugars; like all carbohydrates, they provide the body with glucose.

smog A grayish or brownish fog caused by the presence of smoke and/or chemical pollutants in the air.

social isolation A feeling of unconnectedness with others caused by and reinforced by infrequency of social contacts.

social phobia A severe form of social anxiety marked by extreme fears and avoidance of social situations.

specificity principle Each part of the body adapts to a particular type and amount of stress placed upon it.

sperm The male gamete produced by the testes and transported outside the body through ejaculation.

spermatogenesis The process by which sperm cells are produced.

spinal block An injection of anesthesia directly into the spinal cord to numb the lower body during labor and childbirth.

spiritual health The ability to identify one's basic purpose in life and to achieve one's full potential; the sense of connectedness to a greater power.

spiritual intelligence The capacity to sense, understand, and tap into ourselves, others, and the world around us.

static flexibility The ability to assume and maintain an extended position at one end point in a joint's range of motion.

static stretching A gradual stretch held for a short time of 10 to 30 seconds.

sterilization A surgical procedure to end a person's reproductive capability.

stimulant An agent, such as a drug, that temporarily relieves drowsiness, helps in the performance of repetitive tasks, and improves capacity for work.

strength Physical power; the maximum weight one can lift, push, or press in one effort.

stress The nonspecific response of the body to any demands made upon it; may be characterized by muscle tension and acute anxiety, or may be a positive force for action.

stressor Specific or nonspecific agents or situations that cause the stress response in a body.

stroke A cerebrovascular event in which the blood supply to a portion of the brain is blocked.

subcutaneous Under the skin.

suction curettage A procedure in which the contents of the uterus are removed by means of suction and scraping.

sudden infant death syndrome (SIDS) The unexplained death of an apparently healthy baby under one year of age during sleep.

synapse A specialized site at which electrical impulses are transmitted from the axon terminal of one neuron to a dendrite of another.

synergistic Characterized by a combined effect that is greater than the sum of the individual effects.

syphilis A sexually transmitted disease caused by the bacterium *Treponema pallidum*, and characterized by early sores, a latent period, and a final period of life-threatening symptoms including brain damage and heart failure.

systemic disease A pathologic condition that spreads throughout the body.

systole The contraction phase of the cardiac cycle.

systolic blood pressure Highest blood pressure when the heart contracts.

tachycardia An abnormally rapid heart rate, over 100 beats per minute.

tamoxifen An estrogen-based medication that can help reduce the likelihood of developing cancer.

tar A thick, sticky dark fluid produced by the burning of tobacco, made up of several hundred different chemicals, many of them poisonous, some of them carcinogenic.

target heart rate Sixty to eighty-five percent of the maximum heart rate; the heart rate at which one derives maximum cardiovascular benefit from aerobic exercise.

tendons The connective tissues that attach muscle to bone.

teratogen Any agent that causes spontaneous abortion or defects or malformations in a fetus.

terminal illness An illness in which death is inevitable.

testes (singular, **testis**) The male sex organs that produce sperm and testosterone.

testosterone The male sex hormone that stimulates male secondary sex characteristics.

thallium scintigraphy A diagnostic test in which radioactive isotopes are injected into the bloodstream, and images of the rays emitted by the isotopes are captured and then translated into images of the heart as it pumps.

thanatology The discipline of humanitarian caregiving for critically ill patients and their grieving family members and friends.

toxic shock syndrome (TSS) A disease characterized by fever, vomiting, diarrhea, and often shock, caused by a bacterium that releases toxic waste products into the bloodstream.

toxicity Poisonousness; the dosage level at which a drug becomes poisonous to the body, causing either temporary or permanent damage.

traditional marriage A marital relationship in which the roles of the partners are distinct; defined by gender-based cultural norms and expectations.

transcendence The sense of passing into a foreign region or dimension, often experienced by a person near death.

trans-fatty acids Fats formed when liquid vegetable oils are processed to make table spreads or cooking fats, and also found in dairy and beef products; considered to be especially dangerous dietary fats.

transgendered Having a gender identity opposite one's biological sex; transsexual.

transient ischemic attack (TIA) A cerebrovascular event in which the blood supply to a portion of the brain is blocked temporarily; repeated attacks are predictors of more severe strokes.

Transtheoretical Model of Change A model of behavioral change that focuses on the individual's decision making; it states that an individual progresses through a sequence of six stages as he or she makes a change in behavior.

trichomoniasis An infection of the protozoan *Trichomonas vaginalis*; females experience vaginal burning, itching, and discharge, but male carriers may be asymptomatic.

triglyceride A blood fat that flows through the blood after meals and is linked to increased risk of coronary artery disease.

tubal ligation The suturing or tying shut of the fallopian tubes to prevent pregnancy.

tubal occlusion The blocking of the fallopian tubes to prevent pregnancy.

tuberculosis A highly infectious bacterial disease that primarily affects the lungs and is often fatal.

tumor suppressor gene Gene that normally controls cell growth. Many cancers are linked to defects in a tumor suppressor gene.

twelve-step programs Self-help group programs based on the principles of Alcoholics Anonymous.

ulcer A lesion in, or an erosion of, the mucous membrane of an organ.

unsaturated fat A chemical term indicating that a fat molecule contains fewer hydrogen atoms than its carbon skeleton can hold. These fats are normally liquid at room temperature.

urethra The canal through which urine from the bladder leaves the body; in the male, also serves as the channel for seminal fluid.

urethral opening The outer opening of the thin tube that carries urine from the bladder.

urethritis Infection of the urethra.

uterus The female organ that houses the developing fetus until birth.

vagina The canal leading from the exterior opening in the female genital area to the uterus.

vaginal contraceptive film (VCF) A small dissolvable sheet saturated with spermicide that can be inserted into the vagina and placed over the cervix.

vaginal spermicide A substance that kills or neutralizes sperm, inserted into the vagina in the form of a foam, cream, jelly, or suppository.

vaginismus A sexual difficulty in which a woman experiences painful spasms of the vagina during sexual intercourse.

values The criteria by which one makes choices about one's thoughts and actions and goals and ideals.

vas deferens Two tubes that carry sperm from the epididymis into the urethra.

vasectomy A surgical sterilization procedure in which each vas deferens is cut and tied shut to stop the passage of sperm to the urethra for ejaculation.

vector A biological or physical vehicle that carries the agent of infection to the host.

vegans People who eat only plant foods.

ventricle Either of the two lower chambers of the heart, which pump blood out of the heart and into the arteries.

video display terminal (VDT) A screen or monitor that emits electromagnetic fields from all sides; these fields may lead to increased reproductive problems, miscarriages, low birthweights, and cataracts.

virus A submicroscopic infectious agent; the most primitive form of life.

visualization An approach to stress control, self-healing, or motivating life changes by means of guided, or directed, imagery.

vital signs Measurements of physiological functioning; specifically, temperature, blood pressure, pulse rate, and respiration rate.

vitamins Organic substances that are needed in very small amounts by the body and carry out a variety of functions in metabolism and nutrition.

waist-hip ratio The proportion of one's waist circumference to one's hip circumference.

wellness A state of optimal health.

withdrawal Development of symptoms that cause significant psychological and physical distress when an individual reduces or stops drug use.

zygote A fertilized egg.

References

Chapter 1

1. "Constitution of the World Health Organization." *Chronicle of the World Health Organization,* Geneva, Switzerland: WHO, 1947.
2. Travis, John, and Regina Sara Ryan. *The Wellness Workbook,* 3rd ed. Berkeley, CA: Celestial Arts, 2004.
3. Travis, John. Personal interview.
4. Travis and Ryan, *The Wellness Workbook.*
5. Matthews, Dale. Personal interview.
6. "Study Finds Art Majors Are Most Religious." *U.S. Catholic,* Vol. 69, No. 9, August 2004, p. 10.
7. Hale, Cara, et al. "Social Support and Physical Health: The Importance of Belonging." *Journal of American College Health,* Vol. 53, No. 6, May–June 2005, p. 276.
8. Zimmer, Christine, et al. "A Scope-of-Practice Survey Leading to the Development of Standards of Practice for Health Promotion in Higher Education." *Journal of American College Health,* Vol. 51, No. 6, May 2003, p. 247.
9. Kochanek, Kenneth, and Betty Smith. "Deaths: Preliminary Data for 2002." *National Vital Statistics Reports,* Vol. 52, No. 13, February 11, 2004.
10. Reeves, Mathew. "Healthy Lifestyle Characteristics Among Adults in the United States, 2000." *Archives of Internal Medicine,* Vol. 165, April 2005, pp. 854–857.
11. *Healthy People 2010,* www.healthy people.gov.
12. *Healthy Campus 2010,* University of Southern California, Health Promotion and Prevention Services, www.usc.edu/student-affairs/Health_Center/hpps.hp2010.shtml.
13. American College Health Association, "The American College Health Association National College Health Assessment."
14. American College Health Association. "The American College Health Association National College Health Assessment (ACHA-NCHA), Spring 2003 Reference Group Report." *Journal of American College Health,* Vol. 53, No. 5, March–April 2005, p. 199, www.acha.org.
15. Ibid.
16. Terry, Anna. *Osteoporosis May Threaten Young Women,* Press release, University of Arkansas, June 21, 2004.
17. Bylund, Carma, et al. "Accuracy of Parents' Perceptions of Their College Student Children's Health and Health Risk Behaviors." *Journal of American College Health,* Vol. 54, No. 1, July–August 2005, p. 31.
18. Escoffery, Cam, et al. "Internet Use for Health Information Among College Students." *Journal of American College Health,* Vol. 53, No. 4, January–February 2005, p. 183.
19. Yoon, Paula. Personal interview.
20. "Health Disparities Experienced by Black or African Americans—United States." *Morbidity and Mortality Weekly Report,* Vol. 54, No. 1, January 14, 2005, p. 1(3).
21. Tashiro, Cathy. "The Meaning of Race in Health Care and Research—Part 1: The Impact of History." *Pediatric Nursing,* Vol. 31, No. 3, May–June 2005, p. 208(3).
22. "Health Disparities Experienced by Black or African Americans—United States."
23. Tashiro, "The Meaning of Race in Health Care and Research."
24. National Eye Institute, Press release, *U.S. Latinos Have High Rates of Eye Disease and Visual Impairment,* www.nei.nih.gov/latinoeyestudy/.
25. "Treatments, Outcomes Differ Widely Among Women of Different Races, Ethnicities." *Women's Health Weekly,* February 13, 2003, p. 14.
26. "Cancer Facts for Minorities in the United States." National Center for Chronic Disease Prevention and Health Promotion, www.cdc.gov/cancer/minorityawareness.htm.
27. Jha, Ashish, et al. "Racial Trends in the Use of Major Procedures among the Elderly." *New England Journal of Medicine,* Vol. 353, No. 7, August 18, 2005, pp. 683–691.

Chapter 2

1. Prochaska, James, et al. *Changing for Good.* New York: Quill, 1994.
2. Armitage, C. J., et al. "Stages of Change or Changes of Stage? Predicting Transitions in Transtheoretical Model Stages in Relation to Healthy Food Choice." *Journal of Consulting Clinical Psychology,* Vol. 72, No. 3, June 2004, p. 491.
3. DiClemente, C. C., et al. "Readiness and Stages of Change in Addiction Treatment." *American Journal of Addiction,* Vol. 13, No. 2, March–April 2004, pp. 103–119.
4. van Sluijs, E. M., et al. "Stage-based Lifestyle Interventions in Primary Care: Are They Effective?" *American Journal of Preventive Medicine,* Vol. 26, No. 4, May 2004, p. 330.
5. Dalton, C. C., and L. N. Gottlieb. "The Concept of Readiness to Change." *Journal of Advances in Nursing,* Vol. 42, No. 2, April 2003, pp. 108–117.
6. Jacobs, A. D., et al. "Effects of a Tailored Follow-up Intervention on Health Behaviors, Beliefs, and Attitudes." *Journal of Women's Health,* Vol. 13, No. 4, June 2004. p. 557.
7. Prokhorov, A., et al. "Self-Reported Health Status, Health Vulnerability, and Smoking Behavior in College Students: Implications for Intervention." *Nicotine and Tobacco Research,* Vol. 5, No. 4, August 2003, p. 545.
8. Steinman, K. J. "College Students' Early Cessation from Episodic Heavy Drinking: Prevalence and Correlates." *Journal of American College Health,* Vol. 51, No. 5, March 2003, p. 197.
9. Seligman, Martin. Personal interview.
10. Fadiman, James. Personal interview.
11. "More Than Good Intentions: Realistic Goals Help You Lose Weight

and Get Fit." *Healthy Women,* January 2005.

12. Christian, Kenneth W. Personal interview.

13. Eisenberg, M., and H. Wechsler. "Substance Use Behaviors Among College Students with Same-Sex and Opposite-Sex Experience: Results from a National Study." *Addictive Behaviors,* Vol. 28, No. 6, 2003, p. 899.

14. Yacoubian, George, et al. "Correlates of Ecstasy Use Among Students Surveyed Through the 1997 College Alcohol Study." *Journal of Drug Education,* Vol. 33, No. 1, January 2003, p. 61.

15. Mayers, L. B., et al. "Tattooing and Body Piercing." *Pediatrics,* Vol. 111, May 2003, p. 1126.

Chapter 3

1. Kessler, Ronald, et al. "Lifetime Prevalence and Age-of-Onset Distributions of *DSM-IV* Disorders in the National Comorbidity Survey Replication." *Archives of General Psychiatry,* Vol. 62, No. 6, June 2005, p. 593.

2. Wang, Philip, et al. "Failure and Delay in Initial Treatment Contact After First Onset of Mental Disorders in the National Comorbidity Survey Replication." *Archives of General Psychiatry,* Vol. 62, No. 6, June 2005, p. 603.

3. Shapiro, Deane, and Roger Walsh. *Beyond Health and Normalcy.* New York: Van Nostrand Reinhold, 1983.

4. Satcher, David. "Executive Summary: A Report of the Surgeon General on Mental Health." *Public Health Reports,* Vol. 115, No. 1, January 2000.

5. Russinova, Zlaytka, et al. "Use of Alternative Health Care Practices by Persons with Serious Mental Illness: Perceived Benefits." *American Journal of Public Health,* Vol. 92, March 2003, p. 1600.

6. Bradberry, Travis, and Jean Greaves. *The Emotional Intelligence Quickbook.* New York: Fireside Books, 2005.

7. Mayer, John. Personal interview.

8. Seligman, Martin. *Authentic Happiness.* New York: Free Press, 2002.

9. Robins, Richard, and Jennifer Beer. "Positive Illusions about the Self: Short-term Benefits and Long-term Costs." *Journal of Personality & Social Psychology,* Vol. 80, No. 2, February 2001, p. 340.

10. Seligman, *Authentic Happiness.*

11. Flora, Carlin. "Happy Hour." *Psychology Today,* Vol. 38, No. 1, January–February 2005, p. 40.

12. Lucas, R. F., et al. "Reexamining Adaptation and the Set Point Model of Happiness: Reactions to Changes in Marital Status." *Journal of Personality and Social Psychology,* Vol. 84, No. 3, March 2003, p. 527.

13. Seligman, *Authentic Happiness.*

14. Flora, "Happy Hour."

15. Levy, B. C. E., et al. "Longitudinal Benefit of Positive Self-Perceptions of Aging on Functional Health." *Journals of Gerontology. Series B Psychological Sciences and Social Sciences.* Vol. 57, No. 5, September 2002, pp. 409–417.

16. Larsen, Randy. Personal interview.

17. Ornish, Dean. *Love & Survival: The Scientific Basis for the Healing Power of Intimacy.* New York: HarperCollins, 1999.

18. Hales, Dianne. "Can Prayer Really Heal?" *Parade,* March 23, 2003, p. 4.

19. Storch, Eric, et al. "Religiosity and Depression in Intercollegiate Athletes." *College Student Journal,* Vol. 36, No. 4, December 2002, p. 526.

20. Koenig, Harold. Personal interview.

21. McCaffrey A. M., et al. "Prayer for Health Concerns: Results of a National Survey on Prevalence and Patterns of Use." *Archives of Internal Medicine,* Vol. 164, No. 8, April 26, 2004, pp. 858–862.

22. Johnson, M. R., "Faith, Prayer, and Religious Observance." *Clinical Cornerstone,* Vol. 6, No. 1, 2004, p. 17.

23. Krucoff, Mitchell, et al. "Music, Imagery, Touch, and Prayer as Adjuncts to Interventional Cardiac Care: The Monitoring and Actualisation of Noetic Trainings (MANTRA) II Randomised Study." *Lancet,* Vol. 366, July 15, 2005, pp. 211–217.

24. McCullough, Michael. Personal interview.

25. Hale, Cara, et al. "Social Support and Physical Health: The Importance of Belonging." *Journal of American College Health,* Vol. 53, No. 6, May–June 2005, p. 276.

26. Hermann, Karen, and Nancy Betz. "Path Models of the Relationships of Instrumentality and Expressiveness to Social Self-Efficacy, Shyness, and Depressive Symptoms." *Sex Roles: A Journal of Research,* Vol. 51, No. 1–2, July 2004, pp. 55(12).

27. Ibid.

28. Kamdar, B. B., et al. "The Impact of Extended Sleep on Daytime Alertness, Vigilance and Mood." *Sleep Medicine,* Vol. 5, No. 5, September 2004, p. 441.

29. Vorona, R. D., et al. "Overweight and Obese Patients in a Primary Care Population Report Less Sleep than Patients with a Normal Body Mass Index." *Archives of Internal Medicine,* Vol. 165, No. 1, January 10, 2005, p. 25.

30. "Wake Up Call for Better Sleep." *Harvard Health Letter,* August 2004.

31. Lambert, Craig. "Deep into Sleep." *Harvard Magazine,* July–August 2005, p. 25.

32. Lambert, Craig. "Unsound Sleep." *Harvard Magazine,* July–August 2005, p. 25.

33. *National Institutes of Health State-of-the-Science Conference Statement: Manifestations and Management of Chronic Insomnia in Adults.* Bethesda, MD: NIH, 2005.

34. "Wake Up Call for Better Sleep."

35. Kelly, William. "Sleep-Length and Life Satisfaction in a College Student Sample." *College Student Journal,* Vol. 38, No. 3, September 2004, p. 428(3).

36. Howell, A. J., et al. "Sleep Quality, Sleep Propensity and Academic Performance." *Perception and Motor Skills,* Vol. 99, No. 2, October 2004, p. 525.

37. Millman, Richard. "Excessive Sleepiness in Adolescents and Young Adults: Causes, Consequences, and Treatment Strategies." *Pediatrics,* Vol. 115, No. 6, June 2005, p. 774.

38. Lambert, "Deep into Sleep."

39. Kobau, R., et al. "Sad, Blue, or Depressed Days, Health Behaviors and Health-Related Quality of Life, Behavioral Risk Factor Surveillance System, 1995–2000." *Health Quality of Life Outcomes.* Vol. 2, No. 1, p. 40, July 30, 2004.

40. *Diagnostic & Statistical Manual IV TR*(electronic). Washington, DC:

American Psychiatric Publishing, 2003.

41. Kessler, "Lifetime Prevalence and Age-of-Onset Distributions of *DSM-IV* Disorders in the National Comorbidity Survey Replication."

42. Insel, Thomas, and Wayne S. Fenton. "Psychiatric Epidemiology: It's Not Just About Counting Anymore." *Archives of General Psychiatry,* Vol. 62, No. 6, June 2005, p. 590.

43. Wang, "Failure and Delay in Initial Treatment Contact After First Onset of Mental Disorders in the National Comorbidity Survey Replication."

44. Kessler, Ronald, et al. "Prevalence, Severity, and Comorbidity of 12-Month *DSM-IV* Disorders in the National Comorbidity Survey Replication." *Archives of General Psychiatry,* Vol. 62, No. 6, June 2005, p. 617.

45. Jonas, B. S., and A. C. Looker. "More College Students Seeking MH Services." *Mental Health Weekly,* Vol. 14, No. 13, March 29, 2004, p. 7(1).

46. American College Health Association. "The American College Health Association National College Health Assessment (ACHA-NCHA), Spring 2003 Reference Group Report." *Journal of American College Health,* Vol. 53, No. 5, March–April 2005, p. 199.

47. Voelker, Rebecca. "Stress, Sleep Loss, and Substance Abuse Create Potent Recipe for College Depression." *Journal of the American Medical Association,* Vol. 291, No. 18, May 12, 2004, p. 2177.

48. Benton, Sherry, et al. "Changes in Counseling Center Client Problems Across 13 Years." *Professional Psychology: Research and Practice,* Vol. 34, No. 1, January 2003, p. 66.

49. Bray, Steven, and Heidi Born. "Transition to University and Vigorous Physical Activity: Implications for Health and Psychological Well-Being." *Journal of American College Health,* Vol. 52, No. 4, January–February 2004. p. 181.

50. Wart, Paula. "Why Be Happy?" *Health Plus,* Vanderbilt University, January 3, 2005.

51. "Mounting Evidence Indicates Heart Disease Link." *Medical Letter on the CDC & FDA,* July 21, 2002, p. 14.

52. Johns Hopkins University Evidence-Based Practice Center. *Post-Myocardial Infarction Depression.* Rockville, MD: Agency for Healthcare Research and Quality, May 2005.

53. Mussolino, M. E., et al. "Depression and Bone Mineral Density in Young Adults: Results from NHANES III." *Psychosomatic Medicine,* Vol. 66, No. 4, July–August 2004, pp. 533–537.

54. Tucker, Miriam. "History of Depression Predicts Physical Problems in Women: Current Depression Not Required." *Family Practice News,* Vol. 34, No. 12, June 15, 2004, p. 46(1).

55. Miller, Michael Craig. "Is Exercise a Good Treatment for Depression?" HEALTHBeat, July 6, 2005, www.health.harvard.edu/mental.

56. Turner, R. J., and D. A. Lloyd. "Stress Burden and the Lifetime Incidence of Psychiatric Disorder in Young Adults: Racial and Ethnic Contrasts." *Archives of General Psychiatry,* Vol. 61, No. 5, May 2004, p. 481.

57. "Depression Is Up for College Students." *Getting Paid in Behavioral Healthcare,* Vol. 10, No. 5, May 2005, p. 7.

58. Tija, Jennifer, et al. "Factors Associated with Undertreatment of Medical Student Depression." *Journal of American College Health,* Vol. 53, No. 5, March–April 2005, p. 219.

59. Jensen, Peter. Personal interview.

60. Spence, S. H., et al. "Mother's Depression in Early Childhood Increases the Risk of Adolescent Anxiety and Depression." *Evidence-Based Mental Health,* Vol. 6, No. 1, February 2003, p. 15.

61. Lenz, Brenda. "Tobacco, Depression, and Lifestyle Choices in the Pivotal Early College Years." *Journal of American College Health,* Vol. 52, No. 5, March–April 2004, p. 213.

62. McChargue, Dennis, et al. "Attachment and Depression Differentially Influence Nicotine Dependence among Male and Female Undergraduates: A Preliminary Study." *Journal of American College Health,* Vol. 53, No. 1, July–August 2004, p. 5.

63. Andreasen, Nancy. "Vulnerability to Mental Illnesses: Gender Makes a Difference, and So Does Provid-ing Good Psychiatric Care." *American Journal of Psychiatry,* Vol. 162, No. 2, February 2005, p. 211.

64. Kendler, Kenneth, et al. "Sex Differences in the Relationship between Social Support and Risk for Major Depression: A Longitudinal Study of Opposite-Sex Twin Pairs." *American Journal of Psychiatry,* Vol. 162, No. 2, February 2005, p. 250.

65. Schatzberg, Alan, et al. "Medication (Nefazodone) or Psychotherapy (CBASP) Is Effective When the Other Is Not." *Archives of General Psychiatry,* Vol. 62, No. 6, June 2005, p. 513.

66. Greden, John. Personal interview.

67. "What Are the Real Risks of Antidepressants?" *Harvard Mental Health Letter,* Vol. 21, No. 11, May 2005.

68. "FDA Reviews Data for Antidepressant Use in Adults." *FDA Talk Paper,* July 1, 2005.

69. "What Are the Real Risks of Antidepressants?"

70. Kennedy, Noel, et al. "Gender Differences in Incidence and Age at Onset of Mania and Bipolar Disorder over a 35-Year Period in Camberwell, England." *American Journal of Psychiatry,* Vol. 162, No. 2, February 2005, p. 257.

71. *Coping with Anxiety and Phobias.* Cambridge, MA: Harvard Health Publications, 2005.

72. Ibid.

73. Cropper, Carol. "The Lingering Legacies of ADHD." *BusinessWeek Online,* May 27, 2005.

74. Sherman, Carl. "Adult ADHD: Drug Choice Includes Timing Issues." *Clinical Psychiatry News,* Vol. 33, No. 6, June 2005, p. 22.

75. Ibid.

76. Wolraich, Mark, et al. "Attention-Deficit/Hyperactivity Disorder Among Adolescents: A Review of the Diagnosis, Treatment, and Clinical Implications." *Pediatrics,* Vol. 115, No. 6, June 2005, p. 1734.

77. Teter, Christian, et al. "Prevalence and Motives for Illicit Use of Prescription Stimulants in an Undergraduate Student Sample." *Journal of American College Health,* Vol. 53, No. 6, May–June 2005, p. 253.

78. Treatment for Adolescents with Depression (TADS) Team. "Fluoxe-

tine, Cognitive-Behavioral Therapy, and Their Combination for Adolescents with Depression." *Journal of the American Medical Association,* Vol. 292, No. 7, July 28, 2004, p. 861.

79. Wilburn, Victor, and Delores Smith. "Stress, Self-Esteem, and Suicidal Ideation in Late Adolescents." *Adolescence,* Vol. 40, No. 157, Spring 2005, p. 33.

80. Gould, Madelyn. Personal interview.

81. Horton, Leslie. "Social, Cultural and Demographic Factors in Suicide." In Simon, Robert and Robert Hales (eds.), *Textbook of Suicide Assessment and Prevention.* Washington, DC: American Psychiatric Press (in press).

82. Webster, D. W., et al. "Association Between Youth-Focused Firearm Laws and Youth Suicides." *Journal of the American Medical Association,* Vol. 292, No. 5, August 4, 2004, p. 594.

83. Jick, Hershel, et al. "Antidepressants and the Risk of Suicidal Behaviors." *Journal of the American Medical Association,* Vol. 292, No. 3, July 21, 2004, p. 339.

84. Kessler et al., "Prevalence, Severity, and Comorbidity of 12-Month *DSM-IV* Disorders in the National Comorbidity Survey Replication."

85. Frankenberger, Kristi, et al. "Effects of Information on College Students' Perceptions of Antidepressant Medication." *Journal of American College Health,* Vol. 53, No. 1, July–August 2004, p. 35.

86. Walsh, Nancy. "St. John's Wort for Depression." *Family Practice News,* Vol. 33, No. 1, January 1, 2003, p. 25.

Chapter 4

1. Segerstrom, Suzanne, and Gregory E. Miller, "Psychological Stress and the Human Immune System: A Meta-Analytic Study of 30 Years of Inquiry." *Psychological Bulletin,* Vol. 130, No. 4, July 2004, p. 601.

2. Lazarus, R., and R. Launier. "Stress-Related Transactions Between Person and Environment." In *Perspectives in Interactional Psychology.* New York: Plenum, 1978.

3. Young, D. R., et al. "Health Status Among Urban African American Women: Associations Among Well-Being, Perceived Stress, and Demographic Factors." *Journal of Behavioral Medicine,* Vol. 27, No. 1, February 2004, p. 63.

4. Bovier, P. A., et al. "Perceived Stress, Internal Resources, and Social Support as Determinants of Mental Health Among Young Adults." *Quality of Life Research,* Vol. 13, No. 7, February 2004, p. 161.

5. Epel, Elisa, et al. "Accelerated Telomere: Shortening in Response to Life Stress." *Proceedings of the National Academy of Sciences,* Vol. 101, No. 49, December 7, 2004, p. 17312.

6. "Stress Takes the Edge Off." *Harvard Mental Health Letter,* May 2005.

7. Schmeelk-Cone, K. H., et al. "The Buffering Effects of Active Coping on the Relationship Between SES and Cortisol Among African American Young Adults." *Behavioral Medicine,* Vol. 29, No. 2, Summer 2003, p. 85.

8. Dickerson, Sally, and Margaret Kemeny. "Acute Stressors and Cortisol Responses: A Theoretical Integration and Synthesis of Laboratory Research." *Psychological Bulletin,* Vol. 130, No. 3, May 2004, p. 355.

9. Ketterer, Mark. "Stressed Out Men May Have Inherited Risk for Early Heart Disease." Presentation, American Psychosomatic Society, March 2003.

10. Matthews, Karen, et al. "Blood Pressure Reactivity to Psychological Stress Predicts Hypertension in the CARDIA Study." *Circulation,* Vol. 110, No. 1, July 6, 2004, p. 74.

11. "Stress and the Heart." *Harvard Men's Health Watch,* February 2005.

12. Ibid.

13. Wittstein, llan, et al. "Neurohumoral Features of Myocardial Stunning Due to Sudden Emotional Stress." *New England Journal of Medicine,* Vol. 352, No. 6, February 10, 2005, p. 539–548.

14. Segerstrom and Miller, "Psychological Stress and the Human Immune System."

15. Freeman, L. M., and K. M. Gil. "Daily Stress, Coping, and Dietary Restraint in Binge Eating." *International Journal of Eating Disorders,* Vol. 36, No. 2, September 2004, p. 204.

16. Sax, Linda, et al. *The American Freshman: National Norms for Fall 2004.* Los Angeles, CA: University of California, Los Angeles Higher Education Research Institute, December 2004.

17. "Stressed Out: A New Study Explains Why Female Professors Have Added Stress." *University Business,* Vol. 8, No. 4, April 2005, p. 26.

18. Park, Crystal, et al. "The Daily Stress and Coping Process and Alcohol Use Among College Students." *Journal of Studies on Alcohol,* Vol. 65, No. 1, January 2004, p. 126.

19. "In Case You Haven't Heard. . . ." *Mental Health Weekly,* Vol. 15, No. 3, January 17, 2004, p. 8.

20. Rosenthal, Beth Spenciner, and Arleen Cedeno Schreiner. "Prevalence of Psychological Symptoms Among Undergraduate Students in an Ethnically Diverse Urban Public College." *Journal of American College Health,* Vol. 49, No. 1, July 2000.

21. Ibid.

22. Sax, et al., *The American Freshman: National Norms for Fall 2004.*

23. Evans, Sybil. Personal interview.

24. Bushman, Brad. Personal interview.

25. Hall, Cathy, et al. "Motivational and Attitudinal Factors in College Students With and Without Learning Disabilities." *Learning Disability Quarterly,* Vol. 25, No. 1, Spring 2002, p. 79.

26. Spalding, T. W., et al. "Aerobic Exercise Training and Cardiovascular Reactivity to Psychological Stress in Sedentary Young Normotensive Men and Women." *Psychophysiology,* Vol. 41, No. 4, July 2004, p. 552.

27. "Three for 2003: Reducing the Burden of Stress." *Harvard Women's Health Watch,* Vol. 10, No. 5, January 2003, p. 1.

28. Wilburn, Victor, and Delores Smith. "Stress, Self-esteem, and Suicidal Ideation in Late Adolescents." *Adolescence,* Vol. 40, No. 157, Spring 2005, p. 33.

29. Foley, Kevin. "PTSD in African Americans." *Clinical Psychiatry News,* Vol. 33, No. 4, April 2005, p. 20.

30. McLean, L. M., and R. Gallop.

"Implications of Childhood Sexual Abuse for Adult Borderline Personality Disorder and Complex Posttraumatic Stress Disorder." *American Journal of Psychiatry,* Vol. 160, No. 2, February 2003, p. 369.

31. Duncan, Renae. "Childhood Maltreatment and College Drop-out Rates: Implications for Child Abuse Researchers." *Journal of Interpersonal Violence,* Vol. 15, No. 9, September 2000, p. 987.

Chapter 5

1. Suminski, Richard, et al. "Physical Activity Among Ethnically Diverse College Students." *Journal of American College Health,* Vol. 51, September 2002, p. 75.

2. "Biology Shows Women and Men Are Different." *Mayo Clinic Women's Healthsource,* September 2002.

3. Lavie, C., et al. "Exercise Capacity in Adult African-Americans Referred for Exercise Stress Testing: Is Fitness Affected by Race?" *Chest,* Vol. 126, No. 6, December 2004, pp. 1962–1968.

4. Hunter, G. R., et al. "Aerobic Fitness, Physiologic Difficulty and Physical Activity in Black and White Women." *International Journal of Obesity and Related Metabolic Disorders,* Vol. 28, No. 9, September 2004, pp. 1111–1117.

5. "A Report of the Surgeon General: Physical Activity and Health, Adults." 2004, USDHHS, CDC, President's Council on Physical Fitness and Sports, http://fitness.gov/adults.pdf.

6. Mokdad, A., et al. "Actual Causes of Death in the United States, 2004." *Journal of the American Medical Association,* Vol. 291, 2004, p. 1238.

7. Wallace, Lorraine, et al. "Promoting Physical Activity in the Family Practice Setting." *American Family Physician,* Vol. 67, No. 6, March 15, 2003, p. 1196.

8. Racette, Susan, et al. "Weight Changes, Exercise, and Dietary Patterns During Freshman and Sophomore Years of College." *Journal of American College Health,* Vol. 53, No. 6, May–June 2005, p. 245.

9. American College Health Association. "The American College Health Association National College Health Assessment (ACHA-NCHA) Spring 2003 Reference Group Report." *Journal of American College Health,* Vol. 53, No. 5, March–April 2005, p. 199.

10. Buckworth, Janet, and Claudio Nigg. "Physical Activity, Exercise, and Sedentary Behavior in College Students." *Journal of American College Health,* Vol. 53, No. 1, July–August 2004, p. 28.

11. Suminski, "Physical Activity Among Ethnically Diverse College Students."

12. Mack, Mick, et al. "Changes in Short-term Attitudes Toward Physical Activity and Exercise of University Personal Wellness Students." *College Student Journal,* Vol. 38, No. 4, December 2004, p. 587.

13. Reed, Julian, and D. Allen Phillips. "Relationship between Physical Activity and the Proximity of Exercise Facilities and Home Exercise Equipment Used by Undergraduate University Students." *Journal of American College Health,* Vol. 53, No. 6, May–June 2005, p. 285.

14. Mack et al., "Changes in Short-Term Attitudes Toward Physical Activity and Exercise of University Personal Wellness Students."

15. DeVahl, Julie, et al. "Academic Incentives for Students Can Increase Participation in and Effectiveness of a Physical Activity Program." *Journal of American College Health,* Vol. 53, No. 6, May–June 2005, p. 295.

16. Sparling, Phillip, and Teresa Snow. "Physical Activity Patterns in Recent College Alumni." *Research Quarterly for Exercise and Sport,* Vol. 73, No. 2, June 2002, p. 200.

17. "Poor Fitness in Young Adults Associated with Later Cardiovascular Problems." *FDA Consumer,* Vol. 38, No. 1, January–February 2004, p. 7.

18. Thomas, D. Q., et al. "Physiologic Profile of the Fitness Status of Collegiate Cheerleaders." *Journal of Strength Conditioning Research,* Vol. 18, No. 2, May 2004, p. 252.

19. Hussey, J. M., et al. "Physical Activity Behavior and Knowledge of Effects of Physical Activity and Exercise Recommendations among University Students." *Journal of Sports Sciences,* Vol. 22, No. 3, March 2004, p. 282.

20. Bauman, A. E., et al. "Updating the Evidence That Physical Activity Is Good for Health: An Epidemiological Review 2000–2003." *Journal of the Science of Medicine and Sport,* Vol. 7, No. 1 (Suppl.), April 2004, pp. 6–19.

21. Aronson, D., et al. "C-Reactive Protein Is Inversely Related to Physical Fitness in Middle-aged Subjects." *Atherosclerosis,* Vol. 176, No. 1, September 2004, pp. 173–179.

22. Katzmarzyk, P. T., et al. "Cardiorespiratory Fitness Attenuates the Effects of the Metabolic Syndrome on All-cause and Cardiovascular Disease Mortality in Men." *Archives of Internal Medicine,* Vol. 164, No. 10, May 24, 2004, p. 1092.

23. Ortlepp, J. R., et al. "Relationship Between Physical Fitness and Lifestyle Behaviour in Healthy Young Men." *European Journal of Cardiovascular Prevention and Rehabilitation,* Vol. 11, No. 3, June 2004, p. 192.

24. Bauman, "Updating the Evidence That Physical Activity Is Good for Health."

25. Holmes, M. D., et al. "Physical Activity and Survival after Breast Cancer Diagnosis." *Journal of the American Medical Association,* Vol. 293, No. 20, May 25, 2005, p. 2479.

26. Stevens, J., et al. "Fitness and Fatness as Predictors of Mortality From All Causes and From Cardiovascular Disease in Men and Women in the Lipid Research Clinics Study." *American Journal of Epidemiology,* Vol. 156, No. 9, November 1, 2002, p. 832.

27. Bauman, "Updating the Evidence That Physical Activity Is Good for Health."

28. Sigal, Ronald, et al. "Physical Activity/Exercise and Type 2 Diabetes." *Diabetes Spectrum,* Vol. 18, No. 2, Spring 2005, p. 88.

29. Miller, Michael Craig. "Is Exercise A Good Treatment for Depression?" HEALTHBeat, July 6, 2005, www.health.harvard.edu/mental.

30. van Gelder, B. M., et al. "Physical Activity in Relation to Cognitive Decline in Elderly Men: The FINE Study." *Neurology,* Vol. 63, No. 12,

December 28, 2004, pp. 2316–2321.

31. Colcombe, S. J., et al. "Neurocognitive, Aging and Cardiovascular Fitness: Recent Findings and Future Directions." *Journal of Molecular Neuroscience,* Vol. 24, No. 1, 2004, pp. 9–14.

32. Podewils, L. J., et al. "Physical Activity, APOE Genotype, and Dementia Risk: Findings from the Cardiovascular Health Cognition Study." *American Journal of Epidemiology,* Vol. 161, No. 7, April 2005, p. 639.

33. "Keys to Healthy Bones: A New Surgeon General's Report Warns of a Coming Osteoporosis Crisis." *Tufts University Health & Nutrition Letter,* Vol. 22, No. 11, January 2005, p. 4.

34. Ford, M. A., et al. "Past and Recent Physical Activity and Bone Mineral Density in College-aged Women." *Journal of Strength and Conditioning Research,* Vol. 18, No. 3, August 2004, p. 405.

35. "Step Up to Denser Bones." *Science News,* Vol. 167, No. 17, April 23, 2005, p. 270.

36. "Physical Activity for Lifelong Bone Health: The American College of Sports Medicine Promotes Osteoporosis Prevention." *Journal of Musculoskeletal Medicine,* Vol. 22, No. 1, January 2005, p. 6.

37. Mayo, M. J., et al. "Exercise-Induced Weight Loss Preferentially Reduces Abdominal Fat." *Medicine and Science in Sports and Exercise,* Vol. 35, No. 2, 2003, pp. 207–213.

38. Penhollow, Tina, and Michael Young. "Sexual Desirability and Sexual Performance: Does Exercise and Fitness Really Matter?" *Electronic Journal of Human Sexuality,* Vol. 7, October 5, 2004, www.ejhs.org.

39. Molaison, E. F. "Linking Decisional Balance to Participation in Physical Activity in College Students." *Journal of the American Dietetic Association,* Vol. 104, No. 8, August 2004, p. A57(1).

40. Yu, S., et al. "What Level of Physical Activity Protects Against Premature Cardiovascular Death? The Caerphilly Study." *Heart,* Vol. 89, April 2003, p. 502.

41. *Dietary Guidelines for Americans 2005,* U.S. Department of Health and Human Services (USDHHS), U.S. Department of Agriculture (USDA), www.healthierus.gov/dietaryguidelines.

42. Mayo Clinic staff. "Fitness Myths: Separate Fact from Fiction," www.mayoclinic.com.

43. Wessel, Timothy, et al. "Relationship of Physical Fitness vs. Body Mass Index with Coronary Artery Disease and Cardiovascular Events in Women." *Journal of the American Medical Association,* Vol. 292, No. 10, September 8, 2004, p. 1179.

44. Weinstein, Amy, et al. "Relationship of Physical Activity vs. Body Mass Index with Type 2 Diabetes in Women." *Journal of the American Medical Association,* Vol. 292, No. 10, September 8, 2004, p. 1188.

45. Blair, S. N., et al. "The Evolution of Physical Activity Recommendations: How Much is Enough?" *American Journal of Clinical Nutrition,* Vol. 79, No. 5, May 2004, p. 913S.

46. *Dietary Guidelines for Americans 2005,* USDHHS, USDA.

47. Janol, Jeffrey. "Comparing Intensity-Monitoring Methods: What Are the Most Effective Ways to Control Exercise Intensity?" *IDEA Fitness Journal,* Vol. 2, No. 4, April 2005, p. 38.

48. "Variety of Preparticipation Activities, Not Just Stretching, Recommended to Prevent Injuries in Sports." *American College of Sports Medicine,* News Release, March 3, 2004.

49. Bauman, A. E. "Updating the Evidence that Physical Activity is Good for Health." *Journal of Science and Medicine in Sport,* Vol. 7, No. 1 (Suppl.), April 2004, p. 6.

50. Lange, R. M., and M. A. Nies. "Benefits of Walking for Obese Women in the Prevention of Bone and Joint Disorders." *Orthopedic Nursing,* Vol. 23, No. 3, May–June 2004, p. 211.

51. "College Students Walk Less than Younger Children." American College of Sports Medicine, News Release, June 2, 2004.

52. "Number of Daily Steps Impacts Obesity Factors in Women." American College of Sports Medicine, News Release, May 5, 2004.

53. "Pedometer-Based Walking Programs Can Help Achieve Physical Activity Recommendations." American College of Sports Medicine, News Release, January 12, 2004.

54. "Women with Pedometers Step Up Exercise Levels." American College of Sports Medicine, News Release, April 5, 2005.

55. "Spin it." *Fit Facts,* American Council on Exercise, www.acefitness.org.

56. "Kick Your Way to Fitness." *Fit Facts,* American Council on Exercise, www.acefitness.org.

57. Molaison, "Linking Decisional Balance to Participation in Physical Activity in College Students."

58. Harne, Amanda, and Walter Bixby. "The Benefits of and Barriers to Strength Training Among College-Age Women." *Journal of Sport Behavior,* Vol. 28, No. 2, June 2005, p. 151.

59. Ormsbee, Michael, and Matt Vukovich. "Performance-Enhancing Drugs: Who's Taking Them, and What Are the Benefits and Risks?" *IDEA Fitness Journal,* Vol. 2, No. 5, May 2005, p. 60.

60. "The Truth About Steroids." *Fit Facts,* American Council on Exercise, www.acefitness.org.

61. Adams, Jacqueline. "The Incredible Bulk." *Science World,* Vol. 61, No. 12, March 28, 2005, p. 18.

62. Mayo Clinic staff. "Performance-Enhancing Drugs: Dangerous, Damaging, and Potentially Deadly." www.mayoclinic.com.

63. Ibid.

64. Schilling, Brian, et al. "Creatine Supplementation and Health Variables: A Retrospective Study." *Medicine and Science in Sports and Exercise,* Vol. 33, No. 2, February 2001, p. 183.

65. Keller, Joy. "Does Stretching Improve Performance?" *IDEA Fitness Journal,* Vol. 2, No. 1, January 2005, p. 16.

66. Cannavan, D., and A. J. Blazevich. "The Acute Effects of Stretching on Athletic Performance Indicators." *Journal of Sports Sciences,* Vol. 23, No. 2, February 2005, p. 107.

67. Nelson, Arnold, et al. "Acute Effects of Passive Muscle Stretching

on Sprint Performance." *Journal of Sports Sciences,* Vol. 23, No. 5, May 2005, p. 449.

68. Keller, "Does Stretching Improve Performance?"

69. "Yoga Becomes Big Business." *Sporting Good Business,* Vol. 38, No. 3, March 2005, p. 16.

70. McCall, Timothy, "Count on Yoga." *Yoga Journal,* January–February 2005, p. 96.

71. "Pilates Research Offers New Information on Popular Technique." News Release, American College of Sports Medicine, March 30, 2005.

72. "Tai Chi Training Improves Balance Control in Elderly." News Release, American College of Sports Medicine, April 5, 2004.

73. Cutts, Steven. "Back Pain—and Its Management." *Practice Nurse,* December 17, 2004, p. 38(5).

74. Malanga, Gerard, and Robin Dennis. "Treatment of Acute Low Back Pain: Use of Medications: Reduction and Control of Pain and Return of Function Are the Goals." *The Journal of Musculoskeletal Medicine,* Vol. 22, No. 2, February 2005, p. 79.

75. Hu, F. B., et al. "Adiposity as Compared with Physical Activity in Predicting Mortality Among Women." *New England Journal of Medicine,* Vol. 351, No. 26, December 23, 2004, pp. 2694–2703.

76. "Hydration Tips for Runners: American College of Sports Medicine Clarifies Balancing of Fluid Loss/Intake." *Journal of Musculoskeletal Medicine,* Vol. 22, No. 6, June 2005, p. 320.

77. Williams, M. H. "Dietary Supplements and Sports Performance: Introduction and Vitamins." *Journal of the International Society of Sports Nutrition,* Vol. 1, No. 2, December 2004, pp. 1–6.

78. Williams, M. H. "Dietary Supplements and Sports Performance: Minerals." *Journal of the International Society of Sports Nutrition,* Vol. 2, No. 1, 2005, pp. 43–49.

79. "Energy Bars: Need a Prepackaged Pick-Me-Up? Here's How to Crack the Snack Bar Code." *Natural Health,* Vol. 35, No. 2, February 2005, p. 20.

80. Glazer, James. "Management of Heatstroke and Heat Exhaustion." *American Family Physician,* Vol. 71, No. 11, June 1, 2005, p. 2133.

81. Glazer, James. "Heat Exhaustion and Heatstroke: What You Should Know." *American Family Physician,* Vol. 71, No. 11, June 1, 2005, p. 2141.

82. White, K., et al. "EMG Power Spectra of Intercollegiate Athletes and Anterior Cruciate Ligament Injury Risk in Females." *Medicine and Science in Sports and Exercise,* Vol. 35, No. 3, 2003, pp. 371–376.

83. Fagenbaum, R., and W. G. Darling. "Jump Landing Strategies in Male and Female College Athletes and the Implications of Such Strategies for Anterior Cruciate Ligament Injury." *American Journal of Sports Medicine,* Vol. 31, No. 2, March–April 2003, p. 233.

84. Garman, F., et al. "Occurrence of Exercise Dependence in a College-Aged Population." *Journal of American College Health,* Vol. 52, No. 5, March–April 2004, p. 221.

Chapter 6

1. Panel on Micronutrients, Subcommittees on Upper Reference Levels of Nutrients and Interpretation and Uses of Dietary Reference Intakes, and the Standing Committee on the Scientific Evaluation of Dietary Reference Intakes. *Dietary Reference Intakes for Energy, Carbohydrates, Fiber, Fat, Protein and Amino Acids.* Washington, DC: National Academy of Sciences Press, 2002.

2. Grandjean, Ann, et al. "The Effect on Hydration of Two Diets, One with and One without Plain Water." *Journal of the American College of Nutrition,* Vol. 22, April 2003, p. 165.

3. Gross, Lee, et al. "Increased Consumption of Refined Carbohydrates and the Epidemic of Type 2 Diabetes in the United States: An Ecologic Assessment." *American Journal of Clinical Nutrition,* Vol. 79, 2004, pp. 774–779.

4. *Dietary Guidelines for Americans 2005,* U.S. Department of Health and Human Services (USDHHS), U.S. Department of Agriculture (USDA), www.healthierus.gov/dietaryguidelines.

5. Harder, B. "Wholesome Grains: Insulin Effects May Explain Healthful Diet." *Science News,* Vol. 161, No. 20, May 18, 2002, p. 308.

6. University of Sydney, Australia, Glycemic Index Testing Service, Human Nutrition Unit, www.glycemicindex.com.

7. Mozaffarian, Dariush, et al. "Cereal, Fruit, and Vegetable Fiber Intake and the Risk of Cardiovascular Disease in Elderly Individuals." *Journal of the American Medical Association,* Vol. 289, No. 13, April 2, 2003, p. 1659.

8. Liu, Simin. "Whole-Grain Foods, Dietary Fiber, and Type 2 Diabetes: Searching for a Kernel of Truth." *American Journal of Clinical Nutrition,* Vol. 77, 2003, pp. 527–529.

9. Panel on Micronutrients, Subcommittees on Upper Reference Levels of Nutrients and Interpretation and Uses of Dietary Reference Intakes, and the Standing Committee on the Scientific Evaluation of Dietary Reference Intakes. *Dietary Reference Intakes for Energy, Carbohydrates, Fiber, Fat, Protein and Amino Acids.*

10. "Position of the American Dietetic Association: Health Implications of Dietary Fiber." *Journal of the American Dietetic Association,* Vol. 102, No. 7, July 2002, p. 993.

11. Erkkila, Arja, et al. "Fish Intake is Associated with a Reduced Progression of Coronary Artery Atherosclerosis in Postmenopausal Women with Coronary Artery Disease." *Journal of Clinical Nutrition,* Vol. 80, No. 3, September 2004, p. 626.

12. McKenna, Dolores, et al. "Intake of Omega-3 Polyunsaturated Fatty Acids Among College-Age Women." *Topics in Clinical Nutrition,* Vol. 19, No. 2, April–June 2004, p. 107(10).

13. Keys to Healthy Bones: A New Surgeon General's Report Warns of a Coming Osteoporosis Crisis. *Tufts University Health & Nutrition Letter,* Vol. 22, No. 11, January 2005, p. 4.

14. *Dietary Guidelines for Americans 2005,* USDHHS, USDA.

15. Zemel, Michael. "Role of Calcium and Dairy Products in Energy Partitioning and Weight Management." *American Journal of Clinical Nutri-*

tion, Vol. 79, No. 5, May 2004, p. 907S.

16. "African-American Health and Dairy Foods." *Journal of the American Dietetic Association,* Vol. 104, No. 3, March 2004, p. 500a.

17. "Read the Fine Print: Recent Calcium Supplement Studies." *Harvard Health Letter,* July 2005, p. 6.

18. Greer, Frank. "Bone Health: It's More than Calcium Intake." *Pediatrics,* Vol. 115, No. 3, March 2005, p. 792.

19. *Dietary Guidelines for Americans 2005,* USDHHS, USDA.

20. Keinan-Bok, Lital, et al. "Dietary Phytoestrogens and Breast Cancer Risk." *American Journal of Clinical Nutrition,* Vol. 79, 2004, p. 282.

21. I-Min, Lee, et al. "Vitamin E in the Primary Prevention of Cardiovascular Disease and Cancer." *Journal of the American Medical Association,* Vol. 294, No. 1, July 6, 2005, p. 56.

22. Redberg, Rita. "Vitamin E and Cardiovascular Health: Does Sex Matter?" *Journal of the American Medical Association,* Vol. 294, No. 1, July 6, 2005, p. 107.

23. Neff, Matthew. "Antioxidant Vitamin Supplements and Cardiovascular Disease Risk Reduction." *American Family Physician,* Vol. 71, No. 7, April 1, 2005, p. 1433.

24. "Vitamin E Gets an F." *Harvard Health Letter,* June 2005.

25. Jacobs, Eric, and Michael Thun. "Low-Dose Aspirin and Vitamin E: Challenges and Opportunities in Cancer Prevention." *Journal of the American Medical Association,* Vol. 294, No. 1, July 6, 2005, p. 105.

26. "America's New "Food Pyramid." *The Lancet,* Vol. 365, No. 9470, April 30, 2005, p. 1516.

27. Brooks, George, et al. "Chronicle of the Institute of Medicine Physical Activity Recommendation: How a Physical Activity Recommendation Came to Be Among Dietary Recommendations." *American Journal of Clinical Nutrition,* Vol. 79, No. 5, May 2004, p. 921S.

28. Djoussé, Luc, et al. "Fruit and Vegetable Consumption and LDL Cholesterol: The National Heart, Lung, and Blood Institute Family Heart Study." *American Journal of Clinical Nutrition,* Vol. 79, No. 2, February 2004, p. 213.

29. Slattery, Martha, et al. "Plant Foods, Fiber, and Rectal Cancer." *American Journal of Clinical Nutrition,* Vol. 79, No. 2, February 2004, p. 274.

30. Moorman, P. G., and P. D. Terry. "Consumption of Dairy Products and the Risk of Breast Cancer: A Review of the Literature." *American Journal of Clinical Nutrition,* Vol. 80, 2004, p. 5.

31. Schulze, M. B., et al. "Sugar-Sweetened Beverages, Weight Gain, and Incidence of Type 2 Diabetes in Young and Middle-Aged Women." *Journal of the American Medical Association,* Vol. 292, No. 8, August 25, 2004, p. 927.

32. "Rebuilding the Pyramid: The Government's New Food Pyramid Replaces 'One Size Fits All' with a Customizable Eating and Exercise Plan." *Tufts University Health & Nutrition Letter,* Vol. 23, No. 4, June 2005, p. 1.

33. Racette, Susan, et al. "Weight Changes, Exercise, and Dietary Patterns During Freshman and Sophomore Years of College." *Journal of American College Health,* Vol. 53, No. 6, 2005, p. 245.

34. Gray, L. E., et al. "Assessment of Dietary Fiber Intake Among University Students." *Journal of the American Dietetic Association,* Vol. 104, No. 8, August 2004, p. A26.

35. *Dietary Guidelines for Americans 2005,* USDHHS, USDA.

36. Conklin, Martha, et al. "College Students' Use of Point of Selection Nutrition Information." *Topics in Clinical Nutrition,* Vol. 20, No. 2, April–June 2005, p. 97(12).

37. "Going Nuts Over the Benefits of Healthy Snacks: Items Such as Trail Mix and Yogurt Are Finding Their Niche with Consumers." *DSN Retailing Today,* Vol. 44, No. 8, April 25, 2005, p. F4.

38. Lofshult, Diane. "More Natural Snacks." *IDEA Fitness Journal,* Vol. 2, No. 5, May 2005, p. 77.

39. *Dietary Guidelines for Americans 2005,* USDHHS, USDA.

40. Schlosser, Eric. *Fast Food Nation.* New York: Simon & Schuster, 2001.

41. Conklin, Martha, et al. "Nutrition Information at Point of Selection Could Benefit College Students." *Topics in Clinical Nutrition,* Vol. 20, No. 2, April–June 2005, p. 90(7).

42. Tanja, V. E. Kral, et al. "Combined Effects of Energy Density and Portion Size on Energy Intake in Women." *American Journal of Clinical Nutrition,* October 2004, Vol. 79, No. 6, p. 962.

43. "Future Ingredients and Challenges of Functional Products." *The Food Institute Report,* No. 17, May 2, 2005, p. 3.

44. Partnership for Food Safety, www.fightbac.org.

45. Crespo, J. F., and J. Rodriguez. "Food Allergy in Adulthood." *Allergy,* Vol. 58, March 2003, p. 98.

Chapter 7

1. Fontaine, K. R., et al. "Years of Life Lost Due to Obesity." *Journal of the American Medical Association,* Vol. 289, No. 2, April 9, 2003, p. 183.

2. Goel, Mita Sanghavi, et al. "Obesity Among U.S. Immigrant Subgroups by Duration of Residence." *Journal of the American Medical Association,* Vol. 292, No. 23, December 13, 2004, p. 2860.

3. "Global Strategy on Diet, Physical Activity and Health." World Health Organization, www.who.int/dietphysicalactivity/publications/facts/obesity/en/.

4. Wald, Nicholas, and Walter Willett. "Reversing the Obesity Epidemic." *Lancet,* Vol. 364, July 10, 2004, p. 1040.

5. American Obesity Association, www.obesity.org.

6. Goel et al. "Obesity Among U.S. Immigrant Subgroups by Duration of Residence."

7. *Preventing Childhood Obesity: Health in the Balance* (2005). Washington, DC: Institute of Medicine, 2005.

8. National Center for Health Statistics, www.hhs.gov.

9. Ludwig, David, and S. Gortmaker. "Programming Obesity in Childhood." *Lancet,* Vol. 364, No. 9430, July 17, 2004, p. 226.

10. "State Efforts to Control Obesity." University of Baltimore, www.ubalt.edu/experts/obesity/index.html.

11. Prince, J. R. "Why All the Fuss About Portion Size? Designing the

New American Plate." *Nutrition Today,* Vol. 39, No. 2, March 2004, p. 59.

12. Pereira, M. A., et al. "Fast-food Habits, Weight Gain, and Insulin Resistance (The CARDIA Study): 15-year Prospective Analysis." *Lancet,* Vol. 365, No. 9453, January 1, 2005, pp. 36–42.

13. Bray, Steven, and Heidi Born. "Transition to University and Vigorous Physical Activity: Implications for Health and Psychological Well-Being." *Journal of American College Health,* Vol. 52, No. 4, January–February 2004, p. 181.

14. Hu, Frank, et al. "Television Watching and Other Sedentary Behaviors in Relation to Risk of Obesity and Type 2 Diabetes Mellitus in Women." *Journal of American Medical Association,* Vol. 289, No. 14, April 9, 2003, p. 1785.

15. Pereira, Mark. Presentation, American Heart Association, Miami Beach, FL, February 2003.

16. Frank, L. D., et al. "Obesity Relationships with Community Design, Physical Activity, and Time Spent in Cars." *American Journal of Preventive Medicine,* Vol. 27, No. 2, August 2004, p. 87.

17. U.S. Department of Health and Human Services, Press Release, "Citing Dangerous Increase in Deaths, HHS Launches New Strategies Against Overweight Epidemic."

18. Whitaker, R. C. "Predicting Preschooler Obesity at Birth: The Role of Maternal Obesity in Early Pregnancy." *Pediatrics,* Vol. 114, No. 1, July 2004, p. 29.

19. Ludwig, David, and S. Gortmaker. "Programming Obesity in Childhood."

20. Elliott, M. A., et al. "Pediatric Obesity Prevention and Management." *Minerva Pediatrics,* Vol. 56, No. 3, June 2004, p. 265.

21. Delrue, M., and J. Michaud. "Fat Chance: Genetic Syndromes with Obesity." *Clinical Genetics,* Vol. 66, No. 2, August 2004, p. 83.

22. McLaren, L., and L. Gauvin. "The Cumulative Impact of Being Overweight on Women's Body Esteem: A Preliminary Study." *Eating and Weight Disorders,* Vol. 7, No. 4, December 2002, p. 324.

23. DiGioacchino, Rita, et al. "Body Dissatisfaction Among White and African American Male and Female College Students." *Eating Behaviors,* Vol. 2, December 2001, p. 39.

24. Davison, Tany, and Marita McCabe. "Relationships Between Men's and Women's Body Image and Their Psychological, Social, and Sexual Functioning." *Sex Roles: A Journal of Research,* Vol. 52, No. 7–8, April 2005, p. 463.

25. Sabiston, Catherine, et al. "Examining Current-Ideal Discrepancy Scores and Exercise Motivations as Predictors of Social Physique Anxiety in Exercising Females." *Journal of Sport Behavior,* Vol. 28, No. 1, March 2005, p. 68.

26. Cohen, Diane, and Trent Petrie. "An Examination of Psychosocial Correlates of Disordered Eating Among Undergraduate Women." *Sex Roles: A Journal of Research,* Vol. 52, No. 1–2, January 2005, p. 29.

27. Davison and McCabe, "Relationships Between Men's and Women's Body Image and Their Psychological, Social, and Sexual Functioning."

28. American College Health Association. "The American College Health Association National College Health Assessment (ACHA-NCHA), Spring 2003 Reference Group Report." *Journal of American College Health,* Vol. 53, No. 5, March–April 2005, p. 199.

29. Huang, Terry, et al. "Overweight and Components of the Metabolic Syndrome in College Students." *Diabetes Care,* Vol. 27, No. 12, December 2004, p. 3000.

30. Graham, Melody, and Amy Jones. "Freshman 15: Valid Theory or Harmful Myth?" *Journal of American College Health,* Vol. 50, No. 4, January 2002, p. 171.

31. Lakdawalla, Darius, et al. "Are the Young Becoming More Disabled?" *Health Affairs,* Vol. 23, No. 1, January–February 2004, p. 168.

32. Moreira-Andres, M. N., et al. "Comparison of Anthropometric Parameters as Predictors of Serum Lipids in Premenopausal Women." *Journal of Endrocrinology Investigation,* Vol. 27, No. 4, April 2004, p. 340.

33. Deen, Darwin. "Metabolic Syndrome: Time for Action." *American Family Physician,* Vol. 69, No. 2, June 15, 2004, p. 2875.

34. U.S. Preventive Services Task Force (USP-STF), www.ahrq.gov/clinic/uspstfix.htm.

35. "More Evidence on the Cost of Obesity." *Occupational Health Management,* Vol. 15, No. 2, February 2004, p. 19.

36. USDHHS, Press Release, "HHS Announces Revised Medicare Obesity Coverage Policy: Policy Opens Door to Coverage Based on Evidence," July 15, 2004.

37. Ford, Gregory, et al. "Associations of Body Mass Index with Meniscal Tears." *American Journal of Preventive Medicine,* Vol. 28, No. 4, May 2005, p. 364.

38. Taylor, Eric, et al. "Obesity, Weight Gain, and the Risk of Kidney Stones." *Journal of the American Medical Association,* Vol. 293, No. 4, January 26, 2005, p. 459.

39. Conklin, Martha, et al. "College Students' Use of Point of Selection Nutrition Information." *Topics in Clinical Nutrition,* Vol. 20, No. 2, April–June 2005, p. 97(12).

40. Conklin, Martha, et al. "Nutrition Information at Point of Selection Could Benefit College Students." *Topics in Clinical Nutrition,* Vol. 20, No. 2, April–June 2005, p. 90(7).

41. Calle, Eugenia, et al. "Overweight, Obesity, and Mortality from Cancer in a Prospectively Studied Cohort of U.S. Adults." *New England Journal of Medicine,* Vol. 348, No. 17, April 24, 2003, p. 1625.

42. Ibid.

43. Lahmann, P. H., et al. "Breast Cancer Risk in Overweight Postmenopausal Women." *Cancer Epidemiol Biomarkers Prev.,* Vol. 15, No. 8, August 2004, p. 1414.

44. Vorona, Robert, et al. "Overweight and Obese Patients in a Primary Care Population Report Less Sleep Than Patients with a Normal Body Mass Index." *Archives of Internal Medicine,* Vol. 165, No. 1, January 10, 2005, p. 25.

45. Flegal, Katherine, et al. "Excess Deaths Associated with Underweight, Overweight, and Obesity." *Journal of the American Medical Association,* Vol. 293, No. 15, April 20, 2005, p. 1861.

46. Gregg, Edward, et al. "Secular

Trends in Cardiovascular Disease Risk Factors According to Body Mass Index in U.S. Adults." *Journal of the American Medical Association,* Vol. 293, No. 15, April 20, 2005, p. 1868.

47. Mark, David. "Deaths Attributable to Obesity." *Journal of the American Medical Association,* Vol. 293, No. 15, April 20, 2005, p. 1918.

48. Johnston, E., et al. "The Relation of Body Mass Index to Depressive Symptoms." *Canadian Journal of Public Health,* Vol. 95, No. 3, May–June 2004, p. 179.

49. Teixeira, P. J., et al. "Pretreatment Predictors of Attrition and Successful Weight Management in Women." *International Journal of Obesity Related Metabolic Disorders,* July 20, 2004.

50. Hensrud, D. D. "Tackling Obesity in a 15-Minute Office Visit: Physicians Can Start Patients on an Effective Weight-Loss Program, Despite Time Constraints." *Postgraduate Medicine,* Vol. 115, No. 1, January 2004, p. 59.

51. U.S. Department of Health and Human Services, U.S. Department of Agriculture, *Dietary Guidelines for Americans 2005,* www.healthierus.gov/dietaryguidelines.

52. American Obesity Association, www.obesity.org.

53. Klein, Samuel, et al. "Weight Management Through Lifestyle Modification for the Prevention and Management of Type 2 Diabetes: Rationale and Strategies." *Diabetes Care,* Vol. 27, No. 8, 2004, pp. 2067–2073.

54. Slawson, David. "Popular Diets Equally Effective for Losing Weight." *American Family Physician,* Vol. 71, No. 9, May 1, 2005, p. 1783.

55. Tsai, Adam, and Wadden, Thomas. "Systematic Review: An Evaluation of Major Commercial Weight Loss Programs in the United States." *Annals of Internal Medicine,* Vol. 142, No. 1, January 4, 2005, p. 56.

56. McTigue, Kathleen, et al. "Screening and Interventions for Obesity in Adults: Summary of the Evidence for the U.S. Preventive Services Task Force." *Annals,* Vol. 139, 2003, p. 930.

57. Dansinger, Michael, et al. "Comparison of the Atkins, Ornish, Weight Watchers, and Zone Diets for Weight Loss and Heart Disease Risk Reduction: A Randomized Trial." *Journal of the American Medical Association,* Vol. 293, No. 1, January 5, 2005, p. 43.

58. Tsai and Wadden, "Systematic Review."

59. Eckel, Robert. "The Dietary Approach to Obesity." *Journal of the American Medical Association,* Vol. 293, No. 1, January 5, 2005, p. 96.

60. Yancy, W. S., et al. "A Low-Carbohydrate, Ketogenic Diet Versus a Low-Fat Diet to Treat Obesity and Hyperlipidemia: A Randomized, Controlled Trial." *Annals of Internal Medicine,* Vol. 140, No. 10, May 18, 2004, p. 769.

61. Stern, Linda, et al. "The Effects of Low-Carbohydrate versus Conventional Weight Loss Diets in Severely Obese Adults: One-Year Follow-up of a Randomized Trial." *Annals of Internal Medicine,* Vol. 140, No. 10, May 18, 2004, p. 778.

62. "The Skinny on Popular Diets." *Harvard Heart Letter,* February 2003, p. 1.

63. Willett, Walt. "Reduced-Carbohydrate Diets: No Roll in Weight Management?" *Annals of Internal Medicine,* Vol. 140, No. 10, May 18, 2004, p. 836.

64. Levine, James, et al. "Interindividual Variation in Posture Allocation: Possible Role in Human Obesity." *Science,* Vol. 307, No. 5709, January 28, 2005, p. 584.

65. Ibid.

66. Helmering, Doris, and Dianne Hales. *Think Thin, Be Thin.* New York: Broadway Books, 2005.

67. White, M. A., et al. "Mediators of Weight Loss in a Family-Based Intervention Presented over the Internet." *Obesity Research,* Vol. 12, No. 7, July 2004, p. 1050.

68. Womble, L. G., et al. "A Randomized Controlled Trial of a Commercial Internet Weight Loss Program." *Obesity Research,* Vol. 12, 2004, p. 1011.

69. National Weight Control Registry, www.lifespan.org/services/bmed/wt_loss/nwcr/.

70. White, M. A., et al. "Gender, Race, and Obesity-Related Quality of Life at Extreme Levels of Obesity." *Obesity Research,* Vol. 12, No. 6, June 2004, p. 949.

71. Encinosa, W. E., et al. "Use and Costs of Bariatric Surgery and Prescription Weight-Loss Medications." *Health Affairs,* Vol. 24, No. 4, July–August 2005, p. 1039.

72. American Obesity Association. www.obesity.org.

73. Buchwald, Henry, et al. "Bariatric Surgery." *Journal of the American Medical Association,* Vol. 292, No. 14, October 13, 2004, p. 1724.

74. Cohen and Petrie, "An Examination of Psychosocial Correlates of Disordered Eating Among Undergraduate Women."

75. O'Dea, Jennifer, and Suzanne Abraham. "Eating and Exercise Disorders in Young College Men." *Journal of American College Health,* Vol. 50, No. 4, May 2002, p. 273.

76. National Eating Disorders Center, www.nationaleatingdisorders.org.

77. Kirn, Timothy. "Four Factors Useful in Identifying Eating Disorders in Girls." *Clinical Psychiatry News,* Vol. 33, No. 1, January 2005, p. 42.

78. Hales, Robert, and Stuart Yudofsky (eds.). *Textbook of Clinical Psychiatry,* 4th ed. Washington, DC: American Psychiatric Publishing, 2003, p. 975.

79. Frank, Guido, et al. "Increased Dopamine D2/D3 Receptor Binding After Recovery from Anorexia Nervosa Measured by Positron Emission Tomography and [(11)C] Raclopride." *Biological Psychiatry,* June 28, 2005 (Epub ahead of print).

80. Ibid.

81. Wilson, G. Terence, and Roz Shafran. "Eating Disorders Guidelines from NICE." *Lancet,* Vol. 365, No. 9453, January 1, 2005, p. 79.

82. Cummings, Sue, et al. "Position of the American Dietetic Association: Weight Management." *Journal of the American Dietetic Association,* Vol. 102, No. 8, August 2002, pp. 11, 1145.

Chapter 8

1. Hale, Cara. "Social Support and Physical Health: The Importance of Belonging." *Journal of American College Health,* Vol. 53, No. 6, May–June 2005, p. 276.

2. Maple, Marilyn. Personal interview.

3. McGinty, Kristen, et al. "Nonverbal

and Verbal Communication in 'Involved' and 'Casual' Relationships Among College Students." *College Student Journal,* Vol. 37, No. 1, March 2003, p. 68.

4. Goulston, Mark. Personal Interview.

5. Hall, Judith. Personal interview.

6. Lito, Mie. "Self-Disclosure in Romantic Relationships and Friendships Among American and Japanese College Students." *The Journal of Social Psychology,* Vol. 145, No. 2, April 2005, p. 127.

7. Billingham, Robert. Personal interview.

8. Yager, Jan. Personal interview.

9. American College Health Association. "The American College Health Association National College Health Assessment (ACHA-NCHA), Spring 2003 Reference Group Report." *Journal of American College Health,* Vol. 53, No. 5, March–April 2005, p. 199, www.acha.org.

10. Laumann, Edward. Personal interview.

11. Sprecher, Susan. "Insiders' Perspectives on Reasons for Attraction to a Close Other." *Social Psychology Quarterly,* Vol. 61, No. 4, December 1998.

12. Luo, Shanhong, and Eva Klohnen. "Assortative Mating and Marital Quality in Newlyweds: A Couple-Centered Approach." *Journal of Personality and Social Psychology,* Vol. 88, No. 2, February 2005.

13. Buss, David. *The Evolution of Desire.* New York: Basic Books, 1994.

14. Singh, Devendra. "Mating Strategies of Young Women: Role of Physical Attractiveness." *The Journal of Sex Research,* Vol. 41, No. 1, February 2004, p. 43.

15. Fisher, Helen. Personal interview.

16. Knox, David, et al. "College Students Attitudes and Behaviors Toward Ending an Unsatisfactory Relationship." *College Student Journal,* Vol. 36, No. 4, December 2002, p. 630.

17. U.S. Census Bureau, Washington, DC, www.census.gov.

18. Poponoe, David, and Barbara Dafoe Whitehead. *The State of Our Unions 2005.* Rutgers, NJ: National Marriage Project, 2005, http://marriage.rutgers.edu.

19. "Cohabitation, Marriage, Divorce, and Remarriage in the United States." Series Report 23, No. 22. Hyattsville, MD: National Center for Health Statistics, 2002.

20. Wellner, Alison. "Mapping the Unmarried: Cohabiting Couples are Found in Clusters Around the Country." *Forecast,* Vol. 23, No. 4, April 2003, p. 5.

21. Hymowitz, Kay. "The Cohabitation Blues." *Commentary,* Vol. 115, No. 3, March 2003, p. 56; Alternatives to Marriage Project, www.unmarried.org.

22. Blonna, Richard, and Jean Levitan. *Healthy Sexuality.* Belmont, CA: Wadsworth, 2005, p. 193.

23. The Gottman Institute, Seattle, WA, www.gottman.com.

24. Poponoe and Whitehead, *The State of Our Unions 2005.*

25. Crooks, Robert, and Karla Baur. *Our Sexuality,* 8th ed. Pacific Grove, CA: Wadsworth, 2002.

26. Sternberg, Robert. Personal interview.

27. National Center for Health Statistics, Washington, DC, www.cdc.gov/nchs.

28. "Does Togetherness Equal Happiness?" *Marriage Partnership,* Vol. 20, No. 1, Spring 2003, p. 13.

29. Crooks and Baur. *Our Sexuality.*

30. The Gottman Institute.

31. Neff, L. A., and B. R. Karney. "Gender Differences in Social Support: A Question of Skill or Responsiveness?" *Journal of Personality and Social Psychology,* Vol. 88, 2005, p. 79.

32. Poponoe and Whitehead, *The State of Our Unions 2005.*

33. Kornbluh, Karen. "The Parent Trap." *Atlantic Monthly,* Vol. 291, No. 1, January–February 2003, p. 111.

34. Wyn, Roberta, and Victoria Ojeda. *Women, Work, and Family Health: A Balancing Act.* Menlo Park, CA: Kaiser Family Foundation, April 2003.

Chapter 9

1. Herman-Giddens, Marcia. Personal interview.

2. Funkhouser, Ellen, et al. "Vaginal Douching Practices Among Women Attending a University in the Southern United States." *Journal of American College Health,* Vol. 50, No. 4, p. 177.

3. Rempel, J. K., and B. Baumgartner. "The Relationship Between Attitudes Towards Menstruation and Sexual Attitudes, Desires, and Behavior in Women." *Archives of Sexual Behavior,* Vol. 32, No. 2, April 2003, p. 155.

4. Dell, Diana. "What's New in PMS?" *Contemporary OB/GYN,* Vol. 50, No. 1, January 2005, p. 48.

5. Ibid.

6. Bertone-Johnson, Elizabeth, et al. "Calcium and Vitamin D Intake and Risk of Incident Premenstrual Syndrome." *Archives of Internal Medicine,* Vol. 165, June 2005, p. 1246.

7. "Just the Facts . . . Circumcision." American Academy of Pediatrics, www.aap.org/mrt/factscir.htm.

8. Kinkade, Scott, et al. "Does Neonatal Circumcision Decrease Morbidity?" *Journal of Family Practice,* Vol. 54, No. 1, January 2005, p. 81.

9. Ibid.

10. Crooks, Robert, and Karla Baur. *Our Sexuality,* 8th ed. Pacific Grove, CA: Wadsworth, 2002.

11. Centers for Disease Control and Prevention, Washington, DC, www.cdc.gov.

12. "National Survey of Adolescents and Young Adults: Sexual Health Knowledge, Attitudes, and Experiences." Menlo Park, CA: Kaiser Family Foundation, 2003.

13. Ibid.

14. Blonna, Richard, and Jean Levitan. *Healthy Sexuality.* Belmont, CA: Wadsworth, 2005.

15. Prinstein, M. J., et al. "Adolescent Oral Sex, Peer Popularity, and Perceptions of Best Friends' Sexual Behavior." *Journal of Pediatric Psychology,* Vol. 28, No. 4, June 2003, p. 243.

16. National Center for Health Statistics, Centers for Disease Control and Prevention, Washington, DC, www.cdc.gov/nchs.

17. Duncan, Greg, et al. "Peer Effects in Drug Use and Sex Among College Students." *Journal of Abnormal Child Psychology,* Vol. 33, No. 3, June 2005, p. 375.

18. "Smarter Sex Survey," www.SmarterSex.org.

19. Netting, N. S., and Matthew Burnett. "Twenty Years of Student Sexual Behavior: Subcultural Adaptations to a Changing Health Environment." *Adolescence,* Vol. 39, No. 153, Spring 2004, p. 19.

20. Johnson, Thomas, and Courtney Stahl. "Sexual Experience Associated with Participation in Drinking Games." *Journal of General Psychology,* Vol. 131, No. 3, July 2004, p. 304.

21. Apostolopoulos, Y., et al. "HIV-Risk Behaviours of American Spring Break Vacationers: A Case of Situational Disinhibition?" *International Journal of STDs and AIDS,* Vol. 13, No. 11, November 2002, p. 733.

22. Raffaelli, Marccela, et al. "Acculturation Status and Sexuality among Female Cuban American College Students." *Journal of American College Health,* Vol. 54, No. 1, July–August 2005, p. 7

23. Ibid.

24. Robinson, John, and Geoffrey Godbey. "No Sex, Please . . . We're College Graduates." *American Demographics,* February 1998.

25. Bailey, J. V., et al. "Sexual Behavior of Lesbians and Bisexual Women." *Sexually Transmitted Infections,* Vol. 79, No. 2, April 2003, p. 147.

26. Crooks and Baur, *Our Sexuality.*

27. Eisenberg, M. E. "The Association of Campus Resources for Gay, Lesbian, and Bisexual Students with College Students' Condom Use." *Journal of American College Health,* Vol. 51, No. 3, November 2002, p. 109.

28. Kenagy, Gretchen. "Transgender Health: Findings from Two Needs Assessment Studies in Philadelphia." *Health and Social Work,* Vol. 30, No. 1, February 2005, p. 19.

29. Goodson, P., et al. "Defining Abstinence: Views of Directors, Instructors, and Participants in Abstinence-Only-Until-Marriage Programs in Texas." *Journal of School Health,* Vol. 73, No. 3, March 2003, p. 91.

30. Witkin, A., et al. "Comprehensive Versus Abstinence-Only Sex Education: What Works?" *Focus,* Vol. 18, No. 2, January 2003, p. 1.

31. Crooks and Baur, *Our Sexuality.*

32. Blonna and Levitan, *Human Sexuality.*

33. "It's Smart to Carry Condoms but. . . ." *Chain Drug Review,* Vol. 26, No. 13, August 16, 2004, p. 49.

34. Eisenberg, M. E. "The Association of Campus Resources for Gay, Lesbian, and Bisexual Students with College Students' Condom Use." *Journal of American College Health,* Vol. 51, No. 3, November 2002, p. 109.

35. Duncan, C., et al. "Barriers to Safer Sex Practices Among African American College Students." *Journal of National Medical Association,* Vol. 94, No. 11, November 2002, p. 944.

36. Gurman, Tilly, and Dina Borzekowski. "Condom Use Among Latino College Students." *Journal of American College Health,* Vol. 52, No. 4, January–February 2004, p. 169.

37. Tulloch, Heather, et al. "Partner Communication Skills and Condom Use Among College Couples." *Journal of American College Health,* Vol. 52, No. 6, May–June 2004, p. 263.

38. "Erectile Dysfunction: The Viagra Revolution." *Harvard Men's Health Watch,* April 2005.

39. Ibid.

40. Jannini, E. A., et al. "Disorders of Ejaculation." *Journal of Endocrinology Investigation,* Vol. 25, No. 11, December 2002, p. 1006.

41. Chen, J., et al. "Efficacy of Sildenafil as Adjuvant Therapy to Selective Serotonin Reuptake Inhibitor in Alleviating Premature Ejaculation." *Urology,* Vol. 61, No. 1, January 2003, p. 197.

42. Ragucci, K. R., and N. S. Culhane. "Treatment of Female Sexual Dysfunction." *Annals of Pharmacotherapy,* Vol. 37, No. 4, April 2003, p. 546.

43. Berman, L., et al. "Seeking Help for Sexual Function Complaints: What Gynecologists Need to Know About the Female Patient's Experience." *Fertility and Sterility,* Vol. 79, No. 3, March 2003, p. 57.

44. Bancroft, J. "Distress About Sex: A National Survey of Women in Heterosexual Relationships." *Archives of Sexual Behavior,* Vol. 32, No. 3, June 2003, p. 193.

Chapter 10

1. Coles, Clifton. "Contraception Rises Among U.S. Women." *The Futurist,* Vol. 39, No. 3, May–June 2005, p. 15.

2. Murray, Steven, and Jessica L. Miller. "Birth Control and Condom Usage Among College Students." *Research Quarterly for Exercise and Sport,* Vol. 71, No. 1, March 2000.

3. "Emergency Contraceptive Pills." *Women's Health Policy Fact Sheet,* Kaiser Family Foundation, February 2004.

4. Hansen, Laura, and Joseph Saseen. "New Contraceptive Options: Patient Adherence and Satisfaction." *American Family Physician,* Vol. 69, No. 4, February 15, 2004, p. 811.

5. "Stroke Risk Low in Women Using Birth Control Pills." *Clinical Reviews,* Vol. 14, No. 7, July 2004, p. 28.

6. Apter, D., et al. "Effect of an Oral Contraceptive Containing Drospirenone and Ethinylestradiol on General Well-Being and Fluid-Related Symptoms." *European Journal of Contraception and Reproductive Health Care,* Vol. 8, No. 1, March 2003, p. 37.

7. Davis, Ann, et al. "Oral Contraceptives for Dysmenorrhea in Adolescent Girls: A Randomized Trial." *Obstetrics & Gynecology,* Vol. 106, No. 1, July 2005, p. 97.

8. "Is Ortho Evra Right for You?" Planned Parenthood, www.plannedparenthood.org

9. "FDA Says Internet Site is Selling Counterfeit Versions of Birth Control Patch." *Medical Letter on the CDC & FDA,* February 29, 2004, p. 16.

10. "Is NuvaRing Right for You?" www.plannedparenthood.org

11. "Is Lunelle Right for You?" www.plannedparenthood.org

12. Bock, Robert. "Depo Provera Appears to Increase Risk for Chlamydial and Gonococcal Infections." National Institute of Child Health and Human Development News Release, August 23, 2004.

13. Steiner, M. J. "Contraceptive Effectiveness of a Polyurethane Condom and a Latex Condom: A Randomized Controlled Trial." *Obstetrics and Gynecology,* Vol. 101, No. 3, March 2003, p. 539.

14. Michaels Opinion Research. "In the Heat of the Moment." Menlo Park, CA: Henry J. Kaiser Family Foundation, June 2001.

15. Macaluso, M., et al. "Efficacy of the Female Condom as a Barrier to Semen During Intercourse." *American Journal of Epidemiology,* Vol. 157, No. 4, February 15, 2003, p. 289.

16. Tucker, Miriam. "Emergency

Contraception: Better Education Urged." *Family Practice News,* Vol. 35, No. 11, June 1, 2005, p. 69.

17. Vastag, Brian. "Plan B for 'Plan B'?" *Journal of the American Medical Association,* Vol. 291, No. 23, June 16, 2004, p. 2805.

18. "Questions for Recommendations for Clinical Practice Emergency Contraception." *Journal of Family Planning and Reproductive Health Care,* Vol. 29, No. 2, April 2003, p. 16.

19. "Emergency Contraception: Increasing Public Awareness." *Issues Brief,* Vol. 2, February 2003, p. 1. Alan Guttmacher Institute, www.guttmacher.org.

20. "Emergency Birth Control (Information from Your Family Doctor)." *American Family Physician,* Vol. 70, No. 4, August 15, 2004, p. 717.

21. McCarthy, Susan. "Availability of Emergency Contraceptive Pills at University and College Student Health Centers." *Journal of American College Health,* Vol. 51, No. 1, July 2002, p. 15.

22. "No Reason for Limiting Use of Emergency Contraception." *Reproductive Health Matters,* Vol. 13, No. 25, May 2005, p. 200.

23. Baill, Cori, et al. "Counseling Issues in Tubal Sterilization." *American Family Physician,* Vol. 67, April 15, 2003, p. 1287.

24. "Sterilization: Is Your Practice Up to Date?" *Contraceptive Technology Update,* Vol. 25, No. 7, July 2004, p. 79.

25. "Trends in Abortion in the United States, 1973–2000." New York, Alan Guttmacher Institute, January 2003.

26. Henshaw, Stanley. "U.S. Teenage Pregnancy Statistics with Comparative Statistics for Women Aged 20–24." New York, Alan Guttmacher Institute, May 2003.

27. Finer, Lawrence, and Stanley Henshaw. "Abortion Incidence and Services in the United States in 2000." *Perspectives on Sexual and Reproductive Health,* Vol. 35, No. 1, January–February 2003, p. 6.

28. "Abortion Not Implicated in Carcinogenesis." *Women's Health Weekly,* July 22, 2004, p. 21.

29. "FDA Issues Public Health Advisory for Mifepristone." *FDA News,* July 19, 2005.

30. Lafayette, Leslie. Personal interview.

31. Hueston, W. J. "Delayed Prenatal Care and the Risk of Low Birth Weight Delivery." *Journal of Community Health,* Vol. 28, No. 3, June 2003, p. 199.

32. Spinelli, A., et al. "Do Antenatal Classes Benefit the Mother and Her Baby?" *Journal of Maternal and Fetal Neonatal Medicine,* Vol. 13, No. 2, February 2003, p. 94.

33. Devine, K. S. "Caring for the Infertile Woman." *American Journal of Maternal and Child Nursing,* Vol. 28, No. 2, March–April 2003, p. 100.

34. "Assisted Reproductive Technology Statistics." *American Family Physician,* Vol. 71, No. 3, February 1, 2005, p. 615.

Chapter 11

1. National Institute on Drug Abuse, National Institutes of Health, www.nida.nih.gov/about/welcome/aboutdrugabuse/trends/.

2. Kirn, Timothy. "Adolescent Use of Drugs, Tobacco Continues Decline: More Are Abusing Painkillers, Inhalants." *Clinical Psychiatry,* Vol. 33, No. 2, February 2005, p. 1.

3. Johnston, L. D., et al. *Monitoring the Future.* Bethesda, MD: National Institute on Drug Abuse, 2005.

4. Brunk, Doug. "Report Finds Dire Substance Abuse Risks at Home: Nearly Half of U.S. Children Are Exposed." *Family Practice News,* Vol. 35, No. 10, May 15, 2005, p. 1.

5. "'Coming-out' Process Related to Substance Use Among Gay, Lesbian, and Bisexual Teens." *Brown University Digest of Addiction Theory and Application,* Vol. 24, No. 6, June 2005, p. 3.

6. Boyd, C. J., et al. "Ecstasy Use Among College Undergraduates: Gender, Race, and Sexual Identity." *Substance Abuse Treatment,* Vol. 24, No. 3, April 2003, p. 209.

7. Engwall, Douglas, et al. "Gambling and Other Risk Behaviors on University Campuses." *Journal of American College Health,* Vol. 52, No. 6, May–June 2004, p. 245.

8. Turchi, Renee, et al. "Gambling and Children." *Contemporary Pediatrics,* Vol. 22, No. 1, January 2005, p. 45.

9. Platz, Laurie, et al. "Gambling by Underage College Students: Preferences and Pathology." *College Student Journal,* Vol. 39, No. 1, March 2005, p. 3.

10. Ibid.

11. Turchi, "Gambling and Children."

12. Institute for Safe Medication Practices, www.ismp.org.

13. "National Institutes of Health State-of-the-Science Conference Statement: Manifestations and Management of Chronic Insomnia in Adults." Bethesda, MD: National Institutes of Health, 2005.

14. "More on Sleeping Pills." *Harvard Health Letter,* Vol. 30, No. 5, March 2005, p. 7.

15. "Lessons to Learn from the COX-2 Saga." *Harvard Health Letter,* Vol. 30, No. 5, March 2005, p. 1.

16. "Stepping into the Vioxx Void." *Harvard Health Letter,* Vol. 30, No. 3, January 2005, p. 6.

17. Hall, Kristina, et al. "Illicit Use of Prescribed Stimulant Medication Among College Students." *Journal of American College Health,* Vol. 53, No. 4, January–February 2005, p. 167.

18. McCabe, S. E., et al. "Nonmedical Use of Prescription Opioids Among U.S. College Students: Prevalence and Correlates from a National Survey." *Addiction Behavior,* May 2005, Vol. 30, No. 4, pp. 789–805.

19. Wu, Tianying, et al. "Caffeinated Coffee, Decaffeinated Coffee, and Caffeine in Relation to Plasma C-Peptide Levels, A Marker of Insulin Secretion, in U.S. Women." *Diabetes Care,* Vol. 28, No. 6, June 2005, p. 1390(7).

20. "Caffeine Doesn't Raise Risk of Colorectal Cancer." *HealthFacts,* Vol. 30, No. 3, March 2005, p. 4.

21. "Caffeine and Atrial Fibrillation." *Nutrition Research Newsletter,* Vol. 24, No. 4, April 2005, p. 15.

22. Adams, Jacqueline. "Venti." *Science World,* Vol. 61, No. 9–10, February 7, 2005, p. 27(2).

23. United Nations Office on Drugs and Crime. *2004 World Drug Report.* Vienna, Austria: Vienna International Centre, 2004.

24. Johnston, L. D., P. M. O'Malley, J. G. Bachman, and J. E. Schulenberg. *Monitoring the Future National Results on Adolescent Drug*

Use: Overview of Key Findings, 2004, Bethesda, MD: National Institute on Drug Abuse, 2005.

25. "Most Adolescents in Treatment Also Need Psychiatric Care." *Alcoholism & Drug Abuse Weekly,* Vol. 17, No. 22, June 6, 2005, p. 6.

26. "Do 12-Step Programs Aimed at Dually Diagnosed Patients Increase Drug Abstinence?" *The Brown University Digest of Addiction Theory and Application,* Vol. 24, No. 1, January 2005, p. 1(3).

27. Nestler, Eric. "Historical Review: Molecular and Cellular Mechanisms of Opiate and Cocaine Addiction." *Trends in Pharmacological Sciences,* Vol. 25, No. 4, April 2004, p. 210.

28. Wilens, T. E., et al. "Does Stimulant Therapy of Attention-Deficit/Hyperactivity Disorder Beget Later Substance Abuse? A Meta-Analytic Review of the Literature." *Pediatrics,* Vol. 111, No. 1, 2003, p. 179.

29. Duncan, Greg, et al. "Peer Effects in Drug Use and Sex Among College Students." *Journal of Abnormal College Psychology,* Vol. 33, No. 3, June 2005, p. 375.

30. "A Third of 21–25-Year-Old Drivers Drank or Used Drugs in First Year." *Alcoholism & Drug Abuse Weekly,* Vol. 17, No. 26, July 11, 2005, p. 7(1).

31. "Marijuana and Mental Health Problems." *Drug Detection Report,* Vol. 15, No. 13, June 30, 2005, p. 104.

32. Duncan, et al. "Peer Effects in Drug Use and Sex Among College Students."

33. "Reefer Rx: Marijuana as Medicine." *Harvard Health Letter,* September 2004.

34. "Depression and Marijuana Use." *Family Practice News,* Vol. 35, No. 12, June 15, 2005, p. 64(1).

35. National Institute on Drug Abuse, www.nida.nih.gov.

36. Stephenson, Joan. "Cannabis Consequences." *Journal of the American Medical Association,* Vol. 291, No. 23, June 16, 2004, p. 2809.

37. Henry, John, et al. "Comparing Cannabis with Tobacco: Smoking Cannabis, Like Smoking Tobacco, Can be a Major Public Health Hazard." *British Medical Journal,* Vol. 326, No. 7396, May 3, 2003, p. 942.

38. Partnership for a Drug-Free America, "Marijuana," www.drugfreeamerica.org.

39. "Club Drugs: Study Explores Reasons for Use by Young Adults." *Brown University Digest of Addiction Theory and Application,* Vol. 24, No. 2, February 2005, p. 1(3).

40. Sim, Tiffanie, et al. "Psychosocial Correlates of Recreational Ecstasy Use by College Students." *Journal of American College Health,* Vol. 54, No. 1, July–August, p. 25.

41. Ricuarte, George, and Una McCann. "Recognition and Management of Complications of New Recreational Drug Use." *The Lancet,* Vol. 365, No. 9477, June 18, 2005, p. 2137(9).

42. Ibid.

43. Reitman, David. "'Club' Drugs 101: Substance Use and Abuse for 21st Century Clinicians." *Consultant,* Vol. 45, No. 7, June 2005, p. 753(5).

44. Ricuarte and McCann, "Recognition and Management of Complications of New Recreational Drug Use."

45. Reitman, "'Club' Drugs 101.

46. Ricuarte and McCann, "Recognition and Management of Complications of New Recreational Drug Use."

47. "Prescription Narcotics: Methamphetamine Tops List of Treatment Admissions." *Alcoholism & Drug Abuse Weekly,* Vol. 17, No. 28, July 25, 2005, p. 1(2).

48. "Instant Pleasure, Instant Ageing: Methamphetamine," *The Economist,* Vol. 375, No. 8431, June 18, 2005, p. 31US.

49. Ibid.

50. "Effects of Methamphetamine: Brain Region Recovery Possible in Former Users." *The Brown University Digest of Addiction Theory and Application,* Vol. 24, No. 5, May 2005, p. 5(2).

51. Reitman, "'Club' Drugs 101."

52. Teter, Christian, et al. "Prevalence and Motives for Iliicit Use of Prescription Stimulants in an Undergraduate Student Sample." *Journal of American College Health,* Vol. 53, No. 6, May–June 2005, p. 253.

53. Hall, Kristina, et al. "Illicit Use of Prescribed Stimulant Medication Among College Students." *Journal of American College Health,* Vol. 53, No. 4, January–February 2005, p. 167(8).

54. Teter, et al. "Prevalence and Motives for Illicit Use of Prescription Stimulants in an Undergraduate Student Sample."

55. "Mechanisms of Opiate and Cocaine Addiction Reviewed." *Obesity, Fitness & Wellness Week,* July 17, 2004, p. 27.

56. "Scientists May Use Existing Drugs to Stop Addiction." *Health & Medicine Week,* September 20, 2004, p. 1186.

57. "Heroin." National Institute on Drug Abuse, www.nida.nih.gov.

58. McCabe, et al. "Nonmedical Use of Prescription Opioids Among U.S. College Students."

59. Torpy, Janet. "Opioid Abuse." *Journal of the American Medical Association,* Vol. 291, No. 10, September 15, 2004, p. 1213.

60. Wu, L. T., et al. "Inhalant Abuse and Dependence Among Adolescents in the United States." *Journal of the American Academy of Child and Adolescent Psychiatry,* Vol. 43, No. 10, October 2004, p. 1206.

61. National Institute on Drug Abuse, www.nida.nih.gov.

62. *Behavioral Change Through Treatment,* NIDA InfoFacts, www.drugabuse.gov.

Chapter 12

1. White, A. M., et al. "College Students Lack Knowledge of Standard Drink Volumes: Implications for Definitions of Risky Drinking Based on Survey Data." *Alcoholism, Clinical and Experimental Research,* Vol. 29, No. 4, April 2005, pp. 631–63.

2. Nelson, T. F., et al. "'Binge' Drinking and Blood Alcohol Concentration." *Journal of Studies on Alcohol,* Vol. 66, No.3, May 2005, pp. 438–439.

3. Moore, Alison, et al. "Longitudinal Patterns and Predictors of Alcohol Consumption in the United States." *American Journal of Public Health,* Vol. 95, No. 3, March 2005, p. 458.

4. American College Health Association. "The American College Health Association National Col-

lege Health Assessment (ACHA-NCHA), Spring 2003 Reference Group Report." *Journal of American College Health,* Vol. 53, No. 5, March–April 2005, p. 199.

5. Shinew, Kimberly, and Diana Parry. "Examining College Students' Participation in the Leisure Pursuits of Drinking and Illegal Drug Use." *Journal of Leisure Research,* Vol. 37, No. 3, Summer 2005 p. 364.

6. Brewer, Robert, and Monica Swahn. "Binge Drinking and Violence." *Journal of the American Medical Association,* Vol. 294, No. 5, August 3, 2005, p. 616.

7. Ibid.

8. Sullivan, Michelle, "Maternal Binge Drinking Tied to Childhood Problems: Risk of Behavior Problems Is 2.5 Times Higher for Bingers' Babies Than for Those Exposed to Less." *Clinical Psychiatry News,* Vol. 32, No. 4, April 2004, p. 74.

9. Hingson, Ralph, et al. "Magnitude of Alcohol-Related Mortality and Morbidity among U.S. College Students Ages 18–24." *Annual Review of Public Health,* Vol. 26, April 2005, pp. 259–279.

10. Wechsler, Henry, et al. "Drinking and Driving Among College Students: The Influence of Alcohol-Control Policies." *Journal of American College Health,* Vol. 53, No. 14, January–February 2005, p. 192.

11. Neal, Dan, et al. "It's All Fun and Games . . . or Is It? Collegiate Sporting Events and Celebratory Drinking." *Journal of Studies on Alcohol,* March 2005, Vol. 66, No. 2, p. 291.

12. Shinew and Parry, "Examining College Students' Participation in the Leisure Pursuits of Drinking and Illegal Drug Use."

13. "The American College Health Association National College Health Assessment."

14. Ibid.

15. Shinew and Parry, "Examining College Students' Participation in the Leisure Pursuits of Drinking and Illegal Drug Use."

16. Siebert, Darcy Clay, et al. "Differences in African American and White College Students' Drinking Behaviors: Consequences, Harm Reduction Strategies, and Health Information Sources." *Journal of American College Health,* Vol. 52,

No. 3, November–December 2003, p. 123.

17. "The American College Health Association National College Health Assessment."

18. Shinew and Parry, "Examining College Students' Participation in the Leisure Pursuits of Drinking and Illegal Drug Use."

19. Wilson, Gregory, et al. "Athletic Status and Drinking Behavior in College Students: The Influence of Gender and Coping Styles." *Journal of American College Health,* Vol. 52, No. 6, May–June 2004, p. 269.

20. Neal et al., "It's All Fun and Games . . . or Is It?"

21. McKinnon, Sarab, et al. "Increased Risk of Alcohol Abuse Among College Students Living on the U.S.-Mexico Border: Implications for Prevention." *Journal of American College Health,* Vol. 51, No. 4, January 2003, p. 149.

22. Park, Crystal, et al. "The Daily Stress and Coping Process and Alcohol Use Among College Students." *Journal of Studies on Alcohol,* Vol. 65, No. 1, January 2004, p. 126.

23. Weitzman, Elissa. "Poor Mental Health, Depression, and Associations with Alcohol Consumption, Harm, and Abuse in a National Sample of Young Adults in College." *The Journal of Nervous and Mental Disease,* Vol. 192, No. 4, April 2004, p. 269.

24. Nelson, T.F., et al. "The State Sets the Rate: The Relationship of College Binge Drinking to State Binge Drinking Rates and Selected State Alcohol Control Policies." *American Journal of Public Health,* Vol. 95, No. 3, 2005, pp. 441–446.

25. Vickers, Kristin, et al. "Binge Drinking in Female College Students: The Association of Physical Activity, Weight Concern, and Depressive Symptoms." *Journal of American College Health,* Vol. 53, No. 3, November–December 2004, p. 133.

26. Moore, Michele Johnson, et al. "Feasibility and Efficacy of a Binge Drinking Prevention Intervention for College Students Delivered via the Internet versus Postal Mail." *Journal of American College Health,* Vol. 54, No. 1, p. 38.

27. Chiauzzi, Emil, et al. "My Student Body: A High-Risk Drinking Prevention Web Site for College Students." *Journal of American College Health,* Vol. 53, No. 6, p. 263.

28. Hingson, et al. "Magnitude of Alcohol-Related Mortality and Morbidity Among U.S. College Students Ages 18–24."

29. Ibid.

30. Delva, Jorge, et al. "A Study of the Relationship Between Protective Behaviors and Drinking Consequences Among Undergraduate College Students." *Journal of American College Health,* Vol. 53, No. 1, July–August 2004, p. 19.

31. Mohler-Kuo, M., et al. "Correlates of Rape While Intoxicated in a National Sample of College Women." *Journal of Studies on Alcohol,* Vol. 65, No. 1, February 2004, p. 37.

32. Delva et al., "A Study of the Relationship Between Protective Behaviors and Drinking Consequences Among Undergraduate College Students."

33. "The American College Health Association National College Health Assessment."

34. Rhodes, Warren, et al. "Does Knowledge of College Drinking Policy Influence Student Binge Drinking?" *Journal of American College Health,* Vol. 54, No. 1, p. 45.

35. Foote, Jeffrey, et al. "A National Survey of Alcohol Screening and Referral in College Health Centers." *Journal of American College Health,* Vol. 52, No. 4, January–February 2004, p. 149.

36. Weitzman, Elissa, et al. "Reducing Drinking and Related Harms in College: Evaluation of the 'A Matter of Degree' Program." *American Journal of Preventive Medicine,* Vol. 27, No. 3, October 2004, p. 187.

37. "Alcohol Consumption and Waist Circumference." *Nutrition Research Newsletter,* Vol. 22, No. 5, May 2003, p. 5.

38. "Regular Alcohol Consumption is Good for the Heart." *Harvard Health Letter,* Vol. 28, No. 6, April 2003, p. 1.

39. Jancin, Bruce. "Cardiovascular Benefits of Alcohol Challenged." *Family Practice News,* Vol. 33, No. 6, March 15, 2003, p. 12.

40. "Alcohol and Hormone Therapy Increase the Risk of Breast Cancer." *OB/GYN Clinical Alert,* January 2003, p. 68.

41. "Drinking Increases Risk." *Women's Health Weekly,* February 6, 2003, p. 2.

42. Robb-Nicholson, Celeste. "Alcohol and Breast Cancer." *Harvard Women's Health Watch,* Vol. 10, No. 9, May 2003, p. 1.

43. Mukamai, Kenneth, et al. "Prospective Study of Alcohol Consumption and Risk of Dementia in Older Adults." *Journal of the American Medical Association,* Vol. 289, No. 11, March 19, 2003, p. 1405.

44. "Fetal Alcohol Syndrome Is Still a Threat." *Harvard Mental Health Letter,* September 2004.

45. Sempos, C. T., et al. "Average Volume of Alcohol Consumption and All-Cause Mortality in African Americans: The NHEFS Cohort." *Alcoholism, Clinical and Experimental Research,* Vol. 27, No. 1, 2003, p. 88.

46. "Drug Treatment for Alcoholism Today." *Harvard Mental Health Letter,* July 2005, p. 3.

47. Ibid.

48. Kirkpatrick, Jean. Personal interview.

49. "Helping Others Stay Sober Leads to Positive Outcomes for Recovering Alcoholics." *The Brown University Digest of Addiction Theory and Application,* Vol. 24, No. 6, June 2005, p. 2(2).

50. Students Against Destructive Decisions, www.sadd.org/contract.htm#collegecfl

Chapter 13

1. "Lower Adult Smoking Rates with More Adults Quitting," Press Release. CDC Office of Communication. November 10, 2005.

2. Rogers, Richard, et al. "Mortality Attributable to Cigarette Smoking in the United States." *Population and Development Review,* Vol. 31, No. 2, June 2005, p. 259(35).

3. Troschair et al., "Cigarette Smoking Among Adults—United States, 2003."

4. American College Health Association. "The American College Health Association's National College Health Assessment (ACHA-NCHA), Spring 2003 Reference Group Report." *Journal of American College Health,* Vol. 53, No. 5, March–April 2005, p. 199.

5. "Nicotine: It May Have a Good Side." *Harvard Health Letter,* May 2005.

6. Silverman, Jennifer. "Smoking Cessation Counseling." *Family Practice News,* Vol. 35, No. 10, May 1, 2005, p. 78(1).

7. Kropp, Rhonda, et al. "Adolescents' Beliefs About the Risks Involved in Smoking 'Light' Cigarettes." *Journal of the American Academy of Child and Adolescent Psychiatry,* Vol. 44, No. 5, May 2005, p. 469(1).

8. Mahoney, Diana. "One Smoke Before Age 11 Predicts a Later Habit." *Pediatric News,* Vol. 39, No. 7, July 2005, p. 26(1).

9. Kirn, Timothy. "Tobacco Addiction: Teens More Susceptible." *Pediatric News,* Vol. 39, No. 6, June 2005, p. 6(1).

10. Fiske, Susan. "Butt Out?" *Psychology Today,* March–April 2003, p. 41.

11. "The American College Health Association's National College Health Assessment, Spring 2003 Reference Group Report."

12. Patterson, Freda. "Cigarette Smoking Practices Among American College Students: Review and Future Directions." *Journal of American College Health,* Vol. 52, No. 5, March–April 2004, p. 203(8).

13. Ibid.

14. Lenz, Brenda. "Tobacco, Depression, and Lifestyle Choices in the Pivotal Early College Years." *Journal of American College Health,* Vol. 52, No. 5, March–April 2004, p. 213.

15. Ibid.

16. Rigotti, N., et al. "U.S. College Students' Exposure to Tobacco Promotions: Prevalence and Association with Tobacco Use." *American Journal of Public Health,* Vol. 95, No. 138, January 2004.

17. Moran, Susan, et al. "Social Smoking Among U.S. College Students." *Pediatrics,* Vol. 4, No. 4, October 11, 2004, pp. 1028–1034.

18. Wechsler, Henry, et al. "College Smoking Policies and Smoking Cessation Programs: Results of a Survey of College Health Center Directors." *Journal of American College Health,* Vol. 49, No. 5, March 2001, p. 205.

19. Bacon, C. G., et al. "Sexual Function in Men Older than 50 years of Age: Results from the Health Professionals Follow-up Study." *Annals of Internal Medicine,* Vol. 139, No. 3, August 5, 2003, p. I22.

20. "Smoking During Pregnancy Lowers Not Only Birthweight But IQ." *Contemporary OB/GYN,* Vol. 50, No. 7, July 2005, p. 17(1).

21. "Nicotine Replacement Use on the Rise." *Alcoholism & Drug Abuse Weekly,* Vol. 17, No. 31, August 15, 2005, p. 7(1).

22. Breslau, Naomi, et al. "Smoking and the Risk of Suicidal Behavior: A Prospective Study of a Community Sample." *Archives of General Psychiatry,* Vol. 62, No. 3, March 2005, pp. 328–334.

23. Parmet, Sharon. "Smoking and the Heart." *Journal of the American Medical Association,* Vol. 290, No. 1, July 2, 2003, p. 146.

24. Sutherland, G. "Smoking: Can We Really Make a Difference?" *Heart,* Vol. 89, No. 5, May 2003, p. 25.

25. Yap, Ronald, and Kevin McVary. "Smoking and Erectile Dysfunction: How Strong a Link?" *Contemporary Urology,* Vol. 15, No. 3, March 2003, p. 34.

26. "Smokeless Tobacco Threatens Heart Health." *Medical Update,* Vol. 30, No. 111–112, May–June 2005, p. 6(1).

27. Smith, Kenesha, et al. "What Interventions Can Help Patients Stop Using Chewing Tobacco?" *Journal of Family Practice,* Vol. 54, No. 4, April 2005, p. 368(2).

28. Troschair et al. "Cigarette Smoking Among Adults—United States, 2003."

29. Mitchell, Amy, and Thomas Parish. "Using Combination Therapy for Smoking Cessation." *Clinician Reviews,* Vol. 15, No. 5, May 2005, p. 39(8).

30. Centers for Disease Control and Prevention, www.cdc.gov.

31. Ramsay, Jim, and Anne Hoffmann. "Smoking Cessation and Relapse Prevention Among Undergraduate Students: A Pilot Demonstration Project." *Journal of American College Health,* Vol. 53, No. 1, July–August 2004, p. 11(8).

32. Ibid.

33. "Study Finds Online Smoking Cessation Treatments Fall Short." *The Brown University Digest of Addiction Theory and Application,* Vol. 24, No. 5, May 2005, p. 5(1).
34. "Nicotine Replacement Use on the Rise."
35. Mitchell and Parish, "Using Combination Therapy for Smoking Cessation."
36. Nicotrol, www.nicotrol.com.
37. "Cigarettes: The Lung Cancer Risk Lingers." *Harvard Health Letter,* July 2005.
38. Chriqui, J., et al. "State Smoking Restrictions for Private-Sector Worksites, Restaurants, and Bars—United States, 1998 and 2004." *Morbidity and Mortality Weekly Report,* Vol. 54, No. 26, July 8, 2005, p. 649(5).
39. Oh, Sang Woo, et al. "Association Between Cigarette Smoking and Metabolic Syndrome." *Diabetes Care,* Vol. 28, No. 8, August 2005, p. 2064(3).
40. "Tobacco Settlement States' Allocations of Fiscal Year 2004 and Expected Fiscal Year 2005 Payments." *Medical Benefits,* Vol. 22, No. 9, May 15, 2005, p. 6(2).
41. Chriqui et al. "State Smoking Restrictions for Private-Sector Worksites, Restaurants, and Bars."

Chapter 14

1. Centers for Disease Control and Prevention, www.cdc.gov.
2. Arbes, Jr., S. J., et al. "Prevalences of Positive Skin Test Responses to 10 Common Allergens in the U.S. Population: Results from the Third National Health and Nutrition Examination Survey." *Journal of Allergy and Clinical Immunology,* Vol. 116, No. 2, August 2005, p. 377–383.
3. Howland, Jonathan, et al. "Prevalence of Allergy Symptoms and Associated Medication Use in a Sample of College Seniors." *Journal of American College Health,* Vol. 51, No. 2, September 2002, p. 67.
4. Cohen, S., et al. "Emotional Style and Susceptibility to the Common Cold." *Psychosomatic Medicine,* Vol. 65, No. 4, July–August 2003, p. 652.
5. Barrett, B. P., et al. "Treatment of the Common Cold with Unrefined Echinacea. A Randomized, Double-Blind, Placebo-Controlled Trial." *American Family Physician,* Vol. 67, No. 7, April 1, 2003, p. 1589.
6. Little, Paul, et al. "Information Leaflet and Antibiotic Prescribing Strategies for Acute Lower Respiratory Tract Infection." *Journal of the American Medical Association,* Vol. 293, No. 24, June 22–29, 2005, p. 3029.
7. Thompson, William, et al. "Influenza-Associated Hospitalizations in the United States." *Journal of the American Medical Association,* Vol. 292, No. 11, September 15, 2004, p. 1333.
8. Nichol, Kristin, et al. "Colds and Influenza-Like Illnesses in University Students: Impact on Health, Academic and Work Performance, and Health Care Use." *Clinical Infectious Diseases,* Vol. 40, No. 9, May 1, 2005, p. 1263(8).
9. Allred, Norma, et al. "Responses of U.S. College and University Student Health Services to the 2004 Influenza Vaccine Shortage." *Journal of American College Health,* Vol. 53, No. 6, May–June 2005, p. 291.
10. "CDC Recommendations to Prevent Influenza." *Journal of the American Medical Association,* Vol. 291, No. 1, January 7, 2004, p. 34.
11. Bruce, Michael, et al. "Risk Factors for Meningococcal Disease in College Students." *Journal of the American Medical Association,* Vol. 286, No. 6, August 8, 2001, p. 286.
12. Ringold, Sarah. "Hepatitis A Virus." *Journal of the American Medical Association,* Vol. 294, No. 2, July 13, 2005, p. 270.
13. "Hepatitis C Fact Sheet." CDC, Washington, DC: www.cdc.gov/hepatitis.
14. Torpy, Janet. "Body Piercing." *Journal of the American Medical Association,* Vol. 291, No. 8, February 24, 2004, p. 1024.
15. Ringold, Sarah. "Tuberculosis." *Journal of the American Medical Association,* Vol. 293, No. 22, June 8, 2005, p. 2820.
16. Kuehn, Bridget. "CDC: New Repellents for West Nile Fight." *Journal of the American Medical Association,* Vol. 293, No. 21, June 1, 2005, p. 2583.
17. Parmet, Sharon, et al. "Vaginal Symptoms." *Journal of the American Medical Association,* Vol. 291, No. 11, March 17, 2004, p. 1406.
18. American College Health Association. "The American College Health Association's National College Health Assessment (ACHA–NCHA), Spring 2003 Reference Group Report." *Journal of American College Health,* Vol. 53, No. 5, March–April 2005, p. 199.
19. Koumans, Emilia, et al. "Sexually Transmitted Disease Services at U.S. Colleges and Universities." *Journal of American College Health,* Vol. 53, No. 5, March–April 2005, p. 211.
20. "The American College Health Association's National College Health Assessment, Spring 2003 Reference Group Report."
21. Koumans et al., "Sexually Transmitted Disease Services at U.S. Colleges and Universities."
22. "Check Your Sexually Transmitted Disease Screening: More Young Adults Are at Risk for Chlamydia: One in 25 Young Americans are Infected with Chlamydia, Research Shows." *Contraceptive Technology Update,* Vol. 25, No. 8, August 2004, p. S1.
23. Ibid.
24. Miller, William, et al. "Prevalence of Chlamydial and Gonococcal Infections among Young Adults in the United States." *Journal of the American Medical Association,* Vol. 291, No. 18, May 12, 2004, p. 2229.
25. Golden, Matthew, et al. "Effect of Expedited Treatment of Sex Partners on Recurrent or Persistent Gonorrhea or Chlamydial Infection." *New England Journal of Medicine,* Vol. 352, No. 7, February 17, 2005, p. 676.
26. Weinstock, H., et al. "Sexually Transmitted Disease Among American Youth: Incidence and Prevalence Estimates, 2000." *Perspectives on Sexual and Reproductive Health,* Vol. 36, 2004, p. 6.
27. McPartland, Tara, et al. "Men's Perceptions and Knowledge of Human Papillomavirus (HPV) Infection and Cervical Cancer." *Journal of American College Health,* Vol. 53, No. 5, March–April 2005, p. 225.
28. Weinstock, H., et al. "Sexually Transmitted Disease Among American Youth."
29. Ibid.

30. "Fluoroquinolone-Resistant Gonorrhea Rates on the Rise in the U.S." *Clinical Infectious Diseases,* Vol. 38, No. 12, June 15, 2004, p. iii(1).

31. "The Global HIV/AIDS Epidemic." *Kaiser Family Foundation HIV/AIDS Policy Fact Sheet,* December 2004.

32. "The HIV/AIDS Epidemic in the United States." *Kaiser Family Foundation HIV/AIDS Policy Fact Sheet,* September 2005.

33. Voelker, Rebecca. "Women Shoulder Growing HIV/AIDS Burden." *Journal of the American Medical Association,* Vol. 293, No. 3, January 19, 2005, p. 281.

34. Stephenson, Joan. "Researchers Report Findings on HIV Drug Resistance, New Infections." *Journal of the American Medical Association,* Vol. 291, No. 12, March 24–31, 2004, p. 1431.

35. Leone, P., et al. "HIV Transmission Among Black Women—North Carolina, 2004." *Morbidity and Mortality Weekly Report,* Vol. 54, No. 4, February 4, 2005, p. 89.

36. "HIV Testing in the United States." *Kaiser Family Foundation HIV/AIDS Policy Fact Sheet,* June 2005.

37. Marelich, William, and Tonya Clark. "Human Immunodeficiency Virus (HIV) Testing and False Disclosures in Heterosexual College Students." *Journal of American College Health,* Vol. 53, No. 3, November–December 2004, p. 109.

Chapter 15

1. "Exercise, C-reactive Protein, and Your Heart." *Harvard Men's Health Watch,* Vol. 9, No. 12, July 2005, p. 1.

2. "The Bigger Worry: Heart Disease or Cancer?" *Harvard Health Letter,* February 2005.

3. Daviglus, Martha, et al. "Favorable Cardiovascular Risk Profile in Young Women and Long-term Risk of Cardiovascular and All-Cause Mortality." *Journal of the American Medical Association,* Vol. 292, No. 13, October 6, 2004, p. 1588.

4. "Young Adults Who Maintain Their Weight, Even if Overweight, Have Lower Risk Factor Levels for Heart Disease in Early Middle Age." *NIH News,* November 8, 2004.

5. Collins, Kristina, et al. "Heart Disease Awareness Among College Students." *Journal of Community Health,* Vol. 29, No. 5, October 2004, p. 405.

6. Green, John, et al. "Heart Disease Risk Perception in College Men and Women." *Journal of American College Health,* Vol. 51, No. 5, March 2003, p. 207.

7. Spencer, Leslie. "Results of a Heart Disease Risk-Factor Screening Among Traditional College Students." *Journal of American College Health,* Vol. 50, No. 6, May 2002, p. 291.

8. Gordon, Neil, et al. "Effectiveness of Therapeutic Lifestyle Changes in Patients with Hypertension, Hyperlipidemia, and/or Hyperglycemia." *American Journal of Cardiology,* Vol. 94, No. 12, December 15, 2004, p. 1558.

9. *Dietary Guidelines for Americans,* 2005. Washington, DC: U.S. Department of Health and Human Services, U.S. Department of Agriculture, **www.health.gov/dietaryguidelines/**

10. Gulati, Martha, et al. "The Prognostic Value of a Nomogram for Exercise Capacity in Women." *New England Journal of Medicine,* Vol. 353, No. 5, August 4, 2005, pp. 517–519.

11. Jensen, M. K., et al. "Intakes of Whole Grains, Bran, and Germ and the Risk of Coronary Heart Disease in Men." *American Journal of Clinical Nutrition,* Vol. 80, No. 6, December 2004, p. 1492.

12. Dallongeville, Jean, et al. "Fish Consumption Is Associated With Lower Heart Rates." *Circulation,* Vol. 108, 2003, pp. 820–825.

13. Panagiotakos, D. B., et al. "Fish consumption and the risk of developing acute coronary syndromes." *International Journal of Cardiology,* Vol. 102, No. 3, July 20, 2005, pp. 403–409.

14. Neff, Matthew. "Antioxidant Vitamin Supplements and Cardiovascular Disease Risk Reduction." *American Family Physician,* Vol. 71, No. 7, April 1, 2005, p. 1433.

15. "Declining Prevalence of No Known Major Risk Factors for Heart Disease and Stroke Among Adults." *Journal of the American Medical Association,* Vol. 291, No. 17, May 5, 2004, p. 2069.

16. "Heart Disease and Stroke Statistics—2004." American Heart Association, 2004.

17. Wessel, Timothy, et al. "Relationship of Physical Fitness vs. Body Mass Index with Coronary Artery Disease and Cardiovascular Events in Women." *Journal of the American Medical Association,* Vol. 292, No. 10, September 8, 2004, p. 1179.

18. Blair, Steven, and Tim Church. "The Fitness, Obesity, and Health Equation." *Journal of the American Medical Association,* Vol. 292, No. 10, September 8, 2004, p. 1232.

19. Bauer, Jeff. "Intensity of Exercise Is What Counts When It Comes to Reducing Heart Disease Risk." *RN,* Vol. 66, No. 1, January 2003, p. 97.

20. Mitka, Mike. "Secondhand Smoke an Acute Heart Risk?" *Journal of the American Medical Association,* Vol. 291, No. 22, June 9, 2004, p. 3690.

21. Critchley, Julia, and Simon Capewell. "Mortality Risk Reduction Associated with Smoking Cessation in Patients with Coronary Artery Disease." *Journal of the American Medical Association,* Vol. 290, No. 1, July 2, 2003, p. 86.

22. Darwin, Deen. "Metabolic Syndrome: What Is It and What Can I Do About It?" *American Family Physician,* Vol. 69, No. 12, June 2004, p. 2887.

23. "Young Adults Who Maintain Their Weight."

24. Huang, Terry, et al. "Overweight and Components of the Metabolic Syndrome in College Students." *Diabetes Care,* Vol. 27. No. 12, December 2004, p. 3000.

25. Tzou, Wendy, et al. "Increased Subclinical Atherosclerosis in Young Adults with Metabolic Syndrome: The Bogalusa Heart Study." *Journal of the American College of Cardiology,* Vol. 46, No. 3, August 2, 2005, pp. 457–463.

26. "Diagnosis and Management of the Metabolic Syndrome: A Scientific Statement for Health Care Professionals." *Circulation: Journal of The American Heart Association,* Vol. 112, September 12, 2005, pp. 2735–2752.

27. Orchard, T. J., et al. "The Effect of Metformin and Intensive Lifestyle Intervention on the Metabolic Syndrome: The Diabetes Prevention

Program Randomization Trial." *Archives of Internal Medicine,* Vol. 142, 2005, pp. 611–619.

28. Lawson, Willow. "The Emotional Life of the Heart." *Psychology Today,* Vol. 38, No. 1, January–February 2005, p. 24(1).

29. Mitka, Mike. "Depression-Heart Disease Link Probed." *Journal of the American Medical Association,* Vol. 293, No. 3, January 19, 2005, p. 283.

30. "Type D Personality and Cardiovascular Risk." *Harvard Health Letter,* August 2005.

31. Schiffer, A., et al. "The Distressed (Type D) Personality Is Independently Associated with Impaired Health Status and Increased Depressive Symptoms in Chronic Heart Failure." *European Journal of Cardiovascular Prevention and Rehabilitation,* Vol. 12, No. 4, August 2005, p. 341.

32. "Type D for Distressed." *Harvard Health Letter,* August 2005.

33. Fitzgerald, Garret, et al. "Vioxx." *Circulation,* January 17, 2005.

34. Hampton, Tracy. "Experts Point to Lessons Learned from Controversy over Rofecoxib Safety." *Journal of the American Medical Association,* Vol. 293, No. 3, January 19, 2005, p. 413.

35. Dubois, Anne. "Advancements in the Control, Prevention of Hypertension, Related Disease." Press Release. International Society on Hypertension in Blacks, July 8, 2005.

36. Forman, John, et al. "Folate Intake and the Risk of Incident Hypertension Among US Women." *Journal of the American Medical Association,* Vol. 293, No. 3, January 19, 2005, p. 320.

37. Robertson, Rose Marie. Personal interview.

38. Hu, Frank, et al. "Hypertension: Overweight and Increased Cardiovascular Mortality: No French Paradox." *Journal of the American Heart Association,* Vol. 96, No. 7, October 2005, p. 695.

39. Chobanian, A. V., et al. "Seventh Report of the Joint National Committee on Prevention, Detection, Evaluation, and Treatment of High Blood Pressure." *Hypertension,* Vol. 42, No. 6, December 2003, p. 1206.

40. Forman, et al. "Folate Intake and the Risk of Incident Hypertension among US Women."

41. Riehle J. F., et al. "Ethnic Differences in the Treatment and Control of Hypertension in Patients with Diabetes." *Journal of Clinical Hypertension,* Vol. 7, No. 8, August, 2005, pp. 445–454.

42. LaRosa, John, et al. "Intensive Lipid Lowering with Atorvastatin in Patients with Stable Coronary Disease." *New England Journal of Medicine,* Vol. 352, No. 14, April 7, 2005, p. 1425.

43. "Exercise, C-reactive Protein, and Your Heart."

44. Ridker, Paul, et al. "C-reactive Protein Levels and Outcomes After Statin Therapy." *New England Journal of Medicine,* Vol. 352, No. 1, January 6, 2005, pp. 29–38.

45. Ridker, Paul, et al. "Non-HDL Cholesterol, Apolipoproteins A-1 and B100, Standard Lipid Measures, Lipid Ratos, and CRP as Risk Factors for Cardiovascular Disease in Women." *Journal of the American Medical Association,* Vol. 294, No. 3, July 20, 2005, p. 326.

46. "Inflammation Information." *Harvard Health Letter,* July 2005, p. 3.

47. "Exercise, C-reactive Protein, and Your Heart."

48. "CPR: Are We Doing It Wrong?" *Harvard Health Letter,* Vol. 30, No. 7, May 2005, p. 1.

49. Sanders, Arthur, and Gordon Ewy. "Cardiopulmonary Resuscitation in the Real World: When Will the Guidelines Get the Message?" *Journal of the American Medical Association,* Vol. 293, No. 3, January 19, 2005, p. 363.

50. "CPR: Are We Doing It Wrong?"

51. Ridker, et al. "C-reactive protein levels and outcomes after statin therapy."

52. Stone, G. W., et al. "Percutaneous Recanalization of Chronically Occluded Coronary Arteries: Procedural Techniques, Devices, and Results." *Catheter Cardiovascular Intervention,* September 9, 2005 (E-pub ahead of print).

53. Women's Health Initiative Steering Committee. "Effects of Conjugated Equine Estrogen in Postmenopausal Women with Hysterectomy." *Journal of the American Medical Association,* Vol. 291, No. 14, April 14, 2004, p. 1701.

54. White, Halina, et al. "Northern Manhattan Study Interim Report." International Stroke Conference, January 2005.

55. Chimowitz, M. I., et al. "Comparison of Warfarin and Aspirin for Symptomatic Intracranial Arterial Stenosis." *New England Journal of Medicine,* Vol. 352, No. 13, March 31, 2005, pp. 1305–1316.

Chapter 16

1. *Cancer Facts and Figures 2005.* Atlanta: American Cancer Society, 2005.

2. Mitka, Mike. "New Cancer Figures Released." *Journal of the American Medical Association,* Vol. 291, No. 5, February 4, 2004, p. 552.

3. Kaklamani, Virginia. "TGFBR1*6A and Cancer Risk." *Journal of Clinical Oncology,* Vol. 21, No. 17, September 1, 2003, p. 3236.

4. "Cancer in Racial and Ethnic Minorities." *Cancer Facts and Figures 2005.* Atlanta: American Cancer Society, 2005.

5. Calle, Eugenia, et al. "Overweight, Obesity, and Mortality from Cancer in a Prospectively Studied Cohort of U.S. Adults." *New England Journal of Medicine,* Vol. 348, No. 17, April 24, 2003, p. 1625.

6. *Fulfilling the Potential of Cancer Prevention and Early Detection.* Washington, DC: National Academy of Sciences, 2003.

7. "Cancers Linked to Infectious Diseases." *Cancer Facts and Figures 2005.* Atlanta: American Cancer Society, 2005.

8. Cook, Nancy, et al. "Low-Dose Aspirin in the Primary Prevention of Cancer." *Journal of the American Medical Association,* Vol. 294, No. 1, July 6, 2005, p. 47.

9. Lee, I-Min, et al. "Vitamin E in the Primary Prevention of Cardiovascular Disease and Cancer." *Journal of the American Medical Association,* Vol. 294, No. 1, July 6, 2005, p. 56.

10. Willett, Walter. "Diet and Cancer." *Journal of the American Medical Association,* Vol. 293, No. 2, January 12, 2005, p. 233.

11. van Gils, C. H., et al. "Consumption of Vegetables and Fruits and Risk of Breast Cancer." *Journal of the American Medical Association,* Vol. 293, No. 2, January 12, 2005, p. 183.

12. Chao, A., et al. "Meat Consumption and Risk of Colorectal Cancer." *Journal of the American Medical Association,* Vol. 293, No. 2, January 12, 2005, p. 172.

13. Takkouche, Bahi, et al. "Personal Use of Hair Dyes and Risk of Cancer." *Journal of the American Medical Association,* Vol. 293, No. 20, May 25, 2005, p. 2516.

14. Poochareon, V. N., and Cockerell, C. J. "The War Against Skin Cancer: The Time for Action is Now." *Archives of Dermatology,* Vol. 141, No. 4, April 2005, pp. 499–501.

15. Mahler, Heike, et al. "Effects of UV Photographs, Photoaging Information, and Use of Sunless Tanning Lotion on Sun Protection." *Archives of Dermatology,* Vol. 141, March 2005, p. 373, www.archdermatol .com.

16. Hamant, E.S., and B.B. Adams. "Sunscreen Use Among Collegiate Athletes." *Journal of the American Academy of Dermatology,* Vol. 53, No. 2, August 2005, pp. 237–241.

17. Christenson, Leslie, et al. "Incidence of Basal Cell and Squamous Cell Carcinomas in a Population Younger than 40 Years." *Journal of the American Medical Association,* Vol. 294, No. 6, August 10, 2005, p. 681.

18. Warthan, M. M., et al. "UV Light Tanning as a Type of Substance-Related Disorder." *Archives of Dermatology,* Vol. 141, No. 8, August 2005, pp. 963–966.

19. "Drinking Increases Risk." *Women's Health Weekly,* February 6, 2003, p. 2.

20. Li, Christopher, et al. "Relationship Between Long Durations and Different Regimens of Hormone Therapy and Risk of Breast Cancer." *Journal of the American Medical Association,* Vol. 289, No. 24, June 25, 2003, p. 3254.

21. Holmes, Michelle, et al. "Physical Activity and Survival after Breast Cancer Diagnosis." *Journal of the American Medical Association,* Vol. 293, No. 20, May 25, 2005, p. 2479.

22. "American Cancer Society Issues Updated Breast Cancer Screening Guidelines," News Release, May 15, 2003.

23. Yu Shen, et al. "Role of Detection Method in Predicting Breast Cancer Survival: Analysis of Randomized Screening Trials." *Journal of the National Cancer Institute,* Vol. 97, August 17, 2005, pp. 1195–1203.

24. American College of Radiology Imaging Network (ACRIN) Presentation. Arlington, VA, September 2005.

25. Hampton, Tracy. "Monoclonal Antibody Therapies Shine in Breast Cancer Clinical Trials." *Journal of the American Medical Association,* Vol. 293, No. 24, June 22–29, 2005, p. 2985.

26. Chao et al. "Meat Consumption and Risk of Colorectal Cancer."

27. Hampton, Tracy. "NSAID Studies Abound in Cancer Research." *Journal of the American Medical Association,* Vol. 293, No. 21, June 1, 2005, p. 2579.

28. "Vitamin B$_6$ May Help Prevent Colorectal in Women." *Harvard Women's Health Watch,* Vol. 12, No. 11, July 2005, p. 1.

29. Fletcher, Robert. "Screening Sigmoidoscopy—How Often and How Good?" *Journal of the American Medical Association,* Vol. 290, No. 1, July 2, 2003, p. 106.

30. Schoenfeld, Phillip, et al. "Colonoscopic Screening of Average-Risk Women for Colorectal Neoplasia." *New England Journal of Medicine,* Vol. 352, No. 20, May 19, 2005, pp. 2061–2068.

31. Cote, Michele, et al. "Risk of Lung Cancer among White and Black Relatives of Individuals with Early-Onset Lung Cancer." *Journal of the American Medical Association,* Vol. 293, No. 24, June 22–29, 2005, p. 3036.

32. Johansson, Jan-Erik, et al. "Natural History of Early, Localized Prostate Cancer." *Journal of the American Medical Association,* Vol. 291, No. 22, June 9, 2004, p. 2713.

33. *Cancer Facts & Figures 2005.*

34. Hampton, Tracy. "Cancer Treatment's Trade-off." *Journal of the American Medical Association,* Vol. 294, No. 2, July 13, 2005, p. 167.

35. American Diabetes Association, www.diabetes.org.

36. Peters, Anne. *Conquering Diabetes.* New York: Hudson Street Press, 2005.

37. American College of Endocrinologists. "Implementation Conference for ACE Outpatient Diabetes Mellitus Consensus Conference Recommendations: Position Statement." July 8, 2005, www.aace .com.

38. Beaser, Richard, and Amy Campbell. *The Joslin Guide to Diabetes.* New York: Simon & Schuster, 2005.

39. National Diabetes Education Program, www.ndep .nih.gov.

40. Keymeulen, B., et al. "Insulin Needs After CD3-Antibody Therapy in New-Onset Type 1 Diabetes." *New England Journal of Medicine,* Vol. 352, No. 25, June 23, 2005, pp. 2642–2644.

41. Theodore, William. Personal interview.

42. Engel, Jerome. Personal interview.

43. Hales, Dianne. "Their Best Chance for a Normal Life." *Parade,* September 18, 2005.

44. Cutts, Steven. "Back Pain—and Its Management." *Practice Nurse,* December 17, 2004, p. 38(5).

45. Malanga, Gerard, and Robin Dennis. "Treatment of Acute Low Back Pain: Use of Medications: Reduction and Control of Pain and Return of Function Are the Goals." *The Journal of Musculoskeletal Medicine,* Vol. 22, No. 2, February 2005, p. 79.

46. Margo, Katherine. "Spinal Manipulative Therapy for Low Back Pain." *American Family Physician,* Vol. 71, No. 3, February 1, 2005, p. 464.

47. Wendling, Patrice. "Surgery No Better Than Rehab for Low Back Pain." *American Family Physician,* Vol. 71, No. 3, February 1, 2005, p. 558.

Chapter 17

1. Rothstein, William, and Sushama Rajapaksa. "Health Beliefs of College Students Born in the United States, China, and India." *Journal of American College Health,* Vol. 51, No.5, March 2003, p. 189.

2. Arnold, Matthew. "83 Million Consumers Go Online First for Health Info." *Medical Marketing & Media,* Vol. 39, No. 2, February 2004, p. 22.

3. Bard, Mark. Personal interview.

4. Escoffery, Cam, et al. "Internet Use for Health Information among College Students." *Journal of Amerian College Health,* Vol. 53, No. 4, January–February 2004, p. 183.

5. Baker, Laurence, et al. "Use of the

Internet and E-mail for Health Care Information." *Journal of the American Medical Association,* Vol. 289, No. 18, May 14, 2003, p. 2400.

6. Hales, Dianne. "The Best Medical Help Online." *Parade,* September 19, 2004, p. 9.

7. Mold, J. W., et al. "Evidence-Based Medicine Meets Goal-Directed Health Care." *Family Medicine,* Vol. 35, No. 5, May 2003, p. 360.

8. Wynia, Matthew, et al. "Do physicians Not Offer Useful Services Because of Coverage Restrictions?" *Health Affairs,* Vol. 22, No. 4, July–August 2003.

9. Prochazka, Allan, et al. "Support of Evidence-Based Guidelines for the Annual Physical Examination: A Survey of Primary Care Providers." *Archives of Internal Medicine,* Vol. 165, No. 12, June 27, 2005, pp. 1347–1352.

10. American Society of Plastic Surgeons, www.plasticsurgery.org.

11. "Fact Sheet: Protecting the Privacy of Patients' Health Information." U.S. Department of Health and Human Services, April 14, 2003.

12. "In-Hospital Medical Errors Cause 195,000 Deaths in 2002, Study Shows." *Health & Medicine Week,* August 16, 2004, p. 949.

13. "Doctors and Other Health Professionals Report That Fear of Malpractice Has a Big, and Mostly Negative, Impact on Medical Practice, Unnecessary Defensive Medicine, and Openness in Discussing Medical Errors." *Health Care News,* February 7, 2003, p. 3.

14. *NCCAM,* http://nccam.nih.gov.

15. Barnes, P., E. Powell-Griner, K. McFann, and R. Nahin. "Complementary and Alternative Medicine Use Among Adults: United States, 2002." *CDC Advance Data Report #343,* May 27, 2004.

16. Rieder, M. J., and D. Matsui. "Complementary and Alternative Medicine: How Do We Know If It Works?" *Healthcare Papers,* Vol. 3, No. 5, 2003, p. 62.

17. Giordano, James, et al. "Complementary and Alternative Medicine in Mainstream Public Health: A Role for Research in Fostering Integration." *Journal of Alternative and Complementary Medicine,* Vol. 9, No. 3, June 2003, p. 441.

18. National Center for Complementary and Alternative Medicine, http://nccam.nih.gov/health/backgrounds/mindbody.htm

19. Zepf, Bill. "Evidence Basis for Four Commonly Used Herbs." *American Family Physician,* Vol. 67, No. 7, April 1, 2003, p. 1607.

20. Gold, Paul, et al. "The Lowdown on Ginkgo Biloba: This Popular Herbal Supplement May Slightly Improve Your Memory, But You Can Get the Same Effect by Eating a Candy Bar." *Scientific American,* Vol. 288, No. 4, April 2003, p. 86.

21. Rados, Carol. "Ephedra Ban: No Shortage of Reasons." *FDA Consumer Magazine,* March–April 2004.

22. Federal Drug Administration, www.cfsan.fda.gov/%7Edms/ds-warn.html.

23. Bitton, Asaf, and James Kahn. "Government Share of Health Care Expenditures." *Journal of the American Medical Association,* Vol. 289, No. 9, March 5, 2003, p. 1165.

24. Harrison, Bridget. "A Historical Survey of National Health Movements and Public Opinion in the United States." *Journal of the American Medical Association,* Vol. 289, No. 9, March 5, 2003, p. 1163.

25. Hoffman, Catherine, et al. "Holes in the Health Insurance System—Who Lacks Coverage and Why." *Journal of Law, Medicine & Ethics,* Vol. 32, No. 3, Fall 2004, p. 390.

26. Vastag, Brian. "Universal Health Coverage." *Journal of the American Medical Association,* Vol. 291, No. 6, February 11, 2004, p. 684.

27. Harrell, Joseph, and Olveen Carrasquillo. "The Latino Disparity in Health Coverage." *Journal of the American Medical Association,* Vol. 289, No. 9, March 5, 2003, p. 1167.

28. Reed, Vita. "Many College Students Required to Have Insurance: Study Shows Unexpected Medical Expenses Were a Leading Cause of Students Dropping out of School." *San Diego Business Journal,* Vol. 26, No. 115, April 11, 2005, p. 17(2).

29. Board on Health Care Services. *Hidden Costs, Value Lost: Uninsurance in America.* Washington, DC: Institute of Medicine, 2003.

30. Goold, S. D., et al. "Will Insured Citizens Give Up Benefit Coverage to Include the Uninsured?" *Journal of General Internal Medicine,* Vol.19, No.8, August 2004, p. 868.

31. Vastag, Brian. "Insure Everyone Now, Urges IOM." *Journal of the American Medical Association,* Vol. 291, No. 6, February 11, 2004, p. 681.

Chapter 18

1. U.S. Census Bureau.

2. Dausch, Judith. "Aging Issues Moving Mainstream." *Research Quarterly for Exercise and Sport,* Vol. 74, No. 2, June 2003, p. 136.

3. "Scientists Find What Type of Genes Affect Longevity." *Genomics & Genetics Weekly,* August 1, 2003, p. 4.

4. Knox, David, et al. "College Student Views of the Elderly: Some Gender Differences." *College Student Journal,* Vol. 39, No. 1, March 2005, p. 14(3).

5. Roizen, Michael. Personal interview.

6. Hardy, Susan, and Thomas Gill. "Recovery from Disability Among Community-Dwelling Older Persons." *Journal of the American Medical Association,* Vol. 291, No. 13, April 7, 2004, p. 1596.

7. "Facts About Older Americans." National Council on Aging, www.aoa.gov.

8. Gregg, Edward, et al. "Relationship of Changes in Physical Activity and Mortality Among Older Women." *Journal of the American Medical Association,* Vol. 289, No. 18, May 14, 2003, p. 2379.

9. Dausch, "Aging Issues Moving Mainstream."

10. Leveille, Susan, et al. "Trends in Obesity and Arthritis Among Baby Boomers and Their Predecessors, 1971–2002." *American Journal of Public Health,* Vol. 95, No. 9, September 2005, p. 1607–1613.

11. Gazzaley, Adam, et al. "Top-Down Suppression Deficit Underlies Working Memory Impairment in Normal Aging." *Nature Neuroscience,* September 11, 2005, online issue.

12. Sherman, Sherry. Personal interview.

13. Speller, Marsha. Personal interview.

14. Lyndaker, C., and L. Hulton. "The Influence of Age on Symptoms of Perimenopause." *Journal of Obstetrical Gynecology and Neonatal Nurs-

ing, Vol. 33, No. 3, May–June 2004, p. 347.

15. Avis, Nancy, et al. "Quality of Life in Diverse Groups of Midlife Women: Assessing the Influence of Menopause, Health Status and Psychosocial and Demographic Factors." *Quality of Life Research,* Vol. 13, No. 5, June 2004, p. 933.

16. Hales, Dianne. "Embrace the Change." *Parade,* October 10, 2004, p. 4.

17. Pinkerton, JoAnn. Personal interview.

18. Hulley, Stephen, and Deborah Grady. "The WHI Estrogen-Alone Trial: Do Things Look Any Better?" *Journal of the American Medical Association,* Vol. 291, No. 14, April 14, 2004, p. 1769.

19. Hersh, Adam, et al. "National Use of Postmenopausal Hormone Therapy." *Journal of the American Medical Association,* Vol. 291, No. 1, January 7, 2004, p. 47.

20. Women's Health Initiative Steering Committee. "Effects of Conjugated Equine Estrogen in Postmenopausal Women with Hysterectomy." *Journal of the American Medical Association,* Vol. 291, No. 14, April 14, 2004, p. 1703.

21. Ockene, Judith, et al. "Symptom Experience after Discontinuing Use of Estrogen Plus Progestin." *Journal of the American Medical Association,* Vol. 294, No. 2, July 13, 2005, p. 183.

22. Pettiti, Diana. "Some Surprises, Some Answers, and More Questions about Hormone Therapy." *Journal of the American Medical Association,* Vol. 294, No. 2, July 13, 2005, p. 245.

23. *Facts about Menopausal Hormone Therapy.* Washington, DC: U.S. Department of Health and Human Services, 2005.

24. Birge, Stanley. "The WHI and the Brain: What Have We Learned?" *Sexuality, Reproduction & Menopause,* Vol. 2, No. 2, June 2004, p. 71.

25. "Osteoporosis Overview," The NIH Osteoporosis and Related Bone Diseases ~ National Resource Center, www.osteo.org.

26. Slovik, David (ed.). *Osteoporosis: A Guide to Prevention and Treatment.* Cambridge, MA: Harvard Medical School, 2005.

27. "Increasing Evidence That Osteo-porosis Begins in the Womb." *Medical Letter on the CDC and FDA,* June 29, 2003, p. 32.

28. *Facts about Menopausal Hormone Therapy.*

29. Ibid.

30. Tulsky, James. "Beyond Advance Directives." *Journal of the American Medical Association,* Vol. 294, No. 3, July 20, 2005, p. 359.

31. "Living Wills and Health Care Proxies." *Harvard Health Letter,* Vol. 30, No. 8, June 2005, p. 1.

32. "Lesson of the Terri Schiavo Case: Living Wills No Panacea for End of Life." *Healthcare Risk Management,* May 1, 2005.

33. Kübler-Ross, Elisabeth. *Death: The Final Stage of Growth.* Englewood Cliffs, NJ: Prentice Hall, 1975.

34. Jemal, Ahmedin, et al. "Trends in the Leading Causes of Death in the United States, 1970–2002." *Journal of the American Medical Association,* Vol. 294, No. 10, September 14, 2005, p. 1255.

35. Teno, Joan, et al. "Family Perspectives on End-of-Life Care at the Last Place of Care." *Journal of the American Medical Association,* Vol. 291, No. 1, April 7, 2004, p. 88.

36. Ganzini, Linda. "Nurses' Experiences with Hospice Patients Who Refuse Food and Fluids to Hasten Death." *New England Journal of Medicine,* Vol. 349, No. 4, July 24, 2003, p. 359–365.

37. Jacobs, Sandra. "Death by Voluntary Dehydration—What the Caregivers Say." *New England Journal of Medicine,* Vol. 349, No. 4, July 24, 2003, p. 325.

38. Parmet, Sharon. "Suicide in Older Persons." *Journal of the American Medical Association,* Vol. 291, No. 9, March 3, 2004, p. 1158.

39. Brown, Gregory, et al. "Cognitive Therapy for the Prevention of Suicide Attempts." *Journal of the American Medical Association,* Vol. 294, 2005, p. 563.

40. Kayashima, R., and K. L. Braun. "Examining the Variance in Support for Assisted Death Among Physicians, Patients, and the General Public." *Gerontologist,* October 15, 2001, p. 166.

41. Braun, Kathryn, et al. "Support for Physician-Assisted Suicide: Exploring the Impact of Ethnicity and Attitudes Toward Planning for Death." *Gerontologist,* Vol. 41, No. 1, February 2001, p. 51.

42. Marcoux, I., et al. "Withdrawing an Explicit Request for Euthanasia or Physician-Assisted Suicide: A Retrospective Study on the Influence of Mental Health Status and Other Patient Characteristics." *Psychological Medicine,* Vol. 35, No. 9, September 2005, p. 1265.

43. Shojania, Kaveh, et al. "Changes in Rates of Autopsy-Detected Diagnostic Errors Over Time: A Systematic Review." *Journal of the American Medical Association,* Vol. 289, No. 21, June 4, 2003, p. 2849.

44. Shear, Katherine, et al. "Treatment of Complicated Grief." *Journal of the American Medical Association,* Vol. 293, No. 21, June 1, 2005, p. 2601.

45. Glass, Richard. "Is Grief a Disease? Sometimes." *Journal of the American Medical Association,* Vol. 293, No. 21, June 1, 2005, p. 2658.

46. Ringold, Sarah. "Grief." *Journal of the American Medical Association,* Vol. 293, No. 21, June 1, 2005, p. 2686.

47. Shear et al., "Treatment of Complicated Grief."

Chapter 19

1. National Safety Council, www.nsc.org.

2. Villaveces, A. "Association of Alcohol-Related Laws with Deaths Due to Motor Vehicle and Motorcycle Crashes in the United States, 1980–1997." *American Journal of Epidemiology,* Vol. 157, No. 2, January 15, 2003, p. 131.

3. Tyson, Rae. "DOT Announces Record Low Highway Fatality Rate in 2004." *In the News,* NHTSA, August 1, 2005.

4. "National Safety Council Announces Motor Vehicle Safety Initiative." *Safety Compliance Letter,* No. 2441, May 2004, p. 15.

5. "CAA Reminds All Canadians to Buckle Down to Road Safety Use Child Car Seats and Vehicle Seat Belts." *Canadian Corporate News,* April 6, 2004.

6. Paschall, M. J. "College Attendance and Risk-Related Driving Behavior in a National Sample of Young Adults." *Journal of Studies of Alcohol,* Vol. 64, No. 1, January 2003, p. 43.

7. Agency for Healthcare Research and Quality, www.meps.ahrq.gov.

8. "Young Americans Still Shunning Seat Belts." *Health and Medicine Week,* August 25, 2003, p. 638.

9. Cummings, Peter, and Frederick Rivara. "Car Occupant Death According to Restraint Use of Other Occupants." *Journal of the American Medical Association,* Vol. 291, No. 3, January 21, 2004, p. 343.

10. "Risk of Death in Car Crashes Reduced If All Occupants Wear Seat Belts." *Health & Medicine Week,* February 2, 2004, p. 408.

11. Ferguson, Susan. "The Blue Ribbon Panel on Depowered and Advanced Airbags—Status Report on Airbag Performance." *Annual Proceedings/Association for the Advancement of Automotive Medicine,* Vol. 47, September 2003, p. 79.

12. Nerenberg, Arnold. Personal interview.

13. McEvoy, Suzanne, et al. "Role of Mobile Phones in Motor Vehicle Crashes Resulting in Hospital Attendance: A Case-Crossover Study." *British Medical Journal,* Vol. 331, No. 7514; August 20, 2005, p. 428.

14. Seo, Dong-Chui, and Mohammad Torabi. "The Impact of In-Vehicle Cell Phone Use on Accidents and Near-Accidents Among College Students." *Journal of American College Health,* Vol. 53, No. 3, November–December 2004, p. 101.

15. Strayer, David, et al. "Cell Phone Use Can Lead to Inattention Blindness Behind the Wheel." *Injury Insight,* February–March 2003.

16. Ludwig, Timothy, et al. "Using Social Marketing to Increase the Use of Helmets among Bicyclists." *Journal of American College Health,* Vol. 54, No. 1, July–August 2005, p. 51.

17. Ibid.

18. National Center for Health Statistics (NCHS).

19. Reichard, John. "Report Cites One Million Annual Ergonomics Injuries." *Medicine and Health,* Vol. 55, No. 5, January 29, 2001, p. 3.

20. Fitzgerald, Nancy. "Safety on Campus." *Careers & Colleges,* Vol. 22, No. 18, March 2002, p. 18.

21. Health, Iona. "Treating Violence As a Public Health Problem: The Approach Has Advantages But Diminishes the Human Rights Perspective." *British Medical Journal,* Vol. 325, No. 7367, October 5, 2002, p. 726.

22. Centers for Disease Control and Prevention (CDC).

23. Carr, Joetta. *Campus Violence White Paper.* Baltimore, MD: American College Health Association, February 5, 2005.

24. Baum, Katrina, and Patsy Klaus. "Violent Victimization of College Students, 1995–2002." *Bureau of Justice Statistics Special Report,* January 2005.

25. Ibid.

26. Carr, *Campus Violence White Paper.*

27. DeSouza, Eros, and A. Gigi Fansler. "Contrapower Sexual Harassment: A Survey of Students and Faculty Members." *Sex Roles: A Journal of Research,* June 2003, p. 529.

28. Carr, *Campus Violence White Paper.*

29. Ibid.

30. American College Health Association, National College Health Assessment.

31. Hughes, Patricia, et al. "Self-Defense and Martial Arts Evaluation for College Women: Preliminary Validation of Perceptions of Dangerous Situations Scale." *Research Quarterly for Exercise and Sport,* Vol. 74, No. 2, June 2003, p. 153.

32. Isely, P. J. "Sexual Assault of Men: College Age Victims." *National Association of Student Personnel Administrators Journal,* Vol. 35, No. 4, pp. 305–317. (Reported at webits3.appstate.edu.)

33. Hensley, Laura. "Treatment for Survivors of Rape: Issues and Interventions." *Journal of Mental Health Counseling,* Vol. 24, No. 4, October 2002, p. 330.

34. Mohler-Juo, M., et al. "Correlates of Rape while Intoxicated in a National Sample of College Women." *Journal of Studies on Alcohol,* Vol. 65, No. 1, 2004, p. 37.

35. McDonald, Theodore, and Linda Kline. "Perceptions of Appropriate Punishment for Committing Date Rape: Male College Students Recommend Lenient Punishments." *College Student Journal,* Vol. 38, No. 1, March 2004, p. 44.

36. Ibid.

Chapter 20

1. YES! (Youth for Environmental Sanity), www.yesworld.org.

2. Sax, Linda. *The American Freshman: National Norms for Fall 2004.* Los Angeles, CA: UCLA Higher Education Research Institute, 2004.

3. "Diesel Fumes in Particulate Air Pollution Linked to Increased Atopy and Allergy." *Health and Medicine Week,* September 1, 2003, p. 652.

4. Environmental Protection Agency, global warming page, www.epa.gov/globalwarming/.

5. "A Wake-Up Call of Environmental Health." *The Lancet,* Vol. 362, No. 9384, August 23, 2003, p. 587.

6. Environmental Protection Agency, www.epa.gov.

7. "Renewables Are So Right." *Energy & Environmental Management,* September–October 2004, p. 15.

8. "Air Pollution: Particularly Offensive to the Heart." *Harvard Heart Letter,* August 2005, p. 1.

9. Gregg, Jillian, et al. "Urbanization Effects on Tree Growth in the Vicinity of New York City." *Nature,* Vol. 10, No. 424, July 2003, p. 183.

10. "Renewables Are So right."

11. *Second National Report on Human Exposure to Environmental Chemicals.* Atlanta, GA: Centers for Disease Control and Prevention, 2003, www.cdc.gov/exposurereport.

12. "American Radon Scientists Call on EPA to Act on Radon Exposure." *Health and Medicine Week,* June 9, 2003, p. 36.

13. Portnoy, Jay, et al. "Health Effects of Indoor Fungi." *Annals of Allergy, Asthma & Immunology,* Vol. 94, No. 3, March 2005, p. 313.

14. "Major Developments to Improve Hearing Health Reported." *Health & Medicine Week,* January 19, 2004, p. 543.

15. "Old Ears on Young Bodies May Affect College Students' Learning." Press Release, Purdue University, July 28, 2005.

16. Voelker, Rebecca. "Access to Clean Water and Sanitation Pose 21st Century Challenge for Millions." *Journal of the American Medical Association,* Vol. 292, No. 3, July 21, 2004, p. 318.

17. "After 60 Years of Success, Water Fluoridation Still Laking in Many

Communities." Press Release, American Dental Association, July 11, 2005.

18. "Environmental Cancer Risks." *Cancer Facts & Figures 2004,* American Cancer Society, 2004.

19. Stephenson, Joan. "CDC Report on Environmental Toxins." *Journal of the American Medical Association,* Vol. 289, No. 10, March 12, 2003, p. 1230.

20. "U.N. Organization Warns That Pesticide Waste Is Time Bomb in Poor Countries." *Health & Medicine Week,* October 4, 2004, p. 486.

21. "Occupational Use of Pesticides May Be Implicated in Prostate Cancer." *Health and Medicine Week,* September 8, 2003, p. 669.

22. "Parental Exposure to Pesticides Is Not Likely Linked to Childhood Brain Cancer." *Health and Medicine Week,* August 18, 2003, p. 64.

Index

Page numbers beginning with the letter "A" indicate topics in Hales Health Almanac.